D1556189

Tumors of the Pediatric Central Nervous System

Edited by

Robert F. Keating, MD
Associate Professor of Neurosurgery and Pediatrics
Department of Neurosurgery
Children's National Medical Center
The George Washington University School of Medicine
Washington, DC

James Tait Goodrich, MD, MPhil, PhD, FRSM (London)
Professor of Clinical Neurosurgery, Pediatrics, Plastic and Reconstructive Surgery
Leo Davidoff Department of Neurological Surgery
Albert Einstein College of Medicine/Montefiore Medical Center
Bronx, New York

Roger J. Packer, MD
Professor of Neurology and Pediatrics
Executive Director, Neuroscience and Behavioral Medicine
Chairman, Department of Neurology
Children's National Medical Center
The George Washington University School of Medicine
Washington, DC

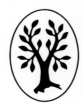

2001
Thieme
New York • Stuttgart

Thieme New York
333 Seventh Avenue
New York, NY 10001

Editor: Kathleen Lyons
Assistant Editor: Michelle Schmitt
Director of Production and Manufacturing: Anne Vinnicombe
Production Editor: Regina C. Paleski
Marketing Director: Phyllis Gold
Sales Manager: Ross Lumpkin
Chief Financial Officer: Peter von Woerden
President: Brian D. Scanlan
Cover Designer: Kevin Kall
Designer: Jose Fonfiras
Compositor: Prepare
Printer: Grafiche Fover

Library of Congress Cataloging-in-Publication Data

Tumors of the pediatric central nervous system / edited by Robert F. Keating, James Tait
Goodrich, Roger J. Packer.
    p. ; cm.
  Includes bibliographical references and index.
  ISBN 0-86577-848-5 (alk. paper)
   1. Central nervous system--Cancer. 2. Cancer in children. I. Keating, Robert F. II.
Goodrich, James T. III. Packer, Roger J., 1951-
   [DNLM: 1. Central Nervous System Neoplasms--therapy--Child. 2. Central Nervous
System Neoplasms--therapy--Infant. WL 358 T927 2001]
  RC280.N43 T85 2001
  618.92'9948--dc21

                                   00-053279

Important note: Medical knowledge is ever changing. As new research and clinical experience broaden our knowledge, changes in treatment and drug therapy may be required. The authors and editors of the material herein have consulted sources believed to be reliable in their efforts to provide information that is complete and in accord with the standards accepted at the time of publication. However, in view of the possibility of human error by the authors, editors, or publisher of the work herein, or changes in medical knowledge, neither the authors, editors, publisher, nor any other party who has been involved in the preparation of this work, warrants that the information contained herein is in every respect accurate or complete, and they are not responsible for any errors or omissions or for the results obtained from use of such information. Readers are encouraged to confirm the information contained herein with other sources. For example, readers are advised to check the product information sheet included in the package of each drug they plan to administer to be certain that information contained in this publication is accurate and that changes have not been made in the recommended dose or in the contraindications for administration. This recommendation is of particular importance in connection with new or infrequently used drugs.

Some of the product names, patents, and registered designs referred to in this book are in fact registered trademarks or proprietary names even though specific reference to this fact is not always made in the text. Therefore, the appearance of a name without designation as proprietary is not to be construed as a representation by the publisher that it is in the public domain.

Compositor: Prepare   Printer: Grafiche Fover

5 4 3 2 1

TNY ISBN 0-86577-848-5

GTV ISBN 3-13-126951-0

Dedications

Robert F. Keating

To my wife, Susan, and my boys, Douglas and Gregory, many thanks for the never-ending support and countless laughs along the way.

To Dr. David McCullough (1935–1992), whose inspiration and tireless devotion to his patients left an undying impression. His work continues today for his extended family.

James Tait Goodrich

In infinito vacuo, ex fortuitâ atomorum collisione!
[Fortunately the gods have allowed me more than just one fortunate collision!]

Reflecting back over a career in education, I have often thought back on the teachers who have had the most influence on me. Recognizing that this book has been put together by a group of educators, myself included, I thought it appropriate to dedicate my portion to a group of educators who have had a special influence on my life:

Donald Collins, Professor of Biological Sciences, Orange Coast College
A natural educator, one who was able to instill in a young and rather immature individual's mind the love for science and biology. You provided the first and most significant spark in a high school dropout; you ignited the flame, and its brilliance has never died!

James L. McGaugh, Professor of Psychobiology, University of California at Irvine
I came to UCI fresh out of a community college. I spent many pleasurable hours in your lab studying the intricacies of learning and memory. I learned from you that to be an educator one needs to not only know a subject well, one must be able to deliver it in a fashion that all can understand—of this you are truly the master!

Paul L. Kornblith, former Chairman of Neurosurgery, Albert Einstein College of Medicine,
Montefiore Medical Center, Bronx, New York

As a young, graduating resident of a neurosurgery program I had little idea of where to go or what field to pursue in neurosurgery. My initial thoughts were vascular neurosurgery. At a counter in a small, fish restaurant in Washington, DC, you said, "pediatric neurosurgery is where it is at"—wonderful foresight on your part. For during the following five years we developed a most remarkable and vibrant program at Montefiore. What wonderful and halcyon days they were!

Judy L. Goodrich, Wife and Mentor
In December of 1968, I was discharged from the U.S. Marine Corps after having completed a tour of duty in Vietnam. My only goal at that point was hedonism—to find the finest wave on the Southern California coast and end the day with a great bottle of wine (albeit one with a screw top). I did all this well, and then I came to the point when I had to wake up to reality. Whatever made you decide to join me on this voyage I will never know. You have been a very special and constant companion, a unique person in your understanding of the complexities of this job that I have. After 30-plus years, you are truly my greatest treasure and mentor. Thanks for always being there.

Roger J. Packer

I would like to thank my wife, Bernice, and my children, Zehava and Michael, for all their support.

Contents

Section I. Current Diagnosis and Therapeutic Approaches

Section II. Intracranial Tumors

Section III. Spinal Cord Tumors

Section IV. Outcomes and Complications

Contributors

Marc S. Arginteanu, MD
Clinical Assistant Professor
Department of Neurosurgery
Mount Sinai Hospital
New York, New York

Casilda M. Balmaceda, MD
Professor of Neurology
Department of Neurology
Columbia University
*   College of Physicians and Surgeons*
The Neurological Institute
Columbia Presbyterian Medical Center
New York, New York

Mitchel S. Berger, MD
Professor and Chairman
Department of Neurological Surgery
University of California, San Francisco
San Francisco, California

Helaine F. Bertsch, MD
Department of Radiation Oncology
Hartford Hospital
Hartford, Connecticut

Marc Bestak, MD
Associate Professor of Pediatrics
Department of Pediatrics
Albert Einstein College of Medicine
Montefiore Medical Center
Bronx, New York

Keith S. Blum, DO
Department of Neurosurgery
Beaumont Hospital
Royal Oak, Michigan

Timothy N. Booth, MD
Assistant Professor of Radiology
Department of Radiology
University of Texas Southwestern
Dallas, Texas

Gavin Wayne Britz, MD
Acting Instructor
Department of Neurological Surgery
University of Washington
Seattle, Washington

Jeffrey N. Bruce, MD
Associate Professor of Neurosurgery
Department of Neurological Surgery
Columbia University College of Physicians and Surgeons
New York, New York

Russell Buchanan, MD
Clinical Instructor
Department of Neurosurgery
The George Washington University
*   Medical Center*
Washington, DC

Dennis R. Burholt, PhD
Scientific Director for Clinical Services
Precision Therapeutics, Inc.
Pittsburgh, Pennsylvania

Robert W. Butler, PhD
Associate Professor
Department of Pediatrics
Oregon Health Sciences University
Portland, Oregon

Philip H. Cogen, MD, PhD
Professor and Chairman, Neurosurgery and Pediatrics
Department of Pediatric Neurosurgery
Children's National Medical Center
The George Washington University
Washington, DC

Shlomi Constantini, MD
Division of Pediatric Neurosurgery
Department of Neurosurgery
Dana Children's Hospital
Tel Aviv-Sourasky Medical Center
ISRAEL

Edward E. Conway, Jr, MD, MS, FAAP, FCCP, FCCM
Associate Professor of Pediatrics, Critical Care Medicine,
*   and Anesthesiology*
Albert Einstein College of Medicine
Bronx, New York
Associate Chairman of Pediatrics
Medical Director, Singer Division
Beth Israel Medical Center
New York, New York

Concezio Di Rocco, MD
Professor of Pediatric Neurosurgery
Department of Neurosurgery
Head, Section of Pediatric Neurosurgery
Catholic University Medical School
Rome
ITALY

Daniel J. Donovan, MD
Chief, Neurosurgery Service
Tripler Army Medical Center
Honolulu, Hawaii

Sarita Duchatelier, MD
Chief Pediatric Neurologist
Department of Pediatric Neurology
Good Samaritan Hospital Medical Center
West Islip, New York

Richard G. Ellenbogen, MD
Theodore S. Roberts Endowed Chair in Pediatric
*   Neurological Surgery*
Associate Professor
Department of Neurological Surgery
University of Washington
Children's Hospital and Regional Medical Center
Seattle, Washington

Fred J. Epstein, MD
Division of Pediatric Neurosurgery
Department of Neurosurgery
Beth Israel Medical Center, North Division
Institute for Neurology and Neurosurgery
New York, New York

Margaret Ekstein, MD
Senior Anesthesiologist
Tel Aviv University Medical Center
Tel Aviv
ISRAEL

Neil A. Feldstein, MD
Associate Professor of Pediatric Neurosurgery
Department of Neurological Surgery
Columbia University College of Physicians and Surgeons
New York, New York

Michael R. Fetell, MD
Professor of Neurology
Department of Neurology
Columbia University
*   College of Physicians and Surgeons*
The Neurological Institute
Columbia Presbyterian Medical Center
New York, New York

John C. Flickinger, MD
Professor of Radiation Oncology and Neurological Surgery
Department of Radiation Oncology
University of Pittsburgh
Pittsburgh, Pennsylvania

Henry S. Friedman, MD
James B. Powell, Jr, Professor of Neuro-oncology
Department of Surgery
Duke University Medical Center
Durham, North Carolina

Joel W. Goldwein, MD
Associate Professor of Radiation Oncology
Department of Radiation Oncology
University of Pennsylvania
Philadelphia, Pennsylvania

Robert Goodkin, MD
Associate Professor
Department of Neurological Surgery
University of Washington
Seattle, Washington

James Tait Goodrich, MD, PhD, MPhil, FRSM (Lond)
Professor of Clinical Neurosurgery, Pediatrics, Plastic
*   and Reconstructive Surgery*
Leo Davidoff Department of Neurological Surgery
Albert Einstein College of Medicine
Montefiore Medical Center
Bronx, New York

Harold J. Hoffman, MD, FRCSC, FACS
Emeritus Professor of Surgery
Department of Surgery
University of Toronto
*   and The Hospital for Sick Children*
Toronto, Ontario
CANADA

Robin P. Humphreys, MD, FRCSC, FACS, FAAP
Professor of Surgery and Division Head
Harold J. Hoffman/Shoppers Drug Mart Chair
University of Toronto
Division of Neurosurgery, Department of Surgery
The Hospital for Sick Children
Toronto, Ontario
CANADA

Aldo Iannelli, MD
Assistant Professor
Department of Neurosurgery
Section of Pediatric Neurosurgery
Catholic University Medical School
Rome
ITALY

Salvatore A. Insinga, DO
Chief Resident in Neurosurgery
NYCOM-Long Island Jewish Medical Center
New Hyde Park, New York

David F. Jimenez, MD
Associate Professor
Department of Neurosurgery
University of Missouri
Columbia, Missouri

Robert F. Keating, MD
Associate Professor of Neurosurgery and Pediatrics
Department of Neurosurgery
Children's National Medical Center
The George Washington University School of Medicine
Washington, DC

Michel Kliot, MD
Associate Professor of Neurological Surgery
Department of Neurological Surgery
University of Washington
Seattle, Washington

Douglas Kondziolka, MD, MSc, FRCSC, FACS
Professor of Neurological Surgery and Radiation Oncology
Department of Neurological Surgery
University of Pittsburgh
Pittsburgh, Pennsylvania

Paul L. Kornblith, MD
Adjunct Professor
School of Health and Rehabilitation Services
University of Pittsburgh
President and Chief Executive Officer
Precision Therapeutics, Inc.
Pittsburgh, Pennsylvania

Jang-Chul Lee, MD
Associate Professor
School of Medicine
Keimyung University
Taegu
KOREA

L. Dade Lunsford, MD, FACS
Professor of Neurological Surgery, Radiology,
and Radiation Oncology
Department of Neurological Surgery
University of Pittsburgh
Pittsburgh, Pennsylvania

David Magill, MD
Resident
Department of Physical Rehabilitation and Department
of Pediatrics
Montefiore Medical Center
Bronx, New York

Michael D. Medlock, MD
Department of Neurosurgery
Massachusetts General Hospital
Boston, Massachusetts

Douglas C. Miller, MD, PhD
Associate Professor of Neuropathology and Neurosurgery
Division of Neuropathology
Department of Pathology
New York University School of Medicine
New York, New York

Lieutenant Colonel Leon E. Moores, MD
Assistant Professor of Neurosurgery
Director, Pediatric Neurosurgery
Department of Neurosurgery
National Capital Area Consortium
Neurosurgery Program
Uniformed Services University of the Health Sciences
Washington, DC

Lisa Mulligan, MD
Department of Neurosurgery
National Naval Medical Center
Bethesda, Maryland

Cheryl A. Muszynski, MD
Assistant Professor of Neurosurgery
Department of Neurosurgery
Albert Einstein College of Medicine
Bronx, New York
and Beth Israel Medical Center
New York, New York

H. Stacy Nicholson, MD, MPH
Associate Professor of Pediatrics
Department of Pediatric Hematology-Oncology
Oregon Health Sciences University
Portland, Oregon

Subhadra L. Nori, MD
Associate Professor of Clinical Rehabilitation Medicine
Department of Physical Medicine
and Rehabilitation
Albert Einstein College of Medicine
North Bronx Healthcare Network
Jacobi Medical Center
Bronx, New York

Irene Osborn, MD
Department of Anesthesia
Mount Sinai Medical Center
New York, New York

Roger J. Packer, MD
Professor of Neurology and Pediatrics
Executive Director, Neuroscience
and Behavioral Medicine
Chairman, Department of Neurology
Children's National Medical Center
The George Washington University
School of Medicine
Washington, DC

Fabio Papacci, MD
Department of Neurosurgery
Section of Pediatric Neurosurgery
Catholic University Medical School
Rome
ITALY

Andrew T. Parsa, MD, PhD
Resident
Department of Neurological Surgery
Columbia University
College of Physicians and Surgeons
The Neurological Institute
Columbia Presbyterian Medical Center
New York, New York

Giorgio Perilongo, MD
Professor of Pediatrics
Department of Pediatric Hematology-Oncology
University of Padova
Padova
ITALY

David W. Pincus, MD, PhD
Assistant Professor of Pediatric Neurosurgery
Department of Neurological Surgery
University of Florida
Gainesville, Florida

Ian F. Pollack, MD
Department of Neurosurgery
Children's Hospital of Pittsburgh
Pittsburgh, Pennsylvania

Kalmon D. Post, MD
Department of Neurosurgery
Mount Sinai Hospital
New York, New York

Charles L. Rosen, MD
Department of Neurosurgery
The George Washington University
Medical Center
Washington, DC

Alan D. Rosenthal, MD, FACS
Associate Clinical Professor
Department of Neurosurgery
Albert Einstein College of Medicine
Bronx, New York
and The Long Island Jewish Medical Center
New Hyde Park, New York

Steven J. Schneider, MD, FACS
Clinical Assistant Professor of Neurosurgery
Department of Neurosurgery
New York University Medical Center
New York, New York
and North Shore University Hospital
Manhasset, New York

Michael E. Seiff, MD
Department of Neurosurgery
Park Plaza Hospital
Houston, Texas

Caple A. Spence, MD
Department of Neurosurgery
The George Washington University
Medical Center
Washington, DC

Richard Sposto, MD
Associate Professor of Research
Department of Preventive Medicine
University of Southern California
Arcadia, California

Richard Teff, MD
Staff Neurosurgeon
Army Medical Department
William Beaumont Army Medical Center
El Paso, Texas

Philip V. Theodosopoulos, MD
Chief Resident
Department of Neurological Surgery
University of California, San Francisco
San Francisco, California

Gilbert Vézina, MD
Associate Professor of Radiology and Pediatrics
Department of Diagnostic Imaging and Radiology
Children's National Medical Center
The George Washington University
Washington, DC

Eugenio Vines, MD
Instructor in Radiotherapy
Department Instituto de Radiomedicina
Universidad de Santiago de Chile
Santiago, Chile

David M. Weitman, MD, PhD
Chief Resident
Department of Neurosurgery
The George Washington University Medical Center
Washington, DC

Jeffrey H. Wisoff, MD
Associate Professor of Neurosurgery
Director, Division of Pediatric Neurosurgery
New York University Medical Center
New York, New York

Steven M. Wolf, MD
Assistant Professor of Neurology and Pediatrics
Albert Einstein College of Medicine
Bronx, New York
and Director of Pediatric Neurology
St. Lukes-Roosevelt Hospital
New York, New York

Ann-Marie Yost, MD
Central Washington Neurosurgery
Yakima, Washington

"Don't do something! Stand there and observe the child," were the words of wisdom I heard from a respected former university chairman of pediatrics. For the young patient with a 9-month history of symptoms suggesting intracranial hypertension, which is associated with gait ataxia, observe was about the most one could do when one suspected an intracranial neoplasm. After a period of observation, a procedure was performed in which air was instilled into the patient's lateral ventricle, which was presumably expanded from the tumor's blockade downstream, and, eventually, the air capped the front edge of a mass residing partly (or completely) within the fourth ventricle. An operation was planned—one about which a surgeon often would feel at a disadvantage. What were the actual dimensions of the tumor and into what critical structures had it become insinuated? Was it surgical skill alone that would be the major determinant of the child's outcome? Was there any other reasonable postoperative treatment option? How naïve we were.

In many respects, the publishing date of this text marks the thirty-first anniversary of the beginning of the expansion of researchers and clinicians' knowledge about brain and spinal cord tumors that occur specifically in children. At least since 1955, neurosurgeons dedicated full-time to the care of children had been established in major pediatric hospitals around the world. By 1970, some had reported their case experiences with central nervous system tumors, as typified by the texts of Donald Matson, and two years later, by those of Wolfgang Koos and Meredith Miller. By today's standards, those writings might be considered rather pro forma. The tumor diagnosis was reached often intuitively, the principles of operation were applicable as much to one tumor type as to the next, and, in the end, only the anatomical and pathological features were relied on when assigning a specific identity to a child's brain or spinal cord neoplasm. Also, by 1970, the concept of multidiscipline patient care, at least as it pertained to the management of cerebellar medulloblastoma, had been introduced.

In 1969, five major publications from different countries (none of them to be found in the traditional neurosurgical literature) had examined the usefulness of radiation therapy in the treatment of cerebellar medulloblastoma. C. H. Chang was the lead author of one of those papers; in it he presented the classification of tumor staging to which reference is made at tumor-board patient conferences regularly today. As time has passed, we have accepted that the care of a child's central nervous system neoplasm is dependant on a team of individuals who contribute their expertise in clinical diagnosis, imaging, anesthesia, surgery, neuropathology, oncology and radiation therapy, and outcome measures. It is fitting that the thoughts of these allied health-care professionals occupy sections of this text. Information and input from the skilled individuals in these various fields provide the physician responsible for a child's care with a complete definition of the patient's tumor type and the various nonoperative strategies that will best assist the patient.

"Do you want to see the scan first or the patient?" This question, a prelude to the "new" consultation, echoes repeatedly throughout hospital corridors today and reveals our infatuation with—and, admittedly, reliance on—contemporary imaging information. But first, we must not neglect the patient's or family's version of the facts. For example, in a child with a suspected posterior fossa tumor, headache that appeared long before vomiting began suggests a tumor type other than a fourth ventricular ependymoma (for which vomiting is often the earliest symptom). A child's altered gait that is characterized as "a loss of spinal rhythm" and that is associated with back pain that awakens the child from sleep can only mean an intradural spinal cord tumor. How appropriate it is, then, that the chapter alignments in Section I of this text honor these principles of patient assessment. From these principles, one moves to the operating suite.

During the last three decades, the extent of the surgical removal of a child's brain tumor has been identified repeatedly as the most important determinant of disease control. Maximum bulk excision of the tumor tissue offers the best outcome. The surgeon is under pressure! But he or she now has incredible preoperative imaging and intra-operative technologies that provide a measure of reassurance. Additionally, the surgeon relies on a skilled neuro-anesthetist in the operating theater. This expert individual tracks vital data using real-time monitoring equipment. The neuro-anesthetist also actively performs checks for covert evidence of bleeding beneath the drapes, trapped monitoring or infusion lines, or, for example, a "tight" brain (the causes of which are outlined in Chapter 6). Brain surgery is a partnership.

On the other hand, did one ever suspect that there could be a tumor located in a surgically approachable region of the brain that would not require operative removal or even biopsy? The first evidence of such a tumor was discovered following several years of retrospective studies of patients with neurofibromatosis type 1 (NF-1) who had isolated optic nerve gliomas. The research showed that this NF group seemed to have a better prognosis than the patients without NF-1 (Chapter 21). Furthermore, at least half of the patients with optic pathway gliomas and NF-1 require no treatment for their tumors, which will remain quiescent. No surgery is required. And, it has only been 18 years since we learned of the distinct "pencil glioma" of the aqueduct of Sylvius that produces hydrocephalus that, currently, is easily remedied via a third ventriculostomy. In most instances, that is all that is required as this particular neoplasm has "a particularly indolent course and good long-term outcome" (see Chapter 13). Is the surgeon slowly becoming disenfranchised? Hardly.

Consider that in 1970 the diagnosis of a "brain stem tumor" represented a dark corner in our management of brain neoplasms in children. We were often forced to recognize the futility of our treatment options for a child with a diffuse intrinsic brain stem tumor. At most, an operation would consist of a biopsy, the results of which might occasionally leave the surgeon and pathologist confused. To the extent that this type of tumor is diffuse within the pons, as is demonstrated so exquisitely on magnetic resonance imaging, a poor prognosis remains true now as it did 30 years ago. But modern imaging techniques have influenced positively the outcomes for some children with brain stem tumors. The ability to obtain presurgical knowledge of a tumor's anatomical categorization—that is, focal or exophytic, or other characteristics—can urge operative exploration and decompression of a brain stem tumor that may be followed by dramatic recoveries and long-term survival in pediatric patients (see Chapter 13).

When striving to treat children who have central nervous system tumors, surgeons may occasionally question their own efforts. Consider the dilemma presented by the diagnosis of a pediatric craniopharyngioma, arguably a tumor distinct from that which occurs in adults. The history of surgical treatment for this type of tumor has, in part at least, been reactionary. In the beginning, the goal of surgery was the preservation of a child's vision, perhaps combined with the goal of modulation of the degree of the associated endocrinopathy. In some instances, these goals were achieved. But visual failure, usually related to tumor cyst reexpansion, could recur, and the surgeon might find him- or herself on a "treadmill" of cyst drainages, innovative shunts, recurrent solid disease, increased visual failure, and so on. Radiation or various intra-cavitary therapies were introduced, and, for some patients, they provided a lasting solution. But critics of these modalities argued in favor of radical, microscopic tumor removal—a recommendation that, in the end, was instituted in perhaps 60% of cases. However, the potential morbidity—such as panhypopituitarism, personality and memory disorders, or morbid obesity—was substantial. Not surprisingly, the author of this text's chapter on craniopharyngioma cautions that, "the cognitive and psychosocial sequelae may be functionally devastating, interfering with education, limiting independence, and adversely affecting the quality of life as these children approach adulthood" (see Chapter 19). Hence, if there is one type of pediatric brain tumor above all others that should be the focus of a detailed multi-center study, it is the craniopharyngioma because of the tumor's impact on multiple body systems (see Chapters 35, 37, and 39).

Great challenges and questions remain with regard to tumors of the pediatric central nervous system. For example, contrast the choroid plexus papilloma with the choroid plexus carcinoma. The former, at operation, is a tumor that can be lifted out from its ventricular cavity, whereas the latter is a tumor for which even the simplest of biopsies can result in exsanguinating hemorrhage in an infant. Why are the outcomes for lesions designated as primitive neuroectodermal tumors so much worse when they occupy the cerebral hemispheres as opposed to the subtentorial cerebellar vermis? What is the best operative approach for the fourth ventricular ependymoma that surrounds cranial nerves and is invasive of the brain stem? And, perhaps most intriguing, just where will gene therapy take us in the next 30 years?

Confirming what some neurosurgeons have suspected for the last decade, sufficient evidence exists indicating that the incidence of brain tumors in children is increasing. Pediatric patients with central nervous system tumors first present for neurosurgical intake at a much earlier stage in the course of their illnesses than was the case 3 decades ago, but the diagnosis of a brain tumor creates no less anxiety for a family now than it did 30 years ago. More information about opportunities for treatment is available than ever before, but today's electronic information overload can heighten expectations. Much is demanded of the pediatric neurosurgeon, who is expected to be the "complete" physician. Fortunately, today's surgeon is part of a complete and expert health-care team, as the various sections of this text so ably depict.

Robin P. Humphreys, MD
Neurosurgeon-in-Chief
Harold J. Hoffman/Shoppers Drug Mart
Chair in Pediatric Neurosurgery
The Hospital for Sick Children
The University of Toronto
Toronto, Ontario, Canada

Preface

Although pediatric central nervous system tumors are, fortunately, uncommon, they, nevertheless, are the second most common form of cancer in childhood and the leading cause of cancer-related death in children. Despite their relative infrequency, they, nonetheless, contribute to a large share of uncertainty and misery for the practicing clinician, whether oncologist or family physician.

The variability in histological type and location of the tumors as well as their proclivity to occur in very young children makes management difficult. Yet with modern therapeutic approaches more than half of the children who have central nervous system tumors can expect to be cured of their diseases.

A central nervous system tumor and the treatment that a young patient requires as a result may cause brain injury and long-term neurological, intellectual, hormonal, and psychological damage. By necessity, treatment is often multidisciplinary, and it is challenging to the neurosurgeon, neurologist, oncologist, and radiation therapist.

In today's rapidly changing medical arena, the diagnosis and treatment of a child with a central nervous system neoplasia has become increasingly complex. Improved radiological diagnosis, less invasive surgical methods, revised pathological classifications as well as a greater understanding of the roles of radiotherapy and chemotherapy in the battle for saving children's lives continue to redefine the "state-of-the-art." In addition, one must consider the advances and new horizons in the world of immunotherapy and genetic engineering, ethical issues, efficacy, and cost effectiveness in the contemporary realm of fiscal accountability.

This volume was conceived as an attempt to bridge the wide divide between primary care and the specialist's focus. In addition to overviews on diagnosis, epidemiology, pathology, and radiology as well as clinical insight into neurosurgical, anesthetic, and critical care considerations, attention is focused on adjuvant therapies including chemotherapy, radiotherapy, and genetic intervention. Individual tumor types are reviewed with respect to diagnosis and current therapeutic strategies, and the text concludes with an examination of outcomes and complications.

The treatment paradigm facing the clinician today revolves around a complex and often confusing interplay between patient, parents, primary care individuals, and numerous specialists. We have produced this work to simplify these relationships and to enlighten those involved. This, in turn, should offer greater promise for the individuals who need it most—the children.

Robert F. Keating, MD
James Tait Goodrich, MD, PhD, MPhil, FRSM [Lond]
Roger J. Packer, MD

Current Diagnosis and Therapeutic Approaches

Chapter 1

Pediatric Neuro-oncology
A Historical Perspective

James Tait Goodrich

To provide some perspective on the development of modern pediatric oncology practices, the editors thought it useful to open with a historical overview of this relatively new field. Oncologic treatment of central nervous system (CNS) lesions is also a relatively new modality, with most of the development occurring in the period since World War I. Review of the earlier historical literature reveals little understanding of what constituted a "cancer." Subsequent chapters in this volume will deal with the recent treatments with some 20th century historical reviews. This chapter will focus on the general views and contemporary medical and surgical treatment of cancer of the CNS through the first quarter of the 20th century. This review is meant to be very general in origin and scope, with the purpose of illustrating how far we have come in the management of pediatric neuro-oncologic lesions, as well as showing how much further we have to go.

BEFORE THE RENAISSANCE

The earliest medical literature on oncologic lesions appears in the Edwin Smith (1832–1906) Papyrus, which dates from 1600 BC. In this early treatise, only swellings, injuries, and inflammations are discussed, some of which might have been cancerous though little in the way of detail is provided with which to confirm this. A second papyrus, dating from 1552 BC, called the Ebers Papyrus because it was acquired by Georg Ebers in Thebes in 1872, includes mention of a case of a large tumor of the limb. However, the admonition is made against surgery as that type of treatment could prove fatal. A review of the early Greek literature, in particular the writings of Hippocrates (460–370 BC), reveals a number of interesting and thorough clinical observations, though few examples exist of what might be called oncologic description.[1] Hippocrates does provide what appear to be descriptions of breast cancer, cancer of the rectum and uterus, and skin and stomach lesions. Treatment offered in the way of surgical excision or medical therapies was minimal at best as the prognosis for these lesions was almost always dismal. Bedside care and comfort to the patient in the final days were the best and only treatments offered during this period.

The concept of a disease process now known as cancer dates from the early hippocratic schools. The word cancer was derived from "carcinos," meaning "crab"—a term used to medically describe chronic ulcerations and swellings and any eating types of sores; in retrospect, these lesions were most likely tumors of malignant origin.[2,3] Celsus (25 BC–AD 50), the great medical encyclopedist, translated the word "carcinos" to "cancer" and introduced the term "carcinoma."[4] He described a number of cancerous-type lesions, mostly involving breast, skin, nose, and lips, and he rarely recommended surgery (which typically included only caustic medicants or cautery application). Galen of Pergamon (AD 130–200), the great Alexanderian surgeon, brought us "oncos" to describe a tumor or swelling. Galen also developed the humoral theory and its effect on the development of cancer.[5] According to this theory, cancerous lesions developed as a result of buildup of "black bile," one of the four humors, which solidified and formed lesions. Treatment involved the administration of purgatives to dissolve the collection, and, when that failed, the lesion was excised. Such was Galen's influence on medicine that this humoral view of cancer was to remain the dominant theme of medical oncology for more than 1600 years. The general use of the word "cancer" as a medical term for a disease began to appear regularly in the English literature in the early 17th century when it replaced the term "canker."[3]

The period of late antiquity (approximately AD 600–1000) shows medical practice to be heavily under the influence of the Arabic schools of medicine. The Arabic schools and their educators were great codifiers of the earlier Greek and Latin writings, translating virtually all existing writings into Arabic to form the then-current corpus of medical texts. Because these individuals were compilers and not innovators, it is not surprising that a review of the Arabic literature shows little in the way of new advances in medical or surgical treatments. However there are in these writings some interesting perspectives as to surgical treatment of oncologic diseases. In his great *Canon of Medicine* descriptions of cancer invasion, Avicenna (AD 980–1037) described the destruction of adjoining tissues, loss of sensation in and use of the affected part, and eventual death secondary to widespread disease.[6] Albucasis (939–1013), one of the most elite of Arabic surgeons, wrote on the surgical excision of cancerous lesions.[7,8] These cancerous lesions had to be at an accessible site, such as the breast or on a limb, and for such he recommended complete excision. Albucasis's surgical excision technique involved a circular cauterization with a hot iron, and the lesion was literally burned out; the edges of the cancerous lesion were allowed to ulcerate. For advanced lesions he appropriately recommended no surgical treatment. Medical management of cancerous lesions envoked the galenic view of purgatives and bleeding to remove the sequestered black bile. At no point in these early writings, whether from the Greek, Latin, or Arabic schools, are there any recommendations for operating on the brain for cancerous lesions. Except for the rare case of head trauma, there are almost no recommendations for opening the dura and excising an intracranial lesion. Because the risk of hemorrhage, cerebrospinal fluid leaks, and infections led to an almost 100% mortality, it was very rare for a surgeon to even consider operating on the brain.

THE RENAISSANCE

Further review of the medieval and renaissance literature shows no further innovations or new techniques for oncologic treatment of any type. The galenic view of purging and the use of purgatives remained the main form of medical treatment.[9] Tumors and/or swellings (i.e., cancers) were only treated to the extent that they were accessible. Hence tumors of the breast, limbs, rectum, and uterus were typically accessible and could be considered for treatment. Treatment involved surgical excision initially with cautery (i.e., burned out) followed by administration of purgatives. Later, 16th century European surgeons excised lesions with sharp knives, followed by administration of purgatives to break up and move along the sequestered black bile. In effect, the persisting views of the galenic humoral theory remained in force some 14 centuries later.

The Renaissance led to a number of new surgical concepts, in particular the routine introduction and development of the anatomical dissection. During this era, surgeons again realized that to understand internal anatomy one needed to perform hands-on anatomical dissections—a teaching technique that had been virtually dead for religious and secular reasons since before the time of the Arabic schools. In Italy the great schools of medicine, such as those in Padua and Bologna, introduced anatomical theaters where routine dissections of executed criminals were performed. Under great personages such as Andreas Vesalius (1519–1564) and Berengario da Carpi (1460–1530?), dissections became a routine part of the medical school curiculum.[10-12] However, a review of the 16th century surgical texts still shows a very heavy influence of the galenic humoral theories, and again cancerous lesions were removed only to the extent that they were accessible and fairly discrete. In an era before antisepsis and anesthesia (concepts not introduced until the mid-19th century), these must have been extraordinarily painful procedures with a high incidence of death due to infection and generalized sepsis.

In the 17th century there appeared numerous surgical manuals with excellent anatomical and surgical illustrations showing techniques for removal of superficial cancerous lesions. However, the approach to and understanding of cancerous lesions in the brain were not even attempted until the 19th century. Some examples of the early surgical techniques are given below to provide a short overview of what our early surgical brethren offered in terms of treatment. Medical treatment still consisted of purgatives, caustics, and bleeding.

Johannes Scultetus (1595–1645) provided one of the best illustrated surgical manuals of the 17th century.[13] This volume gave several examples of surgical excisions of cancerous lesions, particularly of the breast (Fig. 1–1). In an era before

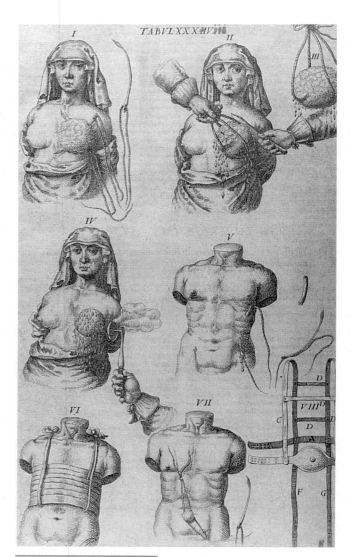

Figure 1–1 Gruesome 17th century techniques for removal of cancerous lesions of the breast, carried out on unanesthetized patients. (From Scultetus, Johannes. *Armamentarium chirurgicum XLIII. Typis and impensis*. Ulm: Balthasari Kühnen; 1655.)

antisepsis and anesthesia, the then-prevalent techniques of burning out, cauterizing, and excising lesions must have been a horrendous experience. Postoperative treatment followed galenic humoral theory in that the patient would be given foul-tasting emetics and purgatives, with venous bleeding then applied—all done in an effort to keep the four humors in balance. One can only imagine the high morbidity and mortality associated with these somewhat coarse and brutal, by today's standards, techniques.

THE 18TH CENTURY

Henri Francois LeDran (1685–1770), a leading figure in the early French school of medicine, introduced a new and innovative view of cancer when he proposed that cancer began as a local disease that later spread via the lymphatic chain to lymph nodes and then to the general circulation. This revolutionary view led to the concept of metastasis and its pathogenesis. As a result of these new and novel observations, LeDran was among the first to argue for early surgical intervention to prevent metastasis. LeDran also argued against the use of caustic pastes and purgatives, believing that surgery was the better option.[14,15]

At the age of 79 years, Giovanni Battista Morgagni (1682–1771) published a remarkable work on the "seat and causes of diseases" (*De Sedibus et Causis Morborum*, 1761).[16] This work was a culmination of a lifetime of work using autopsy material and clinically correlating autopsy findings with the medical history, an exercise that is very common today but was virtually unheard of in the 18th century. Morgagni's work contains about 70 letters reviewing more than 700 cases. A number of different cancers are reviewed, including those involving the breast, stomach, rectum, and pancreas. Unfortunately, Morgagni had no concept of the origins or pathology of different cancers. He did, however, provide some very interesting and early examples of cancerous lesions and speculated on the cancer's effect on the patient's outcome.

Matthew Baillie (1761–1823), of the English school of medicine, continued the pathologic studies of diseases and published his gross pathology findings in his landmark work *The Morbid Anatomy of Some of the Most Important Parts of the Human Body* (1793).[17] An atlas followed in 1799–1802 called *A Series of Engravings with Explanations Which Are Intended to Illustrate the Morbid Anatomy of Some of the Most Important Parts of the Human Body*.[18] The atlas provides the first illustrations of the appearance of specimens showing different tumors affecting the brain and its membranes. The drawings were of the highest caliber and are the first to reflect some, albeit minimal, understanding of cancerous lesions (Fig. 1–2).

The development of a scientific approach to oncologic surgery has been historically a late phenomenon and occurred in the same period as the works and writings of the great English surgeon John Hunter (1728–1793). Hunter is considered the father of modern surgery because few individuals have been as productive as he in the field of original surgical research. Hunter offered some interesting views on cancer that were published posthumously in his *Lectures on the Principles of Surgery* (1839).[19] Hunter believed that there were three conditions that influenced the development of cancer: age, heredity, and, perhaps, climate. From his clinical observations it was apparent to Hunter that cancers occurred between the ages of 40 and 60 years; pediatric lesions were not discussed. Hunter noted that the earlier the cancer appeared (an example used was breast cancer), the worse the outcome. Cancers described by Hunter were typically solid lesions of the breast, uterus, lips, nose, pancreas, and so forth. It appears that Hunter did not have an understanding of, or at least did not describe, cancers that we now know as leukemias or lymphomas. Hunter appreciated the fact that the involvement of lymph nodes was a sign that the cancer had spread and cure was unlikely. If the lesion was well circumscribed and mobile, the lesion was easily removed and Hunter considered the patient to be curable.

THE 19TH CENTURY

Astley Paston Cooper (1768–1841), a pupil of John Hunter's, carried on the great hunterian tradition of surgery, combining surgical research and anatomical dissections. Cooper was very interested in diseases of the breast, publishing his findings in a book on diseases of the breast.[20] Cooper performed a number of anatomical dissections, combined these findings with his clinical experiences, and provided some of the earliest "modern" technical advances in the surgical treatment (i.e., excision) of localized cancer lesions.

From among the extraordinary school of surgeons in England came the Scotsman Charles Bell (1774–1842). Bell is remembered for a number of original contributions to

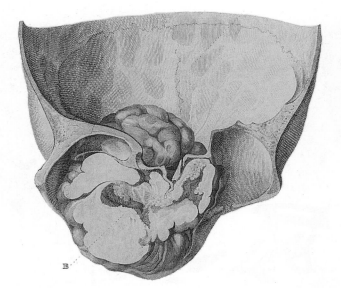
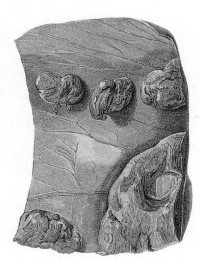

Figure 1–2 Early illustrations of intracranial meningiomas from Baillie's illustrated atlas. (From Baillie M. *A Series of Engravings Accompanied with Explanations, Which Are Intended to Illustrate the Morbid Anatomy of Some of the Most Important Parts of the Human Body.* London: W. Bulmer & Co.; 1799–1803.)

surgery, in particular the discovery of the physiologic functions of motor and sensory nerves. Germane to this chapter is an illustration by Bell showing the earliest illustrated example of a cerebellopontine angle tumor; this illustration appeared in Bell's 1830 book *The Nervous System of the Human Body*, 2nd edition[21] (Fig. 1–3). Bell described a cerebellopontine angle tumor arising from the trigeminal nerve in a patient who had developed severe facial pain. While the case is described as a postmortem finding, it is nevertheless one of the earliest examples of a clinical finding (facial pain) being collaborated with the pathologic finding of an intracranial tumor.

John Abercrombie (1780–1844), Lord-Rector of Marischal College, Aberdeen, Scotland, published the first work devoted solely to pathologic disorders of the brain and spine, albeit a work with many misconceptions about the origins of tumors and pathologic processes of the brain and spinal cord. Abercrombie had published a number of articles on neuropathology in the *Edinburgh Medical and Surgical Journal* and then summarized these findings in a monograph entitled *Pathological and Practical Researches on Diseases of the Brain and Spinal Cord* (1828).[22] This work of 476 pages contains more than 150 case reports, although no illustrations, describing various pathologic conditions of the brain, spinal cord, and peripheral nerves. In the third and fourth sections of this book are early gross clinical descriptions of tumors and mass lesions involving the brain and spinal cord. Abercrombie noted that, clinically, masses in the head could cause "long-continued severe headaches" (headaches that typically occurred in the morning and were exacerbated by motion).

Severe headaches could also be accompanied by impairment or loss of vision. Vomiting and convulsions were also appreciated and described as part of the clinical picture of brain tumor. Clinical findings such as hemiplegia were detailed. Of particular note were some of the first clinical and pathologic descriptions of tumors of the spinal cord. Abercrombie's clinical descriptions included tumors, cysts, abscesses, and tuberculomas. He also pointed out that these tumors anatomically could arise from both within and external to the spinal cord. The final section of the book is an appendix in which Abercrombie noted that tumors and other pathologic lesions also occurred in nerves. He described softening, discoloration, swelling, shrinking, and compression of nerves by tumors. This volume by Abercrombie is considered by most medical writers to be the earliest definitive work (albeit with many inaccuracies) to discuss tumors and cancers of the brain and spinal cord.

In the early part of the 19th century there appeared a number of excellent pathology atlases with beautifully illustrated engravings of lesions of the brain and spinal cord. The first neuropathology atlas of note was by Robert Hooper (1773–1835) who authored a remarkable work entitled *The Morbid Anatomy of the Human Brain, Illustrated by Coloured Engravings of the Most Frequent and Important Organic Diseases to Which That Viscus Is Subject*.[23] Hooper was a London practitioner who was also interested in pathology. His work was based on his 4000-plus autopsies performed at the St. Marylebone Infirmary over a 30-year period (Fig. 1–4). In this work, along with descriptions of hemorrhage, abscess, and the like,

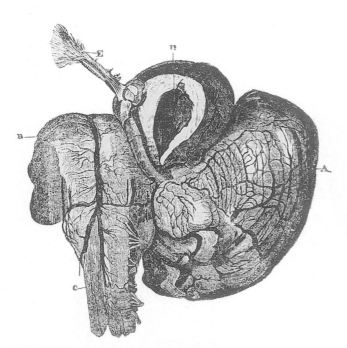

Figure 1–3 Earliest illustrations of a cerebellopontine angle in a patient who presented with facial pain. (From Bell C. *The Nervous System of the Human Body*. 2nd ed. London: Longmans and Co.; 1830.)

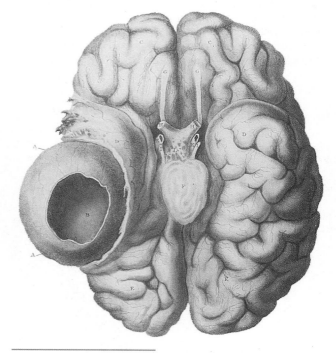

Figure 1–4 An encysted tumor of the brain presented in Hooper's monograph. (From Hooper R. *The Morbid Anatomy of the Human Brain, Illustrated by Coloured Engravings of the Most Frequent and Important Organic Diseases to Which That Viscus Is Subject*. London: printed for the Author; 1828.)

are some of the earliest descriptive examples of tumors of the brain, which Hooper described as "cephaloma," "chondroma," "osteoma," "melanoma," and so forth. Tumors are described as either circumscribed or "so blended with the surrounding cerebral substance they could not be easily traced." Terms such as "soft," "hard," "solid," and "cystic" were used to characteristically describe tumors. Hooper also recognized the single versus multilocular nature of cysts, though it is not always clear whether he is discussing tumors or abscesses. Tumors such as gliomas and meningiomas are easily ascertained from his gross descriptions. Microscopic descriptions were not provided. Interestingly, the text contains no clinical descriptions, just descriptions of gross morphology and pathology of the human brain. It is of interest that Hooper was also the first to illustrate an example of multiple sclerosis.

In 1828, Robert Carswell (1793–1857) became the first professor of pathology at University College Hospital in London.[24] Ten years later (1838), this artist-pathologist published an atlas entitled *Pathological Anatomy: Illustrations of the Elementary Forms of Disease*, in which he included a large number of examples of neuropathologic lesions, along with examples of metastatic melanoma (melanosis) and other carcinomas of the brain.[25] Carswell was an accomplished artist in both watercolors and etching, and he provided more than 2000 watercolor plates ("my coloured delineations") of different pathologic processes. In addition, these plates were then engraved on stone (for lithographic purposes) by Carswell himself. According to William Osler, "these illustrations have, for artistic merit and for fidelity, never been surpassed, while the matter represents the highest point which the science of morbid anatomy had reached before the introduction of the microscope."[26]

One of the most beautifully illustrated neuropathology atlases to appear in this period was issued by Richard Bright (1789–1858). Bright's atlas on diseases of the brain and spinal cord was issued as the second part of a two-part work. It appeared in 1831 as *Diseases of the Brain and Nervous System*, published as Volume 2 under the general title *Reports of Medical Cases*.[27] Although Bright is best remembered for his description of glomerulonephritis (Bright's disease), he also provided a number of original graphic and clinical descriptions of diseases of the CNS. Within this volume are 25 elegant colored plates and more than 200 autopsy cases of neuropathologic diseases. Bright categorized these conditions into five pathologic phenomena: (1) inflammation and febrile illness; (2) mass lesions causing surrounding pressure, hemorrhage, or stroke; (3) concussion from outside phenomena; (4) irritation; and (5) deficient blood circulation leading to insufficient blood supply. In this volume is the first description of a pediatric pontine glioma with hydrocephalus, which would appear to be one of the earliest discussions of a primary pediatric neuro-oncologic lesion. Bright also described a number of other interesting clinical histories of patients with brain lesions. He noted that patients with increased intracranial pressure could develop paresis and, eventually, coma. Cases were described with premorbid clinical findings of screaming, agitation, and convulsions. Clinical complaints of headaches (typically dull), tinnitus, visual loss, loss of consciousness, and, eventually, coma were outlined in his clinical histories. Case CLXIV (see ref. 27, p. 349) is a typical example wherein he describes a "tumour in the brain" in a 45-year-old

man who initially presented with a headache and then numbness of the right arm. This progressed to a complete right hemiplegia, loss of speech, and eventually death on his 26th hospital day. On autopsy, Bright found a lesion in the left cerebral hemisphere. Bright illustrated the gross anatomical findings of the patient in this work. Despite these elegant findings, clinicians would wait another 30-plus years before Paul Broca (1824–1880) and Carl Wernicke (1848–1905) provided the definitive anatomical and clinical association of the left hemisphere lesions with expressive (Broca's) and receptive (Wernicke's) aphasia.[28,29] To Richard Bright we owe an extraordinary debt of gratitude for a work that was clinically quite advanced and to this day contains some of the most beautifully illustrated examples of brain lesions ever published.

Another striking atlas illustrating pathologic diseases, in a similar style as that of Bright, published in Paris, France, by Jean Cruveilhier (1791–1874) was entitled *Anatomie Pathologique du Corps Humain* (1829–1842).[30] Cruveilhier was the first professor of pathologic anatomy at the Paris School of Medicine. He worked at the Salpêtrière, which was originally built as a hospital, but is described as more of a prison for female destitutes and incurables. By 1822 it was a "grand asylum of human misery" containing 3900 incurables, 800 insane people, and 360 sick people.[31] To this hospital Cruveilhier was proudly attached (or so he states in his preface!) and from this institution came his abundant autopsy material. His atlas was issued in a series of fascicles dealing with all parts of the human body. Of interest to us are several illustrated examples of meningiomas, cerebellopontine angle tumors, epidermoid tumors *(tumeur perlée)*, along with several spinal cord pathologic specimens (Fig. 1–5). The illustrations, done in exquisite watercolors, have rarely been exceeded in the accuracy of graphic detail. This work has remained a benchmark with which all other pathologic atlases are compared.

A work important in the early period of neuropathology, unfortunately not illustrated, was that by the Frenchman Claude Francois Lallemand (1790–1853). As an intern at the Hôtel Dieu he had seen a great deal of pathology, and it was his goal to classify this material into a useful medical handbook. To do this, Lallemand issued a three-volume work (1820–1825) of more than 1500 pages entitled *Recherches anatomico-pathologiques sur l'encéphale et ses dépendences*.[32] It was Lallemand's goal to present a work that classified diseases of the brain solely on pathologic grounds. To do this he used the Morgagni style of presenting a series of clinical cases with autopsied material that documented the cases. He presented the clinical histories with the autopsied material of 1818 cases. Important to us are the numerous early descriptions of brain tumors that he described as fibrous, fibrocartilaginous, cartilaginous, or osseous. Unfortunately, microscopic demonstrations were not done. Nevertheless this is an important work, accomplished in the prelocalization era, on the nature and clinical types of tumors in a vast number of cases.

C. P. Ollivier D'Angers (1796–1845) produced a monograph entitled *De La Moelle épinière et de ses maladies* that focused more on disorders of the spinal cord.[33] He believed that disorders of the spinal cord were oftened ignored at autopsy, and it was his intention to correct this oversight. D'Angers presents 65 cases with two illustrated examples. He

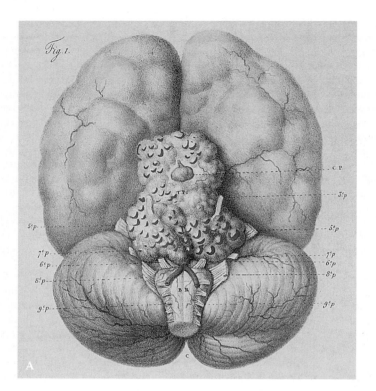
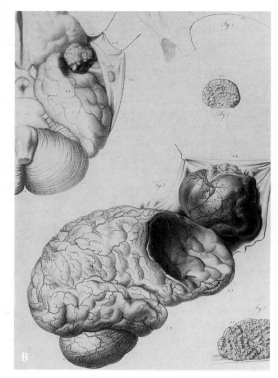
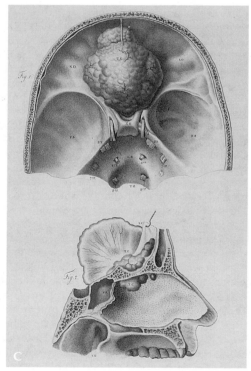
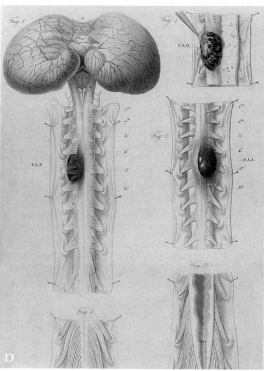

Figure 1–5   Examples of epidermoid tumors of the skull base, called "tumeur perlée," from Cruveilhier's atlas on morbid conditions. (B) Examples of different dural-based meningiomas, including a large frontal meningioma, from Cruveilhier's atlas on morbid conditions. (C) Examples of subfrontal and olfactory groove meningiomas, from Cruveilhier's atlas on morbid conditions. (D) A rare example of a spinal cord tumor, most likely a meningioma or perhaps a neurofibroma, from Cruveilhier's atlas on morbid conditions. (From Cruveilhier J. *Anatomie pathologique du corps humain, décriptions avec figures lithographiees et coloriées; des diverses alterations morbides don't le corp humain est susceptible.* Paris: J. B. Bailliere; 1835–1842.)

classifed the numerous spinal disorders under several headings, including congenital malformations, atrophy, trauma, compression, commotion, induration, tumors (*tissus morbides développés*), and so forth. Of particular importance in this volume is the earliest illustrated example of spinal root tumor (Fig. 1–6). This tumor originated from the T1 vertebra, causing 2 years of severe pain in the patient, who eventually committed suicide. At autopsy the tumor was found to be soft and solid, and contained a concentric arrangement of fibers on cross section (neurofibroma?).

Modern histologic pathology as we now know it developed in the 19th century. The science of histology was inaugurated with the work of Xavier Bichat (1771–1802). His studies revealed that organs did not exist solely as basic units but rather are composed of tissues.[34] This was further elaborated in the writings of Theodor Schwann (1810–1882), who elaborated the cellular theory.[35] These new concepts were applied to cellular disease by the great German pathologist Rudolf Virchow (1821–1902) who postulated the fundamental concept of *Omnis cellula e cellula* (each cell comes from a cell).[36] The importance of this work can scarcely be overstated; it is not only the cornerstone but the very foundation of cellular pathology. Virchow's theory that the seat of disease, as well as any developed tissue, could be traced back to the cell prompted his dictum *Omnis cellula e cellula* to be added to William Harvey's (1578–1657) *Omne vivum ex ovo* (Every living thing from an egg). From this viewpoint came the new concept that from the cell can come both normal and abnormal processes. Virchow published approximately 35 papers on neuropathology, including several on tumors of the brain and congenital anomalies. These new concepts firmly put to rest the age old doctrine of the humoral theory that had been in existence since the 2nd century AD when first postulated by Galen of Pergamon.

These new findings and concepts prompted a number of innovative investigations of the CNS. A prominent figure from this period and one best remembered for some of the earliest accurate neurology contributions was Jean Marie Charcot (1825–1893). Charcot assumed the chair of pathologic anatomy at the Faculty of Medicine in Paris in 1872 and went on to have one of the most productive careers of any figure in the history of medicine. Charcot believed very strongly in the postmortem examination, and, using some very simple staining techniques, he described a number of neurologic diseases, including amyotrophic lateral sclerosis, bulbar paralysis, multiple sclerosis, tabes dorsalis, and several muscular dystrophies.[37] Building on the recently developed views of pathologic diseases, Charcot provided a number of accurate descriptions of pathologic processes involving the CNS.

There were a number of prominent physicians in the latter half of the 19th century who contributed to the then-evolving views of cancer of the nervous system. Space does not allow a full discussion of all the personages involved, but several do merit mention. Alois Alzheimer (1864–1915) was the founder of the Munich school of neuropathology. He is remembered eponomically for his work on the organic mental diseases, arteriosclerosis, and senility. Alzheimer's talent for illustrating lesions is evident throughout his work, and his profusely illustrated works contain some of the earliest and finest examples of cancerous lesions of the brain. Franz Nissl (1860–1919) of Heidelberg, a contemporary of Alzheimer, was a pioneer in the techniques of histopathology, without which little understanding of what is normal in the brain could be understood. Nissl devised a number of histologic stains that he then used to delineate the various pathologic processes of the CNS.[38] In 1904, Alzheimer and Nissl published a remarkable six-volume work entitled *Histologische und histopathologische Arbeiten über dis Grosshirnrinde*.[39] In this work are detailed some of the earliest and finest examples of pathologic processes of the brain. The German schools were exceptionally productive at this time, with techniques and stains for study of the CNS being developed by Alfons Maria Jakob (1884–1931), Max Bielchowsky (1869–1940), Carl Weigert (1845–1904), and Walter Spielmeyer (1879–1935). With the combination of the microscope and special stains that revealed both normal and abnormal pathologic processes, the CNS was being explored to determine what constitutes cancers of the brain. With the introduction of anesthesia in the 1840s, antisepsis in the 1860s, and cerebral localization in the 1870s, the medical team could now make a preoperative determination of where the lesions might be localized in the brain, put a patient to a sleep for painless surgery, and remove the lesions with a markedly reduced risk of infection.

In the 19th century surgeons were becoming more adventurous, developing a better understanding of the cause and subsequent removal of cancerous lesions. However, surgical morbidity remained exceptionally high. Joseph Lister (1827–1912) continued the fine English tradition of surgery and made one of the greatest advances to surgery ever: the introduction of the antiseptic technique. The control of infection and its reduction led to profound changes in surgery and dramatically influenced postsurgical outcome. Surgical

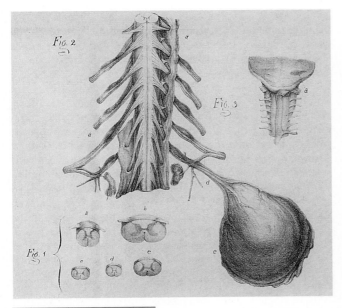

Figure 1–6 An example of a large neurofibroma (?) from Ollivier's monograph on maladies of the spine. (From Ollivier D'Angers CP. *De la moelle épinière et de ses maladies*. Paris: Crevot; 1824.)

mortality dropped from as high as 95% to as low as 10% with the reduction of infection. One cannot underestimate the profound effect that Lister's antiseptic techniques had on surgery: Without this contribution the situation was almost always hopeless when cerebral or spinal tumor surgery was involved.

The new developments of anesthesia, antisepsis, and cerebral localization encouraged the Scottish surgeon William Macewen (1848–1924) to successfully remove the first dural lesion on July 27, 1879.[40] Macewen was a surgeon and lecturer in surgery at the Royal Infirmary, Glasgow, and surgeon at the Hospital for Sick Children in Glasgow. The patient was a 14-year-old girl who had presented with supraorbital periosteal tumor a year previously, which had been removed. She presented again with progressive headaches, swelling over the eye, and seizures involving the right side. A large trephine was applied and a dural-based lesion was found and removed from under the skull flap. The patient recovered rapidly and returned to normal health. When Macewen published his collected cases in 1888, he had operated on 21 cerebral cases with only 3 deaths and 18 recoveries—a remarkable accomplishment for this period.[41,42]

A well-known and celebrated case of an intraparenchymal brain tumor and the first brain tumor to be successfully removed by surgical means occurred in 1884 when A. H. Bennett (1848–1901), a general surgeon, removed a lesion diagnosed and localized by Rickman J. Godlee (1849–1925)[43] (Fig. 1–7). The case involved a 25-year-old man who, for 3 years, had had a succession of focal motor seizures. They started as seizures of the left face and progressed down the arm and leg. Six months prior to surgery he presented with weakness of the arm. Eye examination just prior to surgery revealed papilledema and hemorrhages. In addition, the patient had developed severe headaches and vomiting. On November 25, 1884, at the Hospital for Epilepsy and Paralysis (now known as Maida Vale Hospital), a trephination was done over the fissure of Rolando, a cortical incision made, and a tumor found at the depth of $\frac{1}{8}$ in. It was encapsulated and enucleated piecemeal and found to be a glioma. Unfortunately, the patient died a month later from complications of meningitis.

In 1888 another English surgeon, Victor A. H. Horsley (1857–1916), removed a spinal cord tumor that had been diagnosed by the neurologist William Gowers (1845–1915).[44] These innovative individuals not only laid the foundation work for neurosurgery but also for modern neuro-oncology.

The first textbook to contain "modern" views of neuropathology and brain tumors was that of Byrom Bramwell (1847–1931) published in 1888.[45] Many of the illustrations were done by Bramwell himself (Fig. 1–8). Bramwell graduated from the University of Edinburgh in 1869. He entered into private practice with his father and then went on to teach medical jurisprudence at Durham University. In 1880 he returned to Edinburgh and became the appointed pathologist and physician to the Royal Infirmary. A superb clinician and expert diagnostician, he was a popular teacher with large, well-attended classes. Bramwell developed a strong interest in diseases of the nervous system and published two classics, one of which focused on diseases of the spinal cord (1882)[46] and the other on intracranial tumors (1888).[45] The intracranial tumor book immediately became a classic standard work of the 19th century. This work appeared shortly after the classic localization studies of Charcot, Broca, Ferrier, and others that had localized neurologic symptoms to specific areas of the brain. Bramwell

CASE OF CEREBRAL TUMOUR.

BY

A. HUGHES BENNETT, M.D., F.R.C.P.,
PHYSICIAN TO THE HOSPITAL FOR EPILEPSY AND PARALYSIS, AND
ASSISTANT PHYSICIAN TO THE WESTMINSTER HOSPITAL.

THE SURGICAL TREATMENT

BY

RICKMAN J. GODLEE, M.S., F.R.C.S.,
SURGEON TO UNIVERSITY COLLEGE HOSPITAL.

Received January 13th—Read May 12th, 1885.

THE chief features of interest in the case, to which the attention of the Society is directed, are, that during life the existence of a tumour was diagnosed in the brain, and its situation localised, entirely by the signs and symptoms exhibited, without any external manifestations on the surface of the skull. This growth was removed without any immediate injurious effects on the intelligence and general condition of the patient. Although he died four weeks after the operation, the fatal termination was due, not to any special effects on the nervous centres, but to a secondary surgical complication. The case, moreover, teaches some important physiological, pathological, and clinical lessons, and suggests practical reflections which may prove useful to future medicine and surgery.

Figure 1–7 The initial leaf of the classic Bennett and Godlee paper on a successful removal of a cerebral tumor. (From Bennett AH, Godlee RJ. Case of cerebral tumor. *Med Chir Trans* 1885;68:243.)

built on their findings, using pathologic brain tumors as evidence of regional brain function. Bramwell was the first author to describe the effects of pituitary tumors on the hypothalmus. He was also an early advocate for neurosurgery and quite excited about the work of Horsley and Macewen. From a case report came the following observations (ref. 45, see pp. 249–250): "The brilliant results which Macewen has obtained in cerebral surgery, and which Victor Horsley has recently published, seem to prove that the expectations which Hughes Bennett formed when he first advocated the operation were well founded. And, thanks to antisepsis, the dangers of trephining are now so slight, that in all cases of intracranial tumour in which substantial improvement is not obtained by the administration of iodide of potassium [early chemotherapy?], the possibility of removing the new growth by operative procedure must be carefully considered." Bramwell then outlines what he believed were the most important conditions for successful operative interference: "1. Successful localization of the tumour.... 2. The tumour must be assessible.... 3. The tumour must be single and of such a pathological character as to permit of complete enucleation or removal.... In the case of multiple tumours, such as secondary deposits of cancer or melanotic sarcoma, operative measures for the removal of the tumour are of course quite out of the question. Hence the great importance of exact diagnosis, not only as regards the position of the

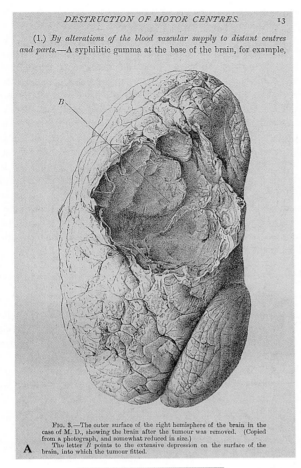

(1.) *By alterations of the blood vascular supply to distant centres and parts.*—A syphilitic gumma at the base of the brain, for example,

B

Fig. 3.—The outer surface of the right hemisphere of the brain in the case of M. D., showing the brain after the tumour was removed. (Copied from a photograph, and somewhat reduced in size.)
    The letter *B* points to the extensive depression on the surface of the brain, into which the tumour fitted.

A

SYMPTOMS DUE TO ASSOCIATED LESIONS. 17

In Figs. 5 and 6, the swollen condition of the hemisphere in which the tumour is situated is well shown.

A

B

D

C

E

Fig. 6.—Transverse vertical section through the brain, showing a large glio-sarcomatous tumour in the left hemisphere, which is markedly larger than the right.
    The letter *A* points to the nucleus caudatus; *B*, to the optic thalamus; and *C*, to the lenticular nucleus of the right side.
    The letter *D* points to the left or internal capsule, which was compressed, and to some extent invaded by the new growth; the letter *E* points to the tumour.

(3.) Cerebral symptoms in cases of intracranial tumour may be due to associated meningitis, hæmorrhage into the substance of the tumour and surrounding nerve tissue, or other accidental complications.

B (4.) The presence or absence of constitutional disturbance, and the

Figure 1–8 (A) An illustration by Bramwell of an intraparenchymal lesion that had been removed by surgery. (B) An intraparenchymal lesion, most likely a glioblastoma multiforme, described as a gliosarcomatous lesion in Bramwell's monograph on brain tumors. (From Bramwell B. *Intracranial Tumours*. Edinburgh: YJ Pentland; 1888.)

tumour, but also as regards the pathological character of the new growth." These are indeed very prophetic comments made at the beginning of the modern era of neurosurgery and neuropathology.

The present-day classification of brain tumors was initiated by the great American neurosurgeon Harvey Cushing (1870–1939). Cushing began the classification of brain tumors with his work on tumors of the pituitary gland (1912),[47] followed by his work on acoustic nerve tumors published in 1917.[48] Cushing continued his classifications of tumors of the CNS with his landmark work published in collaboration with P. Bailey (1892–1973) in 1926. With this work we have the first classification of tumors of the CNS based on a histologic profile[49] (Fig. 1–9). Cushing further classified another group of tumors with his seminal work on meningiomas, published in 1938 in collaboration with the brilliant neuropathologist Louise Eisenhardt (1891–1966).[50]

A technical achievement introduced in the 1890s that revolutionized the concept of how we deal with brain tumors was the application of the X ray to physical diagnosis. Up to this point the nervous system was totally inaccessible to direct examination without dire consequences. Roentgen's discovery of the X ray dramatically changed our ability to examine and

diagnose brain tumors. For the first time, internal structures could be visualized by noninvasive techniques. Roentgen's work was further refined with a serendipitous finding by William H. Luckett (1872–?) who studied a patient with a frontal skull fracture and spontaneous pneumoencephaly.[51] The air within the ventricles provided the contrast necessary to see internal structures, such as a tumor. In 1918–1919, Walter Dandy (1886–1946), a neurosurgeon, and Kenneth D. Blackfan (1883–1947), a pediatrician, took this one step further and introduced ventriculography/encephalography whereby air was introduced by a lumbar puncture.[52–56] Originally designed to permit a better understanding of hydrocephalus, this technique became the diagnostic standard for CNS examinations until the introduction of computed tomography (CT). By analyzing shifts and defects within the pneumoencephalogram the surgeon could now better localize the deeper lesions.

Feeling that the brain remained a "dark continent," the Portuguese physician and statesman Antonio Caetano de Abrev Friere Egas Moniz (1874–1955) adopted the concept of introducing a nontoxic contrast dye into the arteries[57] this technique made visible vessels that could be now contrasted on X ray. His book, published in 1931, contained 189 arteriograms and laid the foundation for modern arteriography.[58]

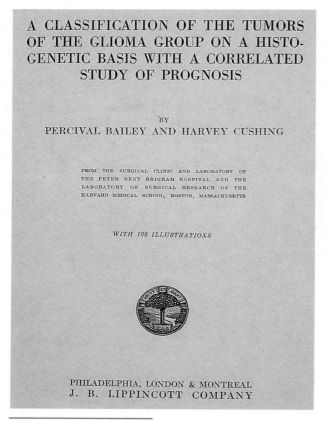

A CLASSIFICATION OF THE TUMORS
OF THE GLIOMA GROUP ON A HISTO-
GENETIC BASIS WITH A CORRELATED
STUDY OF PROGNOSIS

BY
PERCIVAL BAILEY AND HARVEY CUSHING

FROM THE SURGICAL CLINIC AND LABORATORY OF
THE PETER BENT BRIGHAM HOSPITAL AND THE
LABORATORY OF SURGICAL RESEARCH OF THE
HARVARD MEDICAL SCHOOL, BOSTON, MASSACHUSETTS

WITH 108 ILLUSTRATIONS

PHILADELPHIA, LONDON & MONTREAL
J. B. LIPPINCOTT COMPANY

Figure 1–9 The first monograph to provide an early and detailed classification of brain tumors based on their histogenetic correlation by P. Bailey and H. Cushing. (From Bailey P, Cushing HW. *A Classification of the Tumors of the Glioma Group on a Histogenetic Basis with a Correlated Study of Prognosis.* Philadelphia: JB Lippincott; 1926.)

Moniz was awarded the Nobel Prize in 1949, not for this work but for his studies on the development of frontal lobotomy.

One of the single greatest contributions to the diagnosis of brain lesions was the introduction of CT by Sir Godfrey N. Hounsfield (1919–).[59] Hounsfield was working for the EMI Ltd and was interested in pattern recognition, that is, how to acquire patterns and reproduce them in detailed images. His initial concept was a simple one: how to describe objects within a closed box.[60] He solved this problem by generating γ rays or X rays through the box in a series of different angles, taking a large quantity of measurements at different angles (i.e., tomograms). From these multiple multiplanar images he could reconstruct the internal object. The original experiment took 9 days to complete; Hounsfield quickly reduced that to 5 minutes, and today modern machines produce these images in seconds. The first clinical picture of the brain was taken in October 1971; the brain was selected because it does not move with respirations (movement blurs images). Hounsfield was awarded the Nobel Prize in medicine in 1979 for this work. He was the first engineer to receive a Nobel Prize in the medicine category. This technique of CT, along with the more recent magnetic resonance imaging (MRI), has revolutionized how we look at the brain and other internal structures.

SUMMARY

With this brief introduction the reader can appreciate how far we have come; at the same time, one must appreciate how far we have yet to go. For 1600 years we stagnated in the humoral theories of Galen; however, in the last century we have managed to advance several new concepts. The cell was discovered; anesthesia and antisepsis were introduced; and, thanks to the pioneering work of Cushing, Horsley, and others, the CNS could be approached and operated on with success. However, the "cure" of pediatric neuro-oncologic lesions remains not in the hands of surgeons but rather in the hands of oncologists and pediatricians. We can locate the lesions, remove them, and make a diagnosis, but the final cure resides in turning off that malignant cell, eliminating its immortality, and stabilizing the cellular system. Subsequent chapters in this volume will delineate some of these important neuro-oncologic concepts and techniques.

REFERENCES

1. Hippocrates. *Magni Hippocratis Medicorum Omnium Facile Principis, Opera Omnia quae extant ... nunc denuo Latina Interpretations and Annotatioibus illustrata Anutio Foesio.*Genevae: S. Chouet; 1657–1662.
2. Raven RW. *The Theory and Practice of Oncology. Historical Evolution and General Principles.* Park Ridge, NJ: Parthenon Publishing Group; 1990.
3. Bett WR. Historical aspects of cancer. In: Raven RW, ed. *Cancer.* Vol. 1. London: Butterworths; 1957:1–5.
4. Celsus. *Medicinae Libri VIII.* In aedibus Aldi et Andreae Asulani soceri, Venice, 1528.
5. Galen of Pergamon. *Omnia quae extant opera in Latinum sermonem conversa.* 5th ed. Venice: Apud Juntas, 1576–1577.
6. Avicenna. *Liber canonis, De medicinis cordialibus et Cantica.* Basel: Per Joannes Heruagios, 1556.
7. Albucasis [Abu Al-Quasim]. *Liber theoricae necnon practicae Alsaharavii.* Augsburg: Impensis Sigismundi Grimm and Marci Vuirsung, 1519.
8. *Albucasis on Surgery and Instruments.* A definitive edition of the arabic text with English translation and commentary by M. S. Spink and G. L. Lewis. Berkeley: University of California Press, 1973:170–172, 812–819.
9. *Medicae Artis Principes, post Hippocratem and Galenum.* Geneva: Henri Estienne, 1567.
10. Vesalius, Andreas. *De Humani Corporis Fabrica Libri Septum.* Basel: Ex officina Joannis Oporini; 1543.
11. Singer, Charles. *Vesalius on the Human Brain.* Introduction, translation of text. London: Oxford University Press, 1952.
12. Berengario da Carpi, Jacobi. *Tractatus de fractura calvae sive cranei.* Bologna: Impressum per Hieronymum de Benedictus; 1518.
13. Scultetus, Johannes. *Armamentarium chirurgicum XLIII. Typis and impensis.* Ulm: Balthasari Kühnen, 1655.
14. LeDran H. *Consultations sur la pluspart des maladies qui sont du ressort de la chirurgie.* Paris: Chez P. Fr. Didot le jeune; 1765.
15. LeDran H. *Traité des operations de chirurgie.* Paris: Charles Osmont; 1742.
16. Morgagni GB. *De sedibus et causis morborum per anatomen indagatis libri quinque.* Vienna: ex trypographica Remondiana; 1761.

17. Baillie M. *The Morbid Anatomy of Some of the Most Important Parts of the Human Body.* London: Printed for J. Johnson and G. Nicol; 1793.
18. Baillie M. *A Series of Engravings with Explanations Which Are Intended to Illustrate the Morbid Anatomy of Some of the Most Important Parts of the Human Body.* London: W. Bulmer & Co.; 1799–1803.
19. Hunter J. *Lectures on the Principles of Surgery.* Philadelphia: Haswell, Barrington & Haswell; 1839.
20. Cooper A. *Illustrations of Diseases of the Breast.* London: Longman & Rees; 1829.
21. Bell C. *The Nervous System of the Human Body.* 2nd ed. London: Longman and Co.; 1830.
22. Abercombie J. *Pathological and Practical Researches on Diseases of the Brain and the Spinal Cord.* Edinburgh: Printed for Waugh and Innes; 1828.
23. Hooper R. *The Morbid Anatomy of the Human Brain, Illustrated by Coloured Engravings of the Most Frequent and Important Organic Diseases to Which That Viscus Is Subject.* London: printed for the Author; 1828.
24. Behan PO, Behan WMH. Sir Robert Carswell: Scotland's pioneer pathologist. In: Rose FC, Bynum WF, eds. *Historical Aspects of the Neurosciences. A Festschrift for Macdonald Critchley.* New York: Raven Press; 1982:273–292.
25. Carswell R. *Pathological Anatomy: Illustrations of the Elementary Forms of Disease.* London: Longman and Co.; 1838.
26. Bibliotheca Osleriana. *A Catalogue of Books Illustrating the History of Medicine and Science.* Collected, arranged, and annotated by Sir William Osler. Montreal: McGill–Queen's University Press, 1969. See citation Osler 2250.
27. Bright R. *Reports of Medical Cases Selected with a View of Illustrating the Symptoms and Cure of Diseases by Reference to Morbid Anatomy. Diseases of the Brain and Nervous System.* Vol. 2. London: Longman and Co.; 1831.
28. Broca P. Perte de la parole; ramollissement chronique et destruction partielle du lobe antérieur gauche du cerveau. *Bull Soc Anthrop Paris* 1861;2:235.
29. Wernicke C. *Der aphasische Symptomenkomplex.* Breslau: M. Cohn & Weigert, 1874.
30. Cruveilhier J. *Anatomie pathologique du corps humain, décriptions avec figures lithographiées et coloriées; des diverses altérations morbides dont le corp humain est suseptible.* Paris: J. B. Bailliere;1829–1842.
31. Spillane JD. *The Doctrine of the Nerves. Chapters in the History of Neurology.* Oxford: Oxford University Press, 1981; see p. 195.
32. Lallemand F. *Recherches anatomico-pathologiques sur l'encéphale et ses dépendances.* Paris: J. Baudouin Fréres; 1820–1825.
33. Ollivier D'Angers CP. *De la moelle épinière et de ses maladies.* Paris: Crevot; 1824.
34. Bichat MFX. *Recherches physiologiques sur la vie et la mort.* Paris: Brosson, Gabon et Cie; 1800.
35. Schwann T. Mikroskopische Untersuchungen über die Struktur der Tiere und Pflanzen. *Fororiep's Neue Notizen.* 1838;5:228.
36. Virchow R. *Die Cellularpathologie in ihrer Begründung auf physiologische und pathologische Gewebelehre.* Berlin: A. Hirschwald; 1858.
37. Charcot JM. *Lectures on the Diseases of the Nervous System.* Delivered at the Salpêtrière, translated by G. Sigerson. London: The New Sydenham Society; 1877–1889.
38. Nissl F. *Histologische und histopathologische Arbeiten über die Grosshirnrinde.* Vol 1. Jena: G. Fischer; 1904.
39. Alzheimer A, Nissl F. *Histologische und histopathologische Arbeiten über die Grosshirnrinde.* Jena: G. Fisher; 1904.
40. Macewen W. Tumour of the dura mater—convulsions—removal of tumour by trephining—recovery. *Glasgow Med J* 1879;12:210–213.
41. Macewen W. An address on the surgery of the brain and spinal cord. Delivered at the annual meeting of the British Medical Association held in Glasgow, August 9, 1888. BMJ 1888;302–309.
42. Pearce JMS. The first attempts at removal of brain tumors. In: Rose FC, Bynum WF, eds. *Historical Aspects of the Neurosciences. A Festschrift for Macdonald Critchley.* New York: Raven Press, 1982:239–242.
43. Bennett AH, Godlee RJ. Case of cerebral tumor. *Med Chir Trans* 1885;68:243.
44. Gowers WR, Horsley VAH. A case of tumour of the spinal cord. Removal; recovery. *Med Chir Trans* 1888;71:377.
45. Bramwell B. *Intracranial Tumours.* Edinburgh: YJ Pentland; 1888.
46. Bramwell B. *The Diseases of the Spinal Cord.* Edinburgh: Maclachland & Stewart; 1882.
47. Cushing H. *The Pituitary Body and Its Disorders: Clinical States Produced by Disorders of the Hypophysis Cerebri.* Philadelphia: JB Lippincott; 1912.
48. Cushing HW. *Tumors of the Nervus Acusticus and the Syndrome of the Cerebellopontine Angle.* Philadelphia: WB Saunders, 1917.
49. Bailey P, Cushing HW. *A Classification of the Tumors of the Glioma Group on a Histogenetic Basis with a Correlated Study of Prognosis.* Philadelphia: JB Lippincott; 1926.
50. Cushing HW, Eisenhardt L. *Meningiomas: Their Classifications, Regional Behaviour, Life History, and Surgical End Results.* Springfield, IL: Charles C Thomas; 1938.
51. Luckett WH. Air in the ventricles, following a fracture of the skull. *Surg Gynecol Obstet* 1913;17:237–240.
52. Dandy WE, Blackfan KD. An experimental and clinical study of internal hydrocephalus. *JAMA* 1913;61:2216–2217.
53. Dandy WE, Blackfan KD. Internal hydrocephalus: an experimental, clinical and pathologic study. *Am J Dis Child* 1914;8:406–482, 1914; 1917;14:424–443.
54. Dandy WE. Ventriculography following the injection of air into the cerebral ventricles. *Ann Surg* 1918;68:5–11.
55. Dandy WE. Roentgenography of the brain after the injection of air into the spinal canal. *Ann Surg* 1919;70:397–403.
56. Dandy WE. Localization or elimination of cerebral tumors by ventriculography. *Surg Gynecol Obstet.* 1920;30:329–342.
57. Moniz CE. L'encéphalographie artérielle, son importance dans la localisation des tumeurs cérébrales. *Rev Neurol* 1927;2:72–90.
58. Moniz CE. *Diagnostic des tumeurs cérébrales et épreuve de l'encéphalographie artérielle.* Paris: Masson & Cie, 1931.
59. Hounsfield GN. Computerized transverse axial scanning (tomography) *Br J Radiol* 1973;46:1016–1022.
60. Bull JWD. The history of neuroradiology. In: Rose FC, Bynum WF, eds. *Historical Aspects of the Neurosciences. A Festschrift for Macdonald Critchley.* New York: Raven Press; 1982;255–264.

Chapter 2

Epidemiology of Brain Tumors

Marc Bestak

Among children younger than 15 years, more than 7000 new cases of cancer are diagnosed each year. Although leukemia is the most common malignancy of childhood, central nervous system (CNS) tumors are second in frequency, representing approximately 20% of all childhood cancers in the United States (Table 2–1).[1]

Although the past 30 years has seen improvement in the prognosis for all malignancies of childhood, from 25% in 1970 to 70% in 1991,[2,3] brain tumors continue to be a cause of excess mortality. The morbidity caused by CNS tumors and their therapy exceeds that of most other childhood cancers.

In 1990, the overall incidence rate of brain tumors in the United States was reported by the Surveillance Epidemiology and End Results (SEER) program as 6.3 primary malignant brain tumors per 100,000 individuals, whereas in children under the age of 15 years the incidence was 2.8 per 100,000 individuals.[4] Although the incidence of astrocytomas is the same in boys and girls younger than 15, the sex ratio of brain tumors among children under 15 is approximately 1.1 : 1, with male predominance.[5,6] A 1995 update of the SEER program showed that rates of brain tumor development stabilized for all age groups except for individuals 85 years and older. Mortality rates continued to decline for the younger age groups, and slowed substantially.[7]

Bunin et al,[8] reporting their experience from the Greater Delaware Valley Pediatric Tumor Registry, noted that whereas the incidence of acute lymphoblastic leukemia and acute myelogenous leukemia did not change significantly over the past 20 years, that of CNS tumors rose 2.7% per year. In this report, brain tumors of children were divided into three groups: glioma, primitive neuroectodermal tumor (PNET)/medulloblastoma (MB), and other. Neither the rate nor the change in rate differed among white males, who experienced a 3.6% annual increase in incidence. The incidence in white females ages 0 to 4 increased by 6.2% annually. There was no significant change in incidence over time in older white females or in blacks. The incidence of PNET/MB increased an estimated 4.3% per year. Blacks experienced slightly lower rates of gliomas and PNET/MB than whites. The PNET/MB incidence in males was 1.7 times that in females.

Brain tumors are the cause of one-fourth of all cancer deaths among children, according to many U.S. and international sources and registries.[9–11]

Treatment of children with brain tumors has changed substantially over the last half century. The use of computed tomography (CT) and magnetic resonance imaging (MRI) facilitates early diagnosis, planning for surgery, and the surgical approach to the tumor. The intraoperative microscope makes it possible for the surgeon to distinguish between tumor and normal brain. These developments have resulted in a greater likelihood that complete surgical resection of the tumor will be accomplished.

Effective chemotherapy has been shown to improve the survival of many patients with CNS tumors, and external-beam radiotherapy remains an important modality of treatment for all but the youngest patients with these tumors. Intensive chemotherapeutic programs to which autologous stem cell reconstitution following bone marrow ablative chemotherapy is added have somewhat replaced radiother-

TABLE 2–1   Annual Incidence of Cancer in Children under Age 15, per Million Members of the Population

Diagnosis	No. of Cases per Year	Rate per Million
Brain and other CNS tumors	1095	45.8
Neuroblastoma	387	16.1
Wilms' tumor	363	17.7
Rhabdomyosarcoma and embryonal sarcoma	215	8.8
Retinoblastoma	154	7.6
Osteosarcoma	139	6.9
Ewing's sarcoma	112	3.1

Adapted from Young J, Ries L, Silverberg E, et al. Cancer incidence, survival, and mortality for children younger than 15 years. *Cancer* 1986;58:598–602.

apy for the 15% of brain tumor patients who are diagnosed prior to their second birthday. The effects of radiotherapy for such young and developing brains are prohibitive; they carry a high probability of failure of growth, failure of emotional and intellectual development, as well as a significantly increased risk of secondary malignancy. In fact, the level of adult resistance to the untoward effects of intensive radiation therapy is not present in children until the ninth year of life.

BOX 2–1
Risks of Cranial Radiotherapy

- **Secondary malignancy**
- **Diminished cognitive development**
- **Diminished social development**
- **Hormonal deficiency**

Jenkin[12] described some of the problems of long-term outcome following survival of treatment for CNS tumors of childhood. Among the greatest concerns are those of early relapse, late relapse, and secondary malignancy. Patients with high-grade tumors are most likely to relapse within 5 years of diagnosis. Such patients include those with high-grade gliomas and those with unresectable MBs. Patients with low-grade tumors, such as those with optic gliomas or low-grade astrocytomas, are at risk for both late relapse and mortality. The incidence of secondary malignant tumors in patients treated with radiotherapy during the 30 years after treatment is 2.5% at 10 years, 13% at 20 years, and 19% at 30 years. The most common secondary malignant tumors are gliomas, meningiomas, acute leukemia, and sarcomas.

An important issue in long-term outcome is the cognitive and social development of children who survive treatment for brain tumor. Are these children successfully educated? Do they obtain good jobs? Do they marry and have children? What is their final height, and are hormonal deficiencies present? Although the exact incidence of such problems is not known, it is clear that many young children have serious cognitive and hormonal impairment following whole-brain irradiation.

Eighty-five percent of brain tumors in patients 2 to 12 years of age are posterior fossa (infratentorial) tumors. In this age group, embryonal tumors, such as MB and ependymoma, predominate. In patients older than 70 years, a second peak of brain tumors occurs, consisting predominantly of gliomas.[13–15] Supratentorial brain tumors are more common in children younger than 2 years and in adolescents.[16]

Although the exact incidence of individual tumors of the CNS in childhood is not known, Figure 2–1 presents an approximation.

Two percent of intracranial neoplasms in children are rhabdoid tumors arising in the brain. Five percent of childhood CNS tumors arise in the spinal cord. These are primarily ependymomas and oligodendrogliomas.

Although primary brain tumors are far more common in children than brain metastases, it should be noted that the most common sources of brain metastases in persons younger than 21 years are sarcomas (rhabdomyosarcoma, Ewing's sarcoma, and so forth) and germ cell tumors.[17] In children younger than 3 years, the most common tumors are primitive neuroectodermal tumors in those under 1 year, astrocytomas and ependymomas in those under 2 years, and astrocytomas in those under 3 years.[18]

ETIOLOGIC STUDIES OF PRIMARY BRAIN TUMORS

The causes of brain tumors have been studied for several years. They can be placed into two broad categories: those causes that have been confirmed and those that have not. *Among the confirmed etiologies, hereditary causes and exposure to ionizing therapeutic radiation are proven.* Occupational and dietary exposures, though possibly related, have not yet been shown to be unique causes of brain tumors. Over the past several years, studies of mutations of oncogenes and tumor suppressor genes have indicated an association with the development of malignancies of the brain.[19,20]

Levine describes the differences between oncogenes and tumor suppressor genes and their relationship to tumorigenesis in his review of the *p53* tumor suppressor gene.[21]

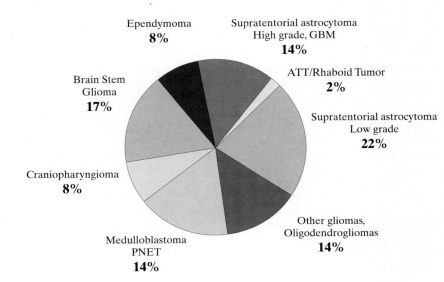

Ependymoma
8%

Supratentorial astrocytoma
High grade, GBM
14%

Brain Stem
Glioma
17%

ATT/Rhaboid Tumor
2%

Supratentorial astrocytoma
Low grade
22%

Craniopharyngioma
8%

Other gliomas,
Oligodendrogliomas
14%

Medulloblastoma
PNET
14%

Figure 2–1   Relative frequency of childhood brain tumors (PNET, primitive neuroectodermal tumor; GBM, glioblastoma multiforme.)

Oncogenes and tumor suppressor genes regulate the growth and proliferation of cells. Mutations in oncogenes typically occur in one allele of the gene and act in a dominant capacity toward the normal, nonmutated allele. Thus, they constitute an increase in function that may temporarily or permanently result in a signal for cells to divide. These mutations do not occur naturally, and they are not inherited. There is some degree of tissue preference for particular oncogenes. Either tumor suppressor genes have mutations in both alleles or, more often, the mutation is followed by a loss of the normal allele (termed reduction to homozygosity in that allele). They act as negative regulators of cell proliferation. These mutated genes can occur in either germ cells or somatic cells. When in germ cells, the predisposition to cancer is often inherited as a dominant trait. Somatic mutations in tumor suppressor genes often show a tissue preference with regard to the type of cancers in which they are found.

BOX 2–2
Syndromes Associated with CNS Tumors

- **Neurofibromatosis type 1**
- **Neurofibromatosis type 2**
- **Tuberous sclerosis type 1**
- **Tuberous sclerosis type 2**
- **von Hippel-Lindau syndrome**
- **Li-Fraumeni syndrome**
- **Nevoid basal cell carcinoma syndrome**
- **Turcot's syndrome**
- **Ataxia-telangiectasia syndrome**
- **Gardner's syndrome**
- **Down syndrome**

Several syndromes have been shown to be associated with the development of brain tumors, the most common of which is neurofibromatosis type 1 (NF-1), an autosomal dominant disorder in which there is a high frequency of de novo germline mutations. Its incidence is approximately 1 per 3000 in the population. The most commonly seen features of this syndrome are neurofibromas, café au lait spots, and Lisch nodules. The NF-1 tumor suppressor gene is located on chromosome 17q12-22. This syndrome is associated with hematologic malignancies and solid tumors, including CNS tumors. In children, gliomas of the optic pathway are most common, although other glial tumors and meningiomas can be seen as well. Optic glioma pathway tumors arise in children younger than 7 years and behave in a significantly more benign fashion than those occurring in children without NF-1.[22] Neurofibromatosis type 2 (NF-2), the gene for which is located on chromosome 22q12, is associated with vestibular schwannoma, ependymoma, and meningioma. The incidence of NF-2 is 1 per 30,000.

Another phakomatosis is tuberous sclerosis, an autosomal dominant disorder in which the patient has multiple hamartomas of the skin, brain, heart, kidney, and other organs. In type 1 tuberous sclerosis (TSC-1) (incidence 1 in 10,000), the tumor suppressor gene is on chromosome 9q32-34, whereas for type 2 tuberous sclerosis (TSC-2) (incidence 1 in 150,000) it is on 16p13.3. The CNS lesions are most often cortical tubers. Subependymal giant cell astrocytomas are unique to this disorder. Five percent of tuberous sclerosis patients have malignant brain tumors, including astrocytoma, ependymoma, and glioblastoma multiforme.[23,24]

The von Hippel-Lindau syndrome, an autosomal dominant disorder with a high degree of penetrance, has been associated with cerebellar hemangioblastoma, pheochromocytoma, paraganglioma, papillary cystadenoma of the epididymis, clear-cell carcinoma of the kidney, glioma, and retinal tumors. The gene is on the short arm of chromosome 3 (3p25-26). In Poland, the incidence is estimated at 1 in 30,000 to 1 in 50,000.[25]

Li-Fraumeni syndrome is the name given to the syndrome of families with multiple cancers.[26–29] Li and Fraumeni described such families between 1969 and 1988. Li-Fraumeni syndrome is linked to mutations of *p53* (normally a tumor suppresser gene), located on the short arm of chromosome 17. Multiple childhood solid tumors, including CNS tumors and, in young adults, tumors of the breast, bone, brain, lung, and other sites, have been seen. The most common CNS tumor seen in patients with Li-Fraumeni syndrome is astrocytoma. Familial cases of glioblastoma multiforme and astrocytoma inherited in autosomal dominant fashion may represent part of this syndrome.[30,31]

MB has been described in patients with autosomal dominant nevoid basal cell carcinoma syndrome, the gene for which is located on chromosome 1q22; Turcot's syndrome (polyposis of the colon in association with a CNS malignancy; glioblastoma and MB have been reported), the gene for which is located on chromosome 5q21-22; and ataxia-telangiectasia syndrome (telangiectases, degeneration of the cerebellum, and hematologic and other malignancies). Gardner's syndrome is also associated with MB.

Brain tumors are sometimes associated with other childhood cancers. Pituitary adenomas occur in children with multiple endocrine adenomatosis syndrome. Embryonal CNS tumors can be seen in patients with renal tumors.[32] Pineoblastoma has been associated with retinoblastoma in a syndrome known as trilateral retinoblastoma.[33]

Hereditary cancer occurs at a younger age than expected, suggesting that the occurrence of brain tumors in children may represent hereditary susceptibility in some families.[34] Siblings may be at a 3- to 10-fold increased risk of brain tumors, and the risk for other childhood cancers, in particular tumors of bone and the hematopoietic/lymphatic system, is also increased.[35] In a study of childhood astrocytoma, patients were more likely than controls to have a first- or second-degree relative with cancer, most frequently a brain tumor or breast cancer. This was especially true for children whose brain tumors were diagnosed before age 5 years. Persons with a genetic predisposition to cancer are not only expected to develop cancer at younger-than-usual age but also to develop multiple tumors more frequently.

A recent report from China suggests that an increased incidence of intracranial germ cell tumors is seen in children with Down syndrome and that children with this syndrome, who often manifest subtle neurologic changes, should be evaluated with α-fetoprotein and β-human chorionic gonadotropin assays.[36]

An unusual tumor that may arise in a large number of body sites, the most common of which is the brain, is the atypical teratoid/rhabdoid tumor. The median age of presentation is 20 months, and the male/female ratio is 1.6:1.[37] The disease is usually fatal, and aggressive chemotherapy/stem cell reconstitution is recommended in view of the risks of radiotherapy in this age group. This tumor is associated with monosomy or deletion of chromosome 22. The major problem in diagnosis is differentiating it from PNET/MB, in which an isochromosome (17q) is present in 50% of cases.

Patients with hereditary retinoblastoma often have bilateral disease and develop second primary tumors more frequently than sporadic retinoblastoma patients.[34] Patients with multifocal brain tumors or second primary tumors after a brain tumor may signal the presence of a hereditary syndrome. Children with brain tumors are also at increased risk for secondary tumors, although the late effects of therapy for the first tumor probably account for a large fraction of the secondary malignancies.

However, the genetic loci for the more common juvenile pilocytic or low-grade diffuse astrocytoma have not yet been identified.

Biegel[38] recently described the current knowledge about the cytogenetics of pediatric brain tumors. Fifty percent of PNET/MBs have an isochromosome (17q) abnormality. It is probable that this site contains a tumor suppressor gene, which is important to the development of this tumor. Another tumor suppressor gene in chromosome band 22q11.2 may play a role in the atypical teratoid/rhabdoid tumor. Meningiomas, rare in children, have been shown to contain chromosome 22 deletions, and such deletions have also been seen in ependymomas. Malignant anaplastic astrocytomas and glioblastoma multiforme have abnormalities, including loss of alleles on 1p, 19q,[39] and 17p13, and TP53 mutations, trisomy 7, epidermal growth factor receptor rearrangements, and loss of chromosomes 10 and 22, similar to what is seen in these tumors in adults. However, the

genetic loci for the more common juvenile pilocytic or low-grade diffuse astrocytoma have not been identified yet (Table 2–2).

It is hoped that as more is learned about genetic aberrations associated with oncogenesis, new therapies can be developed to antagonize the products of those genetic aberrations. As an example, Chen et al[40] evaluated the ability of a tumor suppressor gene, when bound to an adenovirus vector, to inhibit an astrocytoma cell line by causing cell cycle arrest in G1. (The tumor suppressor gene *p27KIP1* is a downstream effector of transforming growth factor β and a universal cyclin-dependent kinase inhibitor). By showing inhibition of tritiated thymidine uptake in the cell line and marked diminution of aneuploid cells in the culture, it became clear that *p27KIP1* is a candidate for the gene therapy of human brain tumors. New therapies may also be directed against tumor angiogenesis or against the deep neuronal extensions of glial tumors.

BOX 2–3
Nongenetic Factors Associated with Brain Tumor Development

- **Therapeutic radiation**
- **In utero exposure to an atomic explosion**
- **Immunologic deficiency states**
  - **HIV-1**
  - **Posttranplantation immunodeficiency**
- **Tobacco smoke**
- **Organic compound exposure**
- **Nitrosamine exposure**

TABLE 2–2   Genetic Loci Implicated in Some Pediatric Brain Tumors

Tumor	Chromosome	Disorder	Gene
PNET/MB	5q21-22	Turcot's syndrome	APC
	9q22.3	NBBCS	PTC
	17p13		
	17q		?ERB2
Astrocytoma, grade III to IV	7p12		EGFR
	17p13.1	Li-Fraumeni syndrome	TP53
	17q11.2	Neurofibromatosis-1	NF1
Subependymal giant cell tumor	9q34, 16q13	Tuberous sclerosis	TSC1, TSC2
Meningioma	22q		Unknown tumor suppressor
	22q12	Neurofibromatosis-2	NF2
ATT/Rh tumor	22q11.2		Unknown tumor suppressor

NBCCS, nevoid basal cell carcinoma syndrome; PNET/MB, primitive neuroectodermal tumor/medulloblastoma; ATT/Rh, Atypical teratoid/rhabdoid tumor; APC, adenomatous polyposis coli gene; PTC, mutation of homologue of *Drosophila* patched gene, a transmembrane tumor suppressor gene; EGFR, epidermal growth factor receptor. Blank spaces = unknown.
Adapted from Biegel J. Genetics of pediatric central nercous system tumors. *J Pediatr Hematol/Oncol* 1997;19:492–501.

NONOCCUPATIONAL RISK FACTORS

An association between diagnostic X rays in utero and the development of cancer was reported in 1956 by Stewart et al[41,42] and again in 1962 by McMahon.[43] There was a 1.5- to 2-fold increased risk of childhood cancer in these studies. Animal studies have failed to show that in utero irradiation is more carcinogenic than irradiation of adult animals.[44]

There was no excess of cancer deaths in Japanese children under the age of 10 after in utero irradiation from the atomic bombs. The atomic bomb radiation did, however, have a delayed effect, and the cancer incidence in adults who were exposed in utero is increased in a dose-response fashion.[45]

Although Preston-Martin[46] reported an increased risk for childhood brain tumors among children who received diagnostic X rays prior to 1964, and full-mouth X rays were shown to be a risk factor for brain tumors among adults who received full mouth X rays prior to 1946,[47] there is a much lower dose of radiation used today for such X rays. This current dose seems unlikely to pose a risk for childhood brain tumors.[48]

Exposure to therapeutic X rays in childhood is a more likely cause of childhood brain tumors. Tinea capitis in childhood was once treated with 1 to 2 Gy radiotherapy and was associated with a sevenfold increased risk of brain and other CNS tumors that occurred 6 to 29 years after therapy.[49] Studies of patients treated for childhood cancer observed an excess of second cancers in the brain; a large fraction of these tumors were thought to be radiation-associated.[50-52]

In summary, it can now be said that children who are exposed to therapeutic doses of X rays to the head are at increased risk for the development of brain tumors. Modern diagnostic X rays, because of their low dose and short exposure time, do not increase the risk for the fetus or the child.[48]

BIRTH-RELATED FACTORS

Higher birth weight may be associated with childhood brain tumors. Heavier infants have a greater number of cells. The cells would result from more cell divisions, which would increase the accumulation of genetic errors, leading to a higher probability of neoplastic transformation. Perhaps a greater number of cells might provide more targets for carcinogens. Although other childhood cancers, including Wilms' tumor, leukemia, and neuroblastoma, have been associated with higher birth weight, studies of high birth weight have been inconclusive regarding brain tumor development.[53,54]

ELECTROMAGNETIC FIELDS

For the past 15 years, studies have investigated the possibility that children living in homes near power lines or other electric transmission facilities or in homes with elevated magnetic fields have an increased risk of cancer. The studies involving CNS tumors in children evaluated the configurations of power-line wiring near the homes in which children who had developed brain tumors lived. How close children lived to the wires, the size of the wires, and the proximity to the origin of electrical current were studied. Wertheimer and Leeper[55] found a 2.4-fold increased risk of brain tumors associated with living in a home whose power line wiring configurations were in the two highest current categories at birth or at death of the index child. Tomenius[56] found a relative risk of 3.7 to 3.94 CNS tumors for those children living within 150m of a visible electric construction, especially if the power lines were 200 kV, and for those living in a home with a 50-Hz magnetic field of at least 3.0 mG (for which the relative risk was 2.1). Savitz[57] in an attempt to overcome the weaknesses of the previous studies employed a panel of independent electrical experts. A twofold increase in risk was associated with high current configuration.

Wiring configuration may be a better indicator of long-term past exposure than one or a few measurements taken many years after the presumed development of the cancer. It is also possible that other risk factors for CNS tumors in children may be present in patients' environments simultaneously with electromagnetic fields. Nine studies of electromagnetic fields based on wire codes, distance, measurements, and modeling, and six studies that examined the use of appliances by children or their mothers during pregnancy, and the association of these factors with brain tumor development in children, were carefully examined by Kheifets et al.[58] No support was found for an association of electromagnetic field exposure and brain cancer.

IMMUNOLOGIC RISK FACTORS

Patients receiving intensely immunosuppressive therapy as preparation for organ transplantation have had an increased risk of CNS malignancies; these have almost universally been malignancies of the lymphoid system rather than primary CNS tumors.[59,60]

Inherited immunodeficiency states, such as Wiskott-Aldrich syndrome (eczema, thrombocytopenia, and immunodeficiency) and ataxia-telangiectasia syndrome (cerebellar hypoplasia, telangiectases of the sclerae and ear pinnae), have been associated with lymphoid malignancies and, rarely, with primary CNS tumors.[30] Similarly, HIV type 1 has been associated with the development of CNS lymphoma. The incidence of primary brain lymphoma has begun to decrease as more effective anti-HIV therapy has become available.[61]

ENVIRONMENTAL AND CHEMICAL RISK FACTORS

When experimental animals are exposed to certain organic compounds in utero or shortly after birth, the development of CNS tumors is commonly seen. These compounds include N-nitroso compounds, such as N-methyl N-nitrosourea hydrazo and azoxy compounds, nitrosamines, nitrosoureas, hydrazines, triazines, alkyl sulfates and sulfanates, propane sulfone, propylene imine, acrylonitrile vinyl chloride, ethylene oxide, and polycyclic aromatic hydrocarbons (although these last mentioned must be directly implanted to induce brain tumors because they do not readily cross the blood-brain barrier).[62-64] Whether children born to parents who are often exposed to such chemicals at work are also at risk for the development of CNS tumors is not yet proven, but reports of such occurrences provide us with suspicion (Table 2–3).[65]

TABLE 2–3 Environmental Risk Factor for Primary Malignant Brain Tumors

Factor	Evidence of Increased Risk in Adults	Evidence of Increased Risk in Children
Occupational and industrial chemicals		
N-Nitroso compounds	Positive	?
Synthetic rubber production	Positive	?
Vinyl chloride	Positive	?
Petroleum refining/petrochemical production	Equivocal	?
Pesticides	Equivocal	?
Formaldehyde	Equivocal	?
Parental exposures to ionizing radiation:		Equivocal
Therapeutic	Positive	Positive
Prenatal exposures		Slightly positive
Diagnostic/dental		Equivocal
Industrial, parental	Slightly positive	Equivocal
Extremely low-frequency electromagnetic fields		
Residential wire codes	Negative	Negative
Occupational	Negative	
Viral and protozoal infections		
Simian virus 40		Positive
Chickenpox, prenatal		Positive
Toxoplasma gondii infection	Positive	Positive
Medications		
Anticonvulsants	Equivocal	
Barbiturates, prenatal		Negative
Antinausea medications, prenatal		Equivocal
Head injuries	Slightly positive	
Dietary		
N-nitroso compounds	Slightly positive	Slightly positive
Aspartame	Negative	Negative
Hair dyes and sprays	Equivocal	
Smoking, maternal	Negative	Negative
Alcohol, maternal	Negative	Equivocal
Home appliances		
Microwave exposure	Negative	Negative
Electric blankets	Negative	Negative
Electrically heated water beds	Negative	Negative
Cellular telephones	Negative	Negative

Positive, preponderance of studies showing a positive association; equivocal, both positive and negative studies; negative, most studies show a negative association; slightly positive, there are more positive than negative studies. Blanks and ? = no data available. Adapted from Sasco and Vainio,[67] Peters et al,[68] and Hemmininki et al.[69]

Tobacco and tobacco smoke are the most important sources of nitrosoamines; there has, however, been no definite association made between maternal smoking and childhood brain tumors.[35,46,66] Nor has there been adequate confirmation of risk regarding maternal exposure to smoke during gestation. A recent analysis in France suggests a twofold risk of brain tumors in fetuses exposed to intrauterine smoke and possibly a greater risk in fetuses exposed to paternal smoke in utero.[67]

Foods containing nitrosamines, nitrates, and nitrites comprise cured meats and fish products. Frying changes nitrites to nitrosamines. The highest levels of these chemicals are found in bacon, but ham and hot dogs are significant sources as well.[48] Some brands of beer contain nitrosamines. Consumption of each of these foods during pregnancy (by his-

tory), with the surprising exception of fried bacon, has been shown to increase the risk of development of childhood brain tumors.[35,46,66] Childhood consumption of cured meats does not appear to be a risk for brain tumor development.[46,66]

Kuijten and Bunin[48] suggest that more important carcinogens may be present among the yet-to-be-identified compounds in foods containing N-nitroso compounds.

Studies of parental occupations in relation to the development of brain tumors in children have similarly raised interesting etiologic possibilities. Fathers working in the aircraft industry who were often exposed to solvents had a high association with childhood brain cancer diagnosed under age 10.[68] Suggestive associations have been made between the development of brain tumors and fathers who work with or are exposed to the following: paint,[68,69] agricultural chemicals,[70] ionizing radiation,[71] electromagnetic fields,[71,72] paper and pulp mill materials,[65] printing materials,[72] graphic arts materials,[73] machine repair equipment and materials,[69] petroleum,[72] construction materials,[70] and metals.[70,74]

A Swedish study showed an increase in low-grade astrocytomas and leukemia in relation to increased parental age, and suggested that accumulated chromosomal aberrations and mutations during the maturation of germ cells is the cause.[75]

A report of a 6.7-fold increased risk of astrocytomas among people living in proximity to a cranberry bog[76] highlights one of the unique aspects of CNS neoplasia for which the underlying principle is yet to be determined.

There is much to learn about the causes of brain tumors. Such knowledge will provide us with the methods to find more effective and less toxic therapies for children afflicted with a CNS neoplasm, as well as to determine preventable causes of these tumors in our environment, and even in our genes and their products, which might then be inhibited or eliminated.

SUMMARY

The past decade of research has produced much information about the etiology of CNS tumors of children and adolescents. Methods to prevent many of these tumors are not yet available. However, concern about the increasing incidence of brain tumors has lead to new insights. There remains a crucial need for less toxic and more effective therapy for tumors occurring in the developing brain; hope for such treatment may come from gene and gene product investigations.

REFERENCES

1. Young J, et al. Cancer incidence, survival, and mortality for children younger than 15 years. *Cancer* 1986;58(Suppl 2): 598–602.
2. Pui C. Childhood leukemias. *N Engl J Med* 1995;332: 1618–1630.
3. Crist W, Kun L. Common solid tumors of childhood. *N Engl J Med* 1991;324:461–471.
4. Miller B, et al. *SEER Cancer Statistics Review: 1973–1990*. NIH Publication. No. 93,1993:2789.
5. Wrench M, Barger F. Environmental risk factors for primary malignant brain tumors: a review. *J Neuro-oncol* 1993;17:47–64.
6. Greenberg R, Shuster JL. Epidemiology of cancer in children. *Epidemiol Rev* 1985;7:22–48.
7. Legler JM, et al. Brain and other central nervous system cancers: recent trends in incidence and mortality. *J Natl Cancer Inst* 1999;91(16):1382–1390.
8. Bunin G, et al. Increasing incidence of childhood cancer: report of 20 years experience from the Greater Delaware Valley Pediatric Tumor Registry. *Pediatr Perina Epidemiol* 1996;10:319–338.
9. Cutler S, Young JL. *Third national cancer survey—incidence data*. NCI monograph, 1975.
10. Waterhouse J, Muir C, Correa P. *Cancer incidence in five continents*. Lyons: International Agency for Research on Cancer; 1976.
11. Young J, Percy C, Assire A. *Cancer Incidence and Mortality in the United States 1973–1977*. Washington, DC: National Cancer Institute; 1981.
12. Jenkin D, et al. Brain tumors in children: long term survival after radiation treatment. *Int J Radiat Oncol Biol Phys* 1995;31:445–451.
13. Schoenberg B, Christine B, Wishnant J. The epidemiology of primary intracranial neoplasms: the Connecticut experience. *Am J Epidemiol* 1976;104:499.
14. Schoenberg B, et al. The epidemiology of primary intracranial neoplasms of childhood: a population study. *J Epidemiol* 1976;104:499.
15. Gurney J, et al. Incidence of cancer in children in the United States. *Cancer* 1995;75:2186.
16. Kadota R, et al. Brain tumors in children. *J Pediatr* 1989; 114(4):511–519.
17. Johnson J, Young B. Demographiccs of brain metastasis. *Neurosurg Clin North Am* 1996;7(3):337–344.
18. Rickert CH. Epidemiological features of brain tumors in the first 3 years of life. *Childs Nerv Syst* 1998;14(10): 547–550.
19. Brugge J, Curran T, Harlow E. *The Origins of Human Cancers: A Comprehensive Review*. Cold Spring Harbor, NY: Cold Spring Harbor Press; 1991.
20. Tumour suppressor genes, the cell cycle and cancer. *Cancer Surv.* 1992:12.
21. Levine A. The p53 Tumor-Suppressor Gene. *N Engl J Med* 1992;326(20):1350–1352.
22. Listernick R, Charrow J, Gutmann DH. Intracranial gliomas in neurofibromatosis type 1. *Am J Med Genet* 1999;89(1):38–44.
23. Fryer A, et al. Evidence that the gene for tuberous sclerosis is on chromosome 9. *Lancet* 1987;1:659–661.
24. Kandt R, Haines J, Smith M. Linkage of an important gene locus for tuberous sclerosis to a chromosome 16 marker for polycystic kidney disease. *Nature Genet* 1992;2:37–41.
25. Krzystolik K, Cybulski C, Lubinski J. [Hippel-Lindau disease]. *Neurol Neurochir Pol* 1998;32(5):1119–1133.
26. Li F, Fraumeni JF. Soft tissue, breast cancer and other neoplasms. *Ann Inter Med* 1975;83:833–834.
27. Li F, Fraumeni JF. Prospective study of a family syndrome. *J Am Med Women's Assoc* 1982;247:2692–2694.
28. Li F, Winston K, Gimbrere K. Follow-up of children with brain tumors. *Cancer* 1984;54:135–138.
29. Li F, Fraumeni JF, et al. A cancer family syndrome in 24 kindreds. *Cancer Res* 1988;48:5358–5362.
30. Schoenberg B, Glista G, Reagan T. The familial occurrence of glioma. *Surg Neurol* 1975;3:139.
31. Russell D, Rubinstein L. *Pathology of Tumors of the Nervous System*. 5th ed. Baltimore: Williams & Wilkins; 1989.
32. Bonnin J, et al. An association of embryonal tumors originating in the kidney and in the brain. *Cancer* 1984;54:2137.
33. Bader J, et al. Bilateral retinoblastoma with ectopic intracranial retinoblastoma: trilateral retinoblastoma. *Cancer Genet Cytogenet* 1982;5:203.
34. Knudson A, Jr. Mutation and cancer: statistical study of retinoblastoma. *Proc Natl Acad Sci* USA 1971;68:820–823.
35. Kuijten R, et al. Gestational and familial risk factors for childhood astrocytoma: results of a case-control study. *Cancer Res* 1990;50:2608–2612.

36. Chik K, et al. Intracranial germ cell tumors in children with and without Down syndrome. *J Pediatr Hematol Oncol* 1999;21(2):149–151.

37. Rorke L, Packer R, Biegel J. Central nervous system atypical teratoid/rhabdoid tumors of infancy and childhood: definition of an entity. *J Neurosurg* 1996;85:56–65.

38. Biegel J. Genetics of pediatric central nervous system tumors. *J Pediatr Hematol Oncol*, 1997;19(6):492–501.

39. Maruno M, et al. Chromosomal aberrations detected by comparative genomic hybridization (CGH) in human astrocytic tumors. *Cancer Lett*, 1999;135(1):61–66.

40. Chen J, et al. Tumor suppression and inhibition of aneuploid cell accumulation in human brain tumor cells by extopic overexpression of the cyclin-dependent kinase inhibitor p27KIP1. J Clin Invest, 1996;97(8):1983–1988.

41. Stewart A, et al. Malignant disease in childhood and diagnostic irradiation in utero. *Lancet* 1956;2:447–448.

42. Stewart A, Webb J, Hewitt D. A survey of childhood malignancies. *BMJ* 1958;1:1495–1508.

43. McMahon B. Prenatal x-ray exposure and childhood cancer. *J Natl Cancer Inst* 1962;28:1173–1191.

44. Radiation, U.N.S.C.o.t.E.o.A. *Sources and Effects of Ionizing Radiation*. New York: United Nations; 1977.

45. Yoshimoto Y. Cancer risk among children of atomic bomb survivors: a review of RERF epidemiologic studies. *JAMA* 1990;264:596–600.

46. Preston-Martin S, et al. N-Nitroso compounds and childhood brain tumors: a case-control study. *Cancer Res.* 1982;42:5240–5245.

47. Preston-Martin S, et al. Risk factors for meningiomas in men in Los Angeles County. *J Natl Cancer Inst* 1983;70: 863–866.

48. Kuijten R, Bunin G. Review: risk factors for childhood brain tumors. *Cancer Epidemiol Biomark Prev* 1993;2: 277–288.

49. Ron E, et al. Tumors of the brain and nervous system after radiotherapy in childhood. *N Engl J Med* 1988;319: 1033–1039.

50. Meadows A, et al. Second malignant neoplasms in children: an update from the late effects study group. *J Clin Oncol* 1985;3:532–538.

51. Kingston J, et al. Patterns of multiple tumors in patients treated for cancer during childhood. *Br J Cancer* 1987;56: 331–338.

52. Neglia J, et al. Second neoplasms after acute lymphoblastic leukemia in childhood. *N Engl J Med* 1991;325:1330–1336.

53. Mole R. Antenatal irradiation and childhood cancer: causation or coincidence? *Br J Cancer* 1974;30:199–208.

54. Gold E, et al. Risk factors for brain tumors in children. *Am J Epidemiol* 1979;109:309–319.

55. Wertheimer N, Leeper E. Electrical wiring configurations and childhood cancer. *Am J Epidemiol* 1979;109:273–284.

56. Tomenius L. 50–Hz electromagnetic environment and the incidence of childhood tumors in Stockholm County. *Bioelectromagnetics* 1986;7:191–207.

57. Savitz D, et al. Case-control study of childhood cancer and exposure to 60-Hz electric and magnetic fields. *Am J Epidemiol* 1988;128:10–20.

58. Kheifets LI, Sussman SS, Preston-Martin S. Childhood brain tumors and residential electromagnetic fields (EMF). *Rev Environ Contam Toxicol* 1999;159:111–129.

59. Hoover R, Fraumeni J. Risk of cancer in renal transplant recipients. *Lancet* 1973;2:55.

60. Schneck S, Penn I. De novo brain tumors in renal transplant recipients. *Lancet* 1971;2:55f.

61. Jones JL, et al. Effect of antiretroviral therapy on recent trends in selected cancers among HIV-infected persons. Adult/Adolescent Spectrum of HIV Disease Project Group. *J Acquir Immune Defic Syndr* 1999;21(Suppl 1): S11–7.

62. Zeller W, et al. Experimental chemical production of brain tumors. *Ann NY Acad Sci* 1982;381:250.

63. Rice J, Ward J. Age dependence of susceptibility to carcinogenesis in the nervous system. *Ann NY Acad Sci* 1982;381:274.

64. Maekawa A, Mitsumori K. Spontaneous occurrence and chemical induction of neurogenic tumors in rats—influence of host factors and specificity of chemical structure. *Crit Rev Toxicol* 1990;20:287–310.

65. Kwa S, Fine L. The association between parental occupation and childhood malignancy. *J Occup Med* 1980; 22:792.

66. Howe G, et al. An exploratory case-control study of brain tumors in children. *Cancer Res* 1989;49:4349–4352.

67. Sasco AJ, Vainio H. From in utero and childhood exposure to parental smoking to childhood cancer: a possible link and the need for action. *Hum Exp Toxicol* 1999;18(4): 192–201.

68. Peters J, Preston-Martin S, Yu M. Brain tumors in children and occupational exposure of parents. *Science* 1981; 213:235.

69. Hemmininki K, et al. Childhood cancer and parental occupation in Finland. *J Epidemiol Comm Health* 1981;35: 235–237.

70. Wilkins J, Koutras R. Paternal occupation and brain cancer in offspring: a mortality-based case-control study. *Am J Ind Med* 1988;14:299–318.

71. Nasca P, et al. An epidemiologic case-control study of central nervous system tumors in children and parental occupational exposures. *Am J Epidemiol* 1988;128: 1256–1265.

72. Johnson C, Spitz M. Childhood nervous system tumours: an assessment of risk associated with paternal occupations involving use, repair or manufacture of electrical equipment. *Int J Epidemiol* 1989;18:756–762.

73. Kuijten R, et al. Parental occupation and childhood astrocytoma: results of a case-control study. *Cancer Res* 1992;52: 782–786.

74. Wilkins J, Sinks T. Parental occupation and intracranial neoplasms of childhood. *Am J Epidemiol* 1990;132:275–292.

75. Hemminki K, Kyyronen P, Vaittinen P. Parental age as a risk factor of childhood leukemia and brain cancer in offspring. *Epidemiology* 1999;10(3):271–275.

76. Aschengrau A, et al. Cancer risk and residential proximity to cranberry cultivation in Massachusetts. *Am J Public Health* 1996;86(9):1289–1296.

Chapter 3

Diagnostic Principles

Sarita Duchatelier and Steven M. Wolf

Early diagnosis of central nervous system (CNS) tumors in children is a major factor in determining treatment and outcome. The prognosis of CNS tumors is based on histologic stage of malignancy and response to therapy. Frequently the tumor's response to therapy is dependent on its location and impingement on adjacent structures and tissues. The differences between supratentorial, infratentorial, and spinal cord tumors can be detected based on the patient's presenting symptoms and physical examination. Most clinical presentations can be localized to a specific region of the brain; however, some signs are nonlocalizing or falsely localizing. Many investigators have tried to categorize some of the common presentations of brain tumors as seen in Table 3–1. This chapter will outline the major signs and symptoms that are beneficial in the detection and localization of tumors of the CNS and spinal cord.

TABLE 3–1   Focal Manifestation of Primary Brain Tumors

Tumor Location	Neurologic Signs
Frontal lobe	Dementia, personality changes, gait disturbances, generalized or focal seizures, expressive aphasia
Parietal lobe	Receptive aphasia, sensory loss, hemianopsia, spatial disorientation
Temporal lobe	Complex partial or generalized seizures, quadrantanopsia, behavioral alterations
Occipital lobe	Contralateral hemianopsia
Thalamus	Contralateral sensory loss, behavioral changes, language disorder
Cerebellum	Ataxia, dysmetria, nystagmus
Brain stem	Cranial nerve dysfunction, ataxia, pupillary abnormalities, nystagmus, hemiparesis, autonomic dysfunction

CLINICAL PRESENTATIONS

Vomiting

Vomiting is one of the most common presentations of childhood CNS tumors.[1] It is not unusual for a child with frequent vomiting to be misdiagnosed as having a gastrointestinal disease or a migraine headache variant.[2] In the series of Bailey and associates,[3] vomiting occurred in 84% of pediatric patients with intracranial tumors. Vomiting is considered a nonlocalizing sign of increased intracranial pressure, (ICP) presenting either alone or in association with nausea, headache, and behavioral changes. It is thought to be secondary to a generalized increase of ICP, caused by direct irritation of the vagal nuclei or the vomiting centers in the floor of the fourth ventricle (area prostema). Vomiting is most commonly the initial symptom of ependymoma in the posterior fossa. Since ependymomas usually begin in the fourth ventricle, they may cause early obstructive hydrocephalus or direct irritation of the brain stem involving the vomiting center.

The severity and duration of vomiting can fluctuate before the diagnosis of a brain tumor is made. Vomiting can present alone, with mild or intermittent symptoms in the early-morning hours. It can also present abruptly and daily with headaches. These symptoms may abate early in the young child if the intracranial sutures are open and capable of accommodating the increased volume and thus decrease ICP. This waxing and waning of symptoms may mistakenly be attributed to a viral illness. Parents often report that immediately following emesis the headaches improve. This is thought to be attributed to changes in the patient's pCO_2 with associated hyperventilation. This is another potential finding that may confuse the physician about whether the child is suffering from a migraine or a tumor.

Headache

Headache, which is a constant feature of increased ICP in adults, is less common in children with mass lesions. The typical history is one of worsening headaches that often awaken the patient in the early morning or during the night. Depending on the child's age and ability to localize the headaches, the common complaint is that of bifrontal, steady pain that improves later in the day. This description rarely helps the clinician to localize the site of the tumor. Associated signs that accompany headaches, such as a head tilt or visual disturbance, often help in tumor localization. Commonly, physicians believe that only constant headache is an ominous sign of increased ICP whereas intermittent episodes are more indicative of migraines. In 1992, a headache study conducted by Chu and Shinnar with 104 children under the age of 7 years concluded that, in the absence of other symptoms, neuroimaging studies for headaches yield little diagnostic information.[4] In cases where there are signs of focality by examination or history, neuroimaging is mandatory in young children.

Posterior fossa tumors can produce more localized headaches than supratentorial lesions by eliciting irritation of the posterior roots of the cervical cord, which results in pain at the occipital area as well as the neck. Benign cerebellar astrocytomas are more insidious in their presentation than malignant medulloblastomas. Here the headaches may be paradoxically frontal. When occipital headaches occur, patients may show other signs of tonsilar herniation, such as neck stiffness and opisthotonus.

Supratentorial headaches are frequently unlocalizable, but a persistent focus correlates with true localization in more than 90% of patients.[5] The duration of symptoms before diagnosis is longer with supratentorial gliomas than with tumors of the posterior fossa. The early onset of hydrocephalus is more commonly associated with infratentorial tumors. The grade of the tumor and duration of symptoms are inversely related. The longer duration of symptoms before diagnosis tends to carry a better prognosis.[6] This is based on the assumption that low-grade tumors are slow growing, with a prolonged symptomatic course.

Seizures

In children, seizures may be a rare early indication of a mass lesion. In one series (Low et al),[7] an initial presentation of seizures occurred in about 15% of children with supratentorial lesions. The temporal lobe is the most common site for tumors producing seizures as an early sign. A tumor that has a predilection for the medial temporal lobe is the ganglioglioma. Children harboring a ganglioglioma usually present with a long history of poorly controlled seizures and behavioral abnormalities. A well-demarcated, cystic temporal lobe mass without edema on magnetic resonance imaging (MRI) in a child is almost pathognomatic for ganglioglioma. Oligodendrogliomas can also present with refractory seizures, but these slow-growing tumors appear most frequently in the frontal lobes, and the patient usually has focal neurologic deficits. Even a large craniopharyngioma from the suprasellar area that impinges on the medial aspect of the temporal lobe can cause seizures. These patients may also present with visual complaints and endocrine abnormalities.

Seizure types can range from generalized to complex partial seizures, either alone or in combination with generalized seizures. Complex partial seizures are the most common type seen with intracranial masses. Patients with olfactory or gustatory hallucinations may have an associated temporal lobe glioma.[8]

Ataxia/Dysmetria

Gait disturbances may suggest either a brain stem or a cerebellar process that can present early at any stage with or without associated signs. The triad of long-tract signs, cranial neuropathies, and ataxia usually suggests brain stem pathology, whereas scanning speech, dysmetria, and ataxia is more often consistent with a cerebellar process. A detailed history will be helpful in localizing the lesion as well as in differentiating acute versus chronic symptoms. Complaints of increased difficulty walking, hopping, or running with a stiffening of gait over several months would suggest a chronic process, in contrast to awakening in the morning and abruptly falling to one side with a hemiparesis. On examination, upper motor neuron signs, such as increased tone, hyperactive reflexes, and extensor plantar responses, place the lesion centrally. Up to 95% of children with a cerebellar astrocytoma may present with ataxia. However, lesions that are supratentorial may also present with ataxia, as seen in 39% of the patients in Ludwig's series.[9] In these examples the ataxia was secondary to frontal lobe dysfunction due to an oligodendroglioma.

Different types of ataxia have also been shown to help in localizing a lesion. Both appendicular and limb ataxia reflect signs of cerebellar hemisphere dysfunction or, more specifically, compromised pathways through the cerebellar peduncles. In addition, slow-coarse nystagmus may be directed to the hemisphere that is involved, whereas a more midline tumor may present with truncal ataxia, limited problems of coordination, and little or no nystagmus.

Visual Disturbance

Visual changes, such as blurry vision, loss of vision, or diplopia, may reflect direct or indirect involvement of the visual pathway. The symptomotology varies depending on the location and extent of the mass lesion. The visual pathway may be compromised from the optic nerve or chiasm posterior to Brodmann's area 17 of the occipital lobe. In infants, nystagmus and strabismus may be the first indication of a visual deficit.[10] Pathologic strabismus, particularly esotropia due to abducens nerve paresis from a brain stem glioma, must be distinguished from the more common forms of benign esotropia (congenital accommodative and nystagmus-blocking syndromes). Older children with strabismic disorders usually do not complain of diplopia owing to a sensory adaptive mechanism called suppression, whereas patients with new onset of paralytic strabismus do complain of diplopia. Objectively this may be observed during testing for optokinetic nystagmus (OKN).

Nystagmus can result from lesions of the vestibular system, brain stem, or cerebellum. *Many varieties of nystagmus have been found to help localize to a particular area in the brain. The presence of downbeating, small-amplitude nystagmus and ocular myoclonus localizes the pathology to the medullary region, whereas upbeat nystagmus is more-often associated with tumors of the pontine-mesencephalic junction. Convergence retraction nystagmus suggests localization to the midbrain, leading to a median longitudinal fasciculus syndrome. Diencephalic lesions may manifest seesaw-like nystagmus.*[11]

Optic gliomas confined to the optic nerve often present with unilateral visual abnormalities and proptosis. A more infiltrating and expanding mass that affects the optic chiasm or hypothalamus may cause bitemporal hemianopia and endocrine abnormalities. In one retrospective study by Pierce et al,[12] a variety of signs and symptoms were reported in patients with optic chiasm gliomas (Table 3–2). This study found no direct correlation with computed tomography (CT) or MRI tumor characteristics and presenting signs and symptoms, or with the occurrence or absence of neurofibromatosis type 1 (NF-1). In addition, 50% of patients from this study

TABLE 3–2 Visual Symptoms with Optic Gliomas

	No. Patients	%Patients
Visual abnormality	23	96
Visual acuity	11	46
Field cuts	6	25
Both	5	21
Diplopia	1	4

had NF-1, which stressed the importance of the neurocutaneous examination in the pediatric patient.

Pineal tumors are another type of mass lesion in children that may present with visual disturbances. These germ cell tumors occur predominantly in males. In the series of Kageyama et al.[13] the most common symptoms of patients with pineal germinomas of decreasing incidence included Parinaud's sign (paralysis of conjugated upward gaze), increased ICP, Argyll Robertson pupil (impaired pupillary light reaction with intact accommodative response), diplopia, diabetes insipidus, and hypopituitarism. Pressure on the corpora quadrigemina (quadrigeminal plate) is thought to cause a limited conjugated upward gaze, as well as impaired pupillary response. This may also be called *Parinaud's syndrome*, which specifically includes paralysis of upward gaze usually associated with convergence-retraction nystagmus, lid retraction, and light-near dissociation of the pupils.

BOX 3–1
Signs of Pineal Tumor

- **Parinaud's sign**
- **Increased intracranial pressure**
- **Argyll Robertson pupil**
- **Diplopia**
- **Diabetes insipidus**
- **Hypopituitarism**

Other midline neoplasms that present with visual disturbances are pituitary adenomas and craniopharyngiomas. The prolactin-secreting adenomas are more common in adolescent girls and may manifest with amenorrhea or galactorrhea. Craniopharyngioma may also produce various types of field deficits, depending on the location and extent of mass. Usually unilateral or bilateral temporal field cuts are seen.

A common finding on the visual examination that represents increased ICP is papilledema. Up to 90% of patients with cerebellar astrocytoma present with papilledema. Papilledema is actually a late finding of increased ICP; loss of venous pulsations can be seen earlier. Optic pallor on examination suggests longstanding papilledema, which in turn leads to optic atrophy.

Macrocephaly

A striking clinical finding in young children is the ability to accommodate large tumors and present with minimal signs of increased intracranial pressure. It is imperative that an infant's head circumference be measured when there are any signs of a change in mental status, including irritability or lethargy. The presence of open sutures or frontal bossing is a longstanding sign of increased ICP. Percussion of the head may give a high-pitched sound, termed the "cracked-pot" or Macewen's sign.[14]

Altered Mental Status and Altered Consciousness

The brain stem contains the reticular formation, which is important in arousal, wakefulness, and sleep. An isolated change in mental status is rarely seen in children yet is common in adults with frontal or temporal lobe lesions. However, a brain stem lesion that affects the reticular formation may present with lethargy and behavioral changes. This compression can occur in the upper brain stem from downward uncal or transtentorial herniation. Lower thalamic compression can also present with drowsiness if there is midbrain involvement.[15, 16]

Endocrine

Children with CNS tumors may have endocrine dysfunctions ranging from short stature, amenorrhea, precocious puberty, and hypothyroidism to diabetes insipidus. Rodriguez and associates noted that 42% of their patients with chiasmatic hypothalmic gliomas presented with a hormonal deficiency, such as diabetes insipidus and precocious or delayed puberty. In patients with endocrinopathies, it is crucial to obtain a detailed ophthalmologic examination because patients rarely complain of visual disturbance. Subtle visual field cuts are commonly found on detailed examination.

BOX 3–2
Endocrine Signs Indicating Tumor

- **Growth disturbances**
- **Precocious puberty**
- **Amenorrhea**
- **Hypothyroidism**
- **Diabetes insipidus**

Craniopharyngiomas are another type of midline neoplasm that frequently presents with endocrine disturbances. Imura et al[17] found that 91% of their patients with craniopharyngiomas had hypopituitarism. There are often multiple hormonal deficiencies; however, upon review, more than half of patients with craniopharyngiomas present with growth hormone deficiency.

Cranial Neuropathies

Cranial neuropathies are seen in multiple types of brain tumors. They are produced either directly by compression/ invasion or indirectly by increased ICP. *The most common cranial nerve involvement seen with elevated ICP is the abducens or sixth-nerve palsy.* The patient usually complains of diplopia or presents with a compensatory head tilt or strabismus. Brain stem gliomas often present with unilateral or bilateral abducens nerve palsy either by direct compression of the nerve or, less commonly, by hydrocephalus. Maria et al[18] reviewed the clinical features of brain stem gliomas and reported that most children could be placed into one of seven groups of clinical associations Table 3–3.

Other cranial nerve palsies, in order of decreasing frequency, are cranial nerve VII presenting as a lower motor neuron defect with facial weakness; and cranial nerves IX and X as paralysis of the soft palate, depressed palatal sensation, and dysphagia. Rarely do long-tract sensory findings occur in children with gliomas, but occasionally the fifth cranial nerve sensory component is involved.

TABLE 3–3   Clinical Presentation of Brain Stem Gliomas with Typical Signs and Symptoms

1. Diplopia, asymmetrical cranial nerve deficits, and difficulty walking **(most common syndrome)**
2. Headaches, vomiting, and ventriculomegaly with early aqueduct occlusion **(hydrocephalus syndrome)**
3. Apathy, depression, decline in school performance, and memory loss **(psychiatric syndrome)**
4. Significant behavioral change, nightmares, and enuresis **(3 and 4 often occur together)**
5. Failure to thrive, intractable vomiting, and hydrocephalus (in infants) **(failure-to-thrive syndrome)**
6. Acute strokelike onset of hemiplegia, quadriparesis, internuclear ophthalmoplegia, and upbeat nystagmus **(stroke or hemorrhagic syndrome)**
7. Cerebellopontine angle presentation with involvement of cranial nerves V, VII, and ataxia **(cerebellopontine angle syndrome)**

Pain

Back pain in a child may be a warning sign of an underlying spinal cord lesion and therefore warrants a thorough neurologic examination and history. Spinal cord tumors are divided anatomically by the location of the tumor, either intramedullary or extramedullary. The most common initial symptom of an extramedullary tumor is pain, either spinal or radicular. Spinal pain is usually a dull ache that typically is worse at night and often awakens the child from sleep. Tumors such as neurinomas and meningiomas typically present with a radicular symptomatology due to the compression of the nerve roots. These tumors are seen more frequently in adults; hence, radicular pain is an uncommon sign in children. Radicular pain might be caused by distortion of the roots by edema, tumor infiltration of the root entry zone, and direct infiltration of the root if the intramedullary tumor is exophytic into the subarachnoid space.[19] In a study by Lewis et al in 1986,[20] back pain was the most common symptom of spinal cord compression, occurring in 17 of 21 patients (80%) with systemic cancer. On neurologic examination, localized back pain was the most reliable clinical finding in 14 of 21 patients (67%). Table 3–4 summarizes the pattern of neurologic deficits seen with epidural cord compression. The diagnosis of infectious diskitis can also produce similar findings but will be differentiated by MRI.

Weakness

Weakness of an extremity is commonly seen with supratentorial tumors; however, it can also be the presenting sign of spinal cord compression. In the series reported by Baten and Vannucci,[21] 72% of patients with spinal cord compression presented with weakness. Other associated signs from the history must be elicited to differentiate the two types of presentation. For example, bladder or bowel dysfunction with lower-limb weakness places a lesion in the spinal cord. On examination, looking for upper versus lower motor findings or asymmetry can further aid in localizing the lesion. The Brown–Sequard syndrome, which is caused by hemisection of the spinal cord, is most frequently observed after spinal cord trauma but can also be found with spinal cord tumors. It is defined as (1) impaired motor function on the ipsilateral side below the level of the lesion, (2) diminished or loss of vibration, pressure, and

TABLE 3–4   Epidural Cord Compression: Clinical Localization

Sign	Location		
	Spinal Cord	Conus Medullaris	Cauda Equina
Weakness	Symmetrical; profound	Symmetrical; variable	Asymmetrical; may be mild
Tendon reflexes	Increased or absent	Increased knee decreased ankle;	Decreased; asymmetrical
Babinski	Extensor	Extensor	Plantar
Sensory	Symmetrical; sensory level	Symmetrical; saddle	Asymmetrical; radicular
Sphincter abnormality	Spared until late	Early involvement	May be spared
Progression	Rapid	Variable, may be rapid	Variable; may be slow

position sense on the ipsilateral side of the body below the level of the lesion, and (3) loss of pain and temperature sense on the contralateral side below the lesion.[22]

BOX 3–3
Signs of Brown-Sequard Syndrome

- **Loss of motor function ipsilaterally**
- **Diminished sensations of vibration, pressure, and positioning ipsilaterally**
- **Decreased pain and temperature sensation contralaterally**

Sensory Loss

Sensory disturbances are commonly seen with CNS tumors and spinal cord lesions; however, this may be the most difficult parameter to determine in a young child. Careful manual testing is necessary to indicate a sensory loss.

Bowel/Bladder Disturbances

Sphincter disturbances appear early when a mass is located in the lumbosacral area but late if the compression is higher. If the tumor directly involves the conus medullaris, urinary retention or constipation may be the earliest sign of spinal cord compression (Table 3–4). Lesions above T12 usually cause bladder incontinence and bowel constipation. Lesions below T12 frequently cause bladder flaccidity with fecal incontinence and loss of anal sphincter function. Clearly, rectal examination and catheterization of the bladder are indicated in all children under evaluation.[19]

SUMMARY

A thorough knowledge of the signs and symptoms of patients presenting with tumors is the best weapon for early diagnosis and treatment. Frequently, the neurologic findings lead to localization of the tumor. This aids in determining the proper neuroimaging test without wasting time and money. Physicians should rely on the history and physical examination, and use other tests to corroborate their clinical suspicions.

REFERENCES

1. Farwell JR, Dorhmann GJ, Flannery JT. Intracranial neoplasm in infants. *Arch Neurol* 1978;35:533.

2. Papadakis N, Millan J, Grady DF. Medulloblastoma of the neonatal period and early infancy. *J Neurosurg* 1971: 34:88.

3. Bailey P, Buchanan DN, Bucy PC. *Intracranial Tumors of Infancy and Childhood.* Chicago: University of Chicago Press; 1939:445.

4. Chu ML, Shinnar S. Headaches in children younger than 7 years of age. *Arch Neurol* 1992;49:79–82.

5. Jelsma RK, Bucy PC. The treatment of glioblastoma multiforme of the brain. *J Neurosurg* 1967;27(5):388–400.

6. Walker MD. Adjuvant therapy for brain tumor. *Int Adv Surg Oncol* 1980;3:351–369.

7. Low NL, Correll JW, Hammill JF. Tumors of the cerebral hemisphere in children. *Arch Neurol* 1965;13:547–554.

8. Howe JG, Gibson JD. Uncinate seizures and tumors: a myth reexamined. *Ann Neurol* 1982;12:227.

9. Ludwig A. A clinicopathological study of 323 patients with oligodendrogliomas. *Ann Neurol* 1986;19(1):15–27.

10 Bradbury PG, Levy IS, McDonald WI. Transient uniocular visual loss on development of the eye in association with intracranial tumors. *J Neurol Neurosurg Psychiatr* 1987;50:615.

11. Brazis P, Masdeu JC, Biller J. *Localization in Clinical Neurology: The Localization of Lesions that Affect the Visual Pathway.* 2nd ed. Little, Brown & Co; 1990:99–125.

12. Pierce SM, Barnes PD, Loeffler JS, et al. Definitive radiation therapy in the management of symptomatic patients with optic glioma. *Cancer* 1990;65;45–52.

13. Kageyama N, et al. Intracranial germinal tumors. *Prog Exp Tumor Res* 1987;30:255–267.

14. Albright L. Posterior fossa tumors. *Neurosurg Clin North Am* 1992;3(4):881.

15. Cohen ME, Duffner PK. *The International Review of Child Neurology: Brain Tumors in Children—Principles of Diagnosis and Treatment.* 2nd ed. New York: Raven Press; 1994.

16. Ropper AH. Lateral displacement of the brain and level of consciousness in patients with a hemispheric mass. *N Engl J Med* 1986;314:953.

17. Imura H, Kato Y, Nakai Y. Endocrine aspects of tumors arising from suprasellar, third ventricular regions. *Prog Exp Tumor Res* 1987;30:313–324.

18. Maria BL, Rehder K, Eskin TA et al., Brainstem glioma. I: Pathology, clinical features, and therapy, *J Child Neurol* 1993;8(2):112–128.

19. Steinbok P, Cochrane D, Poskitt K. Intramedullary spinal cord tumors in children. *Neurosurg Clin North Am* 1992;3(4):931–945.

20. Lewis DW, Packer RJ, Raney B, et al. Incidence, presentation, and outcome of spinal cord disease in children with systemic cancer. *Pediatrics* 1986;78(3):438–446.

21. Baten M, Vannucci RC. Intraspinal metastatic disease in childhood cancer. *J Pediatr* 1977;90:207–212.

22. Menke JH, ed. *Tumors of Nervous System: Textbook of Child Neurology.* Baltimore: Lippincott, Williams & Wilkins, 1995:635–701.

Chapter 4

Neuroradiology

Gilbert Vézina and Timothy N. Booth

Dramatic improvements in the imaging of patients with primary central nervous system (CNS) neoplasms have occurred in the past two decades. The advent of computed tomography (CT, 1973) and, more recently, magnetic resonance imaging (MRI, 1977) have revolutionized the diagnosis, staging, and follow-up of tumors of the brain and spinal cord. MRI is clearly the modality of choice in brain imaging. Absence of beam-hardening artifacts, greater tissue contrast, and multiplanar capabilities make MRI more sensitive than CT in detection of cerebral tumors (especially small lesions, and tumors in the posterior fossa). In the spine, MRI has become the optimal modality for the study of patients with suspected intramedullary lesions.[1] Inherent motion of body tissues, especially cerebrospinal fluid (CSF), can be overcome with the use of gradient moment nulling techniques, cardiac gating, and appropriate selection of phase and frequency directions.

The addition to MRI of gadolinium as an intravenous contrast agent has been invaluable. Gadolinium accumulates in CNS tissues that lack an intact blood-brain barrier, a situation found in most neoplastic lesions. Contrast enhancement (CE) better localizes a tumor nidus but does not necessarily imply tumor grade. Although tumoral enhancement often does not delineate the true boundaries of a tumor, the presence of enhancement can guide the neurosurgeon to the more biologically active portion of the tumor.

Enhanced MRI has also become the gold standard in the evaluation of postoperative tumor residual. The presence and volume of residual tumor impacts on decisions regarding early reoperation and therapeutic protocols. However, like CT, MRI may not be able to distinguish postoperative changes (hemorrhage, edema, surgical trauma) and nonneoplastic CE (secondary to neovascularization, blood-brain barrier breakdown, or direct extravasation of contrast) from residual tumor. Surgically induced postoperative CE can mimic residual tumor and can be observed within 24 hours of surgery. The former is usually linear and thin in the first few days after surgery; then it thickens and can become more nodular. Thus, though the ideal timing of the postoperative MRI examination is still being debated, it remains prudent to image within days of surgery (less than 3 to 5 days); immediate (less than 24 hours) imaging may not appreciably increase the potential to completely exclude residual tumor.[2, 3]

NEW IMAGING TECHNIQUES

Until recently, MRI was used to characterize cerebral neoplasms by demonstrating anatomy in various planes, by displaying differences in relaxation times (T1 and T2) between normal and abnormal tissues, and by detecting breakdown in the blood-brain barrier on T1-weighted images with the use of intravenous paramagnetic CE. In the past few years, advances (rapid imaging techniques, novel pulse sequences, improved hardware configuration) have significantly improved our ability to image/resolve tumors and to characterize them. Familiarity with their basic concepts will help physicians to understand their usefulness and limitations.

Rapid imaging and improved resolution are now possible using more powerful millitesla gradients. Techniques that utilize either string of spin echos (turbo SE, fast SE) or hybrid combinations of gradient and spin echos allow faster image acquisition. The cranium can be imaged in 1 or 2 minutes per imaging series, compared with 6 to 8 minutes for traditional spin echo acquisitions. Greater spatial resolution can be achieved without compromise in signal to noise (512×256–512 image matrix instead of 256×192–256, for an improved pixel size of 0.1 to 0.2 mm^2 from 0.6 to 1 mm^2 previously). Magnetic resonance images can also be acquired individually in as little as 0.5 second (single-slice or HASTE [half-Fourier aquisition single-shot turbo spin-echo] techniques), very much like CT images, thus allowing imaging of less cooperative patients with reduced sedation needs.

The latest innovations in hardware includes magnetic field gradients that are strong enough and switch rapidly enough that an entire imaging plane can be acquired in a single radiofrequency excitation. *This technique, called echo planar imaging (EPI), allows image acquisition in a fraction of a second (as short as 50 milliseconds), or repeated multislice acquisitions on the order of 1 second.* The decreased imaging time permits aquisition of images of higher temporal resolution. Potential advantages include decreased sedation needs; the subsecond temporal resolution allows for the evaluation of cortical physiologic events, such as cerebral tissue perfusion and cortical activation.

New techniques have been introduced that suppress the normal tissue signal and improve tumor-to-background contrast, thus improving lesion detection.

Fluid attenuated inversion recovery (FLAIR) is a heavily T2-weighted pulse sequence that nulls the bright signal from cerebrospinal fluid (CSF), allowing improved lesion conspicuity. FLAIR images can now be obtained in relatively short imaging times (1 to 6 minutes) and have become a popular addition to the standard T1-, T2-, and gadolinium-enhanced T1-weighted imaging. Suppression of signal from free water in CSF is achieved using an inversion pulse that nulls signal from tissues with long T1 relaxation (free, unrestricted water protons). This pulse sequence maintains the hyperintense lesion contrast of T2-weighted spin echo imaging. *Small lesions that do not enhance, especially those on the cortex or next to the ventricles, and lesions in the ventricles or subarachnoid spaces are seen with much greater conspicuity with FLAIR imaging than with conventional spin echo imaging.*[4]

Magnetization transfer (MT) imaging increases visualization of contrast enhancement by suppressing the signal intensity of the normal brain tissue. This is based on the fact that biologic tissues contain two separate groups of hydrogen protons: a highly mobile water proton pool [unrestricted, or "free" hydrogen (H_f)]; and a relatively immobile hydrogen pool ["restricted" hydrogen (H_r) molecules bound to macromolecules such as those found in cellular membranes]. Free protons (H_f) have long T1 and T2 relaxation times; restricted hydrogens (H_r) have very short T2 decay and cannot be imaged. Though H_r cannot be imaged, they exert a significant influence on H_f due to constant transfer of magnetic spins between the hydrogen molecules of these two pools (i.e., MT).

The addition of an off-resonance radiofrequency pulse that saturates bound protons eliminates their contribution to the free-proton pool. By saturating H_r, the net magnetization of the H_f pool is decreased due to the transfer of the saturated H_r to H_f. A decrease in the net magnetization of the H_f results in a decrease in tissue signal intensity.

This MT-related decrease in signal intensity lowers the background signal of cerebral tissue and therefore increases the conspicuity of gadolinium CE by increasing the contrast-to-noise ratio. This is advantageous in the detection of tumor CE. Enhancement of small tumors not otherwise visualized can be achieved. Improved detection of lesion enhancement also helps in guiding tumor biopsy sites.[5]

Tumor characterization is dependent on biologic/metabolic properties of CNS tissues. These techniques aim to identify molecular biologic factors that are potentially able to guide clinical management decisions. Long the sole domain of positron emission tomography (PET) scanning, novel techniques include magnetic resonance spectroscopy and cerebral blood volume mapping. Spectroscopic and hemodynamic data can be obtained in a clinical setting and can help in the differentiation of active tumor, normal brain tissue, and necrosis. Thus, one can noninvasively monitor the success or failure of tumor control during therapy.[6]

Magnetic resonance spectroscopy is sensitive to the biochemical changes that occur in neoplasia by identifying markers of cellular proliferation. Spectroscopy provides information about the presence and amount of hydrogen molecules attached to different cerebral molecular compounds. The presence and concentration of these compounds can be estimated.

Hydrogen atoms located on different molecular compounds have intrinsic differences in resonant frequencies (or chemical shift) due to their differing molecular environment. A spectrum can be generated that corresponds to a scale of resonant frequencies (chemical shift) versus amplitude (concentration). Molecular compounds identified within cerebral tissue include *N*-acetyl aspartate (NAA, a neuronal marker), choline (a marker of membrane-associated compounds), creatinine andphosphocreatinine (energy metabolites), and lactate (a by-product of cerebral metabolism).

Magnetic resonance spectroscopy is useful in characterizing glial tumors. *Compared with more benign tumors, malignant glial tumors have an increased rate of membrane turnover (increased level of choline) and a decreased or absent NAA peak.* In children, spectroscopy has been successfully used to differentiate posterior fossa medulloblastoma, low-grade astrocytomas, and ependymomas.[7] Spectroscopy can separate tumor from necrosis; in necrosis, there is a depression of neuronal and membrane markers but elevation of lactate and lipid peaks as a result of metabolic acidosis and tissue breakdown.

Spectroscopy also allows for noninvasive monitoring of the response of unresected tumor to therapy, as tumor response is associated with decreasing levels of choline.

BOX 4–1
Advantages of MR Spectroscopy

- **Helpful in characterizing gliomas**
- **Differentiates tumor regrowth from necrosis**
- **Monitors a tumor's response to therapy**

Hemodynamic magnetic resonance imaging can demonstrate the neovascularization associated with tumor growth. Cerebral tissue perfusion can be assessed following a dynamic injection of a gadolinium chelate if a first-pass transit of contrast can be identified. During the first-pass transit through the cerebrovascular bed (which lasts 5 to 15 seconds), gadolinium is restricted to the intravascular space. The restricted intravascular presence of highly paramagnetic contrast molecules (gadolinium) alters the effective magnetic susceptibility of the blood. (Magnetic susceptibility is a measure of the magnetic field resulting within a medium in response to the application of the external magnetic field.) Thus, the dynamic injection of gadolinium creates microscopic field gradients around the cerebral microvasculature, resulting in local alterations in magnetic susceptibility. These alterations cause a shortening of T2 relaxation and signal loss. From the amount of signal loss, the concentration of gadolinium in each pixel can be calculated and a pixel-by-pixel relative estimate of blood volume can be inferred. Maps of cerebral blood volume (CBV) and cerebral blood flow (CBF) can be generated. In adults, high-grade glial tumors have higher CBV values than low-grade tumors, and these correlate with grade of vascularity and mitotic activity.[8]

Knowledge of tumoral vascularity is helpful in improving tumor grading, identifying optimal biopsy site in tumors with heterogeneous vascularity, monitoring for malignant degeneration and treatment efficacy, and differentiating tumor recurrence from radiation necrosis.

Single photon emission computed tomography (SPECT) has recently made significant gains in resolution with the use of state-of-the-art high-resolution gamma camera computer systems. Compared to PET, SPECT is more widely available and is utilized in tumor grading, prognosis, and selection of biopsy sites.

Of pediatric tumors, 80% show uptake of thallium 201 ^{201}Tl chloride. The mechanism of thallium uptake in tumor is unknown, though may be in proportion to the tumor's metabolic activity. *Uptake of thallium is highly specific for brain tumors, and can be used to differentiate high-grade tumors from tumoral necrosis, identify foci of higher grade tumors in histologically heterogenous tumors, differentiate residual tumor from postoperative changes, and differentiate demyelinating processes from tumors.*[9] In nonpilocytic glial tumors, there appears to be some correlation between the amount of thallium accumulation and the grade of malignancy or biologic behavior.

Like SPECT, PET is a biochemical and physiologic imaging technology. Fluorine 18 ^{18}F fluorodeoxyglucose (FDG) and carbon 11 ^{11}C methionine (MET) PET are the most widely used tracers for evaluation of brain tumors. FDG uptake is increased in malignant tumors, as these utilize more glucose than normal tissue due to a preferential shift to anaerobic glycolysis. MET uptake is increased in tumors as MET is incorporated into lipids and RNA.

With the exception of pilocytic astrocytomas, low-grade gliomas show little or no difference in FDG uptake compared with surrounding brain; such a hypometabolic tumor may not be differentiated from radiation necrosis.[10] ^{11}C-MET is useful in evaluation of a hypometabolic lesion identified on FDG PET because accumulation of the ^{11}C activity is noted in low-grade (hypometabolic) lesions, whereas little or no accumulation is seen necrotic tissue.[11]

CORTICAL LOW-GRADE TUMORS

Unlike the adult situation, the benign/low-grade glioma is the most common form of childhood brain tumor. Astrocytomas, oligodendrogliomas, and gangliogliomas are the most common histologic varieties, though rarer tumors have recently been described, including desmoplastic infantile gangliogliomas (DIGs), dysembryoplastic neuroepithelial tumors (DNETs), and pleomorphic xanthoastrocytomas (PXAs). All of these lesions are slow growing and well demarcated. They are accompanied by little or no edema, and can cause remodeling of the adjacent skull.

Cortical *astrocytomas* can be pilocytic or fibrillary. Typical presentation includes either a biphasic mass with an enhancing solid nodule and a tumor cyst, or a more homogeneous, primarily solid lesion. Low-grade astrocytomas demonstrate hypodensity on unenhanced CT and bright T2 signal. Most low-grade gliomas are slow growing and well demarcated. They are accompanied by little or no edema.

Ten to twenty percent of pilocytic astrocytomas are calcified on CT. Cysts are seen in 80% of pilocytic tumors; their solid portions almost always enhance (Fig. 4–1). Diffuse/fibrillary low-grade astrocytomas are not readily differentiated from pilocytic tumors; they originate more commonly from the white matter, have a more homogeneous structure, and are less often cystic (Fig. 4–2). Poorly defined borders and lack of enhancement suggest the diagnosis of a fibrillary astrocytoma.[12]

Gangliogliomas occur most frequently in the frontal and temporal lobes and are cortically based (Fig. 4–3). The typical ganglioglioma shows very low T1 and very bright T2 signal,

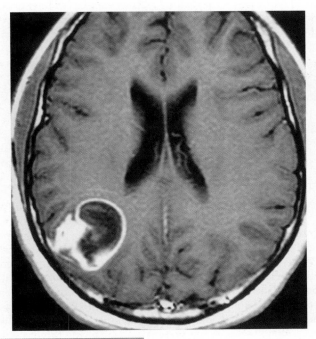

Figure 4–1 Cortical pilocytic astrocytoma. Gadolinium-enhanced T1-weighted image shows a parietal, cortically based tumor with enhancing nodule and cyst.

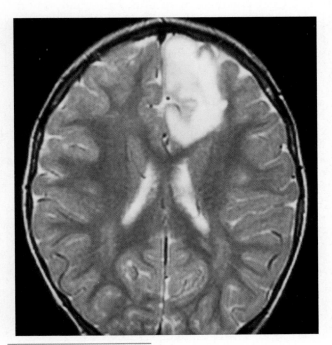

Figure 4–2 Low-grade fibrillary astrocytoma. A 2-year-old boy with history of focal seizures has a mass occupying the cingulate and superior frontal gyri, which is well delineated and has no edema on this T2-weighted image. The mass did not enhance.

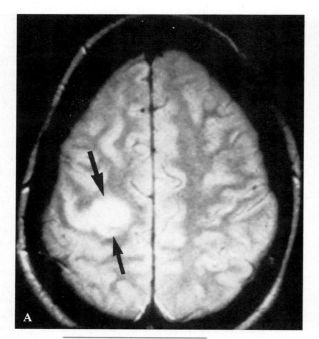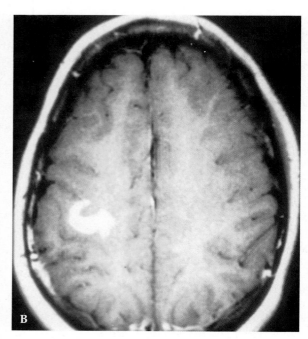

Figure 4–3   Posterior right frontal ganglioglioma. Axial proton density (A) and enhanced T1-weighted (B) images show an enhancing mass (arrows) infiltrating the primary motor cortex. The lesion is well circumscribed with no surrounding edema.

BOX 4–2
Imaging Characteristics of Low-Grade Astrocytoma

- CT is hypodense with minimal enhancement, minimal or no edema, and well-demarcated borders
- Bright T2 signal on MRI

---

exerts little mass effect despite its size, and occasionally enhances; peritumoral edema is rare. Thus, gangliogliomas can be confused with cystic encephalomalacia or even arachnoid cysts.[13] Lesions that enhance are less characteristic; they are more often solid, with poorly defined margins, mixed hypo- and isoattenuation on CT, and display more mass effect and peritumoral edema.[14]

BOX 4–3
MRI Appearance of Cortical Ganglioglioma

- Very low T1 signal; very bright T2 signal
- Enhancement uncommon
- Minimal mass effect

DNETs are intra- or subcortical tumors showing well-demarcated lobular margins, increased signal intensity on T2-weighted images, little or no peritumoral edema, little mass

effect, and minimal or no CE. Most are based in the cerebral cortical mantle, primarily in the temporal or frontal lobe. On CT they are hypointense, occasionally calcified. The tumor characteristically takes a gyriform or multinodular configuration with low T1 and high T2 signal. Partial CE is seen in 20 to 30% of cases.[15] *An identical MRI appearance can be encountered in gangliogliomas and occasionally in childhood oligodendrogliomas or low-grade astrocytomas.*

BOX 4–4
MRI Appearance of DNET

- Located in the temporal or frontal cortical mantle
- High T2 signal; low T1 signal
- Minimal to no edema
- Well-demarcated borders

PXA is an uncommon, histologically distinctive, benign, supratentorial astrocytoma occurring in young patients, typically in the second and third decades of life.[16] The typical PXA is superficially located, involving the leptomeninges and superficial cortex, and most frequently encountered in the parietal and temporal lobes. This superficial component is solid, well demarcated, has a heterogeneous T2 appearance, and shows intense enhancement; meningeal enhancement is occasionally seen. When present, nonenhancing tumor cysts are located deep to the enhancing cortical component. Histologically, the tumor can be mistaken for a high-grade glioma, though the distinction is important as PXA generally has a favorable prognosis.

BOX 4–5
PXA

- Located in leptomeninges and superficial cortex, frequently in the parietal and temporal lobes
- Nonenhancing tumor cysts may be seen
- Heterogeneous T2 appearance
- Intense enhancement

Intracranial *oligodendrogliomas* are usually supratentorial and peripheral in location; low- and high-grade histologies are encountered. Tumors are hypo- or isodense on noncontrast CT; up to 50% enhance, but enhancement tends to be mild. Highergrade or mixed tumors tend to enhance more than low-grade lesions. In older patients, calcification is common (40%), hemorrhage and cyst formation less so (20%). Peripheral lesions occasionally have associated calvarial erosion. In the pediatric age group, oligodendrogliomas are usually not calcified, and they present as cortically based tumors (or occasionally intraventricular) showing low T1 signal, varied CE, and increased T2 signal.[17]

BOX 4–6
Imaging Characteristics of Oligodendroglioma

- CT shows a supratentorial tumor that is hypointense to isointense; 50% enhance; 40% show calcification in older patients; 20% show cysts or hemorrhage
- MRI shows low T1 signal; high T2 signal; variable contrast enhancement

---

Desmoplastic infantile astrocytomas and *DIGs* are massive, supratentorial tumors of infants. These rare lesions feature large size, involvement of the superficial cortex and leptomeninges, dural attachment, and cysts. On T1-weighted images, the superficial solid component enhances intensely and displays irregular borders due to leptomeningeal infiltration. The cystic component is large, deep to the cortical solid component, does not enhance, and has T1 and T2 signal slightly brighter than that of CSF (Fig. 4–4).[18, 19]

BOX 4–7
MRI Appearance of DIG

- Supratentorial tumor with large cystic components
- Involves superfical cortex and leptomeninges, dural attachment, and cysts
- Solid component enhances intensely
- Irregular borders

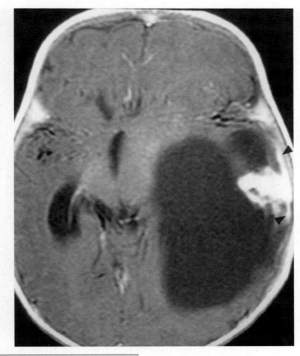

Figure 4–4 Desmoplastic infantile ganglioglioma. Axial enhanced T1-weighted image reveals a superficial enhancing solid cortical nodule with a large deep cystic component that does not enhance. Superficial infiltration of the meninges is seen (arrowheads).

SUPRATENTORIAL MALIGNANT TUMORS

High-grade tumors tend to infiltrate the surrounding cerebral tissues, resulting in more marked mass effect and greater surrounding edema than that seen with low-grade tumors. Enhancement is varied but is generally present. The two most common malignant cerebral tumors in children are malignant gliomas and PNETs; the latter include cerebral neuroblastoma, ependymoblastoma, and pineoblastoma). Choroid plexus carcinomas are less common, followed by metastases and lymphoma.

High-grade astrocytomas in children have an appearance similar to that in the adult population. They tend to infiltrate the surrounding cerebral tissues, resulting in more marked mass effect and greater surrounding edema than that seen with low-grade tumors (Fig. 4–5). High-grade gliomas—especially glioblastoma multiforme—demonstrate prominent heterogeneity on T2–weighted images. *Glioblastomas* demonstrate enhancement within the tumor (partial, often ringlike with thick,irregular, nodular walls), as well as heterogeneity due to the presence of necrosis and intratumoral hemorrhage. *Anaplastic astrocytoma* usually shows less enhancement, and low-grade fibrillary *astrocytoma* rarely enhances—though there is considerable overlap between the degree of CE observed in lower and higher grade astrocytomas.[20]

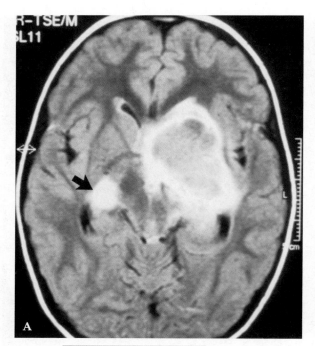 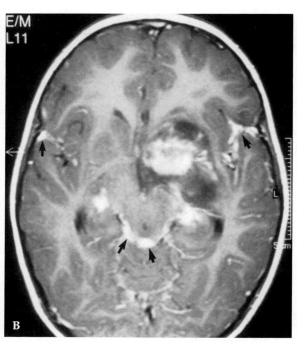

Figure 4–5 Metastatic deep hemispheric malignant astrocytoma. Axial fluid attenuated inversion recovery (A) and contrast-enhanced T1 (B) images reveal a large mass in the left basal ganglia. The mass enhances centrally (B), has metastasized to the opposite deep right hemisphere (arrow, A) and shows extensive leptomeningeal enhancement, indicative of leptomeningeal spread (arrows, B).

BOX 4–8
Glioblastoma

- **Prominent heterogeneity on T2-weighted images**
- **Partial enhancement**
- **Edema, marked mass effect**
- **Infiltrate surrounding cerebral tissues**

BOX 4–9
Supratentorial PNET

- **MRI shows large, well-defined tumor**
- **Hemorrhage, necrosis, calcifications, and cysts are common**
- **Features are heterogeneous**
- **Modest edema despite tumor size**
- **50% of lesions show calcification on CT**

Imaging differentiation between the various grades of malignant gliomas is best achieved by analysis of mass effect and heterogeneity. The larger mass effect of the more malignant tumors reflects their greater tendency to infiltrate the surrounding brain tissue and their greater vasogenic edema; extension across the corpus callosum is a sure sign of malignant infiltration.

PNETs are typically large, well-defined tumors of younger children, most often located in the frontoparietal region, that can arise either cortically or in the deep, periventricular white matter. Hemorrhage, necrosis, calcifications, and cyst formation are common (Fig. 4–6). Thus, MRI features are heterogeneous, and can include areas of high T1 signal (hemorrhage), high T2 signal (cysts, necrosis), and intermediate to low T2 signal (reflecting the high cellularity and the increased nuclear-to-cytoplasmic ratio). Peritumoral edema is common, though often minimal given the large size of the tumor. The solid portion of PNET characteristically enhances intensely, sometimes little or not at all. CT reveals calcifications in up to 50% of lesions; these are not well appreciated on magnetic resonance images.[21]

Choroid plexus carcinomas readily invade the ependyma and extend to the parenchyma; they often contain central T2 bright foci (necrosis), are accompanied by marked vasogenic edema, and disseminate readily within the ventricular and subarachnoid spaces.[22] *Once there is extensive parenchymal invasion, accurate diagnosis may not be possible; tumors with similar appearance include the malignant glioma, the malignant ependymoma (Fig. 4–7), PNET and metastasis (Fig. 4–8).*

BOX 4–10
Choroid Plexus Carcinomas

- **Mixed T2 signal**
- **Invade ependyma into surrounding parenchyma**
- **Ventricular and subarachnoid dissemination**

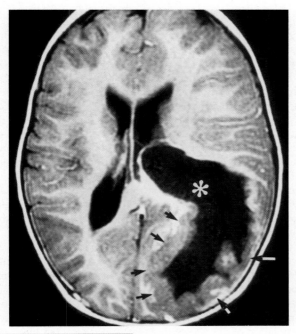

Figure 4–6 Cortical primitive neuroectodermal tumor in a 14-month-old girl. Axial enhanced T1-weighted image reveals a large mass with minimal enhancement (arrows) occupying most of the left parietal lobe. A large cystic/necrotic component (asterisk) extends deep into the mass toward the left lateral ventricle.

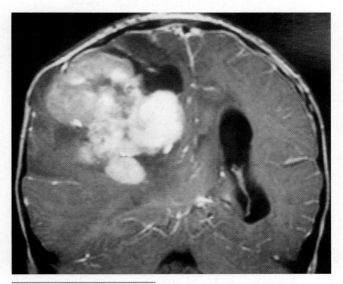

Figure 4–7 Malignant hemispheric ependymoma in a 4-year-old boy. Coronal enhanced T1-weighted image reveals a large, irregularly enhancing mass occupying most of the superior right hemisphere. The adjacent calvarium shows evidence of remodeling.

Primary CNS *lymphoma* presents either as a solitary mass or with multifocality (in 10 to 50% of cases). Of the lesions, 60% are periventricular in location. Half occur in the deep cerebral white matter; other locations include the deep central gray matter, the posterior fossa, rarely the spine. There is relatively little mass effect, and significantly less than that associated with malignant gliomas. Most are isodense to hyperdense on noncontrast CT. The T2 signal on MRI is mixed; both hypo- and hyperintense signal areas are identifiable. Up to 80% show enhancement. Enhancement tends to be solid and homogeneous in immunocompetent patients, as opposed to irregular and heterogeneous, often with a ring pattern, in the immunocompromised group.[23]

BOX 4–11
Lymphoma

- **May be either a solid mass or multiple lesions (10 to 50%)**
- **Periventricular location (60%)**
- **50% found in the deep white matter**
- **Minimal mass effect**
- **Mixed T2 signal**
- **Solid enhancement, often with a ring pattern**

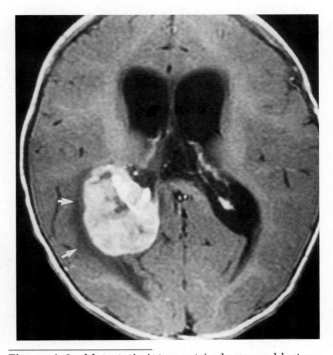

Figure 4–8 Metastatic intraventricular neuroblastoma. Axial enhanced T1-weighted image shows an enhancing mass centered in the atrium of the right lateral ventricle. The adjacent brain parenchyma shows T1 dark signal consistent with edema (arrows), suggestive of ependymal invasion.

OTHER SUPRATENTORIAL TUMORS

Intraventricular Tumors

Choroid plexus papillomas are the most common intraventricular tumors in children. Most originate in the atria of the lateral ventricles; the fourth ventricle is an unusual site of origin in children but is more common in adults. On noncontrast CT, they are iso- to hyperdense, well-marginated masses that fill and then expand the ventricle of origin; the ventricular wall is rarely invaded. Intense enhancement is seen. Calcifications are uncommon. MRI typically demonstrates a homogeneous lesion with lobulated, frondlike borders that is isointense on T1- and T2-weighted images (Fig. 4–9); larger masses can contain T2 bright areas representing cystic degeneration.[24] *Other intraventricular tumors encountered in children include papillary ependymoma, meningioma, PNET, metastatic lesions, choroid plexus carcinoma, subependymal giant cell astrocytoma, and malignant glioma.*

BOX 4–12
Choroid Plexus Papillomas

- **Most originate in the atria of the lateral ventricles**
- **Intense enhancement**
- **Hyperdense on CT**
- **Isointense on T1- and T2-weighted MRI**

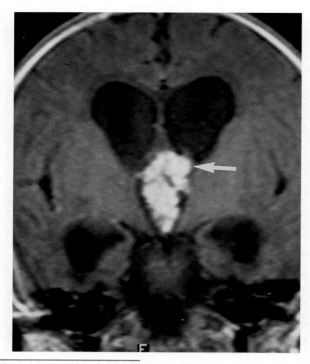

Figure 4–9 Four-month-old with macrocrania due to obstruction of the third ventricle by a choroid plexus papilloma. Coronal enhanced T1-weighted image reveals a tumor occupying the third ventricle, with a peduncle extending toward the left foramen of Monroe (arrow). The lateral ventricles are markedly enlarged.

Diencephalic Gliomas

Gliomas of the chiasm, hypothalamus, and thalamus compose 20 to 30% of all pediatric gliomas. Ninety percent are of low-grade histology.

In the thalamus, lesions are usually well marginated, bright on T2-weighted images, and variably enhanced. Tumor cysts can be present (Fig. 4–10).

Astrocytomas may involve the visual pathways from the optic disks to the optic radiations (Fig. 4–11). Tumors originating in the optic nerve often extend into the chiasm, though extension into the optic tracts is less common. Identification of the site of origin of tumors originating in the chiasm and hypothalamus can be difficult unless there is clear involvement of the optic nerves or tracts; hypothalamic tumors may grow inferiorly to involve the chiasm, and chiasmatic tumors may grow superiorly to involve the hypothalamus.

CT and MRI both demonstrate optic nerve and chiasmatic involvement. MRI better delineates extension of abnormal signal into the optic tracts and, at times, into the temporal lobes, thalamus, internal capsules, and upper brain stem. These areas of high T2 signal may represent tumoral infiltration, edema, or, in children with neurofibromatosis type 1, vacuolation of the deep white matter and gray matter nuclei that is characteristic of this patient population.[25]

Enhancement is most common in the chiasm or in portions of the optic nerves, less so in the retrochiasmatic component. Cysts and calcifications are unusual in untreated tumors, more so following radiation.[12]

Sellar/Suprasellar Tumors

Craniopharyngioma is the most common suprasellar mass in the pediatric age group. Often it involves the sella turcica, though it is rarely confused with the pituitary adenoma. Germinomas occasionally present in the suprasellar cistern and the adjacent hypothalamus; they commonly extend superi-

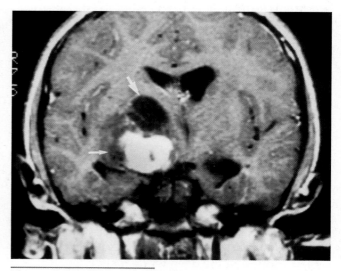

Figure 4–10 Diencephalic pilocytic astrocytoma. Coronal enhanced T1-weighted image reveals an intensely enhancing mass occupying the lateral thalamus, with nonenhancing cystic components (arrows).

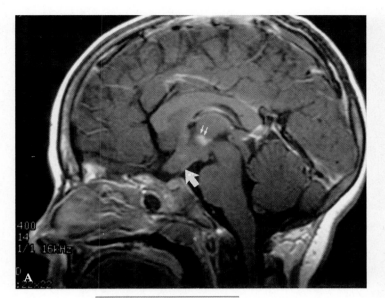
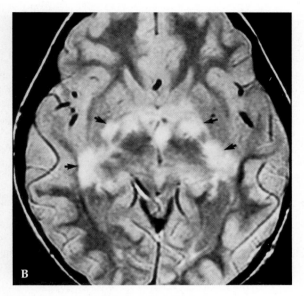

Figure 4–11   Infiltrative chiasmatic glioma in a 3-year-old girl with neurofibromatosis type 1. Sagittal enhanced T1 (A) and axial proton density (B) images reveal a mass occupying the chiasm (arrow, A), with abnormal enhancement in the superior hypothalamus (double arrow, A). Extensive involvement of the optic tracks is present to the level of the lateral geniculate bodies (arrows, B).

orly along the septum pellucidum or present with a concurrent, separate pineal mass. Histiocytosis often presents as a mass involving the pituitary stalk and the floor of the third ventricle. Large tumors of the diencephalon (chiasm, hypothalamus) can also present as suprasellar masses.

Two types of *craniopharyngioma* have been described: a childhood version, with frequent cysts, calcification, and an adamantinomatous histology; and an adult version, generally without calcification or cyst formation and a papillary squamous histology. *However, there appears to be a continuum of mixed histologies across all age groups; adamantinomatus epithelium is present in the majority of cases (80%),* squamous epithelium in 25%.[26]

Craniopharyngiomas in children tend to be larger, with more sizable cysts, more frequent calcification, and more frequent infiltration of the hypothalamus and the third ventricle than the adult entity. Tumors are almost always suprasellar in location, with intrasellar extension in half of cases. Infants and young children can have huge lesions due to late clinical presentation.[26]

Due to their high protein content, the cystic components tend to be of higher signal on unenhanced T1 images than the solid components. Following contrast administration, the solid components and the walls of the cysts enhance intensely (Fig. 4–12). The contents of the cysts do not enhance. The T2 signal overall is bright, although larger calcification will appear as hypointense T2 foci.

Pituitary adenomas arise from the anterior lobe of the pituitary gland. They have similar radiographic features in children as in adults.

Pineal Region Tumors

Pineal region masses in children are usually germ cell/mixed germ cell tumors or pineoblastomas. These are not radiographically distinguishable. Other tumor types (pineocytoma, astrocytoma, oligodendroglioma) are less common.

BOX 4–13
Craniopharyngiomas

- **Large tumors, containing large cysts, often calcified**
- **Suprasellar location, often with intrasellar extension**
- **Cysts show high signal on unenhanced T1-weighted images**
- **Solid components show high signal on enhanced T1-weighted images**
- **High signal on T2-weighted images**

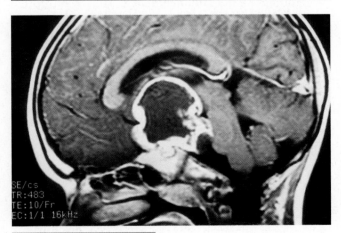

Figure 4–12   Suprasellar craniopharyngioma. Sagittal postcontrast image reveals a large mass occupying the suprasellar cistern, invaginating the floor of the third ventricle and displacing the pons posteriorly. The periphery of the mass shows irregular nodular enhancement.

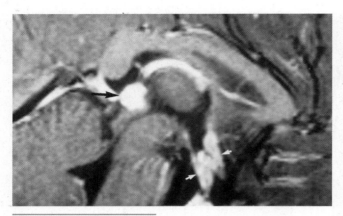

Figure 4–13 Pineal germinoma with anterior third-ventricle extension. Post gadolinium sagittal T1-weighted image reveals an enhancing mass in the pineal gland (long arrow) and coating of the infundibular and chiasmatic recesses of the third ventricle (short arrows).

Germ cell tumors occur most commonly in the pineal region, though 20 to 30% will arise in the suprasellar area. On MRI, germ cell tumors (with the exception of teratomas) tend to have signal intensity equal to that of gray matter on T2-weighted images. They are relatively homogeneous, though small intralesional cysts can be seen. T2 hypointense foci often reflect the presence of calcification, seen in up to 50% of cases on CT. Homogeneous enhancement is usually demonstrated on both CT and MRI (Fig. 4–13). Choriocarcinomas may harbor areas of subacute hemorrhage demonstrated on MRI.[27]

BOX 4–14
Germ Cell Tumors

- Signal intensity on T2-weighted images is similar to gray matter
- T2 hypointense foci reflect calcification, which is seen in up to 50% of cases on CT
- Homogeneous enhancement is shown on both MRI and CT
- MRI may show subacute hemorrhage (choriocarcinoma)

Teratomas tend to be heterogeneous, with multilocular mixed and solid elements. Areas of lipid characteristics (signal identical to fat on T1 and T2 sequences, low/fatty attenuation on CT) are pathognomonic. Calcifications are common. Enhancement is heterogeneous, usually limited to the solid tissue or the walls lining cystic spaces.

POSTERIOR FOSSA TUMORS

Half of brain tumors in children originate in the posterior fossa. Medulloblastomas, cerebellar astrocytomas, brain stem gliomas, and ependymomas account for 95% of tumors in the posterior fossa

Medulloblastoma/PNET

Medulloblastoma is the most common malignant brain tumor of childhood, accounting for approximately 20% of pediatric CNS neoplasms. It grows aggressively and has a high propensity to metastasize throughout the CNS.

Medulloblastomas usually arise in the inferior medullary velum and grow anteriorly into the fourth ventricle; they are typically homogeneous, well-defined tumors, iso- to hyperdense to cortex on unenhanced CT; they have low T1 and T2 signals that are similar or lower than those of the cerebellar cortex. Calcification is present in 10 to 20% of cases, and peritumoral edema is uncommon.[28] Occasionally, intratumoral cysts or necrosis are seen. Hydrocephalus is usually present.[29] Most medulloblastomas enhance following contrast administration. Few (5 to 10%) do not enhance; in this situation, detection of subarachnoid metastatic disease is difficult by MRI, as the metastatic nodules often do not enhance either (Fig. 4–14). Detection of nonenhancing metastatic nodules is improved with the use of FLAIR in the brain and myelographic T2 sequencing in the spine, but "sugar-coating" metastatic disease will go unnoticed.

BOX 4–15
Medulloblastoma

- Arise from inferior medullary velum
- Appear isointense to hyperintense on CT
- Low T1 and T2 signal intensity
- Show enhancement following contrast administration
- Calcification is seen in 10 to 20% of tumors
- Cysts occur occasionally
- Metastatic disease is common

A special type of teratoma that can be misdiagnosed both radiologically and histologically as a PNET has recently been described. The *atypical teratoid/rhabdoid tumor* (ATT/RhT) occurs in younger patients than the PNET (medium age 16.5 months versus 3 to 5 years) and carries a grim prognosis, with few survivors past 1 year of diagnosis.[30] These tumors can be intra-axial, extra-axial, or both because they often invade through the meningeal and ependymal boundaries. Leptomeningeal spread occurs in one-third of cases at presentation. ATT/RhT is most commonly located in the cerebellum, followed by the cerebral hemispheres and pineal region. It can be multicentric. Radiologic features include heterogeneity due to the frequent presence of necrosis, cystic change, calcifications, and hemorrhage. Marked enhancement is common. CT features include increased density on unenhanced scans, inhomogeneous CE, and commonly cysts or foci of hemorrhage. The MRI appearance includes hyperintensity on T1-weighted images (due to the frequent hemorrhagic components), iso- to hypointensity on T2-weighted images, and enhancement with gadolinium (Fig. 4–15).

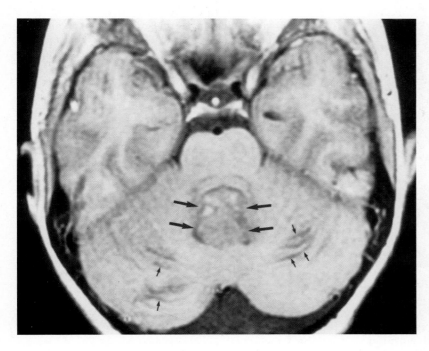

Figure 4–14 Fourth-ventricle medulloblastoma with extensive leptomeningeal metastatic disease. Axial enhanced T1-weighted image reveals a mass occupying the fourth ventricle (long arrows). The mass shows minimal enhancement. Multiple cerebellar folia are enlarged (short arrows), which at surgery were occupied by (nonenhancing) subarachnoid leptomeningeal metastases.

BOX 4–16
ATT/Rht

- Patients are very young at presentation and prognosis is grim
- Metastases are common
- Common locations are cerebellum and cerebrum
- Radiologic features are heterogeneous
- Increased density on CT
- Foci of increased signal on T1 images
- T2-weighted images: isointense to hypointense signal
- Enhancement with contrast

Cerebellar Astrocytomas

Cerebellar astrocytomas account for 30 to 40% of posterior fossa tumors in childhood. Benign and anaplastic lesions are encountered. Benign tumors predominate and are subdivided into two categories: juvenile pilocytic astrocytoma (JPA, 80%) and diffuse/fibrillary astrocytoma (20%). The tumors are either solid or mixed solid and cystic, well demarcated, and demonstrate hypodensity on unenhanced CT. On T2-weighted images, the solid elements tend to be hyperintense to gray matter, a feature that differentiates this tumor from medulloblastoma.[31]

The typical appearance of a JPA is that of a predominantly cystic lesion with a mural nodule and wall that does not enhance. Cysts are seen in 80% of pilocytic tumors; the cyst can be round or ovoid, and is almost always unilocular. The tumor nodule is either rounded or plaque-like, and enhances homogeneously and intensely. MRI is superior to CT in demonstrating the geography of the mural nodule; the latter

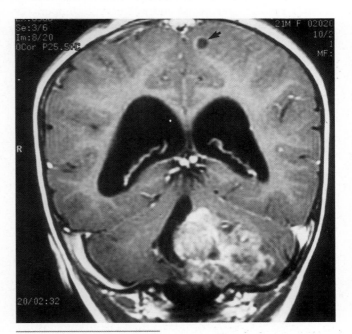

Figure 4–15 Atypical teratoid/rhabdoid tumor and incidental parenchymal cysticercosis gadolinium-enhanced T1-weighted coronal image in a 2-year-old girl from Central America reveals a large, irregularly enhancing mass occupying the lateral aspect of the fourth ventricle and the left cerebellar hemisphere. A nonenhancing cystic lesion is also identified near the vertex in the left parietal cortex (arrow), which proved to be a cysticercosis in the colloid stage.

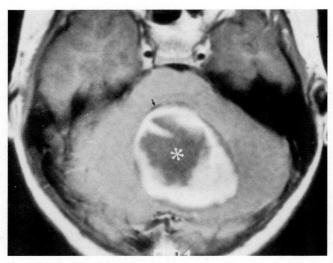

Figure 4–16   Cerebellar pilocytic astrocytoma in a 5-year-old presenting with headache, vomiting, and ataxia. Gadolinium-enhanced axial T1-weighted image reveals a large mass occupying the vermis, extending into the left cerebellar hemisphere. Note the enhancing periphery of the lesion, with a central nonenhancing microcystic portion (asterisk). The fourth ventricle is draped around the anterior portion of the tumor (arrow).

enhances intensely with gadolinium. Other tumors will be solid or present mixed solid and microcystic components (Fig. 4–16). Ten to twenty percent are calcified.[12]

BOX 4–17
JPA

- **Cystic lesion containing a mural nodule**
- **Cyst wall may or may not enhance**
- **10 to 20% calcified on CT**

Diffuse/fibrillary low-grade astrocytomas are not readily differentiated from pilocytic tumors; ill-defined borders and lack of enhancement suggest the diagnosis of a diffuse/fibrillary astrocytoma. Highly anaplastic astrocytomas and glioblastomas occasionally encountered in the cerebellum. These lesions tend to have more mass effect than their benign counterpart, be widely infiltrative, and show various areas of necrosis; most enhance.

Ependymomas

In children, 60 to 70% of intracranial ependymomas are infratentorial. Infratentorial ependymomas arise in the fourth ventricle or one of its lateral outlets (foramen of Lushka). They characteristically spread extensively along the subarachnoid spaces surrounding the fourth ventricle, including the foramen magnum and the upper cervical spine, the prepontine cistern, and the cerebellopontine angle cisterns. Fifty percent show calcifications on CT. Supratentorial ependymomas tend to be parenchymal in location. MRI features of posterior fossa lesions include a heterogeneous appearance

(mix of solid elements, small cysts, calcification, and hemorrhagic by-products) and a typical "melted-wax" morphology, as the tumor insinuates itself along the fourth ventricle, ventricular outlets, and basal cisterns (Fig. 4–17). Mass effect is usually moderate.[32] Supratentorial lesions often harbor cystic components, sometimes large, whereas infratentorial ependymomas may contain small cysts or no cysts. The solid portion in both locations most commonly shows incomplete, patchy enhancement. Homogeneous enhancement or absence of enhancement is less commonly observed.

Subependymomas can mimic intraventricular ependymomas and are not differentiated by imaging criteria.[33]

BOX 4–18
Ependymoma

- **Subarachnoid spread is common**
- **50% calcified on CT**
- **Heterogeneous appearance on MRI**
- **"Melted-wax" appearance**
- **Cysts common in supratentorial lesions**

Brain Stem Gliomas

Brain stem gliomas are viewed not as a single entity but as a heterogeneous group, with some subgroups having better prognosis for survival. A classification scheme based on the primary level of origin and the pattern of growth as determined by MRI findings has been proposed.[34]

1. *Diffuse pontine tumors (traditionally referred to as "brain stem gliomas") represent over half of brain stem tumors.* These are

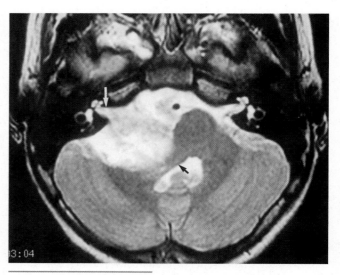

Figure 4–17   Posterior fossa ependymoma in an 11-year-old boy. Axial T2-weighted image reveals a mass in the right cerebellar pontine angle cistern. The middle cerebellar peduncle is displaced posteromedially (short arrow). The basilar artery is surrounded by tumor, which extends into the right internal auditory canal (long arrow).

large, homogeneous, infiltrating masses that usually involve most of the pons and extend readily in the midbrain, medulla, or cerebellar peduncles (Fig. 4–18). Extension into the thalamus, cerebellum, and upper spinal cord is also seen, though less commonly. Exophytic extension is most common in the basilar subarachnoid spaces and less common in the fourth ventricle. Leptomeningeal spread is unusual. These tumors are of low density on CT and have bright T2 signal on MRI. Enhancement and hydrocephalus are present at diagnosis in approximately 25% of cases. This radiologic picture almost always corresponds to a fibrillary histology of intermediate to high-grade malignancy.[35] *Caution is needed not to confuse diffuse brain stem gliomas from the diffuse brain stem "hamartomas" occasionally encountered in children with neurofibromatosis type 1.* The latter are characterized by diffuse enlargement, isointensity to the uninvolved portions of brain stem on T1-weighted images, iso- or mild hyperintensity on T2-weighted images, and lack of CE (Fig. 4–19).

BOX 4–19
Imaging Characteristics of Diffuse Pontine Glioma

- **Low density on CT, bright T2 signal on MRI**
- **Inflitrates most of pons, into adjacent structures**
- **Patchy enhancement in 25% of cases**

---

2. *Focal dorsal (tectal) midbrain tumors.* These tumors present as well-demarcated enlargement of the tectum that almost always causes acqueductal stenosis and hydrocephalus. Benign tectal tumors may extend to the adjacent posterior thalamus and usually do not enhance. These lesions are usually small (rarely larger than 15 to 20 mm) and restricted

to their site of origin. Sagittal MRI best demonstrates the enlarged tectum. Their diagnosis on CT studies is difficult; severe chronic obstructive hydrocephalus and fullness in the region of the tectum are often the only findings. Therefore, it is inadequate to perform only CT in children presenting past infancy with unexplained hydrocephalus.[36]

BOX 4–20
Imaging Characteristics of Tectal Glioma

- **Well demarcated**
- **Usually do not enhance**
- **Small (less than 15 to 20 mm)**
- **Difficult to visualize on CT**
- **Hydrocephalus secondary to stenosis**

---

3. *Focal (benign) cervicomedullary masses with dorsal exophytic components projecting in the fourth ventricle.* These tumors present as an intramedullary solid lesion occupying the upper cervical spinal cord. Due to their benign growth pattern, their upward extension is physically limited at the junction of the upper spinal cord and the medulla (by crossing pyramidal decussation fibers). In this location, the obex of the fourth ventricle is the point of least resistance. Therefore, growth within the medulla is primarily along a dorsal vector, producing a dorsally exophytic mass that ultimately extends to the fourth ventricle (Fig. 4–20).[37] Enhancement of the solid tissue is usually present. Histology is frequently pilocytic, and partial to complete surgical resection may be feasible.

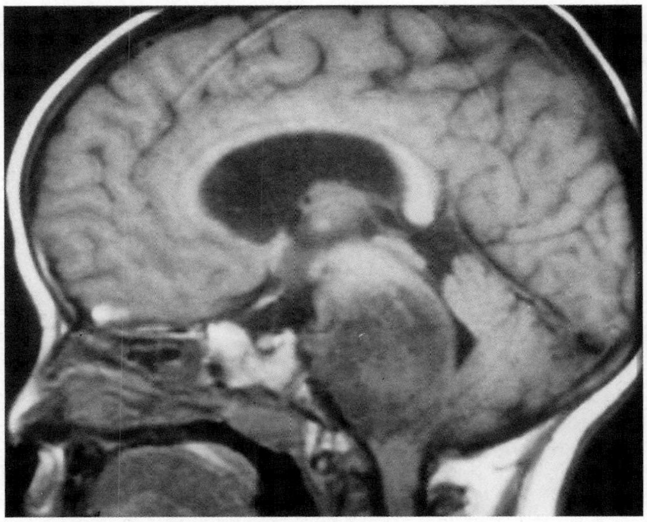

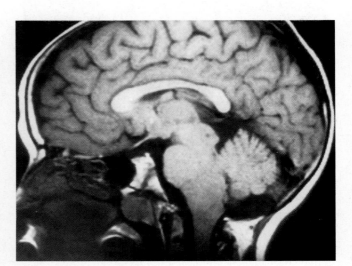

Figure 4–18 Diffuse infiltrative brain stem glioma. Sagittal T1-weighted image reveals a large, low-signal, intrinsic mass within the expanded pons.

Figure 4–19 Brain stem hamartoma in 10-year-old boy with neurofibromatosis type 1. Sagittal nonenhanced T1-weighted image reveals marked enlargement and deformity of the entire brain stem. The signal intensity is identical to that of the remainder of the white matter. This lesion has been stable for more than 10 years.

4. *Focal midbrain (nontectal) and focal pontine lesions.* These tumors present as a focal mass or a mural nodule within a cyst. Histology is usually benign (pilocytic).

5. *Diffuse midbrain and medullary lesions.* These tumors have a greater tendency to show CE than diffuse pontine tumors.

A tumor is considered *focal* if it is sharply marginated and occupies less than half of the involved brain stem segment; longitudinal extension into a single adjacent segment is allowed provided the mass remains sharply marginated and appears to compress and displace, rather than infiltrate, adjacent brain parenchyma. A focal tumor can have exophytic components of any size. In contradistinction, *diffuse* brain stem tumors are poorly marginated, involve more than half of the involved brain stem segment, or infiltrate above and below.

Using this MRI-based classification, clear prognostic differences can be established: 72% cumulative 5-year survival for focal tumors versus 20% for diffuse lesions.[34] Such outcome prediction supports results of previous studies[35, 37, 38] and helps to determine appropriate treatment of the child with a brain stem glioma.

SPINAL CORD TUMORS

Intraspinal tumors in children are relatively rare, occurring at a frequency of 5 to 10 times less than that of intracranial neoplasms. The most common location of intraspinal neoplasms is within the intramedullary compartment. Gliomas are the predominant histologic diagnosis, with astrocytomas and ependymomas described most frequently.[39] However, in a recent series, gangliogliomas were reported to be more common than ependymomas[40] and also have been found with increasing frequency in the literature. Other tumor types, including PNETs, hemangioblastomas, germinomas, oligodendrogliomas, and glioblastomas, are less common.

Patients with intramedullary neoplasms can present with nonspecific symptoms, and plain radiographs often are obtained initially due to availability and relative low cost. Abnormalities on radiographs are seen in a significant percentage of cases. Findings include widened interpedicular distance, flattening of pedicles, and erosion of the vertebral bodies or lamina. Myelography can localize a lesion to the intramedullary compartment if cord expansion is present, but it is nonspecific and invasive. A cervical puncture is often required to delineate the superior extent of the tumor. Increased specificity is achieved with the addition of CT and administration of intravenous iodinated contrast material. MRI nevertheless remains the most sensitive and effective means of elucidating intramedullary spinal cord tumors.

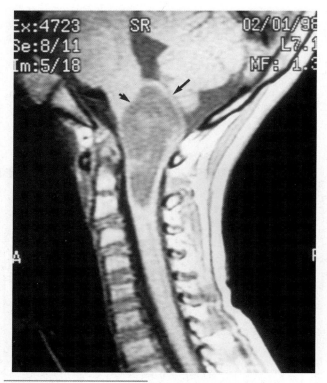

Figure 4–20 Cervicomedullary pilocytic astrocytoma. Unenhanced sagittal T1-weighted image reveals a well-defined mass occupying the upper cervical cord, the low medulla, and extending posteriorly toward the fourth ventricle (long arrow). There is a sharp cutoff between the tumor and the lower medulla (short arrow).

Astrocytomas, the most common intramedullary tumor in children, are commonly found in the thoracic cord followed by the cervical cord.[1] Astrocytomas tend to arise eccentrically in the cord and infiltrate into the adjacent cord. Two morphologic types are encountered. A focal astrocytoma extends over four to six spinal segments and is solid, but may contain intratumoral cysts (Fig. 4–21). The second type is a holocord astrocytoma, which involves the entire cord with extensive cyst formation both rostral and caudal to the solid portion of the tumor.[1, 41] Cyst formation is common, and if complete cystic degeneration is present the tumor is likely to be an astrocytoma. Cord astrocytomas are usually low grade but can be more malignant, with high-grade astrocytomas and glioblastomas reported.[41]

Astrocytomas on MRI are hypo- to isointense relative to normal cord on T1-weighted images, with increased signal present on T2-weighted images. Cord expansion is often present but should be differentiated from the normal enlargement of the cord in the cervical and lumbar regions. Associated cysts are hypointense on T1-weighted images and markedly hyperintense on T2-weighted images, paralleling the signal intensity of CSF. Protein within the cysts can alter their imaging characteristics, causing cysts to appear similar to solid tumor.[1] Most but not all astrocytomas enhance after administration of gadolinium. Irregular nodular enhancement is typical in astrocytomas. The enhancement is usually eccentric and may be localized to a specific quadrant in the spinal cord, thus aiding surgical excision.[42] Tumor cysts are characterized by peripheral enhancement and require complete surgical excision. Associated benign cysts do not demonstrate surrounding enhancement and can be treated by simple drainage.

BOX 4–23
Spinal Astrocytomas

- **Thoracic spine most common location, followed by cervical spine**
- **Arise eccentrically and infiltrate adjacent cord**
- **Two types: focal, which is solid and involves four to six spinal segments but may contain cysts; and holocord, which involves the entire cord with extensive cyst formation**
- **Hypointense to isointense on T1-weighted images, increased signal on T2-weighted images**
- **Irregular enhancement**

Ependymomas are the second most common intramedullary tumor encountered in children and are found in relatively older children, most commonly in the lumbar region.[1] Congenital tumors are also located in this area, but

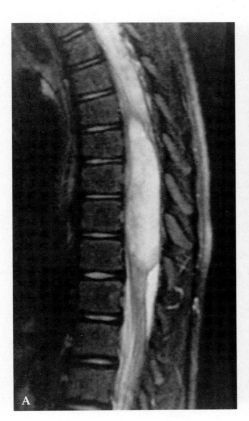
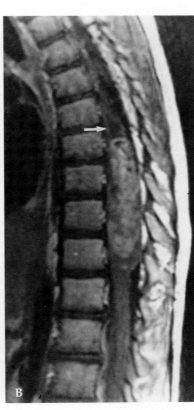

Figure 4–21 Thoracic pilocytic astrocytoma in a 5-year-old with back pain. Sagittal T2 (A) and enhanced T1 (B) images reveal a T2 hyperintense intramedullary mass extending over four spinal segments. Heterogeneous contrast enhancement is present (B). A small cyst is identified at the superior margin of the tumor (arrow, B).

they present at a younger age and are usually associated with dysraphism. Ependymomas are typically focal and usually limited to five vertebral segments, with holocord lesions occurring rarely.[43] Cyst formation is frequently present. Ependymomas arise from the ependyma lining the central canal and therefore are located centrally in the spinal cord. These tumors are better defined than astrocytomas and are more amenable to surgical resection.[43]

MRI reveals decreased T1 and increased T2 signal in the spinal cord. Homogeneous intense enhancement is characteristic (Fig. 4–22).[44] Evidence of prior hemorrhage has been noted with ependymomas with significant frequency (20 to 30%). On MRI hemosiderin is hypointense on T1-weighted images and markedly hypointense on T2-weighted images. Gradient echo images allow better definition of prior hemorrhage, with blood products exhibiting blooming due to magnetic susceptibility artifact. Hemorrhage can be central due to intratumoral bleeding or peripheral as a result of a resolving hematoma and pseudocapsule formation. Ependymomas are thought to be prone to hemorrhage because they are well-demarcated lesions without intervening normal neural tissue. This allows motion between the tumor and cord, especially in the cervical region where hemorrhage is more common.[45]

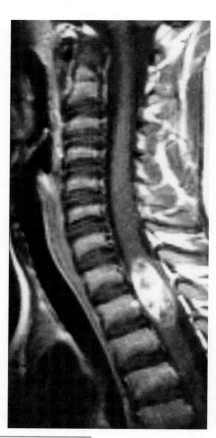

Figure 4–22 Ependymoma of the cervicothoracic cord in a 10-year-old with lower-extremity weakness and back pain. Sagittal enhanced T1-weighted image demonstrates a well-defined, enhancing intramedullary mass.

The myxopapillary lesion is a subtype of ependymoma and can have unique imaging features. It always involves the filum terminale and the distal cord. The distal spinal canal can be completely filled with tumor; at times, tumor in this location can be difficult to appreciate on MRI due to relatively similar signal to CSF.[46] Due to the presence of intracellular and perivascular mucin, increased signal on T1, proton density, and FLAIR images can be observed and can help to distinguish these tumors from CSF.

SUMMARY

Several modalities are available for imaging and diagnosing pediatric CNS tumors. Although MRI has become the standard modality, newer modalities, including EPI, FLAIR, spectroscopy, SPECT, and PET, have improved our ability to image, characterize, and thereby treat these tumors. It is the physician's responsibility to understand and apply both the techniques and the imaging characteristics of various tumor types to properly diagnose and treat these young patients.

REFERENCES

1. Blaser S, Harwood-Nash D. Pediatric spinal neoplasms. *Top Magn Reson Imaging* 1993;5:190–202.
2. Oser AB, Moran CJ, Kaufman BA, Park TS. Intracranial tumor in children: MR imaging findings within 24 hours of craniotomy. *Radiology* 1997;205:807–812.
3. Rollins NK, Nisen P, Shapiro KN. The use of early postoperative MR in detecting residual juvenile cerebellar pilocytic astrocytoma. *Am J Neuroradiol* 1998;19:151–156.
4. Tsuchiya K, Mizutani Y, Hachiya J. Preliminary evaluation of fluid-attenuated inversion-recovery MR in the diagnosis of intracranial tumors. *Am J Neuroradiol* 1996;17;1081–1086.
5. Mehta RC, Pike GB, Haros SP, Enzmann DR. Central nervous system tumor, infection, and infarction: detection with gadolinium-enhanced magnetization transfer MR imaging. *Radiology* 1995;195:41–46.
6. Tzika AA, Vajapeyam S, Barnes PD. Multivoxel proton MR spectroscopy and hemodynamic MR imaging of childhood brain tumors: preliminary observations. *Am J Neuroradiol* 1997;18:203–218.
7. Wang Z, Zimmerman RA, Sauter R. Proton MR spectroscopy of the brain: clinically useful information obtained

in assessing CNS diseases in Children. *AJR* 1996;167: 191–193.

8. Aronen HJ, Gazit IE, Louis DN, et al. Cerebral blood volume maps of gliomas: comparison with tumor grade and histologic findings. *Radiology* 1994;191:41–51.

9. Nadel HR. Thallium-201 for oncological imaging in children. *Semin Nucl Med* 1993;23:243–254.

10. DiChiro G, De La Paz RL, Brooks RA, et al. Glucose utilization of cerebral gliomas measured by ^{18}F-fluorodeoxyglucose and positron emission tomography. *Neurology* 1982;32:1323–1329.

11. Ogawa T, Shishido F, Kanno I, et al. Cerebral glioma: evaluation with methionine PET. *Radiology* 1993;186:45–53.

12. Lee YY, Van Tassel P, Bruner JM, et al. Juvenile pilocytic astrocytomas: CT and MR characteristics. *Am J Roentgenal* 1989;152:1263–1270.

13. Castillo M, Davis PC, Takei Y, et al. Intracranial ganglioglioma: MR, CT, and clinical findings in 18 patients. *Am J Neuroradiol* 1990; 11:109–114.

14. Chintagumpala MM, Armstrong D, Miki Sc, et al. Mixed neuronal-glial tumors (gangliogliomas) in children. *Pediatr Neurosurg* 1996;24:306–313.

15. Reiche W, Feiden W, Eymann R, et al. Dysembryoplastic neuroepithelial tumor: neuroradiologic findings in common and uncommon sites. *Int J Neuroradiol* 1997;3:428–434.

16. Lipper MH, Eberhard DA, Phillips CD, et al. Pleomorphic xanthoastrocytoma, a distinctive astroglial tumor: neuroradiologic and pathologic features. *Am J Neuroradiol* 1993;14:1397–1404.

17. Tice H, Barnes PD, Goumnervoa L, et al. Pediatric and adolescent oligodendrogliomas. *Am J Neuroradiol* 1993; 14:1293–1300.

18. Martin DS, Levy B, Awwad EE. Desmoplastic infantile ganglioglioma: CT and MR features. *Am J Neuroradiol* 1991;12:1195–1197.

19. Taratuto AL, Rorke LB. Desmoplastic cerebral astrocytoma of infancy and desmoplastic infantile ganglioglioma. In: Kleihues P, Cavenee WK, eds. *Pathology and Genetics of Tumors of the Nervous System*. International Agency for Research on Cancer; 1997:70–72.

20. Dean B, Drayer BP, Bird CR, Flom R. Gliomas: classification with MR imaging. *Radiology* 1990;174:411–415.

21. Figueroa RE, Gammal TE, Brooks BS, et al. MR findings on primitive neuroectodermal tumors. *J Comput Assist Tomogr* 1989;13:773–778.

22. Packer RJ, Perilongo G, Johnson D, Sutton L. Choroid plexus carcinoma of childhood. *Cancer.* 1992;69:580–585.

23. Koeller KK, Smirniotopoulos JG, Jones RV. Primary central nervous system lymphoma: radiologic–pathologic correlation. *RadioGraphics* 1997;17:1497–1526.

24. Coates TL, Hinshaw DB, Peckman N, et al. Pediatric choroid plexus neoplasms: MR, CT, and pathologic correlation. *Radiology* 1989;173:81–88.

25. DiPaolo DP, Zimmerman RA, Rorke LB, et al. Neurofibromatosis type 1: pathologic substrate of high-signal intensity foci in the brain. *Radiology* 1995;195:721–724.

26. Eldevik OP, Blaivas M, Gabrielsen TO, et al. Craniopharyngioma: radiologic and histologic findings and recurrence. *Am J Neuroradiol* 1996;17:1427–1439.

27. Smirniotopouls JG, Rushing EJ, Mena H. Pineal region masses: differential diagnosis. *RadioGraphics* 1992;12: 577–596.

28. Sandhu A, Kendall B. Computed tomography in management of medulloblastomas. *Neuroradiology* 1987;29: 444–452.

29. Meyers SP, Kemp SS, Tarr RW. MR Imaging Features of Medulloblastomas. *Am J Roentgenal* 1992 (April);158: 859–865.

30. Rorke LB, Packer RJ, Biegel JA. Central nervous system atypical teratoid/rhabdoid tumors of infancy and childhood: definition of an entity. *J Neurosurg* 1996;85: 56–65.

31. Zimmerman RA, Bilaniuk LT, Rebsamen S. Magnetic resonance imaging of pediatric posterior fossa tumors. *Pediatr Neurosurg* 1992;18:58–64.

32. Kun LE, Kovnar EH, Sanford RA. Ependymomas in children. *Pediatr Neurosci* 1988;14:57–63.

33. Hoeffel C, Boukobza M, Polivka M, et al. MR Manifestations of Subependymomas, *Am J Neuroradiol* 1995;16: 2121–2129.

34. Fischbein NJ, Prados, Wara W, et al. Radiologic classification of brain stem tumors: correlation of magnetic resonance imaging appearance with clinical outcome. *Pediatr Neurosurg* 1996;24:9–23.

35. Packer RJ, Nicholson HS, Vezina LG, et al. Brainstem gliomas. *Neurosurg Clin North Am* 1992;3:863–879.

36. Sherman J, Citrin C, Barkovich A, et al. MR imaging of the mesencephalic tectum. *Am J Neuroradiol* 1987;8:59–64.

37. Epstein F, Wisoff J. Intra-axial tumors of the cervicomedullary junction. *J Neurosurg* 1987;67:483–487.

38. Squires LA, Allen JC, Abbott R, et al. Focal tectal tumors: management and prognosis. *Neurology* 1994;44:953–956.

39. Di Lorenzo N, Giuffre R, Fortuna A. Primary spinal neoplasms in childhood: analysis of 1234 published cases (including 56 personal cases) by pathology, sex, age, and site. Differences from adults. *Neurochirurgia* 1982;25: 153–164.

40. Constantini S, Epstein FJ. Intraspinal tumors in infants and children. In: Youmans JR, ed. *Neurological Surgery: A Comprehensive Guide to the Diagnosis and Management of Neurosurgical Problems*. Philadelphia: WB Saunders; 1996: 3123–3133.

41. Epstein F. Spinal cord astrocytomas of childhood. *Prog Exp Tumor Res* 1987;30:135–153.

42. Parizel PM, Baleriaux D, Rodesch G, et al. Gd-DTPA-enhanced MR imaging of spinal tumors. *Am J Neuroradiol* 1989;10:249–258.

43. Gangemi M, Maiuri F, Donati PA, et al. Giant spinal cord ependymoma in a child. *J Neurosurg Sci* 1996;40:71–75.

44. Fine MJ, Kricheff II, Freed D, Epstein FJ. Spinal cord ependymomas: MR imaging features. *Radiology* 1995; 197:655–658.

45. Nemoto Y, Inoue Y, Tashiro T, et al. Intramedullary spinal cord tumors: significance of associated hemorrhage at MR imaging. *Radiology* 1992;182:793–796.

46. Epstein NE, Bhuchar S, Gavin R, et al. Failure to diagnose conus ependymomas by magnetic resonance imaging. *Spine* 1989;14:134–137.

Chapter 5

Surgical Neuropathology

Douglas C. Miller

Pathologic classification and description of tumors of the central nervous system (CNS) remains a complex and inexact science. Competing classification schemes, based more or less on histogenetic principles, continue to be promulgated, both in individual papers or chapters and in major texts or tumor atlases.[1–5] In part, this reflects true progress: "new" entities are regularly being identified, debated, and eventually accepted into major classifications (although often not without considerable controversy). Among the more recently identified tumor types now widely accepted (and this is not an inclusive list) are intraventricular ("central") neurocytoma,[6–8] pleomorphic xanthoastrocytoma (PXA)[9–11] dysembryoplastic neuroepithelial tumor (DNT),[12–15] desmoplastic infantile astrocytoma (DIA)[16] the related desmoplastic infantile ganglioglioma (DIG)[17] and clear cell ependymoma.[18] Tumor entities recently proposed but not yet codified in an agreed-on nosology or with fully accepted diagnostic criteria include parenchymal tumor with neurocytic elements, which is variably referred to as "ganglioglioneurocytoma,"[19, 20] "glioneurocytoma,"[21] "malignant neurocytic tumor,"[22] and "parenchymal neurocytic tumor."[23] Though widely used and included in the revised World Health Organization (WHO) classification,[3, 3A] even now there remains controversy over the scope and use of the category of primitive neuroectodermal tumors (PNETs). This chapter on the neuropathology of pediatric nervous system tumors will of necessity take a point of view within these various controversies.

The problems of classifying and describing pediatric CNS tumors are more complex than those of adult tumors, as has been pointed out for example by Rorke et al.[24] A plurality, if not a majority, of primary CNS neoplasms in adults are glioblastomas (highest grade fibrillary astrocytomas), whereas in children there is a higher proportion of mixed gliomas, low-grade glial tumors of various types, and PNETs. Among children, the proportion of intracranial tumors that are ependymomas is higher than for adults; on the other hand, although spinal cord intramedullary neoplasms are rare in all age groups, in adults ependymomas predominate whereas in children they are not among the three most common diagnoses. Pediatric tumors more often have foci with characteristics that do not easily fit the usual features of the diagnostic category to which the predominant features would suggest it belongs, so that they are more often difficult to pigeon-hole.

When one adds to this the different emphases that different expert neuropathologists are likely to place on a given set of features, it becomes completely understandable (if no less frustrating) that the same set of slides of an individual neoplasm can receive more than one diagnosis from a panel of such experts. Faced with these problems, some have sought "objective" data to subclassify tumors; principally, this has involved immunohistochemistry such that the use of multiple antibodies in panels to characterize neoplasms is essentially the standard of care for neuropathologists whose principal activity is tumor diagnosis. Another approach has been one that can be described (perhaps uncharitably) as categorical nihilism: rather than make tumors fit established pigeon-holes, one can catalog a large number of features from large numbers of tumors and seek statistical correlations both between features and between sets of correlated features and prognosis. This approach has been championed by Floyd Gilles,[25–31] and he has demonstrated its potential power. Problems with this approach have more to do with the reluctance of most tumor neuropathologists to learn an entirely new approach, of clinicians to adapt to a new nomenclature that avoids almost any resemblance to the standard diagnostic terms in general use, and the failure of Gilles et al to substantially incorporate data from immunostains into the diagnostic features used to categorize tumors. This chapter will not resolve these issues, although it may aspire to at least illuminate some of them.

A final introductory point is that in adults about half of the clinically apparent intracranial neoplasms, and perhaps up to 80% of all intracranial neoplasms found in life and at autopsy, are metastatic deposits from primary tumors outside the nervous system. In children, metastatic involvement of the CNS from extra-CNS sites is much less common, in part because CNS primary tumors are the most common solid cancers of childhood. This difference in incidence reflects greatly on the pathologic diagnostic approach in pediatric neuro-oncology, as it does on clinical management.

GROSS NEUROPATHOLOGY OF INTRACRANIAL TUMORS: SPECIAL CONSIDERATIONS FOR PEDIATRIC BRAIN TUMORS

Many of the gross pathologic considerations of intracranial mass lesions of adults apply equally to children with such tumors, except perhaps in early infancy when the skull is thin and less mineralized, with open fontanelles, making fatal downward herniations less likely. However, a fair proportion of pediatric tumors are clearly of congenital origin and therefore have grown together in the skull with the brain; thus, cerebral compression and tissue shifts or herniations are less likely to be life-threatening emergencies in children, as compared with most adults with large intracranial tumors. The presence of a longstanding congenital mass lesion in a child's brain, particularly in supratentorial lobar sites, is often accompanied by a thinning of the overlying calvarium, which is readily identified by magnetic resonance imaging (MRI) and is indicative of the chronicity of the neoplastic process. Another difference between pediatric and adult CNS tumors is that the former include a higher proportion of entities with a propensity for dissemination through cerebrospinal fluid (CSF) pathways. Most notably, these include PNETs, which are in part virtually defined by this propensity (Fig. 5–1), but this is recognized as a common outcome in typical brain stem diffuse astrocytomas ("brain stem gliomas")[32] and is a recognized, if less common, eventuality with ependymomas.[33]

SYSTEMATIC CLASSIFICATION AND DESCRIPTION OF PEDIATRIC CNS TUMORS

Most of the remainder of this chapter will proceed sequentially through a version of CNS tumor classification modified for pediatric entities. Obviously, many tumor types are common to both children and adults, but the prognostic associations of particular features or diagnoses and the images provided will all be taken from pediatric cases. The broad outlines of the classification are presented in Table 5–1. *In general, intraaxial neoplasms, whether of neuroepithelial origin or from nonneuroepithelial elements, are "malignancies" as conventionally defined by the potential for metastatic dissemination. Many are low-grade malignancies, including most classically pilocytic astrocytomas, but none of these tumors are truly benign. In contrast, most extra-axial neoplasms are benign, with no metastatic potential, even when the locally aggressive behavior of the tumor can have severe neurologic consequences.* Craniopharyngiomas are classical examples of such benign tumors with frequent adverse outcomes.

NEUROEPITHELIAL TUMORS

Gliomas

Astrocytomas

Diffuse Fibrillary Astrocytomas—Grades I–III (II–IV WHO)

In most large series, fibrillary astrocytomas are either the most common or the second most common of all pediatric brain tumors. (In adults, by most accounts these are by far the most common of primary brain tumors.) Fibrillary ("ordinary") astrocytomas are composed of cells that by their cytoplasmic content of intermediate filaments, which are usually composed of glial fibrillary acidic protein (GFAP) and, less characteristically (although quite frequently) of vimentin, by their extensive stellate fine cytoplasmic processes, and by their lack of junctional attachments or close spatial relationships to neighboring tumor cells, are recognizably astrocytes.

These tumors are usually highly infiltrative. Although by MRI they may have discernible borders, histologic investigations in and beyond that border virtually always reveal single tumor cells spreading well beyond the gross border. In consequence, these are literally unresectable; unlike cancers elsewhere in the body, the margins can never be made free of residual tumor cells by any neurosurgical technique. Thus, even low-grade examples have a tendency to recur, and high-grade examples recur relatively rapidly.

Although the infiltrative nature of fibrillary astrocytomas is most commonly seen as a diffuse if insidious process, it has long been known that some demonstrate a propensity for distinctive patterns of infiltration. Three such patterns were extensively described in detailed autopsy studies by Scherer[34–36] and are known as the "secondary structures of Scherer": perineuronal satellitosis, perivascular satellitosis, and subpial nodular growth and spread.

Fibrillary astrocytomas are the only astrocytic neoplasms that properly and classically are graded. While the well-known extant grading systems were all more or less explicitly constructed from adult patients with fibrillary astrocytomas of the cerebral hemispheres,[3, 3A, 37–44] the prognostic associations of those grades are fairly accurately projected to children with similar tumors (with specific exceptions based on site).

All of the modern grading systems are, in effect, three-grade systems, although the Daumas-Duport and revised WHO systems theoretically contain four grades. (In practice, there are so few grade I/IV fibrillary astrocytomas, as defined by these classifications, that such tumors are all grade II, III, or IV.) Grade I/III neoplasms are of low to moderate cell density, with mild to moderate nuclear pleiomorphism (variability in nuclear size, shape, and staining density), little or no mitotic activity apparent on histologic sections, and neither vascular hyperplasia nor necrosis (Fig. 5–2). In the WHO classification even one mitotic figure is sufficient to push an otherwise low-grade tumor into the category of anaplastic astrocytoma (grade II/III or III/IV), but at New York University (NYU) Medical Center, where we typically see large resection specimens (not small biopsies), we do not alter the grade of such a low-grade astrocytoma based on the finding of one or two mitotic figures, and our follow-up data[45] support this conclusion. Immunostains for the nuclear proliferation–associated antigen Ki67 (for paraffin sections, using the antibody MIB1) show a low labeling index in low-grade astrocytomas, in most laboratories under 5% (Fig. 5–2E). The MIB1 antibody recognizes, in sections of formalin-fixed paraffin-embedded tissue, the nuclear antigen Ki67. This antigen is expressed throughout the cell cycle except in G_O. Thus all labeled nuclei in such a stained section are engaged in proliferation.

In children, such low-grade fibrillary astrocytomas are the most common single diagnosis among intramedullary spinal cord neoplasms.[46, 47] In the brain, they are relatively rare in the cerebellum (where pilocytic tumors predominate) but are seen with some frequency in the white matter of the frontal lobes, temporal lobes, and parietal lobes. *Small biopsies of brain stem tumors are sometimes thought to represent low-grade fibrillary astrocytomas, but with diffuse brain stem tumors this most often is a misinterpretation of a low-cell-density infiltration from a higher grade tumor not reached in the biopsy.*

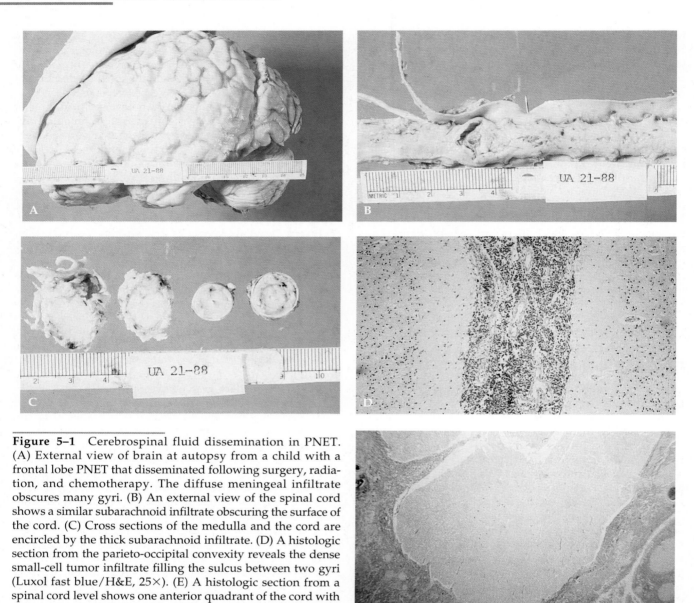

Figure 5–1 Cerebrospinal fluid dissemination in PNET. (A) External view of brain at autopsy from a child with a frontal lobe PNET that disseminated following surgery, radiation, and chemotherapy. The diffuse meningeal infiltrate obscures many gyri. (B) An external view of the spinal cord shows a similar subarachnoid infiltrate obscuring the surface of the cord. (C) Cross sections of the medulla and the cord are encircled by the thick subarachnoid infiltrate. (D) A histologic section from the parieto-occipital convexity reveals the dense small-cell tumor infiltrate filling the sulcus between two gyri (Luxol fast blue/H&E, 25×). (E) A histologic section from a spinal cord level shows one anterior quadrant of the cord with the nerve roots and subarachnoid space extensively infiltrated by the small neoplastic cells (Luxol fast blue/H&E 6.25×).

This last point can be generalized: small samples from the periphery of higher grade astrocytomas are usually composed of normal parenchyma infiltrated by scattered single tumor cells, and the low cell density should not be interpreted (as it often is by nonexpert pathologists) as synonymous with low-grade tumor. Correlation with MRI features will often offer one important clue to the erroneous nature of such a conclusion; but careful attention to the degree of nuclear hyperchromasia and the atypicality of the nuclei in general will usually alert the expert pathologist to the proper diagnosis.

The next grade of fibrillary astrocytoma, the anaplastic astrocytoma (grade II/III, WHO grade III/IV), is marked by an increase in cellularity, pleomorphism, and mitotic activity (Fig. 5–3). In the modified Ringertz three-grade classifica-

tions, such tumors often show some degree of vascular hyperplasia (Fig. 5–3C, D) which is "allowed" within this grade. The WHO revised CNS tumor classification[3,3A] mandates that any such example with vascular hyperplasia be called glioblastoma, a conclusion that ignores the abundant data on the prognostic importance of necrosis separating anaplastic astrocytoma from glioblastoma, and which is therefore not used in this chapter—or by this author. The vascular hyperplasia may take the form of fully developed glomeruloid complexes (Fig. 5–3D), or may simply be indicated by a redundancy of enlarged vascular cells (endothelial and pericytic) with enlarged nuclei, with consequent thickening of vessel walls, and by an increase in vascular density (Fig. 5–3C). Such early manifestations of vascular hyperplasia are more

TABLE 5–1   Classification of Primary Pediatric CNS Tumors

I. NEUROEPITHELIAL TUMORS

A. Gliomas
  1. Astrocytoma
    a) Diffuse fibrillary astrocytoma—graded I–III (II–IV WHO) (includes variants such as "giant cell glioblastoma," "small cell glioblastoma," "gemistocytic astrocytoma")
    b) Juvenile pilocytic astrocytoma (JPA)
    c) Pleiomorphic xanthoastrocytoma (PXA)
    d) Desmoplastic infantile astrocytoma (DIA)
  2. "Oligodendroglioma"
    a) Oligodendroglioma (ordinary, or "low grade")
    b) Anaplastic oligodendroglioma
  3. Ependymoma
    a) Cellular ependymoma
    b) "Anaplastic" cellular ependymoma
    c) Clear cell ependymoma
    d) Myxopapillary ependymoma
    e) Subependymoma
    f) Mixed cellular ependymoma and subependymoma
  4. Neuronal and mixed glial-neuronal tumor
    a) Ganglioglioma
      i) Desmoplastic infantile ganglioglioma (DIG)
    b) Gangliocytoma
    c) Intraventricular neurocytoma
    d) Ganglioglioneurocytoma
      i) Diffuse "oligodendroglioma"-like
      ii) Cortical "DNT"-type (includes all DNT)
      iii) Mixed diffuse and DNT types
      iv) Mixed lipomatous/neurocytic tumors
  5. Mixed "pure" glioma
    a) Mixed astrocytoma/oligodendroglioma (and oligodendroglioma/astrocytoma)
    b) Mixed astrocytoma/ependymoma
    c) Complex mixed glioma: Astrocytoma/ ependymoma/oligodendroglioma
  6. Mixed glial/mesenchymal tumor
    a) Gliosarcoma (high-grade astrocytoma or, less frequently, other glioma, with mesenchymal metaplasia to fibrosarcoma, myosarcoma, osteogenic sarcoma, chondrosarcoma, or other malignant mesenchymal pattern
    b) Gliofibroma ("glioneurofibroma")
B. Primitive neuroectodermal tumors (includes entities otherwise called "medulloblastoma," "pineoblastoma," "cerebral neuroblastoma," as well as others listed below)
  1. Undifferentiated PNET
  2. PNET with differentiation
    a) PNET with neuroblastic differentiation
    b) PNET with neuronal differentiation (includes desmoplastic/insular variants
    c) PNET with spongioblastic differentiation
    d) PNET with astrocytic differentiation
    e) PNET with ependymal differentiation ("ependymoblastoma")
    f) PNET with "oligodendroglial" differentiation
    g) PNET with rhabdomyoblastic differentiation)
    h) PNET with rhabdoid differentiation ("atypical teratoid tumor")
    i) PNET with other mesenchymal differentiation (particularly bone, cartilage differentiation)
    j) PNET with neural tube differentiation ("medulloepithelioma")
    k) PNET with mixed differentiation (any combination of any of the above)

II. NONNEUROEPITHELIAL INTRA-AXIAL NEOPLASMS

A. Germ cell tumors
  1. Germinoma
  2. Nongerminoma germ cell tumor
    a) Yolk sac tumor/entodermal sinus tumor
    b) Embryonal carcinoma
    c) Choriocarcinoma
    d) Teratoma
      i) Mature teratoma
      ii) Immature teratoma
B. Primary CNS lymphomas (very rare in pediatric age groups)
C. Choroid plexus neoplasm
  1. Papilloma
  2. Carcinoma

III. EXTRA-AXIAL NEOPLASMS

A. Craniopharyngioma
B. Pituitary adenoma (classified by hormone content with immunostains)
C. Nerve sheath tumors
  1. Schwannomas (in children mostly in association with NF-2)
  2. Neurofibromas (in children mostly in association with NF-1)
  3. Variants of schwannoma and neurofibroma
  4. Atypical, "cellular," and malignant Schwann cell tumors
  5. Miscellaneous other nerve sheath tumors: perineurioma, neurothekeoma
D. Meningiomas (rare in children)
  1. Spontaneous meningiomas (very rare in children)
    a) "Ordinary" meningiomas
    b) Atypical meningiomas
    c) Malignant meningiomas
  2. Radiation-associated meningiomas
  3. Meningiomas in NF-2
E. Hemangioblastomas (and von Hippel-Lindau disease)
F. Miscellaneous primary CNS intra-axial sarcomas and other mesenchymal tumors

IV. MISCELLANEOUS EXTRA-AXIAL NEOPLASMS OR NONNEOPLASTIC MASSES

Includes arachnoid cysts; glial-ependymal cysts; Rathke's cleft cysts

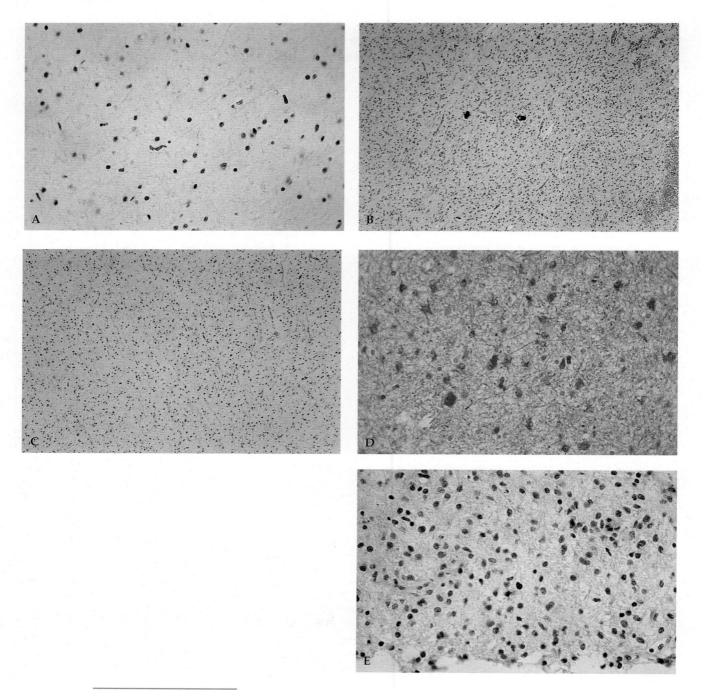

Figure 5–2   Low-grade fibrillary astrocytoma. (A) The white matter is subtly infiltrated by irreg-ular elongate single tumor astrocytes (H&E, 100×). (B) The tumor cells may occasionally accu-mulate to a higher cell density without provoking a suspicion of a higher grade tumor; this is close to the upper limit of tumors likely to remain low grade. Note the scattered microcalcifications (H&E, 25×). (C) The extent of the infiltrative nature of the neoplasm can be better appreciated when the residual myelinated axons are demonstrated (Luxol fast blue/H&E, 25×). (D) The astro-cytic character of the cells is indicated not only by their overall morphology but also by the expres-sion of glial fibrillary acidic protein. Here, the tumor cells that are positive (brown) have more irregular nuclei; positive cells with round or ovoid pale nuclei and more extensive processes are reactive astrocytes in the gliosis within and around the tumor [glial fibrillary acidic protein (GFAP) 100×]. (E) The tumor has a low proliferation rate; few nuclei are positive (brown) in this immunos-tain for the nuclear proliferation–associated antigen Ki67 (MIB1 immunostain for Ki67, 100×).

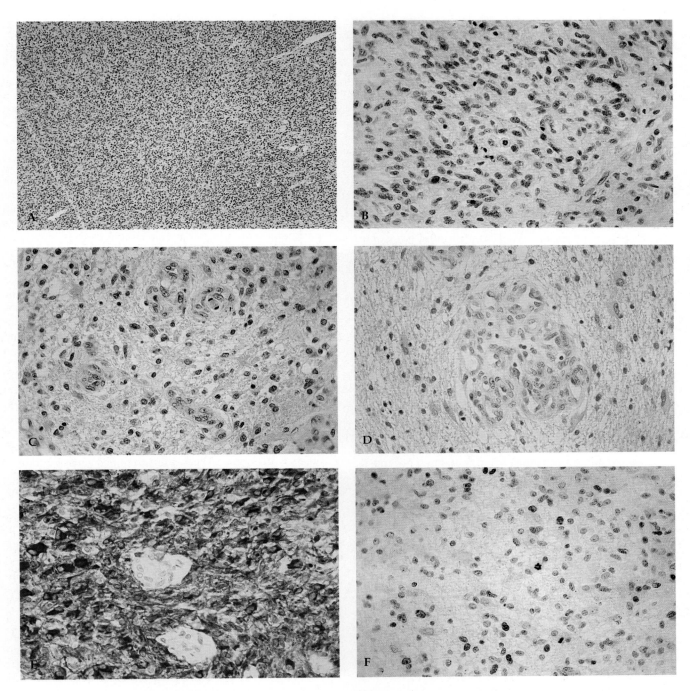

Figure 5–3 Anaplastic astrocytoma. (A) The cell density of these tumors can vary from about the same as that seen in Figure 4–2B up to high densities, as seen here (H&E, 25×). (B) A higher power view of this same tumor shows the irregular, mostly elongated nuclei with considerable hyperchromatism and much greater pleiomorphism than is seen with low-grade astrocytomas. There are multiple pyknotic (apoptotic) nuclei and at least one mitotic figure in this field (H&E, 100×). (C) Vascular hyperplasia in anaplastic astrocytomas may be manifest only by an increased microvascular density with crowded endothelial cells (H&E, 100×). (D) Alternatively, the vascular hyperplasia often includes structures with a full-fledged glomeruloid character (H&E, 100×). (E) The astrocytic nature of the cells is demonstrated by their immunopositivity for GFAP; note that the hyperplastic vessels are immunonegative (GFAP, 100×). (F) The proliferation index of anaplastic astrocytomas can be highly variable but is typically more than low-grade astrocytomas. Note the stained mitotic figures in addition to the positive nuclei (MIB1, 100×).   *(Continued on next page)*

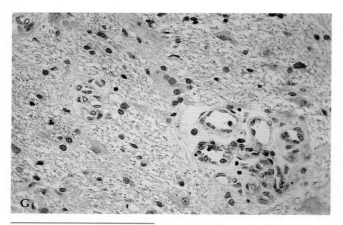

Figure 5–3 *(continued)* (G) The infiltrating edge of an anaplastic astrocytoma with cells among considerable residual myelin includes a hyperplastic vessel as the growth factors secreted by the tumor act at its advancing front (Luxol fast blue/H&E, 100×).

commonly found in or even beyond the apparent edge of the infiltrating tumor (Fig. 5–3G).

The highest grade of fibrillary astrocytoma is the glioblastoma (grade III/III, WHO grade IV/IV). The tumors in this category share all of the features of anaplastic astrocytomas and also have foci of necrosis (Fig. 5–4). The necrosis may have a surrounding zone of high cell density, known as a pseudopalisade (Fig. 5–4A, B).

In addition to the above features, certain fibrillary astrocytomas contain other features that may have prognostic importance and thus merit special mention. Tumors that have a substantial proportion of tumor cells with large amounts of cytoplasm containing the tumor nuclei at one edge, parodying the appearance of large reactive astrocytes, are often known as gemistocytic astrocytomas. (Large reactive astrocytes with a rounded or ovoid "bag" of eosinophilic cytoplasm and an eccentrically placed nucleus—giving an almost plasmacytoid appearance—are also known as gemistocytes.) Such gemistocytic cells are commonly found in anaplastic astrocytomas and glioblastomas, but are not a feature of low-grade fibrillary astrocytomas. In the rare instance in which an astrocytoma has no other high-grade features but contains more than a rare gemistocyte, the diagnosis of low-grade fibrillary astrocytoma becomes inappropriate because the presence of these gemistocytic tumor cells heralds an anaplastic behavior (Fig. 5–5A). These cells overexpress the antiapoptosis protein bcl2[48] and thus are resistant to tumoricidal therapies. They may also be rich in various growth factors [basic fibroblast growth factor (FGF), vascular endothelial growth factor (VEGF), platelet-derived growth factor (PDGF)], so that they persist and nourish other tumor constituents, perhaps accounting for the aggressive clinical behavior of these neoplasms.

On the other hand, glioblastomas with a large proportion of very large cells that often contain multiple nuclei with marked pleomorphism, are usually accepted as giant cell glioblastomas (Fig. 5–5B, C). These tumors are associated

with longer average survivals than glioblastomas with a more conventional cytologic composition.

At the opposite end of the cytologic spectrum are high-grade astrocytic neoplasms composed nearly exclusively of small cells with scant cytoplasm and hyperchromatic small nuclei (Fig. 5–5D). Such small-cell glioblastomas are thought to be more aggressive than the average glioblastoma, in part because recurrent glioblastomas frequently have a high proportion of small cells.[49] In any patient with such a tumor as a primary neoplasm (rather than a recurrence of a previously characterized fibrillary astrocytoma), the differential diagnosis of PNET must be considered. In adults, this is often controversial because PNET is thought to be rare in patients much beyond adolescence, but in children as well there can be significant disagreement among experts as to whether a particular example is better characterized as small-cell glioblastoma or as PNET. If divergent differentiation (to neuronal, ependymal, or nonneuroepithelial lineages) can be demonstrated, then the case for a diagnosis of PNET is strong; however, in the absence of such differentiation the diagnostic dilemma may not be resolved by objective tests, and the diagnosis rendered by any individual expert neuropathologist may depend more on training, experience, and prejudices (what I have termed a matter of "religion") than on objective facts.

In adults, extensive studies have demonstrated a variety of genetic changes in tumor suppressor genes and in cell cycle/growth control genes in astrocytomas, particularly glioblastomas.[48, 50–59] (For reviews, see refs. 54 and 60.) It is known that glioblastomas arise within diverse and distinct genetic pathways, some with *p53* gene mutations,[50, 52, 54–56, 58] others with normal *p53* genes but amplified genes for the epidermal growth factor receptor (EGFR),[52, 54, 56–58] and still others with mutations or deletions of other genes, (including *p16*,[53, 54, 57] *mdm2*,[52, 54, 59] and *PTEN*.[61] It is clear from chromosomal analyses that other unidentified tumor suppressor genes exist on chromosome 10 and are frequently deleted or mutated in adult glioblastomas, particularly those with EGFR amplification.[62] Much less is known about the spectrum and frequencies of particular genetic alterations in pediatric fibrillary astrocytomas, although it is clear that some examples have *p53* mutations.[51, 63, 64]

Juvenile Pilocytic Astrocytomas

The term "juvenile pilocytic astrocytoma" (JPA) was originally meant to convey a contrast with "piloid" astrocytic tumors typically found in adults. The latter were regarded as aggressive high-grade neoplasms, not different from other anaplastic astrocytomas or glioblastomas, whereas the juvenile pilocytic tumors were almost without exception indolent neoplasms curable with surgery alone.[65] This distinction has been largely abandoned, and the term "pilocytic astrocytoma" is reserved for tumors with the distinctive histologic features formerly ascribed to JPA. "Adult"-type pilocytic tumors are no longer recognized as separate entities; but rather, are regarded as one of the variant growth patterns of high-grade fibrillary astrocytomas.

JPAs, in contrast, remain a distinctive entity, which, depending on location, carry separate clinicopathologic syn-

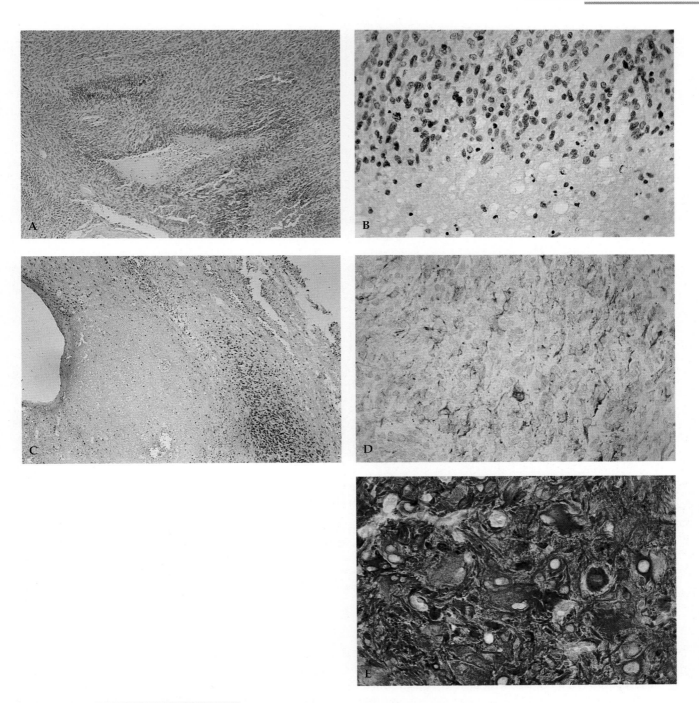

Figure 5–4   Glioblastoma. (A) This example has a fairly high cell density and multiple areas of necrosis with surrounding pseudopalisades. The nonnecrotic areas otherwise resemble an anaplastic astrocytoma (H&E, 25×) (B) A close view of a necrotic zone and its surrounding pseudopalisade. The cells in the pseudopalisade include some in mitosis, many undergoing apoptosis, and are in general oriented with the long axis of their nuclei arrayed radially around the necrosis (H&E, 100×). (C) Other necrotic zones in some glioblastomas lack pseudopalisades. Whether the mechanisms of necrosis in these zones is fundamentally different from those with such surrounding patterns remains uncertain (H&E 25×). (D) In some glioblastomas the cells express GFAP only in limited areas; the astrocytic nature of these cells is reaffirmed by their GFAP-immunopositive fine linear processes (GFAP, 100×). (E) In other glioblastomas there is strong and diffuse GFAP immunopositivity (GFAP, 100×).

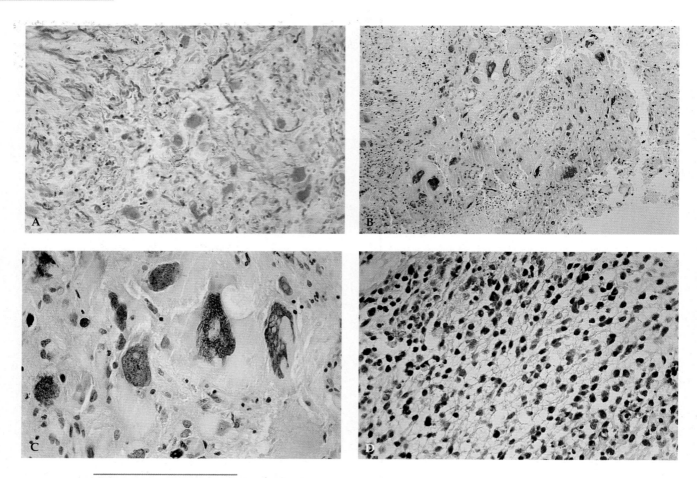

Figure 5–5 Cytologic subtypes of high-grade astrocytoma. (A) Astrocytomas with a prominent component of gemistocytes, here seen as cells with large amounts of GFAP-immunopositive cytoplasm, usually behave as anaplastic astrocytomas even if they lack all other high-grade features (GFAP, 100×). (B) Giant cell glioblastomas have very large cells with large bizarre nuclei; these cells often aggregate into epithelioid masses (H&E, 25×). (C) The hyperchromatic and highly pleiomorphic nuclei of the giant cell glioblastoma are distinctive (H&E, 100×). (D) Small-cell glioblastomas are characterized by a monotonous population of small cells with small hyperchromatic nuclei and scanty cytoplasm, an appearance that may overlap with that of primitive neuroectodermal tumors (H&E, 100×).

dromes and correlations. The most common site for a JPA is in the cerebellum; next is the general region of the hypothalamus, third ventricle, optic chiasm and nerves, and the suprasellar cistern; after that, a certain number are recognized in the thalamus, and less commonly pilocytic tumors are found at almost any level of the neuraxis. Although descriptions of JPAs in the spinal cord exist, the large series of radically excised spinal cord intramedullary neoplasms in children described from NYU Medical Center[46, 47] had no pilocytic tumors and showed that the gliosis surrounding other cord tumors—ependymomas, gangliogliomas, even fibrillary astrocytomas—could be confused with JPA in small biopsies, perhaps accounting for the other reports.

The classical JPA of the cerebellum or chiasmatic-hypothalamic region is a tumor with a solid nodule and a large cyst. The nodule histologically consists of neoplastic fibrillary glial tis-

sue with alternating zones of loose, spongy tissue and compact solid tissue, the latter often limited to perivascular zones (Fig. 5–6A). Within these zones there are bipolar astrocytes with elongated or spindle-shaped nuclei, which occasionally are highly pleomorphic but more typically are somewhat similar in size and shape. When assembled into parallel bundles these cells may caricature parallel strands of combed hair (Fig. 5–6B).

The loose or spongy zones have a somewhat mucinous or myxoid extracellular matrix, and a similar secretion is found in microcysts lined by tumor cells in the more solid portions (Fig. 5–6C). Associated with the tumor cells, particularly in the compact zones, are darkly eosinophilic rodlike structures, [Rosenthal fibers (Fig. 5–6D)], which are ultrastructurally demonstrably located within small astrocytic processes and which are known to be composed largely of the heat shock protein α-B crystallin. Other structures of similar significance

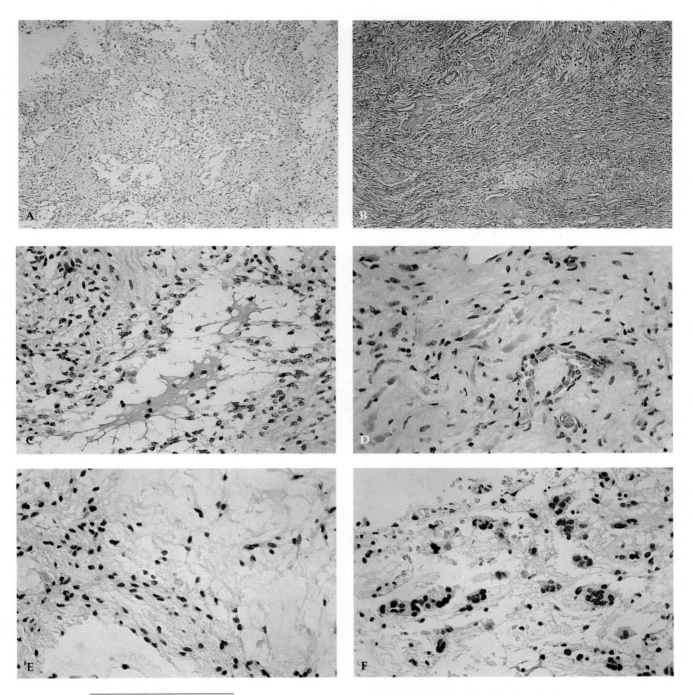

Figure 5–6   Pilocytic astrocytoma. (A) The most prototypical growth pattern for a pilocytic astrocytoma is one with alternating solid ("compact") and loose ("spongy") areas (H&E, 25×). (B) Bundles of parallel elongated bipolar cells give rise to the term pilocytic in that they resemble combed hair (H&E, 25×). (C) Microcysts are common in pilocytic tumors (and in certain other low-grade gliomas); they contain an eosinophilic secretion and often also some "floating" tumor cells. There is a granular body in the wall of the microcyst in this example (H&E, 100×). (D) Rosenthal fibers are eosinophilic rod-shaped intra-astrocytic inclusions, commonly found in pilocytic astrocytomas but also in the gliosis around other lesions in certain sites (H&E, 100×). (E) Eosinophilic granular bodies are intra-astrocytic inclusions common in pilocytic tumors and certain other low grade gliomas (H&E, 100×). (F) Multinucleated giant cells are not uncommon in pilocytic astrocytomas; they should not be used to invoke a higher grade diagnosis (H&E, 100×).   *(Continued on next page)*

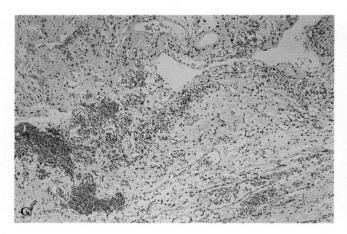

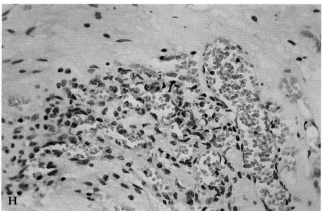

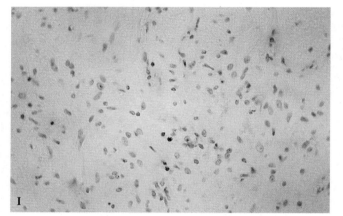

Figure 5–6 *(continued)* (G) Pilocytic astrocytomas often have arcades of hyperplastic vessels underlying the walls of macroscopic cysts (H&E, 25×). (H) A closer examination of the hyperplastic vessels reveals glomeruloid structures identical to those seen in high-grade fibrillary astrocytomas (H&E, 100×). (I) An MIB1 immunostain shows the typical low level of proliferative activity in the average pilocytic astrocytoma.

but very different structure include hyaline droplets (not illustrated) and granular bodies (Fig. 5–6E).

Some of these features are usually present in nonclassical examples. How much pattern is necessary to distinguish a JPA from a low-grade fibrillary astrocytoma composed of bipolar spindle cells is controversial; this author prefers to limit the diagnosis of JPA to tumors that have most of the classical features. Clearly, the presence of a few Rosenthal fibers or granular bodies is insufficient. Occasional examples of JPA are composed of more pleomorphic cells, with larger and more variable nuclei, and may include multinucleated giant cells. These cells, with their nuclei distributed at the periphery of the cytoplasmic mass, have been called "coins-on-a-plate cells" by Scheithauer[66] and, while hardly diagnostic, can be a helpful guide to the correct diagnosis (Fig. 5–6F). Also, many pilocytic astrocytomas have foci with vascular hyperplasia (Fig. 5–6G, H); when the tumors are excised in large pieces or intact, thereby allowing an appreciation of their anatomy, the vascular hyperplasia is usually close to the wall of a macroscopic cyst.

The danger is in misdiagnosing a pilocytic tumor as anaplastic astrocytoma, based on the presence of pleomorphism, giant cells, and vascular hyperplasia, leading to overly aggressive radiation or chemotherapy. It may seem just as bad to call an aggressive anaplastic astrocytoma a pilocytic tumor, but, given the lack of highly effective therapies available for high-grade astrocytomas, such a mistake, while not trivial, may have fewer long-term consequences.

Most pilocytic astrocytomas are slow-growing, indolent, low-grade malignancies. Rarely do these tumors result in death or significant permanent neurologic disability, related to their occurrence or recurrence in vital structures, including the optic nerves, chiasm, or brain stem. A few cases involving widespread dissemination (metastasis) along CSF pathways have been described.[67–70]

Less is known about the genetic changes in pilocytic astrocytomas than is known about such changes in pediatric fibrillary astrocytomas. Rare examples of *p53* mutations have been documented.[51, 71] Larger numbers accumulate wild-type *p53* protein abnormally without a *p53* gene mutation; the underlying basis for this accumulation is not well established and may be multifactorial.[51]

Pleomorphic Xanthoastrocytomas

PXA is a relatively newly described entity. It was first recognized as a distinctive superficially located cerebral hemispheric tumor in children and young adults by Kepes et al,[72] who regarded them as sarcomas with abundant lipid-filled (xanthoma) cells, and who called attention to the relatively good clinical outcome, which contrasted with the apparent highly malignant histologic appearance.[72] Shortly after this initial description, Kepes, in association with Eng and Rubinstein, utilized the then new technique of immunoperoxidase staining to identify the tumor cells as GFAP-positive and therefore astrocytic, giving rise to the seminal report discussing the entity of PXA.[9] This is now a well-recognized tumor type, which most often is, as originally described, a tumor of low malignant potential occurring at the interface of the cerebral hemispheres and the leptomeninges, and thus involving both. Occasional examples occur in unusual sites (cerebellum, brain stem), contain nonastrocytic elements (ganglioglioma), or are more clinically aggressive.[10, 73-79]

The correct diagnosis of PXA starts with neuroimaging because the recognition of the superficial cortical/meningeal location and of the usual mixture of cystic and solid components suggests this diagnostic possibility to the pathologist (Fig. 5–7A). Histologically there is usually a striking pleomorphism with large astrocytic tumor cells, with large, pleomorphic, even bizarre nuclei (Fig. 5–7B). There is an obvious resemblance to, and thus differential diagnosis with, giant cell glioblastoma. In the margins of the mass in the brain there is usually an infiltrative border identical to that seen in fibrillary astrocytomas. In the solid portions of the mass, both in the leptomeninges and the cortex, the tumor cells often assume an epithelioid configuration, with cells in clusters closely packed together; furthermore, the cells are surrounded by a basal lam-

ina detectable by silver reticulin staining, whereas ordinary fibrillary astrocytomas lack reticulin (Fig. 5–7C). Whereas reticulin staining is often necessary to prove the diagnosis, it can be suggested from the initial hematoxylin -cosin (H&E) stains, in part from a disparity between the marked pleomorphism and the absence (in most examples) of other high-grade features, including mitotic figures in any considerable number, vascular hyperplasia, or necrosis. Indeed, many experts would deny that a previously untreated unoperated example with an appearance suggestive of PXA but with a high mitotic rate or with necrosis should be accepted as PXA; it is clear that some glioblastomas mimic PXA, but the clinical behavior of these unusual tumors is that of glioblastoma. Therefore the necessary diagnostic features for a diagnosis of PXA include the presence of pleomorphic astrocytic cells and single-cell reticulin deposits, and the absence of other high-grade features. Interestingly, neither the absence or scarcity of xanthomatous cells (Fig. 5–7D), nor their presence, is crucial to the diagnosis, as these are very rare in some PXAs and such cells may also occur in true aggressive glioblastomas.[80]

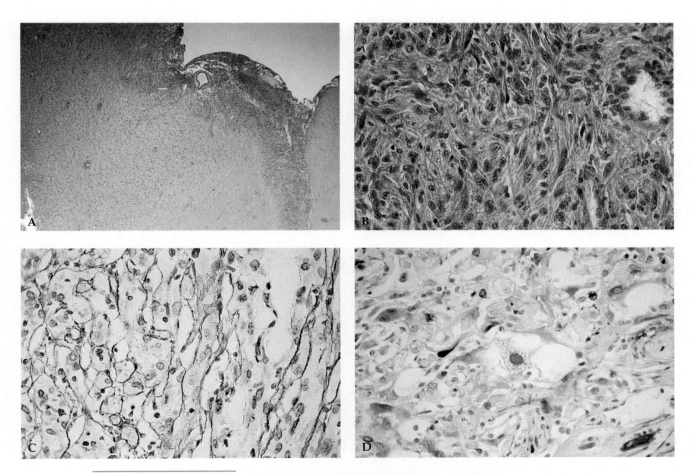

Figure 5–7 Pleomorphic xanthoastrocytoma (PXA). (A) PXAs are superficial tumors that involve the leptomeninges and the underlying cortex (H&E, 6.25×). (B) The cells of a PXA are generally large and pleiomorphic, with large, even bizarre nuclei (H&E, 100×). (C) Reticulin stains outline individual cells in PXA, whereas ordinary fibrillary astrocytomas lack basal lamina and do not stain with reticulin in this fashion (reticulin silver, 100×). (D) Lipid-filled astrocytes, the source of the "xantho" in the name of this tumor type, are not always present. This example has GFAP immunopositivity (GFAP, 100×).

PXAs may be related to a far less common neoplasm, gliofibroma (or glioneurofibroma).[81-84] Both are tumors in the general category of astrocytoma but having some epithelial and mesenchymal character, including reticulin deposits, and both occur mostly at the brain-leptomeningeal interface. Gliofibromas occur in the spinal cord as well as the brain,[84-86] unlike PXA.

Desmoplastic Infantile Astrocytoma

DIA was first described by Taratuto et al,[16] who noted the existence in infants 18 months or younger of large, often cystic, supratentorial masses with a dural attachment that somewhat resembled meningioma. Histologically these tumors had a variably loose to dense collagenous stromal background in which there were spindle cells in wavy fascicles, often closely mimicking spindle cell meningiomas. (Fig. 5–8). The tumors, despite an often ominous computed tomography (CT) or MRI appearance, usually had a bland histologic aspect and appeared benign or low grade; their astrocytic nature was demonstrable with GFAP immunostains (Fig. 5–8C). As with PXAs and gliofibromas, these tumors (despite their initial resemblance to meningiomas) are not sharply demarcated from the brain tissue; there is no arachnoidal plane between the dural-based tumor and the cerebral tissue, and histologically these tumors infiltrate to some depth in the manner of fibrillary astrocytomas.

As experience with this diagnosis has accumulated, rare examples have been encountered in the infratentorial compartment, cases have been seen in adults,[87] and at least one example has been described with CSF metastases at presentation.[88] However, the overwhelming majority of reported cases retain the clinical characteristics from the original report (i.e., they are supratentorial tumors in infants). A related tumor, the desmoplastic infantile ganglioglioma, has subsequently been described (see below).

Oligodendrogliomas

Oligodendrogliomas (Ordinary, or "Low Grade")

The term "oligodendroglioma" was first used by Bailey and Cushing[89] in their classic monograph on brain tumor classification to describe tumors composed of cells with centrally placed round nuclei and relatively modest amounts of perinuclear cytoplasm, with minimal cell processes demonstrable by metallic impregnation techniques. The first definitive paper on these tumors followed from Bailey and Bucy.[90] There was a presumption that these cells, so clearly different from tumor astrocytes, arose from the other major glial cell type, namely oligodendrocytes, which also had round nuclei and relatively scanty short processes. In modern H&E stains, these tumors have a characteristic appearance in which the perinuclear cytoplasm (in sections of formalin-fixed,

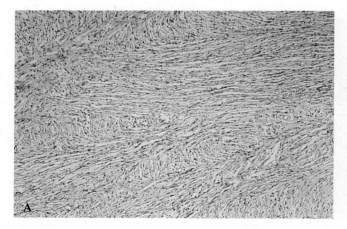

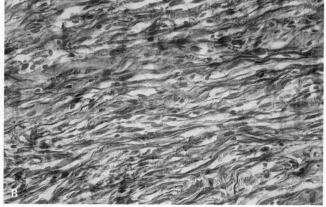

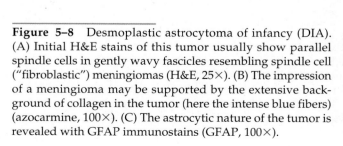

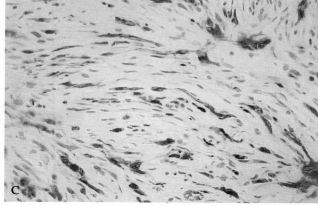

Figure 5–8 Desmoplastic astrocytoma of infancy (DIA). (A) Initial H&E stains of this tumor usually show parallel spindle cells in gently wavy fascicles resembling spindle cell ("fibroblastic") meningiomas (H&E, 25×). (B) The impression of a meningioma may be supported by the extensive background of collagen in the tumor (here the intense blue fibers) (azocarmine, 100×). (C) The astrocytic nature of the tumor is revealed with GFAP immunostains (GFAP, 100×).

paraffin-embedded tissue) fails to stain with eosin and thus appears optically clear. (Fig. 5–9) The borders of these tumor cells are generally distinct, and the tumors are either infiltrative among normal parenchymal elements or, when more solid, have an almost epithelial appearance. The solid portions of these tumors have also been described as having a honeycomb appearance, based on the sheets of closely packed empty cytoplasm separated by distinct cell borders. The tumors often exhibit the same secondary structures of Scherer as they infiltrate, as do fibrillary astrocytomas; in fact, they may do so more often than astrocytomas. In classical examples, there is a delicate capillary vascular network dividing the solid sheets of tumor cells into lobules; the vessels have an almost right-angle branching pattern, which has been likened to chicken wire (Fig. 5–9). In many tumors of this type there is extensive microcalcification in viable tissue and even in normal-appearing cerebral tissues adjacent to the tumor.

The true incidence of oligodendrogliomas is unknown; reports vary from less than 1% to as much as 15% or even approaching 20% of all CNS primary tumors.[91] One difficulty in arriving at such estimates is that different pathologists have used different diagnostic criteria to define these tumors as distinct from mixed gliomas with apparent oligodendroglial elements. Depending on the sensitivity one has for astrocytic elements, one may diagnose a majority of tumors with this histologic appearance as "oligodendroglioma" or as "mixed oligodendroglioma/astrocytoma." Another difficulty

is that, despite intensive studies, no immunohistochemical marker that selectively stains normal oligodendrocytes (of which there are several) reliably and specifically stains tumor with this appearance; either many tumors with astrocytic or neuronal elements are also stained, or most examples are not marked by the candidate antibodies. Similarly, no ultrastructural feature consistently and reliably identifies a tumor as a true oligodendroglioma. In recent years, several tumor types have been identified that have the H&E appearance of an oligodendroglioma but that are provably of other cytologic lineage or differentiation. These include clear cell ependymomas,[18, 92] intraventricular neurocytomas,[6–8] and parenchymal neurocytic tumors[19–23] (see below). In addition, the tumor most commonly identified as dysembryoplastic neuroepithelial tumor (DNT)[12–15] was often originally misdiagnosed as oligodendroglioma. *Thus, the modern histopathologic diagnosis of oligodendroglioma is, or ought to be, one of exclusion: these are the "clear cell" CNS tumors that are not demonstrably ependymal or neuronal.* Studies based solely on the H&E appearance or supplemented only with GFAP immunostains clearly overstate the frequency of this diagnosis.

In children, tumors with an oligodendrogliomatous appearance (whatever their true lineage) are relatively rare[93]; these tumors are more commonly found in younger adults, especially when neurocytic and DNT examples are excluded.

Oligodendrogliomas are usually more indolent than fibrillary astrocytomas and have even been termed "benign";

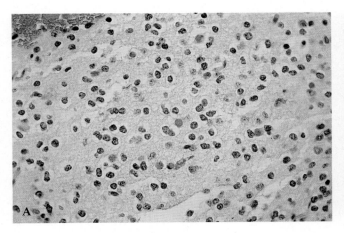
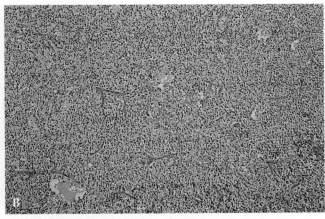
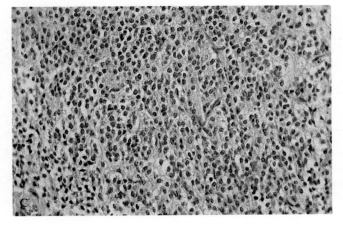

Figure 5–9 Oligodendroglioma. (A) The typical appearance of the cells of tumors called "oligodendroglioma" is as seen here: medium size cells with centrally placed, mostly round nuclei, surrounded by a "halo" of cytoplasm that does not stain with H&E, giving a clear-cell appearance (H&E, 100×). (B) Oligodendrogliomas are infiltrative neoplasms, resembling in this regard fibrillary astrocytomas, but they often reach higher cell densities than low-grade astrocytomas. Such tumors have sheets of clear cells closely abutting each other, giving what is classically described as a honeycomb pattern (H&E, 25×). (C) In many such tumors the honeycomb is separated into lobules by ramifying fine capillaries with roughly right-angle branches, a so-called "chicken wire" vascular pattern (H&E, 100×).

this is clearly a misnomer given that the median survival in most series for patients with a diagnosis of oligodendroglioma is less than 10 years. Attempts to identify histologic prognostic factors have been problematical, as there is little agreement from series to series.[91] Recently, several studies of proliferation indices using immunostains for the nuclear proliferation-associated antigen Ki67 or for proliferating cell nuclear antigen (PCNA) have suggested that there exist thresholds of labeling index (LI) above which the tumors are clearly more aggressive,[94–96] although there is not unanimity on this[97] and the proposed thresholds are not easily transferable from one laboratory to another with the current technology for determining LI.[96]

Anaplastic Oligodendrogliomas

The diagnosis of "anaplastic" oligodendroglioma identifies a tumor with the same cytologic character as the ordinary oligodendroglioma (with the same problems regarding mixed tumors and tumors of other lineage that implies), but with greater pleomorphism, plus a high level of mitotic activity, vascular hyperplasia, and even glioblastoma-like necrosis. There has long been a debate over the nosology of these neoplasms, leaving aside the question of true oligodendrocyte lineage *versus* other lineages because glioblastoma has in the past been variably defined as including any glial neoplasm with all of the described high-grade features; more recently, it has been defined as including only "pure" fibrillary astrocytomas with these features. Following modern practice, including that codified in the latest WHO classification,[3,3A] elaborate grading systems of supposed oligodendrogliomas include low-grade ("ordinary") and high-grade ("anaplastic") categories without room for a pure "oligodendroglial" glioblastoma. Most recently, it was suggested that the most crucial indicator of anaplastic grade (and corresponding aggressive clinical behavior) in such tumors is the presence of vascular hyperplasia (or its MRI counterpart of enhancement).[98, 99] Once again, it is difficult to estimate the frequency with which such tumors occur in children, but it is likely to be low in comparison with an adult population.

Tumors conventionally identified as oligodendrogliomas occasionally have *p53* mutations, but these are less common than in fibrillary astrocytomas. Cytogenetic studies have shown that classical oligodendrogliomas have a high frequency of chromosomal losses from chromosomes 19q and 1p,[100–103] but the crucial gene changes in the chromosomal regions affected have not yet been identified. The presence of these cytogenetic abnormalities, which closely correlate with classical oligodendroglioma histologic features, has been shown to predict chemosensitivity of the tumors to the "PCV" (procarbazine, CCNU, vincristine) regimen.[104] There is frequent overexpression of EGFR in these tumors, but the *EGFR* gene is not usually amplified.[105]

Ependymomas

Ependymomas are tumors with the cytologic features of differentiated ependymal cells and thus are recognizably tumors of the cells that line the brain's ventricular spaces and the spinal cord central canal. Despite this, almost half of all ependymomas arise outside of a ventricular cavity, with

no demonstrable connection to a normal ependymal epithelium. These are, in general, uncommon tumors, but in children, particularly those under the age of 3 years, a significant fraction of primary CNS tumors are ependymal, particularly in the posterior fossa; it has been estimated that more than 10% of all pediatric CNS tumors are fourth ventricular ependymomas.[106]

Cellular Ependymoma

The most common histologic variant of ependymoma is often termed the "cellular" ependymoma. In this tumor, there are sheets of fairly closely packed cells of small to moderate size, arranged in distinctive patterns indicative of their differentiation (Fig. 5–10A). These patterns include the formation of rosettes with central lumens (virtually miniature ventricles) (Fig. 5–10B), the formation of less regular canals and surfaces with neoplastic epithelial lining patterns (again resembling ventricular spaces and surfaces) (Fig. 5–10C), and perivascular pseudorosettes (in which the central structure is a vessel, not a lumen lined by the tumor cells themselves) (Fig. 5–10D). In all of these structures the tumor cells are unipolar elongate cells with their nuclei at one pole of the cell; the other pole consists of an extended process pointing to the lumen (of rosettes and canals) or the vascular wall (of pseudorosettes). These processes within the rosettes and pseudorosettes are most often well filled with intermediate filaments and thus are clearly delineated by stains for GFAP or vimentin.

Although the presence of these features is necessary for a diagnosis of ependymoma, other features are often present that can help guide a pathologist to the correct diagnosis. These include the presence of thick-walled hyalinized blood vessels, some with fibrinoid breakdown of their walls and with hemosiderin accumulations indicative of prior microhemorrhages. In CNS sites where Rosenthal fibers are commonly found in gliosis, the edges of ependymomas often elicit a strong gliotic reaction, with abundant Rosenthal fibers. Small biopsies (as are most frequently encountered in specimens from the brain stem or spinal cord) may catch these gliotic areas and lead to an erroneous diagnosis of pilocytic astrocytoma. Most ependymomas have circumscribed, almost sharp borders against adjacent brain parenchyma (Fig. 5–10E), which is quite different from the infiltrative borders characteristic of astrocytomas and tumors with "oligodendrogliomatous" morphology. However these other glial tumor types occasionally have sharp pseudoborders, and rare ependymomas have more infiltrative patterns, so that the border with the adjacent parenchyma can be suggestive but is not diagnostic. *Without the diagnostic pseudorosettes or the less common epithelial formations (central-lumen rosettes, canals), many ependymomas resemble astrocytomas, and they may contain gemistocytic cells that are indistinguishable from gemistocytes in anaplastic astrocytomas or glioblastomas. This confusion occurs more often in ependymomas, which have other atypical features and fit the historical definition of anaplastic ependymoma.*

"Anaplastic" Cellular Ependymoma

When ependymomas of the classical type just described accumulate zones with more than a few mitotic figures, have foci

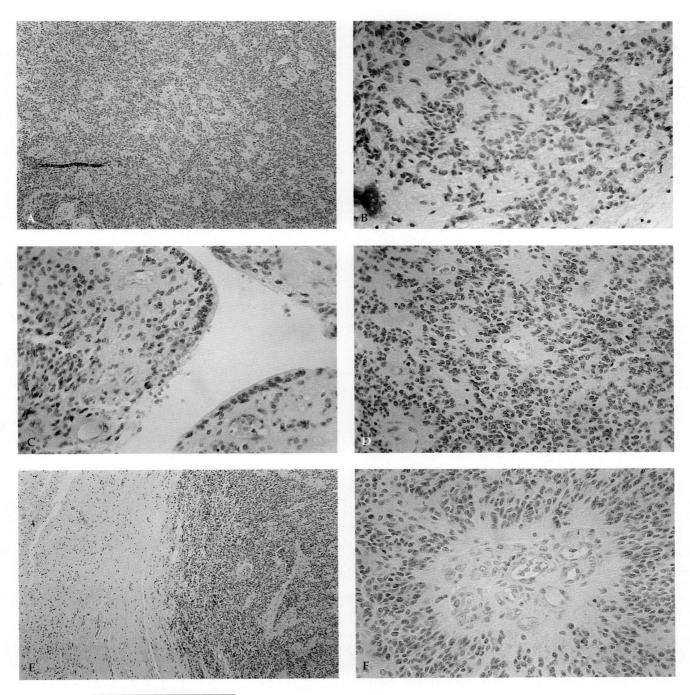

Figure 5–10   Ependymomas. (A) Cellular ependymoma with a distinctive pattern of closely packed cells surrounding pale-staining spaces; at higher power these are seen to be perivascular pseudorosettes (H&E, 25×). (B) Central lumen rosettes are central lumens surrounded by radially disposed tumor cells whose processes define the lumen (H&E, 40×). (C) In some ependymomas, larger and more irregular canals are lined by neoplastic ependymal cells, creating miniature ventricle–like spaces (H&E, 100×). (D) Pseudorosettes are the commonest architectural arrangement in ependymomas. Here each central vessel is surrounded by radially disposed tumor cells, with a nucleus-free zone of fibrillary tumor cell processes between the vessel wall and the ring of surrounding nuclei. The tumor, like many cellular ependymomas, is composed essentially of a monotonous collection of back-to-back pseudorosettes (H&E, 100×). (E) Sharp border between highly cellular ependymoma and slightly gliotic brain (H&E, 25×). (F) Some pseudorosettes contain hyperplastic vessels (H&E, 100×).   *(Continued on next page)*

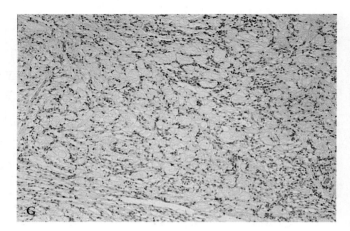

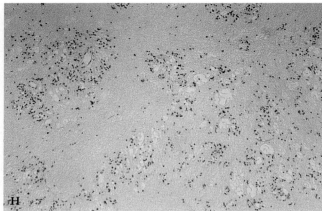

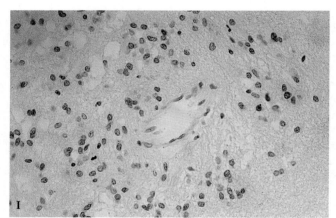

Figure 5–10 *(continued)* (G) Myxopapillary ependymomas often lack distinctive pseudorosettes because the zone between the tumor cell bodies containing the nuclei and the vessel wall is distended and replaced by the mucinous secretion that characterizes the tumors (H&E, 25×). (H, I) Subependymomas are tumors of low cell density with a distinctive pattern with clusters of nuclei and broad fibrillary anuclear zones.

of necrosis, or have vascular hyperplasia (Fig. 5–10F), neuropathologists have traditionally rendered a diagnosis of higher grade ependymoma. As with alleged oligodendrogliomas, most such grading schemes have had poor clinical correlations; they do not reliably predict recurrence after surgery or response to radiation or chemotherapy, and they do not reliably indicate average survival times. Consequently, most modern accounts use only two grades of "cellular" ependymoma, low and high grade, the latter usually termed "anaplastic" ependymoma.

While some controversy remains, the accumulated literature strongly suggests that such a grading system is still highly unreliable and therefore not justifiable; no histologic feature or combination of features has been clearly demonstrated to impact on response to therapy, time to recurrence, or survival.[1–4, 107–114] A study by this author of a cohort of children enrolled in Children's Cancer Group ependymoma clinical trials emphasized this with rigorous statistical analysis.[115] In children, it is clear that for the most common ependymomas, those of the posterior fossa in the fourth ventricle, age at diagnosis and perhaps extent of resection are the most crucial indicators of subsequent clinical course, with children whose tumors are detected before the age of 3 years or are not clearly resected (to a "gross total resection" as confirmed by MRIs) faring the worst.

Clear Cell Ependymoma

The existence of either focal areas or whole tumors of provable ependymal lineage or differentiation but with an H&E appearance of "oligodendroglioma" with clear cells has already been alluded to in the discussion of oligodendroglial tumors. The original explicit demonstration of the existence of these tumors relied on ultrastructural evidence of the ependymal nature of the tumor cells,[18, 116] and this was emphasized in a subsequent description.[92] However in common practice many or most such examples can be recognized by the combination of close examination of large resection specimens for a few rosettes or pseudorosettes, and the use of GFAP and vimentin immunostains to highlight perivascular radially oriented processes. Small samples will probably continue to require electron microscopic examination for demonstration of the diagnostic features. Tumors of this type demostrate clinical behavior no different from that of other cellular ependymomas.

Myxopapillary Ependymoma

Myxopapillary ependymomas are distinctive neoplasms that occur almost exclusively in the spinal cord and cauda equina. There are no more than two cases alleged to have arisen as primary cerebral tumors. As these tumors have a significant, indeed high incidence of CSF dissemination, especially but not exclusively after surgery, any alleged cerebral example must be regarded as a potential secondary implant from a spinal cord primary tumor until careful MRI examinations prove otherwise.

These tumors are most commonly found affecting the conus and filum of the cord or even "free" within the cauda equina. Histologically they may be difficult to recognize as ependymal, until it is realized that the papillary structures with tumor cells enclosing lakes of mucin and myxoid matrix represent pseudorosettes in which the space between the tumor cell bodies and the vascular walls is distended by the accumulation of the secreted extracellular matrix (Fig. 5–10G). In some cases, the nuclei seem to form lines reminiscent of nuclear palisades in schwannomas, and indeed that is one of the more common diagnostic errors associated with this tumor type.

Like other spinal cord ependymomas, myxopapillary ependymomas are relatively rare in children and are mostly found in adults. In the intramedullary spinal cord tumors radically resected from 174 children at NYU Medical Center between 1977 and 1994, only 20 ependymomas were found, and of these only 6 were myxopapillary.[117]

Subependymoma

Subependymoma has at various times been regarded as a special type of subependymal astrocytoma or as a variant of ependymoma; a variety of features point to the latter characterization as more accurate. These tumors are slow growing and rarely present in childhood, although once diagnosed in adults it is often clear that the tumor must have been present during childhood. Occasionally such tumors surface in patients within the pediatric age group. The tumors were originally described within the fourth ventricle but are now well documented in other sites, including the spinal cord and the brain parenchyma distant from any ventricular cavity.

Subependymomas have a distinctive histologic pattern; they have low cell density, with extensive areas of dense finely fibrillary glial matrix within which there are loose clusters of small, often round nuclei (Fig. 5–10H, I). Careful examination at low power reveals that the clusters usually represent very wide and loose perivascular arrangements approximating pseudorosettes. As with cellular ependymomas, thick-walled hyalinized vessels are very common in these tumors.

Mixed Cellular Ependymoma and Subependymoma

One of the points that emphasizes that subependymomas are essentially ependymal and not astrocytic in lineage is that composite or mixed examples of cellular ependymoma and subependymoma are well described. Interestingly, these tumors, at least from anecdotal evidence, behave more like the cellular variants than like "pure" subependymomas. The border between the two elements is usually abrupt (hence "composite") rather than there being an intimate admixture of the two patterns.

Neuronal and Mixed Glial-Neuronal Tumors

The category of neuronal or mixed glial-neuronal neoplasms is of particular interest in pediatric neuro-oncology, as these tumor types are more frequently recognized in children. The category includes well-established entities, such as gangliogliooma; one of the newer accepted entities, namely, intraventricular neurocytoma; and one of the entities about which there remains considerable controversy, the parenchymal neurocytic neoplasm or ganglioglioneurocytoma.

Gangliogliomas

Gangliogliomas are neoplasms that are composed of two histologically disparate elements: a glial component, almost always astrocytic, and sometimes resembling pilocytic astrocytoma or pleiomorphic xanthoastrocytoma, and a neuronal component, consisting of large ganglion cells (Fig. 5–11). Most examples have a low-grade appearance without necrosis, vascular hyperplasia, or significant nuclear atypism, although the mixture of smaller astrocytic nuclei and large neuronal nuclei can give an impression of pleomorphism, which then can lead to an erroneous diagnosis of anaplastic astrocytoma if the pathologist does not recognize the neuronal component as such. Neoplasms of this type have been recognized at least since the 1930s.[118] Most examples described in the literature have been temporal lobe neoplasms associated with chronic seizure disorders, although it has long been clear that examples from other cerebral lobes, and from all other portions of the CNS, including the spinal cord, have been encountered. The revolution in histopathology brought about in the last three decades by the development and maturation of immunohistochemistry has altered this perspective on gangliogliomas: in particular, studies for the synaptic vesicle protein synaptophysin have assisted in the recognition of gangliogliomas such that many more examples in all sites are now recorded.[20,119–126] In gangliogliomas there is a dense perikaryal surface immunopositivity for synaptophysin, synaptic vesicle protein 2 (SV2), synapsin I, and synaptobrevin, in a pattern that is virtually diagnostic for abnormality of the ganglion cells (Fig. 5–11C): cortical neurons trapped within "pure" glial tumors do not exhibit this immunoreactivity, nor do cells in other gray matter structures, with limited exceptions in the spinal cord, brain stem, and cerebellar Purkinje cells.[20,119, 120, 122–126] Although the specificity and hence the utility of this pattern has been challenged[127, 128] with careful attention to anatomical site, to the presence or absence of a normal surrounding neuropil (as seen in the anterior horn of the cord, the hippocampal Ammon's horn, the brain stem nuclei, and the cerebellar cortex), and to whether the staining is truly on the perikaryon or on the apical dendrites (more common, for example, on Purkinje cells), this remains a very useful adjunct to the standard diagnostic criteria for a diagnosis of ganglion cell neoplasia. Based on the examination of large resection samples (as compared to small biopsy samples) and with the use of these immunohistochemical stains we have found that among pediatric intramedullary spinal cord tumors, which admittedly are rare neoplasms, gangliogliomas are the second most common type of tumor after fibrillary astrocytomas.[117]

Occasionally gangliogliomas have "aggressive" histologic features: the astrocytic component has more nuclear atypism, and there may be more than rare mitotic figures, vascular hyperplasia, or even necrosis (Fig. 5–11D). The prognostic

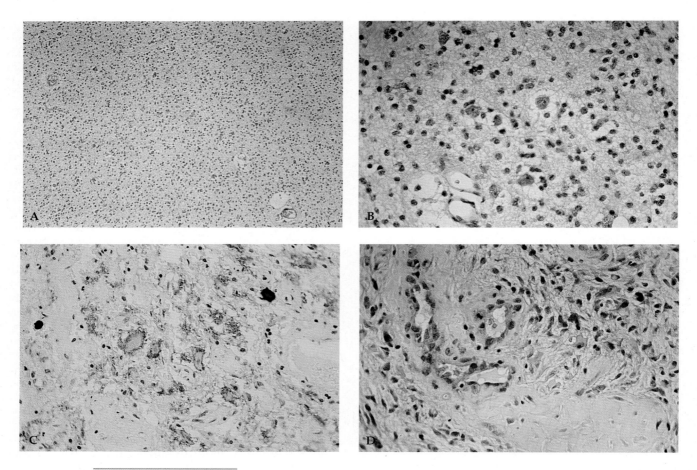

Figure 5–11   Gangliogliomas. (A) These tumors are composed of a mixture of small to mid-size astrocytes, occasionally with pilocytic characteristics, and large ganglion cells. The ganglion cells may vary in size, and with the small astrocytes an overview of the tumor gives an impression of considerable pleomorphism (H&E, 25×). (B) The neuronal cells may appear similar to normal large neurons, but are not arranged in layers or columns as in cortex, and they often include a few with "dysplastic" features or which are binucleated (H&E, 100×). (C) Stains for synaptic vesicle antigens reveal dense perikaryal surface immunoreactivity indicating numerous synapses on the neoplastic neuronal cell bodies, a strong indication that the neurons in question (with certain specific exceptions—see text) are neoplastic and not trapped normal cells (synaptophysin, 100×). (D) This cauda equina anaplastic ganglioglioma has both marked atypicality of its astrocytic component and vascular hyperplasia; elsewhere, not shown, there was necrosis. The tumor progressed despite surgery, radiation therapy, and chemotherapy (H&E, 100×).

significance of these changes, which in fibrillary astrocytomas are clear indicators of high-grade malignant neoplasms, is much diminished in gangliogliomas. Several studies have found no statistically sound associations of such histologic features with prognosis and have suggested that because the grading of gangliogliomas into ordinary and "anaplastic" categories is not clinically relevant, it should not be done.[121, 129] However, individual cases with these features and with aggressive clinical behavior culminating in death are recorded,[130–132] so this remains somewhat controversial.

There are descriptions of gangliogliomas in which the glial element is "oligodendroglioma." Our own series of gangliogliomas included some examples, but we found that the "oligo-like" cells were associated with a tumor neuropil of

synaptophysin-immunopositive processes, indicating that these were in fact small neurons (neurocytoma cells).[20] We proposed that such tumors were better termed "gangliglioneurocytomas," which will be discussed later in this chapter.

The occurrence of gangliogliomas, as with other tumors apparently composed of two different cell types, raises provocative questions as to the cellular origins (histogenesis) of these tumors. A common assumption is that these tumors (and other mixed tumors; see later in this chapter) arise from a clone of bipotential or multipotential progenitor cells, which then differentiate into the apparent astrocytic and neuronal components. The fact that such immature, uncommitted cells are not seen histopathologically or in tissue cultures that yield both astrocytic and neuronal tumor cells[20] suggests that this might not be true; however, the demonstration that gangliogliomas are clonal neoplasms in which both the neuronal and the astrocytic cells have the same pattern of X-chromosome inactivation is strong support for a progenitor cell hypothesis.[133]

Desmoplastic Infantile Gangliogliomas

In 1987, VandenBerg et al[17] described a series of infants with large supratentorial tumors that were easily interpreted as meningeal sarcomas or high-grade gliomas involving the leptomeninges and the brain; the tumors were often cystic and had considerable collagenous matrix. With immunohistochemistry and electron microscopy, these authors identified a neuronal (ganglion cell) component and an astrocytic component in these tumors, proving that these were a distinct subcategory of gangliogliomas, for which they proposed the term *desmoplastic infantile ganglioglioma* (DIG). Importantly, children with these tumors were shown to have a surprisingly good clinical outcome; with extensive surgical resection alone, most survived tumor-free, although incomplete resections were associated with recurrences and at least one death.[17] The tumors had an obvious relationship to the desmoplastic dural-based astrocytomas described in a similar age group by Taratuto et al,[16] and in a follow-up article Vandenberg discussed the histopathologic spectrum of all of these infantile meningeal and cerebral neoplasms, which could include foci resembling PNET without (apparently) altering the good prognosis.[134] Others have since described similar cases,[135–137] and this is now a fairly well-accepted entity, included in the WHO revised classification.[3,3A]

The clinical spectrum of cases of DIG may be broader than originally suspected (rare instances being found in posterior fossa sites, or in older children or adults,[138–140]), but the essential clinicopathologic core message remains that these are usually found in infants and are typically large, cystic, and solid supratentorial neoplasms with dural, leptomeningeal, and cerebral parenchymal components, and that with resection alone there is usually a good oncologic outcome. The cases described in older patients have been claimed to better represent examples of mixed ganglioglioma and pleomorphic xanthoastrocytoma.[2] Recognition of the ganglion cell elements can be difficult, but synaptophysin or a similar immunostain is effective in revealing these crucial yet "obscure" elements. We have briefly described one case (in our larger series of all gangliogliomas) in which multiple recurrences culminated in a transformation to glioblastoma, with the death of the patient 13 years after the initial presentation at the age of less than 1 year.[20]

Gangliocytomas

In contrast to gangliogliomas, the term "gangliocytoma" identifies a CNS neoplasm composed wholly of large neuronal cells, without any astrocytic component. Such tumors are much less common than gangliogliomas. In some instances, it is difficult to determine if the astrocytic cells seen in a ganglion cell tumor are reactive (leading to a diagnosis of gangliocytoma) or neoplastic (leading to a diagnosis of ganglioglioma). Some neuropathologists prefer not to make these distinctions and use the generic term "ganglion cell tumor."

A true gangliocytoma is as close to a benign intraparenchymal CNS tumor as can exist; recurrence or dissemination after surgical resection is essentially unknown. Some tumors once considered hypothalamic or intrasellar gangliocytomas are now known to be pituitary adenomas with gangliocytic differentiation.[141] Another difficulty is that hamartomas containing large neuronal elements are difficult or impossible to reliably and nonarbitrarily separate from gangliocytomas in the most common type of neurosurgically obtained tissue (i.e., small fragments). In this regard, one should note that the hypothalamus is one of the chief sites in which both gangliocytomas and neuronal-glial hamartomas are said to occur. Here, as elsewhere in pediatric neuro-oncology, we are truly in the "borderland of embryology and pathology."[142]

Special mention must be made of the distinctive cerebellar lesion known as "dysplastic gangliocytoma of Lhermitte and Duclos" (Lhermitte-Duclos disease). This is a malformation of the cerebellar foliar cortex in which large ganglion cells, representing abnormal neuronal elements, replace the internal granular layer of the cortex in a chaotic but focal fashion. By most accounts these are not neoplasms, although examples of recurrence after surgical excision have been described.[143–145]

Intraventricular Neurocytomas

Intraventricular neurocytomas were first definitively identified by Hassoun and colleagues,[6] although in retrospect examples had earlier been described as neuronal tumors in these sites.[146, 147] The entity, while relatively new, in fact replaces the diagnostic terminology previously applied to tumors whose clinical and pathologic characteristics had been described as ependymomas of the foramen of Monro[148] or oligodendrogliomas of the interventricular septum.[149, 150] As the name and the prior discussion suggest, these tumors are typically found in the lateral or third ventricle close to and in one of the foramina of Monro and attached medially to the interventricular septum. We have seen several of these arise at other ventricular sites.[19]

These are tumors whose histopathologic appearance is more or less that of the classical oligodendroglioma (Fig. 5–12A): a sheetlike proliferation of fairly closely packed, medium-size cells with round, centrally placed nuclei lying in clear or pale-staining cytoplasm; alternatively, the same appearance has been described as a honeycomb arrangement of such cells. The initial recognition of these cells as neuronal depended on electron microscopy, which showed primarily extensive fine processes forming a neuropil and containing presynaptic endings with dense-core neurosecretory vesicles, clear synaptic vesicles, or both.[6–8, 146–147] More recently, immunohistochemical staining, particularly for synaptophysin, has shown that the vesicles in the neuropil have the expected immunoreactivity for neuronal/synaptic markers (synaptophysin, SV2, synapsin 1), allowing diagnosis by easier means (Fig. 5–12B). Occasionally tumors are synaptophysin-poor but stain for chromogranin, and by electron microscopy these tumors have synaptic endings rich in dense-core neurosecretory vesicles. While it is often said that with H&E stains these tumors are indistinguishable from oligodendroglioma, there are often anuclear zones of fibrillary neuropil surrounded by tumor cells in a fashion resembling neuroblastic (central fibrillary or Homer Wright) rosettes, but larger. These have been termed "neurocytic" rosettes or "giant Homer Wright" rosettes.[2, 8] They are

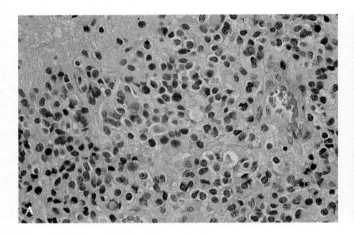

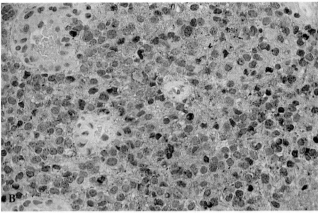

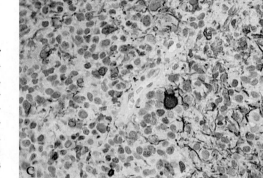

Figure 5–12 Intraventricular neurocytoma. (A) In H&E (or similar) stains, these tumors are very similar to "oligodendrogliomas" and consist of variably densely packed clear cells, often in a honeycomb pattern (hematoxylin/phloxine/saffranin, 100×). (B) The neuronal nature of these tumors is indicated by a granular neuropil–like immunoreactivity for synaptophysin (and other synaptic antigens) apparently between the cells (and actually within fine synaptic endings from them) (synaptophysin, 100×). (C) In some neurocytomas many cells are immunoreactive for GFAP (GFAP, 100×).

essentially identical to the large rosettes seen in pineocytoma (see below), a tumor that may in fact ultimately be recognized as "pineal neurocytoma."

While neurocytoma was originally thought of as a pure neuronal neoplasm, it was subsequently shown that some, or even most, of the cells also had GFAP expression and thus were clearly bipotential stem cells with both astrocytic and neuronal characteristics[151–153] (Fig. 5–12C). This was further confirmed by tissue culture studies.[154] Examples with ganglion cells are also described.[155] Most intraventricular neurocytomas have bland histopathologic characteristics, with few mitotic figures; low proliferation rates, as measured by immunostains for proliferation markers such as Ki67 (Fig. 5–12C); and an absence of significant pleomorphism, vascular hyperplasia, or necrosis. Occasionally, an aggressive appearance has been described,[153, 156] and the terms "malignant neurocytoma" or "anaplastic neurocytoma" have been suggested. The clinical correlate of such grading is still unclear, although cases with CSF dissemination are described[157]; this author has autopsied one patient with such dissemination from a bland, ordinary-appearing intraventricular neurocytoma.

Ganglioglioneurocytomas

Following on our observation of gangliogliomas with oligodendroglioma-like elements that were demonstrably neurocytic by immunostaining and electron microscopy, we pro-posed that such tumors be identified descriptively by their elements: "ganglio-" (large neurons), "glio-" (astrocytoma cells), "neurocytoma" (neurocytoma cells).[19,20] Some examples lack detectable ganglion cells but have the neurocytomatous and astrocytic components; we use the term "glioneurocytoma" to describe such tumors, as has Min.[158] With this observation and with the perspective of the descriptions of intraventricular neurocytomas as easily confused with oligodendroglioma with H&E stains, we undertook a study of parenchymal (non-intraventricular) CNS neoplasms composed wholly or in part of oligo-like elements. We found that about half of such tumors had synaptophysin immunoreactivity and, less frequently, neurofilament protein immunoreactivity, suggestive of neurocytic rather than glial differentiation.[159-160] Frequently, as with intraventricular neurocytoma, there was concurrent GFAP expression, often in cells identical to those usually termed "minigemistocytes" in conventional descriptions of oligodendroglioma. In a few cases, electron microscopy confirmed that the synaptophysin immunopositivity represented neurites with bouton-like endings containing synaptic vesicles. More recently, we used antibodies to other synaptic vesicle antigens (synaptobrevin; SV2) and to neurofilament protein components to confirm the neuronal nature of some or all of the cells in these tumors.[160] With the immunostains it also became easier to recognize that many of these tumors had ganglion cell elements and were, again, "ganglioglioneurocytomas" (GGNs).

As might be expected, because most of these tumors would have conventionally been classified as oligodendroglioma, a tumor less commonly found in children than in adults, GGN is less commonly found in children than in adults, although we have seen multiple pediatric examples. A few examples have such prominent rosette formation that a diagnosis of oligodendroglioma is implausible[160A]; such tumors may be misdiagnosed as clear cell ependymomas (see above), especially if there are perivascular pseudorosette-like structures as well. One of the first cases we encountered that led us to propose the nosologic category of GGN was a frontal lobe tumor in a 7-year-old boy, which we initially called ependymoma; a recurrence a year later had obvious ganglion cells, leading to the use of synaptophysin staining for both the recurrence and the original, in turn leading to a corrected diagnosis of GGN.

Diffuse "Oligodendroglioma"-like Ganglioglioneurocytomas

The majority of tumors to which we assign the controversial diagnostic term "diffuse oligodendroglioma-like GGN" are diffuse tumors involving white matter and gray matter (usually cortex) that would conventionally be termed "oligodendroglioma" or mixed glioma. More of our cases have occurred in adults than in children, but we have seen pediatric examples as well. Similar observations and conclusions have been made by Ng et al,[161] Nishio et al,[162] Min et al,[158] and Giangaspero et al.[163]

Cortical "DNT"-Type Ganglioglioneurocytomas (Includes All DNT)

Some of our cases have been more restricted to the cortex in their growth, rather than being diffuse lesions spreading through the white matter. These have also had the distinctive multinodular architecture, clusters of microcysts, and other features described by Daumas-Duport as "dysembryoplastic neuroepithelial tumor" (DNT).[12, 13] Although the original descriptions of DNT suggested that the majority component of the tumors was oligodendrogliomatous, our observations and those of others[14, 15, 164] suggest that these cells are often identifiable as neuronal (neurocytomatous). It has been suggested that the cerebral neurocytomas described by Nishio et al[162] are, in fact, DNTs[8, 165]—a suggestion we could agree on if we acknowledge that "DNT" describes a particular architecture and pattern found in some ganglioglioneurocytomas, and that descriptive terminology of the components of a DNT lead to the other nomenclature.

DNTs were originally described as tumors, almost all of temporal lobe origin, that are cortically based, multinodular masses associated with interspersed zones of cortical dysplasia. The original cases were all described in children or young adults with chronic seizures, mostly complex partial epilepsy.[12, 13] *Histologically these tumors contain the three cellular elements typical of GGN: a majority component of small to midsize "oligo-like" cells; astrocytes; and large neurons (ganglion cells)* (Fig. 5–13A). In the most typical areas (the "specific component" of Daumas-Duport), the oligo-like cells are closely associated in almost linear arrays along the axons of the ganglion cells. There are clusters of microcysts within the nodular masses, and ganglion cells are found floating in the eosinophilic or mucinous fluid that occupies these cystic spaces (Fig. 5–13A); there is often a myxoid/mucinous background in the neuropil as well. Immunostaining reveals granular synaptophysin (and other SV antigen) immunoreactivity in the neuropil and decorating the surfaces of the ganglion cell perikarya, as in gangliogliomas (Fig. 5–13B).

Tumors with all of the gross (or neuroradiologic) and histologic characteristics of DNT have subsequently been described in children and adults without a long history of epilepsy, often after a single seizure leading to an MRI. This presumably reflects changes in clinical practice and improved imaging rather than a difference in tumor biology, although patients who have demonstrated prolonged survival with chronic partial seizures without the benefit of such clinical investigations will clearly be "self-selected" for a nonprogressive variant of this tumor. Whereas in the original descriptions of DNT in patients with chronic seizure disorders radical surgical excision was curative, there is now in our patient populations (and in anecdotes not yet published beyond abstracts) increasing recognition of cases in which these tumors have recurred locally or, in rare instances, behaved more aggressively, either with CSF dissemination or with transformation to aggressive, high-grade neoplasms of either retained mixed glial-neuronal character or of pure glial character, including typical glioblastomas. *At present, there is no suggestion of a way to recognize which examples of ordinary-appearing DNT/GGN will recur or be aggressive and which will be cured by excision, although high-proliferation indices and vascular hyperplasia are suggestive features that we are considering as candidates for such indicators.*

Mixed Diffuse and DNT Types

In addition to the two types of GGN just described, we have seen examples in which the two patterns are combined. There is a cortically based multinodular component, usually with microcysts, but this blends into a more diffusely infiltrative component that spreads widely through the white matter—one that, as discussed for diffuse GGN above, would more conventionally (and without special investigation, such as synaptophysin staining or electron microscopy) be diagnosed as oligodendroglioma or mixed glioma.

Mixed Lipomatous/Neurocytic Tumors

There have been several reports of tumors in children (and adults) composed of bland, oligo-like components with admixed astrocytes and zones with mature adipose cells.[166, 167] These lesions resemble closely the cerebellar tumors originally described as lipomatous PNET ("lipomatous medulloblastomas")[168, 169] and, like those tumors, are more indolent neoplasms than typical PNETs (see below).

Mixed "Pure" Gliomas

As should be implicit in the foregoing discussions of oligodendroglioma and parenchymal neurocytic neoplasms, there are gliomas with no demonstrable recognizable neuronal elements even when immunohistochemical and electron microscopic techniques are utilized. These tumors, if pure oligo-like neoplasms, are either clear cell ependymomas or are best

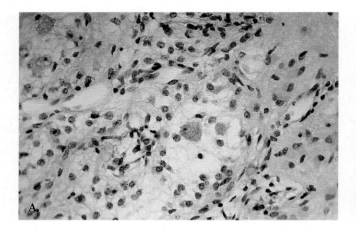

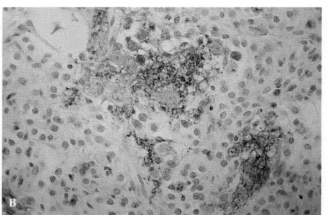

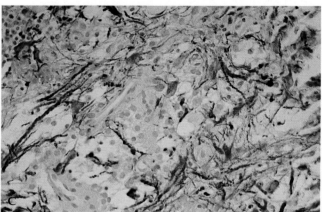

Figure 5–13 Dysembryoplastic neuroepithelial tumor type of ganglioglioneurocytoma. (A) The most characteristic histologic feature of these tumors consists of nodules of fibrillary tumor tissue with multiple microcysts; within and around the microcysts the majority of cells are small, round, "oligodendroglioma-like" cells, admixed with less frequent astrocytes and with large ganglion cells, some of which "float" in the microcysts (H&E, 100×). (B) Synaptophysin stains show patchy but strong immunoreactivity coating the surfaces of the ganglion cells and in the neuropil around the small "oligodendrocyte"-like cells (synaptophysin, 100×). (C) GFAP stains show no immunoreactivity in the small oligodendrocyte-like cells or the large neurons but reveal prominent GFAP-positive processes and scattered positive astrocytes.

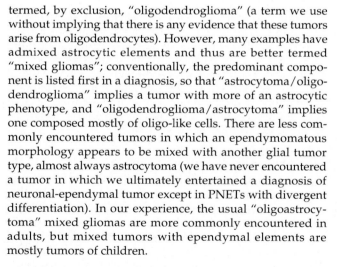

termed, by exclusion, "oligodendroglioma" (a term we use without implying that there is any evidence that these tumors arise from oligodendrocytes). However, many examples have admixed astrocytic elements and thus are better termed "mixed gliomas"; conventionally, the predominant component is listed first in a diagnosis, so that "astrocytoma/oligodendroglioma" implies a tumor with more of an astrocytic phenotype, and "oligodendroglioma/astrocytoma" implies one composed mostly of oligo-like cells. There are less commonly encountered tumors in which an ependymomatous morphology appears to be mixed with another glial tumor type, almost always astrocytoma (we have never encountered a tumor in which we ultimately entertained a diagnosis of neuronal-ependymal tumor except in PNETs with divergent differentiation). In our experience, the usual "oligoastrocytoma" mixed gliomas are more commonly encountered in adults, but mixed tumors with ependymal elements are mostly tumors of children.

Mixed Astrocytoma/Oligodendroglioma (and Oligodendroglioma/Astrocytoma)

The criteria for a diagnosis of mixed astrocytic and oligodendrogliomatous tumor have never been firmly established (as discussed under "Oligodendroglioma," above), and various proposals remain in competition for diagnostic authority. The controversies range from what to call tumors with a mostly glioblastomatous phenotype with small foci of cells having round, centrally placed nuclei lying in clear

cytoplasm to how to classify tumors with a mostly bland, classical oligodendrogliomatous phenotype in which there are intimately admixed cells of astrocytic phenotype with eccentrically placed ovoid, elongated, and irregular nuclei associated with larger amounts of brightly eosinophilic cytoplasm (usually GFAP-immunopositive) and with some degree of multipolar process formation. The first of these dichotomous problems has considerable clinical importance because survival in glioblastomas with as little as an estimated 5% of an oligo component is thought to be better,[170] and the response of such tumors to a specific chemotherapy regimen (PCV) is thought to be considerably better than the response of pure glioblastomas to this or any other chemotherapy.[171] Not long ago several neuropathologists of note advocated calling any tumor with any oligo component of 5% or more simply "oligodendroglioma," but this was never widely accepted.

The problems of how to classify tumors with mostly oligo features and a scattering of astrocytic cells involves questions regarding whether the astrocytes are reactive or neoplastic, and if they are the latter whether they alter the prognosis, particularly if they appear more anaplastic than the oligo component. These questions remain unanswered. An additional problem is posed by the use of GFAP immunohistochemical staining because some cells in oligodendrogliomas are GFAP-negative, some retain an ordinary round oligo-like phenotype with a central nucleus but have a zone of cytoplasmic GFAP-immunopositivity next to the nucleus

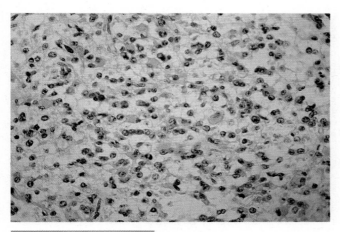

Figure 5–14 "Oligodendroglioma" with minigemistocytes. These are insufficient to justify a diagnosis of mixed glioma, as they are not astrocytes (H&E, 100×).

("gliofibrillary oligodendrocytes"),[172] and some have an appearance with eccentrically placed (but still round) nuclei with eosinophilic GFAP-immunopositive cytoplasm and are termed "minigemistocytes" or "minigemistocytic oligodendrocytes"[172] (Fig. 5–14). The presence of these two types of GFAP-immunopositive cells is insufficient to justify a diagnosis of mixed glioma; to call a tumor "mixed," we require more typically astrocytic tumor cells without round nuclei and with cellular processes.

Mixed Astrocytoma/Ependymoma

Mixed astrocytomas/ependymomas are acknowledged to be rare tumors. Ependymomas most typically form rosettes and pseudorosettes in a virtually back-to-back fashion and are sharply demarcated from adjacent brain tissue when they are not wholly within a ventricular cavity, so that some investigators have held that sheets of cells or diffusely invasive patterns always imply a diagnosis of a mixed astrocytic component, or that the tumor is not ependymal at all but rather is an astrocytoma with some pseudorosettes or is a PNET. As with the differential diagnosis of small-cell glioblastoma with PNET, this may be more of a "religious" question than one that is amenable to scientific resolution. In our practice at NYU Medical Center, we have recognized diffusely invasive areas of ependymoma in sheets or other less dense patterns in tumors focally having typical pseudorosettes that, under electron microscopic examination, have the characteristic ependymal features of intracellular lumens and extensive luminal and surface microvilli. Thus, we do not automatically make a diagnosis of mixed ependymoma/astrocytoma when an ependymoma has such diffuse infiltrative or solid sheetlike areas. However, we do recognize such a mixed diagnosis when the putative astrocytic component has different nuclear features, with more elongated or irregular and pleomorphic character than the undoubted ependymal component. We have seen examples of such tumors in children in both cerebral and spinal cord locations. To date, we have not recognized any examples of mixed ependymoma/oligodendroglioma; tumors with pseudorosettes and oligo-like cells have uniformly proved to be either clear cell ependymomas or GGNs.

Complex Mixed Gliomas: Astrocytoma/Ependymoma/Oligodendroglioma

Mixed gliomas comprising astrocytoma, ependymoma, and oligodendroglioma are extremely rare. We have seen one case, which involved a child. The various elements were all typical for their type and require no elucidation. The only differential diagnostic point raised by the existence of all three such glial lineages in a single tumor is whether the tumor is actually a PNET with extensive and divergent differentiation, but in the example we saw a large resection specimen showed no primitive component to allow such an interpretation.

Mixed Glial/Mesenchymal Tumors

A wholly different category of mixed tumor in the CNS is that in which a glial tumor (almost always astrocytic) has a coexisting neoplastic mesenchymal component, usually a sarcoma. Tumors of this type generally fall into two categories: the more or less classical gliosarcoma, and the much less common gliofibroma ("glioneurofibroma"). Gliosarcomas are uncommon in children but will be briefly described here because examples are rarely seen in this age group; gliofibromas are described as congenital tumors found in infants, as newly diagnosed later in childhood, and as tumors of adults. For this portion of the chapter, the combination of sarcomatous elements in primitive or embryonal tumors (PNETs) is not included in this category, since the conceptual origin of the mesenchymal component is somewhat different in PNET from that in "mature" or differentiated glioma types.

Gliosarcoma

Included under the category of gliosarcoma are high-grade astrocytoma or, less frequently, other glioma, with mesenchymal metaplasia leading to fibrosarcoma, myosarcoma, osteogenic sarcoma, chondrosarcoma, or other malignant mesenchymal entity.

Gliosarcomas are glioblastomas with malignant mesenchymal elements either focally present in one portion of a tumor as a distinctly separate growth pattern, or dispersed in the glial component as distinct islands with the separate islands of the glial component, forming what is often described as a mosaic. The latter pattern, in which the sarcomatous component seems to surround hyperplastic blood vessels, whereas the glial component has less conspicuous vascularity, is the classical pattern as described, for example, by Feigin et al[173, 174] (Fig. 5–15). Typically, the spindle cell sarcoma component resembles fibrosarcoma, lacks GFAP immunoreactivity, and is rich in a collagenous extracellular matrix and reticulin fibers, whereas the glial component is largely GFAP-immunopositive, lacks collagen and reticulin, and is composed less homogeneously of spindle cells.

The original modern descriptions of gliosarcoma, particularly those with a mosaic pattern, suggested that these arose from preexisting glioblastomas in which the vascular hyperplasia associated with the high-grade astrocytic proliferation led to the development of a second neoplastic transformation in vascular cells (endothelial, pericytic, or smooth muscle).[173, 174] With more recently developed methods for assessing in situ specific gene mutations, such as *p53* mutations, in the different components of such tumors, it has been shown

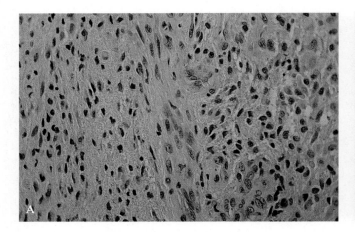

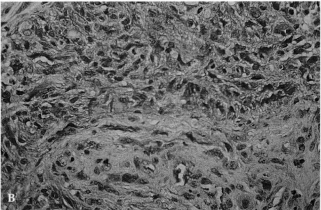

Figure 5–15 Gliosarcoma. (A) H&E stains of these tumors typically reveal spindle cell tumors with some fascicles or areas with a finely fibrillar glioma-like background, and others with a more solid collagenous background (H&E, 100×). (B) Trichrome or similar stains for collagen demonstrate the focal presence of collagen limited to the sarcomatous zones (blue) and its absence from the glial zones (red) (Masson trichrome, 100×). (C) The perivascular "origins" of the sarcomatous components in classical descriptions of gliosarcoma were suggested by appearances such as this one (Masson trichrome, 100×).

that these are clonal neoplasms in which the sarcomatous components arise from the glial component.[175] This process has been termed "neometaplasia" by the eminent surgical pathologist Robert Scully[176]; essentially, it assumes more or less random activation of genes specifying "aberrant" phenotypes in these genetically abnormal cancer cells.

In further support of the latter hypothesis is the constellation of findings of other types of sarcoma in high-grade astrocytomas (and occasionally other gliomas, including oligodendrogliomas, ependymomas, mixed gliomas, and mixed glial-neuronal tumors). Examples making malignant bone, malignant cartilage, smooth- or skeletal muscle neoplasia, and also epithelial tissues with glands and mucin production are well described (see ref. 177 for brief review). We have seen one tumor in a child in which ultrastructural study showed the tubular arrays usually described in cardiac rhabdomyomas. These metaplastic components may occasionally take over a tumor. We have seen a case (in an adult) in which the original biopsy specimen showed only ordinary glioblastoma; a recurrence showed glioblastoma with focal chondrosarcoma and, in the chondroid areas, focal ossification to osteosarcoma; another recurrence was extensively cartilaginous and bony. At autopsy, the very large tumor, which had regrown to occupy about half of one hemisphere, had the consistency of balsa wood, and was wholly composed of chondrosarcoma and focal osteosarcoma; no glial component was recognizable except for rare isolated GFAP-immunopositive cells.

Gliofibroma ("Glioneurofibroma")

Gliofibromas were first described by Friede.[81] These were peculiar cerebral tumors with astrocytic cells located superficially so as to involve the leptomeninges as well as the cerebral parenchyma. As with PXAs, DIAs, and DIGs, which share this superficial location, the tumors were reticulin- and collagen-rich. Friede described the tumors as containing astrocytes with basal lamina, a characteristic of subpial astrocytes of the normal CNS, and presumed that the collagen production was from these astrocytic cells.[81] Subsequent case reports were a mixture of identical suppositions, and suppositions that these were mixed glial and fibroblastic neoplasms in which the collagen production was carried on by the GFAP-negative fibroblastic population. One example was described in the spinal cord of an infant and was clearly a congenital tumor.[86] This tumor has been described in infants, children, and adults. We have recognized at least four such tumors, three of which we analyzed and reported as "glioneurofibromas"[84] because our immunohistochemical and ultrastructural studies suggested that the nonastrocytic component included Schwann cells that were capable of producing myelin even as they invaded the CNS along perivascular spaces; the fourth, identical tumor was encountered subsequent to that publication.

All of our cases involved children and included cerebral and spinal cord examples. The tumors clearly had a malignant potential: one presented with CSF dissemination, and another had fatal diffuse meningeal dissemination after biopsy, radiation, and radical surgery. The congenital tumor described by Iglesias et al[86] was fatal, as was the case described by Friede[81] in which meningeal dissemination also occurred.

Primitive Neuroectodermal Tumors

The term "primitive neuroectodermal tumor" was first coined by Hart and Earle[178] to describe a set of primitive or embryonal tumors found in the cerebral hemispheres of children. These tumors mostly resembled cerebellar "medulloblastoma" and did not fit into the then-established nosologic categories for CNS neoplasms. They had the capacity for differentiation along glial lines but appeared mostly wholly undifferentiated. These rare curiosities became an important terminological issue when Rorke[179] proposed that because of their histologic similarity to medulloblastoma and other embryonal pediatric CNS tumors, such as pineoblastoma and cerebral neuroblastoma, they operationally be regarded as members of a common family, the PNETs. By this suggestion, PNET as a term was transformed from one describing a rare cerebral neoplasm of mostly young children to one describing the most common type of CNS tumor of childhood. *This operational definition was justified by the close histologic similarity between all of the entities thereby encompassed (which included several others; see below); by the propensity of all of the members of this family of neoplasms to have foci with differentiation along neuronal, astrocytic, or other glial lines, and occasionally along other lines such as rhabdomyoblastic cells; and by their similar frequencies of CSF dissemination.* In terms of the first point, it was emphasized that given a slide containing only the tumor with no normal tissue, no pathologist could differentiate the site of origin, so that the diagnoses of "medulloblastoma," "pineoblastoma," "cerebral neuroblastoma," and so forth were indistinguishable histologically.

This proposal set off the most intense controversy yet witnessed in the narrow field of tumor neuropathology. Adherents of Lucien Rubinstein, and Rubinstein himself, condemned the idea as one that abandoned long established and cherished diagnostic entities, that constituted diagnostic nihilism, and that was fundamentally incorrect because the cerebellar examples (i.e., "medulloblastomas") historically carried a far better prognosis than all other members of the proposed nosologic category.[180] Another major part of these arguments hinges on the various beliefs about the histogenesis of these neoplasms, with the concept that cerebellar medulloblastoma must have a unique histogenesis based on the unique developmental programs of the cerebellum.[2] Others supported Rorke's proposal more or less wholeheartedly,[181] and over remarkably few years the clinical community, as represented, for example, in the Children's Cancer Group, largely accepted the idea. In recent years, the concept has received further support as the clinical outcomes for cerebral and pineal examples have improved with advances in neurosurgical technique. The result is that, with equivalent resections and identical adjunctive therapy (combined multidrug chemotherapy and craniospinal radiation, except for the omission of the latter in children under 3 years), these noncerebellar tumors are now associated with survivals identical to those of the cerebellar tumors.[182] There appears to be at least some consensus that outside of the cerebellum all of these tumors are currently best characterized as PNETs, and

the cerebellar examples may remain controversial until other data emerge.[183] Of note, perhaps, is that in the original Bailey and Cushing classification, which essentially introduced the term "medulloblastoma," there was no conception that these tumors were unique to the cerebellum,[89] and in fact the supposed "medulloblast" was thought of as a virtually totipotential neuroepithelial stem cell, more primitive than the "polar spongioblast," and explicitly was linked[89] to the "indifferent cell" concept of Schaper to which Rorke referred in proposing the modern concept of PNET.[179] In a modern perspective, the Bailey and Cushing account of these tumors reads very much more like Lucy Rorke than like Lucien Rubinstein.

One criticism of the PNET concept, as put forth by Rorke, is that it encourages pathologists to lump any tumor under this diagnosis when it contains small densely packed cells and is difficult to diagnose, whether or not there is evidence of another, more differentiated tumor type. In this regard certain features are thought by some to represent evidence for a mature glioma tumor type and not PNET; these include "geographic" foci of necrosis with surrounding tumor cell pseudopalisades, and vascular hyperplasia, both of which have been invoked to favor a diagnosis of glioblastoma.[2] In fact, both of these features occur in otherwise classical PNET (Fig. 5–16C, D), so that this argument is untenable.

Little is known about the genetic changes involved in PNET. Limited studies have examined the presence of alterations in the *MIC2* gene that are characteristic of a similar but distinct group of pediatric embryonal tumors not found (by ordinary definitions) in the CNS: neuroblastoma of the adrenal and other paraganglia, Ewing's sarcoma of bone, extraosseous Ewing's sarcoma, the "Askin tumor," and similar entities regarded as one family of tumors lumped, by deliberate analogy with their CNS look-alikes, as "peripheral PNETs."[184] (Peripheral PNETs are tumors that have a restricted differentiation potential, almost entirely neuronal, and essentially are incapable of differentiation to astrocytes or other glia; rare examples with Schwann cell neoplasia and with skeletal muscle differentiation are recorded.) Early reports of investigations of CNS PNET for *MIC2* gene changes have shown that rare examples have such mutations, but these are a small minority. Peripheral PNETs have a characteristic chromosomal abnormality, the t(11; 14) (q24; q12) translocation, not found in central PNET.

Cytogenetic studies of cerebellar PNET (medulloblastoma) have shown that the most common abnormality found is isochrome 17q,[185] and there are data to suggest that this is less common in noncerebellar PNET. However, many cerebellar PNETs lack this abnormality, so the argument that this cytogenetic difference is sufficient to assert that cerebellar "medulloblastoma" is a different entity from other PNET is inconclusive.

There is some speculation that PNET may often be the result of viral infections, particularly with the Papovaviruses JC, BK, and SV40. These are all DNA tumor viruses that in animal models can produce PNETs in cerebellar and cerebral sites (depending on the model).[186–189] However, which viral DNA of this type has not been detected in several studies in examples of human PNET. It has been found in some other types of brain tumor,[190, 191, 191A] and recently has been reported in some PNET as well.[191B]

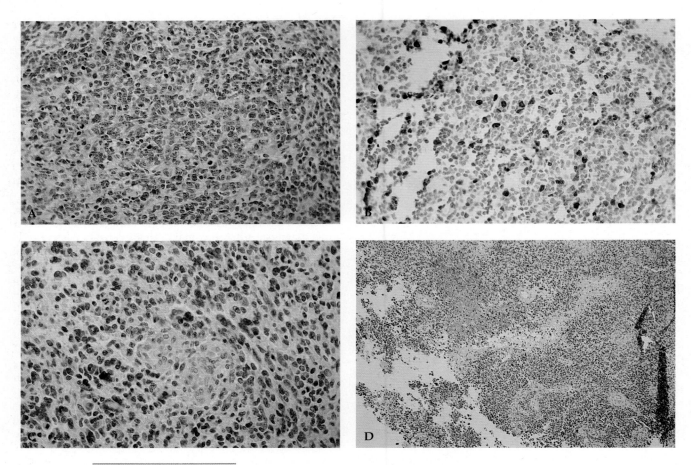

Figure 5–16   Primitive neuroectodermal tumors (PNETs). (A) Undifferentiated PNETs are composed of small cells with negligible cytoplasm with no distinctive histologic growth pattern ("patternless sheets") (H&E, 100×). (B) Most PNETs have a high proliferation rate; this illustration of an MIB1 immunostain is high, but not as high as some examples, which may approach 90 to 100% of tumor cells (MIB1, 100×). (C) PNETs may have features sometimes thought more typical of high-grade gliomas, such as vascular hyperplasia. (D) Foci of necrosis in PNETs occasionally have typical pseudopalisades.

Undifferentiated PNET

Undifferentiated PNET describes a tumor in this group with no evidence of differentiation. By ordinary H&E histologic criteria, these are often said to be the most common of PNETs, although with immunostaining and electron microscopy subtle foci of differentiation are probably present in a majority of PNETs. Nevertheless, undifferentiated PNETs remain an important part of this population. These are usually densely cellular tumors, with cells so closely packed as to virtually overlap in standard 6-μm paraffin sections (Fig. 5–16A). The cells are most typically small, with nuclei perhaps at most twice the size of those of cerebellar granular layer neurons or of small lymphocytes, and they have negligible stainable cytoplasm that contains a densely hyperchromatic nucleus (Fig. 5–16A). The nuclei are most often wedge-shaped but may be spindly or elongated, or more round. These tumors

can, in individual cases, be difficult to separate without special stains from non-Hodgkin's lymphomas, the most cellular of oligodendrogliomas and their look-alikes, and metastatic (or the exceedingly rare primary CNS) embryonal rhabdomyosarcoma. Usually they have high mitotic rates, though in some instances mitotic figures can be exceedingly difficult to find. Evaluation of proliferative capacity with immunostains for nuclear cell cycle–associated antigens, such as Ki67 (antibody MIB1), usually (but surprisingly not invariably) shows a high proportion (LI) of immunolabeled nuclei (Fig. 5–16B). By current definitions, the cells have no immunoreactivity for GFAP, neurofilament epitopes, synaptophysin or other synaptic vesicle antigens, muscle actins, S100 protein, or other markers of astrocytic, other glial, neuronal, or mesenchymal differentiation. They may or may not have cytoplasmic immunoreactivity for vimentin, a lineage-nonspecific intermediate filament; such vimentin expression is common but not invariant. Ultrastructural examination of such tumors reveals minimal cytoplasm with few organelles, none suggestive of differentiation.

PNET with Differentiation

As discussed above, one of the cardinal features of the PNET category of neoplasms is the tendency for the primitive tumor cells, which represent the neoplastic counterparts of multipotential neuroepithelial stem cells, to differentiate along one or more of the pathways to which their normal counterparts are capable of committing. Less commonly, one of these tumors will have focal areas that differentiate along lines not usually regarded as within the usual spectrum of neuroepithelial cells: skeletal muscle, adipose tissue, cartilage, bone, smooth muscle, or true common epithelium. There may also be melanin production. The first and probably numerically most important of all of the potential lines of differentiation is neuronal or neuroblastic differentiation.

PNET with Neuroblastic Differentiation

Neuroblastic differentiation implies the presence of cells that retain a high proliferative capacity and a more or less primitive character with minimal cytoplasm and small dense nuclei, but that exhibit certain patterns of growth or express certain immunohistochemically detectable neuron-specific proteins, allowing their identification as cells committed to a neuronal lineage. The chief histologic pattern that is widely recognized as representing a neuroblastic commitment is the formation of central fibrillary (Homer Wright) rosettes (Fig. 5–17A). These were first described by Wright in adrenal and paraganglion neuroblastomas, but they were subsequently identified as similarly representing a neuronal lineage marker in CNS embryonal tumors. This is a very early-stage marker in the path to neuronal differentiation; cells in these rosettes are most often not immunopositive for synaptophysin or other synaptic vesicle antigens, or for neurofilament protein epitopes. Electron microscopic studies show that the processes in the central fibrillary core of the rosette are primitive neurites. Expression of neuron-specific microtubule or microtubule-associated proteins (class III β-tubulin; MAP2) is often present.[192, 193]

Other forms of neuroblastic expression in PNETs include the focal expression of one or more neuronal lineage-specific molecules in single cells or subclone-like groups of cells. This may be synaptophysin expression (although there are claims that such expression is nonspecific and that all PNETs have it; there are also claims that all PNETs are neuroblastic; our own experience is that synaptophysin is not universally expressed in any category of PNET, and that its presence indicates some commitment to a neuronal phenotype). Interestingly, in PNETs synaptophysin immunopositivity is often intracellular in the small tumor cells' cytoplasm, whereas in more differentiated tumors (e.g., gangliogliomas and neurocytic tumors) the immunopositivity is usually in the neuropil by light microscopy (reflecting the presence of neurites and boutons with synaptic vesicles, below the limits of resolution of conventional light microscopic examination). In PNETs with foci having more advanced neuronal character the synaptophysin

is, as in the more mature neuronal tumor types, in a neuropil pattern, not within cell bodies.

Expression of neurofilament protein epitopes is less common but if present may be for nonphosphorylated low or medium molecular weight neurofilaments or for high molecular weight phosphorylated neurofilaments,[194] which ordinarily implies the presence of relatively mature axonal projections. Many PNETs express retinal-S antigen, a protein once thought specific to retinal neurons.[195–198] As the first PNETs in which this neuronal-specific expression was found were pineal, this was thought to indicate the special phylogenetic and embryologic relationship between the retina and the pineal gland[195]; however, this expression has been found in PNETs of other sites, including cerebellar PNETs.[196–198] This is clearly an argument in favor of the utility of the PNET concept and against the concept of a unique character of cerebellar medulloblastoma.

PNET with Neuronal Differentiation

Some PNETs have patterns or other indications of more advanced neuronal development. This is presented here as a dichotomy between "neuroblastic" and "neuronal" differentiation, but in practice the two may be combined or there may be intermediate stages of differentiation. *One of the classical patterns indicative of neuronal differentiation is the "insular" or "desmoplastic" pattern.* In this pattern, a background of small, densely packed, undifferentiated cells surrounds discrete islands of lower cell density containing less packed larger cells that usually have the H&E appearance of oligo-like neurocytoma cells (Fig. 5–17B, C). In the best known of these tumors, which are cerebellar, the tumors involve the leptomeninges, and the undifferentiated zones contain a collagenous matrix that stains prominently with reticulin stains; the islands of neuronal differentiation are devoid of reticulin, hence the term "reticulin-free" islands. The relatively low cell density in comparison with the surrounding less differentiated background has led to these islands being called "pale islands," and the overall appearance is at low power somewhat reminiscent of the follicles and germinal centers in a reactive lymph node, so that this is also referred to as a "follicular" or "pseudofollicular" pattern. The accumulation of collagen and reticulin (a catch-all histochemical staining term for basement membrane materials, including laminin, collagen IV, and other matrix molecules) is the basis for the established terminology of "desmoplastic medulloblastoma" for the cerebellar examples. However, this pattern in PNET is clearly not limited to the cerebellum; we have seen examples in deep cerebral gray matter, pineal, and cerebral lobar tissues.

That this insular pattern is indicative of neuronal differentiation was first suggested by ultrastructural observations[199] combined with silver stains for axonal processes. The rare but well-established development of larger neurons (ganglion cells) within the pale islands also suggests the nature of the oligo-like cells. More recently, it has been shown that these cells express synaptophysin (Fig. 5–17D), class III β-tubulin, and (often) neurofilament proteins, so that immunohistochemical examination verifies the neuronal differentiation.[119, 192, 200] Whether the pale islands are neuroblastic or neuronal is more of a semantic question, but it seems

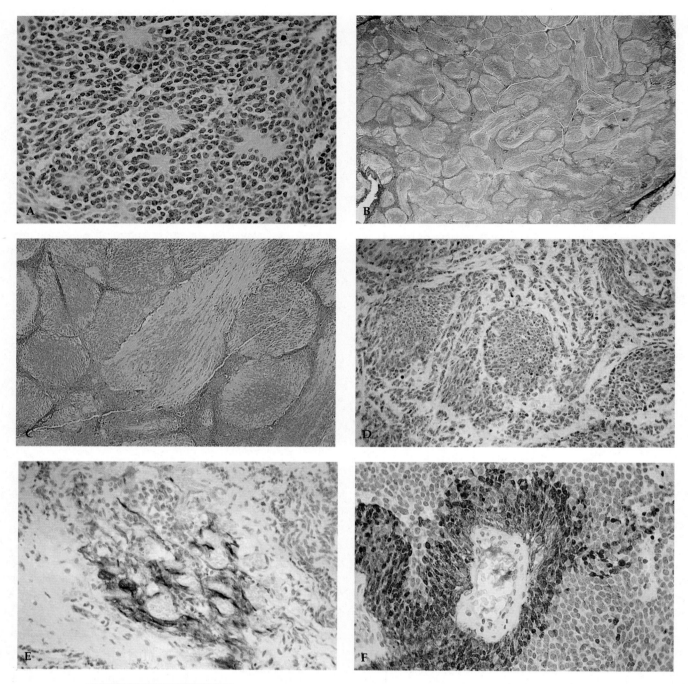

Figure 5–17   Differentiation in PNETs. (A) Neuroblastic PNET with Homer Wright rosettes. Each rosette is an eosinophilic fibrillary solid area surrounded by cells whose processes extend radially inward to produce the fibrillary center (H&E, 100×). (B) Neuronal differentiation in PNET, insular pattern. A low-power view gives an impression of multiple follicles resembling a follicular lymphoma or even a hyperplastic lymph node (H&E, 6.25×). (C) Insular PNET. At higher power the neuronal areas are of lower cell density, with cells with round nuclei in a highly fibrillary neuropil, closely resembling central neurocytomas (H&E, 25×). (D) Insular PNETs have strong neuropil patterns of synaptophysin immunoreactivity within the neuronal pale islands (synaptophysin, 100×). (E) Cells on the periphery of the pale islands are often astrocytic morphologically and express GFAP (GFAP, 100×). (F) Focal astrocytic differentiation in a PNET may be indicated by groups of cells all expressing GFAP, whereas their neighbors are GFAP-negative (GFAP, 100×).

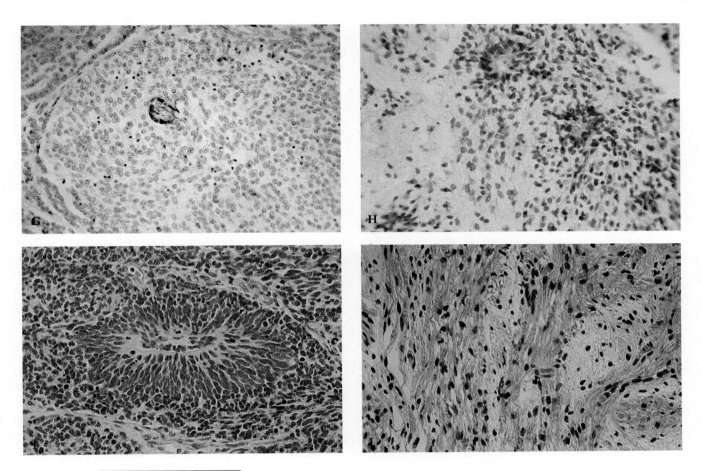

Figure 5–17 *(continued)* (G) In other PNETs astrocytic differentiation may be more limited, with only isolated small tumor cells with all of the characteristics of their neighbors except for GFAP immunopositivity (GFAP, 100×). (H) Focal ependymal ("ependymoblastic") differentiation in a PNET may be seen with central lumen rosettes (H&E, 100×). (I) Other PNETs with ependymal differentiation have that focal development indicated by perivascular pseudorosettes (H&E, 100×). (J) PNET with rhabdomyoblastic differentiation. This pineal example has much lower cell density in the differentiated areas, with large, elongated, neoplastic, striated cells representing the rhabdomyoblasts (H&E, 100×).

logical to use the latter term as these zones are, in isolation, virtually impossible to distinguish in a high-power field from neurocytomas, a tumor regarded as composed of differentiated neuronal cells (although, as discussed, they are better described as at least bipotential because many express GFAP in cells that also contain neuronal markers). Furthermore, proliferation studies show much lower levels of proliferative activity in the pale islands than around them.

Of interest here is that GFAP immunostaining of insular PNET usually, if not always, demonstrates some immunopositive astrocytic tumor cells in the peripheral portions of the pale islands, and sometimes also in the more primitive or undifferentiated components around the islands (Fig. 5–17E). Thus, these are more often PNETs with both neuronal and astrocytic differentiation than PNETs with only neuronal differentiation. Many studies have suggested that PNETs with insular patterns are more likely to be associated with longer

survivals than other PNETs, but this remains uncertain and somewhat controversial.

An unequivocal form of neuronal differentiation in PNET is maturation to recognizable ganglion cells. Care must be taken in making a diagnosis of this type of differentiation not to regard entrapped normal large neurons of the brain as part of the neoplasm. This is rarely difficult. When it is, synaptophysin immunostains can be helpful, as the neoplastic ganglion cells, just as those in gangliogliomas, have a dense perikaryal surface immunopositivity not seen on normal neurons except in rare and selected circumstances. As discussed above (see "Gangliogliomas"), some perikaryal surface staining can be seen in anterior horn cells, on neurons of certain brain stem nuclei, and, to a much lesser extent, on Purkinje cells and hippocampal pyramidal neurons, both of which mostly have dendritic staining. PNETs of the cord and the brain stem occur but rarely; if the question is whether large neuronal cells in a cerebellar PNET are Purkinje cells or tumor neurons, then a low- to medium-power view can usually detect if there is a linear array of such cells (i.e., a row of Purkinje cells in an invaded folium) or a more diffuse and less ordered arrangement.

PNET with Spongioblastic Differentiation

In the classification scheme that was the foundation of modern tumor neuropathology, Bailey and Cushing[89] continued the use of a then current term, "primitive polar spongioblastoma," to describe a tumor of astrocytic lineage thought to arise from a primitive or embryonal stage in astrocytic differentiation. Tumors composed purely of "spongioblastic" tissue patterns are vanishingly rare, but foci with the patterns described under this rubric are well-described in PNET.

In contemporary terms, spongioblastic patterns are represented by palisades or "rhythmic" waves of tumor cell nuclei separated by fibrillary anuclear zones. These striped or striated appearances must not be confused (as indeed they have been, in cases we have reviewed that erroneously carry this diagnosis) with longitudinal sections of perivascular pseudorosettes in ependymomas; in spongioblastoma or spongioblastic areas there are no consistently present and parallel vessels between the palisades of nuclei. These palisaded areas contain bipolar cells with elongated nuclei whose axis is perpendicular to the axis of each nuclear palisade, much as in the nuclear palisades of schwannomas. In most cases, at least some of these cells are immunoreactive for GFAP, consistent with differentiation to a primitive stage of committed astrocytic development; however, a surprising number have coexisting synaptophysin or other neuronal expression.

PNET with Astrocytic Differentiation

This brings up another of the many controversies surrounding the diagnosis of differentiation in PNET. In some PNET, there is unquestionable astrocytic differentiation, with cells having clearly neoplastic nuclear features but with larger amounts of eosinophilic cytoplasm with distinctly apparent processes (Fig. 5–17F). Other typically astrocytic cells are more spindly or bipolar, but are larger than those of undifferentiated PNET, and clearly resemble cells of many high-grade fibrillary astrocytomas (anaplastic astrocytomas and glioblastomas). These morphologic astrocytes virtually always express GFAP as well. Occasionally, large reactive astrocytes are trapped in a PNET as it infiltrates normal tissue; these cells are often also large astrocytes with extensive processes, but their nuclear features are usually distinct from those of the neoplastic cells, and a comparison will quickly resolve the question as to whether such cells are part of the brain or part of the tumor. This is not universally accepted, some authors having asserted that astrocytic differentiation is quite rare[201] and that when seen it represents recruitment of a second neoplastic population from perivascular reactive astrocytes that are secondarily transformed in the presence of the primary PNET.[2, 201] Although ultimate proof or disproof of this hypothesis must await some in situ clonal analysis, the hypothesis strikes this neuropathologist as highly unlikely, as unlikely as the similar older hypotheses as to the origin of gliosarcoma. The specific molecular mechanism(s) for proposed recruitment of reactive cells into a neoplasm to which they are reacting remains to be proposed, and demonstrated.

With GFAP immunostains, one finds in many PNETs small clusters or scattered single cells with strong GFAP immunopositivity (Fig. 5–17F, G). Again, if, as is usually the case, the cells in question have sparse processes and small hyperchromatic nuclei identical to those of their GFAP-negative neighbors, it seems an inevitable conclusion that they are differentiating tumor cells, not reactive cells. Vimentin immunostaining may reveal similar cells with processes, again by their morphology as revealed by the stain suggestive of astrocytic tumor cells. Interestingly, another technique that demonstrates such differentiation is immunostaining with the anticytokeratin cocktail AE1/AE3. It has been known for some time that this cocktail has significant cross-reactivity with GFAP in CNS tissue sections, so that positive staining with this cocktail in a PNET does not indicate (necessarily) true epithelial differentiation; rather, if the cells so stained have multipolar stellate processes and do not form epithelial clusters, they are tumor astrocytes.

PNET with Ependymal Differentiation ("Ependymoblastoma")

In some PNETs one finds small foci with classical pseudorosettes, or with the epithelial-lined canals and central lumen rosettes characteristic of ependymomas (Fig. 5–17H, I). When such features are only focal in a tumor with broad zones of undifferentiated small cells or in a tumor with other foci of neuronal, astrocytic, or other differentiation, then it is clear that the tumor is a PNET with (focal) ependymal differentiation. Such foci in a PNET are likely to have the processes of the tumor cells, whether in rosettes or pseudorosettes, displaying vimentin or GFAP immunopositivity.

Somewhat more problematically, some tumors are mostly composed of such rosettes and pseudorosettes, with relatively small and subtle areas of more diffuse architecture containing primitive cells. Here the differential diagnosis between ependymoma and PNET can be more difficult. This is not made any easier by the fact that in children the most common sites for both tumors are in the posterior fossa. The classical descriptions (or rather refinement of the diagnostic term) "ependymoblastoma" by Rubinstein[202] suggest that when the rosettes or pseudorosettes are multilayered, the tumor is more likely to be an embryonal variant—what most neuropathologists (but not the late Lucien Rubinstein) would call PNET.

PNET with Oligodendroglial Differentiation

There are PNETs with foci in which the cells are not organized into insular patterns but nevertheless have an almost epithelioid pattern with clear cytoplasm, distinct cell borders tightly touching to produce a honeycomb pattern, and centrally placed round nuclei, in short oligo-like cells. The same considerations that apply to the diagnosis of oligodendroglioma *versus* neurocytic tumors *versus* clear cell ependymomas apply to these foci in PNET. In short, if the foci are synaptophysin- and neurofilament protein–immunonegative, and they lack all signs of ependymal differentiation by H&E, immunohistochemical (GFAP and vimentin), and ultrastructural criteria, then the diagnosis by exclusion is one of focal oligodendrogliomatous differentiation in a PNET. *If most of the tumor is composed of these cells, if there is a highly infiltrative pattern in the brain, but if there is still a primitive appearance and all of the above stains and studies are negative, one should also consider a diagnosis of CNS non-Hodgkin's lymphoma (see below) before concluding that the tumor is a PNET.* One such example seen at NYU Medical Center was in a 17-year-old girl; this frontal lobe tumor was originally thought to be a PNET with extensive oligo-like patterns, but immunostaining showed definitively that the tumor was in fact a rare T-cell non-Hodgkin's lymphoma.

PNET with Rhabdomyoblastic Differentiation

The classical literature of medulloblastoma includes a number of case reports in which a cerebellar tumor with the features of medulloblastoma also had foci containing apparent rhabdomyosarcoma, with large eosinophilic cells with discernible cross-striations. These were generally termed "medullomyoblastoma."[203–205] Their relationship to pure primary rhabdomyosarcomas of the cerebellum[206] or other parts of the CNS has never been established, largely because both types of tumor are so rare that modern techniques (other than immunostains) have hardly been applied to any examples of either. In some articles, the development of focal rhabdomyoblastic differentiation in a cerebellar medulloblastoma was "explained" as part of the normal differentiation spectrum of primitive neuroectoderm because there are no somites to give rise to the muscles of the face and head, which receive cranial nerve innervation and those muscles are said to develop from an "ectomesenchyme".[2]

Whether the latter explanation is valid or not, rhabdomyosarcomatous differentiation in PNET is a well-established if rare occurrence and is not limited to PNET from cerebellar sites. Examples in the pineal have been described,[207, 208] and this neuropathologist has personally encountered two definite examples (Fig. 5–17J). In one, the rhabdomyoblastic elements were made apparent by cross-striations in a frozen section performed for intraoperative diagnosis. Immunohistochemical verification, while hardly necessary when the striated cells are so visible, can be obtained with the use of antibodies to muscle-specific actin, muscle myosins, MyoD-1, or other muscle markers. Ordinary histochemical techniques that emphasize the fibrillar proteins of such cells, including phosphotungstic acid–hematoxylin (PTAH), are also often useful.

PNET with Rhabdoid Differentiation ("Atypical Teratoid Tumor")

Rhabdoid tumors were first described as renal neoplasms originally thought to be variants of Wilms' tumor.[209] The tumors were characterized by the presence of cells with eccentrically placed large, pale nuclei with prominent nucleoli, lying in a large cell body with a round eosinophilic inclusion close to the nucleus. The inclusion was found by ultrastructural examination to be composed of a mass of whorled intermediate filaments that with immunostaining were demonstrably vimentin filaments. Subsequently, similar tumors were encountered in nonrenal sites, including other viscera and soft tissue.[210–212] Some tumors with typical features of other diagnoses were found to also contain cells morphologically of rhabdoid character, leading to the suggestion that this is a phenotypic change in tumor cells of diverse origin that was associated with an aggressive clinical course.[212] Some children with renal or extrarenal rhabdoid tumors were found to simultaneously harbor brain tumors, particularly typical PNETs,[213] a finding either of incidental curiosity not other-

wise important to the following discussion, or (as suggested by Biegel) a misinterpretation of metastatic spread of a rhabdoid renal tumor to the brain (personal communication).

As more PNETs were collected or reviewed for various studies, it became clear that there were tumors in children, particularly those younger than 18 months, which had been classified as PNET (or under one of the older site-specific names, such as medulloblastoma) but which were quite different from the usual PNET. These tumors might have foci of typical PNET, but they were mostly composed of larger cells; they frequently had frank mesenchymal differentiation with collagen deposition among spindle cell sarcomatous foci; and they contained cells with the typical morphologic and immunostaining characteristics of rhabdoid cells[194, 214–218] (Fig. 5–18A, B). Cytogenetic studies of a small set of these suggested that they had a chromosomal defect—monosomy 22—which set them apart from most PNETs or other brain tumors.[215] In the initial reports, infants with these tumors all had fatal outcomes despite aggressive therapy directed at the diagnosis of PNET.[216] Given a constellation of unique characteristics (i.e., the chromosomal abnormality, clinical discovery at very young ages, the rhabdoid cells, the frequent mesenchymal differentiation, and the dismal prognosis), Rorke and colleagues proposed that these were a unique clinicopathologic entity that they proposed to name "atypical teratoid tumor."[194, 215, 216, 219] Exceptions to this typical clinicopathologic atypical teratoid tumor scenario are rare, but some have been described, such as tumors in older children[218] or even adults,[219, 220, 221] or with occasional longer than usual survival. Among the examples at NYU Medical Center, one such tumor occurred in the brain stem of a child younger than 2 who has survived for several years.

These tumors have other features: the rhabdoid cells are usually S100 protein–immunopositive and epithelial membrane antigen–immunopositive (Fig. 5–18C). The eosinophilic, round, inclusion-like structure in the cytoplasm of the rhabdoid cell body is vimentin-immunopositive (Fig. 5–18D). These tumors may lack all recognizable PNET elements or may contain classical PNET foci. When these are present they may show focal differentiation, as with any other PNET. There is no suggestion from any data that the tumors are true teratomas or have any relationship to germ cell neoplasms.

At present it is unclear whether these tumors are truly separate from PNETs or represent a peculiar form of differentiation in PNET. Arguments for the latter include the presence in many of foci typical PNET; the argument that there is no "rhabdoid" cell type; that the morphologic entity of rhabdoid cells actually represents a structural pattern that can be assumed by a wide variety of tumor cell types; that the clinical prognosis of children with PNET diagnosed at age 18 months or younger is equally dismal without the rhabdoid elements; and that the particular chromosomal abnormality is seen in a variety of other tumors, including CNS tumors such as ependymomas. More recent genetic investigations suggest that there is a unique rhabdoid gene that is abnormal in those rare "atypical teratoid tumors" that lack the characteristic cytogenetic change (220, and Biegel, personal communication). This remains unsettled, and studies to address these and other relevant points are ongoing. At present this neuropathologist finds it easier to provisionally group the

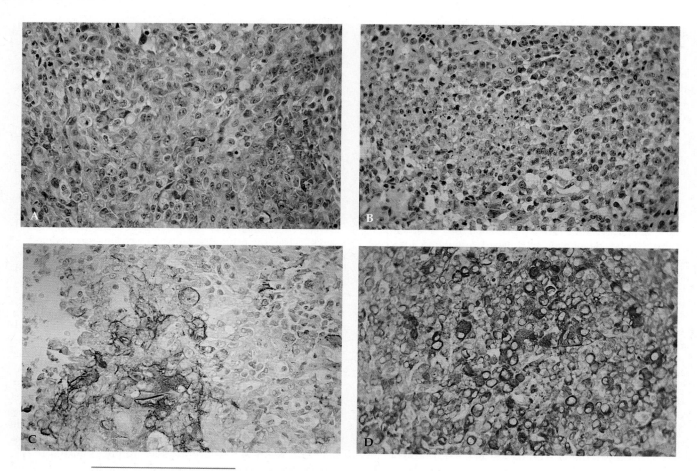

Figure 5–18 PNET with rhabdoid differentiation: "atypical teratoid tumor." (A) The most typical finding that first leads to this diagnosis is the presence in a PNET of large epithelioid cells with large round nuclei, usually with prominent nucleoli. These cells may suggest neuronal differentiation but they fail to stain with any neuronal marker (H&E, 100×). (B) Further search will uncover cells with round eosinophilic cytoplasmic inclusions; these cells are usually smaller than the large cells, with round nuclei shown in Part A (H&E, 100×). (C) The large cells are usually immunopositive for epithelial membrane antigen (EMA) (EMA, 100×). (D) The cells with eosinophilic inclusions are vimentin-immunopositive (vimentin 100×).

"atypical teratoid tumors" with PNET as a recognizable pattern of differentiation.

There are other PNETs composed of larger cells without any classical small-cell undifferentiated components. Some of these have gone by names such as "large-cell medulloblastoma."[221] It is clear that most of the tumors so described do not contain mesenchymal elements or rhabdoid cells.

PNET with Other Mesenchymal Differentiation

As with certain other gliomas, including glioblastoma/gliosarcoma and ependymomas, metaplastic chondrosarcomatous and osteosarcomatous foci may develop in an otherwise typical PNET. No special significance seems to be attached to these very rare observations.

PNET with Neural Tube Differentiation ("Medulloepithelioma")

The term "medulloepithelioma" is another classical nosologic term that delineates an embryonal CNS tumor with a particular pattern of growth, as is the case with spongioblastoma

and, perhaps, ependymoblastoma. In medulloepitheliomas, there are branched curvilinear canal-like structures lined by a neoplastic epithelium composed of stratified or pseudostratified tall columnar cells (Fig. 5–19). Some authors prefer to leave these out of the broad family of PNETs as a special form of neoplasm; others[181] regard this as another form of differentiation in PNET, namely, an attempt to recapitulate the embryonal neural tube. As the cases we have seen have all had concurrent other patterns of differentiation in other foci of the tumor, or recurred as classical PNET without obvious medulloepitheliomatous pattern, this latter point of view seems more accurate.

PNET with Mixed Differentiation

As should be obvious from all of the above descriptions of differentiation in PNETs, there are many instances in which a single PNET exhibits different lineages of differentiation simultaneously. Some of these have already been described as essentially conjoint differentiation within one pattern, such

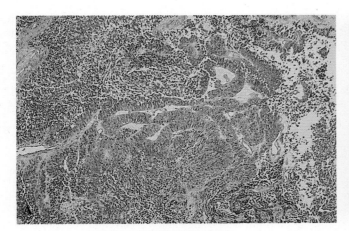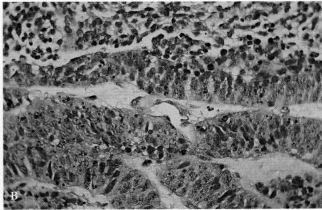

Figure 5–19   PNET with medulloepithelioma. (A) This overview shows a PNET with small undifferentiated cells alternating with epithelial bands of larger, columnar cells lining the channels typical of medulloepithelioma (H&E, 25×). (B) At higher power the complex columnar epithelium of the characteristic channels has distinctive luminal surfaces, with a suggestion of a ciliated or microvillar brush border (H&E, 100×).

as the coexpression of astrocytic and neuronal differentiation in the insular pattern, or the similar coexpression described in some cases with foci of spongioblastomatous differentiation. Others seem largely unrelated: a focus of rhabdomyoblastic differentiation in one part of a tumor, and a focus of neuroblastic differentiation with central fibrillary rosettes in another. There is one last pattern to be described, which is probably best "named" as Rorke would have it, "tumor making brain" (personal communication). Here there can be an extraordinary mixed differentiation of neuronal cells, both ganglion cells and neurocytic cells, with astrocytes, probably true oligodendroglia, and a supporting vascular stroma, so that at first examination such a focus appears to be a portion of cerebral tissue trapped within the tumor, or perhaps a low-grade tumor such as ganglioglioma. It is only with more detailed examination that it becomes apparent that there is no normal order in the structure, no separation of gray matter from white matter, no cortical or other architecture, and no tracts of myelinated white matter (indeed no myelination at all); furthermore, synaptophysin or other synaptic vesicle immunostains show an abnormal pattern of perikaryal surface immunoreactivity on the larger neurons, and the distribution of astrocytes and their nuclear features are more in keeping with neoplastic cells. MIB1 or other immunostains for proliferation-associated antigens also demonstrate that these highly differentiated foci are still neoplastic and proliferative, although the labeling indices are far lower than in undifferentiated portions of the same tumor.

Prognostic Significance of Differentiation in PNET

An as yet unresolved controversy among tumor neuropathologists centers on the question of whether there is any prognostic significance associated with differentiation in PNETs, and if there is whether it is favorable or unfavorable. It has already been mentioned that early descriptions of the insular ("desmoplastic") variant of PNET suggested a favorable prognosis compared

with other PNETs. That this might be so was countered by suggestions that other factors confounded the conclusions: for example, the insular tumors were found more commonly in older children or adults, who in general were thought to have a better prognosis than younger children. A small survey including all age groups that was done at NYU Medical Center found using multivariate statistics that insular differentiation did confer a better prognosis independent of age.[222]

Rorke suggested not long after the modern concept of PNETs became widely accepted that differentiation (in any line) carried a worse prognosis.[223] This was based largely on standard H&E patterns of differentiation without immunostaining. Caputy et al came to an opposite conclusion.[224] In a study that used GFAP immunostaining to identify the relevant differentiation, Goldberg-Stern et al suggested that astrocytic differentiation was prognostically favorable.[225] More recently, using more extensive immunostaining and emphasizing the importance of antigen retrieval techniques to uncover immunohistochemically detectable expression, Rorke and colleagues again found that differentiation, in particular GFAP expression presumed to represent astrocytic differentiation, was unfavorable.[226]

Clearly, the available literature suggests that rhabdoid differentiation is associated with a poor outcome.[216–219] Examples of rhabdomyoblastic differentiation, admittedly all in such small numbers as to invariably represent anecdotes, all have had a poor response to therapy, with poor survival. [203–205, 207, 208]. With these exceptions the prognostic associations of various differentiation patterns remain unclear.

NONNEUROEPITHELIAL INTRA-AXIAL NEOPLASMS

The foregoing discussion has covered all of the intraparenchymal CNS neoplasms of neuroepithelial cells found or described in children. There remain a few intra-axial tumors of nonneuroepithelial origin that require description. Chief among these are the primary germ cell tumors; after these there are CNS lymphomas, which are far less common in children than in adults; and finally, there is a miscellany of primary CNS sarcomas.

Germ Cell Tumors

In the embryo the primordial germ cells originate outside of the embryonic body proper, in the yolk sac; to get to the developing gonads they must undergo a migration, which tends to follow midline guides until the cells approach the urogenital ridges. *The conventional explanation for the origin of extragonadal germ cell tumors has been that under relatively uncommon circumstances some of these primordial cells follow aberrant cues and end up in midline or paramedian sites other than the future gonads, principally the mediastinum and the CNS, where they retain a potential to undergo neoplastic transformation and give rise to germ cell tumors.* Such misplaced but normal germ cells have not been identified in any survey of normal fetal or postnatal brain tissues.[227] In the brain, the two sites at which germ cell neoplasms usually arise are the suprasellar/hypothalamic region and the pineal region. The large majority of CNS germ cell tumors arise in one of these two sites; non-midline sites are unusual, but well documented, particularly for germinomas in the basal ganglia.

In the pineal or hypothalamic/suprasellar region, the putative incorrectly placed primitive germ cells can give rise to the entire spectrum of germ cell neoplasms described in gonadal sites, ranging from the most primitive of such tumors, termed "germinoma" in the CNS and mediastinum but "seminoma" in the testis and "dysgerminoma" in the ovary, to more differentiated patterns, [i.e., embryonal carcinoma, yolk sac tumor (endodermal sinus tumor), choriocarcinoma, and teratomas, the last both immature and mature]. In the non-midline sites, almost all examples are germinomas (basal ganglionic or thalamic sites) or teratomas.

Germinoma

The most common of the intracranial germ cell tumors is the germinoma. This tumor is composed of large, undifferentiated germ cells, which have large, mostly round, pale nuclei with prominent nucleoli (Fig. 5–20). As cells they may be reminiscent of both neoplastic ganglion cells and rhabdoid cells (but without the cytoplasmic vimentin filament inclusion). Some examples also resemble cells of large-cell non-Hodgkin's lymphoma, particularly the highly pleomorphic large pale nuclei of immunoblastic lymphoma, large non-cleaved cell lymphoma, and large cleaved cell lymphoma (all follicular center cell tumors). There may be a confusion with Reed-Sternberg variants of Hodgkin's disease, which with the small lymphocytes in the reactive background (Fig. 5–20B) (see below) can also be included in the differential diagnosis (although the virtual nonexistence of true primary cerebral Hodgkin's Disease (see below) makes this diagnosis so unlikely that it can usually be discounted in the differential diagnosis in a patient with no evidence of extracerebral

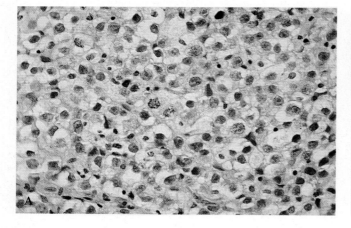
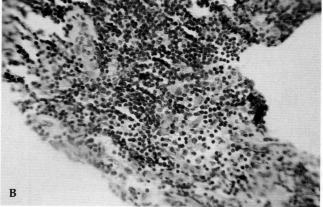
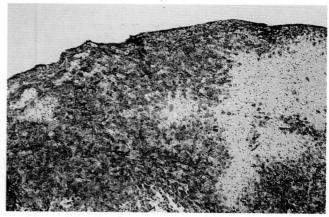

Figure 5–20 Germinoma. (A, B) Germinomas are typically composed of large, "undifferentiated" or primitive germ cells with large round nuclei, admixed with variable densities of reactive small lymphocytes (both H&E, 100×). (C) The cells are immunopositive with antibodies to placental alkaline phosphatase (PLAP, 25×).

tumor). The germinoma cells can be definitively identified as such, if there is doubt, by their immunopositivity for placental Alkaline Phosphatase (PLAP) (Fig. 5–20C). Usually, however, the large cells are intimately admixed with a florid reaction by small lymphocytes, so much so that classical descriptions of this tumor were of a "two-cell tumor" (Fig. 5–20B). There is invariably a high proliferation rate associated with these tumors, easily demonstrated by multiple mitotic figures and verified, if necessary, by MIB1 immunostaining.

Germinomas are among the most treatable of CNS malignancies in children. They are cured by radiation therapy after diagnostic biopsy in more than 90% of cases; more recently, in an effort to spare children the effects of radiation on the brain, multi-agent chemotherapy has been used and with similar effectiveness. Failures, which do occur, are more often refractory to treatment and usually lead to CSF dissemination.

Nongerminoma Germ Cell Tumors

All of the nongerminomatous primary CNS germ cell tumors, which are less common than germinomas, have been historically far more refractory to therapy than germinomas.[228] This trend has more or less continued into the present era, in distinct contrast with the marked improvement in survival of testicular or ovarian germ cell tumors of all types with modern chemotherapy regimens. *There have been no detectable prognostic differences among primary CNS embryonal carcinoma, yolk sac tumor, or choriocarcinoma.* Admittedly, many examples are of mixed type, particularly of embryonal carcinoma and yolk sac tumor with germinomatous areas; choriocarcinoma, either "pure" or as part of a mixed germ cell tumor, is the least common of all of the CNS germ cell tumors.

Embryonal carcinoma is characterized by the formation of solid epithelial nodules and glands lined by neoplastic germ cells that are somewhat similar morphologically to those of germinoma. The glands often are immunopositive for carcinoembryonic antigen (CEA) as well as for cytokeratins and epithelial membrane antigen. Yolk sac tumors have somewhat smaller cells, organized most classically into embryoid bodies and complex ductular or glandlike structures containing a vascular tuft surrounded and lined by neoplastic germ cells, the "Schiller-Duval body" (Fig. 5–21A). These tumors often have foci with differentiation resembling that of hepatocellular carcinomas, and like true hepatocellular carcinoma there is expression detectable by immunostaining of α-fetoprotein (AFP). AFP-positive cells usually contain an eosinophilic hyaline droplet of variable size; such droplets are found (with AFP immunopositivity) without hepatoid differentiation. (Fig. 5–21B).

Occasionally, a yolk sac tumor treated with chemotherapy undergoes a metaplastic transformation into frank adenocarcinoma, usually with tall columnar cells resembling colon carcinoma. This was originally described outside of the CNS but also occurs in the CNS.[229] The cells retain immunopositivity for PLAP and AFP despite their striking resemblance to mucinous colonic adenocarcinoma.

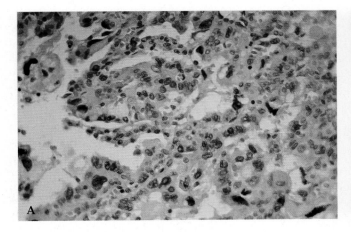

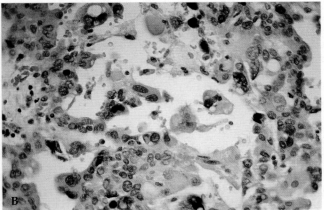

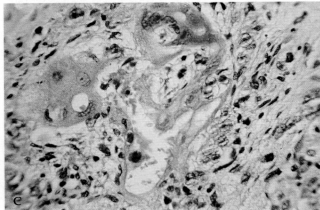

Figure 5–21 Nongerminoma germ cell tumor. (A) Endodermal sinus tumor (EST, yolk sac tumor) with a Schiller-Duval body (H&E, 100×). (B) EST with hyaline intracytoplasmic droplets (H&E, 100×). (C) Multinucleated syncytiotrophoblast cells in a mixed nongerminoma germ cell tumor (H&E, 100×).

Both embryonal carcinoma and yolk sac tumors can have occasional large multinucleated giant cells that both resemble syncytiotrophoblast cells (Fig. 5–21C) (but are clearly malignant tumor cells) and express β-human chorionic gonadotropin (hCG). The presence of such cells does not establish a diagnosis of trophoblastic tumor (i.e., choriocarcinoma); this requires the demonstration of both syncytiotrophoblast and cytotrophoblast cells in the neoplasm. *Primary CNS choriocarcinoma, like its non-CNS counterparts, is highly vascular and has a high frequency of catastrophic intracerebral hemorrhage (as does non-CNS choriocarcinoma when metastatic to the CNS).*

Modern trends in the classification of germ cell neoplasms have tended to lump all nongerminomatous germ cell tumors, including mixed variants, either under the rubric of "nongerminoma GCT" or, particularly for mixed variants, as "teratocarcinomas." The absence of significant treatment or prognostic differences for these different types of germ cell tumor is thought to justify this "lumping."

Because mixed germ cell neoplasms can include a significant component of germinoma, there is at least the theoretical possibility that a biopsy of a pineal or suprasellar/hypothalamic mass may yield apparently "pure" germinoma (carrying a good prognostic expectation) when the tumor in fact contains other, more ominous elements. Preoperative studies of serum and CSF for AFP, hCG, and, to a lesser extent, CEA can be helpful in establishing that the clinical diagnosis ought to be one of teratocarcinoma or mixed germ cell tumor when the limited histologic sample shows only germinoma. Of course, such markers are also of considerable help in following treatment for a tumor known to express them. Occasionally pure germinomas are found to contain scattered large polygonal or irregular multinucleated giant cells, typical of syncytiotrophoblast tumor cells, and these cells are invariably immunopositive for β-hCG. In the absence of cytotrophoblast cells or other nongerminoma germ cell elements, such syncytiotrophoblast elements do not alter the diagnosis of germinoma to one of mixed germ cell tumor, and concomitantly the presence of such cells does not alter the favorable prognosis associated with the diagnosis of pure germinoma.

Teratoma

Teratomas are probably formally within the group of nongerminomatous germ cell tumors, yet they present with such unique pathologic features that they are considered here separately. As with teratomas of the gonads or mediastinum, these are neoplasms that reproduce to various degrees of faithfulness the histologic structure and immunohistochemically detectable expression of normal body tissues. Mature teratomas more faithfully reproduce normal tissues, albeit in significantly abnormal sites. Most commonly, the tissue is skin, which is reproduced with epidermis complete with rete ridges, dermis with dermal papillae, and adnexal structures, including hair, sebaceous and eccrine glands, erector pilae muscles, and nerve bundles (Fig. 5–22A, B). These are usually cystic ("dermoid cysts"), and there is some disagreement as to whether they represent mature teratomas or simply are benign, nonneoplastic cysts formed from embryonal epithelial rests trapped in abnormal sites or implanted by trauma. This is another "religious" question, there being no histologic differences between undoubted neoplasms of this character

in other body sites and these CNS examples. There may be a lymphocytic infiltrate in the dermis, which needs to be carefully proven lymphoid because small neuroblasts are not easily histologically differentiated from lymphocytes. However, the presence of a neuroblastic component would suggest an immature component and a less than benign diagnosis.

Other elements commonly encountered in mature teratomas are islands or nodules of cartilage, sometimes bone, and a variety of other mesenchymal tissues, such as skeletal muscle, and glandular tissues including respiratory epithelium and gastrointestinal epithelium. Some examples are extraordinarily mature, with completely formed bronchi with cartilaginous rings, submucosal glands and lymphoid tissues, and respiratory epithelium. Mature teratomas are considered benign tumors and if totally excised are unlikely to present any clinical problem later in life.

Immature teratomas, on the other hand, are tumors that may have a great deal of mature tissue (Fig. 5–22C) but contain at least some component of more embryonal or fetal tissue, ranging from mildly hypercellular immature cartilage to frankly malignant tissues, including PNET, peripheral neuroblastoma, carcinoma, or sarcoma (Fig. 5–22D–F). *The presence of an immature element, even a limited one, confers a worse prognosis on a teratoma.* While immature CNS tissue is thought to be the most common immature component in gonadal immature teratomas[230] (Fig. 5–22E, F), in the CNS this is less common.

Primary CNS Lymphomas

Until about 1980, primary CNS non-Hodgkin's lymphoma (NHL-CNS) was an exceedingly rare tumor in all age groups, representing far less than 1% of all intra-axial brain and spinal cord tumors. Most cases involved adults, so that the proportion of pediatric brain tumors that were lymphomas was vanishingly small. The only significant exceptions in the pediatric age group were those tumors that arose in the setting of a congenital immunodeficiency syndrome, including ataxia-telangiectasia, Wiskott-Aldrich syndrome, and X-linked immunodeficiency syndrome (Duncan's syndrome). Similarly, in adults immunosuppression associated with organ transplantation or anticancer therapy was a risk factor for NHL-CNS. By 1984, however, it became clear to several groups of investigators that the incidence of NHL-CNS was rising rapidly, in part due to the tendency of these neoplasms to occur in patients with acquired immunodeficiency syndrome (AIDS). It was subsequently shown that an increased frequency of NHL-CNS could be documented in single institutional studies and in national databases.[231–237] Few of these "new" cases occurred in children. We have seen only one case of NHL-CNS in a child with congenital AIDS at NYU Medical Center.[238] At the Massachusetts General Hospital, only 4 of 104 patients with NHL-CNS documented between 1958 and 1994 were children. In addition, at NYU we have seen one teen-aged girl with a brain lesion that ultimately was shown to be a T-cell lymphoma (discussed above with reference to differential diagnosis of PNET).

The older pathologic literature on brain lymphomas includes a number of descriptions of primary cerebral Hodgkin's disease. With modern immunohistologic techniques, these cases, when reevaluated, have virtually all been

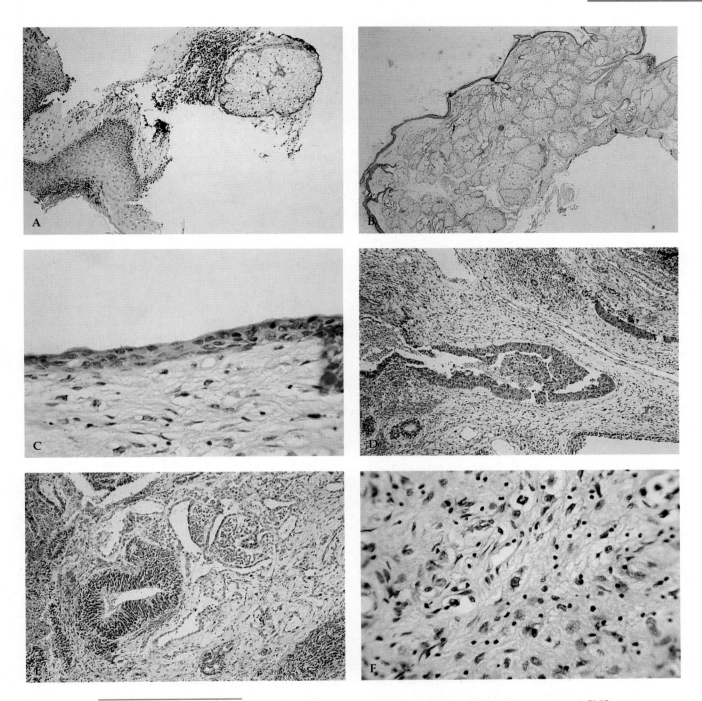

Figure 5–22 Teratomas. (A) Mature cystic teratomas ("dermoid cysts") are the commonest CNS teratomas. They consist of epidermis with dermis, dermal appendages, and hair (H&E, 25×). (B) The mature elements of the skinlike tumor contain no neuroblastic elements (here the sebaceous glands are hyperplastic) (H&E, 6.25×). (C) Immature teratomas may contain relatively mature differentiated tissues, as in this pineal tumor with foci of mature squamous epithelium (H&E, 100×). (D) Disorganized glandular epithelial elements point to some immaturity (H&E, 25×). (E) This example included foci with immature neural tissue, including embryonal elements forming structures resembling the neural tube (H&E, 25×). (F) More differentiated CNS tissues within the tumor resemble ganglioglioma (H&E, 100×).

shown to be primary non-Hodgkin's lymphomas with immunoblastic cells mimicking Reed-Sternberg cells (for review, see refs. 231 and 237). Even in patients known to have systemic Hodgkin's disease, the new discovery of a CNS mass after treatment of the Hodgkin's disease most likely represents a second primary neoplasm, non-Hodgkin's lymphoma, rather than spread of the Hodgkin's disease to the brain.[239]

In children, as in adults, NHL-CNS usually presents as an ill-defined deep-seated or superficial mass, close to ventricular or subarachnoid spaces. Periventricular locations are most common; the lesions may be single or multiple, and in the latter case may raise the differential diagnosis of demyelinating disease on clinical and MRI grounds. Histologically these tumors are often mostly sheetlike, diffuse, highly cellular neoplasms that infiltrate at their advancing edges along perivascular spaces, producing the characteristic perivascular cuffing encompassing redundant concentric deposits of vascular basal lamina (usually seen with reticulin stains). The densely cellular central zones may be mistaken for PNET or, in less usual instances, for an oligo-like tumor. The large majority of NHL-CNS tumors are large-cell B-cell follicular center cell lymphomas (with diffuse, not nodular/follicular, architecture), a fact fairly easily established by immunostaining on paraffin sections for B-cell– and T-cell–specific markers. Conventionally, we and most other laboratories now use CD20 antibodies, such as L26, to mark B cells in such tumors, and CD3 or CD45RO (antibody UCHL1) as pan-T-cell markers. For B-cell tumors the demonstration of light chain restriction, which establishes monoclonality, can be difficult in paraffin sections from formalin-fixed tumor specimens, as the surface immunoglobulin molecules on the neoplastic B cells may be masked or removed during fixation. In the view of many, including this neuropathologist, if the CNS infiltrate consists of large lymphoid cells that are all CD20-positive, whereas there is a scattering or background of smaller T cells that are immunopositive with UCHL1 or CD3, then the neoplastic nature of the infiltrate remains fairly well established. Proof of clonality in T cell tumors in tissue sections is even more difficult and, in effect, depends on methods to establish specific changes in T-cell receptor genes in the tumor cells.

The older literature concerning CNS lymphomas tended to emphasize radiation therapy and noted the rapid, dramatic response on CT scans or MRI images during and after this therapy. Our review[237] and others established the ineffectiveness of radiation for long-term cure, with most patients treated thus having relapsed and died within a year of initial diagnosis. It is now widely acknowledged (for review, see ref. 240) that chemotherapy, usually relying on high doses of methotrexate, is the mainstay of therapy following biopsy verification of the diagnosis of NHL-CNS. Patients so treated often experience durable responses and even apparent "cures."

Choroid Plexus Neoplasms

The choroid plexus is the specialized tissue that resides (mostly) within the brain's ventricular cavities and is responsible for the bulk of CSF production *via* an active process. There are tufts of choroid plexus in the lateral ventricles (at several sites, including the temporal horns, the bodies, and the frontal horns at or near the foramina of Monro), in the third ventricle (hanging from the foramina of Monro), and in the fourth ventricle; at the last location, portions of the choroid plexus usually extend out through the foramina of Luschka into the proximal portions of the cerebellopontine angles. The embryonic origin of the plexus is probably from a specialization of ependymal cells, but histologically and immunohistochemically these tissues behave more as a specialized "common" epithelium than as a neuroepithelial tissue. Rarely, the plexus gives rise to neoplasms, the majority of which are found in children.

Choroid Plexus Papilloma

The most common neoplasm of the plexus is the papilloma. This is a tumor that closely resembles the parent tissue (and indeed may be functional; some cases have been associated with hydrocephalus thought to be due to overproduction of CSF by the tumors, although more usually any hydrocephalus is attributable to obstruction of a crucial foramen by a bulky tumor). They are papillary masses, with each delicate fibrovascular core covered by an epithelium of low columnar or cuboidal cells (Fig. 5–23A, B). Histologically, only the exaggerated exuberantly folded nature of the tumor separates many of these papillomas from normal plexus tissue, although the cells are usually also more crowded than in normal plexus. Because these tumors are usually distinctive histologically, there is little differential diagnosis; the main problem is the occasionally highly papillary ependymoma. As both ependymomas and choroid plexus papillomas may have cells that express GFAP (albeit this is less common in plexus tumors), distinction between these entities, when problematical with H&E staining (which, it should be clear, is rare), usually depends on the demonstration in plexus tumors of transthyretin ("prealbumin").[241, 242] Choroid plexus papillomas are benign tumors, although rare exceptions seed through the CSF; the implants in such dissemination are minimally invasive and also seem to have a benign course.

Choroid Plexus Carcinoma

Occasionally, papillomas have a more crowded appearance than usual and may have an increase in mitotic activity over the negligible mitotic figure counts usual in a choroid plexus papilloma. A category of "atypical" papilloma has been proposed to encompass such tumors, but reliable criteria with adverse prognostic associations have not been shown. However, when a choroid plexus tumor has foci with solid growth patterns, which are invariably associated with greater pleomorphism and higher mitotic counts, and are also often accompanied by foci of necrosis and frank invasion into the brain parenchyma, then the diagnosis of choroid plexus carcinoma is appropriate (Fig. 5–23C, D). These are highly malignant tumors that are usually rapidly fatal despite radical surgery, radiation therapy, and chemotherapy. They may be so solid as to be difficult to recognize as of plexus origin, but many (not all) retain transthyretin expression and so can be identified immunohistochemically (Fig. 5–23E).

Choroid plexus tumors have been produced experimentally in a considerable number of models utilizing SV40 virus or its large T antigen. These models have ranged from intracerebral injections of whole virus to transgenic mouse models

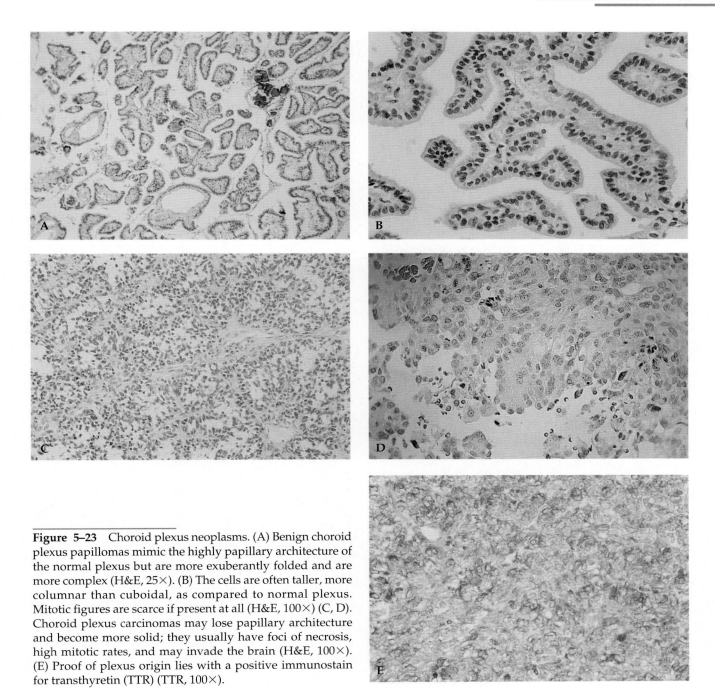

Figure 5–23 Choroid plexus neoplasms. (A) Benign choroid plexus papillomas mimic the highly papillary architecture of the normal plexus but are more exuberantly folded and are more complex (H&E, 25×). (B) The cells are often taller, more columnar than cuboidal, as compared to normal plexus. Mitotic figures are scarce if present at all (H&E, 100×) (C, D). Choroid plexus carcinomas may lose papillary architecture and become more solid; they usually have foci of necrosis, high mitotic rates, and may invade the brain (H&E, 100×). (E) Proof of plexus origin lies with a positive immunostain for transthyretin (TTR) (TTR, 100×).

utilizing the large T-antigen gene alone, with extraneous promoters.[243–245] SV40 DNA has been recovered from a number of different types of brain tumors, but most reliably and regularly from choroid plexus papillomas and carcinomas, and from ependymomas.[190, 191]

Miscellaneous Primary CNS Intra-axial Sarcomas and Other Mesenchymal Tumors

A variety of primary CNS sarcomas that occur within the brain, rather than its coverings, have been described, and most such cases involve children. These include primary

rhabdomyosarcomas, particularly reported in the cerebellum,[206] mesenchymal chondrosarcomas,[246] fibrosarcomas, leiomyosarcomas, angiosarcomas, and a variety of other rare tumors. Each category is remarkably rare. Some of the case reports are so old as to predate the routine use of immunostaining, and there is little to be said about this miscellany of tumors other than that they exist.

Benign masses of adipose tissue (lipomas) are occasionally found in the CNS as incidental lesions either by MRI or at autopsy. These are well-delineated nodules of mature fat cells, often attached to the corpus callosum or the midbrain. So far as can be shown, these represent true lipomatous neoplasms, whereas the "lipomas" found more frequently involving the lower end of the spinal cord in patients with a tethered cord syndrome are more obviously malformative, associated with spinal dysraphism and containing disordered bundles of peripheral nerve roots, skeletal muscle, leptomeninges, and CNS tissue.

EXTRA-AXIAL NEOPLASMS

As mentioned at the outset, most intra-axial brain and spinal cord neoplasms tend to be malignancies, even though some (e.g., pilocytic astrocytomas) only rarely show malignant clinical behavior. In contrast, most extra-axial CNS tumors are benign. This is true in children as well as in adults, although extra-axial tumors in children are distinctly uncommon, even as a proportion of all CNS tumors in these age groups.

Craniopharyngioma

Perhaps the most important numerically of these extra-axial neoplasms are craniopharyngiomas, which are said to be the most common of all nonglial CNS tumors of childhood. Craniopharyngiomas are "common" (in the sense of ordinary) epithelial tumors, not neuroectodermally derived neoplasms; in fact, they are thought to be derived from remnants of the embryonic or fetal pharyngeal epithelium of Rathke's cleft,

which also helps form the adenohypophysis. *There are two histologically distinct patterns of craniopharyngioma: the classical type that closely resembles the tumors of long bones, called "adamantinoma," and the tumor of tooth-forming tissues, called "ameloblastoma."* Tumors with this appearance have a distinctive histologic pattern: a basal layer of small cells, a superimposed layer of stellate cells, and a zone of abrupt maturation at the inner (cyst) surface to large keratinized flat squamous plates, which then desquamate into the cyst in stacks (Fig. 5–24A, B). The squamous debris often calcifies and may undergo osseous metaplasia. Breakdown products of cellular membranes, either of the epithelial cells or of erythrocytes from intratumoral microhemorrhages, lead to the deposition of crystals of cholesterol, which then evoke a foreign body response with giant cells.

The other histologic type of craniopharyngioma is the papillary squamous type (Fig. 5–24C). These tumors rarely calcify, and have a very different histologic appearance, with a true stratified squamous epithelium folded at its outer layers (the base) into papillary formations (Fig. 5–24C). It has been suggested that papillary squamous craniopharyngiomas are found only in adults and may be derived from different source tissues than adamantinomatous craniopharyngiomas,[247, 248] but we and others [249–251] have documented some papillary squamous craniopharyngiomas in children, and also have shown examples with mixed adamantinomatous and papillary squamous craniopharyngioma patterns in the same tumor.

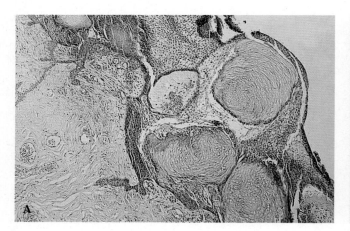

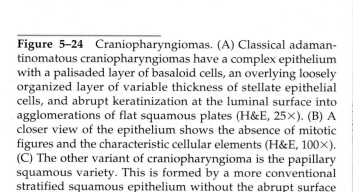

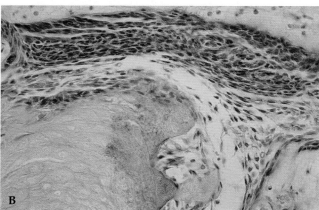

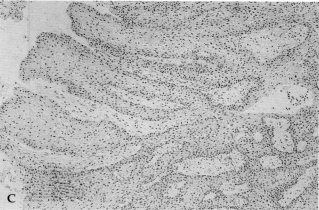

Figure 5–24   Craniopharyngiomas. (A) Classical adamantinomatous craniopharyngiomas have a complex epithelium with a palisaded layer of basaloid cells, an overlying loosely organized layer of variable thickness of stellate epithelial cells, and abrupt keratinization at the luminal surface into agglomerations of flat squamous plates (H&E, 25×). (B) A closer view of the epithelium shows the absence of mitotic figures and the characteristic cellular elements (H&E, 100×). (C) The other variant of craniopharyngioma is the papillary squamous variety. This is formed by a more conventional stratified squamous epithelium without the abrupt surface keratinization (H&E, 25×).

These are tumors that are invariably found in the sella and suprasellar cisterns (with trivially rare exceptions). Portions of the tumor may extend off the midline under one temporal or even frontal lobe, and in other cases there may be extensions through the tentorial notch to impinge on one side of the brain stem. The tumors are usually partially cystic, with a solid nodule. The cyst fluid, particularly of the adamantinomatous type, is usually thick, lipid-rich, and dark brown, and is often described as resembling old motor oil. *Both the adamantinomatous and squamous papillary types, but more often the former, are intimately involved and attached at their superior borders with hypothalamic tissues.* Here there is a zone of dense fibrillary gliosis, usually rich in Rosenthal fibers, which closely mimics the histologic features of the solid portions of pilocytic astrocytomas. Buried in the gliosis, and occasionally beyond into neuronal tissues of the hypothalamus itself, are fingers or islands of craniopharyngiomatous tissue.

Craniopharyngiomas have a significant incidence of local recurrence despite gross total surgical excision.[247, 250, 251] They can be difficult to eradicate when recurrent, particularly because they may involve the optic nerves, chiasm, or tracts, the internal carotid arteries or middle cerebral arteries, or brain stem structures, which prohibits resection without major risk of unacceptable deficits. Furthermore, even when effectively cured, craniopharyngiomas are associated with a variety of devastating endocrinologic and neurologic consequences, including panhypopituitarism with growth retardation, intellectual and memory deficits, and visual impairment, including blindness. Surgical damage to the pituitary stalk, hypothalamus, or neurohypophysis can lead to diabetes insipidus, inappropriate secretion of antidiuretic hormone, or, particularly in young patients (under age 3 years), either the diencephalic syndrome or severe obesity. Nevertheless, there is no described incidence of distant dissemination and these are, at least technically, benign.

There are other masses in the vicinity of the sella that are related to craniopharyngiomas, most notably Rathke's cleft cysts. These are probably not neoplasms but rather developmental rests that enlarge as they accumulate fluid, although some craniopharyngiomas contain foci of cyst lining with all of the characteristics of Rathke's cleft cysts. The cysts are lined by a typical respiratory-type epithelium, formed of low columnar cells with a ciliated luminal border arranged in a pseudostratified array. Some such cysts have undergone squamous metaplasia and resemble unfolded versions of papillary squamous craniopharyngiomas, although the presence of a luminal surface layer of ciliated cells betrays the origin of such squamous linings from Rathke's Cleft epithelia.

Pituitary Adenoma

Pituitary adenomas are among the most classical of tumors found more frequently in adults, but with well-documented pediatric cases. *Pituitary adenomas are conventionally (and usefully) divided by size and clinical presentation into microadenomas, which are essentially entirely intrasellar and present as a result of their producing active hormonal products, and macroadenomas, which are hormonally silent and present when they have mass effect on the optic chiasm, raise ICP and cause headaches, or compress the pituitary and cause hypopituitarism.* While often thought of as

tumors of adults, there is a considerable incidence of pituitary adenomas in children, particularly hormonally active microadenomas secreting growth hormone (GH) (and causing giantism) or adrenal corticotropic hormone (ACTH).

Modern pathologic characterization of pituitary adenomas is based on their size, as indicated above, and on their specific hormonal content as demonstrated immunohistochemically. Older descriptions of "eosinophilic adenomas," "basophilic adenomas," and "chromophobe adenomas" have essentially been abandoned. Conventional commercially available antibodies for immunostains allow the specific identification of all of the usual conventional pituitary hormones, plus a variety of other products occasionally found in these tumors. Thus, an adenoma can be characterized by the presence or absence of immunohistochemically detectable prolactin, GH, ACTH, thyroid-stimulating hormone, follicle-stimulating hormone, and luteinizing hormone; of the α-subunit common to the latter three, all of which are glycoproteins; of components of the secretory vesicle itself, most usually chromogranin but also synaptophysin and related vesicle membrane proteins; and of a variety of other secretory products made as part of larger prohormone molecules, such as enkephalins.

Pituitary adenomas are found histologically in a variety of patterns. These include moderately to densely cellular diffuse sheetlike growths in which the vascular stroma is inconspicuous (Fig. 5–25A); tumors with a more prominent vasculature dividing the sheets of cells into lobules (Fig. 5–25B); tumors with distinctive perivascular arrangements of the cells resembling pseudorosettes and thus simulating ependymomas; and tumors in which the perivascular patterns break up into papillary or pseudopapillary structures. Some adenomas have more than one of these patterns. All of these architectures are distinct from the acinar packets that compose the normal architecture of the adenohypophysis and thus make the diagnosis of adenoma, as compared to normal gland, easy in most cases. At initial inspection, these tumors may resemble malignancies, particularly the more cellular examples, and individual tumors may be easily confused with PNET, lymphoma, ependymoma, oligodendroglioma, and similar tumors, such as neurocytoma; clinical information usually helps the pathologist avoid what will seem like a foolish diagnosis to the submitting surgeon, but if the specimen is submitted without useful clinical data ("brain tumor"), as is true in a dismaying number of instances, the diagnosis is occasionally difficult. The nuclei of an adenoma are usually strikingly bland and regular, and mitotic figures are usually sparse, which can also help. Immunostains that demonstrate the appropriate hormonal content or chromogranin will reassure the pathologist.

Electron microscopy of pituitary adenomas reveals epithelial cells with junctions and a variable content of secretory vesicles. Elaborate classifications based on combinations of the electron microscopic and immunostaining data have been promulgated, correlating hormone content with size of the neurosecretory granules and whether they are numerous or sparse, but these are of limited clinical utility; identifying the hormonal content is the sole important step.[252]

Pituitary carcinoma is exceedingly rare in any age group. Historically it has been identified only when a pituitary "adenoma" has demonstrated metastatic behavior; although

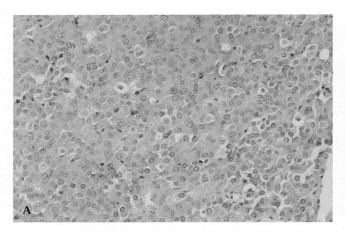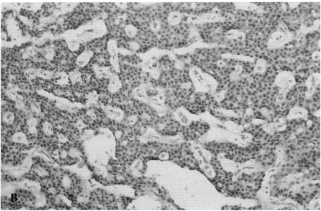

Figure 5–25 Pituitary adenomas. (A) Adenoma with solid, sheetlike growth pattern (H&E, 100×). (B) Adenoma with lobular architecture delineated by a prominent capillary network (H&E, 25×).

recent studies have suggested that measurements of proliferative potential, and of *p53* immunoreactivity, may identify adenomas that might recur or identify carcinomas,[253, 254] there is no definite way to confirm from pathologic examination of the primary pituitary tumor that it represents a carcinoma.

Nerve Sheath Tumors

Neoplasms arising from the cells of the sheaths of peripheral nerves include schwannomas, neurofibromas, and, possibly, granular cell tumors, plus a spectrum of variants such as the combination of skeletal muscle differentiation or rhabdomyosarcoma with schwannoma ("Triton tumor"). *Nerve sheath tumors may occur anywhere in the body where there is peripheral nerve tissue in its broadest sense, including sensory, motor, and autonomic fibers; thus, for example, there are documented rare examples of nerve sheath tumor arising in the dura not associated with a large nerve root, documented examples of intracerebral and intraventricular schwannomas, and documented examples of spinal intramedullary schwannomas.*[255] Most such tumors probably occur in the skin or soft tissue, and are not otherwise relevant to this chapter on the neuropathology of pediatric CNS tumors, but those that occur on or in cranial nerves or spinal nerve roots are usually treated as "CNS tumors" despite the fact that they arise in the portions of the peripheral nervous system closest to the brain or spinal cord.

Schwannoma

Schwannomas are benign neoplasms, presumed on the basis of morphologic characteristics and, more recently, electron microscopic and immunostaining characteristics, to arise from the normal Schwann cells that ensheathe peripheral nerve axons. They are not tumors of perineurial cells or of fibroblasts, although they do make and secrete collagen. Almost all schwannomas arise from sensory nerves, so that in the spinal canal they frequently encompass dorsal root ganglia, and in the cranial cavity they may involve the sensory ganglia of the vestibular branch of the eighth cranial nerve or parts of the trigeminal ganglia (other intracranial ganglionic sites are distinctly uncommon, although described). As CNS tumors they are most commonly encountered in adults as sporadic neoplasms affecting the vestibular branch of one of the eighth nerves, representing so-called acoustic neuromas. In children, schwannomas are rare tumors, and their presence on the eighth nerve, or indeed any cranial or spinal nerve roots, is cause to suspect a genetic tumor syndrome, usually neurofibromatosis type 2 ((NF-2); "central neurofibromatosis"), but sometimes the less well-characterized entity "schwannomatosis."[255] NF-2 patients most often have bilateral acoustic tumors, and they may also have multiple other schwannomas of spinal nerve roots; intramedullary spinal cord ependymomas are also found in many such patients, as are single or multiple meningiomas. Although all of these features individually represent problems most commonly encountered sporadically in adults far more often than in children, patients with NF-2 are often identified (especially now with increased sensitivity for small lesions provided by MRI) in childhood.

Schwannomas, whether found in the setting of NF-2 or otherwise, typically grow from one border of a nerve, in the epineurium, and the normal nerve tissue is separated from the truly encapsulated tumor. The nerve may be progressively stretched over the surface of the enlarging mass, and it may be ultimately so attenuated as to not be dissectable from a large tumor (although this is fairly readily accomplished with smaller tumors). Histologically, therefore, the nerve itself is usually not obviously invaded by tumor cells—a point of difference with neurofibromas (see below). In some schwannomas, the lobular architecture of the tumor may entrap a nerve bundle, which, while still not invaded, is then not readily preserved at surgery if the tumor is to be totally excised. It is suggested that such multilobular schwannomas are more common in NF-2 patients than in those with sporadic single schwannomas.[256] Ganglia that are affected by a schwannoma, however, often have a more infiltrative relationship with tumor cells; furthermore, if one stains for axons with either sensitive silver techniques (Bielschowsky's method) or neurofilament antibody staining techniques, one can occasionally demonstrate axons running through an otherwise ordinary schwannoma.[257]

While the great majority of schwannomas meet the description just given, rare examples arise in the parenchyma of the CNS. Thus, there are descriptions of histologically classical schwannomas in the cerebral hemispheres, in the brain stem, in the brain's ventricular spaces, and in the spinal cord. There is no indication that the existence of such tumors in the CNS tissues is an indication of malignancy. The existence of such intraparenchymal schwannomas can be rationalized (if necessary) by the presence of peripheral (mostly autonomic) nerve fibers in vascular walls and leptomeninges.

Classically, schwannomas have two patterns of growth that are apparent histologically, usually with both types in each tumor. These are referred to as "Antoni A" and "Antoni B" tissues. In the former, the tumor tissue appears solid or compact, and the tumor cells are all bipolar elongated or spindle cells arranged in fascicles (Fig. 5–26A, B). The fascicles are usually short, and there is a complex pattern of intersections between fascicles, often at angles close to 90 degrees. Often

the nuclei of the elongated tumor cells are hyperchromatic, and there can be a significant degree of pleomorphism, which is irrelevant to any judgment as to atypicality or aggressive potential (Fig. 5–26D). Antoni B tissue, in contrast, is loosely structured, with a mucinous or myxoid background in which small cells appear with rounder nuclei and more stellate processes than the cells of the Antoni A pattern (Fig. 5–26B).

The most classical of the classical schwannomas have zones in the Antoni A tissue in which there are parallel lines or palisades of tumor cell nuclei, with an anuclear fibrillary eosinophilic zone between the lines (Fig. 5–26C). This arrangement, referred to as a "Verocay body," is mimicked only by the nuclear palisades of spongioblastic foci of PNETs, although it is occasionally confused with longitudinally sectioned perivascular pseudorosettes of ependymomas. There are no vessels separating the lines of nuclei in a Verocay body. Verocay bodies, which are fairly commonly found in schwannomas of dermal and soft-tissue sites, are found in a

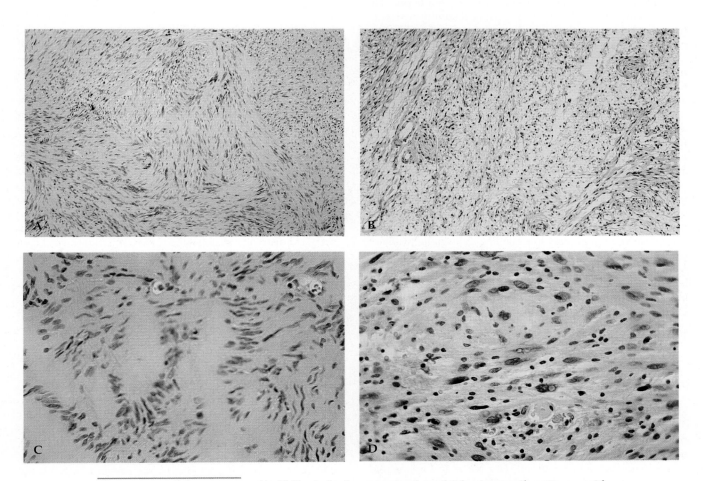

Figure 5–26 Schwannomas. (A, B) Typical schwannomas have biphasic growth patterns, with solid tissue ("Antoni A," Fig. 4–26A) composed of spindle cells in fascicles, and loose tissue ("Antoni B," Fig. 4–26B) with stellate cells with smaller, rounder nuclei (each H&E, 25×). (C) Many schwannomas lack the "textbook" feature of parallel lines or palisades of nuclei—"Verocay bodies"—but when present these aid in the diagnosis even in small fragments supplied with minimal or no clinical data (H&E, 100×). (D) The cells in the Antoni A areas are typically moderately pleomorphic—an appearance with no ominous prognostic import (H&E, 100×).

minority of intracranial and spinal nerve root schwannomas, many of which are predominantly Antoni A with only small Antoni B components. *In cranial nerve schwannomas that are almost entirely composed of Antoni B tissue, with only minimal foci of Antoni A tissue, clinical history is essential to a prompt accurate diagnosis. This is because with H&E staining such tumors may resemble anaplastic astrocytomas, so that if they are submitted as "brain tumor" there is a significant opportunity for a pathologist to err in diagnosis.*

Most schwannomas also have striking, thick-walled vessels; the vessels have somewhat hyalinized walls, with some examples showing fibrinoid breakdown. There is usually considerable hemosiderin deposition, indicating the occurrence of episodes of microhemorrhage prior to tumor resection. There can be considerable accumulation of foamy macrophages in and around the hemosiderin deposits; cholesterol crystal formation with a foreign body giant cell response is less common but is seen. Many schwannomas have microcystic zones, which usually develop in the loose Antoni B tissues; in less common cases there is a macroscopic cyst, lined by loose Antoni B tissues or by a pseudoepithelial pattern of tumor cells. Such cysts must be distinguished from true glandular or epithelioid schwannomas, which are clinically more aggressive (see below).

The cells of a schwannoma are virtually invariably immunopositive for S100 protein, a finding that can be diagnostic in the appropriate differential diagnostic setting although S100 expression is not limited to Schwann cells. The usual schwannoma has each of its cells surrounded by its own basal lamina, which produces a "single-cell" pattern of reticulin staining; this can be a very useful diagnostic point for the pathologist. Some schwannomas have been described as expressing GFAP immunopositivity, and this is thought to occur more often in tumors of cranial nerve or spinal nerve root origin than peripherally. In the vast majority of schwannomas, histologic sections are devoid of apparent mitotic figures, and proliferation markers such as Ki67 (MIB1) show a remarkably low labeling index. (One study of proliferation with the antibody PC10 for the proliferating cell nuclear antigen [PCNA/cyclin] showed a remarkably high level of staining,[258] clearly indicating a separation of true proliferative activity from the labeling index. At NYU Medical Center, we have seen the same phenomenon with PC10 in pituitary adenomas.)

NF-2 is now known to result from mutations in a gene on chromosome 22, the normal gene product of which is called "merlin."[256] The majority of sporadic schwannomas and meningiomas also have a somatic mutation in this gene.

Rarely, schwannomas occur that contain unusual histologic features. These include focal skeletal muscle (rhabdomyoblastic) differentiation, seen as large strap cells with cross-striations; melanin formation (melanotic schwannoma); plexiform architectural patterns ("plexiform schwannoma"), which is not associated with NF-1 or NF-2; and epithelioid patterns with apparent gland formation. The latter is closely associated with malignancy (see below). Melanotic schwannomas with frequent psammoma bodies may be seen as part of the complex genetic syndrome of Carney's complex.[259] (These and other variants of schwannoma are discussed further below.)

Neurofibroma

The other classical variety of nerve sheath tumor is the neurofibroma. Unlike schwannomas, neurofibromas grow by extending inside of and expanding individual nerve fascicles, so that the nerve tissue itself is intimately associated with the neoplastic cells; axon stains will always show trapped axons in neurofibromas up to the time that they have all been destroyed by the tumor. As with schwannomas, sporadic neurofibromas occur most commonly in the skin and subcutaneous tissues, with deep soft-tissue sites and viscera being less commonly involved, and are found most often in adults; *in children, the presence of any neurofibroma should at least raise the question of NF-1, or von Recklinghausen's disease.* Certainly, the finding of any nerve sheath tumor on a cranial nerve or spinal nerve root that is found histopathologically to be a neurofibroma should provoke a concern about this diagnosis. Patients with NF-1 may have a wide variety of abnormalities, some of which are skeletal and not neoplastic, but the most common and characteristic findings are the presence of multiple neurofibromas in the skin, subcutaneous tissues, and nerve roots, together with some hamartomatous lesions of the brain (best recognized with MRI); there is a noncoincidental increased incidence of gliomas in patients with NF1, including optic nerve pilocytic astrocytomas, hypothalamic/chiasmatic pilocytic astrocytomas, and fibrillary astrocytomas of the cerebral hemispheres, brain stem, and spinal cord.

As implied above, neurofibromas differ markedly from schwannomas; it is not entirely clear what normal cell type or types are involved in neurofibromas, as the cells include some with the phenotypes of Schwann cells, perineurial cells, and fibroblasts. The tumors are also composed of spindle cells, and these are usually (but not quite as close to always as schwannomas) S100-immunopositive. These spindle cells are generally loosely packed in a myxoid matrix that replaces the normal connective tissue of the nerve (Fig. 5–27); closely associated with the tumor cells are bundles of collagen, and in standard histologic sections the tumor cells and the collagen both adopt a "wavy" conformation (Fig. 5–27A). Therefore, neurofibromas are more uniform than the biphasic schwannoma, and there is only variation in how myxoid the background gets and how densely cellular the tumors are (varying from low to high). Neurofibromas with higher cell density and with mitotic figures readily identified are suspicious for malignancy.

In patients with NF-1, the most characteristic pattern of neurofibroma is the "plexiform neurofibroma," a lesion in which each separate fascicle of a nerve trunk is individually expanded by a neurofibromatous proliferation. In such tumors, the perineurium of each such fascicle encapsulates its enclosed tumor mass from the adjacent, also involved, fascicles. The resulting appearance has been likened to a "bag of worms" (Fig. 5–27B). It has been alleged that even a single plexiform neurofibroma indicates the presence of NF-1, but this is unlikely to be true. To give one anecdote: This neuropathologist has seen a classical plexiform neurofibroma in the gastric wall of a 67-year-old man with no previous medical history, no family history of neurofibroma or other tumor, and no other evidence of NF-1. (This was in an era prior to the availability of genetic testing.)

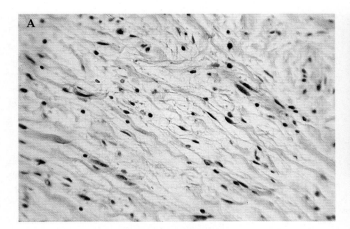

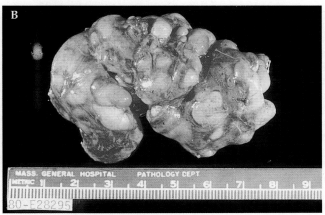

Figure 5–27 Neurofibromas. (A) Benign neurofibromas diffusely expand segments of nerve, with a loose often myxoid matrix containing "wavy" spindle cells in loosely organized fascicles accompanied by similarly wavy collagen bundles (H&E, 100×). (B) Plexiform neurofibromas involve multiple fascicles of nerve trunks, producing this "bag of worms" appearance.

The gene defect underlying NF-1 is a mutation in a gene whose product is now known as "neurofibromin"; as with other, similar gene product names (e.g., dystrophin), it is the absence of the normal gene product that produces the abnormal phenotype. The *NF1* gene is located on chromosome 17.

Variants of Schwannoma and Neurofibroma

As described above, occasional cases of a tumor with a plexiform growth pattern in a nerve are seen histologically to have classical Antoni A structure complete with Verocay bodies. Such tumors have been described as "plexiform schwannomas."[260–262] It has been argued that tumors such as the suggest a spectrum of phenotypes, with schwannoma and neurofibroma at opposite poles along a continuum; this becomes less likely as a general proposition because the genetic defects in schwannomas and neurofibromas are now known to be very different on different chromosomes, although there have been no microdissection studies on the undeniably real cases in which neurofibromas have focal areas closely resembling schwannomas.

Both schwannomas and neurofibromas may occasionally show advanced differentiation resembling sensory end-organs (meissnerian corpuscles). There is no known significance to this architecture. In some patients, "neurotized" nevi may also begin to show this resemblance, raising a differential diagnostic problem that is not always easily resolved. Indeed, some schwannomas contain melanin-producing cells, and both nevus cells and schwannoma cells are S100-immunopositive. As mentioned above, schwannomas can be both grossly and histologically cystic, and the cysts are lined by tumor cells that become more cuboidal and epithelioid as they line the fluid-filled spaces. However, frank epithelial differentiation with gland formation ("epithelioid schwannoma") is rare and thought by some[263] to always be associated with other features of malignancy. Finally, the presence of occasional striated muscle cells in an otherwise ordinary

schwannoma represents a peculiar variant, which again can be "explained" by the rhabdomyoblastic potential of the neural crest cells which ultimately give rise to Schwann cells and thus schwannomas (see p. 75, PNET with Rhabdoid Differentiation); alternatively, this can be regarded as a metaplastic phenomenon. Most described examples have been malignant tumors, but benign variants clearly exist; at NYU Medical Center, even an occasional vestibular nerve schwannoma ("acoustic neuroma") has had focal skeletal muscle differentiation, verified by electron microscopy as well as H&E staining.

Atypical, "Cellular," and Malignant Schwann Cell Tumors

Malignant tumors of peripheral nerve sheath origin have long been recognized; fashions in the nosology of these tumors have changed from "neurofibrosarcoma" through "malignant schwannoma" to the current "malignant peripheral nerve sheath tumor" (MPNST). The literature on MPNST has focused on two issues: recognizing that an undoubted sarcomatous lesion is of nerve sheath origin, and recognizing malignant changes in lesions clearly of nerve sheath origin.

It is more important to deal with the latter issue, as long as specific therapies are not different for spindle sarcomas affecting the nervous system. *Formerly, it was suggested that all MPNST arise either de novo or from preexisting neurofibromas, and that schwannomas do not give rise to malignant lesions.*[264–266] *However, there are case reports and other descriptions of tumors that in part are clearly schwannomas and yet have malignant histologic features and have demonstrated a malignant clinical behavior.*[264, 267–269] There is considerable controversy over what histologic criteria might be used to distinguish benign and malignant tumors sharing schwannomatous features.

Criteria that might suggest malignant progression in a previously benign tumor in other neoplastic types are for the most part not helpful. Pleomorphism and nuclear atypicality with variation in nuclear size and with considerable nuclear hyperchromatism are common in ordinary schwannomas and have no adverse clinical associations. Foci of necrosis in a schwannoma are occasionally seen, usually in association with marked vascular wall thickening and fibrinoid necrosis of the vessels walls, and again this has no ominous prognostic association. Invasive behavior into the parent nerve or ganglion, while uncommon in the case of the former, is again seen in some schwannomas with no suggestion that these are more aggressive tumors, although this feature is so rare that no systematic study has included it as a variable. A loss of the usual architecture of Antoni A and B zones, and an absence of typical Verocay bodies, is not uncommon in cranial nerve schwannomas, which are often predominantly Antoni A tissue and which have Verocay bodies only occasionally, as discussed earlier.

Two histologic features may suggest a more aggressive behavior, although this issue is far from settled. Some schwannomas are more or less exclusively Antoni A, lack distinctive Verocay bodies, are more cellular than their usual counterparts, and contain mitotic figures. These are all features that describe the proposed entity of "cellular schwannoma,"[270–272] which, it is claimed, retains the benign behavior of ordinary schwannomas and should be recognized as a benign tumor to avoid overly aggressive treatment.[1, 3, 4, 270–272] However, the statistical basis of the clinical follow-up with regard to these features is at best weak, and there are distinctive anecdotal reports suggesting that the presence of mitotic figures in a tumor comprising these features are associated with an increased incidence of local recurrence, invasive behavior into the brain (when the tumor is on a cranial nerve), and metastatic spread.[273] We have seen that the usual schwannoma in typical radical excision samples has no mitotic figures detectable at all in routine sections and that proliferation indices in such tumors are very low; for us the presence of even one mitotic figure is somewhat suspicious, and the presence of three or more is so unusual as to require special mention. Others have noted a correlation of mitotic counts, proliferation indices, and malignant versus benign nerve sheath tumors, suggesting that mitotic figures (which ultimately correlate well with Ki67/MIB1 labeling indices) are predictive of aggressive behavior.[274, 275] The importance of mitotic figures as a prognostic indicator was perhaps first systematically suggested for both schwannomas and neurofibromas by Trojanowski et al.[276] We have seen several such tumors recur and at least one metastasize. Unfortunately, we have not yet had the resources to complete a large-scale study of this issue, but provisionally at NYU Medical Center we have regarded schwannomas with two mitotic figures in a single H&E-stained section as "atypical," and those with three or more as "low-grade malignant" (MPNST, grade I/III). Our preliminary data indicate that those we have labeled as low-grade malignant clearly have a higher incidence of recurrence despite apparent gross total excision than do ordinary schwannomas with no apparent mitotic figures. In our view, to withhold a malignant diagnosis unless the tumor is clearly a high-grade spindle cell sarcoma with high mitotic rates and other typically sarcomatous features is to fail to indicate the need for better follow-up and more aggressive

response to early recurrence for these lower grade examples; on the other hand, we are more likely to advocate "watchful waiting" than aggressive radiotherapy following the usual initial radical excision if we make such low-grade malignant diagnoses. It should be clear that this remains a minority view at the present and that the concept of "cellular schwannoma" is, at present, the popular one; however, we and some others clearly disagree. What is needed to settle this controversy is a complete characterization of a large series of putative cellular schwannomas, including mitotic counts done blinded to clinical outcome, proliferation studies with Ki67/MIB1 immunohistochemistry, careful objective image-based (MRI) analysis of extent of resection, and complete clinical follow-up with appropriate statistical correlations. Preliminary results of such a study, restricted to eighth nerve tumors, demonstrate a statistically significant incidence of local recurrence for schwannomas with three or more mitotic figures and a higher MIB1 labeling index. As these have all been local recurrences, perhaps the term "atypical" will prove more appropriate.

The problem of identifying a high-grade spindle cell neoplasm as of nerve sheath origin is often less important because that identification is an academic one: it is clear that the tumor is malignant, and there is at present no different therapeutic approach for "neurogenic" spindle cell sarcomas than for identically located fibrosarcomas, malignant fibrous histiocytomas, leiomyosarcomas, or the like.

Miscellaneous Nerve Sheath Tumors

Two other lesions deserve brief mention. Occasionally a mass attached to a nerve is seen histologically to consist of multiple whorls of spindle cells around vessels or other central foci, including axons. These nearly exactly duplicate the appearance of "onion bulbs" in hypertrophic neuropathies; however, immunohistochemical analysis has shown that the cells of the lesion are not Schwann cells, as in hypertrophic neuropathy, but are S100-negative and EMA-immunopositive, suggesting an origin from perineurial cells. These tumors, occasionally referred to as "localized hypertrophic neuropathy," are now generally recognized as "perineuriomas."[277–279] Some perineuriomas are found with no anatomical relationship to a nerve trunk, and about these there is little controversy. Those attached to nerve are sometimes still thought of as reactive processes rather than neoplasms, but the evidence seems to point to these as identical to the non–nerve-associated examples.[280]

The second entity is neurothekeoma. This was initially described as a nerve sheath myxoma[265]; it was first recognized as a skin tumor of nerve sheath origin and with a distinctive myxomatous histology. With time, it was recognized at other sites, including soft tissue, viscera, and within the spinal canal.[281]

Meningiomas

Meningiomas are among the more common of primary intracranial tumors in adults, representing perhaps 20% or more of all such neoplasms in various series. In children, however, as with the other, mostly benign extra-axial tumors already discussed, they are much less common, and when they occur they do so most often in particular special clinical settings, including NF-2 and after cranial (or craniospinal) radiation therapy. The histologic features of meningiomas, however, are not distinctive either in children in general or in these special settings in particular.

Spontaneous Meningiomas

"Ordinary" Meningiomas

The term "meningioma" encompasses all tumors of meningothelial cell origin, usually presenting as dural-based extra-axial masses within the cranium and, less commonly, in the spinal canal. *"Ectopic" meningiomas also occur, particularly in soft-tissue sites on the head, in the nasal cavities, and in the lungs; in each such ectopic site the possibility of either contiguous spread from an intracranial tumor or of metastatic spread from such a primary tumor must be excluded.*[282–286] Meningiomas are also well recorded as intraventricular neoplasms, although this is an unusual site [287–289]; they are thought to arise from meningothelial cells of the normal tela choroidea (the normal attachment of the choroid plexus), and thus have been found in the frontal and temporal horns of the lateral ventricles, in the third ventricle, and in the fourth ventricle. Intraventricular meningiomas may be more common in children than in adults but are otherwise not distinctive.[289] The published photomicrographs of intraventricular tumors described by Dandy[290] clearly shows that some were meningiomas, although none were described using modern pathologic nosology.

Within this broad category of "ordinary" meningiomas there is a bewildering variety of histologic patterns, which all have been shown to be variants of meningioma, although the large majority of meningiomas present no diagnostic problem to the pathologist as they have, focally or more generally, classical features. One of the best thorough descriptions of most such variants, although frequently couched in terminology not now currently in use, is the classic account of the large personal series of Harvey Cushing with Louise Eisenhardt.[291] A more recent and no less valuable account was produced by Kepes.[292] New variants continue to be recognized, however. Here, necessarily, is a brief account.

The classical features include a lobulated architecture, often with considerable vascularity, and a combination of cellular whorls (Fig. 5–28A), spindle cells in fascicles (Fig. 5–28B), and bland sheetlike areas in which the cell borders are indistinct (Fig. 5–28C) ("syncytial" patterns). Frequently, the whorls calcify in a lamellar fashion, producing psammoma bodies. Many cells in these prototypical variants of meningioma have highly convoluted nuclei in which a substantial finger of cytoplasm has the nucleus folded around it such that in a tissue section the nucleus appears to contain a pale inclusion. These "intranuclear pseudoinclusions" are highly characteristic in meningiomas and so can be a helpful diagnostic sign, although they are by no means found only in meningiomas and therefore their presence does not force a pathologic diagnosis of meningioma in the absence of other histologic or immunohistologic features of meningioma.

Focally, and occasionally more diffusely, some menin-giomas have looser architecture with a myxoid matrix in which there are stellate cells whose processes divide the background into microcystic cavities ("microcystic meningioma"; "meningiome humide" of Masson[293, 294]); tumors with intracellular lumens filled with a periodic acid–Schiff–positive round inclusion of secretion ("secretory meningioma"); tumors with a high vascularity containing numerous capillaries, resembling hemangioblastomas; and so on. All of these variants are meningiomas, with cells retaining the same immunohistochemical and ultrastructural features of those meningiomas that are readily recognized as such. These features include immunopositivity with antibodies to EMA (Fig. 5–28D) and to vimentin. There is often some cytokeratin expression as well. Ultrastructurally, these tumors have extensively interdigitating processes that lack basal lamina and have well-developed desmosomal intercellular junctions.

Atypical Meningiomas

Meningiomas were formerly divided into essentially two categories: benign and malignant. Histopathologic features diagnostic of the latter were classically stated to be brain invasion by the tumor; spontaneous necrosis within the tumor; and an "increased" mitotic rate over more usual meningiomas (with no stated threshold or statistical analysis).[291] Somewhat more recently, other criteria have been proposed, including zones of sheetlike architecture without lobulation or whorls and prominent nucleoli.[291, 295] Until recently, there had been no statistically based studies relating clinical follow-up and outcome to these histologic features.

In the recent era, we and others have attempted to apply modern multivariate statistical techniques to this question. We have found, in agreement with others,[296, 297] that necrosis by itself is not an independent prognostic indicator; that "prominence" of nucleoli is too subjective to analyze, but by the standards used at NYU is found in almost all spindle cell/fibroblastic meningiomas and thus is not a predictor of aggressive behavior; and that mitotic rates that exceed 3 to 6 in the area defined by 50 high-power (400×) fields are strongly indicative of local recurrence. We term such tumors, which recur locally but have little or no tendency for metastatic behavior, "atypical meningiomas,"[296] reserving the term "malignant meningioma" for those meningiomas with a demonstrated metastatic potential. However, others, including the WHO classification, continue to regard brain invasion as a defining characteristic of "malignant meningioma"[1–4]; this appears to be more a matter of definition as the clinical prediction from such invasion is still not metastasis, but local recurrence.

Recent studies have suggested additional criteria for a diagnosis of atypicality in meningiomas or for a prediction of locally aggressive behavior. *In most meningiomas a large proportion of the tumor cells express progesterone receptors in their nuclei, and this is easily demonstrated immunohistochemically*[298]; *the absence of such expression is an independent indicator of local recurrence.*[298] *Another histologic pattern recently described in meningiomas has clear cells, mimicking oligodendroglioma and similar tumors, and tumors with this appearance have also been shown to have an aggressive course.*[299]

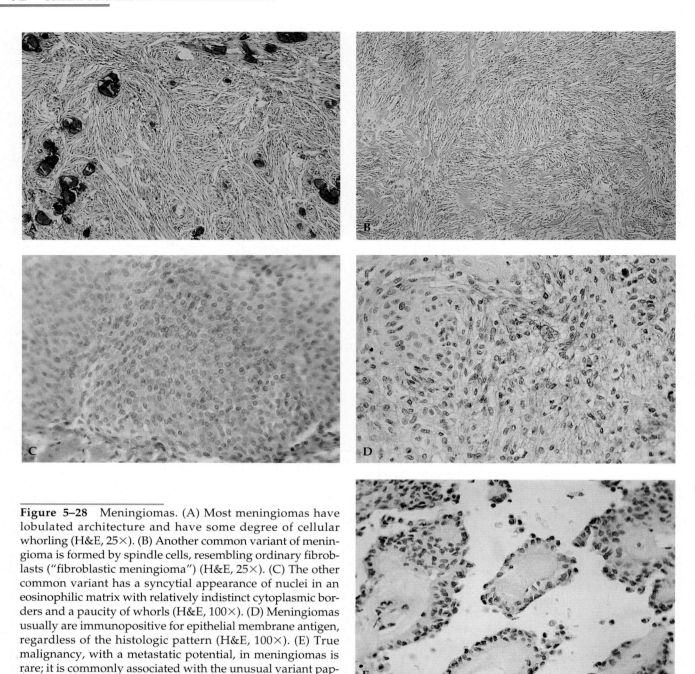

Figure 5–28 Meningiomas. (A) Most meningiomas have lobulated architecture and have some degree of cellular whorling (H&E, 25×). (B) Another common variant of meningioma is formed by spindle cells, resembling ordinary fibroblasts ("fibroblastic meningioma") (H&E, 25×). (C) The other common variant has a syncytial appearance of nuclei in an eosinophilic matrix with relatively indistinct cytoplasmic borders and a paucity of whorls (H&E, 100×). (D) Meningiomas usually are immunopositive for epithelial membrane antigen, regardless of the histologic pattern (H&E, 100×). (E) True malignancy, with a metastatic potential, in meningiomas is rare; it is commonly associated with the unusual variant papillary meningioma (H&E, 100×).

Malignant Meningiomas

True malignant meningiomas are tumors that are still demonstrably meningiomas but that by their particular characteristics are known to have a metastatic potential. Other dural-based malignant tumors ought not to be given this label; this would exclude meningeal hemangiopericytoma (a very rare tumor in children), dural sarcomas such as leiomyosarcoma or mesenchymal chondrosarcoma, and dural lymphomas. The chief histologic pattern in a meningioma that is strongly correlated with malignant behavior is the papillary pattern.[291, 292, 300] Papillary meningiomas are a rare variant of meningioma; they consist of papillary stalks with central vascular cores and tall columnar cells arranged around the central vessels, in a pattern resembling that of papillary ependymoma (Fig. 5–28E). Recognition of these tumors as meningiomas depends on finding characteristic areas with whorls in more solid portions of the tumor. The tumor cells have the usual EMA and vimentin immunoreactivity but may also express GFAP.[301] Because rarely an ependymoma occurs attached to the dura, grossly simulating a meningioma, the diagnosis of papillary meningioma should be made with care to exclude ependymoma, a tumor not otherwise thought to be in the differential diagnosis of meningioma.

There are cases of meningioma in which areas of the tumor are no longer recognizably meningothelial, at least by light microscopy, and instead resemble a spindle cell soft-tissue sarcoma. These tumors, if they retain foci recognizable as meningioma and yet have other areas of outright sarcoma, can be regarded as another type of malignant meningioma.

Radiation-Associated Meningiomas

It is well known that cranial radiation therapy may result in the development within the field of radiation of multiple meningiomas.[292] There is usually a substantial interval between the radiation exposure and the onset of clinical symptoms from the meningiomas, and the large majority of recorded cases therefore have occurred in children or younger adults who received radiation during childhood. This has been recorded after radiation therapy for intracranial primary tumors, usually PNET, ependymoma, or high-grade astrocytoma, but also occasionally for pituitary adenomas or craniopharyngiomas; after prophylactic craniospinal radiation in children with leukemia; and after radiation for head and neck malignancies. In addition, cohorts of children treated with low doses of radiation for tinea capitis had a high incidence of subsequent meningiomas. *Very often the radiation-induced meningiomas are both multiple and individually atypical and aggressive. Both of these features make treatment of the patients difficult, as such patients are prone to recurrences of individual tumors and may need multiple craniotomies to address tumor at different sites.* Histologically, there is nothing distinctive about these radiation-associated tumors other than the high proportion with high mitotic rates or other atypical features.

Meningiomas in Neurofibromatosis Type 2

As mentioned in the discussion of nerve sheath tumors in children with NF-2, meningiomas are another characteristic neoplasm of this syndrome. The tumors may be isolated or multiple, and frequently coexist as clinical problems with the schwannomas, which otherwise are typical of this genetic disorder.

Hemangioblastomas (and von Hippel-Lindau Disease)

Hemangioblastoma is another tumor that is more common in adults than in children but is associated with a genetic syndrome that may lead to a presentation within the pediatric age range. These are tumors with an almost unique gross anatomy; they are usually not dural-based but occur within the leptomeninges, and so remain sharply encapsulated from adjacent brain tissues. The tumors most often are cystic, with one large cyst with a solid mural nodule being the most classical representation, and they occur frequently in the cerebellum, where their appearance might, by MRI or CT, be confused with pilocytic astrocytoma. At surgery, however, the vascular nature of the neoplasm is usually readily apparent.

Histologically, these are tumors with a mixture of two components: a capillary proliferation, with numerous small capillary-size vessels with a single layer of plump endothelial cells lining them, and a "stromal" component between the vessels (Fig. 5–29). Individual tumors may have a more prominent vascular component, with the stromal cells inconspicuous (Fig. 5–29A), or may have a more prominent stromal component, with the vascular component sometimes requiring special techniques to demonstrate its true abundance (Fig. 5–29B). Some tumors vary between these poles from area to area in the same neoplasm.

The nature of the stromal cell remains uncertain after many years of interest. In general, the cells resemble foamy histiocytes or macrophages, albeit often with larger and more pleomorphic nuclei. They may have immunostain characteristics of histiocytes, including HAM56 immunoreactivity. (HAM56 is an antibody that marks all or most macrophage/histiocytic cells and endothelial cells.) Earlier studies had suggested the possibility of a glial origin, with GFAP immunostaining, but

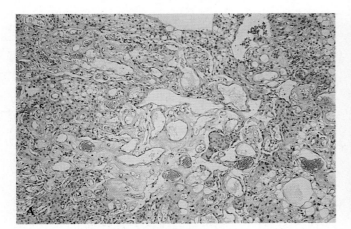 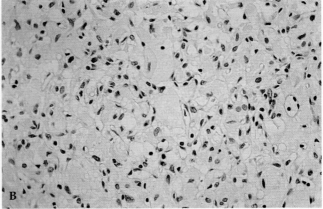

Figure 5–29 Hemangioblastomas. (A) A portion of a hemangioblastoma with a rich capillary component and relatively inconspicuous stromal cells (H&E, 25×). (B) Other portions of hemangioblastomas are composed of prominent stromal cells, and the vascular component is less conspicuous (H&E, 100×).

this is now thought of as either artifact or as phagocytosis of some glial filaments by the stromal cells. The stromal cells do not have immunoreactivity with antibodies to endothelial markers that simultaneously are positive in the vascular cells. They may show immunoreactivity for neuronal markers, and a neuronal origin has recently been suggested (Zagzag, personal communication). Electron microscopy of the stromal cells has not provided evidence to favor any hypothesis regarding a particular lineage. The question is probably more than academic because it is now thought that the stromal cell is the true neoplastic cell in hemangioblastomas: it synthesizes and secretes vascular endothelial growth factor, which presumably drives the capillary proliferation in the tumor, and it is these cells that are deficient in the von Hippel–Lindau gene product in hemangioblastomas.[300] (This reverses the presumptions from 20 or more years ago that these were vascular tumors and the stromal cells were probably a peculiar reactive population.)

Many examples of hemangioblastoma are apparently sporadic, but a substantial minority occur in the setting of von Hippel–Lindau disease, a genetic disorder in which patients have multiple CNS hemangioblastomas, retinal vascular tumors, and renal tumors, including renal cell carcinoma. As the histologic pattern of hemangioblastoma can be confused with that of renal cell carcinoma, it is occasionally crucial to identify whether a given CNS mass in a patient with von Hippel–Lindau disease is a new hemangioblastoma or is a metastasis from a renal cell carcinoma. The carcinomas express cytokeratins and EMA, which hemangioblastomas do not, so that this differential diagnostic problem can be solved with immunostaining. In any event, the development of renal cell carcinoma in the setting of von Hippel–Lindau disease almost always occurs late in the disease, in adults, and not in children.

METASTATIC CANCER IN THE CNS OF CHILDREN

Primary CNS tumors predominate in childhood, and metastatic disease in the nervous system from non-CNS primary sites is uncommon. Nevertheless, it does occur. Principal neoplastic conditions that secondarily involve the CNS include leukemia, non-Hodgkin's lymphoma (rarely, if ever, Hodgkin's disease, as noted previously), neuroblastoma, Ewing's sarcoma, and osteogenic sarcoma.[303] There are recorded cases of other soft-tissue sarcomas, of Wilms' tumor, hepatoblastoma, gonadal germ cell tumors, and melanoma. These tumors may affect the CNS by causing spinal epidural compression, intradural extra-axial mass growth (spinal or cranial), leptomeningeal dissemination (mostly lymphoma and leukemia), or direct intraparenchymal infiltration. The distinctive pathologic pictures presented by the different kinds of metastatic tumor are outside of the scope of this chapter.

SUMMARY

Most primary CNS neoplasms in children are malignancies, though many are low grade and the relative frequencies with which individual CNS tumors are seen differ dramatically in pediatric patients compared with adults. The diversity of histologic appearances is also greater in pediatric examples. Less is known about the underlying genetic and epigenetic molecular abnormalities fundamental to pediatric brain tumors than is known about their adult counterparts. This is now an area of fruitful and intense research. Correct and precise pathologic classification of CNS neoplasms remains the single most important prognostic indicator available, however imprecise or imperfect it may be. Major differences in therapy result from different pathologic diagnoses for tumors in identical sites, with identical clinical presentations, and with similar or identical imaging characteristics.

REFERENCES

1. Burger PC, Scheithauer BW, Vogel FS. *Surgical Pathology of the Nervous System and Its Coverings.* 3rd ed. New York: Churchill Livingstone; 1991.
2. Bigner DD, McLendon RE, Bruner JM, eds. *Russell and Rubinstein's Pathology of Tumors of the Nervous System.* 6th ed. London: Arnold; 1998.
3. Kleihues P, Burger PC, Scheithauer BW. *Histological Typing of Tumours of the Central Nervous System. World Health Organization International Histological Classification of Tumours.* Berlin: Springer-Verlag; 1993.
3A. Kleihues P, Cavenee WP. *Pathology and Genetics of Tumors of the Nervous System. World Health Organization Classification of Tumors.* Lyon: IARC Press; 2000.
4. Burger PC, Scheithauer BW. *Tumors of the Central Nervous System. Atlas of Tumor Pathology,* Third Series, Fascicle 10. Washington, DC: Armed Forces Institute of Pathology; 1993.
5. Divisions of Neuropathology at Brigham and Women's Hospital and Children's Hospital, Boston. Neuropathology. In: Black PM, Loeffler JS. *Cancer of the Nervous System.* Cambridge, MA: Blackwell Scientific; 1997:25–53.
6. Hassoun J, Gambarelli D, Grisoli F, *et al.* Central neurocytoma. An electron microscopic study of two cases. *Acta Neuropathol (Berl)* 1982;56:151–156.
7. Figarella-Branger D, Pellissier JF, Daumas-Duport C, *et al.* Central neurocytomas: critical evaluation of a small-cell neuronal tumor. *Am J Surg Pathol* 1992;16:97–109.
8. Hassoun J, Soylemezoglu F, Gambarelli D, *et al.* Central neurocytoma. A synopsis of clinical and histological features. *Brain Pathol* 1993;3:297–306.
9. Kepes JJ, Rubinstein LJ, Eng LF. Pleomorphic xanthoastrocytoma. A distinctive meningocerebral glioma of young subjects with relatively favorable prognosis. A study of 12 cases. *Cancer* 1979;44:1839–1852.
10. Kepes JJ, Rubinstein LJ, Ansbacher L, Schreiber DJ. Histopathological features of recurrent pleomorphic xanthoastrocytomas: further corroboration of the glial nature of this neoplasm. A study of 3 cases. *Acta Neuropathol (Berl)* 1989;78:585–593.
11. Kros JM, Vecht CJ, Stefanko SZ. The pleomorphic xantho-astrocytoma and its differential diagnosis. A study of five cases. *Hum Pathol* 1991;22:1128–1135.
12. Daumas-Duport C, Scheithauer BW, Chodkiewicz J-P, *et al.* Dysembryoplastic neuroepithelial tumor: a surgically

curable tumor of young patients with intractable partial seizures: report of thirty-nine cases. *Neurosurgery* 1988;23:545–556.

13. Daumas-Duport C. Dysembryoplastic neuroepithelial tumours. *Brain Pathol* 1993;3:283–295.

14. Hirose T, Scheithauer BW, Lopes BS, VandenBerg SR. Dysembryoplastic neuroepithelial tumor (DNT). An immunohistochemical and ultrastructural study. *J Neuropathol Exp Neurol* 1994;53:184–195.

15. Taratuto AL, Pomata H, Sevlever G, *et al*. Dysembryoplastic neuroepithelial tumor: morphological, immunocytochemical and deoxyribonucleic acid analyses in a pediatric series. *Neurosurgery* 1995;36:474–481.

16. Taratuto AL, Monges J, Lylyk P, Leiguarda R. Superficial cerebral astrocytoma attached to dura: report of six cases in infants. *Cancer* 1984;54:2505–2512.

17. VandenBerg SR, May EE, Rubinstein LJ, *et al*. Desmoplastic supratentorial neuroepithelial tumors of infancy with divergent differentiation potential ("desmoplastic infantile gangliogliomas"). *J Neurosurg* 1987;66:58–71.

18. Kawano N, Yada K, Aihara M, Yagishita S. Oligodendroglioma-like cells (clear cells) in ependymoma. *Acta Neuropathol (Berl)* 1983;62:141–144.

19. Miller DC, Kim R, Zagzag D. Neurocytoma: nonclassical sites and mixed elements. *J Neuropathol Exp Neurol* 1992;51:364 [abstr].

20. Miller DC, Lang FF, Epstein FJ. Central nervous system gangliogliomas. Part 1: Pathology. *J Neurosurg* 1993;79:859–866.

21. Min KW, Cashman RE, Brumback RA. Glioneurocytoma: tumor with glial and neuronal differentiation. *J Child Neurol* 1995;10:219–226.

22. Mrak RE. Malignant neurocytic tumor. *Hum Pathol* 1994;25:747–752.

23. Giangaspero F, Cenacchi G, Losi L, *et al*. Extraventricular neoplasms with neurocytoma features. A clinicopathological study of 11 cases. *Am J Surg Pathol* 1997;21:206–212.

24. Rorke LB, Gilles FH, Davis RL, Becker LE. Revision of the World Health Organization classification of brain tumors for childhood brain tumors. *Cancer* 1985;56:1869–1886.

25. Gilles FH, Winston K, Leviton A, Fulchiero A. Histologic features and observational variation in cerebellar gliomas. *J Natl Cancer Inst* 1977;58:175–181.

26. Leviton A, Fulchiero A, Gilles FH, Winston K. Survival status of children with cerebellar gliomas. *J Neurosurg* 1978;48:29–33.

27. Winston K, Gilles FH, Leviton A, Fulchiero A. Cerebellar gliomas in children: clinical considerations and a proposed classification. *J Natl Cancer Inst* 1977;58:833–838.

28. Gilles FH, Leviton AL, Hedley-Whyte ET, Jasnow M. Childhood brain tumor update. *Hum Pathol* 1983;14:834–845.

29. Gilles FH, Sobel EL, Leviton A, *et al*. Quantitative histologic factors for grouping childhood supratentorial neuroglial tumors. *Pediatr Pathol Lab Med* 1997;17:729–754.

30. Sobel EL, Gilles FH, Leviton A, *et al*. Survival of children with infratentorial neuroglial tumors. The Childhood Brain Tumor Consortium. *Neurosurgery* 1996;39:45–54.

31. Gilles FH, Sobel El, Leviton A, *et al*. Quantitative histologic factors for grouping childhood infratentorial neuroglial tumors. *Pediatr Pathol Lab Med* 1997;17:809–834.

32. Packer RJ, Allen J, Nielsen S, *et al*. Brainstem glioma: clinical manifestations of meningeal gliomatosis. *Ann Neurol* 1983;14:177–182.

33. Salazar OM. A better understanding of CNS seeding and a brighter outlook for postoperatively irradiated patients with ependymomas. *Int J Radiat Oncol Biol Phys* 1983;9:1231–1234.

34. Scherer HJ. Cerebral astrocytomas and their derivatives. *Am J Cancer* 1940;40:159–198.

35. Scherer HJ. Structural development in gliomas. *Am J Cancer* 1938;34:333–351.

36. Scherer HJ. The forms of growth in gliomas and their practical significance. *Brain* 1940;63:1–35.

37. Kernohan JW, Mabon RF, Svien HJ, Adson AW. A simplified classification of the gliomas. *Proc Staff Meet Mayo Clin* 1949;24:71–75.

38. Kernohan JW, Sayre GP. *Tumors of the Central Nervous System. Atlas of Tumor Pathology*, Section X, Fascicle 35. Washington, DC: Armed Forces Institute of Pathology; 1952.

39. Ringertz N. Grading of gliomas. *Acta Pathol Microbiol Scand* 1950;27:51–64.

40. Burger PC, Green SB. Patient age, histologic features, and length of survival in patients with glioblastoma multiforme. *Cancer* 1987;59:1617–1625.

41. Burger PC, Vogel SF, Green SB, Strike TA. Glioblastoma multiforme and anaplastic astrocytoma: pathologic criteria and prognostic implications. *Cancer* 1985;56:1106–1111.

42. Nelson DF, Nelson JS, Davis DR, *et al*. Survival and prognosis of patients with astrocytoma with atypical or anaplastic features. *J Neuro-oncol* 1985;3:99–103.

43. Nelson JS, Tsukada Y, Schonfeld D, *et al*. Necrosis as a prognostic criterion in malignant supratentorial, astrocytic gliomas. *Cancer* 1983;52:550–554.

44. Daumas-Duport C, Scheithauer BW, O'Fallon J, Kelly P. Grading of astrocytomas. A simple and reproducible method. *Cancer* 1988;62:2152–2165.

45. McCormack BM, Miller DC, Budzilovich GN, *et al*. Treatment and survival of low-grade astrocytoma in adults—1977–1988. *Neurosurgery* 1992;31:636–642.

46. Constantini S, Houten J, Miller DC, *et al*. Intramedullary spinal cord tumors in children under the age of three years. *J Neurosurg* 1996;85:1036–1043.

47. Miller DC, Rorke LB, Weinberg J, *et al*. Histopathologic diagnoses of intramedullary spinal cord tumors in children. *J Neuropathol Exp Neurol* 1997;56:607 [abstr].

48. Newcomb EW, Bhalla SK, Parrish CL, *et al*. bcl-2 protein expression in astrocytomas in relation to patient survival and *p53* gene status. *Acta Neuropathol (Berl)* 1997;94:369–375.

49. Giangaspero F, Burger PC. Correlations between cytologic composition and biologic behavior in glioblastoma multiforme. *Cancer* 1983;52:2320–2333.

50. Newcomb EW, Madonia WJ, Pisharody S, *et al*. A correlative study of *p53* protein alteration and *p53* gene mutation in glioblastoma multiforme. *Brain Pathol* 1993;3:229–235.

51. Lang FF, Miller DC, Pisharody S, *et al*. High frequency of *p53* protein accumulation without *p53* gene mutation in human juvenile pilocytic, low grade and anaplastic astrocytomas. *Oncogene* 1994;9:949–954.

52. Lang FF, Miller DC, Koslow M, Newcomb EW. Pathways leading to glioblastoma multiforme. A molecular analysis of genetic alterations in 65 astrocytic tumors representing WHO grades I-IV. *J Neurosurg* 1994;81:427–436.

53. Rao LS, Miller DC, Newcomb EW. *p16* gene inactivation in astrocytomas: correlation between *p16* gene deletion and *p16* immunohistochemistry. *Diagnostic Molec Pathol* 1997;6:115–122.

54. Newcomb EW, Cohen H, Lee SR, *et al*. Survival of patients with glioblastoma multiforme is not influenced by altered expression of *p16*, *p53*, *EGFR*, *MDM2* or *Bcl*-2 genes. *Brain Pathol* 1998;8:655–667.

55. Bogler O, Huang HJ, Kleihues P, Cavenee WK. The *p53* gene and its role in human brain tumors. *Glia* 1995;15:308–327.

56. Ohgaki H, Schauble B, zur Hausen A, *et al*. Genetic alterations associated with the evolution and progression of astrocytic brain tumors. *Virchows Arch* 1995;427:113–118.

57. Hayashi Y, Ueki K, Waha A, *et al*. Association of *EGFR* gene amplification and *CDKN2* (*p16/MTS1*) gene deletion in glioblastoma multiforme. *Brain Pathol* 1997;7:871–875.

58. Von Deimling A, von Ammon K, Schoenfeld D, *et al*. Subsets of glioblastoma multiforme defined by molecular genetic analysis. *Brain Pathol* 1993;3:19–26.

59. Biernat W. Kleihuyes P, Yonekawa Y, Ohgaki H. Amplification and overexpression of MDM2 in primary (*de novo*) glioblastomas. *J Neuropathol Exp Neurol* 1997;56:180–185.

60. Kleihues P, Burger PC, Plate KH, *et al*. Glioblastoma. In: Kleihues P, Cavenee WK, eds. *Pathology and Genetics of Tumours of the Nervous System*. Lyon: IARC Press; 1997: 16–24.

61. Tohma Y, Gratas C, Biernat W, *et al*. PTEN (MMAC1) mutations are frequent in primary glioblastomas (de novo) but not in secondary glioblastomas. *J Neuropathol Exp Neurol* 1998;57:684–689.

62. Von Deimling A, Louis DN, von Ammon K, *et al*. Association of epidermal growth factor receptor gene amplification with loss of chromosome 10 in human glioblastoma multiforme. *J Neurosurg* 1992;77:295–301.

63. Louis DN, Rubio M-P, Correa K, *et al*. Molecular genetic alterations in pediatric brain stem gliomas: application of PCR techniques to small and archival brain tumor specimens. *J Neuropathol Exp Neurol* 1993;52:507–515.

64. Pollack IF, Hamilton RI, Finkelstein SD, *et al*. The relationship between TP53 mutations and overexpression of *p53* and prognosis in malignant gliomas of childhood. *Cancer Res* 1997;57:304–309.

65. Rubinstein LJ. *Tumors of the Central Nervous System. Atlas of Tumor Pathology*, second series, Fascicle 6. Washington DC: Armed Forces Institute of Pathology; 1972.

66. Hayostek CJ, Shaw EG, Scheithauer B, *et al*. Astrocytomas of the cerebellum. A comparative clinicopathologic study of pilocytic and diffuse astrocytomas. *Cancer* 1993;72:856–869.

67. Gajjar A, Bhargava R, Jenkins JJ, *et al*. Low-grade astrocytoma with neuraxis dissemination at diagnosis. *J Neurosurg* 1995;83:67–71.

68. Mamelak AN, Prados MD, Obana WG, *et al*. Treatment options and prognosis for multicentric juvenile pilocytic astrocytoma. *J Neurosurg* 1994;81:24–30.

69. Mishima K, Nakamura M, Nakamura H, *et al*. Leptomeningeal dissemination of cerebellar pilocytic astrocytoma. Case report. *J Neurosurg* 1992;77:788–791.

70. Pollack IF, Hurtt M, Pang D, Albright AL. Dissemination of low grade intracranial astrocytomas in children. *Cancer* 1994;73:2869–2878.

71. Willert JR, Daneshvar L, Sheffield VC, Cogen PH. Deletion of chromosome arm 17p DNA sequences in pediatric high grade and juvenile pilocytic astrocytomas. *Genes Chromosomes Cancer* 1995;12:165–172.

72. Kepes JJ, Kepes M, Slowik F. Fibrous xanthomas and xanthosarcomas of the meninges and the brain. *Acta Neuropathol (Berl)* 1973;23:187–199.

73. Lindboe CF, Cappelen J, Kepes JJ. Pleiomorphic xanthoastrocytoma as a component of a cerebellar ganglioglioma: case report. *Neurosurgery* 1992;31:353–355.

74. Glasser R, Rojiani AM, Mickle JP, Eskin TA. Delayed occurrence of cerebellar pleomorphic xanthoastrocytoma after supratentorial pleomorphic xanthoastrocytoma removal. Case report. *J Neurosurg* 1995;82:116–118.

75. Powell SZ, Yachnis AT, Rorke LB, *et al*. Divergent differentiation in pleomorphic xanthoastrocytoma: evidence for a neuronal element and possible relation to ganglion cell tumors. *Am J Surg Pathol* 1996;20:80–85.

76. Allegranza A, Ferraresi S, Bruzzone M, Giombini S. Cerebromeningothelial pleomorphic xanthoastrocytoma. Report on four cases: clinical, radiologic, and pathological features. (Including a case with malignant evolution.) *Neurosurg Rev* 1991;14:43–49.

77. Macauley RJB, Jay V, Hoffman HJ, Becker LE. Increased mitotic activity as a negative prognostic indicator in pleomorphic xanthoastrocytoma. Case report. *J Neurosurg* 1993;79:761–768.

78. Weldon-Linne CM, Victor TA, Groothuis DR, Vick NA. Pleomorphic xanthoastrocytoma: ultrastructural and immunohistochemical study of a case with a rapidly fatal outcome following surgery. *Cancer* 1983;52:2055–2063.

79. Papahill PA, Ramsay DA, Del Maestro RF. Pleomorphic xanthoastrocytoma. A case report and analysis of the literature concerning the efficacy of resection and the significance of necrosis. *Neurosurgery* 1996;38:822–828.

80. Rosenblum MK, Erlandson RA, Budzilovich GN. The lipid-rich epithelioid glioblastoma. *Am J Surg Pathol* 1991; 15:925–934.

81. Friede RL. Gliofibroma. A peculiar neoplasm of collagen forming glia-like cells. *J Neuropathol Exp Neurol* 1978;38:300–3313.

82. Cerdas-Nicolas M, Kepes JJ. Gliofibromas (including malignant forms) and gliosarcomas: comparative study and review of the literature. *Acta Neuropathol (Berl)* 1993; 85:349–361.

83. Reinhardt V, Nahser HCh. Gliofibroma originating from temporoparietal hamartoma-like lesions. *Clin Neuropathol* 1984;3:131–138.

84. Vazquez M, Miller DC, Epstein F, *et al*. Glioneurofibroma: renaming the pediatric "gliofibroma." A neoplasm composed of Schwann cells and astrocytes. *Mod Pathol* 1991;4:519–523.

85. Budka H, Sunder-Plassman M. Benign mixed glial-mesenchymal tumour ("gliofibroma") of the spinal cord. *Acta Neurochir* 1980;55:141–145.

86. Iglesias JR, Richardson EP, Collia F, *et al*. Prenatal intramedullary gliofibroma. A light and electron microscope study. *Acta Neuropathol (Berl)* 1984;62:230–234.

87. Berger MS, Wilson CB. Extent of resection and outcome for cerebral hemispheric gliomas. In: Berger MS, Wilson CB, eds. *The Gliomas*. Philadelphia: WB Saunders; 1999:660–679.

88. Setty SN, Miller DC, Camras L, *et al*. Desmoplastic infantile astrocytoma with metastases at presentation. *Mod Pathol* 1997;10:945–951.

89. Bailey P, Cushing H. *A Classification of Tumors of the Glioma Group on a Histogenetic Basis with a Correlation Study of Prognosis*. Philadelphia: JB Lippincott; 1926.

90. Bailey P, Bucy PC. Oligodendrogliomas of the brain. *J Pathol Bacteriol* 1929;32:735–751.

91. Reifenberger G, Kros JM, Schiffer D, Collins VP. Oligodendroglioma. In: Kleihues P, Cavenee WK, eds. *Pathology and Genetics of Tumours of the Nervous System*, Lyon: IARC Press; 1997:38–42.

92. Min KW, Scheithauer BW. Clear cell ependymoma, a mimic of oligodendroglioma: clinicopathologic and ultrastructural considerations. *Am J Surg Pathol* 1997; 21:820–826.

93. Razack N, Baumgartner J, Bruner J. Pediatric oligodendrogliomas. *Pediatr Neurosurg* 1998;28:121–129.

94. Dehghani F, Schachenmayr W, Laun A, Korf HW. Prognostic implication of histopathological and clinical features of oligodendrogliomas. A study of 89 cases. *Acta Neuropathol (Berl)* 1998;95:493–504.

95. Heegard S, Sommer HM, Broholm H, Broendstrup O. Proliferating cell nuclear antigen and Ki-67 immunohistochemistry of oligodendrogliomas with special reference to prognosis. *Cancer* 1995;76:1809–1813.

96. Coons SW, Johnson PC, Pearl DK. The prognostic significance of Ki-67 labeling indices for oligodendrogliomas. *Neurosurgery* 1997;41:878–884.

97. Wharton SB, Hamilton FA, Chan WK, Chan KK, Anderson JR. Proliferation and cell death in oligodendrogliomas. *Neuropathol Appl Neurobiol* 1998;24:21–28.

98. Daumas-Duport C, Varlet P, Tucker ML, *et al*. Oligodendrogliomas. Part I: Patterns of growth, histological diagnosis, clinical and imaging correlations: a study of 153 cases. *J Neuro-oncol* 1997;34:37–59.

99. Daumas-Duport C, Tucker ML, Kolles H, *et al*. Oligodendorgliomas. Part II: A new grading system based on morphological and imaging criteria. *J Neuro-oncol* 1997;34:61–78.

100. Bello MJ, Leone PE, Vaquero J, *et al*. Allelic loss at 1p and 19q frequently occurs in association and may represent early oncogenic events in oligodendroglial tumors. *Int J Cancer* 1995;64:207–210.

101. Kraus JA, Koopman J, Kaskel P, *et al*. Shared allelic losses on chromosomes 1p and 19q suggest a common origin of oligodendroglioma and oligoastrocytoma. *J Neuropathol Exp Neurol* 1995;54:91–95.

102. Reifenberger J, Reifenberger G, Liu L, *et al*. Molecular genetic analysis of oligodendroglial tumors shows preferential allelic deletions on 19q and 1p. *Am J Pathol* 1994;145:1175–1190.

103. Von Deimling A, Louis DN, von Ammon K, *et al*. Evidence for a tumor suppressor gene on chromosome 19q associated with human astrocytomas, oligodendrogliomas, and mixed gliomas. *Cancer Res* 1992;52: 4277–4279.

104. Cairncross JG, Ueki K, Zlatescu M, *et al*. Specific genetic predictors of chemotherapeutic response and survival in patients with anaplastic oligodendrogliomas. *J Natl Cancer Inst* 1998;90:1473–1479.

105. Reifenberger J, Reifenberger G, Ichimura K, *et al*. Epidermal growth factor receptor expression in oligodendroglial tumors. *Am J Pathol* 1996;149:29–35.

106. Polednak AP, Flannery JT. Histology of cancer incidence and prognosis: SEER population-based data, 1973–1987. Brain, other central nervous system, and eye cancer. *Cancer* 1994;75:330–337.

107. Ringertz H, Reymond A. Ependymomas and choroid plexus papillomas. *J Neuropathol Exp Neurol* 1949; 8:355–380.

108. Kricheff II, Becker M, Schneck SA, Taveras JM. Intracranial ependymomas: factors influencing prognosis. *J Neurosurg* 1964;21:7–14.

109. Barone BM, Elvidge AR. Ependymomas. A clinical survey. *J Neurosurg* 1970;33:428–438.

110. Fokes EC Jr, Earle KM. Ependymomas: clinical and pathological aspects. *J Neurosurg* 1969;30:585–594.

111. Mørk SJ, Løken AC. Ependymoma. A follow-up study of 101 cases. *Cancer* 1977;40:907–915.

112. Pierre-Kahn A, Hirsch JF, Roux FX, *et al*. Intracranial ependymomas in childhood: survival and functional results of 47 cases. *Child's Brain* 1983;10:145–156.

113. Ross GW, Rubinstein LJ. Lack of histopathological correlation of malignant ependymomas with postoperative survival. *J Neurosurg* 1989;70:31–36.

114. Reyes-Mugica M, Chou PM, Myint MM, *et al*. Tomita T. Ependymomas in children: histologic and DNA-flow cytometric study. *Pediatr Pathol* 1994;14:453–466.

115. Miller DC, Li H, Zeltzer P, *et al*. No correlation of anaplastic histologic features with prognosis of pediatric ependymomas [abstract]. *J Neuropathol Exp Neurol* 1997;56:607.

116. Kawano N, Yada K, Yagashita S. Clear cell ependymoma. A histologic variant with diagnostic implications. *Virchows Arch A,* 1989;415:467–472.

117. Miller DC, Rorke LB, Weinberg J, *et al*. Histopathologic diagnoses of intramedullary spinal cord tumors in children [abstract]. *J Neuropathol Exp Neurol* 1997;56:607.

118. Courville CB. Ganglioglioma. Tumor of the central nervous system: review of the literature and report of two cases. *Arch Neurol Psychiatr* 1930;24:439–491.

119. Miller DC, Koslow MK, Budzilovich GN, Burstein DE. Synaptophysin. A sensitive and specific marker for ganglion cells in central nervous system neoplasms. *Hum Pathol* 1990;21:271–276.

120. Wolf HK, Muller MB, Spandle M, *et al*. Ganglioma. A detailed histopathological and immunocytochemical analysis of 61 cases. *Acta Neuropathol* (Berl) 1994;88: 166–173.

121. Lang FF, Epstein FJ, Ransohoff J, *et al*. Central nervous system gangliogliomas, II: Clinical Outcome. *J Neurosurg* 1993;79:867–873.

122. Diepholder HM, Schwechheimer K, Mohadjer M, *et al*. A clinicopathologic and immunomorphologic study of 13 cases of ganglioglioma. *Cancer* 1991;68:2192–2201.

123. Isimbaldi G, Sironi M, Tonnarelli GP, *et al*. Ganglioglioma. A clinical and pathological study of 12 cases. *Clin Neuropathol* 1996;15:192–199.

124. Jaffey PB, Mundt AJ, Baunoch DA, *et al*. The clinical significance of extracellular matrix in gangliogliomas. *J Neuropathol Exp Neurol* 1996;55:1246–1252.

125. Büttner A, Bavbek B, Winkler PA, *et al*. Ganglioglioma. A clinicopathological study of 10 cases. *Neuropathology* 1997;17:94–100.

126. Hirose T, Scheitauer BW, Lopes MBS, *et al*. Ganglioglioma. An ultrastructural and immunohistochemical study. *Cancer* 1997;79:989–1003.

127. Zhang PJ, Rosenblum MK. Synaptophysin expression in the human spinal cord: diagnostic implications of an immunohistochemical study. *Am J Surg Pathol* 1996;20: 273–276.

128. Quinn B. Synaptophysin staining in normal brain: importance for diagnosis of ganglioglioma. *Am J Surg Pathol* 1998;22:550–556.

129. Johannsson JH, Rekate HL, Roessman U. Ganglioglioma: pathological and clinical correlation. *J Neurosurg* 1981;54:58–63.

130. Russell DS, Rubinstein LJ. Ganglioglioma. A case with a long history and malignant evolution. *J Neuropathol Exp Neurol* 1962;21:185–193.

131. Kitano M, Takayama S, Nagao T, *et al*. Malignant ganglioglioma of the spinal cord. *Acta Pathol Jpn* 1987; 37:1009–1018.

132. Rodewald L, Miller DC, Sciorra L, *et al*. Brief clinical report: central nervous system neoplasm in a young man with Martin–Bell syndrome—fra(X)-XLMR. *Am J Med Genet* 1987;26:7–12.

133. Zhu JJ, Leon Sp, Folkerth RD, *et al*. Evidence for clonal origin of neoplastic neuronal and glial cells in gangliogliomas. *Am J Pathol* 1997;151:565–571.

134. VandenBerg SR. Desmoplastic infantile ganglioglioma and desmoplastic cerebral astrocytoma of infancy. *Brain Pathol* 1993;3:275–281.

135. Martin DS, Levy B, Awwad EE, Pittman T. Desmoplastic infantile ganglioglioma: CT and MRI features. *Am J Neuroradiol* 1991;1195–1197.

136. Ng THK, Fung CF, Ma LT. The pathological spectrum of desmoplastic infantile gangliogliomas. *Histopathology* 1990;16:235–241.

137. Paulus W, Schlote W, Perentes E, *et al*. Desmoplastic supratentorial neuroepithelial tumors of infancy. *Histopathology* 1992;21:43–49.

138. Ishida Y, Tamura M. Desmoplastic ganglioglioma. *Brain Tumor Pathol* 1991;8:79–83.

139. Kuchelmeister K, Bergmann M, von Wild K, *et al*. Desmoplastic ganglioglioma: report of two noninfantile cases. *Acta Neuropathol (Berl)* 1993;85:199–204.

140. Galatioto S, Gullotta F. Desmoplastic non-infantile ganglioglioma. *J Neurol Sci* 1996;40:235–238.

141. Horvath E, Kovacs K, Scheithauer BW, *et al*. Pituitary adenoma with neuronal choristoma (PANCH): composite lesion or lineage infidelity? *Ultrastruct Pathol* 1994;18:565–574.

142. Willis RA. *The Borderland of Embryology and Pathology*. 2nd ed. Washington, DC: Butterworths; 1962.

143. Marano SR, Johnson PC, Spetzler RF. Recurrent Lhermitte-Duclos disease in a child: case report. *J Neurosurg* 1988;69:599–603.

144. Banerjee Ak, Gleadhill CA. Lhermitte-Duclos disease (diffuse cerebellar hypertrophy): prolonged post-operative survival. *Irish J Med Sci* 1979;148:97–99.

145. Stapleton SR, Wilkins PR, Bell BA. Recurrent dysplastic cerebellar gangliocytoma (Lhermitte-Duclos disease) presenting with subarachnoid haemorrhage. *Br J Neurosurg* 1992;6:153–156.

146. Ahdevaara P, Kalimo H, Törmä T, Haltia M. Differentiating intracerebral neuroblastoma: report of a case and review of the literature. *Cancer* 1977;40:784–788.

147. Pearl GS, Takei Y, Bakay RAE, Davis P. Intraventricular primary cerebral neuroblastoma in adults: report of three cases. *Neurosurgery* 1985;16:847–849.

148. Zülch, KJ. *Brain Tumors: Their Biology and Pathology*. 3rd ed. Berlin: Springer-Verlag; 1986.

149. Markwalder TM, Huber P, Markwalder RV, *et al*. Primary intraventricular oligodendrogliomas. *Surg Neurol* 1979;11:25–28.

150. Garza-Mercado R, Campa H, Grajeda J. Primary oligodendroglioma of the septum pellucidum. *Neurosurgery* 1987;21:78–80.

151. Miller DC, Kim R, Zagzag D. Neurocytomas: non-classical sites and mixed elements [abstract]. *J Neuropathol Exp Neurol* 1992;51:364.

152. von Deimling A, Janzer R, Kleihues P, Wiestler OD. Patterns of differentiation in central neurocytoma. An immunohistochemical study of eleven biopsies. *Acta Neuropathol (Berl)* 1990;79:473–479.

153. von Deimling A, Kleihues P, Saremaslani P, *et al*. Histogenesis and differentiation potential of central neurocytomas. *Lab Invest* 1991,64:585–591.

154. Westphal M, Stavrou D, Nausch H, *et al*. Human neurocytoma cells in culture show characteristics of astroglial differentiation. *J Neurosci Res* 1994;38:698–704.

155. Nishio S, Takeshita I, Fukui M. Primary cerebral ganglioneurocytoma in an adult. *Cancer* 1990;66:358–362.

156. Yasargil MG, von Ammon K, von Deimling A, *et al*. Central neurocytoma: histopathologic variants and therapeutic approaches. *J Neurosurg* 1992;76:32–37.

157. Eng DY, DeMonte F, Ginsberg L, *et al*. Craniospinal dissemination of central neurocytoma: report of two cases. *J Neurosurg* 1997;86:547–552.

158. Min KW, Cashman RE, Brumback RA. Glioneurocytoma: tumor with glial and neuronal differentiation. *J Child Neurol* 1995;10:219–226.

159. Miller DC, Zhang P. How do we define oligodendrogliomas? An immunohistological study [abstract]. *Brain Pathol* 1994;4:427.

160. Miller DC. New Perspectives on neuronal neoplasms. *Brain Pathol* 1997;7:1139–1140.

160A. Teo JGC, Gultekin H, Bilsky M, Gutin P, Rosenblum MK. A distinctive glioneuronal tumor of the adult cerebrum with neuropil-like (including "rosetted") islands. *Am J Surg Pathol* 1999;23:502–510.

161. Ng H-K, Ko HCW, Tse CCH. Immunohistochemical and ultrastructural studies of oligodendrogliomas revealed features of neuronal differentiation. *Int J Surg Pathol* 1994;2:47–56.

162. Nishio S, Takeshita I, Kaneko Y, Fukui M. Cerebral neurocytoma. A new subset of benign neuronal tumors of the cerebrum. *Cancer* 1992;70:529–537.

163. Giangaspero F, Cenacchi G, Losi L, e*et al*. Extraventricular neoplasms with neurocytoma features. A clinicopathological study of 11 cases. *Am J Surg Pathol* 1997;21: 206–212.

164. Leung SY, Gwi E, Ng HK, *et al*. Dysembryoplastic neuroepithelial tumor. A tumor with small neuronal cells

resembling oligodendroglioma. *Am J Surg Pathol* 1994; 18:604–614.

165. Figarella-Branger D, Soylemezoglu F, Kleihues P, Hassoun J. Central neurocytoma. In: Kleihues P, Cavenee WK, eds. *Pathology and Genetics of Tumours of the Nervous System*. Lyon: IARC Press; 1997:77–79.

166. Ellison DW, Zygmunt SC, Weller RO. Neurocytoma/ lipoma (neurolipocytoma) of the cerebellum. *Neuropathol Appl Neurobiol* 1993;19:95–98.

167. Giangaspero F, Cenacchi G, Roncaroli F, *et al*. Medullocytoma (lipidized medulloblastoma). A cerebellar neoplasm of adults with favorable prognosis. *Am J Surg Pathol* 1996;20:656–664.

168. Bechtel JT, Patton JM, Takei Y. Mixed mesenchymal and neuroectodermal tumor of the cerebellum. *Acta Neuropathol (Berl)* 1978;41:261–263.

169. Chimelli L, Hahn MD, Budka H. Lipomatous differentiation in a medulloblastoma. *Acta Neuropathol (Berl)* 1991;81:471–473.

170. Burger PC. Gliomas: pathology. In: Wilkins RH, Rengachary SS, eds. Neurosurgery. New York: McGraw-Hill; 1985:553–563.

171. Cairncross JG. Oligodendrogliomas and mixed gliomas. In: Black PM, Loeffler JS, eds. *Cancer of the Nervous System*. Cambridge, MA: Blackwell Scientific; 1997:549–557.

172. Kros JM, Van Eden CG, Stefanko SZ, *et al*. Prognostic implications of glial fibrillary acidic protein containing cell types in oligodendrogliomas. *Cancer* 1990;66: 1204–1212.

173. Feigin IM, Gross SW. Sarcoma arising in glioblastoma of the brain. *Am J Pathol* 1955;31:633–653.

174. Feigin IM, Allen LB, Lopkin L, Gross SW. The endothelial hyperplasia of the cerebral blood vessels, and its sarcomatous transformation. *Cancer* 1958;11:264–277.

175. Biernat W, Aguzzi A, Sure U, *et al*. Identical mutations of the *p53* tumor suppressor gene in the glial and sarcomatous part of gliosarcomas suggest a common origin from glial cells. *J Neuropathol Exp Neurol* 1995;54: 651–656.

176. Young Rh, Kleinman GM, Scully RE. Glioma of the uterus. *Am J Surg Pathol* 1981;5:695–699.

177. Biernat W, Hegi M, Aguzzi A, Kleihues P. Gliosarcoma. In: Kleihues P, Cavenee WK, eds. Pathology and Genetics of Tumours of the Nervous System. Lyon: IARC Press; 1997:27–28.

178. Hart MN, Earle KM. Primitive neuroectodermal tumors of the brain in children. *Cancer* 1973;32:890–897.

179. Rorke LB. The cerebellar medulloblastoma and its relationship to primitive neuroectodermal tumors. *J Neuropathol Exp Neurol* 1983;42:1–15.

180. Rubinstein LJ. A commentary on the proposed revision of the World Health Organization classification of brain tumors for childhood brain tumors. *Cancer* 1985;56: 1887–1888.

181. Becker L, Hinton D. Primitive neuroectodermal tumors of the central nervous system. *Hum Pathol* 1983;14:538–550.

182. Rorke LB, Trojanowski JQ, Lee VMY, *et al*. Primitive neuroectodermal tumors of the central nervous system. *Brain Pathol* 1997;7:765–784.

183. Rorke LB, Hart MN. Supratentorial PNET. In: Kleihues P, Cavenee WK, eds. *Pathology and Genetics of Tumours of the Nervous System*. Lyon: IARC Press; 1997:108–109.

184. Shimada H, Brodeur GM. Tumors of peripheral neuroblasts and ganglion cells. In: Bigner DD, McLendon RE, Bruner JM, eds. *Russell and Rubinstein's Pathology of Tumours of the Nervous System*. 6th ed. London: Arnold; 1998:493–533.

185. Biegel JA, Rorke LB, Janss AJ, *et al*. Isochrome 17q demonstrated by interphase fluorescence in situ hybridization in primitive neuroectodermal tumors of the central nervous system. *Genes Chromosomes Cancer* 1995;14:85–96.

186. Zu Rhein GM, Varakis JN. Perinatal induction of medulloblastomas in Syrian golden hamsters by a human polyoma virus (JC). *Natl Cancer Inst Monogr* 1979;51:205–208.

187. Matsuda M, Yasui K, Nagashima K, Mori W. Origins of the medulloblastoma experimentally induced by human polyoma virus JC. *J Natl Cancer Inst* 1987; 79:585–591.

188. Eibl RH, Kleihues P, Jat PS, Wiestler OD. A model for primitive neuroectodermal tumors in transgenic neural transplants harboring the SV40 large T antigen. *Am J Pathol* 1994;144:556–564.

189. Fung K, Trojanowski J. Animal models of medulloblastomas and related primitive neuroectodermal tumors. A review. *J Neuropathol Exp Neurol* 1995;54:285–296.

190. Bergsagel DJ, Finegold MJ, Butel JS, *et al*. DNA sequences similar to those of simian virus 40 in ependymomas and choroid plexus tumors of childhood. *N Engl J Med* 1992;326:988–993.

191. Lednicky JA, Garcea RL, Bergsagel DJ, Butel SJ. Natural simian virus 40 strains are present in human choroid plexus and ependymoma tumors. *Virology* 1995;212:710–717.

191A. Huang H, Reis R, Yonekawa Y, *et al*. Identification in human brain tumors of DNA sequences specific for SV40 large T antigen. *Brain Pathol* 1999;9:33–44.

191B. Krynska B, Del Valle L, Croul S, *et al*. Detection of human neurotropic JC virus DNA sequence and expression of viral oncogenic protein in pediatric medulloblastomas. *Proc Natl Acad Sci USA* 1999;96:11519–11524.

192. Katsetos CD, Liu HM, Zacks SI. Immunohistochemical and ultrastructural observations on Homer Wright (neuroblastic rosettes) and the "pale islands" of human cerebellar medulloblastomas. *Hum Pathol* 1988;19:1219–1227.

193. Katsetos CD, Krishna L, Frankfurter A, *et al*. A cytomorphological scheme of differentiating neuronal phenotypes in cerebellar medulloblastomas based on immunolocalization of class III β-tubulin isotype (βIII) and proliferating cell nuclear antigen (PCNA)/cyclin. *Clin Neuropathol* 1995;14:72–80.

194. Gould VE, Jansson DS, Molenaar WM, *et al*. Primitive neuroectodermal tumors of the central nervous system: patterns of expression of neuroendocrine markers, and all classes of intermediate filament proteins. *Lab Invest* 1990;62:498–509.

195. Perentes E, Rubinstein LJ, Herman MM, Donoso LA. S-antigen immunoreactivity on human pineal glands and pineal parenchymal tumors. A monoclonal antibody study. *Acta Neuropathol (Berl)* 1986;71:224–227.

196. Korf H-W, Czerwionka M, Reiner J, *et al*. Immunocytochemical evidence of molecular photoreceptor markers in cerebellar medulloblastomas. *Cancer* 1987;60: 1763–1766.

197. Bonnin JM, Perentes E. Retinal S-antigen immunoreactivity in medulloblastomas. *Acta Neuropathol (Berl)* 1988;76:204–207.
198. Jaffey PB, To GT, Xu H-J, *et al*. Retinoblastoma-like phenotype expressed in medulloblastomas. *J Neuropathol Exp Neurol* 1995;54:664–672.
199. Rubinstein LJ, Northfield DWC. The medulloblastoma and the so-called "arachnoidal cerebellar sarcoma." A critical re-examination of a nosological problem. *Brain* 1964;87:379–412.
200. Burger PC, Grahmann FC, Bliestle A, Kleihues P. Differentiation in the cerebellar medulloblastoma. A histological and immunohistochemical study. *Acta Neuropathol (Berl)* 1987;73:115–123.
201. Katsetos CD, Burger PC. Medulloblastoma. *Semin Diagn Pathol* 1994;11:85–97.
202. Rubinstein LJ. The definition of the ependymoblastoma. *Arch Pathol* 1970;90:35–45.
203. Marinesco G, Goldstein M. Sur une forme anatomique, non encore decrite, de medulloblastome: medullomyoblastome. *Ann Anat Pathol* 1933;10:513–525.
204. Smith TW, Davidson RI. Medullomyoblastoma. A histologic, immunohistochemical, and ultrastructural study. *Cancer* 1984;54:323–332.
205. Giordana MT, Wiestler OD. Medullomyoblastoma. In: Kleihues P, Cavenee WK, eds. *Pathology and Genetics of Tumours of the Nervous System.* Lyon: IARC Press; 1997: 104–105.
206. Taratuto AL, Molina HA, Diez B, *et al*.Primary rhabdomyosarcoma of the brain and cerebellum. Report of four cases in infants: an immunohistochemical study. *Acta Neuropathol (Berl)* 1985;66:98–104.
207. Schmidbauer M, Budka H, Pilz P. Neuroepithelial and ectomesenchymal differentiation in a primitive pineal tumor ("pineal anlage tumor"). *Clin Neuropathol* 1989; 8:7–10.
208. Raisanen J, Vogel H, Horoupian DS. Primitive pineal tumor with retinoblastomatous and retinal/ciliary epithelial differentiation. An immunohistochemical study. *J Neuro-Oncol* 1990;9:165–179.
209. Weeks DA, Beckwith JB, Mierau GW, Luckey DW. Rhabdoid tumor of kidney. A report of 111 cases from the National Wilms' Tumor Study Pathology Center. *Am J Surg Pathol* 1989;13:439–458.
210. Sotelo-Avila C, Gonzalez-Crussi F, DeMello D, *et al*. Renal and extrarenal rhabdoid tumors in children. A clinicopathological study of 14 patients. *Semin Diagn Pathol* 1986;3:151–163.
211. Parham DM, Weeks DA, Beckwith JB. The clinicopathologic spectrum of putative extrarenal rhabdoid tumors. *Am J Surg Pathol* 1994;18:1010–1029.
212. Weeks DA Jr, Beckwith JB, Mierau GW. Rhabdoid tumor: an entity or a phenotype? *Arch Pathol Lab Med* 1989;113:113–114.
213. Bonnin JM, Rubinstein LJ, Palmer NF, Beckwith JB. The association of embryonal tumors originating in the kidney and in the brain. A report of seven cases. *Cancer* 1984;54:2137–2146.
214. Briner J, Bannwart F, Kleihues P, *et al*. Malignant small cell tumor of the brain with intermediate filaments—a case of primary cerebral rhabdoid tumor. *Pediatr Pathol* 1985;3:117–118.
215. Biegel JA, Rorke LB, Packer RJ, Emanuel BS. Monosomy 22 in rhabdoid or atypical teratoid tumors of the brain. *Neurosurgery* 1990;73:710–714.
216. Rorke LB, Packer RJ, Biergel JA. Central nervous system atypical teratoid/rhabdoid tumors of infancy and childhood: definition of an entity. *J Neurosurg* 1996;85: 56–65.
217. Burger PC, Yu IT, Tihan T, *et al*. Atypical teratoid/rhabdoid tumor of the central nervous system. A highly malignant tumor of infancy and childhood frequently mistaken for medulloblastoma. A Pediatric Oncology Group study. *Am J Surg Pathol* 1998;22:1083–1092.
218. Bhattarcharjee M, Hicks J, Langford L, *et al*. Central nervous system atypical teratoid/rhabdoid tumors of infancy and childhood. *Ultrastruct Pathol* 1997;21: 369–378.
219. Rorke LB. Atypical teratoid/rhabdoid tumours. In: Kleihues P, Cavenee WK, eds. *Pathology and Genetics of Tumours of the Nervous System.* Lyon: IARC Press; 1997: 110–111.
220. Biegel JA, Allen CS, Kawasaki K, *et al*. Narrowing the critical region for a rhabdoid tumor locus in 22q11. *Genes Chromosomes Cancer* 1996;16:94–105.
221. Giangaspero F, Rigobello L, Badiali M, *et al*. Large-cell medulloblastomas. A distinct variant with highly aggressive behavior. *Am J Surg Pathol* 1992;16:687–693.
222. Miller DC, Rezai A, Frempong-Boadu A, Lee M. Levels and pattern of differentiation in PNET with clinical correlation [abstract]. *J Neuropathol Exp Neurol* 1995; 54:423.
223. Packer RJ, Sutton LN, Rorke LB, *et al*. Prognostic importance of cellular differentiation in medulloblastoma of childhood. *J Neurosurg* 1984;61:296–301.
224. Caputy AJ, McCullough DC, Manz HJ, *et al*. A review of the factors influencing the prognosis of medulloblastoma: the importance of cell differentiation. *J Neurosurg* 1987;66:80–87.
225. Goldberg-Stern H, Gadoth N, Stern N, *et al*. The prognostic significance of glial fibrillary acidic protein staining in medulloblastoma. *Cancer* 1991;68:568–573.
226. Janss AJ, Yachnis AT, Silber JH, *et al*. Glial differentiation predicts poor clinical outcome in primitive neuroectodermal tumors. *Ann Neurol* 1996;39:481–489.
227. Rosenblum MK, Ng HK. Germ cell tumours. In: Kleihues P, Cavenee WK, eds. *Pathology and Genetics of Tumours of the Nervous System.* Lyon: IARC Press; 1997: 164–169.
228. Jennings MT, Gelman R, Hochberg FH. Intracranial germ cell tumors: natural history and pathogenesis. *J Neurosurg* 1985;63:155–167.
229. Freilich RJ, Thompson SJ, Walker RW, Rosenblum MK. Adenocarcinomatous transformation of intracranial germ cell tumors. *Am J Surg Pathol* 1995;19:537–544.
230. Scully RE. *Tumors of the Ovary and Maldeveloped Gonads. Atlas of Tumor Pathology*, Second Series, Fascicle 16. Washington, DC: Armed Forces Institute of Pathology; 1979.
231. Hochberg FH, Miller DC. Primary central nervous system lymphoma. *J Neurosurg* 1988;68:835–853.
232. Eby NL, Grufferman S, Flannelly CM, *et al*. Increasing incidence of primary brain lymphoma in the US. *Cancer* 1988;62:2461–2465.

233. O'Sullivan MG, Whittle IR, Gregor A, Ironside JW. Increasing incidence of CNS primary lymphoma in south-east Scotland. *Lancet* 1991;338:895–896.

234. Adams JH, Howatson AG. Cerebral lymphomas. A review of 70 cases. *J Clin Pathol* 1990;43:544–547.

235. Murphy JK, O'Brien CJ, Ironside JW. Morphologic and immunophenotypic characterisation of primary brain lymphomas using paraffin-embedded tissue. *Histopathology* 1989;15:449–460.

236. De Angelis LM. Primary central nervous system lymphoma: a new clinical challenge. *Neurology* 1991;41: 619–621.

237. Miller DC, Hochberg FH, Harris NL, et al. Pathology with clinical correlations of primary CNS lymphoma: the Massachusetts General Hospital experience 1958–1989. *Cancer* 1994;74:1383–1397.

238. Miller DC, Najjar S, Budzilovich GN. Neuropathology of AIDS in surgical biopsies. *Neurosurg Clin North Am* 1994;5:57–70.

239. Miller DC, Knee R, Schonfeld S, et al. Non-Hodgkin's lymphoma of the central nervous system after treatment of Hodgkin's disease. *Am J Clin Pathol* 1989;91: 481–485.

240. Rock JP, Cher L, Hochberg FH, Rosenblum ML. Central nervous system lymphoma in AIDS and non-AIDS patients. In: Black PM, Loeffler JS, eds. *Cancer of the Nervous System.* Cambridge, MA: Blackwell Scientific; 1997;593–606.

241. Herbert J, Cavallaro T, Dwork A. A marker for primary choroid plexus neoplasms. *Am J Pathol* 1990;136: 1317–1325.

242. Albrecht S, Rouah E, Becker LE, Bruner J. Transthyretin immunoreactivity in choroid plexus neoplasms and brain metastases. *Mod Pathol* 1991;4:610–614.

243. Brinster RL, Chen HY, Messing A, et al. Transgenic mice harboring SV40 T-antigen genes develop characteristic brain tumors. *Cell* 1984;37:367–379.

244. Van Dyke TA, Finlay C, Miller DC, et al. The relationship between Simian virus 40 large tumor antigen expression and tumor formation in transgenic mice. *J Virol* 1987;61:2029–2032.

245. Marks J, Lin J, Miller DC, et al. The expression of viral and cellular genes in papillomas of the choroid plexus induced in transgenic mice. In: *Cellular Factors in Development and Differentiation: Embryos, Teratocarcinomas, and Differentiated Tissues.* New York: Alan R. Liss; 1988:163–186.

246. Rushing EJ, Armonda RA, Ansari Q, Mena H. Mesenchymal chondrosarcoma. A clinicopathologic and flow cytometric study of 13 cases presenting in the central nervous system. *Cancer* 1996;77:1884–1891.

247. Adamson TE, Wiestler OD, Kleihues P, Yasargil MG. Correlation of clinical and pathological features in surgically treated craniopharyngiomas. *J Neurosurg* 1990;73:12–17.

248. Giangaspero F, Burger PC, Osborne DR, Stein RB. Suprasellar papillary squamous epithelioma ("papillary craniopharyngioma"). *Am J Surg Pathol* 1984;8: 57–64.

249. Crotty T, Scheithauer BW, Young WF Jr, et al. Papillary craniopharyngioma. A clinicopathological study of 48 cases. *J Neurosurg* 1995;83:206–214.

250. Miller DC. Pathology of craniopharyngiomas: clinical import of pathologic findings. *Pediatr Neurosurg* 1994;21 (Suppl 1): 11–17.

251. Weiner HL, Rosenberg ME, Wisoff JH, et al. Craniopharyngiomas. A clinico-pathological analysis of factors predictive of recurrence and functional outcome. *Neurosurgery* 1994;35:1001–1011.

252. Miller DC. Histopathologic evaluation of pituitary tumors: help for the clinician. In: Cooper PR, ed. *Diagnosis and Management of Pituitary Adenomas.* Park Ridge, IL: American Association of Neurological Surgeons, 1991:37–45.

253. Hsu DW, Hakim F, Biller BMK, et al. Significance of proliferating cell nuclear antigen index in predicting pituitary adenoma recurrence. *J Neurosurg* 1993;78: 753–761.

254. Pernicone PJ, Scheithauer BW, Sebo TJ, et al. Pituitary carcinoma. A clinicopathologic study of 15 cases. *Cancer* 1997;79:804–812.

255. MacCollin M, Woodfin W, Kronn D, Short MP. Schwannomatosis. A clinical and pathologic study. *Neurology* 1996;46:1072–1079.

256. Louis DN, Wiestler OD. Neurofibromatosis type 2. In: Kleihues P, Cavenee WK, eds. *Pathology and Genetics of Tumours of the Nervous System.* Lyon: IARC Press; 1997: 175–178.

257. Hajjaj M, Linthicum FH Jr. Facial nerve schwannoma: nerve fibre dissemination. *J Laryngol Otol* 1996;110: 632–633.

258. Louis DN, Edgerton S, Thor AD, Hedley-Whyte ET. Proliferating cell nuclear antigen and Ki-67 immunohistochemistry in brain tumors: a comparative study. *Acta Neuropathol (Berl)* 1991;81:675–679.

259. Carney JA. Psammomatous melanotic schwannoma. A distinctive, heritable tumor with special associations, including cardiac myxoma and the Cushing syndrome. *Am J Surg Pathol* 1990;14:206–222.

260. Woodruff JM, Marshall ML, Godwin TA, et al. Plexiform (multinodular) schwannoma. A tumor simulating the plexiform neurofibroma. *Am J Surg Pathol* 1983;7: 691–697.

261. Fletcher CD, Davies SE. Benign plexiform (multinodular) schwannoma. A rare tumor unassociated with neurofibromatosis. *Histopathology* 1986;10:971–980.

262. Kleinman GM, Sanders FJ, Gagliardi JM. Plexiform schwannoma. *Clin Neuropathol* 1985;4:265–266.

263. Woodruff JM, Christensen WN. Glandular peripheral nerve sheath tumors. *Cancer* 1993;72:3618–3628.

264. Ashley DJB. Neurilemmoma. *Evans' Histologic Appearances of Tumors.* 3rd ed. Edinburgh: Churchill Livingstone, 1978:482–485.

265. Harkin JC, Reed RJ. *Tumors of the Peripheral Nervous System. Atlas of Tumor Pathology.* Second Series, Fascicle 3. Washington, DC: Armed Forces Institute of Pathology; 1968.

266. Stewart FW, Copeland MM. Neurogenic sarcoma. *Am J Cancer* 1931;15:1235–1320.

267. Woodruff JM, Selig AM, Crowley K, Allen PW. schwannoma (neurilemmoma) with malignant transformation. A rare, distinctive peripheral nerve tumor. *Am J Surg Pathol* 1994;18:882–895.

268. Robson DK, Ironside JW. Malignant peripheral nerve sheath tumor arising in a schwannoma. *Histopathology* 1990;16:295–297.
269. Yousem SA, Colby TV, Urich H. Malignant epitheliod schwannoma arising in a benign schwannoma. A case report. *Cancer* 1985;55:2799–2803.
270. Woodruff JM, Godwin TA, Erlandson RA, *et al.* Cellular schwannoma. A variety of schwannoma sometimes mistaken for a malignant tumor. *Am J Surg Pathol* 1981;5:733–744.
271. White W, Shiu MH, Rosenblum MK, *et al.* Cellular schwannoma. A clinicopathologic study of 57 patients and 58 tumors. *Cancer* 1990;66:1266–1275.
272. Casadei GP, Scheithauer BW, Hirose T, *et al.* Cellular schwannoma. A clinicopathologic, DNA flow cytometric, and proliferation marker study of 70 patients. *Cancer* 1995;75:1109–1119.
273. Muhlbauer MS, Clark WC, Robertson JH, *et al.* Malignant nerve sheath tumor of the facial nerve: case report and discussion. *Neurosurgery* 1987;21:68–73.
274. Kindblom LG, Ahlden M, Meis-Kindblom JM, Stenman G. Immunohistochemical and molecular analysis of *p53*, MDM2, proliferating cell nuclear antigen, and Ki67 in benign and malignant peripheral nerve sheath tumours. *Virchows Arch* 1995;427:19–26.
275. Miracco C, Montesco MC, Santopietro R, *et al.* Proliferative activity, angiogenesis, and necrosis in peripheral nerve sheath tumors. A quantitative evaluation for prognosis. *Mod Pathol* 1996;9:1108–1117.
276. Trojanowski JQ, Kleinman GM, Proppe KH. Malignant tumors of nerve sheath origin. *Cancer* 1980;46:1202–1212.
277. Tsang W, Chan J, Chow L, Tse C. Perineurioma. An uncommon soft tissue neoplasm distinct from localized hypertrophic neuropathy and neurofibroma. *Am J Surg Pathol* 1992;16:756–763.
278. Bilbao J, Khoury N, Hudson A, Briggs S. Perineurioma (localized hypertrophic neuropathy). *Arch Pathol Lab Med* 1984;108:557–560.
279. Tranmer B, Bilbao J, Hudson A. Perineurioma. A benign peripheral nerve tumor. *Neurosurgery* 1986;19:134–138.
280. Emory TS, Scheithauer BW, Hirose T, *et al.* Intraneural perineurioma. A clonal neoplasm associated with abnormalities of chromosome 22. *Am J Clin Pathol* 1995;103:696–704.
281. Paulus W, Jellinger K, Perneczky G. Intraspinal neurothekeoma (nerve sheath myxoma). A report of two cases. *Am J Clin Pathol* 1991;95:511–516.
282. Kershisnik M, Callender DL, Batsakis JG. Extracranial, extraspinal meningiomas of the head and neck (review). *Ann Otol Rhinol Laryngol* 1993;102:967–970.
283. Wilson AJ, Ratliff JL, Lagios MD, Aguilar MJ. Mediastinal meningioma. *Am J Surg Pathol* 1979;3:557–562.
284. Kemnitz P, Spormann H, Heinrich P. Meningioma of lung: first report with light and electron microscopic findings. *Ultrastruct Pathol* 1982;3:359–365.
285. Kaleem Z, Fitzpatrick MM, Ritter JH. Primary pulmonary meningioma: report of a case and review of the literature. *Arch Pathol Lab Med* 1997;121:631–636.
286. Miller DC, Ojemann RG, Proppe KH, *et al.* Benign metastasizing meningioma. A case report and review of the literature. *J Neurosurg* 1985;62:763–766.
287. Sunder-Plassman M, Jellinger K, Kraus H, Rengele H. Intraventriculäre Meningeome im Kindesalter. *Neurochirurgia* 1971;14:54–63.
288. Markwalder TM, Seiler RW, Markwalder RV, *et al.* Meningioma of the third ventricle in a child. *Surg Neurol* 1979;12:29–32.
289. Kandel EI, Filatov YM. Clinical picture and surgical treatment of meningiomas of the lateral ventricle. In: deVet AC, ed. *Proceedings of the Third International Congress of Neurological Surgery.* Copenhagen, 1965; 719–723.
290. Dandy WE. *Benign, Encapsulated Tumors in the Lateral Ventricles of the Brain: Diagnosis and Treatment.* Baltimore: Williams and Wilkins; 1934.
291. Cushing H, Eisenhardt L. *Meningiomas, Their Classification, Regional Behavior, Life History, and End Surgical Results.* Springfield, IL: Charles C Thomas; 1938.
292. Kepes JJ. *Meningiomas: Biology, Pathology, and Differential Diagnosis.* New York: Masson; 1982.
293. Masson P. *Tumeurs Humaines. Histologie Diagnostic et Ethniques.* 2nd ed. Paris: Maloîne; 1968:980.
294. Kleinman GM, Liszcak T, Tarlov E, Richardson EP Jr. Microcystic variant of meningioma. A light-microscopic and ultrastructural study. *Am J Surg Pathol* 1980;4:383–389.
295. De la Monte SM, Flickinger J, Linggood RM. Histopathologic features predicting recurrence of meningiomas following subtotal resection. *Am J Surg Pathol* 1986;10:836–843.
296. Miller DC. Predicting recurrence of intracranial meningiomas: a multivariate clinicopathologic model. An interim report of the New York University Medical Center Meningioma Project. *Neurosurg Clin North Am* 1994;5:193–200.
297. Hsu DW, Pardo FS, Efird JT, *et al.* Prognostic significance of proliferative indices in meningiomas. *J Neuropathol Exp Neurol* 1994;53:247–255.
298. Hsu DW, Efird JT, Hedley-Whyte ET. Progesterone and estrogen receptors in meningiomas: prognostic considerations. *J Neurosurg* 1997;86:113–120.
299. Zorludemir S, Scheithauer BW, Hirose T, *et al.* Clear cell meningioma. A clinicopathologic study of a potentially aggressive variant of meningioma. *Am J Surg Pathol* 1995;19:493–505.
300. Ludwin SK, Rubinstein LJ, Russell DS. Papillary meningioma. A malignant variant of meningioma. *Cancer* 1975;36:1363–1373.
301. Budka H. Non-glial specificities of immunocytochemistry for the glial fibrillary acidic protein (GFAP): triple expression of GFAP, vimentin, and cytokeratins in papillary meningioma and metastasizing renal cell carcinoma. *Acta Neuropathol (Berl)* 1986;72:43–54.
302. Vortmeyer AO, Gnarra JR, Emmert-Buck MR, *et al.* von Hippel-Lindau gene deletion detected in the stromal cell component of a cerebellar hemangioblastoma associated with von Hippel-Lindau disease. *Hum Pathol* 1997;28:540–543.
303. Bouffet E, Doumi N, Thiesse P, *et al.* Brain metastases in children with solid tumors. *Cancer* 1997;79:403–410.

Chapter 6

Anesthetic Considerations

Irene Osborn and Margaret Ekstein

The pediatric neurosurgery patient presents an interesting challenge for the anesthesiologist. One must address the anesthetic considerations for a neurosurgical patient but tailor them to the physiologic and psychological needs of a child. In addition to providing anesthesia for surgery, it is important to allay the fears of the child and parents before that time. Current neuroanesthetic practice is based on our understanding of cerebral physiology and how it can be altered to benefit the patient with intracranial pathologic lesions. From preoperative assessment through postoperative pain management, the anesthesiologist can play an important role in the hospital experience. This chapter will review the anesthetic management of pediatric patients for tumor surgery as well as considerations for diagnostic procedures.

PEDIATRIC NEUROANATOMY AND PHYSIOLOGY

The pediatric brain and central nervous system (CNS) is the largest and fastest developing organ in the body. The neonatal brain at term weighs approximately 335 g and comprises 15 to 20% of total body weight. This more than doubles within the first year. By the age of 2 years, it has reached 80% of the adult weight. The protection afforded the pediatric brain differs from the adult in that the bony skull is incomplete and the skull is pliable.[1] Suture lines, bridged by fibrous connective tissue, are relatively difficult to separate and cannot compensate for acute increases in intracranial volume. Following closure of all cranial sutures, the skull forms a rigid box that contains the neural axis, which is composed of neuronal parenchyma, cerebrospinal fluid, and blood volume. Volume pressure interactions between these three components determine intracranial pressure (ICP). Uncontrolled increases in ICP constitute one of the most serious problems in management, and efforts to control ICP are fundamental.[2]

Cerebral blood flow (CBF) and cerebral metabolic rate ($CMRO_2$) are low in the newborn. In infants older than 6 months and children up to adolescence, CBF values of 90 to 100 mL/100 gm per minute and $CMRO_2$ of 4.5 to 5.0 mL/100 gm per minute have been observed. These values are higher than those reported for normal adults. CBF normally is controlled by the arterial pressure of carbon dioxide ($PaCO_2$), cerebral lactate, and, to a lesser extent, arterial oxygenation. The cere-

bral vasculature of the term newborn and premature infant appears to be more sensitive to the effects of arterial oxygenation.[3] In older children, CBF increases rapidly if arterial oxygenation falls below 50 mm Hg.

Critical CBF below which cerebral function deteriorates ranges between 15 and 20 mL/100 gm per minute. Irreversible structural damage occurs below levels of 10 mL/100 g per minute. This value is lower than the critical level reported for adults. Autoregulation denotes the ability of the brain to maintain CBF at a constant rate over a wide range of perfusion pressures. In newborns and infants, autoregulation probably occurs at lower blood pressure ranges because the mean blood pressure is lower.[4] Maintenance of cerebral perfusion and control of ICP are two of the principal tasks of the neuroanesthetist. To this end, positioning, hyperventilation, and drug therapy are frequently utilized.

PREOPERATIVE ASSESSMENT

The preoperative evaluation of the child undergoing neurosurgery should include the following: (1) assessment of ICP, (2) assessment of respiratory and cardiovascular systems, and (3) evaluation of specific disturbances in the patient's neurologic function. Because many pediatric patients require multiple operations or invasive diagnostic procedures, it is important to establish a good relationship with the child and his or her family. Routine preoperative evaluation is necessary to exclude congenital or familial problems, such as bleeding disorders or malignant hyperthermia.

Some patients may have undergone previous chemotherapy or radiation therapy, which may result in cardiopulmonary abnormalities. Patients with minimal pulmonary reserve may require more vigorous postoperative pulmonary toilet (or prolonged intubation), and parents should be alerted to this possibility. *Although sometimes difficult to assess, gradual ICP increases in infants may be noted by a history of increased irritability, poor feeding, lethargy, and vomiting.* Bulging anterior fontanelles, dilated scalp veins, and motor deficits are also found. Older children may be lethargic and complain of nausea. The preoperative assessment will help the anesthetist prepare for surgery and tailor the induction and management to the patient's condition and pathology.[5]

PREMEDICATION

Although the use of premedication can facilitate the induction of anesthesia, this must be balanced against the risk of exaggerated CNS response. Any evidence of impaired mental function or somnolence should be a contraindication for sedatives. Sedative medication should be used judiciously in children undergoing intracranial surgery. Children with intracranial hypertension may appear well despite the complaint of headaches and vomiting. However, many of these children will have markedly raised ICP, and minor triggers such as sedation may cause difficulty. A decreased respiratory drive caused by most sedatives will increase carbon dioxide tension and hence increase ICP. *Children with intracranial pathologic lesions may be more sensitive to the usual doses of medications.*[6]

If there is no risk from sedation, the extremely anxious child (and his parents) will benefit from premedication. Many patients are afraid of painful procedures and separation from their parents. Others have bad memories of previous operating room visits. There are multiple modalities of premedication that encompass a variety of routes of administration. Agents include benzodiazepines, narcotics, or barbiturates; described routes of administration include oral, intravenous, intramuscular, rectal, and intranasal. Premedication should be administered sufficiently early that there is time for onset of effect. The most appropriate agents should be based on the child's age, general medical condition, and length of the operative procedure. The older child who is less afraid may benefit from the application of EMLA cream to the extremity area for a planned intravenous catheter placement.[7]

INDUCTION OF ANESTHESIA

Induction of anesthesia in pediatric patients with intracranial pathologic lesions presents a unique challenge for the anesthesiologist. Agitated, crying children are more likely to have stormy inductions (breath holding, laryngospasm, tachycardia, and hypertension) than quiet, sedated children. On the other hand, respiratory depression with increased pCO_2 can develop rapidly in patients with increased ICP. *A smooth induction without struggling is the goal, and central to this is rapid control of the airway and hyperventilation.* If an intravenous line is present and functioning, induction should proceed expediently after a pulse oximeter has been placed and oxygen is gently flowing over the child's face. Patients without intravenous access may be induced with a small butterfly catheter, which can often be placed with minimal patient stress or hemodynamic fluctuation. Failing this, a skillful mask induction may be performed, followed by intravenous line placement and progression of intravenous agents.[8]

Effects of Anesthetic Agents

As one of the primary goals of neuroanesthesia is to prevent dangerous increases in ICP, agents that decrease ICP, CBF, and metabolic rate should be chosen. Barbiturates are ideally suited for this purpose and are commonly used for intravenous induction of anesthesia and for (briefly) preventing responses to noxious stimulation.[9] Propofol, a newer intravenous agent, has found multiple uses in neuroanesthesia. It can be used for induction but also as a continuous infusion for maintenance of anesthesia. Its effects on ICP and CBF are similar to those of thiopental but emergence from propofol infusion is more rapid and produces less postoperative nausea. Propofol may lower arterial pressure and should be used with caution in patients with hypovolemia. Etomidate is rarely used in young children but does offer minimal cardiac depression and has cerebral protective effects.[10] Opioids such as fentanyl are also used because of their stable hemodynamic profile, their lack of effect on CBF and ICP, and their blunting of airway responses on intubation and emergence.[11] These synthetic opioids are tolerated in large doses without causing histamine release seen with morphine and demerol. Remifentanil, the newest synthetic opioid, is metabolized by plasma and tissue esterases (not by the liver) and has an extremely short half-life. It appears to have no effect on ICP in adult patients with brain tumors and may be useful for brief but painful procedures in pediatric patients.[12, 13]

Inhalation anesthetics are the mainstay of pediatric anesthesia. However, their known propensity to cause cerebral vasodilation makes them less desirable for neurosurgical anesthesia. However, hyperventilation can minimize the increase in CBF seen with halothane. Isoflurane reduces cerebral oxygen consumption, and, if hyperventilation is added, CBF decreases.[14] It has been the agent of choice for neuroanesthesia for more than 10 years. Two newer agents, desflurane and sevoflurane, are now used in the United States and allow a finer control of anesthetic depth and faster awakening. Desflurane is not a suitable agent for infants and children, as it tends to irritate the airways and produces coughing and laryngospasm.[15] Sevoflurane is not irritating to airways and has demonstrated advantages for inhalation induction.[16] It has also been shown to cause less increase in CBF than isoflurane while producing an equivalent decrease in $CMRO_2$.[17] It is used frequently for pediatric outpatient procedures, and more studies are needed to confirm its safety in more time-consuming procedures.

Endotracheal Intubation

Laryngoscopy and intubation cause intense sympathetic stimulation and are best performed when the child is deeply anesthetized and maximally oxygenated.[18, 19] For procedures involving the forehead or orbits, a preformed endotracheal tube (RAE) is useful because it allows a low profile for connection of the anesthetic circuit and is not easily dislodged. In children younger than 6 years, an uncuffed endotracheal tube should be used that allows an audible leak at 25 to 30 cm H_2O and avoids trauma to the subglottic area.[20] Some anesthetists prefer nasotracheal intubation for the patient in whom postoperative ventilation is expected or in small infants where the tube is better stabilized. When intubation is unexpectedly difficult, it is important to provide assistance if needed. Often the anesthetist must reposition the patient's head, change laryngoscope blades, or administer more anesthetic or relaxant to obtain a better view. Once intubation is established (and carbon dioxide confirmed on the capnograph), the endotracheal tube is secured and breath sounds osculated.

MONITORING

Routine monitoring of all pediatric neurosurgery patients should include a precordial or esophageal stethoscope, electrocardiography (ECG), pulse oximetry, noninvasive blood pressure measurement, and end-tidal carbon dioxide measurement. Most craniotomies and/or cases that involve potential blood loss should include arterial blood pressure monitoring. For volume replacement and monitoring, a central venous catheter is useful, particularly when there is risk of venous air embolism.[21] The intravascular volume of pediatric patients can be minuscule, demanding great expertise in gaining vascular access. This is best done by the most skilled clinician inserting large lines after the induction of anesthesia. Subclavian, external or internal jugular, and femoral lines can be placed but should not be used chronically due to their potential to cause infection and thrombosis. Care should be exercised with the neck lines so as not to compromise venous return from the brain. Urinary catheters or bags are required in time-consuming or complicated cases or when large volumes of urine cause fluid balance problems.

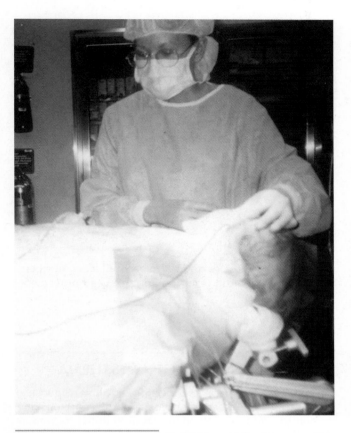

Figure 6–1 Patient in prone position with body covered by "forced-air" warmer. (Photo by I. Osborn.)

Esophageal or rectal temperature monitoring should be used at all times. Provisions to maintain the patient's body temperature include warming the operating room, keeping the patient covered as much as possible during induction and positioning, using radiant heat lamps, warming intravenous fluids and irrigating solutions[22] (Fig. 6–1).

PATIENT POSITIONING

Patient positioning varies in accordance with the location of the lesion and the planned procedure. It is carefully performed after induction and line placement. Elevation of the head by 15 to 30 degrees lowers ICP, but higher elevations may lead to a decrease in cardiac output and cerebral perfusion pressure. The endotracheal tube should be held carefully during positioning, and breath sounds should be rechecked before prepping begins. The eyes must be securely taped and protected, particularly if the patient is to be in the prone or sitting position, and extremities should be carefully padded. Some anesthesiologists advocate the use of nasal rather than oral endotracheal tubes in the prone position, based on their belief that nasal tubes are easier to secure.[23] During positioning of patients, it is important to know that movement of the head can result in kinking or displacement of the tube (Fig. 6–2).

BOX 6–2
Intraoperative Monitoring

- Oxygenation—pulse oximetry
- Ventilation—capnography, precordial/esophageal stethoscope
- Cardiac output—blood pressure, ECG
- Fluid status—urine output, central venous pressure
- Temperature—esophageal or rectal probe
- Muscle relaxation—nerve stimulator
- Neurophysiologic—EEG, evoked potentials

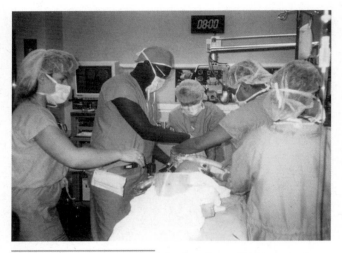

Figure 6–2 Patient positioning involves all team members, with special attention to vital signs and head movement. (Photo by I. Osborn.)

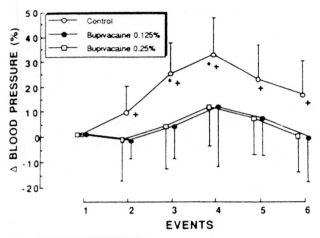

Figure 6–3 Mean percentage changes in arterial blood pressure (mm Hg) above levels before infiltration (baseline) up to the time of opening of the dura. Events: (1) before infiltration; (2) after scalp infiltration; (3) after scalp incision; (4) reflection of scalp flap; (5) craniotomy; (6) dural incision. *Statistically significant differences between control and bupivacaine groups ($p < 0.05$). Statistically significant differences within a group compared with the baseline of that group ($p < 0.05$). (Reproduced with permission from Hartley et al. Scalp infiltration with bupivacaine in pediatric brain surgery. *Anesth Analg* 1991;73:29.)

MAINTENANCE OF ANESTHESIA

The functions of general anesthesia are to blunt response to the surgical stimulus, render the patient unconscious and immobile, and ensure hemodynamic stability as well as optimal brain conditions for surgery. A technique should be selected that will offer a prompt and calm emergence from anesthesia once surgery is completed so that neurologic and follow-up exams can be performed. A combined anesthetic regimen, which utilizes a potent opioid, inhalational agents, and muscle relaxants, offers the advantages of each agent without the problems of large or prolonged doses of a single agent.[24]

Brief periods of painful stimulation and frequently longer periods of minimal pain or no sensation often characterize neurosurgery. *It is important for the patient to be adequately anesthetized during the following intraoperative events: laryngoscopy and intubation, application of pins, skin incision, opening of the dura, and closure of the wound. When scalp and periosteal nerve endings are stimulated, blood pressure (BP) and heart rate (HR) increase. These effects may endanger the patient, particularly in the presence of cerebrovascular anomalies, vascular tumors, or increased ICP.*[25] Additional opioid, thiopental, or propofol is given prior to these anticipated events.

Infiltrating the scalp with a local anesthetic to block nerve endings can prevent or diminish the hemodynamic response to pain.[26] Epinephrine is used to minimize scalp blood loss and will decrease intravascular uptake. Bupivacaine 0.125% with epinephrine 1:400,000 was demonstrated to be as effective as bupivacaine 0.25% with epinephrine 1:400,000 at reducing the hemodynamic response to craniotomy (Fig. 6–3). Because the lower concentration of bupivacaine produces lower blood levels, 0.125% bupivacaine is recommended as a useful, safe adjunct to general anesthesia in children undergoing craniotomy. This or a similar agent should be used whenever possible for wound infiltration prior to incision or closure.

FLUID MANAGEMENT

The purpose of fluid therapy is to maintain hemodynamic stability and tissue perfusion by providing an isovolemic, iso-osmolar, and relatively iso-oncotic intravascular volume. The patient's maintenance fluid requirement (Table 6–1), blood loss, third-space loss, and urine output govern the intraoperative administration of fluids. Balanced salt solutions, such as Ringer's lactate, are preferable to normal saline solution. Normal saline solution has a high chloride content and causes hyperchloremic acidosis, especially in infants.[27, 28] Blood loss during pediatric neurosurgery is often hard to estimate. The surgical drapes and floor may conceal substantial blood loss. Serial hematocrits are the most reliable method to ensure adequate intravascular volume. Normal blood volumes are 100 mL/kg in prematures, 90 mL/kg in newborns, 80 mL/kg in infants, and 70 mL/kg in older children. The lowest safe hematocrit value has not been determined for children; however, values between 30% and 40% in premature infants and newborns and between 20% and 30% in children older than 3 months are

TABLE 6–1 Estimating Pediatric Maintenance Fluid Requirements

Weight	Rate (mL/kg per hour)
For the first 10 kg	4
For the next 10–20 kg	2
For each kg above 20 kg	Add 1

used by most anesthesiologists.[29] Any surgical procedure with blood loss greater than 10% will most likely require a transfusion.

Blood glucose levels should be monitored in all patients having prolonged anesthesia, but neonates and infants are at particular risk. It should be remembered that normal levels for blood glucose are much lower in infants than adults, measuring 80 to 100 mg/dL in adults and only 30 to 40 mg/dL in newborns.[30]

INTRACRANIAL TUMORS

Patients usually receive dexamethasone to reduce swelling around the tumor. Furosemide or mannitol may be necessary to control brain bulk. Intravenous induction, hyperventilation, and a narcotic relaxant or low-dose volatile agent may be utilized. Occasionally, a very "tight" brain is encountered, which requires careful and cooperative management by the anesthesiologist and surgeon. It is important that ventilation be optimal and head position appropriate to facilitate venous drainage. The head of the table should be elevated 30 degrees if tolerated. Additional hyperventilation may be instituted, but one must avoid undue cerebral vasoconstriction (pCO_2 less than 25 to 28 mm Hg), which can lead to ischemia or shift blood flow.[31] Administration of barbiturate or propofol in carefully titrated doses can help to decrease CBF and ICP. It is also important to ensure that adequate muscle relaxation has been achieved.

BOX 6–3
Differential Diagnosis of the "Tight" Brain

- Hypercarbia
- Hypoxemia
- Venous outflow impeded
- Light anesthesia
- Hypertension
- Vasodilators
- Patient disease (mass effect)

Removal of posterior fossa tumors performed in the prone or sitting position requires additional considerations. *Although the use of the sitting position provides surgical advantages for suboccipital craniotomy, the threat of venous air embolism is a serious concern.* The incidence of air embolism in children (33%) is not significantly different from that of adults for this type of surgery.[21, 32] The incidence of hypotension with air entrainment is much greater in pediatric patients, perhaps because the volume of entrained air is larger relative to their cardiac volume. Manipulation of the brain stem may also result in cardiac arrhythmias, which require treatment or brief cessation of the procedure. Normal brain stem function should be ascertained prior to extubation (gag, cough, normal breathing pattern, vocal cord function).

POSTOPERATIVE CONCERNS

The anesthetic considerations for postoperative care are similar to those of any general-anesthetic situation. They include (1) oxygen and respiration, (2) maintenance of body temperature, and (3) analgesia. As with any postsurgical patient, supplemental oxygenation should be implemented and respiratory pattern and adequacy assessed. Hypothermic patients should be rewarmed. Abnormal hemodynamic signs (hypertension/bradycardia) should be carefully assessed. Hypotension may indicate inadequate fluid replacement, which should be corrected. Analgesics should be given judiciously and under close supervision in neurologically impaired patients. Generous use of local anesthetic skin infiltration at the time of surgery can reduce the requirement for postoperative analgesia. Patients without neurologic impairment before surgery can safely be given a routine postoperative pain regimen.[33]

ANESTHESIA FOR DIAGNOSTIC PROCEDURES

Over the past decade, anesthesiologists have increasingly been involved in providing sedation and assistance outside the operating room (Table 6–2). The existence of such remote

---

TABLE 6–2 Pediatric Sedation Agents for Magnetic Resonance Imaging

Agent	Dose	Comments
Chloral hydrate	75–100 mg/kg	Allow 15–20 min onset, best for infants up to 6 mo
Pentobarbital	5 mg/kg p.o.	Mix w. conc. Kool-Aid
Pentobarbital	2-3 mg/kg IV up to 9 mg/kg	Give slowly, sedation in 5–10 min
Ketamine	4–5 mg/kg IM	Fast onset, lasts 20–25 min
Ketamine	1 mg/kg IV, slowly in divided doses	Analgesia, secretions, good for asthmatics
Methohexital	25–30 mg/kg rectally	Onset 8–10 min, duration 25 min–1 h
Methohexital	1–2 mg/kg IV	Give slowly, watch for apnea, incremental doses or infusion
Midazolam	0.25–0.75 mg/kg	Use as premed/supplement, rarely sufficient for entire study
Propofol	2–3 mg/kg IV, dilute w. lidocaine, infusion 50–100 μg/kg/min	Painful injection, may cause repeat bolus or give infusion, most reliable agent

anesthetizing areas helps to avoid repeated trips to the operating room and perhaps helps to reduce medical costs. It is important that both the standard of care and the American Academy of Pediatrics guidelines for sedation[34] be maintained in these areas.

Lumbar Puncture/Bone Marrow Aspiration

Analgesia is an important component of management, along with sedation or amnesia, because the patient must remain still to avoid undue punctures or complications. These procedures may be performed in treatment rooms or in the postanesthesia care unit, while monitoring of blood pressure and pulse oximetry are carried out. A functioning access catheter is often available for the anxious child who must undergo this short, painful procedure. Ketamine was the mainstay of therapy for many years until propofol was introduced and became widely accepted for these procedures.[35] Ketamine is still used in smaller doses as a supplement to propofol. Fentanyl or other short-acting opioids may be used but may cause postoperative nausea. Older children may benefit from the use of EMLA cream applied to the area 1 hour in advance of the procedure.

Magnetic Resonance Imaging

Magnetic resonance imaging (MRI) is now the gold standard for diagnostic imaging and the modality of choice for diagnostic investigation. Although it is noninvasive and painless, a study requires immobility for at least a 20-minute period, which is difficult, if not impossible, for young children and infants (Fig. 6–4). Sedation or general anesthesia usually is required to render patients immobile throughout the scanning period. Anesthetic considerations for MRI include the hazards of working in a magnetic field that disables most monitoring equipment. In addition, some ferromagnetic objects (e.g., stethoscopes, clipboards) can become dangerous projectiles.[36] There are now a wide variety of MRI-compatible monitors and anesthesia machines available that function well within the equipment environment.

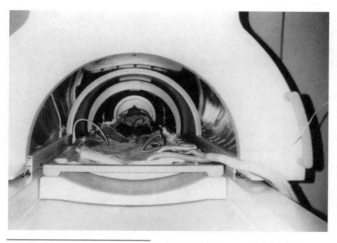

Figure 6–4 Anesthetized patient inside magnetic resonance imager. (Photo by Joseph Lee.)

The anesthetic technique depends on the patient's age, the presence of a functioning intravenous line, and the need for airway control.[37] The anesthetic employed will also depend on the equipment available (a machine and/or ventilator). As this is a painless study, unconsciousness is all that is required, and narcotics are not necessary. Once anesthetized, the patient is virtually inaccessible except by monitor or closed-circuit video image. Following the procedure, patients may be allowed to recover nearby in a monitored setting.[38]

CONCLUSIONS

The anesthesiologist caring for the pediatric neurosurgical patient plays an important role in the child's treatment and well-being. This is an opportunity to become known to the patient and his or her family as a professional who provides information as well as comfort. Understanding the physiologic process of the procedure and its management is essential. In addition, one's interaction with neurosurgeons, neurologists, pediatricians, and nursing staff is critical in promoting continued cooperation and understanding.

REFERENCES

1. Bissonette B, Armstrong DC, Rutka JT. Pediatric neuroanesthesia. In: Albin MS, ed. *Textbook of Neuroanesthesia*. New York: McGraw-Hill; 1997:1186–1187.
2. Shapiro K, Marmaron A. Mechanisms of intracranial hypertension in children. In: McLaurin RL, ed. *Pediatric Neurosurgery: Surgery of the Developing Nervous System*. New York: Grune and Stratton; 1982:255–264.
3. Lassen NA, Christensen MS. Physiology of cerebral blood flow. *Br J Anaesth* 1976;48:719.
4. Hollinger I. *Anesth Clin North Am* 1987;5:3.
5. Osborn IP. *Anesth Clin North Am* 1998;16:683.
6. Weldon BC, Watcha MF, White PF. Oral midazolam in children: effect of time and adjunctive therapy. *Anesthesiology* 1993;75:51.
7. Chang PC, Goresky GV, O'Connoe, et al. A multicenter, randomized study of single-unit dose package of EMLA patch vs. EMLA 5% cream for venipuncture in children. *Can J Anaesth* 1994;41:59.
8. Kleinman SE, Bissonnette B. *Anesth Clin North Am* 1992; 10:3.
9. Shapiro HM, Galindo A, Wyte SR, et al. Rapid intraoperative reduction of intracranial pressure with thiopentone. *Br J Anaesth* 1973;45:1057.
10. Pinaud M, Lebusque J, Chetanneau A, et al. Effects of propofol on cerebral hemodynamics and metabolism in patients with brain trauma. *Anesthesiology* 1990;73:404.
11. Jung R, et al. Cerebrospinal fluid pressures in anesthetized patients with brain tumors: impact of fentanyl vs. alfentanil. *J Neurosurg Anesthesiol* 1988;1:136.
12. Warner DS, Hindman BJ, Todd MM, et al. Intracranial pressure and hemodynamic effects of remifentanil versus alfentanil in patients undergoing supratentorial craniotomy. *Anesth Analg* 1996;83:279.

13. Guy J, Hindman BJ, Baler KZ, et al. Comparison of remifentanil and fantanyl in patients undergoing craniotomy for supratentorial space occupying lesions. *Anesthesiology* 1997;86:514.

14. Frost EAM. Inhalation anaesthetic agents in neurosurgery. *Br J Anaesth* 1984;56:S47–56.

15. Koenig HM. What's up with the new volatile anesthetics, desflurane and sevoflurane, for neurosurgical patients? *J Neurosurg Anesthesiol* 1994;6:229.

16. Black A, Sury MR, Hemington L, et al. A comparison of the induction characteristics of sevoflurane and halothane in children. *Anaesthesia* 1996;51:539.

17. Berkowitz RA, Hoffman WE, Cunningham F, McDonald T. Changes in cerebral blood flow in children during sevoflurane and halothane anesthesia. *J Neurosurg Anesthesiol* 1998;8:194.

18. Raju TNK, Vidyasgar D, Torres C, et al. Intracranial pressure during intubation and anesthesia in infants. *J. Pediatri* 1080;96:860.

19. Friesen RH, Honda AT, Thieme RE. Changes in anterior fontanelle pressure in pre-term neonates with intubation. *Anesth Analg* 1987;66:874.

20. Yemen TA. Pediatric neuroanesthesia. In Stone DJ, Sperry RJ, eds. *The Neuroanesthesia Handbook.* 2nd ed. St. Louis: Mosby; 1996:261.

21. Cucchiara RF, Bowers D. Air embolism in children undergoing suboccipital craniotomy. *Anesthesiology* 1982;57:338.

22. Bissonnette B. Temperature monitoring in pediatric anesthesia. *Int Anesthesiol Clin* 1992;30:63.

23. Pollard RJ, Mickle JP: Pediatric neuroanesthesia. In Cucchiara RF, Black S, eds. *Clinical Neuroanesthesia.* 2nd ed. New York: Churchill Livingstone; 1998.

24. Newfield P. Anesthesia for pediatric neurosurgery. In: Cottrell JE, Smith DS, eds. *Anesthesia and Neurosurgery.* 3rd ed. St. Louis: Mosby; 1994.

25. Hartley EJ, Bissonette B, St-Louis P, et al. Scalp infiltration with bupivacaine in pediatric brain surgery. *Anesth Analg* 1991;73:29.

26. Penfield W. Combined regional and general anesthesia for craniotomy and cortical exploration. *Int Anesth Clin* 1986;24:1.

27. Brown KA, Bissonnette B, MacDonald M, et al. Hyperkalemia during massive transfusion in paediatric craniofacial surgery. *Can J Anaesth* 1990;37:401.

28. Smith DS: Fluid management of the neurosurgical patient. *ASA Refresher Course Lecture* 1986;122:1–7.

29. Cote CJ. Blood, colloid and crystalloid therapy. *Anesth Clin North Am* 1991;9:865.

30. Seiber FE, Smith DS, Traystman RJ. Glucose: a reevaluation of its intraoperative use. *Anesthesiology* 1987;67:72.

31. Leon JE, Bissonette B. Cerebrovascular responses to carbon dioxide in children anesthetized with halothane and isoflurane. *Can J Anaesth* 1991;38:817.

32. Harris M, Yemen T, Strattford M. Venous air embolism during craniectomy in supine infants. *Anesthesiology* 1987;67:816.

33. Tobias JD, Rasmussen GE. Pain management and sedation in the pediatric intensive care unit. *Pediatr Clin North Am* 1994;41:1269.

34. American Academy of Pediatrics Committee on Drugs, Section on Anesthesiology. Guidelines for elective use of conscious sedation, deep sedation and general anesthesia in pediatric patients. *Pediatrics* 1992;89:110.

35. Martin LD, Pasternack LK, Pudimat MA. Total intravenous anesthesia with propofol in pediatric patients outside the operating room. *Anesth Analg* 1992;74:409.

36. Osborn IP, Tarricone S. Anesthesia for neurodiagnostic evaluation. In: Abrams KJ, Grange CM, eds. *Trauma Anesthesia and Critical Care of Neurological Injury.* Armonk: Futura Publishing; 1997:273–280.

37. Frankville DD, Spear RM, Dyk JB. The dose of propofol required to prevent children from moving during magnetic resonance imaging. *Anesthesiology* 1993;79:953.

38. Shellock FG. Guidelines for monitoring and care of children during and after sedation for imaging studies. *Am J Roentgenol* 1993;160:581.

Chapter 7

Critical Care Considerations

Edward E. Conway, Jr

Pediatric patients with tumors of the central nervous system (CNS) require admission to the pediatric intensive care unit (PICU) following surgery, and some may also be admitted prior to surgery for stabilization or for control of elevated intracranial pressure (ICP). Others may be admitted for tumor recurrence or for treatment of complications of therapy. Nonneurosurgical or nonneurologic conditions that may also be present in these patients and necessitate admission include respiratory failure, cardiovascular compromise, metabolic perturbations, hematologic disorders, and infectious processes.

Patients are admitted to the PICU for monitoring. Recent technologic developments, creation of ICUs dedicated exclusively to children, and specific subspecialty training in pediatric intensive care medicine have led to a marked improvement in the outcome for critically ill pediatric patients. Noninvasive monitoring has allowed for better, safer, and more reliable observation for our patients. It must be noted, however, that there is no substitute for a well-trained practitioner observing these patients at the bedside. Vital signs, including temperature, heart rate, respiratory rate, blood pressure, and pulse oximetry (dubbed the fifth vital sign by many), along with a careful neurologic exam either demonstrate the well being of the patient or serve as harbingers of adverse events. Practitioners should be familiar with the unique needs as well as the anatomical and physiologic characteristics of patients in the pediatric age range. It is in the PICU that the oft quoted aphorism "infants and children are small adults" is clearly disproven. Survival figures for pediatric patients with brain tumors are improving despite increasingly toxic treatment protocols. Aggressive supportive care, including the appropriate management of infection, provision of adequate nutrition, and proper use of blood and blood products,[1] has produced a dramatic reduction in mortality during the past 30 years more than any other modality. There is also evidence that children with CNS cancer who are treated at regional centers staffed by experienced multidisciplinary teams had better outcomes than children treated at centers with less experienced staff while receiving identical protocols.[2, 3] It is evident that critically ill infants and children should be cared for by a multidisciplinary team that is experienced and comprehends the unique needs of these patients. We must remember that we are caring not only for a critically ill child, but also for the patient's family.

THE INTRACRANIAL SPACE

To understand many of the postoperative and critical problems seen in pediatric patients with CNS tumors the reader should be familiar with some of the basic neuroanatomical and neurophysiologic principles outlined below.

The Monro-Kellie hypothesis states that the cranial vault contains a fixed volume and consists of three basic components—brain (80%), blood (10%), and cerebrospinal fluid (CSF) (10%)—which are encased by the thick inelastic dura mater and the semirigid cranium. These components exist in a state of volume-pressure equilibrium, and expansion of one component must be compensated for by a reduction in the volume of one or both other components.[4] Figure 7–1 represents a graphic representation of intracranial compliance. The volume-pressure graph demonstrates that between points 1 and 2, despite the increase in intracranial volume (i.e., by tumor, edema, or hemorrhage), a mechanism

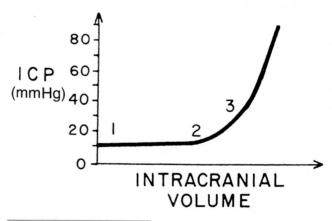

Figure 7–1 The intracranial compliance curve. 1, Compliant portion of curve: large volume shifts may occur with almost no change in intracranial pressure (ICP). 2, Critical volume where small changes in content result in more dramatic rises in ICP. 3, Steep area of compliance curve where minuscule changes in volume result in tremendous elevations in ICP. (Reproduced with permission from Shapiro HM. Intracranial hypertension: therapeutic and anesthetic considerations. *Anesthesiology* 1975;43:445–470.)

exists for the cranial vault to remain at a constant pressure despite an increase in intracranial volume. This is accomplished by the displacement of CSF and cerebral blood into the spinal space. Point 2 on the curve represents an area where despite the ICP being normal, any further increases in volume (such as may be seen with continued tumor growth, edema, obstructive hydrocephalus, or hemorrhage into the tumor) will produce an exponential rise in ICP that may be life threatening. Point 3 represents a decompensated state and a neurosurgical emergency with dangerously high ICP. There is a common misconception that the infant is protected from an increase in ICP by virtue of the open fontanels; however, it must remembered that the brain is encased by inelastic dura mater, which limits the infant's compensatory mechanisms. The infant has a shorter craniospinal axis (measured from the cranial dura down the length of the spinal canal to the lumbosacral area) than the adult. It is evident that less potential space is available to allow for the displacement of CSF or cerebral blood in the pediatric patient. However, certain *slow*-growing brain tumors or other CNS lesions may be better tolerated by the infant because the slow growth allows for eventual splitting and widening of the cranial sutures. This usually occurs over a period of weeks to months.

The compensatory response of the cranial space to an increase in one of the three components of the cranial vault is demonstrated in Figure 7–2. The top diagram demonstrates the three components of the intracranial vault in equilibrium (brain, blood, CSF), and the ICP is normal. The middle diagram represents a state wherein there is an increasing mass (i.e., brain tumor) and the compensatory mechanisms are depicted by the run-off of CSF and venous blood. This corresponds to a move from point 1 to point 2 in Fig. 7–1, and the ICP remains normal. The bottom diagram represents the uncompensated state that occurs following maximal compensatory fluid displacement from the intracranial space and it reflects an elevated ICP. This corresponds to a move from point 2 to point 3 in Fig. 7–1. It is the interaction of these three compartments and the physiologic mechanisms controlling each of them that underlies the framework for neurointensive care.[5]

Brain

Development of the CNS is incomplete at birth. At birth the brain weighs approximately 300 to 400 g and accounts for 10 to 15% of the infant's total body weight. The brain grows rapidly and doubles in weight within 6 months, approaching 900 g at 1 year and acquiring the approximate adult weight of 1200 g by age 12 years.[6, 7] By adulthood the brain accounts for only 2% of the total body weight yet accounts for approximately 15 to 20% of the cardiac output, 20% of the oxygen utilized by the body at rest, and almost 25% of the body's utilization of glucose.[8] It is obvious that the brain's need for energy is substantial; paradoxically, its store of energy-generating substrates is small, making it exclusively dependent on an adequate cerebral blood flow (CBF) for delivery of substrate.

The largest component (80%) of the intracranial vault is the brain. The brain parenchyma is composed of neurons (50%) and glial and vascular elements. There are three types of glial tissue: astroglia (which provides a supporting structure and plays a role in neuronal metabolism), oligodendroglia (which produces myelin around axons), and microglia (which serves as immune cells). Neurons are the basic processing units of the CNS, responsible for the production of neurotransmitters and the conduction of impulses. The energy supplied to the brain is utilized to maintain the neuronal transmembrane potential and support of the membrane (to keep K^+ extracellular and Na^+ and Ca^{2+} intracellular), driving of axonal flow, production of neurotransmitters, and propagation of neural impulses.[9] The metabolic needs of the brain are met by changes in CBF.

Blood

The cerebral blood, including veins, arteries, and capillaries, accounts for approximately 10% of the volume of the intracranial vault. CBF is regulated by brain metabolism, blood pressure, arterial $PaCO_2$, and PaO_2. CBF varies in different regions of the brain, being highest in the gray matter and lowest in the white matter. CBF is also age-dependent, and in

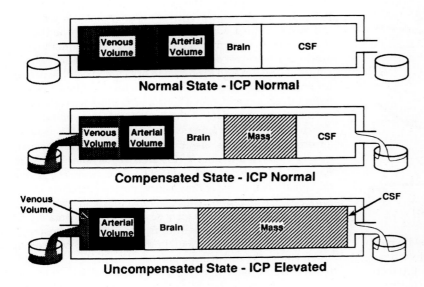

Figure 7–2 Mechanisms for compensation for an expanding intracranial mass lesion. (Reproduced with permission from Kanter MJ, Narayan RK. Intracranial pressure monitoring. *Neurosurg Clin North Am* 1991;2(2):257–265.)

adults the normal CBF is 50 mL/100 g per minute, whereas it is 40 mL/100 g per minute in neonates and 100 mL/100 g per minute in children. The critical blood flow at which ischemia develops and demonstrates electroencephalographic (EEG) changes is 20 mL/100 g per minute in the adult and is approximately 5 to 10 mL/100 g per minute lower in the infant.

Cerebral perfusion pressure (CPP) is defined as the difference between the mean arterial pressure (MAP) and the ICP and is represented by the equation: **$CPP = MAP - ICP$**. CPP is thus the driving pressure that provides substrate (oxygen and glucose) to the brain. The brain possesses a pressure autoregulatory ability that allows it to maintain a stable CBF over a wide range of CPP values by varying the diameter of its arterioles and precapillary vessels. There is also a metabolic autoregulatory mechanism that modulates the diameter of these vessels in response to the cellular metabolic environment. An increase in MAP produces vasoconstriction to maintain a stable CBF, whereas ischemia, hypoxia, or hypercarbia produce vasodilatation to increase CBF.[10] The normal CPP in the adult is approximately 75 to 100 mm Hg, and the accepted lower limit needed to provide adequate CNS perfusion is 50 mm Hg. At a CPP below 20 mm Hg irreversible neuronal damage occurs. In the neonate and infant, the accepted CPP is lower secondary to the lower age-related blood pressure.

Three of the factors governing CBF are frequently monitored and regulated in the PICU: PaO_2 (or oxygen saturations), $PaCO_2$, and arterial blood pressure. Figure 7–3 represents a graphic depiction of the effects of each on CBF. There is a linear relationship between $PaCO_2$ and CBF for values between 20 and 80 mm Hg. There is an approximately 4% increase in CBF for every 1 mm Hg increase in $PaCO_2$. Doubling of the $PaCO_2$ leads to doubling of the CBF.

CBF is ensured by cerebral autoregulation, which maintains the CBF over a wide range of arterial blood pressures between 60 mm Hg and 160 mm Hg in normotensive patients (Fig. 7–3).

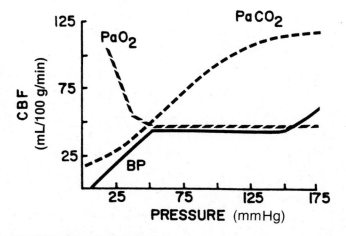

Figure 7–3 Cerebral blood flow (CBF) is affected by mean arterial pressure, PaO_2, and $PaCO_2$. (Reproduced with permission from Shapiro HM. Intracranial hypertension: therapeutic and anesthetic considerations. *Anesthesiology* 1975;43:445–470.)

The brain cannot store oxygen. Under normal conditions there is a margin of safety in that the amount of oxygen delivered exceeds the requirements of a nonstressed brain. CBF is also regulated by the PaO_2, and any events that lead to a decrease in PaO_2 may lead to an increase in CBF and an increase in cerebral blood volume (CBV), and ultimately to an increase in ICP. Events producing hypoxemia may include postoperative hypoventilation, hypotension, seizures, and pulmonary edema. The effect of PaO_2 on CBF is demonstrated in Figure 7–3.

Cerebrospinal Fluid

The CSF is the third component of the intracranial vault and represents approximately 10% of the cranial volume. CSF is a clear, aqueous solution that is an ultrafiltrate of plasma, which bathes the brain and spinal cord. The low specific gravity of CSF in relation to the brain reduces the mass effect of the brain to a minimum and serves as a protective cushion that prevents the brain's full weight from producing traction on nerve roots, blood vessels, and delicate membranes. CSF also provides a chemically appropriate environment that is necessary for neurotransmission and the removal of metabolic by-products. Approximately 70% of the CSF is produced by the choroid plexus located in the lateral, third, and fourth ventricles, and the remainder is formed in the extrachoroidal sites, such as the ventricular ependyma, sylvian aqueduct, subarachnoid pial surface, and brain and spinal cord parenchyma.[11] The rate of formation is approximately 0.35 to 0.40 mL/minute or 500 to 600 mL/day. The turnover time for CSF is approximately 5 to 7 hours. The actual intraventicular volumes are approximately 40 to 60 mL in infants, 60 to 100 mL in young children, 80 to 120 mL in older children, and 100 to 160 mL in adults. CSF moves from the point of production through the CSF pathways via several mechanisms: (1) a pressure gradient that exists between the site of formation (15 mm H_2O) and the site of resorption at the superior sagittal sinus (9 mm H_2O); (2) cilia on the ependymal cells; (3) vascular pulsations; and (4) respiratory variations. After its formation in the lateral ventricles, CSF passes through the paired intraventricular foramina of Monro into the midline third ventricle and through the aqueduct of Sylvius into the fourth ventricle and ultimately into the subarachnoid space via one of two pathways. These include an egress of CSF through the foramen of Magendie or the paired foramina of Luschka of the fourth ventricle. The CSF then bathes the brain and spinal cord and is ultimately resorbed on the superior surface of the brain by the arachnoid villi, which drain into the superior sagittal sinus. CSF is usually absorbed at the same rate at which it is produced (approximately 20 to 25 mL/hour). This pathway is summarized in Figure 7–4. *It is important to realize that displacement of CSF into the spinal canal is one of the compensatory mechanisms for an increasing cerebral vault volume and that any obstruction to the egress of CSF may lead to an increase in ICP.* Approximately 50 to 60% of all pediatric brain tumors arise in the posterior fossa, which is the area located under the tentorium cerebelli and includes the cerebellum, pons, and medulla oblongata.[12] It can be appreciated from Figure 7–4 that tumors in this area can easily compromise CSF outflow, leading to acute hydrocephalus and increased ICP. Figure 7–5A demonstrates a

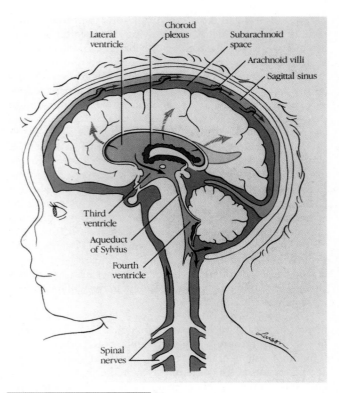

Figure 7–4 The normal cerebrospinal fluid pathways. (Reproduced with permission from Edwards MS, Derechrin M, eds. *About Hydrocephalus: A Book for Parents*. San Francisco: Hydrocephalus Association, 1986.)

normal magnetic resonance image of ventricles, in contrast with Figure 7–5B, which demonstrates massive ventricular dilatation resulting from tumor obstruction of the aqueduct of Sylvius.

RECOGNITION AND MANAGEMENT OF POSTOPERATIVE PROBLEMS

Perioperative complications can be either medical or surgical. Many risks cannot be generalized for all craniotomies because some procedures and approaches have unique problems. The overall risk of postoperative hemorrhage is 0.8–1.1%.[13, 14] *Factors that increase the likelihood of hemorrhage include postoperative hypertension, incomplete tumor resection, and coagulation abnormalities.* Craniotomy in adult patients carries the following risks: anesthetic complications (0.2%); increase in neurologic deficit 24 hours following surgery (10%); and wound infections (2%).[15] The transient increase in neurologic deficit may be attributable to swelling, retraction, or resection.

BOX 7–1
Common Postoperative Problems
• **Delayed emergence from anesthesia**   • **Pain**   • **Nausea and vomiting**   • **Respiratory complications**   • **Cardiovascular instability**   • **Hypo-hyperthermia**   • **Fluid and electrolyte imbalance**   • **Cerebral edema**   • **Intracranial hypertension**

In many hospitals the relationship between the postanesthesia care unit (PACU) and the PICU are interchangeable. At our institution, all children are brought directly to the PICU to recover. Whether children recover in the PACU or

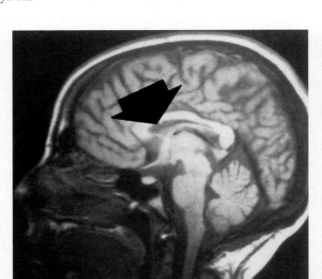
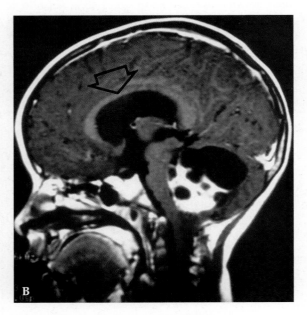

Figure 7–5 (A) Normal ventricular system as seen on magnetic resonance image. (B) Ventricular dilatation secondary to obstruction by tumor.

the PICU, they must be closely monitored for signs that the anesthetic is wearing off and to observe for common postoperative problems (see Box 1). The decision to extubate or to leave the patient's trachea intubated is generally made during the latter stages of the surgery based on the patient's physiologic signs and the scope of the surgery. Once the decision has been made to either extubate or leave the tube in place, the patient is prepared for transport to the PACU or PICU. One must be as vigilant during the transport as during the surgical procedure. *The lateral position is preferred during transport to allow secretions to pool in the side of the mouth rather than in the posterior pharynx.* Airway obstruction, hypoventilation, laryngospasm, aspiration, and hypoxemia may all occur in the patient awakening from anesthesia, and arterial desaturations have been well described in pediatric patients during transport.[16, 17] These events may produce hypoxemia and cause an elevation in CBF.

All arterial, central venous, and peripheral intravenous lines should be secured for transport, and if the patient's trachea is not extubated he or she should be adequately sedated for transport. On arrival a detailed sign-out of the operative procedure, medications, blood loss and replacement, medications, allergies, and anticipated problems should be relayed from the operative team to the team assuming care of the patient postoperatively. The presenting history should also be closely reviewed to identify any potential postoperative problems (e.g., seizure history, allergy). The majority of patients can be safely monitored using an arterial line to continuously monitor central blood pressure, continuous electrocardiography, pulse oximetry, a Foley catheter, and two peripheral intravenous lines.

Delayed Emergence

The CNS effects of anesthetics are complex and may include pupillary changes, sustained clonus, hyperreactive quadriceps reflexes, Babinski's sign (upgoing toes), shivering, and occasional transient worsening of preexisting neurologic deficits.[18, 19] These effects are usually seen with the use of inhalational anesthetics (enflurane and halothane) and resolve in less than an hour following the discontinuance of the anesthetic. Slow awakening or persistent somnolence may be seen following the use of narcotics (morphine, fentanyl). *Patients undergoing craniotomy for large intracranial mass lesions awaken more slowly than patients who have undergone spinal surgery or craniotomy for small brain tumors.*[20] Confusion or drowsiness may result from residual anesthetics or represent cerebral edema or postoperative hemorrhage.

The postoperative neurosurgical patient in the PICU should have neurologic assessments done approximately every 15 minutes for the first 4 hours, then every 30 minutes for the next 8 to 12 hours, and then hourly for the subsequent 12 hours. *The most important clinical sign is the patient's mental status.* The most accepted and reliable tool for evaluating mental status is the Glasgow Coma Scale (GCS) (Table 7-1). Coma is defined as a GCS score lower than 8. Patients with a rapidly increasing headache with vomiting, increasing drowsiness, new hemiparesis or paresthesias, or pupillary changes in a previously awake patient are usually manifesting a neurologic complication.

Common causes of postoperative depressed or altered mental status include hypoxemia, hypercarbia, hypovolemia, hypo- or hyperthermia, hypoglycemia, water or electrolyte imbalance (particularly sodium), postictal state, cerebral edema, increased ICP, or, rarely, ischemia. Other contributing and confounding problems that may occur at the same time include nausea, vomiting, and pain. Goals in the immediate postoperative period are to allow for rapid early emergence, document neurologic improvement, extubate as early as possible, and control pain without causing obtundation of the patient. After consideration of the factors listed above, it may be prudent to obtain an emergent head computed tomography (CT) scan to rule out the possibility of a postoperative hemorrhage or cerebral edema. Recent studies have demonstrated the relatively safe transport of critically ill adult neurosurgical patients for an imaging study with an approximately 10% complication rate.[21] These patients are at risk for airway obstruction, hypoxemia, hypercapnia, and aspiration.

TABLE 7-1

Glasgow Coma Scale			Modified Coma Scale for Infants		
Activity	Best Response		Activity	Best Response	
Eye opening	Spontaneous	4	Eye opening	Spontaneous	4
	To speech	3		To speech	3
	To pain	2		To pain	2
	None	1		None	1
Verbal	Oriented	5	Verbal	Coos, babbles	5
	Confused	4		Irritable	4
	Inappropriate words	3		Cries to pain	3
	Nonspecific sounds	2		Moans to pain	2
	None	1		None	1
Motor	Follows commands	6	Motor	Normal spontaneous movements	6
	Localizes pain	5		Withdraws to touch	5
	Withdraws to pain	4		Withdraws to pain	4
	Abnormal flexion	3		Abnormal flexion	3
	Extension	2		Abnormal extension	2
	None	1		None	1

Common adverse events include neurologic deterioration, psychological distress, hypotension, hypertension, oxygen desaturations, electrocardiographic changes, respiratory distress, and bleeding.

**BOX 7–2
Causes of Postoperative
Altered Mental Status**

- Increased ICP
- Neurologic complications
- Hypo-/hypercarbia
- Hypovolemia
- Hypo-/hyperthermia
- Hypoglycemia
- Electrolyte imbalance
- Postictal state
- Edema

Pain and Sedation

The exact incidence, magnitude, and duration of acute pain experienced by adult neurosurgical patients after various brain operations is not known. There are currently no pediatric studies addressing this issue. A recent adult study demonstrated that postoperative pain occurred more frequently than previously assumed and that the intensity ranged from moderate to severe. It occurred most frequently within the first 48 hours postoperatively and occurred most often following subtemporal and suboccipital surgical approaches.[23] It is suggested that the pain is related to surgical stress in major muscle tissues (i.e., temporal, splenium capitus, and cervical muscles).[23] *It must be remembered that many children are unable or unwilling to complain of pain and therefore the practitioner must have a high index of suspicion.* Pain is a noxious stimuli and may lead to tachycardia, hypertension, anxiety, nausea, and vomiting, which may all produce an elevation in ICP. Failure to provide adequate anesthesia will cause a neuroendocrine response as the result of the aforementioned sympathetic response. Epinephrine, norepinephrine, catecholamines, cortisol, glucagon, growth hormone, vasopressin, and the interleukins are released, leading to a catabolic state with associated problems, including atelectasis, altered gas exchange, fever, immobility, immunosuppression, and psychological changes.

Pain assessment tools are divided into three categories: self-reported, behavioral, and physiologic.[24] In general, patients should be believed and their own rating of the pain should be regarded as the most reliable index. Behavioral responses in children are useful but easily misinterpreted. Common distress behaviors include screaming, grimacing, and thrashing about of the limbs. Physiologic parameters include heart rate, blood pressure, and respiratory rate; however, these may be affected by the underlying CNS lesion.

Fentanyl and morphine are the two most commonly administered opioid agents to provide analgesia. They may be administered by several routes; however, intravenous (bolus, continuous infusion, or patient-controlled by pump)

seems the best route in most cases. Major side effects of these agents include respiratory depression and cardiovascular compromise, and infants younger than 3 months are more susceptible than older children. Tolerance may develop over time, and this means that a higher dosage may be required following prolonged administration. Although many parents fear physical dependence on these agents, the occurrence is exceedingly small. Codeine is an opioid that may be administered orally and is considered to have relatively few unwanted side effects.[25]

**BOX 7–3
Side Effects of Narcotics**

- Respiratory depression
- Cardiovascular compromise
- Ileus
- Nausea/vomiting
- Sedation

Acetaminophen and nonsteroidal anti-inflammatory drugs (NSAIDs) both inhibit prostaglandin synthetase, thus accounting for their analgesic action.[26, 27] *Ketorolac tromethamine is an NSAID that has been reported to provide greater and longer lasting pain relief than morphine, as well as being free of any respiratory depressant effects.*[26] Although initial studies suggested that ketorolac may be as effective as narcotics in treating pain, its actual role appears to be in decreasing total narcotic requirements and limiting narcotic side effects, including ileus, constipation, sedation, nausea, vomiting, and respiratory depression. Adverse effects of NSAIDs include decreased platelet function, peptic ulcer and gastrointestinal bleeding, decreased glomerular filtration rate, and bronchospasm.[28]

**BOX 7–4
Side Effects of NSAIDs**

- Decreased platelet formation
- Peptic ulcer
- Gastrointestinal bleeding
- Decreased glomerular filtration rate
- Bronchospasm

Because many patients in the PICU require invasive procedures, a consideration of topical anesthetics is appropriate. A eutectic mixture of lidocaine, prilocaine, and lidocaine jellies (EMLA) is available and may be used to facilitate the placement of intravenous lines, lumbar punctures, central venous catheters, accessing mediports, arterial punctures, and arterial line placement.

When a patient is restless and agitated, significant life-threatening disturbances must be ruled out, including hypoxia, hypercarbia, acidosis, shock, cerebral ischemia, electrolyte disturbances, infection, temperature dysregulation, or drug intoxication (delayed metabolism, decreased clearance, or decreased protein binding). *The sedation regimen chosen for*

TABLE 7–2 Neurologic Effects of Common Sedative Drugs

Agent	Advantages	Disadvantages
Benzodiazepines	Anxiolysis and amnesia Anticonvulsant action Hemodynamic stability Decrease cerebral metabolism Decrease intracranial pressure Effects are reversible	Respiratory depression Tachyphylaxis Antagonism decreases seizure threshold
Opioids	Analgesia Effects are reversible Minimal alteration of intracranial dynamics	Respiratory depression Addictive Antagonism increases pain
Barbiturates	Sedation and hypnosis Decrease cerebral metabolism Decrease intracranial pressure Anticonvulsant effect	Cardiovascular depression Respiratory depression Alters hepatic drug metabolism Withdrawal phenomenon
Neuroleptics	Antipsychotic action Antiemetic effect	Cardiovascular depression Decrease seizure threshold Neuroleptic malignant syndrome Endocrine changes Anticholinergic effects Hypothermia Extrapyramidal symptoms
Ketamine	Sedation and analgesia Lack of respiratory and cardiovascular depression Amnesia	Increase cerebral metabolism Increase intracranial pressure Proconvulsant Hallucinations and delusions Dissociative state
Propofol	Sedation and hypnosis Ultrashort duration of action Decrease cerebral metabolism Decrease intracranial pressure No drug accumulation	Hypotension Respiratory depression Infection
Clonidine	Sedation and analgesia Blunt sympathetic response	Hypotension Withdrawal hypertension

Reproduced with permission from Mirski MA, et al. Sedation for the critically ill neurologic patient. *Crit Care Med* 1995;23(12):2038–2052.

the agitated pediatric neurosurgical patient must either preserve the neurologic exam for clinical monitoring or have the potential to be discontinued with rapid return of an uncompromised examination.[29] Agents commonly used in the PICU include benzodiazepines, narcotics, barbiturates, and propofol. Propofol is a relatively new nonbarbiturate intravenous anesthetic characterized by rapid induction and awakening from anesthesia. It is a potent cerebral vasoconstrictor and may serve to decrease ICP; however, it is also a myocardial depressant.[30]

Common side effects of sedative agents include altered sensorium, respiratory depression, myocardial and cardiovascular depression, and motor incoordination or dyskinesias (Table 7–2). It must also be remembered that these agents have neurophysiologic side effects (Table 7–3). The presence of a parent may be the best sedative for the child.

Nausea and Vomiting

Nausea and vomiting should be recognized and treated promptly as they may lead to a rise in blood pressure and,

TABLE 7–3 Neurophysiologic Effects of Sedative Drugs

Sedative Agent	CBF	MAP	ICPC	PP	CMRO$_2$
Benzodiazepines	↑	↓	↓	↔	↓
Opioids	↔	↓	↔	↔	↓
Barbiturates	↓↓	↓↓	↓↓	↓	↓↓
Neuroleptics	↓	↓	↑	↓	↔
Propofol	↓↓	↓↓	↓↓	↓	↓↓
Ketamine	↑↑	↑	↑	↔	↔
Clonidine	↓	↓	↔	↓	↔

CBF, cerebral blood flow; MAP, mean arterial pressure; ICP, intracranial pressure; CPP, cerebral perfusion pressure; CMRO$_2$, cerebral metabolic rate of oxygen utilization. ↑, modest increase; ↓, modest decrease; ↔, no clear effect; ↓↓, pronounced decrease; ↑↑, pronounced increase.

Reproduced with permission from Mirski MA, et al. Sedation for the critically ill neurologic patient. *Crit Care Med* 1995;23(12):2038–2052.

ultimately, ICP. Factors that influence postoperative vomiting include age (higher incidence in younger patients), gender (more common in females), obesity, anxiety, history of motion sickness or previous nausea and postoperative vomiting, delayed gastric emptying or air swallowing, medications received (narcotics), duration of surgery, dizziness, postural hypotension, and early administration of fluids. Hunger appears to be a better indicator than thirst that the child is ready for fluids. Treatment consists of administering one of several dopamine antagonists, such as droperidol, promethazine, or metaclopramide. These agents may cause dystonic reactions, which may be difficult to differentiate from the development of new postoperative neurologic findings. *We prefer to administer serotonin antagonists, such as ondansetron, at a dosage of 0.15 mg/kg up to a maximum dose of 4 mg in an adult patient.*[22] Dystonic reactions seen with the dopamine antagonists may be treated with diphenhydramine; however, this agent causes drowsiness and ultimately interferes with the neurologic evaluation.

BOX 7–5
Factors in Postoperative Vomiting

- **Younger age**
- **Female sex**
- **Obesity**
- **Anxiety**
- **Postanesthetic narcotic administration**
- **Increased ICP**

Respiratory Problems

The respiratory system of the neurosurgical patient requires vigilant attentiveness. Inadequate ventilation occurs as a result of respiratory depression, muscle weakness, or airway obstruction. Surgical involvement in areas near the respiratory center or increased pressure on the brain stem may also cause respiratory irregularities.[31] Patients with posterior fossa or brain stem tumors may have lower cranial nerve dysfunction, which causes vocal cord paralysis, swallowing difficulty, and partial airway obstruction. Other causes of respiratory insufficiency include atelectasis, aspiration, pulmonary edema, pneumothorax, and preexisting pulmonary disease. A current or recent upper respiratory infection also increases the risk of postoperative complications.[32] Respiratory insufficiency may present as anxiety, agitation, unresponsiveness, tachycardia, bradycardia, hypertension, dysrhythmia, or respiratory arrest.

The anatomical configuration of the pediatric airway predisposes to upper airway obstruction and hypoventilation. Clinical findings include retractions (suprasternal, intercostal, and subcostal), nasal flaring, inspiratory stridor, paradoxical abdominal breathing (see-saw pattern), and decreased or absent air entry.[33] Complete cessation of gas exchange allows the $PaCO_2$ to increase by 10 to 12 mm Hg in the first minute, 7 to 10 mm Hg in the second minute, and 3 to 6 mm Hg in the third minute; oxygenation drops rapidly as well.[34] Figure 7–3 summarizes the effects of hypoxia and hypercarbia on CBF.

BOX 7–6
Signs of Upper Airway Obstruction

- **Retractions**
- **Nasal flaring**
- **Stridor**
- **Paradoxical abdominal breathing**
- **Decreased or absent air entry**

The tongue is large relative to the size of the oral cavity. Airway obstruction may occur as the tongue falls back into the pharynx and the negative pressure of inspiration causes the airway to collapse. This is usually correctable by a simple jaw thrust. If this maneuver is unsuccessful, then a nasopharyngeal tube should be placed. The tube is inserted gently through the nare whereupon it stents the tongue forward and allows the airway to remain patent. Oral airways are not well tolerated in children and may stimulate gagging, vomiting, or laryngospasm.

Laryngospasm may occur due to secretions or during extubation. The incidence is highest in patients under 9 years of age and is highest in the 1- to 3-month-old group. Therapy includes bag-mask ventilation with 100% oxygen and administration of a short-acting neuromuscular blocker, and continued bag-mask ventilation may be necessary until the laryngospasm resolves. These patients may even require reintubation; however, this is uncommon.

Glottic or laryngeal edema and postoperative croup occurs in 1 to 4% of intubated pediatric patients. The pediatric patient has a smaller larynx, and whereas in the adult patient 1 mm of edema produces only slight hoarseness, in the pediatric patient the airway is reduced by 75% and serious obstruction results.[35] Symptoms include stridor, thoracic retractions, hoarseness, croupy cough ("seal-like"), and possible obstruction. Symptoms usually occur within 30 to 60 minutes of extubation. Treatment includes positioning the patient upright and administering cool mist and inhaled racemic epinephrine, and if the patient is not receiving steroids for the neurologic disorder they should be administered. Other therapeutic options include the use of heliox (a mixture of oxygen and helium), which decreases turbulent flow in the edematous airway and allows for better gas exchange.[36] Bronchospasm may occur secondary to underlying pulmonary disease or as a response to an allergic reaction to a medication, blood, or latex.[37, 38] Therapeutic interventions include oxygen, β_2-agonists, aminophylline, isoproterenol, steroids, and magnesium.[39]

Hypoventilation resulting from residual narcotic effect or inadequate reversal of neuromuscular blockers causes hypercapnia. Patients with underlying neurologic disorders may suffer from a centrally impaired respiratory drive. Cranial nerve dysfunction involving the ninth and tenth nerves may affect the patient's ability to maintain a patent airway. Other upper airway muscles also receive their innervation from the fifth, seventh, ninth, tenth, and twelfth nerves, and during surgery the areas of the brain and brain stem where these nerves and their nuclei arise may be transiently or permanently damaged despite intraoperative monitoring.

Pediatric patients are prone to regurgitation and aspiration of stomach contents for the following reasons: (1) higher intragastric pressure due to small size of stomach, air swallowing, or encroachment of abdominal organs while the patient is in the supine position; (2) relaxation of the gastroesophageal junction and laryngeal incompetence for up to 8 hours following anesthesia; (3) underdeveloped cough reflex; and (4) a discordance of breathing and swallowing in dyspneic infants.[40] Fifty percent of aspirations occur in the postanesthetic period. Aspiration pneumonitis results from the inhalation of acidic fluid, which causes damage of the pulmonary capillary endothelium and inhibition of surfactant production. Bronchospasm and atelectasis develop, and severe hypoxemia and hypercarbia may ensue. Clinical symptoms (respiratory distress) usually occur within 1 to 2 hours and radiographic changes may be delayed for 6 to 12 hours.[41, 42]

Cardiovascular Complications

Postoperative cardiac complications include hypertension, hypotension, and dysrhythmias. The increase in blood pressure is usually caused by pain, hypercapnia, hypoxia, shivering, increased intravascular volume, bladder distention, underlying disease (renal, endocrine, cardiac), increased intracranial pressure, or drug effect.[43] It is essential that the proper size blood pressure cuff be used because use of the wrong cuff size is a common cause of falsely reported hypertension. The blood pressure cuff should cover two-thirds of the length of the patient's upper arm. Treatment of acute hypertension involves administration of adequate analgesia, correction of respiratory problems, and balance of fluids and electrolytes. Most postoperative hypertension resolves in 4 hours; however, one must be diligent in evaluating hypertension in the postoperative neurosurgical patient and a CT scan may be required to rule out a CNS hemorrhage, pneumocephalus, or cerebral edema. Hypertension may be a reflection of Cushing's triad (hypertension, bradycardia, and abnormal breathing patterns). This reflects the body's response to brain stem ischemia, which includes intense peripheral vasoconstriction to improve perfusion to the ischemic brain stem.[44] The cardiovascular response to this vasoconstriction is bradycardia in an attempt to decrease myocardial work. It should be remembered that in pediatric patients the cardiac output is dependent on the heart rate (CO = HR × SV), where CO is cardiac output, HR is heart rate, and SV is stroke volume. Thus, a decrease in heart rate as a compensatory response to hypertension could lead to a deleterious fall in cardiac output. Bradycardia is rarely seen and is actually a late and serious sign of increased ICP. *The most common cause of bradycardia in pediatric patients is hypoxia, and an immediate search for possible causes should be done for the pediatric patient with bradycardia.*

A significant rise in blood pressure may precipitate an increase in ICP, increase the likelihood of hemorrhage at the operative site, and increase edema formation if the blood-brain barrier is disrupted. However, one must remember that *CPP = MAP − ICP*, and the practitioner must decide if the rise in blood pressure is a response to increased ICP or if the elevation in ICP is the result of the hypertension. Cerebral autoregulation occurs over a wide range of cerebral perfusion pressures between 50 to 150 mm Hg (Fig. 7–3). The optimal method for reduction of arterial blood pressure and

agents of choice remains controversial in the setting of an acute brain injury.[45] The major classes of pharmacologic agents used to treat hypertension in pediatric patients are direct vasodilators (smooth-muscle relaxants), α- and β-adrenergic receptor antagonists, calcium channel blockers, and, occasionally, barbiturates. The effects on CBF, ICP, cerebral autoregulation, and on other body organs must be considered.[45] Several of these agents are summarized in Table 7–4. *One must ensure that the patient is adequately sedated as to prevent hypertension.*

BOX 7–7
Causes of Postoperative Hypertension

- **Increased ICP**
- **Pain**
- **Hypercapnia**
- **Hypoxia**
- **Increased intravascular volume**
- **Bladder distention**
- **Drugs**

Hypotension occurs infrequently and is usually caused by hypovolemia, drugs, myocardial depression, increased temperature (vasodilatation), adrenal insufficiency (in the steroid-dependent patient who did not receive adequate perioperative steroid stress coverage), or interference with venous return (tension pneumothorax or cardiac tamponade). The patient's volume status is best assessed by evaluation of end-organ perfusion, including capillary refill time, urine output, and CNS perfusion (mental status). Inadequate replacement of intraoperative fluid losses or ongoing losses may be treated with bolus infusions of non–glucose-containing isotonic fluids, such as 0.9% sodium chloride, or with blood products if required.

BOX 7–8
Causes of Postoperative Hypotension

- **Hypovolemia**
- **Drugs**
- **Myocardial depression**
- **Increased temperature**
- **Adrenal insufficiency**
- **Impaired venous return**

Acute cerebrovascular events may cause CNS-mediated electrocardiographic changes to occur in individuals without coexisting heart disease.[46] *Cerebrogenic cardiac arrhythmias have been described in patients following subarachnoid hemorrhage, stroke, and seizures.*[46, 47] The electrocardiogram (ECG) may demonstrate T-wave inversion or ST depression. The most commonly seen pediatric dysrhythmia is sinus tachycardia. Causes of sinus tachycardia include pain, anxiety, anemia, hypoxia,

TABLE 7–4 Antihypertensive Agents

Drug	Mechanism of Action	Onset of Action	Duration of Action	Drug-Specific Adverse Effects
Sodium nitroprusside	Nitric oxide	Immediate	2–3 min	Cyanide toxicity
Nitroglycerin	Nitric oxide	1–2 min	3–5 min	Methemoglobin production
Hydralazine	Nitric oxide; interferes with calcium mobilization in smooth muscle	15–30 min	3–4 h	Drug-induced lupus syndrome, serum sickness–like illness
Diazoxide	Activates ATP-sensitive potassium channels	1–5 min	1–12 h	Severe hypoglycemia, salt and water retention
Propranolol	β_1- and β_2- receptor antagonist	2 min	1–6 h	Congestive heart failure, bronchospasm, hypoglycemia, drowsiness, bradycardia
Labetalol	α_2-, β_1- and β_2- receptor antagonist	5–10 min	2–12 h	Congestive heart failure, bronchospasm, hypoglycemia, bradycardia
Esmolol	Selective β_1 antagonist	Immediate	≤ 15 min	Bradycaradia, congestive heart failure
Nicardipine	Calcium channel antagonist	1–5 min	3–6 h	Hypotension, reflex tachycardia

Adapted from Tietjen CS, Hurn PD, Ulatowski JA, Kirsch JR. Treatment modalities for hypertensive patients with intracranial pathology: options and risks. *Crit Care Med* 1996;24:311–322.

hypercarbia, hypovolemia, and increased ICP.[46, 47] If other dysrhythmias are present, one should evaluate for a possible metabolic cause, such as an alteration in serum potassium, calcium, or magnesium.

Temperature Perturbations

Hypothermia

Although the actual size and weight of the pediatric patient are considerably smaller, the body surface–to–weight ratio increases as size diminishes, resulting in an increased propensity for heat loss. During prolonged surgery, body heat loss can be extreme. Postoperative hypothermia can be detrimental for several reasons: (1) it prolongs the effects of neuromuscular blockade and may cause hypercarbia, hypoxemia, and delayed extubation; (2) shivering and rewarming cause hypoxia and increased oxygen consumption; (3) vasoconstriction may occur in conjunction with hypertension; (4) prolongation of recovery from anesthesia leads to a delayed assessment of consciousness; and (5) as the temperature increases, the pressure of air trapped intracranially increases.[31] Hypothermia may also result in acidosis and myocardial depression. Therapeutic options include the use of radiant warmers, elevation of ambient temperature, warming of intravenous fluids, and humidification of inspired gases.

BOX 7–9
Causes of Hypothermia

- **Body heat loss secondary to prolonged surgery**
- **Hypothalamic injury**

Fever

Fever is usually the hallmark of an infectious process; however, it can also occur in patients with neurologic disorders, such as hypothalamic damage, intracranial hemorrhage, cerebrovascular accidents, and seizures. Body temperature is regulated through the anterior and posterior hypothalamus. Hypothalamic disease and damage that occurs with head trauma, tumors (craniopharyngioma, astrocytoma), vascular lesions, congenital harmartomas, vasculitis, traumatic hemorrhages, manipulation of the third ventricle, or encephalopathy may produce fever. Hemorrhage into the ventricles or subarachnoid space may produce an inflammatory reaction and fever. Fever has also been seen in almost 25% of all stroke patients. Seizures may cause sustained muscle contractions, which cause an elevation in body temperature. Excessive neuronal discharge may also cause disruption of the thermoregulatory control of the hypothalamus.

Hyperthermia

Hyperthermia (temperature greater than 41°C) may be caused by overwrapping, overwarming, dehydration, sepsis, febrile reaction to an infused blood product, neuroleptic malignant syndrome, or malignant hyperthermia (MH).[48] *MH usually occurs during induction of anesthesia but may occur for several hours following surgery. Prompt recognition is necessary because for each 1°C increase in temperature above 37°C the body increases its metabolic rate by 12%, thus imposing a significant metabolic burden on an individual who is already stressed and necessitating an increase in fluid requirements.* MH is a rare genetic disorder reported to occur in 1 of every 15,000 pediatric anesthetic procedures. The exact pathophysiologic derangement is unknown; however, it is thought to be due to an abnormality of calcium metabolism in skeletal muscle.

Dantrolene is the pharmacologic therapeutic agent for treatment of MH. The elevated temperature is treated with cooling blankets, fans, and ice packs, if necessary, and is not usually responsive to acetaminophen.

Neuroleptic malignant syndrome is another drug-induced disorder that results in muscle stiffness and hyperthermia. Drugs that have been implicated include phenothiazines, thioxanthines, and butyrophenones, which may be used as tranquilizers and antiemetics in addition to their usual use as antipsychotics.

BOX 7–10
Causes of Hyperthermia

- **Overwarming**
- **Dehydration**
- **Sepsis**
- **Transfusion reaction**
- **Malignant hyperthermia**
- **Postictal**
- **Hypothalamic damage**
- **Neuroleptic malignant syndrome (phenothiazines, thioxanthines, butyrophenones)**

Fluid and Electrolyte Balance

Water constitutes 70% of body weight in a newborn infant, which decreases to approximately 60% by age 1 year. Total body water (TBW) in the adult is approximately 60% of body weight and varies with leanness. Approximately two-thirds of TBW is located in the cell, and the remaining one-third is located in the extracellular compartment of the extracellular fluid, 25% is found in the intravascular compartment and the remainder (75%) is located in the interstitial space, which includes plasma and transcellular fluid (pleural, pericardial, peritoneal, and CSF).[49] The CNS plays an integral role in the neuroendocrine regulation of sodium and water homeostasis. Sodium (Na^+) is the predominant extracelluar ion, with 98% of the body's content located in the extracellular compartment. The body's sodium and water content are tightly controlled to maintain a normal osmolarity (285 to 295 mOsm), an adequate intravascular volume, and an adequate blood pressure. Water balance is controlled by thirst and the ability to concentrate urine. Antidiuretic hormone (ADH) increases resorption of water in the collecting tubules, and its release is regulated by serum osmolarity. Release or inhibition of ADH may occur with serum osmolarity changes of only 1 to 2%. Increases in osmolarity are sensed by osmoreceptors in the hypothalamus, which in turn increase the secretion of ADH from the neurohypophysis.

Sodium disturbances are commonly seen in patients with CNS disorders.[50, 51] Hyponatremia (serum sodium less than 130 mmol/L) results most commonly from a problem in the handling of water. Clinical signs include apathy, nausea, vomiting, ataxia, lethargy, coma, seizures, hypovolemia, hypotension, and edema. Common causes include iatrogenic, syndrome of inappropriate secretion of ADH (SIADH), factitious (diabetic) ketoacidosis, gastrointestinal losses, third-space losses, renal loss, congestive heart failure, nephrotic syndrome, and hepatic failure.

BOX 7–11
Causes of Hyponatremia

- **Iatrogenic**
- **SIADH**
- **Gastrointestinal losses**
- **Third-space losses**
- **Congestive heart failure**
- **Nephrotic syndrome**
- **Hepatic failure**
- **Cerebral salt wasting**

The most common cause of hyponatremia in the PICU is SIADH.[50, 51] It occurs in children with CNS infections, tumors, and subarachnoid hemorrhage, and in the postoperative period following intracranial surgery. Other disorders associated with SIADH include pulmonary diseases (pneumonia, asthma), sepsis, postanesthesia-related postoperative pain, and several medications, including barbiturates, carbamazepine, morphine, and vincristine.

BOX 7–12
Causes of SIADH

- **CNS infection**
- **Subarachnold hemorrhage**
- **Intracranial surgery**
- **Pulmonary disease**
- **Sepsis**
- **Postanesthesia**
- **Medications (barbiturates, morphine, tegretal, vincristine)**

The hyponatremia seen in SIADH is due to water retention resulting from excessive ADH release and ongoing sodium loss in the urine. The diagnosis of SIADH is based on the following criteria: low serum sodium (less than 130 mEq/L), low serum osmolarity (less than 280 mOsmol/L), high urine sodium (greater than 18 mEq/L), urine osmolality greater than serum osmolarity, normal endocrine function (thyroid, adrenal), and the absence of dehydration. *The diagnosis should not be made in patients with extreme pain, nausea, or hypotension, or in those who have recently undergone diuretic therapy as all of the above may stimulate ADH release despite serum hypotonicity.*

BOX 7–13
Diagnosis of SIADH

- **Sodium less than 130**
- **Serum osmolarity less than 280**
- **Urine sodium greater than 18 mEq/L**
- **Urine osmolality higher than serum osmolarity**
- **Normal endocrine function**
- **No evidence of dehydration**

Treatment of SIADH consists of fluid restriction, and we usually administer 50 to 70% of the calculated daily maintenance as isotonic fluids (0.9% normal saline). The therapeutic goal is to increase free-water diuresis relative to the sodium concentration. Severe, symptomatic hyponatremia (Na$^+$ less than 120 mEq/L) can be corrected using an infusion of 3% hypertonic saline. Patients who are experiencing a seizure should receive 3 to 5 mL/kg of 3% hypertonic saline to correct the serum Na$^+$ to approximately 125 mEq/L.[52, 53] Correction of the remaining hyponatremia should occur *slowly* at a rate not to exceed a rise rate of 1 to 2 mEq/L per hour to a serum level of 130 mEq/L. Longstanding or more severe hyponatremia should be corrected *more slowly* at a rate of 0.5 mEq/L per hour.

The speed and method of treatment of hyponatremia depend on the severity of symptoms and the state of the extracellular volume. The severity of the symptoms depends on the rate of development as well as on the magnitude of change in the serum sodium level.[51, 54] *Brain edema, which may lead to cerebral herniation and seizures, may occur as the result of hyponatremia; however, too rapid a correction may produce central pontine mylenosis (CPM).* CPM is a syndrome occurring after the rapid correction of hyponatremia; the most characteristic findings are quadriplegia with dysarthria and dysphagia with various levels of consciousness.[54] Demyelination occurs primarily in the central pons, but other areas of the brain have been involved as well.

Another entity that frequently causes hyponatremia in neurosurgical patients is cerebral salt wasting (CSW), which has been documented in neurosurgical patients following head trauma, postoperatively, and in those with infection or tumor.[55, 56] Earlier studies demonstrated that there was much confusion associated with differentiating SIADH from CSW,

and some authors used the terms interchangeably.[51] Patients with CSW have excessive sodium excretion or natriuresis, decreased sodium concentration, decreased extracellular volume, and increased urine volume with hyponatremia. Current studies demonstrate that CSW may occur as often as, or more often than, SIADH.[56] The exact mechanism by which intracranial disease causes renal salt wasting is not understood; however, it is thought that atrial natriuretic peptide (ANP) is involved. *The major difference between SIADH and CSW is the hypovolemia seen in the latter.* The entities are contrasted in Table 7–5. The following are helpful to support the diagnosis of CSW and to demonstrate dehydration: weight loss, clinical signs of dehydration, elevated hematocrit, elevated blood urea nitrogen (BUN)–to–creatinine ratio, and elevated serum protein concentration.

BOX 7–14
Signs of CSW

- **Excessive sodium excretion**
- **Decreased serum sodium**
- **Decreased extracellular volume**
- **Increased urine volume with hyponatremia**

It is important to differentiate between SIADH and CSW as the therapies are in total contrast. *The hallmark of CSW is severe dehydration, and if one is uncertain about differentiating these entities a central venous catheter should be placed.* Patients with CSW who are fluid-restricted will continue to lose sodium in the urine and thus become more dehydrated. Treatment of CSW

TABLE 7–5 **Differential Diagnosis of Cerebral Salt Wasting (CSW) vs. the Syndrome of Inappropriate Antidiuretic Hormone Secretion (SIADH)**

Factor	CSW	SIADH
Plasma sodium conc.	↓	↓
Plasma volume	↓	↑
Signs and symptoms of dehydration	Present	Absent
Salt balance	Negative	Variable
Weight	↓	↑ or no change
Pulmonary capillary wedge pressure	↓	↑ or normal
Central venous pressure	↓	↑ or normal
Hematocrit	↑	↓ or no change
Osmolality	↑ or normal	↓
Blood urea nitrogen/creatinine ratio	↑	Normal
Serum protein conc.	↑	Normal
Urine sodium conc.	↑↑	↑ (Variable)
Urine flow rate	↑↑	↑ (Generally)
Net sodium loss	↑↑↑	↑/↓
Serum potassium conc.	↑ or no change	↓ or no change
Serum uric acid conc.	Normal	↓
Plasma renin activity	↓	↓
Plasma aldosterone conc.+	↓	↑
Plasma ADH conc.+	↓	↑
Plasma ANP conc.	↑	↑

↓, decrease; ↑, increase; ↑↑, significant increase; ADH, antidiuretic hormone; ANP, atrial natriuretic peptide.

consists of correcting the hypovolemia by administering 0.9% sodium chloride for mild and moderate cases, 3% hypertonic sodium chloride for severe cases. Another therapeutic option is to increase the dose of oral salt tablets and oral fludrocortisone, increasing renal sodium and water retention.[57, 58]

BOX 7–15
Treatment of CSW

- **Correct hypovolemia with 0.9% sodium chloride**
- **Salt tablets**
- **Fludrocortisone**

Hypernatremia (serum sodium greater than 150 mmol/L) results from a relative increase in extracellular sodium as compared with extracellular water.[49] Clinical signs are not usually seen until the serum Na$^+$ is approximately 160 to 170 mEq/L. Such signs include irritability, thirst, vomiting, fever, CNS bleeding, lethargy, seizures, coma, doughy skin, and tonic spasms.

Hypernatremia is seen most commonly in postoperative neurosurgical patients who develop centrally acquired diabetes insipidus (DI). DI results from a deficiency in ADH (production or release) and is clinically characterized by the loss of urinary concentrating capacity, resulting in polyuria despite serum hyperosmolarity and even hypovolemia.[59] The severity and duration of symptoms depend on the location and completeness of the CNS lesion. Lesions involving the supraoptic and paraventricular hypothalamic nuclei, or those that interrupt the hypothalamic-neurohypophyseal tract above the level of the median eminence, are more likely to cause permanent DI, as opposed to lesions in the sella turcia.[59] DI also occurs in patients following operative injury to the hypothalamus or the pituitary stalk, or following head injury, bacterial meningitis, or phenytoin use, and in those with elevated ICP and brain death.[60, 61] DI develops postoperatively because of regional brain swelling or disruption of the hypothalamic-posterior pituitary axis. For a patient to develop significant polyuria, there must be a loss of approximately 75% of the ADH-secreting neurons. The most common CNS tumors in pediatric patients causing central DI (decreased ADH production or release) are craniopharyngioma, dysgerminoma, supraoptic glioma, and astrocytoma.[59]

BOX 7–16
Causes of Hypernatremia

- **Diabetes insipidus**
- **Hypothalamic injury**
- **Head trauma**
- **Meningitis**
- **Use of phenytoin**
- **Increased ICP**
- **Brain death**

Clinical diagnosis of DI includes: polyuria (greater than 200 mL/hour in adults and greater than 4–5 mL/hour in pediatric patients), elevated serum Na$^+$ (greater than 145 mEq/L), and low urine specific gravity (less than 1.005). Other potential causes of polyuria must be excluded; these include overhydration, hyperglycemia, and use of diuretics such as mannitol. A triphasic response has been reported in 5 to 10% of pituitary patients postoperatively, consisting of an abrupt cessation of ADH release followed by polyuria that begins within 12 to 24 hours after injury and lasts for 4 to 8 days. An antidiuretic phase that lasts for 5 to 6 days follows, characterized by concentration of the urine and plasma hypo-osmolarity with hyponatremia as a result of free-water absorption. Excessive release of presynthesized ADH from degenerating neurohypophysial tissues represents this finding. Once the release of stored hormone is complete, DI recurs and, though usually persistent, may improve or resolve.[60] DI must be promptly recognized and treated lest the patient rapidly become hypovolemic, hypernatremic, and go into shock.

BOX 7–17
Diagnosis of DI

- **Polyuria greater than 200 mL/hr**
- **Serum sodium greater than 145 mEq/L**
- **Urine specific gravity less than 1.005**

Management of DI includes (1) calculation of the free-water loss based on the following equation:

$$\text{Free water deficit} = 0.6 \times \text{wt (kg)} \times \text{serum Na}^+/140 - 1$$

(2) hourly monitoring and replacement of urinary losses, (3) administration of 0.2% or 0.45% normal saline for maintenance fluids and urinary losses, (4) monitoring of serum electrolytes every 4 to 6 hours, and (5) administration of vasopressin to manage DI in the postoperative pediatric neurosurgical patient. We implement an hourly infusion of maintenance fluids (0.45% NaCl) and replace approximately two-thirds of the urine output from the preceding hour (utilizing 0.45% NaCl). If we are unable to keep up with the urinary losses as they become extreme or there is concern about the patient developing cerebral edema, we utilize a vasopressin infusion and titrate to effect (a urine output of 2 mL/kg per hour). Dosages that have been reported to work are between 1.0 and 3.0 mU/kg/per hour and the half-life of infused vasopressin is approximately 30 minutes.[59, 62] Once the patient has stabilized, usually several days postoperatively, the synthetic analog of ADH, desmopressin acetate (1-deamino-8-D-arginine vasopressin; DDAVP), is utilized intramuscularly, intranasally, or orally.[62, 63]

BOX 7–18
Treatment of DI

- **Calculate free water loss**
- **Monitor urine loss**
- **0.45% sodium chloride maintenance**
- **Serum electrolytes every 4 to 6 h**
- **Vasopressin**

Other electrolyte abnormalities include disorders in potassium, calcium, and magnesium, necessitating that serum levels be obtained postoperatively. Hypokalemia may cause muscle weakness, decreased gastrointestinal motility, and impaired renal water retention.[64] Symptoms of hypocalcemia include hypotension, arrhythmias, laryngospasm, bronchospasm, muscle weakness and spasms, tetany, hyperreflexia, paresthesias, agitation, and seizures.[65] Symptoms of hypomagnesemia are similar to those of hypocalcemia and include muscle weakness, muscle spasms, hypotension, hyperreflexia, paresthesias, agitation, and seizures.[66, 67]

CO_2 crosses the blood-brain barrier (BBB) rapidly, and therefore respiratory acidosis and alkalosis may have profound effects on the CBF in the postoperative neurosurgical patient (Fig. 7–3). Hydrogen (H^+) and bicarbonate (HCO_3^-) cross the BBB poorly; thus, metabolic acidosis and alkalosis have little primary effect on the CNS. *Therapeutic hyperventilation to decrease the $PaCO_2$ may produce respiratory alkalosis and hypokalemia. The most common causes of metabolic alkalosis in the postoperative patient are excessive nasogastric tube drainage or prolonged administration of diuretics. Postoperative metabolic acidosis is usually caused by hypovolemia.*

Hypoglycemia is defined as a blood glucose concentration of less than 50 mg/dL in adults and less than 30 mg/dL in children. Hypoglycemia produces three major effects on the CNS: (1) invokes a stress response,[68, 69] (2) disturbs CBF and (3) alters CNS metabolism, ultimately leading to permanent neurologic damage.[70] The brain has very limited glucose stores and is dependent on CBF to provide glucose. Recent studies have suggested that patients with elevated serum glucose who suffered an ischemic insult had a worse outcome.[71, 72] The explanation commonly given is that in the presence of ischemia glucose is metabolized anaerobically and lactate concentration increases, leading to a decrease in intracellular pH that compromises cellular function. We administer 0.9% sodium chloride to our patients postoperatively, following the serum glucose levels every 4 hours in older patients and every 2 hours in the younger patients. Intraoperative hyperglycemia may occur in patients receiving corticosteroids or in those demonstrating a metabolic stress response. Hyperglycemia may cause an osmotic diuresis and produce electrolyte problems. There are currently no data that demonstrate that the administration of insulin will improve outcome in postoperative pediatric neurosurgical patients with hyperglycemia.

Cerebral Edema

Cerebral edema is an increase in the water content of the brain and may be classified as either cytotoxic or vasogenic. *Cytotoxic edema is the accumulation of primarily intracellular water. This leads to an increase in the size of the brain cell and little change in the extracellular compartment.*[73, 74] *Vasogenic edema occurs as a result of a plasma leak from the vasculature into the brain parenchyma. There is little change in cell volume, and the swelling occurs in the extracellular space.* Vasogenic peritumoral edema is associated with brain tumors.[75] It is a prominent finding both preoperatively (Fig. 7–6) and postoperatively, and may account for more of the neurologic findings than the

lesion itself. Intraoperative manipulation and ischemia may worsen the peritumoral edema. Postoperative cerebral edema peaks at 36 to 72 hours; however, it may be encountered in the first 6 to 12 hours postoperatively.

Vasogenic peritumoral edema is thought to arise from increased capillary permeability and a breakdown of the BBB, allowing macromolecules to leak into the extracellular space and exert an osmotic gradient that permits free water to enter the perivascular space.[76] Putative mediators include histamine, serotonin, glutamate, polyamines, lymphokines, leukotrienes, and vascular permeability factor. Glucocorticoids have been shown to decrease the edema associated with brain tumors. Mechanisms include reduced BBB permeability; increased Na^+, K^+, and water flux across the capillary/tissue interface; and direct inhibition of tumor growth.[77]

Dexamethasone is the drug of choice for treating edema, with 25 times the glucocortocoid strength of cortisol and negligible mineralocorticoid activity. It is a potent anti-inflammatory agent that does not cause sodium or fluid retention. Steroids act quickly; decreased capillary permeability has been shown as early as 1 hour after a single dose.[72] Asymptomatic patients are given steroids orally for several days preoperatively, and symptomatic patients (mass effect or clinical deterioration) are loaded with 10 mg of intravenous dexamethasone and receive 4 mg every 4 to 6 hours. Side effects of steroids include hyperglycemia, gastric ulceration and hemorrhage, psychosis (mood disturbance, irritability, fatigue, argumentativeness, sleep disturbance, excessive talking, and crying), impaired wound healing, and an impaired immune system that predisposes these patients to infectious complications.[78, 79] Withdrawal from corticosteroid therapy can usually be accomplished with few side effects; however, there are no established

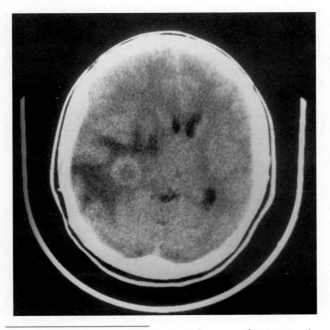

Figure 7–6 Computed tomography scan demonstrating peritumoral edema.

guidelines for their discontinuation. Patients receiving therapy for less than 5 to 7 days can have the steroids abruptly discontinued. Signs of adrenal insufficiency from too rapid a wean include fatigue, weakness, fever, hypotension, hypoglycemia, nausea, anorexia, arthralgias, and skin desquamation. Hypothalamic-pituitary-adrenal (HPA) axis suppression can occur after 5 days of pharmacologic doses of prednisone equal to or greater than 50 mg/day and can last for up to a year in patients who have received steroids for more than a month.

BOX 7–19
Side Effects of Steroids

- Hyperglycemia
- Gastric ulcer
- Psychosis
- Impaired wound healing

Stress coverage to prevent intraoperative or postoperative adrenal crisis should be considered in patients who have been receiving high doses of glucocorticoids (more than 50 mg/m^2 of cortisol daily) for a prolonged period (more than 10 to 14 days).[80] Cortisol is produced in the adrenal cortex, and its release is mediated through adrenocorticotropic hormone (ACTH) from the pituitary gland. A normal adrenal secretes approximately 9 mg/m^2 per day, and stress such as that of a surgical procedure can increase the production 3 to 15 times above the basal level. Patients receiving chronic glucocorticoid therapy may not be able to mount a stress response because the HPA axis is suppressed. It should be remembered that prednisone is four times more potent than cortisol, and dexamethasone is 30 times more potent. This a very important part of the preoperative evaluation, and the decision to administer stress coverage of steroids should be discussed with the anesthesiologist. Patients with adrenal crisis usually become hypotensive, hypoglycemic, hyponatremic, and hyperkalemic. Treatment includes prompt recognition and administration of isotonic fluids and hydrocortisone.[81]

BOX 7–20
Signs of Adrenal Crisis

- Hypotension
- Hypoglycemia
- Hyponatremia
- Hyperkalemia

Intracranial Hypertension

Normal ICP ranges from 5 to 15 mm Hg. Intracranial hypertension (ICH) occurs if the ICP remains elevated above that point for a sustained period of time. Daily fluctuations occur with sneezing, coughing, changes in position, Valsalva maneuvers, and changes in body position but do not result in neurologic deterioration. ICH is a neurologic emergency in the postoperative patient. *ICH should always be*

considered in the postoperative patient who suddenly has a change in the neurologic exam, a decrease in the GCS of more than 2 points, unilateral pupillary dilatation, or posturing. Intracranial compliance is reviewed in Figures 7–1 and 7–2. As an increase occurs in volume of one of the three components of the cerebrospinal axis (brain, CSF, or blood), there must be a compensatory decrease in the volume of one or both of the other components to prevent an increase in ICP. Mass effect may be seen from a hematoma, peritumoral edema may worsen following operative manipulation, or metabolic changes (hypercarbia, hypoxemia) may lead to an altered CBF and an increased ICP.

Management of ICH includes elevating the head of the bed to 30 to 45 degrees; keeping the head midline; inducing hyperventilation to a PaCO$_2$ of 30 to 35 mm Hg; ensuring proper oxygenation; maintaining a normal blood pressure and CPP; implementing removal of CSF if an external drain is present or by CSF shunt tap if a shunt is in place; administering osmotic diuretics such as mannitol and/or furosemide; and inducing sedation, neuromuscular paralysis if necessary, hypothermia, or barbiturate coma.

The ICP in 50 to 70% of patients is approximately 7 to 10 mm Hg higher with no head elevation than with 30 to 50 degrees of elevation.[82, 83] *Mannitol is thought to dehydrate the brain and to improve blood rheology in the CNS microcirculation.* Side effects include dehydration, osmotic diuresis with electrolyte depletion, and possible renal toxicity if the serum osmolarity is above the 330 to 340 mOsm range.[84] *Furosemide is effective when combined with mannitol to lower ICP.* The effects of hyperventilation and proper oxygenation are illustrated in Figure 7–3.[85] *Utilization of pentobarbital coma is controversial, but the mechanism of action is to decrease the cerebral metabolic rate of the injured brain and to obtain electrocerebral silence with burst suppression on the electroencephalogram (EEG).*[86] Side effects include hypotension and myocardial depression, and many patients receiving pentobarbital coma require catecholamine infusions (dobutamine, dopamine) to maintain an adequate blood pressure and CPP. *Moderate hypothermia (33°C) for 24 hours has recently been shown to hasten neurologic recovery in patients with severe traumatic brain injury with GCS scores of 5 to 7 on admission.*[87]

BOX 7–21
Treatment of ICH

- Elevate the head of the bed 30 to 45 degrees
- Keep the head at midline
- Maintain PaCO$_2$ between 30 and 35
- Maintain adequate pO$_2$
- Maintain normal blood pressure and cerebral perfusion pressure
- Drain CSF
- Administer mannitol
- Sedation
- Paralysis
- Barbiturate coma
- Hypothermia

Ischemia

The initial step leading to brain infarction is a reduction in CBF. There is a difference between the amount of blood flow that produces a reversible cessation of physiologic activity and that which causes cell death.[88] Cells that are exposed to a CBF between these two critical values are said to be within the "ischemic penumbra" and may recover function if blood flow is restored. The neuron's tolerance for ischemia is linked to time; a profound decrease in CBF can be tolerated for a short period of time, whereas a moderate decrease over a longer period of time can still allow recovery.[89, 90]

Postoperative cerebral ischemia and infarction are rare in pediatric patients, occuring either as the result of intraoperative vessel ligation during the tumor resection or as the result of excessive retraction leading to postoperative vasospasm. An abnormal increase in brain volume may develop asymmetrically in areas of ischemic infarction, neoplasia, and surrounding a hematoma. This asymmetrical expansion may cause distortion of the normal geometry of the intracranial space and cause vascular compression and/or herniation syndromes.[91] Vessels of the midbrain and diencephalon located at the base of the brain are tethered to the relatively immobile dura and are particularly susceptible. The effect of ischemia on the brain is devastating. Ischemia leads to a decrease in the delivery of substrates (glucose and oxygen) to the neural tissue. Ischemic brain damage occurs when the CBF falls below 15 to 18 mL/100 g per minute in the adult if the metabolic rate is normal. Any increase in the metabolic rate (shivering, fever, hypoxia, etc.) will increase the risk of ischemic damage. Patients should be aggressively hydrated with isotonic fluids, and the blood pressure should be kept in the upper limit of normal for age range. Hypovolemia from aggressive diuresis and fluid restriction should be avoided. Placement of a central venous catheter may be helpful in assessing the patient's hydration status. The administration of catecholamines (dopamine, epinephrine, phenylephrine) should also be considered. The goal is to optimize the CPP.

Pneumocephalus

Pneumocephalus is a pathologic collection of gas in the cranial cavity.[92] Pneumocephalus associated with most craniotomies tends to be small and resolve spontaneously (Fig. 7–7). It is a common consequence of intracranial surgery that occurs in 100% of patients in the first 3 days following craniotomy.[93] Although usually asymptomatic, it has been associated with headache, nausea, vomiting, and lethargy and may lead to tension pneumocephalus and cause ICH. Air enters the intracranial compartment as a result of dural closure after tumor resection or ventriculostomy.[94] Communication must exist between the intracranial and extracranial compartments. The mechanism is similar to an inverted soda bottle, that is, as the soda flows out, air rushes in to equilibrate the pressure differential. A rapid loss of CSF may produce the same effect, with CSF being replaced by air entering through a cranial-dural defect.[95] A second mechanism is the "ball valve" theory whereby a sudden increase in extracranial pressure, such as that caused by sneezing, coughing, or blowing the nose, allows air to enter into the cranial vault

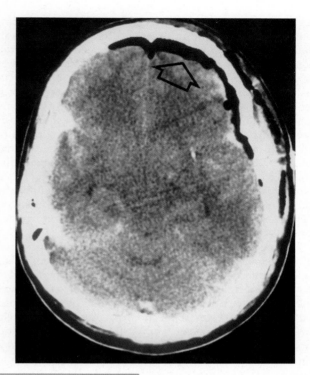

Figure 7–7 Postoperative computed tomography scan demonstrating pneumocephalus.

(via the acute increase in the extracranial-to-intracranial pressure ratio); air is trapped because the baseline intracranial pressure is higher than the extracranial pressure, causing the dura to seal itself and air to become trapped.[91] *In patients undergoing craniotomies, following dural closure expansion of the brain by rehydration, elevation of $PaCO_2$, replacement of CSF, and cerebral edema may make retained air an important contributing factor in ICH.*

To speed the resorption of air some neurosurgeons administer supplemental oxygen to patients following craniotomy.[96] The proposed benefit of this therapy is to replace nitrogen with oxygen, which speeds resorption of intracranial air by increasing the diffusion gradient for nitrogen between the air collection and the surrounding cerebral tissue.[97]

Tension pneumocephalus may occur rarely and produce reduced intracranial compliance and ICH. It is most likely to occur intraoperatively under the following circumstances: administration of N_2O to patients with a recent craniotomy, uncontrolled drainage of CSF from ventricular shunts; traumatic pneumocephalus due to a cranial-dural defect; and unsuspected cranial fistulous tract caused by a tumor or recent neurosurgery. Clinical signs include a deteriorating level of consciousness, hemiparesis, or seizures. Treatment involves prompt recognition and medical management of the ICP and needle aspiration of the trapped air.

Hydrocephalus

Approximately 50 to 60% of pediatric brain tumors arise in the posterior fossa, and presenting signs and symptoms of obstructive hydrocephalus and elevated ICP are not uncommon. Patients who do not respond to administration of steroids and attempts at medical management (fluid restriction and osmotic diuresis) are candidates for placement of an external ventricular drainage (EVD) system (ventriculostomy). Ventriculostomy is effective in treating hydrocephalus, which usually resolves following surgery. (In one series, only 25% of patients required permanent shunts postoperatively.[98]) Upward herniation has been reported to occur in approximately 10% of patients after external drainage, and extreme care must be employed to keep the drainage pressure at approximately 140 to 165 mm H_2O to avoid this.[98, 99] During or following surgery, blood may be introduced into the subarachnoid space and interfere with CSF resorption, and therefore an EVD may be left in place for several days.

Ventriculostomy may be complicated by parenchymal injury, hemorrhage (1.4%), and infection.[100] Ventriculitis is a localized infection that appears to be most directly related to the length of time for which the catheter was left in place, with an incidence of 6% (5 days in place) to 18% (more than 5 days in place). Overall infection rates are approximately 7%.[101] The administration of prophylactic antibiotics and minimal handling and flushing of the system portend a lower infection rate. An EVD may be left in place for up to 2 weeks if (1) antibiotics are administered, (2) the catheter is tunneled at least 4 to 5 cm away from the insertion site, and (3) CSF cultures are performed every 48 to 72 hours and remain negative.

Seizures

Brain tumors are rarely the underlying cause of seizures in children. Nevertheless, they may be the first manifestation of brain tumors in 11 to 50% of children and adults.[102] Adolescents are three times more likely to have a seizure than younger children. Children with supratentorial tumors are more than four times more likely to have seizures than children with infratentorial tumors.[102] Seizures occur in 1 to 6% of patients with infratentorial tumors. Tumors located near the motor or sensory cortex, as well as the temporal lobes, are the most epileptogenic. The causes of seizures in brain tumor patients include tumoral hemorrhage, necrosis, inflammation, and ischemia of neural tissue.

An important element of preoperative evaluation of a patient with brain tumor and seizure disorder is to decide whether or not to prophylactically administer an antiepileptic agent (AED) and if so, which one. Adult data demonstrate a decrease in the incidence of seizures in patients given prophylactic phenytoin.[103] Patients who are receiving AEDs should have a serum level measured preoperatively. Levels should be monitored closely in the postoperative period as there are many pharmacologic interactions between AEDs and other medications commonly administered postoperatively. Prior to surgery, plans should be made to insert a nasogastric tube while the patient is under anesthesia if it is anticipated that the patient may not be able to swallow medications postoperatively.

Seizures must be rapidly recognized and aggressively treated. *Seizure in a patient with cerebral edema, elevated ICP, or*

intracranial hematoma can have devastating effects. The patient with a brain tumor who is experiencing a seizure should have studies done to rule out metabolic causes, including hyponatremia, hypocalcemia, hypomagnesemia, or hypoglycemia. Status epilepticus causes an increase in cerebral metabolic rate and other physiologic alterations (hypertension, hyperglycemia, hyperthermia, increased intrathoracic pressure, hypercarbia, hypoxia) that may be deleterious to the postoperative patient.[104, 105] Lactic acidosis, hyperkalemia, renal failure, myoglobinuria, arrhythmias, pulmonary aspiration, leukocytosis, and CSF pleocytosis occur when seizures last for more than 30 minutes. Postoperative hematoma, pneumocephalus, and brain swelling may also precipitate seizures in these patients, and one should consider obtaining a CT scan if a metabolic explanation for the seizure cannot be immediately found.

BOX 7-22
Causes of Postoperative Seizures

- **Metabolic (hyponatremia, hypocalcemia, hypomagnesemia, hypoglycemia)**
- **Postoperative hematoma**
- **Pneumocephalus**
- **Edema**
- **Infarct**
- **Inadequate antiepeleptic level**

Pulmonary Embolism

Neurosurgical patients are at risk for the development of deep venous thrombosis (DVT) and pulmonary embolism (PE) resulting from prolonged surgery, glucocorticoid administration, osmotic dehydrating agents, release of brain thromboplastin substance during the operation, limb weakness, and immobilization.[106] Patients who are immobilized develop venous stasis because of the lack of the muscle pump effect as well as venous stagnation in the intra-abdominal organs. Although the incidence of DVT is reported to be 10 to 17% in the adult neurosurgical literature, the incidence in pediatric patients is unknown. The location and histologic features of the CNS tumor have been noted as important risk factors for thromboembolism, with the highest incidence in those patients with suprasellar tumors. A recent study of adult patients with brain tumors cited the incidence of PE at 4%.[107, 108]

Risk factors for PE in pediatric patients include central venous catheters, ventriculoatrial shunts, oral contraceptives, infection, dehydration, obesity, recent surgery, and hypercoagulable state.[109] Pleuritic chest pain is the most common symptom of PE, followed by dyspnea, cough, and hemoptysis. Hypoxemia is a commonly found abnormality, and an abnormal chest radiograph may be seen in approximately 50% of patients. *The diagnostic test of choice is a ventilation-perfusion scan* $(\dot{V}/\dot{Q})$; *however, the gold standard is the pulmonary angiogram.*

Management of PE in neurosurgery is problematical because of the potential of intracranial hemorrhage resulting from standard anticoagulant therapy.[110] Therapeutic options include use of streptokinase, urokinase, heparin, low molecular weight heparin, and vena caval interruption with a Greenfield filter; however, there is no adult consensus and no pediatric data are available.[110–112] The best approach to preventing a PE is to prevent the formation of a DVT. Utilization of intermittent pneumatic compression boots and perioperative elastic stockings should be considered in pediatric patients at risk for postoperative DVT and PE until they can ambulate.

Infections

Infections in brain tumor patients may occur either preoperatively or postoperatively and be located either intracranially or extracranially. The patient may be predisposed to infections because of the underlying medical condition. Certain areas of the body, particularly the mouth and skin, are inhabited by microorganisms. Chemotherapy, use of steroids, poor nutritional status, and radiotherapy may render the patient immunosuppressed. Preoperative infections may involve the respiratory and urinary systems, and patients with indwelling catheters may be predisposed to infectious complications of surgery.

Factors that increase the likelihood of postoperative infection include prolonged operative time, reoperations, surgery on previously irradiated wounds, multiple personnel changes in the operating room, breaks in sterile technique, and use of postoperative drains. The incidence of infections after clean craniotomy (no entry into respiratory, gastrointestinal, or genitourinary tract) has been reported as high as 5%.[113] The probability of an infection can be expressed mathematically to demonstrate the relationship between the size of the innoculum, the virulence of the organism, and the host's defense mechanisms.

$$\frac{\text{Probability}}{\text{of infection}} = \frac{(\text{size of innoculum}) \times (\text{virulence})}{\text{host defenses}}$$

It can be seen from this equation that organisms of higher virulence or massive innocula of organisms of lower virulence would be more likely to cause infection, as would a decrease in the host's defenses.[114] Despite strict aseptic technique, quantitative bacteriologic studies of surgical wounds have demonstrated that 35,000 to 60,000 bacteria fall into a surgical wound every hour that it is exposed.[114] It takes approximately 100,000 organisms per gram of tissue to cause a postoperative wound infection; therefore, longer operative times predispose patients to infection. Because the incidence of postoperative infections is low it is obvious that the host's defensive mechanisms (intact mucosal barriers and normal numbers of functioning polymorphonuclear leukocytes) usually provide a barrier to the bacterial inoculum.[114]

> ## BOX 7-23
> ### Factors That Increase
> ### Risk of Infection
>
> - **Prolonged operating time**
> - **Reoperation**
> - **Prior irradiation**
> - **Postoperative drains**

Intracranial infections may result from either hematogenous or direct spread from extracranial sources; however, most neurosurgical infections involve the wound, bone, dura, brain, and the CSF system and commonly result from perioperative contamination. Organisms accounting for almost 87% of postoperative wound infections include the gram-positive *Staphylococcus aureus* and *Staphylococcus epidermidis*, with gram-negative organisms accounting for the remainder.

Antibiotic prophylaxis is controversial; however, studies to date demonstrate that the relative risk of infection without antibiotic prophylaxis is 5.6 times greater than in patients receiving prophylactic antibiotics.[115] No single antibiotic or administration schedule has been shown to be superior to another. The antibiotics should be chosen based on the sensitivities of the most likely infecting organisms at your institution. The most important concept when using prophylactic antibiotics is that administration of the antibiotic long enough in advance prior to the surgical incision ensures adequate tissue levels at the start of the operation. The drug should be readministered at the proper time interval in longer procedures. Postoperative antibiotic administration does not appear necessary in the majority of cases. Some institutions utilize antibiotics while external CSF drainage is being carried out; however, this practice is of uncertain value.[115] Antibiotic concentrations remain low in the CSF; therefore, once bacteria have invaded the CSF, the BBB, which protected the brain, interferes with therapy aimed at eradicating the infection.

Postoperative meningitis, though not very common and usually less devastating than spontaneous meningitis, may be potentially lethal. The pathogenesis is similar to the mechanisms cited for CSF shunt infections, which include direct contamination of the operative field; procedures done through the heavily colonized scalp; occasional need to enter the frontal, sphenoid, or mastoid air sinuses; and incomplete closure of the dura allowing CSF leak.[116] Elevated temperature is commonly seen in postoperative neurosurgical patients, and the fever response may be blunted by administration of steroids. *Bacterial meningitis should be suspected in any postoperative neurosurgical patient if (1) the fever is high, persistent, or rising; (2) a decline in mental status is noted; (3) the patient is experiencing neck stiffness; or (4) a new neurologic deficit is found.* A lumbar puncture should be performed and the CSF evaluated by Gram's stain. Protein and glucose concentration should be measured, and a white blood cell (WBC) count obtained. Assessment of CSF findings in postoperative neurosurgical patients is difficult. CSF protein and cell counts are almost always elevated, and the glucose may be depressed postoperatively. Although the absolute values are not diagnostic, relatively high CSF WBC counts with a polymorphonuclear predominance are suggestive of infection. The Gram stain may show bacteria; however, a negative Gram stain does not rule out meningitis, and bacterial culture growth may take 1 to 2 days. Prior oral antibiotics do not appear to alter the total CSF WBC count, glucose concentration, or the percentage of patients with a positive latex agglutination test. There is, however, a decrease in the percentage of neutrophils in the CSF, a decrease in the protein, and a decrease in the positivity of the Gram stain and culture results.[117] Intravenous antibiotics given 2 to 3 days prior to lumbar puncture also do not alter the CSF cell count or protein and glucose concentrations but do substantially decrease the chance of demonstrating the bacteria on the Gram stain or culturing the organism from the CSF.[117]

Antibiotic selection should include coverage for both gram-positive and gram-negative organisms. We administer vancomycin and a third-generation cephalosporin (good CNS penetration) as empirical coverage in patients with suspected meningitis while the cultures are pending. It is important to tailor the antibiotics once the organism and sensitivity are known to prevent selection of resistant organisms.

Aseptic, or chemical, meningitis may cause a syndrome indistinguishable from bacterial meningitis. It usually presents with spiking fevers, neck stiffness, and headache several days postoperatively and occurs as the steroids are being tapered. A lumbar puncture usually reveals hypoglycorrhachia, an elevated total protein count, and a pleocytosis with a significant mononuclear component.[118] This syndrome has been reported with an incidence between 30% and 70% in children following procedures of the posterior fossa but may occur with operations in other sites.[119, 120] Factors that may explain the increased incidence in pediatric patients include the use of dural grafts and creation of a CSF "dead space" that may leave a CSF pocket resembling a pseudomeningocele.[121] *It can be appreciated from the above that differentiation between aseptic and bacterial meningitis in the postoperative neurosurgical patient can be difficult. Published studies to date have not found any particular laboratory value to be sensitive or specific enough to differentiate between the two.* In patients who look clinically well and are receiving a steroid wean, the steroids are administered in the previous dosage and the patient is observed. If there is any doubt, CSF cultures are obtained and broad-spectrum antibiotics administered. Management of aseptic meningitis with corticosteroids is undertaken to reduce the meningeal inflammation and to prevent long-term complications, such as adhesive arachnoiditis and hydrocephalus.

Empyemas and abscesses are less common than meningitis. The diagnosis may be difficult because postoperative CT changes may mimic infections and the common organisms include *S. aureus* and *S. epidermidis.* The classic triad of fever, headache, and focal neurologic deficit is present in less than 50% of patients with brain abscesses. Subdural empyema can be difficult to distinguish from meningitis or brain abscess on clinical grounds. Headache is present in approximately 75% of patients, and many of these patients also have an alteration in mental status or focal neurologic signs. Superficial wound infections may spread and cause bone flap infection or meningitis. CSF collections under the skin are not uncommon following craniotomy and may allow the formation of a fistula between the CSF spaces and the skin. Attempts to place stitches in these areas may cause ischemia, edema, and inflammation and produce a substratum for infection.[121] These patients may require a lumbar drain to allow the fistula to close. The bone flap after craniotomy is usually devascularized and devitalized, which leads to decreased natural resistance to infection.[121] A superficial wound in this area must be aggressively treated to halt progression of infection.

Nosocomial or hospital-acquired infections are a significant cause of morbidity and mortality. Nosocomial infections are associated with changes in surface flora (broad-spectrum antibiotics), changes in mucosal surfaces (Foley catheters,

central venous and arterial lines, endotracheal tubes), increased adherence of bacteria, bacterial ability to survive and grow on foreign bodies or altered sites, and modification of local host defenses (tracheotomies, indwelling central venous catheters). A prospective study over a 30-month period showed that of approximately 1400 patients who remained in the PICU for 72 hours or more, 6% developed a nosocomial infection.[122] Patients at risk include children under 2 years of age, children in a catabolic state, patients who are chronically malnourished, and patients who are immunocompromised either by a malignancy or as the result of cancer therapy (steroids, chemotherapeutic agents, radiation). Nosocomial infections include urinary tract infections, bacteremias, catheter-related infections, pneumonia, and surgical wound infections.

Catheter-associated urinary tract infections (UTIs) are the most common of all nosocomial infections, accounting for approximately 40% of infections in most adult hospitals[123] *and for approximately 10% of pediatric nosocomial infections.* Risk factors include female gender (periuretheral entry of rectal flora), duration of catheterization, absence of systemic antibiotics, and catheter sterility violations. In one study, between 10% and 33% of short-term (less than 30 days) catheterized patients developed bacteriuria. Even if the catheter is maintained as a closed system the risk of bacteriuria increases by about 3 to 5% per day. Although usually benign, UTIs may cause bacteremia in 2 to 4% of patients.[123]

Bacteremia is defined as a bloodstream infection occurring in a patient with no evidence of localized infection.[124] Most bacteremias occur in association with an intravascular catheter. Organisms isolated most frequently include the coagulase-negative *S. epidemidis, S. aureus,* and enterococci. Factors associated with catheter-related infections include (1) sterility of insertion technique, (2) type of solution being administered (total parenteral nutrition, intralipids, propofol), (3) number of "break-ins" (medications, blood-drawing), (4) presence of surgical wound, and (5) presence of an infection elsewhere in the body.[124]

Nosocomial pneumonia is the second most common hospital-acquired infection in the United States and accounts for 10 to 15% of pediatric nosocomial infections.[125] Bacteria are the usual cause of the pneumonia; however, approximately 20% are of viral cause, with respiratory syncytial virus the predominant viral pathogen. Routes of bacterial contamination include aspiration of microorganisms from the upper airways, hematogenous spread from remote sites of infection, and direct extension from contiguous sites of infection. The lung is the largest epithelial surface of the body, with an area 40 times larger than that of the skin.[126] As respiration occurs, the upper and lower airways are repeatedly exposed to a multitude of airborne particles and microorganisms. Patients with cranial nerve involvement from the CNS tumor and those recovering from anesthesia may be particularly vulnerable to aspiration pneumonia.[41]

Endotracheal tubes contain large numbers of bacteria (colonization), and the tube bypasses the normal mechanical barrier to infection with the vocal cords stented open, thus allowing microaspiration of oropharyngeal secretions. The presence of a cuffed endotracheal or tracheotomy tube does not prevent microaspiration. Patients who receive standard antacids or histamine blockers have been shown to have a higher incidence of nosocomial pneumonia. This results from the elevation of the gastric pH above the normal level of 1 or 2 to 3.5, thus allowing for an increased bacterial load in the stomach. Diagnosis of ventilator-associated pneumonia includes (1) radiographic appearance of a new pulmonary infiltrate, (2) fever, (3) elevated WBC count, (4) purulent tracheobronchial secretions, and (5) tracheal aspirate Gram's stain showing more than 25 leukocytes per high-power field.[126–128]

Pediatric patients with brain tumors may also present to the PICU with overwhelming sepsis resulting from chemotherapy-induced neutropenia. Neutropenia (defined as fewer than 500 granulocytes or band forms per cubic millimeter) and fever carry a greater than 60% likelihood of infection. Common sites of infection in these patients involve the mouth and pharynx (25%), lower respiratory tract (25%), skin, soft tissue, and intravascular catheters (15%), perineal region (10%), urinary tract (5 to 10%), nose and sinuses (5%), and gastrointestinal tract (15%).[129] The cause of the fever is usually only found in 30 to 40% of patients. Common pathogens include gram-negative bacilli (arising from the gastrointestinal tract), such as *Escherichia coli*, *Klebsiella*, and *Pseudomonas aerguinosa*, and gram-positive organisms, such as *S. aureus*, *S. epidermidis*, and β-hemolytic *Streptococcus*. The risk of infection by gram-positive organisms is greater in patients with indwelling catheters. Patients with fever and neutropenia should be rapidly evaluated and empirical antibiotic coverage be instituted. The combination of an antipseudomonal penicillin (tircarcillin-clavulanate, carbenicillin, or piperacillin) or a cephalosporin with antipseudomonal activity (ceftazidime or cefoperazone) and an aminoglycoside (gentamicin, tobramycin, amikacin) is a well-established regimen.[130, 131]

CSF Shunt Complications

Major complications occurring in patients with CSF shunts include mechanical failure (proximal or distal obstruction) and infection. The risk of shunt failure is greatest in the first several months following placement. Many, if not all, of these children are admitted to the PICU for observation preceding the surgical repair. Common signs and symptoms include headache, vomiting, nausea, altered mental status, lethargy, and a general feeling of malise.[11] It should always be remembered in any patient with a shunt in place that the shunt is the source of the problem until proven otherwise.

BOX 7–24
Signs of Shunt Failure

- **Headache**
- **Nausea and vomiting**
- **Altered mental status**
- **Lethargy**
- **Neck pain**
- **Visual changes**

Obstruction is the most common cause of shunt malfunction, with proximal obstruction occurring more frequently than distal. The proximal end of the catheter becomes occluded with choroid plexus, ependymal cells, glial tissue, brain debris, fibrin, or blood, or the tip of the catheter may migrate into the brain parenchyma. Distal obstruction may result from kinking of the tubing, disconnection of the tubing, migration of the catheter outside the peritoneum, intra-abdominal infection, or pseudocyst formation.

The incidence of CSF shunt infections is between 5% and 8%. Infection may involve the shunt equipment, the wound, the CSF, or the distal site where the shunt drains. Approximately 70% of shunt infections occur within the first 2 months following surgery, which increases to almost 90% occurring in the first 6 months postoperatively. The organisms most frequently isolated include *S. epidermidis* (40%) and *S. aureus* (20%), with the remainder being enterococci, streptococci, gram-negative rods, and yeast. Clinical signs of infection depend on the site of the infection: Wound infections manifest with fever, reddening of the incision or shunt tract, and, as they progress, discharge of pus along the incision. Patients with ventriculitis and meningitis have fever, headache, irritability, and neck stiffness or nuchal rigidity. The treatment of choice is removal of the shunt hardware with placement of an EVD and administration of parenteral antibiotics. Infections of temporarily placed EVDs are managed in the same manner.

Gastrointestinal and Nutritional Issues

Nutrition is an essential component to consider in both postoperative and chronically ill patients. Nutrition is a routine part of PICU therapy. Malnutrition is a disorder of body composition in which macronutrient and/or micronutrient deficiencies occur when nutrient intake is less than required, and which results in reduced organ function, abnormal blood chemistries, reduced body mass, and fewer optimal clinical outcomes.[132] With inadequate caloric intake, energy sources are derived from excessive protein breakdown and gluconeogenesis. This protein is derived from muscle and visceral proteins. Weight loss in excess of 10% is suggestive of malnutrition. The general goals in giving nutritional support are to: (1) provide nourishment consistent with the patient's medical condition, nutritional status, and available route of nutrient administration (enteral vs. parenteral), (2) prevent or treat deficiencies (macro- and/or micronutrients), (3) provide nutrients compatible with the patient's existing metabolism, (4) avoid complications associated with technique of delivery, and (5) improve patient outcomes (body composition, tissue repair, and organ function).[132]

The total caloric requirement can either be estimated using predetermined formulas (e.g., Harris-Benedict) or directly measured. Direct measurements of oxygen consumption and carbon dioxide formation are quite difficult to perform in pediatric patients. Estimates of increased caloric intake of 100% or greater over the calculated basal requirement have been previously recommended to account for increased catabolism (fever, sepsis, burns, head injuries, etc.). *The current recommendation is not to allow more than a 50% increase in calories above the basal requirement.* Calorie overload should be avoided, but energy should be supplied to promote anabolic functions.[133]

The pediatric diet should contain the following: 30 to 50% of the total calories given as glucose, 15 to 30% as fat, and 15 to 20% as protein or amino acids. The enteral route is preferred because it allows preservation of gut integrity as well as barrier and immune functions; decreases bacterial translocation; and reduces the overall rate of infectious complications. One must carefully evaluate whether or not a patient will be able to tolerate foods postoperatively. Despite careful preoperative neurologic evaluation and intraoperative cranial nerve monitoring, damage to the cranial nerves may occur, which may be temporary or permanent. As 50% of pediatric brain tumors arise in the posterior fossa, cranial nerves III to XII may potentially be at some risk of injury. Injury to the glossopharyngeal (IX) and the vagus (X) nerves produces loss of palatal elevation, hoarseness, changes in taste, dysphonia, and changes in vocal cord function, making aspiration a significant problem. Injuries to the cranial nerve complex of IX, X, and XI can cause devastating complications of posterior fossa surgery and may require long periods of rehabilitation.

Children with severe neurologic impairment are often malnourished because oropharyngeal incoordination and neurogenic dysphagia result in inadequate oral intake.[134] Choking episodes during meals with hypoxemia and food aspiration are a common problem. Oral feeding of these children can be quite time consuming and frustrating for both patient and caregiver. The provision of a surgical gastrostomy or a percutaneous endoscopic gastrostomy (PEG) may reduce parental stress and decrease the morbidity associated with oral feedings. *It should be remembered that either of these procedures may cause gastroesophageal reflux (GER) and the performance of an antireflux procedure (fundoplication) carries a high surgical morbidity and mortality in neurologically impaired children.*[135] GER occurs in approximately 30% of critically ill patients when they remain supine. Placement of a nasogastric tube may worsen GER in the postoperative patient by interfering with the lower esophageal sphincter and by prolonging esophageal contact with refluxed gastric contents.[136] High gastric residual volumes resulting from gastric distention may also increase the risk of GER and aspiration. Fluids that accumulate in the gastrointestinal tract of a tube-fed patient include formula, saliva, gastric secretions, and regurgitated small-bowel secretions. When gastrointestinal motility is normal, secretions are propelled forward and adsorbed with little problem. Significant gastric dysmotility (delayed emptying, gastroparesis) occurs in patients with sepsis, postsurgical patients, and those with head injuries.[137] A major cause for disruption of enteral feeds is gastric distention, and consideration should be given to utilizing prokinetic agents to facilitate gastric emptying (e.g., metoclopramide or erythromycin.)

A not uncommon PICU dilemma results in the postoperative patient who is to have her or his trachea extubated the following morning and for one reason or another is not extubated or fails a trial of extubation. The patient has not usually received adequate nutrition prior to the attempt at extubation. The plan is then made to reattempt extubation on the following day, and one can quickly see how a viscious cycle of unplanned events leads to the patient not receiving adequate calories for several days. Early aggressive attempts should be made to provide maximal early nutrition either orally or via nasojejunal or nasogastric tube, PEG, or parenterally. Although concern has been expressed that parenteral feedings may cause hyperosmolarity, hyperglycemia, and fluid overload, which may worsen or cause cerebral edema, this has not been shown to occur.[137] Outcome studies performed in adult patients with head injuries demonstrated a significant better survival rate in patients receiving early parenteral feeds than in those who did not receive adequate calories.[138] We currently implement feedings as soon as they are tolerated by the patient by whichever route is available.

Stress ulcers occur frequently in ICU patients with intracranial disease. After major physiologic stress endoscopic evidence of mucosal lesions of the gastrointestinal tract appear within 24 hours of injury; and 17% of these erosions progress to clinically significant bleeding in adult patients.[139] Intracranial diseases of the diencephalon and brain stem may lead to a disinhibition of the medullary vagal system, causing an increase in the production and secretion of acid and pepsin. The pathogenesis of these gastrointestinal lesions is unclear but involves destructive factors, such as pepsin, acid and bile, decreased mucosal blood flow, loss of the mucosal protective layer, decreased epithelial cell replacement, and decreased prostaglandin production. Stress ulcerations are more common in patients with malnutrition and those receiving steroids (due to decreased mucosal blood flow and decreased prostaglandin production). Other medications, such as NSAIDs (e.g., ketorolac), may also contribute. Therapeutic options include antacids, histamine receptor antagonists, and sucralfate. Agents that raise the acidic pH of the stomach above 3.5 have been associated with a higher incidence of nosocomial pneumonia. Side effects of antacids include diarrhea, constipation, hypophosphatemia, and metabolic alkalosis. Histamine blockers (cimetidine, ranitidine, and famotidine) inhibit the release of acid from the gastric parietal cells, and whether they are more protective than antacids is controversial. Sucralfate binds to normal and damaged gastric mucosa, increases the viscosity and mucin content of the gastric mucus, increases mucosal blood flow, and is not associated with an increased incidence of nosocomial pneumonia. Enteral nutrition also plays a role in stress ulcer protection by causing a dilutional alkalinization and by maintaining the positive nitrogen balance important for normal reparative functions of the gastric mucosa.

Although pediatric data are lacking, it is thought that in adult patients who are receiving steroids routine prophylaxis is not warranted except when the following risk factors are present: history of peptic ulcer disease, concurrent use with aspirin or other NSAIDs, renal or hepatic dysfunction, and malnourished state. Only patients who were administered steroids for more than 3 weeks and daily doses of dexamethasone (greater than 40 mg/kg per day) seem to be at risk for gastrointestinal bleeds.[139]

CONCLUSION

Pediatric patients with brain tumors present to the PICU with a myriad of problems arising either from the primary tumor or as a result of surgical or other therapeutic options (chemotherapy, radiotherapy, invasive procedures). It is hoped that after reviewing this chapter the age-old adage "infants and children are small adults" will appear quite untrue. Children with brain tumors need to be cared for by an experienced multidisciplinary team that is familiar with the different physiologic and unique emotional needs of these young patients. The current health care system demands that we continuously evaluate and reevaluate our utilization of these valued resources. Much research is needed to evaluate the health care delivery to and clinical outcomes of these children both during and following their PICU stay. Data collected in adult critical care units is not always applicable to our fragile population, and there is much to be done as we are truly only at the tip of the iceberg of our knowledge base. Scoring systems such as the PRISM (Pediatric Risk of Mortality) and the Fiser Pediatric Cerebral Performance Outcome Category scales need to be applied and validated in these patients.[140, 141] Perhaps new outcome predictors are necessary and "centers of excellence" will help facilitate these studies. It is demanding, exhausting, and truly exciting to be involved in the care of these special children.

REFERENCES

1. Corbally MT. Supportive care of the pediatric cancer patient. *Semin Surg Oncol* 1993;9:461–466.
2. Cohen ME, Duffner PK, Kun Le, et al. The argument for a combined consortium research data base. *Cancer* 1985;56:1897–1901.
3. Bailey C, Gnekow A, Welk S, et al. Prospective randomized trial of chemotherapy given before radiotherapy in childhood medulloblastoma. *Med Pediatr Oncol* 1995;25(3):166–178.
4. Kanter MJ, Narayan RK. Intracranial pressure monitoring. *Neurosurg Clin North Am* 1991;2(2)257–265.
5. Chesnut RM, Marshall LF. Treatment of abnormal intracranial pressure. *Neurosurg Clin North Am* 1991;2(2):267–284.
6. Fletcher JM, Miner ME, Ewing-Cobbs L. Age and recovery from head injury in children. In: Levin H, Grafman J, Eisenberg H, eds. *Neurobehavioral Recovery from Head Injury.* New York: Oxford University Press; 1987:279–291.
7. Yeman TA. Pediatric Neuroanesthesia. In: Stone DJ, Sperry RJ, Johnson JO, Spiekennan BF, Yemen TA, eds. *The Neuroanesthesia Handbook.* St. Louis: Mosby; 1996; 251–274.
8. Ritter AM, Robertson CS. Cerebral metabolism. *Neurosurg Clin North Am* 1994;5(4):633–645.
9. LaManna JC, Lust WD. Nutrient consumption and metabolic perturbations. *Neurosurg Clin North Am* 1997;2(8):145–163.
10. Jordan KG. Neurophysiologic monitoring in the Neuroscience Intensive Care Unit. *Neurol Clin* 1995;(13)3:579–623.
11. Madikians A, Conway EE. CSF shunt problems in pediatric patients. *Pediatr Ann* 1997;26(10):613–620.
12. Duhaime AC, Schut L, Sutton L. Surgery for posterior fossa tumors. In: Packer RJ, Bleyer WA, Pochedly, eds. *Pediatric Neuro-oncology.* Philadelphia: Harwood Academic Publishers; 1991:128–135.
13. Kalfas IH, Little JR. Postoperative hemorrhage: a survey of 4992 Intracranial procedures. *Neurosurgery* 1988;23:343–347.
14. Palmer JD, Sparrow OC, Jannotti, FI. Postoperative Hematoma: A 5 year survey and identification of avoidable risk factors. *Neurosurgery* 1994;35:1061–1065.
15. Mahaley MS, Mettlin C, Natarajan N, et al. National survey of patterns of care for brain-tumor patients. *J Neurosurg* 1989;71:826–836.
16. Chripko D, Bevan JC, Archer DP, et al. Decreases in arterial oxygen saturation in paediatric outpatients during transfer to the postanesthetic recovery room. *Can J Anaesth* 1989;36:128–132.
17. Patel RI, Norden J, Hannallah RS. Oxygen administration prevents hypoxemia during post-anesthetic transport in children. *Anesthesiology* 1988;69:616–618.
18. Rosenberg H, Clofine R, Bialik O. Neurologic changes during awakening from anesthesia. *Anesthesiology* 1981;45:125–130.
19. McCulloch PR, Milne B. Neurological phenomena during emergence from enflurane or isoflurane anesthesia. *Can J Anesth* 1990;37:139–142.
20. Schubert A, Mascha EJ, Bloomfield EL, et al. Effect of cranial surgery and brain tumor size on emergence from anesthesia. *Anesthesiology* 1996;85:513–521.
21. Kalisch BJ, Kalisch PA, Burns SM, et al. Intrahospital transport of neuro ICU patients. *J Neurosci Nursing* 1995;27(2):69–77.
22. Watcha MF, Bras PJ, Cieslak GD, Pennant JH. The dose-response relationship of ondansetron in preventing postoperative emesis in pediatric patients undergoing ambulatory surgery. *Anesthesiology* 1995;87:47–52.
23. DeBenedittis G, Lorenzetti A, Migliare M, et al. Postoperative pain in neurosurgery. A pilot study in Brain Surgery. *Neurosurgery* 1996;38(3):466–470.
24. Von Keuren K, Eland JA. Perioperative pain management in children. *Nursing Clin North Am* 1997;32(1):31–44.
25. Goldsack CS, Scuplak SM, Smith M. A double-blind comparison of codeine and morphine for postoperative analgesia following intracranial surgery. *Anesthesia* 1996;51:1029–1032.
26. Watcha MF, Jones MB, Laqueruela RG, et al. Comparison of ketorolac and morphine as adjuvants during pediatric surgery. *Anesthesiology* 1992;76:368–372.
27. Houck CS, Wilder RT, McDermott JS, et al. Safety of intravenous ketorolac therapy in children and cost savings with a unit dosing system. *J Pediatr* 1996;129:292–296.
28. Tobias JD. Sedation and analgesia for children in the pediatric intensive care unit. *J Inten Care Med* 1995;10:294–314.

29. Mirski MA, Muffelman B, Ulatowski JA, Hanley DF. Sedation for the critically ill neurologic patient. *Crit Care Med* 1995;23:238–253.

30. Chang MA, Theard A, Tempelhoff R. Intravenous agents and intraoperative neuroprotection: Beyond barbiturates. *Crit Care Clin North Am* 1997;13(1):185–200.

31. Roselund RC. Postanesthetic care of the neurosurgical patient. *Anesthesiol Clin North Am* 1987;5(3):639–651.

32. Levy L, Pandit VA, Randal GI, et al. *Anesthesia* 1992; 47:678–682.

33. Hollinger IB. Management of postanesthetic pediatric problems. *Anesthesiol Clin North Am* 1990;8(2):323–353.

34. Emhardt JD, Weisberger EC, Dierdorf SF, et al. The rise of arterial carbon dioxide during apnea in children. *Anesthesiology* 1988;69A:779.

35. Airway and Ventilation In: Chameides L, Hazinski MF, eds. *Textbook of Pediatric Advanced Life Support.* New York: American Heart Association; 1994:4.1–4.22.

36. Kemper KJ, Ritz RM, Benson MS, Bishop MS. Helium-oxygen mixture in the treatment of post extubation stridor in pediatric trauma patients. *Crit Care Med* 1991;19: 356–359.

37. Holzman RS. Latex allergy: an emerging operating room problem. *Anesth Analg* 1993;76:635–641.

38. Hamid RKA. Latex allergy: diagnosis, management and safe equipment. *ASA Refresher Courses in Anesthesiology* 1996;(4)85–96.

39. De Nicola LK, Monem GF, Gayle MD, Kissoon N. Treatment of critical status asthmaticus in children. *Pediatr Clin North Am* 1994;41(6):1293–1316.

40. Salem MR, Wong AM, Collins VJ. The pediatric patient with a full stomach. *Anesthesiology* 1993;39:435–440.

41. Britto J, Demling RH. Aspiration lung injury. *New Horiz* 1993; 1(3):435–439.

42. Cole CJ, Goudsouzian NG, Liu MP. Assessment of risk factors related to the acid aspiration syndrome in pediatric patients. *Anesthesiology* 1982;56:70–72.

43. Frost EA, Gordon R. Complications in the postanesthetic care unit. *Semin Anesthesiol* 1996;15(2):148–158.

44. Cushing H. Some experimental and clinical observations concerning states of increased intracranial tension. *Ann J Med Sci* 1902;124:375–400.

45. Tietjen CS, Hurn PD, Ulatowski JA, Kirsch JR. Treatment modalities for hypertensive patients with intracranial pathology: options and risks. *Crit Care Med* 1996;24(2): 311–322.

46. Davis TP, Alexander J, Lesch M. Electrocardiographic changes associated with acute cerebrovascular disease: a clinical review. *Progre Cardiovasc Dis:* 1993;44(3): 245–260.

47. Oppenheimer S, Cechetto DF, Hachinski VC. Cerebrogenic cardiac arrhythmias. *Arch Neurol* 1990;47:513–519.

48. Conway EE, Zuckerman GB. The long hot summer. *Contemp Pediatr* 1997;14(6):127–136.

49. Khilnani P. Electrolyte abnormalities in critically ill children. *Crit Care Med* 1992;20(2):241–250.

50. Gruskin AB, Baluarte HJ, Prebis JN. Serum sodium abnormalities in children. *Pediatr Clin North Am* 1982; 29:907–932.

51. Diringer MN. Management of sodium abnormalities in patients with CNS disease. *Clin Neuropharmacol* 1992; 15(6)427–447.

52. Sarnaik AP, Meert K. Hackbarth R, et al. Management of hyponatremic seizures in children with hypertonic saline: a safe and effective strategy. *Crit Care Med* 1991;19: 758–762.

53. Andrew RD. Seizure and osmotic change: clinical and neurophysiological aspects. *J Neurol Sci* 1991;101:7–18.

54. Oh MS, Carroll HJ. Disorders of sodium metabolism: hypematremia and hyponatremia. *Crit Care Med* 1992;20: 94–103.

55. Ganong CA, Kappy MS. Cerebral salt wasting in children: the need for recognition and treatment. *Am J Dis Child* 1992;147:167–169.

56. Harrigan MR. Cerebral salt wasting syndrome: a review. *Neurosurgery* 1996;38(1):152–160.

57. Al-Mufti H, Arieff AI. Hyponatremia due to cerebral salt-wasting syndrome. *Am J Med* 1984;77:740–746.

58. Hasan D, Lindsay KW, Wijdicks E, et al. Effect of fludrocortisone acetate in patients with subarachnoid hemorrhage. *Stroke* 1989;9:1156–1161.

59. McDonald JA, Martha PM, Kerrigan J, et al. Treatment of the young child with postoperative diabetes insipidus. *Am J Dis Child* 1989;143:201–204.

60. Blevins LS, Ward GS. Diabetes insipidus. *Crit Care Med* 1992;20:69–79.

61. Outwater KM, Rockoff MA. Diabetes insipidus accompanying brain death in children. *Neurology* 1984;34: 1243–1246.

62. Chanson P, Jedynak CP, Dabrowski G, et al. Ultralow doses of vasopressin in the management of diabetes insipidus. *Crit Care Med* 1987;15(1)44–46.

63. Harri's AS. Clinical experience with desmopressin: efficacy and safety in central DI and other conditions. *J Pediatr* 1989;114(2):711–718.

64. Linshaw MA. Potassium homeostasis and hypokalemia. *Pediatr Clin North Am* 1987;34(3):649–676.

65. Zalaoga GP. Hypocalcemia in critically ill patients. *Crit Care Med* 1992;20:251–262.

66. Whang R. Magnesium deficiency: pathogenesis, prevalence and clinical implication. *Am J Med* 1987;82(Suppl 3A):24–29.

67. Nuytten D, Van Hess J, Meulemars A, et al. Magnesium deficiency as a cause of acute intractable seizures. *J Neurol* 1991;238:262–264.

68. Weisman C. The metabolic response to stress: an overview and update. *Anesthesiology* 1990;73:308–327.

69. Sieber FE, Traystman RJ. Special issues: glucose and the brain. *Crit Care Med* 1991;20:104–114.

70. Malourf R, Brust JC. Hypoglycemia: causes, neurological manifestations and outcome. *Ann Neurol* 1985;17:421–430.

71. Wass CT, Lanier WL. Glucose modulation of ischemic brain injury: review and clinical recommendations. *Mayo Clin Proc* 1996;(71):801–812.

72. Natale JE, Stante SM, D'Alecy LG. Elevated brain lactate accumulation and increased neurologic deficit are associated with modest hyperglycemia in global brain ischemia. *Resuscitation* 1990;19:271–289.

73. Bingaman WE, Frank JI. Malignant cerebral edema and intracranial hypertension. *Neurol Clin* 1995;13(3):479–509.

74. Hariri RJ. Cerebral edema. *Neurosurg Clin North Am* 1994;5(4):687–706.

75. Reuben HJ, Huber P, Ito U, et al. Peritumoral brain edema: a keynote address. *Adv Neurol* 1990;52:307–315.

76. Hossman KA, Wechsler W, Wilmes F. Experimental peritumorous edema: morphological and pathophysiological observations. *Acta Neuropathol* 1979;45:195–200.

77. Glaser AW, Buston N, Walker D. Corticosteroids in the management of central nervous system tumors. *Arch Dis Child* 1997;76:76–78.

78. Chin R, Eagerton DC, Salem M. Corticosteroids. In: Chernow B, ed. *The Pharmacologic Approach to the Critically Ill Patient*. 3rd ed. Baltimore: Williams and Wilkins; 1994; 715–741.

79. Milgron H, Bender B. Psychologic side effects of therapy with corticosteroids. *Am Rev Respir Dis* 1992;147:471–473.

80. Salem M, Tainsh RE, Jr, Branberg J, et al. Perioperative glucocortical coverage: A reassessment 42 years after emergence of a problem. *Ann Surg* 1994;219(4):416–425.

81. Knowlton AI. Adrenal insufficiency in the intensive care setting. *J Intensive Care Med* 1989;4:35–45.

82. Rosner MJ, Coley I. Cerebral perfusion pressure, the ICP and head elevation. *J Neurosurg* 1986;65:636–640.

83. Frank JI. Management of intracranial hypertension. *Med Clin North Am* 1993;77(1):61–76.

84. Paczynski RP. Osmotherapy: basic concepts and controversies. *Crit Care Clin* 1997;13(1):105–129.

85. Yundt K, Kiringer MN. The use of hyperventilation and its impact on cerebral ischemia in the treatment of traumatic brain injury. *Crit Care Clin* 1997;13(1):163–184.

86. Lee MW, Deppe SA, Sipperly E, et al. Efficacy of barbiturate coma in the management of uncontrolled intracrainal hypertension following neurosurgical trauma. *J Neurotrauma* 1994;11(3):325–331.

87. Marion DW, Penrod LE, Kelsey SF, et al. Treatment of traumatic brain injury with moderate hypothermia. *N Engl J Med* 1997;336:540–546.

88. Wityk RJ, Stem BJ. Ischemic stroke: today and tomorrow. *Crit Care Med* 1994;22:1278–1293.

89. Heiss WD, Rosner G. Functional recovery of cortical neurons as related to degree and duration of ischemia. *Am Neurol* 1983;14:294–301.

90. Memezawa H, Smith ML, Siesjo BK. Penumbral tissues salvaged by reperfusion following middle cerebral artery occlusion in rats. *Stroke* 1992;23:552–559.

91. Mayer SA, Thomas CE, Diamond BE. Asymmetry of intracranial hemodynamics as an indicator of mass effect in acute intracerebral hemorrhage. *Stroke* 1996;27:1788–1792.

92. Markham JW. Pneumocephalus. In: Vinken PJ, Brwyn GW, eds. *Handbook of Clinical Neurology*. Amsterdam: North Holland; 1976:201–213.

93. Reasoner DK, Todd MM, Scamman F, et al. The incidence of pneumocephalus after supratentorial craniotomy. *Anesthesiology* 1994;8:1008–1012.

94. Ruge J, Cerullo L, McLaren D. Pneumocephalus in patients with CSF shunts. *J Neurosurg* 1985;63:532–536.

95. Yates H, Hamill M, Borel CO, et al. Incidence and perioperative management of tension pneumocephalus following craniofacial resection. *J Neurosurg Anesthesiol* 1994; 6(1):15–20.

96. Spetzler RF, Zabramski JM. Cerebrospinal fluid fistulae: management and repair. In: Youmans JR, ed. *Neurological Surgery: A Comprehensive Reference Guide to the Diagnosis and Management of Neurosurgical Problems*. 3rd ed. Philadelphia: WB Saunders; 1990:2275–2279.

97. Dexter F, Reasoner DK. Theoretical assessment of normobaric oxygen therapy to treat pneumocephalus: recommendations for dose and duration of treatment. *Anesthesiology* 1996;84:442–447.

98. Papo I, Caruselli G, Luongo A. External ventricular drainage in the management of posterior fossa tumors in children and adolescents. *Neurosurgery* 1982;10:13–15.

99. Epstein F, Murali R. Pediatric posterior fossa tumors: hazards of the pregenative shunt. *Neurosurgery* 1978;3: 348–350.

100. Narayan RK, Kishore PRD, Becker DP, et al. Intracranial pressure: to monitor or not to monitor? *J Neurosurg* 1982;56:650–659.

101. Winfield JA, Rosenthal P, Kanter RK, et al. Duration of intracranial pressure monitoring does not reflect daily risk of infectious complications. *Neurosurgery* 1993;33: 424–431.

102. Gilles FM, Sobel E, Leviton A, et al. Epidemiology of seizures in children with brain tumors. *J Neuro-oncol* 1992;12:53–68.

103. North JB, Penhall RK, Hanieh A, et al. Phenytoin and post-operative epilepsy: a double-blinded study. *J Neurosurg* 1983;58:672–677.

104. Payne JA and Bleck TP. Status epilepticus. *Crit Care Clin* 1997;13(1):17–38.

105. Rubin DM, Conway EE, Caplan SM. Pediatric neurologic emergencies. In: Barkin R, Rosen J, eds. *Emergency Medicine: Concepts and Clinical Practice*. 4th ed. St. Louis: Mosby; 1998:1213–1243.

106. Inci S, Erbengi A, Berker M. Pulmonary embolism in neurosurgical patients. *Surg Neurol* 1995;43:123–129.

107. Constantini S, Karnowski, R, Pomerantz S, et al. Thromboembolic phenomena in neurosurgical patients operated upon for primary and metastatic brain tumors. *Acta Neurochir (Wein)* 1991;109:93–97.

108. Levi ADO, Wallace MC, Bernstein M, et al. Venous thromboembolism after brain tumor surgery: a retrospective review. *Neurosurgery* 1991;28:859–863.

109. King D, Conway EE, Jr. Pulmonary embolus. In: Friedman SB, Fisher M, Schinberg K, Alderman E, eds. *Comprehensive Adolescent Health Care*. 2nd ed. St. Louis: Mosby; 1998:670–673.

110. Hamilton MG, Hull RD, Pineo GF. Venous thromboembolism in neurosurgery and neurology patients: a review. *Neurosurgery* 1994;34(2):280–293.

111. Frim DM, Barker FG, Poletti CE, et al. Postoperative low-dose heparin decreases thromboembolic complications in neurosurgery patient. *Neurosurgery* 1992;30:6:830–833.

112. Wijdicks EF, Scott JB. Pulmonary embolism associated with acute stroke. *Mayo Clin Proc* 1997;72(4):297–300.

113. Dempsey R, Rapp R, Young B, et al. Prophylactic antibiotics in clean neurosurgical procedures: a review. *J Neurosurg* 1988;69:52.
114. Borges LF. Host defenses. *Neurosurg Clin* 1992;3(2):275–278.
115. Haines SJ. Antibiotic prophylaxsis in neurosurgery. *Neurosurg Clin* 1992;3(2):355–357.
116. Kaufman BA, Tunkel AP, Pryor JC, Dacey, RG, Jr. Meningitis in the neurosurgicai patient. *Infecti Dis Clin* 1990;4(4):677–701.
117. Ashwal S, Perkin RM, Thompson JR, et al. Bacterial meningitis in children: current concepts of neurologic management. *Adv Pediat* 1993;40:185–215.
118. Ross P, Rosegay H, Pons V. Differentiation of aseptic and bacterial meningitis in postoperative neurosurgical patients. *J Neurosurg* 1988;69:669–674.
119. Carmel PW, Fraser, RA, Stein BM. Aseptic meningitis following posterior fossa surgery in children. *J Neurosurg* 1974;41:44–48.
120. Carmel PW and Grief LK. The aseptic meningitis syndrome: a complication of posterior fossa surgery. *Pediatr Neurosurg* 1993;19:276–280.
121. Blomstedt GC. Craniotomy infections. *Neurosurg Clin* 1992;3(2)375–383.
122. Milliken J, Tait GA, Ford-Jones, EL, et al. Nosocomial infections in a PICU. *Crit Care Med* 1988;16:233–237.
123. Stamm WE. Catheter-associated urinary tract infections: epidemiology, pathogenesis and prevention. *Am J Med* 1991;91(Suppl 3B):655–715.
124. Stein F, Trevino R. Nosocomial infections in the PICU. *Pediatr Clin* 1994;41(6):1245–1257.
125. Horan TC, White JW, Jarvis WR, et al. Nosocomial infection surveillance. *MMWR CDC Surveill Summ* 1986;35:SS17–SS29.
126. Nelson S, Mason CM, Kolls J and Summer WR. Pathophysiology of pneumonia. *Clin Chest Med* 1995;16(1):1–12.
127. Meduri GU. Diagnosis and differential diagnosis of ventilator-associated pneumonia. *Clin Chest Med* 1995;16(1):61–93.
128. Kirtland SH, Corley DE, Winterbauer RH, et al. The diagnosis of ventilator-associated pneumonia: a comparison of histologic, microbiologic and clinical criteria. *Chest* 1997;112(2):445–458.
129. Giamarellou H. Empiric therapy for infections in the febrile neutropenic compromised host. *Med Clin* 1995;79(3):559–580.
130. Valentino TL, Conway, EE Jr, Maher TS, et al. Pediatric brain tumors. *Pediatr Ann* 1997;26(10):579–587.
130A. Conway Jr EE, Asunction A, Da Rosso R. Diagnosing and managing brain tumors: the pediatrician's role. *Contemp Pediatr* 1999;16(11):84–87.
131. Hathorn JW, Lyke K. Empirical treatment of febrile neutropenia: Evolution of current therapeutic approaches. *Clin Infect Dis* 1997;24(Suppl 2):S256–S265.
132. Cerra FB, Benitez MR, Blackburn GL, et al. Applied nutrition in ICU patients: a consensus statement of the American College of Chest Physicians. *Chest* 1997;111(3):769–778.
133. Chwals WJ. Overfeeding the critically ill child: fact or fantasy? *New Horizons* 1994;2(2):147–155.
134. Heine RG, Reddihough DS, Catto-Smith AG. Gastrooesophageal reflux and feeding problems after gastrostomy in children with severe neurologic impairment. *Dev Med Child Neurol* 1995;37:320–329.
135. Pearl RH, Robie DK, Ein SH, et al. Complications of gastroesophageal antireflux surgery in neurologically impaired versus neurologically normal children. *J Pediatr Surg* 1990;25:1169–1173.
136. Kazi N, Mobarhan S. Enteral feeding associated gastroesophageal reflux and aspiration pneumonia: a review. *Nutr Review* 1996;54(10):324–328.
137. Young B, Ott L, Yingling B, McClain C. Nutrition and brain injury. *J Neurotrauma* 1992;9(Suppl):S375–S383.
138. Twyman D. Nutritional management of the critically ill neurologic patient. *Crit Care Clin* 1997;13(1):39–49.
139. Lu WY, Rohney DH, Boling WB, et al. A review of stress ulcer prophylaxis in the neurosurgical ICU. *Neurosurgery* 1997;41(2):416–426.
140. Pollack MM, Patel KM, Ruttimann VE. PRISM III: an updated pediatric risk of mortality score. *Crit Care Med* 1996;24(5):743–752.
141. Fiser DH. Assessing the outcome of pediatric intensive care. *J Pediatr* 1992;121:68–74.

Chapter 8

Radiotherapy

Eugenio Vines, Helaine F. Bertsch, and Joel Goldwein

HISTORICAL PERSPECTIVE

Radiation therapy has been used in the treatment of childhood central nervous system (CNS) tumors for many decades. Anecdotal reports of radiation therapy for brain tumors go back at least 80 years.[1] Harvey Cushing, who not only established neurosurgery as a modern specialty, also pioneered the use of radiation therapy in the management of these tumors.[2] In 1925, Bailey and Cushing described the posterior fossa medulloblastoma and classified it as a glioma.[3] A year later, Bailey and Cushing reported that four such patients were treated with radiation therapy and survived for 41 to 72 months in "good condition."[4] After analyzing the natural history of medulloblastoma, Ralston Paterson proposed irradiation of "all cerebro-spinal pathways, from the ventricles to the cauda equina."[5] In his textbook, Paterson also stressed the importance of adequate tissue diagnosis and treatment planning. Later, he deemed medulloblastoma to be "curable in about 40 per cent of cases fully treated."[6] Edith Paterson reported a 21% 5-year survival for children with medulloblastoma who were treated with kilovoltage irradiation at the Christie Hospital. A dose of 3000 to 3500 R to the craniospinal axis using 250 kVp was delivered by a three-field technique.[7] Radiation therapy was also used to treat CNS tumors at the Montreal Children's Hospital. Results showed that 42% of 119 children survived longer than 5 years.[8]

Supervoltage equipment became available in the mid-1950s. This technology provided better distribution of radiation throughout the tumor while sparing normal tissue. Survival improvements over these years paralleled those for other pediatric malignancies, such as leukemia, Wilms' tumor, and rhabdomyosarcoma.

The development of computerized isodose treatment planning, simulators, customized blocking, and beams with precisely defined margins has markedly improved our capacity to deliver radiation. New diagnostic techniques, such as computed tomography (CT) and magnetic resonance imaging (MRI), have increased the knowledge of the anatomical patterns of tumor presentation and spread, thereby enhancing our ability to define tumor margins.

However, not all gains are due to radiotherapy technology. Some may have been due to stage migration, earlier diagnosis, more comprehensive means for evaluation, and improved medical management. Evolution in the interpretation of pathology specimens may also have had an effect.

OVERVIEW OF THE PHYSICS OF RADIATION THERAPY

A thorough understanding of the physical and technological aspects of radiotherapy is essential for the design of treatments, as well as for the interpretation of literature. In this section, the basics of radiation physics will be summarized. The reader is referred to standard textbooks for in-depth discussions of these topics.[9, 10]

Radiation energy causes ionization of water molecules, ultimately generating reactive free radicals, which cause damage in multiple macromolecules at the cellular level. The energy of a radiation beam is expressed in electron volts (eV), defined as the energy necessary to move an electron across a gradient of 1 volt. Initial measurements of radiation relied on clinical observation of its effects. Commonly, the dose required to elicit erythema was used to quantify treatments. With increasing technical refinements, this was replaced by measure of ionization in air (exposure) in roentgens (R). *Currently, absorbed dose (energy deposited per unit mass) is measured in gray (Gy = J/kg).* One Gy is equivalent to 100 rads, the legacy dose unit.

Photons and electrons are the most commonly used types of radiation in clinical practice. The deposition of high-energy photons in tissue ($\geq$1.2 MeV) is characterized by sparing of the skin such that the maximum dose is deposited beneath the surface of the irradiated area. Electrons, on the other hand, almost completely lack skin sparing, and their energy is completely deposited in a range of a few centimeters in tissue, with the potential to spare deep structures (Fig. 8–1).

To minimize the radiation deposited outside an intended treatment region, radiation fields are collimated. This is achieved by blocking the beam of radiation using shields inside the treatment machine. Further shaping of the radiation beam is attained by use of secondary blocking, inserted between the head of the machine and the patient (for both electrons and photons) or at the skin surface (for electrons). This is used to protect normal structures from excessive doses of radiation (Fig. 8–2).

Within the energy range of therapeutic use there is little variation in dose absorption between bone and soft tissues. Both approximate the dose distribution characteristics of water. When dose measurements in water are plotted, it becomes evident that different points along a plane perpendicular to the beam in the irradiated field receive the same

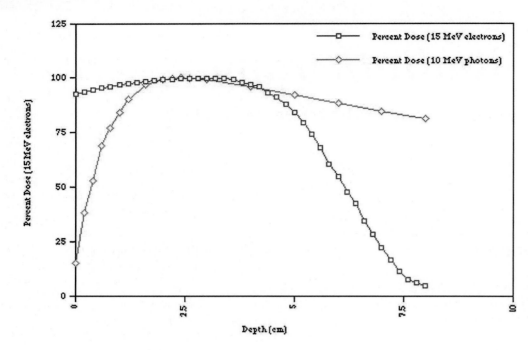

Figure 8–1   Percent depth dose for a 10-MeV photon beam and a 15-MeV electron beam in water. Note that the maximum delivered dose (100%) is at 2.4 cm for the photon beam, compared to 3.0 cm for the electron beam. The relatively low dose delivered by the photon beam at the surface accounts for the skin sparing effect. The limited range of the electron beam is also evident.

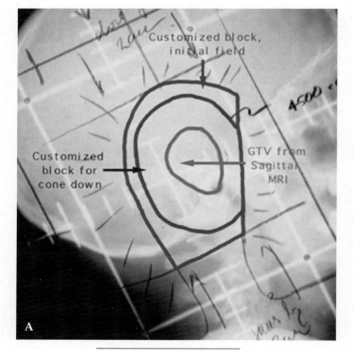

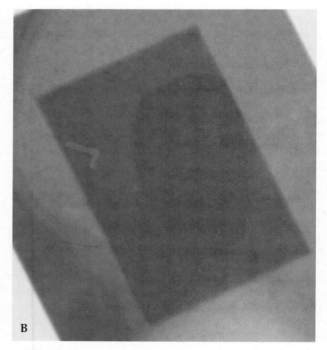

Figure 8–2   (A) Typical simulation film in a brain stem glioma case. The tumor volume is outlined on the film using the technique described in Fig. 8–12. Customized blocking is designed surrounding the tumor and sparing adjacent brain. A cone down field is also represented. This will allow some sparing of normal structures at the periphery of the field, while taking the tumor volume to a higher radiation dose. (GTV: gross tumor volume) (B) Verification portals obtained with the treatment machine. This allows for a direct comparison between planned fields (Fig. 8–2A) and the actual treatment.

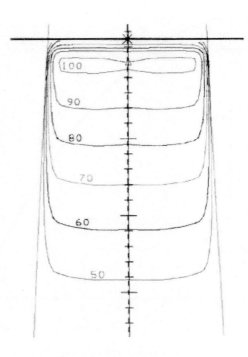

Figure 8–3 Isodose curves in water for a single 6-MeV photon field. Note the inhomogeneous distribution of dose with varying depths. Dose is expressed as a percentage of the maximum dose.

radiation dose. This is represented by *isodose curves* (Fig. 8–3). Treatment with multiple radiation fields improves the dose distribution. Such techniques are used to spare sensitive structures from high doses of radiation (Fig. 8–4).

Brachytherapy uses a sealed radioactive material to deliver radiation. The source is placed at close proximity to the target volume, and the radiation is delivered within a short range. A variety of different sources may be used, with different levels of activity, energies, and half-lives. Brachytherapy treatments may be temporary (i.e., when the

source is removed after a short period of time) or permanent (i.e., when the source is left in place indefinitely).

OVERVIEW OF RADIATION BIOLOGY

Radiation induces the majority of tissue damage through indirect effects on DNA. The interaction of photons and electrons with matter results in disruption of chemical bonds and ionization. Water is the most abundant molecule in living tissue and therefore the most likely to interact with radiation. This interaction generates hydroxyl radicals, which react with oxygen to create highly reactive oxygen species. These radicals, in turn, react with important biologic molecules, causing damage. The most important target for the effect of radiation is thought to be the DNA molecule.

Breaks in the DNA molecule arise from direct or indirect interactions with the incident radiation. Single DNA strand breaks are readily repaired; double-strand breaks result in breaks of chromatin and are more difficult to repair. Ultimately, such breaks may result in permanent damage.

An irradiated cell may experience one of several phenomena:

1. *Repair*: Damaged DNA may be completely repaired. In proliferating cells this is usually accompanied by a cell cycle arrest. Several checkpoints have been described that correspond to critical transitions in the cell cycle. If DNA damage is detected, the cell will not progress to the next stage until the DNA has been repaired.

2. *Mutations*: Mutations are persistent changes in the DNA that do not affect the cell's indemnity.

3. *Reproductive cell death*: The cell may retain its metabolic functions, but it loses its ability to reproduce indefinitely.

4. *Necrosis*: Cell death occurs instantaneously after exposure to extremely high doses of radiation, due to damage to organelles.

5. *Apoptosis*: Also called programmed cell death, apoptosis involves degradation of nuclear and cytoplasmic structures, and phagocytosis of cellular fragments by adjacent cells, without an inflammatory reaction. One mechanism that triggers apoptosis is irreparable DNA damage. Cell cycle checkpoints are involved in this route for apoptosis.

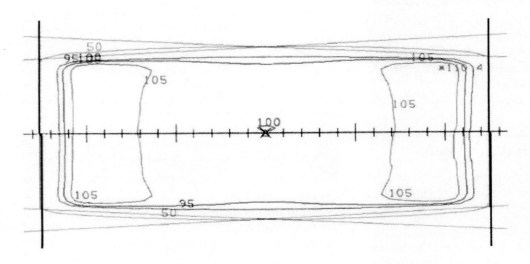

Figure 8–4 Parallel opposed fields, 6-MeV photons. Note how the additional field improves the dose homogeneity throughout the irradiated volume. Dose is expressed as a percentage of the dose delivered to the midplane.

BOX 8–1
Factors That Determine the Radiosensitivity of Cells

- *Oxygenation status:* A well-oxygenated cell is more radiosensitive than a relatively hypoxic cell. This is due to the availability of oxygen to react with free radicals.
- *Relative position in the cell cycle:* Radiosensitivity is known to vary throughout the cell cycle, with late G1, G2, and M being the most radiosensitive phases; and G0, early G1, and S the most radioresistant. This is probably related to the ability of the cell to react to and repair DNA damage.
- *Nutritional and metabolic microenvironment.*
- *Intrinsic radiosensitivity:* Reflects a cell's ability to respond to and repair DNA damage, and its capacity to prevent oxidative damage.

BOX 8–2
Factors That Determine the Effectiveness of Radiation

- *Type of radiation:* For example, neutrons or α particles are more likely to cause lethal damage than photons or electrons.
- *Radiation quality:* X rays of different energies have different efficacies in terms of cell killing, with lower energies (e.g., kilovoltage) being more effective.
- *Linear energy transfer (LET):* (i.e., the probability of energy deposition per track length). The higher the LET, the greater the likelihood of lethal cellular damage.
- *Dose rate:* The time frame in which the radiation dose is deposited in tissue. With a decrease in dose rate, there is an increased chance of repair of radiation damage and a consequent increase in survival. This can be advantageous for protection of normal structures.

RADIATION SURVIVAL CURVE

In cultured cell lines, the reproductive survival of a given cell population after a single fraction of radiation has been delivered can be estimated. A detailed discussion of this and other laboratory techniques is beyond the scope of this chapter. In general, the survival is higher at lower doses of radiation, and vice versa. In a semilogarithmic plot it is apparent that after an initial straight portion, there is a "shoulder" and a final straight

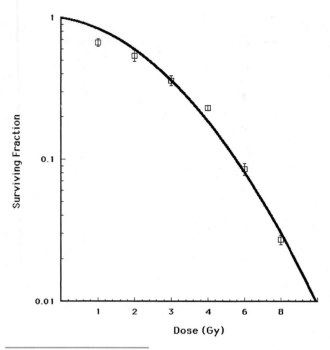

Figure 8–5 In vitro survival of HeLa cells after increasing doses of irradiation. (Courtesy of Eric Bernhard, Ph.D., Department of Radiation Oncology, University of Pennsylvania.)

portion, where the survival tends to be an exponential function of the dose.[11] A cell survival curve is depicted in Figure 8–5. The time frame in which effects of radiation appear varies depending on the type of tissue. Rapidly proliferating tissues, characterized by high cell turnover (e.g., skin, oral mucosa, intestinal epithelium), will manifest radiation injury quickly (within a few weeks). In tissues that do not normally proliferate (e.g., liver, connective, or neural tissue), it may be months or even years before the radiation injury is evident.

EFFECTS OF RADIATION IN NORMAL TISSUES

The effects of radiation in tissue are not specific, perhaps due to the spectrum of cellular reactions to different kinds of injury. There are no pathognomonic changes reflecting radiation injury. However, groups of lesions are highly suggestive of radiation injury, especially with a history of radiation exposure.[12, 13] In general, radiation-induced changes in the CNS include demyelination, degeneration of neurons and glia, and vascular lesions.[14]

BOX 8–3
CNS Radiation-Induced Changes

- **Demyelination**
- **Neural/glial degeneration**
- **Vascular lesions**
- **Perivascular lymphocytic infiltration**

TABLE 8–1   Radiation-Induced Vascular damage.

Vessel Type	Diameter (μm)	Morphologic Changes
Capillaries		Dilatation
Small arteries	Up to 100	Subendothelial fibrosis
		Adventitial fibrosis
		Rarely, fibrinoid necrosis of muscular wall
Medium arteries	100–500	Intimal fibrosis
		Rarely, vasculitis
Large arteries	> 500	Myointimal proliferation, with or without lipid deposits
		Very rarely, perforation
Small veins		Intimal or medial fibrosis
Large veins	> 500	No discernible changes

Adapted from Fojardo LF, Morphology of radiation effects on normal tissues. In: Perez CA, Brady LW, eds. *Principles and Practice of Radiation Oncology*, 3rd ed. Philadelphia: Lippincott-Raven Publishers; 1997.

In the brain, early damage is characterized by demyelination, often with an associated perivascular lymphocytic infiltrate. *Manifestations of delayed damage are almost always limited to the white matter.*[15] These are characterized by extensive demyelination, with associated areas of coagulation necrosis and often with calcification.[12] Fibrinoid exudates can be found around necrotic vessels. Typically, these lesions appear in close proximity to the irradiated tumor. The cortical tissues may appear relatively normal or show glial proliferation (gliosis). In the cerebellum, damage is characterized by formation of empty spaces between the layer of Purkinje cells and the granular layer.[12]

BOX 8–4
Delayed Radiation Changes

- **Extensive demyelination**
- **Associated areas of coagulation necrosis**
- **Calcification**
- **Fibrinoid exudates**
- **Gliosis**

In the brain stem, radiation necrosis is characterized by the presence of small foci in the base of the pons surrounded by eosinophilic swollen axons. The white matter is more frequently affected. These lesions are calcified in the center. They are most commonly seen in patients who have received both chemotherapy and radiation.[16]

Changes in the blood vessels are quite common in the areas of necrosis, consisting of significant intimal proliferation of medium and large arteries and arterioles, with reduction in the caliber of the lumen, sometimes resulting in complete occlusion.[12] Fibrinoid necrosis of arterioles is also common and associated with thrombosis. These vascular lesions have been reportedly associated with cerebral infarction. Capillaries are prone to develop telangiectasia.

The lesions associated with radiation myelopathy are similar to the white matter changes described in the brain, including demyelination and necrosis.[13] *The potential target for radiation damage is thought to be endothelial cells and oligodendrocytes.* Both the white matter and vascular changes are relatively nonspecific. Radiographically, there may be gross atrophy of the cord. These changes may extend beyond the radiation portals as a result of Wallerian degeneration.[12] Radiation-induced vascular changes are variable, depending on blood vessel type and size[17] (Table 8–1).

TREATMENT OF CHILDREN WITH BRAIN TUMORS

The ideal approach to treatment of children with CNS malignancies is multidisciplinary. The neurosurgeon, pediatric neuro-oncologist, and radiation oncologist must communicate at every step of the way. Other clinicians, including neurocognitive specialists, neuroradiologists, endocrinologists, and neuro-ophthalmologists, are no less important.

The initial evaluation should not only determine the extent of disease but should also establish baselines in anticipation of toxicities. These potential toxicities include neurocognitive, auditive, visual, endocrinologic, and growth impairments. Diligent follow-up is critical. Radiographic, ophthalmologic, endocrinologic, and neurocognitive examinations should be performed throughout the patient's life time.

BOX 8–5
Potential Radiation Side Effects

- **Cognitive deficits**
- **Hearing loss**
- **Vision loss**
- **Endocrinopathies**

SIDE EFFECTS OF THERAPY

Morbidity is foremost in the physician's mind when managing pediatric malignancies. The child's normal organs are, in general, more sensitive to radiation than those of adults. *Treatment, therefore, must be designed as much around the potential for toxicity as around the efficacy of therapy.*

Adverse radiation reactions in the CNS can be classified into acute, early-delayed, and late-delayed reactions. [18, 19]

Acute reactions occur during or shortly after radiation therapy; early-delayed reactions appear within a few weeks to months after irradiation; and late-delayed injuries develop months to years after treatment.

The severity of complications is a function of host-, treatment-, and tumor-related factors. For example, young children are more susceptible to chronic radiation injuries than adolescents or young adults. Higher doses of radiation are more likely to result in complications. Impairment secondary to the aggressiveness of the tumor, necrosis, or bleeding is hard to differentiate from treatment complications. Baseline comorbid conditions (e.g., neurofibromatosis) may also affect the patient's cognitive status. [20] The sensitivity of the instruments used to measure the effects is also important. For example, IQ testing has an associated standard error; therefore, differences among patient cohorts cannot be directly extrapolated when estimating the risk of complications for a particular patient. [21]

The anticipation of toxicity is essential in the management of pediatric malignancies. Meticulous optimization of radiation doses and fields should be carried out. Aggressive prophylaxis should be undertaken for expected toxicity. For instance, dental evaluation, fluoride treatment, and continued close dental care are mandatory for children receiving radiation to the teeth and salivary glands. Sometimes this also applies to children being treated with spinal irradiation, where the upper portion of the spinal field may exit through the mandible. Prophylactic use of sucralfate suspension may ameliorate radiation esophagitis in patients receiving craniospinal therapy. Immune-suppressed patients are at risk of developing *Pneumocystis carinii* pneumonia, [22] so that the use of prophylactic trimethoprim-sulfamethoxazole twice weekly should be considered. Antiemetics should likewise be used for the prophylaxis of radiation-induced nausea. [23]

Children who manifest unexpected symptoms during or after therapy, such as irritability or behavioral changes, should be evaluated. Fever, with or without neutropenia, also calls for careful assessment. Headaches may be common during brain radiotherapy, but they should be attributed to radiation only after other causes have been excluded. A high index of suspicion must be maintained in patients with ventriculoperitoneal shunts, and early symptoms should prompt a thorough evaluation. Children on steroids also require close follow-up for related complications.

Acute Side Effects

Acute effects have their onset during or immediately following radiation therapy. Symptoms occurring during treatment generally subside after irradiation has ended and the patient has healed. These effects are a function of age at the time of treatment, volume of tissue irradiated, quality of the radiation, total dose and dose per fraction, developmental potential of the treated site, individual genetic and familial factors, and concurrent treatments (surgery or chemotherapy). Agents such as dactinomycin and doxorubicin can "recall" some

radiation reactions if administered within weeks after radiation therapy has been completed. [24] Such recall reactions may manifest in any organ. [25]

Acute side effects commonly seen with brain irradiation include fatigue, anorexia, nausea, vomiting, headache, dry-skin desquamation, external otitis, and alopecia. Craniospinal irradiation also may result in esophagitis, nausea, and bone marrow suppression. *Neurologic deterioration during therapy, usually an exacerbation of the patient's presenting symptoms, is generally thought to be secondary to radiation-induced edema, although evidence to support this is lacking.* [18] Historically, abrupt neurologic deterioration as well as death has been reported with the use of single large fractions on the order of 7.5 to 10 Gy. [13, 18] In current clinical practice, a daily dose of 1.8 to 2 Gy is well tolerated.

BOX 8–6
Acute Side Effects

- **Fatigue**
- **Anorexia**
- **Nausea/vomiting**
- **Headache**
- **Dry skin**
- **External otitis**
- **Alopecia**

Early-Delayed Side Effects

Early-delayed effects may occur up to 6 months after irradiation. Among such reactions are somnolence syndrome and Lhermitte's sign. The latter is described as the feeling of an electric shock down the spine brought on by flexion of the neck. It is thought to represent transient demyelinization of sensory neurons. [18, 26] *Lhermitte's sign usually appears within 6 to 8 weeks after completion of spinal cord irradiation and tends to resolve spontaneously after 2 to 36 weeks.* [18] The sign has been classically described after mantle irradiation for Hodgkin's disease [27] and after irradiation of the cervical spine. [26] It has no correlation with the development of radiation myelopathy. [28] The somnolence syndrome was reported originally in 1929 in 3% of children irradiated for ringworm of the scalp. [29] Somnolence may last for 10 to 38 days, with no focal neurologic abnormalities. Preceding symptoms include anorexia and irritability. [30] *The somnolence syndrome appears between the fourth and eighth weeks after completion of whole-brain irradiation, with a peak at 5 to 6 weeks.* [30] Although the somnolence syndrome is thought to be primarily related to dose and volume of normal brain irradiated, it has also been described after stereotactic radiosurgery of small lesions. [31] In a prospective series, 79% of children who received 24 Gy of prophylactic radiation to the brain developed some degree of somnolence. [30]

BOX 8–7
Early-Delayed Side Effects

- **Lhermitte's syndrome**
- **Somnolence syndrome**

Late Side Effects

Late effects may occur from months to years after completion of treatment. Relationships between late toxicity and radiation therapy are complex and not simply related to dose and field. Factors such as age, preirradiation condition, other therapies administered, and time at which the analyses are performed may impact treatment toxicity. Sequelae of treatment are not limited to the neural organs; rather, they may present in every irradiated organ. Radiation therapy can prevent any organ from maturing normally beyond its stage of development at the time of treatment. Growth and neurocognitive development are among the most dramatic examples. Endocrine dysfunction secondary to thyroid, pituitary, and/or hypothalamic damage may occur. The development of benign or malignant secondary tumors is also a significant concern in long-term survivors. Other late effects include permanent alopecia, hearing loss, reduced bone marrow reserve, and cataracts.

BOX 8–8
Late Side Effects

- Lack of organ maturation
- Neurocognitive deficits
- Endocrine dysfunction
- Secondary tumors
- Alopecia
- Hearing loss
- Bone marrow changes
- Cataracts

Neurocognitive deficits

The extrauterine development of the brain takes place for the most part during the first 3 years of life, slows down between 3 and 6 years, and begins to plateau after the sixth year of life.[32] During development there is an increase in the size of neurons, axonal growth, dendritic arborization, and synaptogenesis. *Consequently, radiation damage is much more profound in young patients, leading to intellectual deficits.*[33–35] Recent analyses have attempted to account for the multiple factors associated with neurocognitive sequelae. Studies of survivors of medulloblastoma reveal a progressive deterioration of IQ following irradiation.[35–37] It is apparent that one of the most significant predictors of final IQ after whole-brain irradiation is the patient's IQ at the time of treatment.[38] Age and radiation dose also significantly influence the outcome.[38] This suggests that radiation dose is an independent factor in determining the neuropsychological outcome. In retrospective studies, low doses (around 18 Gy) used for prophylactic cranial irradiation in acute lymphoblastic leukemia (ALL) patients resulted in IQ performances not significantly different from those of unirradiated controls.[39] Intelligence impairment after prophylactic cranial irradiation in patients with leukemia seems to be worse in girls than in boys.[40] Also, the specific patterns of IQ deficit differ. Girls surviving ALL had significantly worse generalized IQ impairment, whereas boys had mostly impairment of verbal processes and memory.[40, 41] The volume of irradiated neural tissue is an equally important determinant of neurocognitive morbidity.[42] Patients irradiated to the posterior fossa alone had a lesser deterioration in IQ than patients treated to the whole brain.[43] Surgery may also affect neurocognitive sequelae. Patients having postoperative complications were shown to have worse IQ scores after CNS irradiation.[33, 43] Chemotherapy, especially high-dose methotrexate (MTX), has also been implicated in cognitive deterioration when followed by irradiation.[41] On the other hand, radiation therapy has long been thought to increase the permeability of the blood-brain barrier (BBB), thereby potentially increasing the effects of concomitant or subsequent chemotherapy. A recent study demonstrated an average 2.4-fold increase in BBB permeability to MTX after whole-brain doses of 20 to 40 Gy.[44] This raises the possibility that the sequencing of different treatments may also be important in determining morbidity. Finally, many patients who receive whole-brain irradiation are also treated with moderate to high doses of steroids, either as a part of antileukemic therapy or as part of a primary CNS tumor treatment. Steroids have been associated with neurologic impairment in children with asthma,[45] and there is evidence that glucocorticoids may cause injury to hippocampal neurons.[46, 47]

Hearing Loss

In adults, sensorineural hearing loss starts to manifest after total doses of 30 Gy or more.[48] The addition of cisplatin-based regimes enhances the radiation effect, worsening the risk.[48] As the extent of hearing loss is inversely related to age, the issue is particularly critical in young children, in whom high-frequency hearing loss can result in decreased speech discrimination. A prospective study conducted at St. Jude's Children's Hospital revealed that hearing loss at speech frequencies (500 to 3000 Hz) did not manifest substantially within the cisplatin dose range of 90 to 360 mg/m^2, but reached 25% at 720 mg/m^2. *Substantial hearing loss manifested at doses of 450 mg/m^2 or greater in the frequency range of 6000 to 8000 Hz.* Patients who received cranial irradiation as a part of their treatment developed hearing loss at significantly lower cumulative doses of cisplatin.[49]

Ocular Deficits

Radiation doses of 5000 cGy or higher are associated with significant risk of development of severe dry-eye syndrome.[50] Symptoms include foreign-body sensation, pain, and photophobia. Patients may eventually experience vision loss. These symptoms are rarely encountered in patients treated for CNS malignancies, where doses of radiation to the orbit are significantly lower. One of the most common ocular complications in this population, however, is development of cataracts.[51]

Radiation Necrosis

Radiation necrosis is a severe delayed complication of radiotherapy. Although such necrosis of the brain is rare, it should always be considered in the differential diagnosis when a patient deteriorates several months after completion of therapy. It occurs in 0.1 to 1% of patients who have received 5000 to 6000 cGy in 200-cGy fractions.[52] Above this dose, the incidence increases rapidly. Necrosis usually occurs within 6 months to 5 years after irradiation (most commonly at 1 to 2 years).

Several mechanisms have been proposed as the cause of radiation necrosis of the brain.[53] These include injury to small and medium-sized vessels, damage of glial cells, and immune reaction to antigens released from damaged cells. Cellular debris is thought to promote local inflammation, causing edema and mass effect. Patients present with intracranial hypertension (ICH) and may have focal neurologic deficits.[54] Radiation necrosis appears as a mass lesion with surrounding edema on CT scans and often is hard to distinguish from recurrent tumor. Focal lesions can be treated surgically, with removal of necrotic debris. Partial mass removal or biopsy has little effect on symptoms, and complete removal is recommended whenever possible.[54] Steroids are usually effective in the treatment of these patients.[55] Recently, hyperbaric oxygen treatments have been described to stabilize and improve brain lesions secondary to radiation injury in children.[56, 57]

BOX 8–9
Radiation Necrosis

- **Presents from 6 months to 5 years postirradiation**
- **Increased incidence with increased radiation dose**
- **ICP is increased**
- **Inflammation causes edema and mass effect**
- **Difficult to distinguish from recurrent tumor**
- **Treated by steroids, surgical excision, or hypobaric oxygen**

Necrotizing Leukoencephalopathy

Necrotizing leukoencephalopathy was originally described in 1972 in children with acute leukemia treated with MTX. Leukoencephalopathy denotes white matter necrosis in the absence of demonstrable microorganisms.[58] It is associated with combined radiation therapy and chemotherapy to the CNS (intravenous and intrathecal MTX), radiation doses of 2000 cGy or more, and CNS relapse of ALL. Histologically, there are multiple necrotic foci containing cellular debris, as well as reactive astrocytosis. In more severe cases, diffuse demyelinization is present.[58] In one retrospective study, 9% of patients irradiated with less than 24 Gy to the brain plus intrathecal MTX developed leukoencephalopathy. This contrasts dramatically with 22% of patients receiving radiation doses higher than 24 Gy.[59] As a general rule, the hemispheric gray matter and basal ganglia are spared. Later, cerebral atrophy and ventricular enlargement develop. Clinically, necrotizing leukoencephalopathy is characterized by the insidious development of dementia, commonly accompanied by drooling, dysarthria, or dysphagia. Further deterioration follows, with seizures, spasticity, paresis, and ataxia. Most patients sustain permanent neurologic damage.[60] Mineralizing microangiopathy may accompany this process. Dystrophic calcification of the CNS has been described in children who died of ALL. The lenticular nucleus is almost always involved. The cerebral gray matter and, less frequently, the cerebellar cortex

may also be involved.[61] Calcification of the basal ganglia after cranial irradiation alone has been occasionally described.[62] The functional sequelae of mineralizing microangiopathy are usually mild.[60]

Moyamoya Syndrome

Moyamoya syndrome encompasses stenosis of large and intermediate cerebral arteries, abnormal netlike vessels, and transdural anastomoses. Typically, the syndrome is idiopathic.[63] Moyamoya syndrome has been described as secondary to several nonspecific conditions, such as arteriosclerosis, thromboembolic events, inflammatory conditions, and, rarely, irradiation.[64] Often, the syndrome appears related to irradiation of a tumor near the sella, particularly optic gliomas,[64] and is also associated with neurofibromatosis.[65] The most common symptoms are the result of focal ischemic lesions.[66] Other complaints at presentation include headache, altered consciousness, vertigo, speech disturbance, and seizures. The symptoms tend to persist or worsen in a majority of patients.[64]

Radiation Myelopathy

Radiation myelopathy is one of the most dreaded toxicities associated with spinal radiotherapy. It is characterized by sensory and motor symptoms. Sensory symptoms include decreased thermal sensation, weakness, and decreased proprioception. Motor findings include foot drop, gait disturbances, spasticity, weakness, and paralysis. Abnormal plantar reflex and hyperreflexia are also found.[13] The diagnosis is made by exclusion because a more common cause of myelopathy in a cancer patient is tumor. Also, the diagnosis of radiation myelitis is less likely when the latency period is less than 6 months following irradiation or when spinal cord doses are less than 50 Gy given with standard fractionation.[13] Myelography is usually negative, as is CT of the spine. MRI findings include enlargement of the spinal cord, decreased T1 signal intensity, contrast enhancement, and increased T2 signal intensity.[67] Larger fractional doses of radiation and chemotherapy also seem to lower the threshold for the development of radiation myelopathy.[68]

BOX 8–10
MRI Findings of Radiation Myelopathy

- **Cord enlargement**
- **Decreased T1 signal intensity**
- **Increased T2 signal intensity**
- **Contrast enhancement**

Bone Development

Disturbances of bone development after kilovoltage irradiation have been reported since the early 1930s. *Partial irradiation of vertebral bodies is known to result in bone asymmetry, wedging of vertebral bodies, and scoliosis.*[69] Neuhauser et al described the effects of irradiation in vertebral body contour and development.[70] They found that radiation doses higher than about 2000 R resulted in vertebral contour irregularities in almost all cases. The effect on growth arrest secondary to spine irradiation was also found to be dependent on the length of irradiated spine. Finally, Neuhauser et al recommended homogeneous irradiation of vertebrae in the radiation field to minimize future deformities.[70] Younger age and higher radiation doses have been found to be associated with the greatest loss in sitting height in children who received spinal irradiation for lymphoma, medulloblastoma, and leukemia.[71] Silber et al analyzed a group of 49 irradiated patients followed at the Children's Hospital of Philadelphia.[72] They proposed a multiple regression model to predict eventual adult stature based on gender, patient's height and age at radiation therapy, ideal stature, radiation therapy doses, and irradiated segment (length of cervical, thoracic, or lumbar spine, pelvis, and femur).

Cardiovascular Deficits

Spinal irradiation is the standard of care in the treatment of medulloblastoma, and it is also used in the treatment of CNS leukemia. *In this situation, the heart receives an inhomogeneous radiation dose incidental to the spinal radiation field* (Fig. 8–6). In one study, 31% of patients treated with spinal irradiation had abnormal Q waves in the resting electrocardiogram (ECG). In the same study, 75% of these patients had abnormal exercise capacity measured both subjectively and objectively. The posterior left ventricle wall was abnormally thin in almost all irradiated patients; however, cardiac chamber sizes were not, leading to a high estimated ventricular wall stress. The authors postulated that an inhomogeneous dose of irradiation may have resulted in these findings because they were not observed in patients who received a more homogeneous cardiac dose.[73]

In craniospinal or spinal irradiation, there is some dose exit through the lungs in the spinal portals. In one report, approximately 60% of patients treated with craniospinal irradiation, with or without chemotherapy, displayed some degree of restrictive lung disease, compared with 14% of patients treated with chemotherapy and no spinal radiotherapy.[74]

Endocrine Dysfunction

Endocrine sequelae may likewise be a consequence of cranial radiotherapy. *It is important to note that the incidence of radiation-related endocrinologic sequelae seems to increase with time; therefore, prolonged follow-up in these patients is important.*[75] The pituitary gland is included in whole-brain fields and may receive some dose when the posterior fossa is irradiated. The degree of pituitary hormonal deficiency is related to the radiation dose, and the effect is usually seen in 2 to 5 years. Low doses of radiation may produce isolated growth hormone deficiency, and higher doses, panhypopituitarism. Diabetes insipidus may occur, but this is very unusual and is generally associated with underlying damage to the pituitary gland. Hypothyroidism may be a result of the exit dose of the spinal field through the thyroid, as well as hypothalamic/pituitary dysfunction from direct irradiation. Delayed puberty and precocious puberty are both associated with radiation therapy and affect girls more commonly than boys.

The effects of radiotherapy on the hypothalamic-pituitary axis were reported by Constine et al in a group of adults and children treated for brain tumors.[76] With doses to the hypothalamus/pituitary ranging from 39.6 to 70.2 Gy, endocrine deficiencies were encountered in 55 to 74% of the patients, with almost 75% of patients having more than one hormonal defect.

Deficiency in growth hormone secretion has been detected as early as 3 months after completion of treatment. In a prospective evaluation of endocrine function after cranial irradiation for brain tumor, the incidence of growth hormone deficiency rose from 28% at 3 months to 87% at 12 months.[77] It is estimated that after cranial doses of 20 to 30 Gy, approximately 65% of children with ALL will have some degree of growth hormone deficiency.[78] There is a marked effect of age on growth retardation after radiotherapy: the younger the child, the worse the growth impairment.[79] These observations underscore the need for continued follow-up. The effect of therapy on the patient's growth seems to be less for patients treated with cranial irradiation only, higher for patients

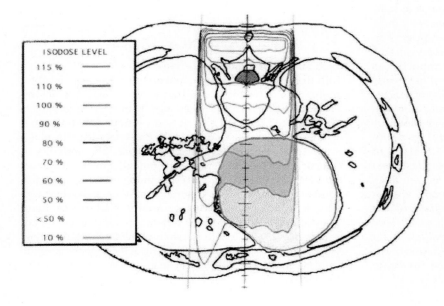

Figure 8–6 Dose distribution of a typical spinal radiation field in the midthorax. An inhomogeneous dose distribution is appreciated (see also Fig. 8–3). The dose delivered to the posterior wall is higher than the dose received by the remainder of the organ.

treated with craniospinal irradiation, and highest when treatment included both craniospinal irradiation and chemotherapy.[80] *Chemotherapy has resulted in impaired growth and growth hormone deficiency even in the absence of cranial irradiation.*[81] In prepubertal patients, growth percentile closely parallels the adequacy of growth hormone secretion,[77] thus making it a good parameter for clinical monitoring. When the growth percentile changes significantly, then endocrinologic evaluation is indicated. Almost without exception, children who receive craniospinal irradiation for medulloblastoma will require growth hormone replacement. Despite the fact that growth hormone replacement therapy will increase the growth rate in these patients, they will consistently fail to reach their expected height, even when the spine has not been irradiated.[80]

Secondary Tumors

Secondary neoplasms are a major concern in long-term survivors of childhood cancer. *Second malignant tumors become a significant cause of death in long-term survivors of childhood brain tumors during the second decade of follow-up.*[82] The actual incidence of second malignancies is difficult to establish because follow-up of survivors is still ongoing and there is significant heterogeneity in the populations at risk. Jenkin analyzed 1034 children treated with irradiation between 1958 and 1995, and found an incidence of second malignant tumors of 13% at 20 years, and 19% at 30 years.[83] Patients with the longest follow-up were treated at a time when the index malignancy was the highest cause of mortality. On the other hand, current treatments have resulted in higher cure rates (although follow-up of these patients is obviously shorter term). This is not a trivial issue because development of a second malignancy can take years or decades.

Not all second malignancies are related to therapy. Clearly, some patients suffering from pediatric malignancies have an inherited predisposition to cancer, which may result in the development of a second tumor in cured children.[84] Radiation has a definite causative role in these patients. *Most of the radiation-related second malignancies seem to occur in or immediately adjacent to the radiation portals.* With continued follow-up past 15 years, the relative risk of radiation-induced solid tumors initially increases, subsequently reaches a plateau, and eventually appears to decrease.[85] In a large retrospective series, the 5-year survival after a second malignant tumor was reported as 58%.[83] *Patients with a carcinogenic genotype are at higher risk for developing a second malignancy. Such is the case in patients with retinoblastoma and phakomatoses.*[86] Often, the second malignant tumor is a sarcoma,[87] *but leukemia and lymphoma are also found.*[86] *Malignant gliomas have been reported after pituitary radiotherapy in children and adults.*[88] Malignant melanoma arising in the radiated field has been described in two long-term survivors of brain tumors, as well as in survivors of a variety of childhood cancers treated with or without radiotherapy.[89] *Meningiomas arising in the irradiated areas have also been described following treatment of childhood brain tumors or after prophylactic brain irradiation for leukemias.* Of note, the latent period for manifestation of the radiation induced meningioma seems to be inversely related to the dose of radiation.[90]

INFORMED CONSENT

As in many other areas of medicine, careful discussion of the diagnosis, treatment, and expected results is of paramount importance to the success of a doctor-patient relationship. Underlying the concept of informed consent is the exchange of information that leads to an agreement.[91] Legally, the parents exercise the child's right to self-determination and informed consent. However, potentially harmful decisions should be challenged.[92] An effective approach needs to incorporate the family's cultural background, coping skills, and concerns regarding the treatment and its side effects. The prior experiences of family members, incomplete or erroneous information provided by other health care professionals, and the common perception of radiation therapy as a "last-ditch effort" may negatively influence the parents' attitude toward treatment. Changes in physical appearance, such as hair loss, can also cause significant distress. Parents are naturally concerned about side effects of treatment, and there is often a desire not to intervene, especially if the child "appears well."[93]

The use of elaborate terminology in the discussion may result in frustration.[93] Likewise, consent forms that may be difficult to understand or are inappropriate for the family's educational level do not lead to effective communication. The importance of a thorough and mutually understandable discussion cannot be overemphasized.

Enrollment of children in clinical research protocols should be encouraged, as it represents the de facto standard of care for children in the United States. In general, the same considerations apply when obtaining consent for participation in a clinical trial. In one survey, parents were willing to discuss experimental chemotherapy with their terminally ill children but were not prepared to discuss the issues related to the advanced stages of the disease.[94] Parents may underestimate the child's understanding of his or her condition.[94] Careful discussion of experimental treatments is therefore critical because the issues of increased toxicity, including mortality, and potential lack of therapeutic benefit must be addressed (Table 8–2).

BASELINE STUDIES

Both malignancy and the adverse effects of therapy may disturb the normal physiologic functioning of a child. Furthermore, nowadays more children with cancer are reaching adulthood, and their full potential detriment from therapy is yet to unfold. In the 1980s, it was estimated that approximately 1 in every 1000 adults in the third decade of life was a survivor of childhood cancer.[95] Therefore, late morbidity of pediatric cancer treatment has the potential to become a significant social issue. Careful evaluation of the patient's performance and physiologic status at baseline is the best tool with which to quantify the eventual impact of treatment. Some clinicians recommend baseline IQ and achievement testing in every child with a brain tumor.[77] Such studies allow for continued evaluation of the effects of therapy and provide information that is potentially useful in the design of less morbid treatment approaches.

TABLE 8–2   Helping Families Understand Radiation Therapy

1. *Explain diagnostic and therapeutic procedures.* This should be done in lay terms to ensure understanding. A careful step-by-step discussion of every procedure (e.g., simulations and daily treatments) is very helpful in relieving the anxieties regarding radiation therapy.
2. *List the purposes and expected benefits from the treatment.*
3. *Outline morbidity from both procedures and treatment.* We routinely discuss potential side effects of irradiation comprehensively. A clear distinction is made between acute and late effects, incidence, and intensity of complications.
4. *Discuss treatment options.* This requires familiarity with allied treatment modalities (e.g., surgery and chemotherapy), current research protocols, and alternative treatments. The radiation oncologist should also be familiar with some of the sources of information that are available to parents, such as news, books, discussion groups, and the World Wide Web.
5. *Respond to questions and concerns.* The physician should be ready to address the family's thoughts and emotions.
6. *Clarify the voluntary nature of the treatment.* However, parental decisions that are potentially harmful to the child can and should be challenged.
7. *Carefully discuss the right to withdraw treatment,* including situations considered "against medical advice."
8. *Adequately document the patient's chart* to include a summary of the discussion, date, time, and those present when informed consent is obtained.
9. *Obtain written consent forms.* We ask children older than 12 years to "assent" to treatment, thus fostering their participation in the decision-making process. It is our practice to provide the parents with signed copies of the consent forms. Dialogue regarding consent issues, risks vs. benefits, and withdrawal from treatment continue throughout planning and therapy.[91]

Audiologic, visual, neurocognitive, and endocrinologic testing should be considered as baseline studies in all patients thought to be at risk for toxicity to some or all of those systems.

SEQUENCING OF CHEMOTHERAPY AND RADIATION

There are several potential advantages to the use of radiation and chemotherapy in combination (Table 8–3).

Results in some cases have been discouraging. Hartsell et al reviewed the outcome of 23 children with medulloblastoma who were younger than 3 years at diagnosis. These patients received primary chemotherapy after surgical resection in several treatment protocols conducted at the Saint Jude Children's Research Hospital. Only 26% of these patients completed planned chemotherapy without evidence of disease progression. Of the remaining children, 60% had progressive disease in spite of craniospinal irradiation.[98]

The Pediatric Oncology Group conducted a trial of chemotherapy and delayed irradiation in children younger than 3 years with brain tumors. Diagnoses included medulloblastoma, ependymoma, primitive neuroectodermal tumor, malignant glioma, and brain stem glioma. Chemotherapy consisted of vincristine and cyclophosphamide alternated with cisplatin and etoposide for 12 to 24 months. Response to chemotherapy varied between 0% (brain stem glioma)

TABLE 8–3   Potential Advantages of Combining Chemotherapy and Radiation

1. *Aiming chemotherapy at subclinical matastatic disease may improve the chance of cure.* Distant recurrence of tumors may be secondary to metastatic deposits present prior to local treatment; in this setting, *effective chemotherapy aimed at subclinical metastatic disease* may improve the chance of cure.[96] In the CNS, extra-CNS relapse is generally not an issue, with the exception of medulloblastoma.
2. *The combination of chemotherapy and radiation may allow for preservation of an organ that would otherwise have to be resected.* This is of no benefit to the patient unless both anatomy and function are preserved.[96]
3. *The combination of chemotherapy and irradiation may result in better rates of local control than either alone.* In a randomized trial comparing radiotherapy alone with chemotherapy plus irradiation in 58 children with high-grade gliomas, 5-year survival was 43% for the combined modality group, vs. 17% for the radiotherapy-alone group.[97] Chemotherapy consisted of weekly vincristine administration during the 6 weeks of irradiation, followed by vincristine, CCNU, and prednisone. This combined modality approach is generally considered to be the standard of care for these patients.
4. *Preradiation chemotherapy may prevent disease progression.* There have been several attempts to use postoperative chemotherapy alone in infants and very young children with brain tumors. The morbidity of CNS irradiation in these patients is significant, and chemotherapy is delivered in an attempt to allow for further development of the CNS before irradiation. *Preradiation chemotherapy* administered to infants and very young children can prevent disease progression in less than 50% of cases.

and 60% (malignant glioma). Progression-free survival was approximately 40% at completion of scheduled chemotherapy.[99] Neuropsychometric testing was not systematically performed in these patients. The authors concluded that irradiation could be delayed in a substantial proportion of these patients.

TECHNICAL ISSUES

Immobilization

Reproducible positioning and immobilization are critical to minimize variation in treatment delivery. In the pediatric population, this is not only obtained with state-of-the-art immobilization methods; it also frequently requires the use of conscious sedation or anesthesia in the young and uncooperative patient. Most frequently, we use Aquaplast for the manufacture of immobilization devices. In our hands, this provides excellent stability and reproducibility.

Sedation and Anesthesia

Getting children to cooperate and helping them to remain in the treatment position may present a significant challenge. *In general, children 3 years or older are able to lie still during procedures.*[100] Nurses and radiation therapists must devote a great deal of time and effort to preparing patients for simulation and treatment.

At our institution, the assessment for sedation is made through a multidisciplinary approach. The patient's parents and caregivers provide key elements in the history. *The need for sedation or general anesthesia during a former diagnostic or therapeutic procedure is a very important indication of whether a patient will need it for irradiation.* Clinical evaluation by the nurse and radiation therapist is also necessary in making the decision to sedate a child. A tour of the radiation oncology department is offered to the child and parents to allow familiarity with treatment rooms and equipment. This may help to decrease the patient's anxiety and, ultimately, circumvent the need for sedation. In general, we attempt conscious sedation before considering general anesthesia because the former is easier to administer and has fewer potential complications. Longer procedures, such as simulation, planning CT scans, and setups, are more likely to require sedation than daily treatments. The pediatric conscious sedation guidelines for radiation oncology in use at the Hospital of the University of Pennsylvania are depicted in Table 8–4).

Children who cannot be adequately sedated require general anesthesia for simulation and treatments. More than 30 years ago, Harrison and Bennett enunciated the basic principles of anesthesia for radiotherapy: The method must be effective to attain proper immobilization, and a rapid induction and recovery are necessary to avoid drowsiness and irritability after the procedure has been completed.[101] Efficient coordination with the pediatric anesthesiologist is invaluable for these patients. Of the many anesthetic drugs in use, propofol is preferred because of its favorable side-effect profile and relatively short duration of action.[102] In our experience, anesthesiologists have used different forms of general anesthesia on different occasions in the same patient. This can result in changes in the patient's position in such a way as to affect

therapy. It is important to make the anesthesiologist aware of the importance of positioning. These changes in anesthetic techniques must be closely monitored throughout therapy.

TREATMENT PLANNING

In clinical radiotherapy, the treatment planning is driven by anatomical and biologic factors. The clinician must be aware of several factors during the treatment planning process:[103]

1. *Thorough knowledge of the natural history and pathologic characteristics of the tumor.* This information is not always readily accessible to the clinician. Critical review of the literature is of prime importance in this assessment because some of the data derive from inherently flawed historical series. Autopsy and reoperation series, as well as analysis of patterns of failure, are important in understanding the natural history of the disease.

2. *Adequate evaluation of the patient and staging procedures to determine the full extent of the tumor.* In the past two decades, the introduction of CT and MRI has resulted in significant improvement in our ability to define tumor extent for treatment planning purposes. Software that allows a tridimensional reconstruction of tumor and normal structures is also useful for optimization of treatment planning.

3. *Selection of a treatment strategy.* Once again, this mandates an accurate understanding of the literature and knowledge of current clinical trials.

4. *Radiation treatment planning, with precise definition of the target volume and radiation ports.* This is arguably the simplest step in adequate planning. Classically, several techniques and field arrangements have been described, depending on diagnosis and anatomical location. The selection of treatment technique today is driven not only by the requirement for adequate treatment to the tumor but by the necessity of sparing healthy structures. New techniques designed to improve healthy-organ sparing while maintaining irradiation to the areas at risk are becoming increasingly important.[48]

5. *Computations to determine the distribution of radiation within the volume of interest.*

6. *Accurate and reproducible repositioning and immobilization techniques for daily treatment delivery.*

7. *Applicable dosimetry, portal localization, and verification procedures to ensure quality control throughout the therapeutic process.*

8. *Periodic evaluation of the patient during and after therapy to assess the effects of irradiation on the tumor and patient tolerance.*

According to the International Commission on Radiological Units and Measurements (ICRU), specification of volumes and doses is necessary for prescribing, documenting, and reporting therapy.[104] The purpose of the treatment (palliative or curative) should be specified. The gross tumor volume (GTV) and clinical target volume (CTV) are defined prior to the treatment planning process.[104] The definition of GTV is intuitively obvious and is made based on clinical examination and available imaging studies. For CTV, the clinician must consider the areas at risk for subclinical extension, such as adjacent tissues and lymph nodes. Such information is not necessarily available for all tumors and is often

TABLE 8–4   Conscious Sedation Guidelines for Radiation Oncology at the Hospital of the University of Pennsylvania

Drug	Route	Dose	Onset	Duration	Antidote	Comments
Sedatives						
Chloral hydrate	PO/rectal	60 mg/kg 30–60 min additional before procedure, 30 mg/kg 10 min before (if needed)	30–60 min	4–8 h		Neonatal dose 25 mg/kg maximum dose procedure 120 mg/kg, or 2 g. May combine with benadryl.
Diphenhydramine (Benadryl)	PO/IV/IM	5 mg/kg/day, divided doses q 8–6 h; max dose 300 mg/d	1–3 h	4– h		Peak at 2–4 h IV infusion over 10–15 min (maximum concentration 25 mg/ml). Not recommended under 2 years.
Pentobarbital (Nembutal)	IV	2 mg/kg, followed by 2 mg/kg×2, 5–10 min before procedure (if needed)	0–1 minute	15 min		Patients older than 6 months
Morphine sulfate	IV	0.05–0.1 mg/kg	Within 5 min	3–5 h	Naloxone	IV infusion over 5 min. May combine with pentobarbital
Midazolam (Versed)	IV	0.08–0.15 mg/kg; max dose 10 mg IV	1–5 min	1–2 h	Flumazenil	IV infusion over 1–2 min (maximum concentration 1 Mg/mL)
Antidotes						
Flumazenil (Mazicon)	IV	Initial dose 0.01 mg/kg (max dose 0.2 mg), followed by 0.005 mg/kg q 1 min ft max dose 0.2 mg	1–3 min	<1 h (may need to repeat)		Peak effect at 6–10 min. May cause phlebitis.
Naloxone (Narcan)	IV/endotracheal	0.01 mg/kg, may repeat q 1–2 min as needed	0–2 min	20–60 min (may need to repeat)		IV infusion over 30s. For continuous IV infusion, dilute to 4 μg/mL

defined empirically. Most primary CNS neoplasms infiltrate for a considerable distance into surrounding normal CNS tissue,[105] and their borders are poorly demarcated, even by CT or MRI. Therefore, it is often necessary to irradiate a substantial amount of normal tissue within the target volume. Tolerance of these tissues to irradiation may become a dose-limiting factor.

In addition, provisions must be made to ensure adequate coverage of CTV. This is accomplished by adding a margin to account for patient movement, breathing, and internal-organ motion, as well as inaccuracies resulting from variations in setup and positioning. The resulting index is the planning target volume (PTV). Although organ motion has been studied to some extent in certain anatomical areas, the variations in setup and immobilization are extremely complex and depend partially on immobilization methods. The experience of technicians at different institutions is also a factor. This particular issue has not been well studied and may be a significant element leading to imprecise planning in children.

The treated volume includes the PTV. This is determined by the radiation oncologist as the volume encompassed by the isodose appropriate for the treatment. The volume that receives a significant dose of radiation depends on the particular treatment technique and is called the irradiated volume (Fig. 8–7).[104]

Simulation requires the use of a specially designed diagnostic X-ray machine to duplicate what must be done with the therapy unit. This ensures that the treatment beam accurately encompasses the region that must be treated while avoiding the irradiation of normal structures that need not be included in the treatment zone. Occasionally, dedicated CT units, similar to those in diagnostic departments, are used for treatment planning purposes. The resultant images may be fed into computerized treatment planning systems and

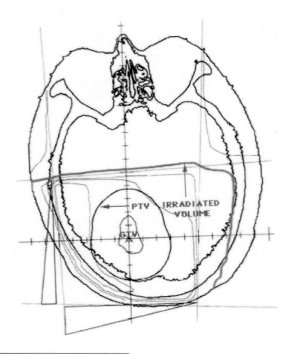

Figure 8–7 Schematic representation of a posterior fossa tumor treated by two orthogonal radiation fields. Gross tumor volume (GTV), planning target volume (PTV), and irradiated volume are represented.

used to develop dose-volume histograms (treatment templates for fields treated in unusual configurations) and, ultimately, to optimize therapy.

THREE-DIMENSIONAL CONFORMAL RADIOTHERAPY

Classically, radiation therapy of diverse malignancies has been carried out with a limited number of field arrangements. These are defined at the time of simulation, and the dosimetry is subsequently verified with the aid of isodose displays. The dosimetry is displayed in a single axial plane, usually at the central axis of the radiation beam. Optionally, off-axis planes can be evaluated. This approach does not take into account the patient's tridimensional geometry because it assumes ideal conditions for the purpose of calculations. The limitations were partly due to constraints in computer processing power necessary to perform the millions of calculations required for treatment planning. In contrast, three-dimensional treatment planning relies on three-dimensional display of the anatomy, radiation beams, and dosimetry, thereby rendering a more accurate representation of the treatment. Such planning has become commonplace, the result of access to inexpensive and powerful computers necessary to calculate and plan such therapy. Useful technical innovations that help in treatment planning include the beam's eye view display, which helps in assessing adequate coverage of the target volume, isosurface displays, and dose-volume his-

tograms. The dose-volume histogram is a graphic representation of the irradiated volume. The structure (e.g., normal organ, tumor) to be analyzed is outlined on the planning CT scan. Once beam arrangements and doses are entered, the dose is plotted against treated volume. This approach is most useful in comparing different treatment plans and in assigning them a relative merit. Spatial information is lost, however, as it cannot provide the anatomical location of a given dose level.

Conformal therapy seeks to shape the radiation portals and, more importantly, the isodose volume to closely approximate the contours of the target volume. Accurate positioning, immobilization, and reliable setup reproducibility are key to success. The underlying assumptions are that the daily variations in setup are known and measurable, as is the extent of subclinical tumor. Implied benefits of this approach are the ability to maximize sparing of normal structures while opening the possibility of moderate tumor dose escalation.

INTENSITY MODULATION

Intensity modulation is a novel technique that relies on delivery of a dose gradient throughout the target volume, with the potential of dose escalation in the tumor. Simultaneously, the dose to normal structures is maintained within the tolerance range. The technique can be performed either with multiple static fields, or dynamically, with the treatment machine moving while dose is being delivered. Intensity modulation techniques rely heavily on computerized and automated radiotherapy equipment, which is not readily available in the radiotherapy community and is still considered investigational.

DOSING CONSIDERATIONS

During radiotherapy treatment planning, the treatment dose is selected following consideration of the optimal tumoricidal dose, normal tissue to be irradiated, and potential associated toxicity. The tumoricidal dose, in turn, depends on the tumor burden and the intrinsic radiosensitivity of the tumor cells. It is commonly accepted that areas harboring small numbers of tumor cells (subclinical disease) can be sterilized with lower doses of radiation than the gross tumor.[106] Normal organ toxicity is an important constraint that is dependent on the toxicity end point (e.g., necrosis, ototoxicity, cataracts, neurocognitive impairment, etc.) and its potential for correction (e.g., cataracts.) Our knowledge of these parameters is incomplete and based on primarily empirical data that cannot easily be extrapolated to individual patients.

FRACTIONATION

Early in the development of the field of radiation oncology, it was appreciated that the delivery of large single doses of radiation was associated with significant toxicity to normal tissues.[107] Indeed, a single dose of radiation cannot sterilize a tumor without causing unacceptable side effects in normal tissues. This toxicity can be avoided, at least partially, by

TABLE 8–5   Summary of Phase I/II Hyperfractionation Trials in Diffuse Brain Stem Gliomas.[117–120]

Trial	Patients	Dose/Dose per Fraction	Median Survival	Long-Term Survival
POG Phase I/II[117]	38 entered 34 eligible	66 Gy/1.1 Gy bid	11 mo	<20% at 18 mo
POG #8495, Phase I/II[118]	57 entered 57 eligible	70.2 Gy/1.17 Gy bid	10 mo	23% at 24 mo
CCG Phase I[119]	16 entered 15 evaluable	64.8 Gy/1.2 Gy bid	≈7 mo	≈20 mo
CCG Phase I/II[120]	54 entered 53 eligible	72 Gy/1 Gy bid	9 mo	8% at 3 y

delivering several smaller doses over an extended period of time. Fractionated courses of treatment were associated with improved tumor control rates and acceptable early and late normal-tissue complications.[108] Multiple fractionation schedules were empirically designed at different centers to accommodate the basic objective of tumor control with acceptable toxicity. In addition, constraints of patient logistics and availability of equipment were considered. In the United States, conventionally fractionated radiotherapy (1.8 to 2 Gy/day, 5 days a week) has become the standard against which other radiotherapy schedules are measured.

The protraction of treatment over several weeks allows acutely reacting tissues (e.g., skin or mucosa) to recover during treatment, thus ameliorating the severity of acute side effects. A daily fraction size of approximately 2 Gy also results in adequate preservation of late-responding tissues (e.g., brain, spinal cord, or connective tissues). However, tumors with very short doubling times may also proliferate during a protracted treatment course, resulting in less overall cell death.[109] Possible changes in fractionation schedules aimed at improving tumor control in this setting have been proposed,[110] that is, accelerated fractionation and hyperfractionated radiotherapy.

In accelerated fractionation, a conventional dose of radiation is delivered in a shorter time. This requires somewhat higher doses per fraction or more than five treatments in a week. Accelerated hyperfractionated schedules deliver more than one treatment per day.

In hyperfractionated radiotherapy, smaller radiation fractions are delivered two or three times a day. Total treatment dose is moderately increased, and overall treatment time is similar to, or slightly shorter than, a conventional course. The effectiveness in tumor cell kill would be higher by increasing the total dose. Since there is no increase in overall treatment time, unwanted tumor proliferation is avoided. This has been postulated to be due to redistribution of some cell populations in the cell cycle, from relatively radioresistant phases to relatively radiosensitive ones.[111] Although the biological mechanism remains elusive, hyperfractionated radiotherapy has resulted in better tumor control in some head and neck cancers.[112]

A corollary of the effect of fractionation in sparing of normal tissues is that the severity of side effects is related to fraction size. Therefore, use of fractions smaller than conventional (i.e., 180 to 200 cGy) should be associated with even better tissue tolerance than conventional irradiation. Theoretically, this is another potential advantage of hyperfrac-

tionated treatments. However, there is little clinical evidence that hyperfractionated radiotherapy results in late tissue effects that are less than or equal to those of conventional irradiation.[113] In some hyperfractionation trials in head and neck radiotherapy, however, high late tissue complication rates have been observed.[114] It has become apparent that a critical interval between fractions must be respected to allow for completion of damage repair in normal tissues. In general, this time interval has been estimated at 4 to 6 hours. However, animal evidence suggests that radiation damage repair in the spinal cord may take longer than 6 hours,[115] and there are not enough experimental or clinical data to estimate the optimum interval between fractions in the CNS.

In pediatric neuro-oncology, hyperfractionated radiotherapy had been the most widely used modality for treatment of diffuse brain stem gliomas. Conventional irradiation, to doses of 50 to 55 Gy, results in a 5-year survival of approximately 5%, with a suggestion of a dose-response relationship.[116] Higher total doses with lower fraction sizes delivered twice a day were projected to result in improved tumor control, improved survival, and milder or similar late effects. A number of trials have been conducted to test this hypothesis (Table 8–5). *However, no advantage over conventional irradiation has been demonstrated.*[117–120]

TREATMENT TECHNIQUES

Craniospinal Irradiation

The target volume encompasses the whole craniospinal axis. This poses several technical challenges because it is not possible to encompass the entire neuraxis in a single radiotherapy field. Dose inhomogeneity results from variations in anatomical contour and depth of structures of interest. Abutment of adjacent fields not only results in dose variations but, more importantly, creates the risk of overdose or underdose at the junctions. Physical characteristics of the radiation beam, such as energy, "depth dose," flatness, and penumbra, must be considered to optimize treatment.

The cranial or helmet field is designed to encompass the cranial meninges,[121] sometimes including the posterior half of the orbit. Adequate margin should be used in the region of the cribriform plate and in the temporal fossa to achieve the desired dose distribution. Custom blocking is mandatory to prevent excessive dosage to normal structures. The bottom of the field is usually placed at the bottom of C2. We favor an elongated helmet field, with the bottom placed as low as possible without irradiating through the patient's shoulders. That leaves ample margin for the junction move every 900 cGy of treatment (see below.)

In a lateral radiograph of the skull, the cribiform plate lies inferior to the orbital roof. Careless blocking in this area to protect the eye and the retina will result in underdose to the cribiform plate. Several reports suggest that recurrences in the subfrontal area and cribiform plate may be due to inadequate design of treatment portals.[122]

The bottom of the spinal field should provide adequate margin around the dural sac. This is at the level of the bottom of S3 in 96% of children. The most accurate determination of this level for the individual patient is from the sagittal MRI images.[123] Laterally, the subarachnoid space extends to the spinal ganglia. The spinal ganglia, in turn, closely correspond with the vertebral pedicles and with the sacral foramina, thus making unnecessary the inclusion of the sacroiliac joints in the spinal radiation field.[122]

The junction of cranial and spinal fields is set up to eliminate geometrical divergence and overlap between fields. The cranial field is rotated to parallel the divergence of the spinal field in the sagittal plane. At the same time, the lateral fields are angled to avoid divergence into the spine (Fig. 8–8). Even a perfect geometrical match does not preclude areas of high dose at the junction, as scattered radiation from adjacent fields cannot be avoided. Some authors advocate the use of a gap between adjacent fields to avoid overdose. However, a 5-mm gap between the cranial and the spinal fields will result in a "cold spot," with delivery of approximately 90% of the prescribed dose.[122]

It is also customary to move the junctions ("feather") periodically during treatment, thus minimizing "hot spots" and "cold spots" due to motion or setup uncertainty. With this technique, hot spots may be inadvertently created at the junction if doses per fraction are different in the two adjacent fields[124] (Table 8–6).

The spine is irradiated with one or two posterior fields, depending on the total length of the segment to be treated and the constraints on the treatment machine. Abutting spinal fields result in dose inhomogeneity at the junction. Fields are matched to avoid overdose at critical structures, namely, the spinal cord. Nevertheless, small areas of overdose are created below the depth of the match. These areas cannot be avoided with conventional techniques (Fig. 8–9).

Posterior Fossa

A commonly used technique relies on anatomical landmarks (Fig. 8–10). This technique can be traced to radiologic studies published in the 1930s.[7, 125] We routinely use the sagittal MRI images to define the location and borders of the posterior fossa, as well as the primary tumor volume (Fig. 8–11). Using this technique,[126] we have encountered significant discrepancies between individual patients' anatomy and anatomical landmarks (Fig. 8–12).

Proton Therapy

The first clinical use of proton irradiation was carried out in 1954 for pituitary suppression in patients with metastatic

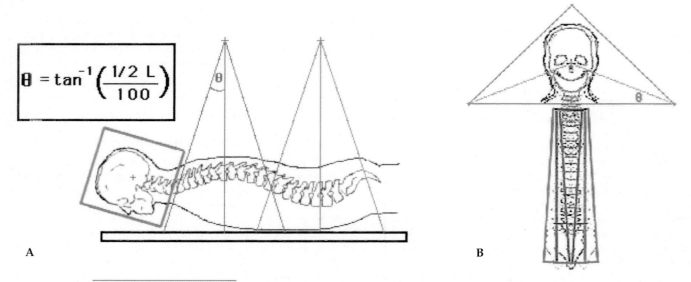

$$\theta = \tan^{-1}\left(\frac{1/2\ L}{100}\right)$$

A

B

Figure 8–8 (A) Craniospinal irradiation setup, sagittal view. The lateral cranial fields (box) are matched to the upper spinal field by clockwise rotation around the axis. The angle of rotation (θ) equals the angle of divergence for the upper spinal field. It is calculated using the formula in the insert, where *L* is the length of the upper spinal field defined at 100 cm from the radiation source. (B) Craniospinal irradiation setup, coronal view. The upper spinal field (triangle) is matched to the lateral cranial fields by lateral rotation of the treatment table. The angle of rotation (θ) equals the angle of divergence for the cranial field. It is calculated using the formula in the insert, where *L* is the length of the cranial field defined at 100 cm from the radiation source.

TABLE 8–6 Schematic representation of two adjacent fields treated at different doses per fraction. The junctions are moved every week, so the upper field shortens while the lower field elongates. The total volume covered by the two fields remains constant. The bold area indicates a progressive "hot spot" across the junction due to the unequal dose contributions of both fields.

Week 1		Week 2		Week 3	
Weekly dose	Cummulative dose	Weekly dose	Cummulative dose	Weekly dose	Cummulative dose
				900 cGy	2700 cGy
		900 cGy	1800 cGy	*1000 cGy*	*2800 cGy*
900 cGy	900 cGy	*1000 cGy*	*1900 cGy*	*1000 cGy*	*2900 cGy*
1000 cGy	*1000 cGy*	*1000 cGy*	*2000 cGy*	*1000 cGy*	*3000 cGy*

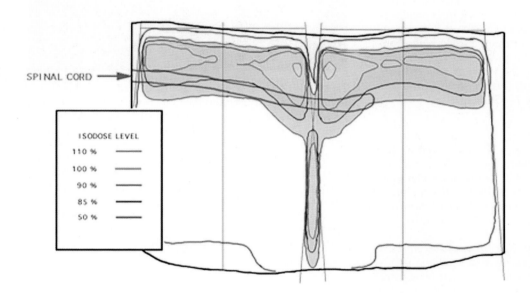

Figure 8–9 Schematic representation of two adjacent fields treated at different doses per fraction. The junctions are moved every week, so the upper field shortens while the lower field elongates. The total volume covered by the two fields remains constant. The shaded area indicates a progressive "hot spot" across the junction due to the unequal dose contributions of both fields.

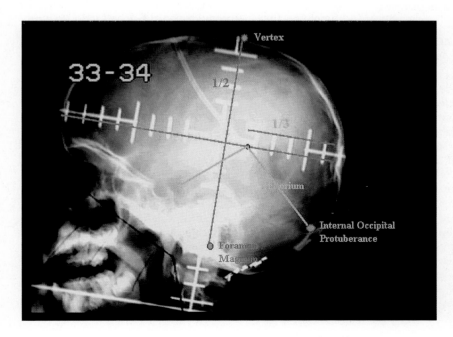

Figure 8–10 Matching of adjacent spinal fields. Treatment has been designed to deliver at least 90% of the prescribed dose to the spinal canal at the junction of both fields. Note that the area distal to the matching depth receives up to 110% of the delivered dose.

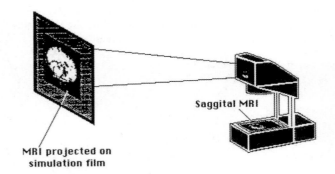

Figure 8–11 Popular technique used to outline the posterior fossa in the lateral X ray of the skull. The green lines represent the *tentorium cerebelli*, or the cephalad limit of the posterior fossa. To estimate it, a line is drawn from the foramen magnum to the vertex of the skull. Then a perpendicular is drawn, bisecting it. A point (X) is identified on the perpendicular line, one-third of the way from the back. Lines from the internal occipital protuberance and the posterior clinoid to point X approximate the roof of the *tentorium*. (Reproduced with permission from Oncolink (http://www.oncolink.upenn.edu), Radiation Oncology Teaching Section.)

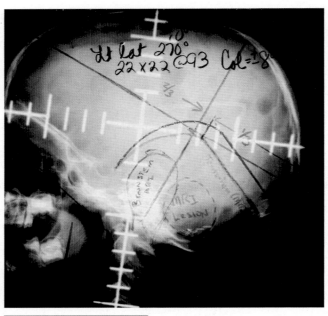

Figure 8–12 Use of a projector to superimpose structures identified from MRI on simulation fields.[126] A midplane sagittal MRI is necessary to implement this technique. At the time of simulation, a lateral skull X ray is obtained. The borders of the skull, sella, and brain stem are traced in the simulation film. In a dark room, the midplane sagittal MRI is projected onto the simulation X ray, visually correcting to match the adequate magnification. The tumor volume is drawn on the simulation film following the MRI outline. The process can be iterated for off-axis sagittal planes. (Adapted with permission from Oncolink (http://www.oncolink.upenn.edu), Radiation Oncology Teaching Section.)

breast cancer.[127] Proton irradiation is characterized by the "Bragg peak," a highly constricted dose distribution in tissue, with the potential of enhanced tissue sparing when compared with photon irradiation. *As charged particles, protons deliver large amounts of energy within a small range before stopping completely.* Biologically, proton cell killing is equivalent to photon cell killing.[128]

The advantage of proton irradiation in children is its inherent ability to spare normal tissue from irradiation, thus ameliorating late sequelae, especially in the neurocognitive area.[129] The improved spatial dose localization necessitates high precision in the treatment delivery, aggressive immobilization and reproducibility, and accurate treatment planning.

Radioprotectors and Sensitizers

Radioprotectors have also been conceived as means for improving the therapeutic ratio. *Such substances could be selectively absorbed by normal tissues, and would decrease the toxicity of radiation, while allowing for delivery of higher radiation doses to the tumor without increased side effects.* The administration of *cysteine* confers protection against radiation in laboratory animals. *Sulfhydril compounds,* such as cysteine, cysteamine, and glutathione, block the reaction of oxygen and free radicals, thus diminishing oxidative damage to the DNA molecule. The most effective radioprotector is *amifostine,* currently in use for prevention of chemotherapy side effects.[130]

Radiosensitizers, on the other hand, increase the sensitivity of tumor cells to radiation. Their application in clinical practice stems from a potential widening of the therapeutic ratio (i.e., increase in tumor cell death with no increase in normal tissue complications). The most studied radiosensitizers are the nitroimidazoles, related to metronidazole, which act as electron donors and can replace oxygen in the generation of free radicals in hypoxic cells.[131] However, clinical trials with

diverse nitroimidazoles have been disappointing.[132] Other radiosensitizers that are under clinical evaluation include thymidine analogs (bromodeoxyuridine and iododeoxyuridine), fluoropyrimidines (5-fluorouracil or 5-FU, fluorodeoxyuridine). The combination of 5-FU and radiotherapy has become part of the standard therapy in rectal cancer.[133]

Currently, no radioprotectors or sensitizers are in routine use in clinical pediatric radiotherapy.

SUMMARY

During the past 50 years there have been major improvements in the treatment of children with brain tumors. Mortality and treatment-related morbidity are still a significant concern in these patients. During that time period, radiation therapy has played a leading role in the management of these children. Further technical improvements in radiation delivery and dose localization may enhance local tumor control and normal tissue sparing, with the potential for somewhat higher cure rates with diminished complications. More effective future treatments will stem from a better understanding of tumor and normal tissue biology and their interaction with radiation.

REFERENCES

1. Pohle EA. *Clinical Roentgen Therapy.* Philadelphia: Lea & Febiger; 1938.
2. Schulder M, Black PM, Alexander E, Loeffler JS. The influence of Harvey Cushing on neuroradiologic therapy. *Radiology* 1996;201:671–674.
3. Bailey, P, Cushing H. Medulloblastoma cerebelli: common type midcerebellar glioma of childhood. *Arch Neurol Psychiat* 1925;14:192–224.
4. Bailey, P, Cushing H. *Tumors of the Glioma Group.* Philadelphia: JB Lippincott; 1926.
5. Paterson R: *The Treatment of Malignant Disease by Radium and X-rays Being a Practice of Radiotherapy.* London: Edward Arnold and Co.; 1948.
6. Paterson R: *The Treatment of Malignant Disease by Radiotherapy.* Baltimore: Williams & Wilkins; 1963.
7. Paterson E, Parr RF. Medulloblastoma. Treatment by irradiation of the whole central nervous system. *Acta Radiol* 1953;39:323–336.
8. Bouchard J. *Radiation Therapy of Tumors and Diseases of the Nervous System.* Philadelphia: Lea & Febiger; 1966.
9. Johns HE, Cunningham JR. *The Physics of Radiology.* 4th ed. Springfield, IL: Charles C. Thomas; 1983.
10. Khan FM. *The Physics of Radiation Therapy.* 2nd ed. Baltimore: Williams & Wilkins; 1994.
11. Andrews JR. *The Radiobiology of Human Cancer Radiotherapy.* Philadelphia: WB Saunders; 1968.
12. Fajardo LF. *Pathology of Radiation Injury.* Chicago: Masson; 1982.
13. Schultheiss TE, Kun LE, Ang KK, Stephens LC. Radiation response of the central nervous system. *Int J Radiat Oncol Biol Phys* 1995;31:1093–1112.
14. Zeman W, Samorajski T. Effects of irradiation on the nervous system. In: Berdjis CC, ed. *Pathology of Irradiation.* Baltimore: Williams & Wilkins; 1971.
15. Rubin P, Cassaret GW. *Pathology of Radiation Injury.* Philadelphia: WB Saunders, 1968.
16. Burger PC, Boyko OB. The pathology of central nervous system radiation injury. In: Gutin PH, Leibel SA, Sheline GE, eds. *Radiation Injury to the Central Nervous System.* New York: Raven Press; 1991.
17. Fajardo LF. Morphology of radiation effects on normal tissues. In: Perez CA, Brady LW, eds. *Principles and Practice of Radiation Oncology.* 3rd ed. Philadelphia: Lippincott-Raven Publishers; 1997.
18. Sheline GE, Wara WM, Smith V. Therapeutic irradiation and brain injury. *Int J Radiat Oncol Biol Phys* 1980;6:1215–1228.
19. Levin VA, Leibel SA, Gutin PH. Neoplasms of the central nervous System. In: De Vita VT, Hellman S, Rosenberg SA, eds. *Cancer: Principles and Practice of Oncology.* Philadelphia: Lippincott-Raven Publishers; 1997.
20. Hofman KJ, Harris EL, Bryan RN, Denckla MB. Neurofibromatosis type 1: the cognitive phenotype. *J Pediatr* 1994;124:S1–S8.
21. Goldwein JW. Radiotherapy for pediatric brain tumors. Standards of care, current clinical trials, and new directions. ASTRO refresher course, 37th annual ASTRO meeting, 1995.

22. Schiff D. Pneumocystis pneumonia in brain tumor patients: risk factors and clinical features. *J Neuro-oncol* 1996;27:235–240.
23. Lippens RJ, Broeders GC. Ondansetron in radiation therapy of brain tumor in children. *Pediatr Hematol Oncol* 1996;13:247–252.
24. Cassady JR, Richter MP, Piro AJ, Jaffe N. Radiation-adriamycin interactions: preliminary clinical observations. *Cancer* 1975;36:946–949.
25. Ma LD, Taylor GA, Wharam MD, Wiley JM. "Recall" pneumonitis: adriamycin potentiation of radiation pneumonitis in two children. *Radiology* 1993;187:465–467.
26. Jones A. Transient radiation myelopathy (with reference to Lhermitte's sign of electrical paresthesia). *Br J Radiol* 1964;37:727–744.
27. Carmel RJ, Kaplan HS. Mantle irradiation in Hodgkin's disease. An analysis of technique, tumor eradication, and complications. *Cancer* 1976;37:2813–2825.
28. Michalski JM, Garcia DM. Spinal canal. In: Perez CA, Brady LW, eds. *Principles and Practice of Radiation Oncology.* 3rd ed. Philadelphia: Lippincott-Raven Publishers; 1997.
29. Druckmann A. Schlafsucht als Folge der Röntgenbestrahlung. Beitrag zur Strahlenempfindlichkeit des Gehirns. *Strahlen-therapie* 1929;33:382–384.
30. Freeman JE, Johnston PGB, Voke JM. Somnolence after prophylactic cranial irradiation in children with acute lymphoblastic leukaemia. *BMJ* 1973;4:523–525.
31. Dunbar SF, Tarbell NJ, Kooy HM, et al. Stereotactic radiotherapy for pediatric and adult brain tumors: preliminary report. *Int J Radiat Oncol Biol Phys* 1994;30:531–539.
32. Rubin P, Van Houtte P, Constine L. Radiation sensitivity and organ tolerances in pediatric oncology: a new hypothesis. *Front Radiat Ther Oncol,* 1982;16:62–82.
33. Kao GD, Goldwein JW, Schultz DJ, et al. The impact of perioperative factors on subsequent intelligence quotient deficits in children treated for medulloblastoma/posterior fossa primitive neuroectodermal tumors. *Cancer* 1994;74:965–971.
34. Packer RJ, Bruce DA, Atkins TA, et al. Factors impacting on neurocognitive outcome in long-term survivors of PNET/MB. *Ann Neurol* 1986;20:396–397.
35. Packer RJ, Sutton LN, Atkins TE, et al. A prospective study of cognitive function in children receiving whole-brain radiotherapy and chemotherapy: 2-year results. *J Neurosurg* 1989;70:707–713.
36. Hoppe-Hirsch E, Renier D, Lellouch-Tubiana A, et al. Medulloblastoma in childhood: progressive intellectual deterioration. *Child's Nerv Sys* 1990;6:60–65.
37. Packer RJ, Sposto R, Atkins TE, et al. Quality of life in children with primitive neuroectodermal tumors (medulloblastomas) of the posterior fossa. *Pediatr Neurosci* 1987;13:169–175.
38. Silber JH, Radcliffe J, Peckham V, et al. Whole brain irradiation and decline in intelligence: the influence of dose and age on IQ score. *J Clin Oncol* 1992;10:1390–1396.
39. Halberg FE, Kramer JH, Moore IM, Wara WM, Mathay KK, Ablin AR. Prophylactic cranial irradiation dose effects on late cognitive function in children treated for acute lymphoblastic leukemia. *Int J Radiat Oncol Biol Phys* 1991;22:13–16.
40. Waber DP, Tarbell, NJ Kahn CM, et al. The relationship of sex and treatment modality to neuropsychologic outcome

in childhood acute lymphoblastic leukemia. *J Clin Oncol* 1992;10:810–817.

41. Waber DP, Tarbell NJ, Fairclough D, et al. Cognitive sequelae of treatment in childhood acute lymphoblastic leukemia: cranial radiation requires an accomplice. *J Clin Oncol* 1995;13:2490–2496.

42. Garcia-Perez A, Sierrasesumaga L, Narbona-Garcia J, et al. Neuropsychological evaluation of children with intracranial tumors: impact of treatment modalities. *Med Pediatr Oncol* 1994;23:116–123.

43. Hoppe-Hirsch E, Brunet L, Laroussinie F, et al. Intellectual outcome in children with malignant tumors of the posterior fossa: influence of the field of irradiation and quality of surgery. *Child's Nerv Syst* 1995;11:340–346.

44. Qin D, Ma J, Xiao J, Tang Z. Effect of brain irradiation on blood-csf barrier permeability of chemotherapeutic agents. *Am J Clin Oncol* 1997;20:263–265.

45. Bender BG, Lerner JA, Kollasch E. Mood and memory changes in asthmatic children receiving corticosteroids. *J Am Acad Child Adolesc Psychiatry* 1988;6:710–715.

46. Sapolsky RM. A mechanism for increased glucocorticoid toxicity in the hippocampus: increased neuronal vulnerability to metabolic insults. *J Neurosci* 1985;5:1227–1231.

47. Packan DR, Sapolsky RM. Glucocorticoid endangerment of the hippocampus: tissue, steroid, and receptor specificity. *Neuroendocrinology* 1990;51:613–618.

48. Fukunaga-Johnson N, Sandler HM, Marsh R, Martel MK. The use of 3D conformal radiotherapy (3D CRT) to spare the cochlea in patients with medulloblastoma. *Int J Radiat Oncol Biol Phys* 1998;41:77–82.

49. Schell MJ, McHaney VA, Green AA, et al. Hearing loss in children and young adults receiving cisplatin with or without prior cranial irradiation. *J Clin Oncol* 1989;7:754–760.

50. Parsons JT, Bova FJ, Fitzgerald CR, et al. Tolerance of the visual apparatus to conventional therapeutic irradiation. In: Gutin PH, Leibel SA, Sheline GE, eds. *Radiation Injury to the Central Nervous System.* New York: Raven Press; 1991.

51. Pakisch B, Langmann G, Langmann A, et al. Ocular sequelae of multimodal therapy of hematologic malignancies in children. *Med Pediatr Oncol* 1994;23:344–349.

52. Danoff BF, Cowchock S, Marquette C, et al. Assessment of the long term effects of primary radiation therapy for brain tumors in children. *Cancer* 1982;49:1580–1586.

53. Santoni R, Liebsch N, Finkelstein DM, et al. Temporal lobe (TL) damage following surgery and high-dose photon and proton irradiation in 96 patients affected by chordomas and chondrosarcomas of the base of skull. *Int J Radiat Oncol Biol Phys* 1998;41:59–68.

54. Edwards MS, Wilson CB. Treatment of radiation necrosis. In: Gilbert HA, Kagan AR, eds. *Radiation Damage to the Nervous System. A Delayed Therapeutic Hazard.* New York: Raven Press; 1980.

55. Gutin PH. Treatment of radiation necrosis of the brain. In: Gutin PH, Leibel SA, Sheline GE, eds. *Radiation Injury to the Central Nervous System.* New York: Raven Press; 1991.

56. Ashamalla HL, Thom SR, Goldwein JW. Hyperbaric oxygen therapy for the treatment of radiation-induced sequelae in children: the University of Pennsylvania experience. *Cancer* 1996;77:2407–2412.

57. Chuba PJ, Aronin P, Bhambhani K, et al. Hyperbaric oxygen therapy for radiation-induced brain injury in children. *Cancer* 1997;80:2005–2012.

58. Price RA, Jamieson PA. The central nervous system in childhood leukemia II: subacute leukoencephalopathy. *Cancer* 1975;35:306–318.

59. Matsumoto K, Takahashi S, Sato A, et al. Leukoencephalopathy in childhood hematopoietic neoplasm caused by moderate-dose methotrexate and prophylactic cranial radiotherapy—an MR analysis. *Int J Radiat Oncol Biol Phys* 1995;32:913–918.

60. Bleyer WA, Griffin TW. White matter necrosis, mineralizing microangiopathy, and intellectual abilities in survivors of childhood leukemia: associations with central nervous system irradiation and methotrexate therapy. In: Gilbert HA, Kagan AR, eds. *Radiation Damage to the Nervous System. A Delayed Therapeutic Hazard.* New York: Raven Press; 1980.

61. Price RA, Birdwell DA. The central nervous system in childhood leukemia III: mineralizing microangiopathy and dystrophic calcification. *Cancer* 1978;35:717–728.

62. Harwood-Nash DCF, Reilly BJ. Calcification of the basal ganglia following radiation therapy. *Am J Roentgenol Rad Ther Nuclear Med* 1970;108:392–395.

63. Suzuki J, Kodama N. Moyamoya disease: a review. *Stroke* 1983;14:104–109.

64. Bitzer M, Topka H. Progressive cerebral occlusive disease after radiation therapy. *Stroke* 1995;26:131–136.

65. Erickson RP, Woolliscroft J, Allen RJ. Familial occurrence of intracranial arterial occlusive disease (moyamoya) in neurofibromatosis. *Clin Genet* 1980;18:191–196.

66. Rajakulasingam K, Cerullo LJ, Raimondi AJ. Childhood moyamoya syndrome: postradiation pathogenesis. *Child Brain* 1979;5:467–475.

67. Koehler PJ, Verbiest H, Jager J, Vecht CJ. Delayed radiation myelopathy: serial MR-imaging and pathology. *Clin Neurol Neurosurg* 1996;98:197–201.

68. Watterson J, Toogood I, Nieder M, et al. Excessive spinal cord toxicity from intensive central nervous system-directed therapies. *Cancer* 1994;74:3034–3041.

69. Arkin AM, Pack GT, Ransohoff NS, Simon N. Radiation-induced scoliosis. *J Bone Joint Surg* 1950;32:401–404.

70. Neuhauser EBD, Wittenborg MH, Berman CZ, Cohen J. Radiation effects of roentgen therapy on the growing spine. *Radiology* 1952;59:637–650.

71. Probert JC, Parker BR, Kaplan HS. Growth retardation in children after megavoltage irradiation of the spine. *Cancer* 1973;32:634–639.

72. Silber JH, Littman PS, Meadows AT. Stature loss following skeletal irradiation for childhood cancer. *J Clin Oncol* 1990;8:304–312.

73. Jakacki RI, Goldwein JW, Larsen RL, et al. Cardiac dysfunction following spinal irradiation during childhood. *J Clin Oncol* 1993;11:1033–1038.

74. Jakacki RI, Schramm CM, Donahue BR, et al. Restrictive lung disease following treatment for malignant brain tumors: a potential late effect of craniospinal irradiation. *J Clin Oncol* 1995;13:1478–1485.

75. Tao ML, Barnes PD, Billett AL, et al. Childhood optic chiasm gliomas: radiographic response following radiotherapy and long-term clinical outcome. *Int J Radiat Oncol Biol Phys* 1997;39:579–587.

76. Constine LS, Woolf PD, Cann D, et al. Hypothalamic-pituitary dysfunction after radiation for brain tumors. *N Engl J Med* 1993;323:87–94.

77. Duffner PK, Cohen ME, Voorhess ML, et al. Long-term effects of cranial irradiation on endocrine function in children with brain tumors: a prospective study. *Cancer* 1985;56:2189–2193.

78. Rappaport R, Brauner R. Growth and endocrine disorders secondary to cranial irradiation. *Pediatr Res* 1989;25;561–567.

79. Shalet SM, Gibson B, Swindell R, Pearson D. Effect of spinal irradiation on growth. *Arch Dis Child* 1987;62: 461–464.

80. Ogilvy-Stuart AL, Shalet SM. Growth and puberty after hormone treatment after irradiation for brain tumors. *Arch Dis Child* 1995;73:141–146.

81. Roman J, Villaizan CJ, Garcia-Foncillas J, et al. Growth and growth hormone secretion in children with cancer treated with chemotherapy. *J Pediatr* 1997;131:105–112.

82. Jenkin D, Greenberg M, Hoffman H, Hendrick B, Humphreys R, Vatter A. Brain tumors in children: long-term survival after radiation treatment. *Int J Radiat Oncol Biol Phys* 1995;31:445–451.

83. Jenkin D. Long-term survival of children with brain tumors. *Oncology* 1996;10:715–719.

84. Brada M, Hawkins M. Brain tumors in children–lifetime for patients and investigators. *Int J Radiat Oncol Biol Phys* 1995;31:671–672.

85. De Vatahire F, Shamsaldin A, Grimaud E, et al. Solid malignant neoplasms after childhood irradiation: decrease of the relative risk with time after irradiation. *CR Acad Sci Paris Life Sci* 1995;318:483–490.

86. Meadows AT, D'Angio GJ, Mike V, et al. Patterns of second malignant neoplasms in children. *Cancer* 1977;40: 1903–1911.

87. Koot RW, Tan WF, Dreissen JJR, et al. Irradiation induced osteosarcoma in the posterior cranial fossa six years after surgery and radiation for medulloblastoma. *J Neurol Neurosurg Psychiatry* 1996;61:429–430.

88. Tsang RW, Laperriere NJ, Simpson WJ, et al. Glioma arising after radiation therapy for pituitary adenoma. *Cancer* 1993;72:2227–2233.

89. Corpron CA, Black CT, Ross MI, et al. Melanoma as a second malignant neoplasm after childhood cancer. *Am J Surg* 1996;171:459–462.

90. Salvati M, Cervoni L, Puzzilli F, et al. High-dose radiation induced meningiomas. *Surg Neurol* 1997;47:435–442.

91. Berry DL, Dodd MJ, Hinds PS, Ferrell BR. Informed consent: process and clinical issues. *Oncol Nursing Forum* 1996;23:507–512.

92. Monaco GP, Smith G, Fiduccia D. Pediatric cancer: advocacy, legal, insurance, and employment issues. In Pizzo PA, Poplack DG, eds. *Principles and Practice of Pediatric Oncology*. 3rd ed. Philadelphia: Lippincott-Raven; 1997.

93. Hersch SP, Wiener LS, Figueroa V, Kunz JF. Psychiatric and psychosocial support for the child and the family. In: Pizzo PA, Poplack DG, eds. *Principles and Practice of Pediatric Oncology*. 3rd ed. Philadelphia: Lippincott-Raven; 1997.

94. Kamps WA, Akkerboom, Kingma A, Humphrey GB. Experimental chemotherapy in children with cancer—a parent's view. *Pediatr Hematol Oncol* 1987;4:117–124.

95. Meadows AT, Krejmas NL, Belasco JB. The medical cost of cure: sequelae in survivors of childhood cancer. In: van Eys J, Sullivan M, eds. *Status of the Curability of Childhood Cancers: The University of Texas System Cancer Center, MD Anderson Hospital and Tumor Institute 24th Annual Clinical Conference on Cancer, 1979*. New York: Raven Press; 1980.

96. Tannock IF. Treatment of cancer with radiation and drugs. *J Clin Oncol* 1996;14:3156–3174.

97. Sposto R, Ertel IJ, Jenkin RDT, et al. The effectiveness of chemotherapy for treatment of high grade astrocytoma in children: results of a randomized trial: a report from the Children's Cancer Study Group. *J Neuro-oncol* 1989;7:165–177.

98. Hartsell WF, Gajjar A, Heideman RL, et al. Patterns of failure in children with medulloblastoma: effects of preirradiation chemotherapy. *Int J Radiat Oncol Biol Phys* 1997;39:15–24.

99. Duffner PKF Horowitz ME, Krischer JP, et al. Postoperative chemotherapy and delayed radiation in children less than three years of age with malignant brain tumors. *N Engl J Med* 1993;328:1725–1731.

100. Bucholtz JD. Issues concerning the sedation of children for radiation therapy. *Oncol Nursing Forum* 1992;19: 649–655.

101. Harrison GG, Bennett MB. Radiotherapy without tears. *Br J Anaesth* 1963;35:720–721.

102. McDowall RH, Scher CS, Barst SM. Total intravenous anesthesia for children undergoing brief diagnostic or therapeutic procedures. *J Clin Anesth* 1995;7:273–280.

103. Perez CA, Purdy JA. Rationale for treatment planning in radiation therapy. In: Levitt SH, Khan FM, Potish RA, eds. *Levitt and Tapley's Technological Basis of Radiation Therapy: Practical Clinical Applications*. 2nd ed. Philadelphia: Lea & Febiger; 1992.

104. *ICRU Report 50: Prescribing Recording, and Reporting Photon Beam Therapy*. Bethesda, MD: International Commission on Radiation Units and Measurements, 1993.

105. Matsukado Y, MacCarty CS, Kernohan JW. The growth of glioblastoma multiforme (astrocytomas grades 3 and 4) in neurosurgical practice. *J Neurosurg* 1961;18:636.

106. Fletcher GH. Basic clinical parameters. In: Levitt SH, Khan FM, Potish RA, eds. *Levitt and Tapley's Technological Basis of Radiation Therapy: Practical Clinical Applications*. 2nd ed. Philadelphia: Lea & Febiger; 1992.

107. Thames HD. On the origin of dose fractionation regimens in radiotherapy. *Semin Radiat Oncol* 1992;2:3–9.

108. Coutard H. Roentgentherapy of epitheliomas of the tonsillar region, hypopharynx and larynx from 1920–1926. *Am J Roentgenol* 1932;28:313.

109. Withers HR, Taylor JM, Maciejewski B. The hazard of accelerated tumor clonogen repopulation during radiotherapy. *Acta Oncologica* 1988;27(2):131–146.

110. Peters LJ, Ang KK, Thames HD. Altered fractionation schedules. In: Perez CA, Brady LW, eds. *Principles and Practice of Radiation Oncology*. 2nd ed. Philadelphia: JB Lippincott; 1992.

111. Shukovsky LJ, Fletcher GH, Montague ED, Withers HR. Experience with twice-a-day fractionation in clinical radiotherapy. *Radiology* 1976;126:155–162.

112. Horiot JC, Le Fur R, N'Guyen T, et al. Hyperfractionation versus conventional fractionation in oropharyngeal

carcinoma: final analysis of a randomized trial of the EORTC cooperative group of radiotherapy. *Radiother Oncol,* 1992;25(4):231–241.

113. Beck-Bornholdt H-P, Dubben H-H, Liertz-Petersen C, Willers H. Hyperfractionation: where do we stand? *Radiother Oncol* 1997;43:1–21.

114. Meoz RT, Fletcher GH, Peters LJ, et al. Twice-daily fractionation schemes for advanced head and neck cancer. *Int J Radiat Oncol Biol Phys* 1984;10:831–836.

115. Withers HR, McBride WH. Biologic basis of radiation therapy. In: Perez CA, Brady LW, eds. *Principles and Practice of Radiation Oncology.* 3rd ed. Philadelphia: Lippincott-Raven Publishers; 1997.

116. Halperin EC, Constine LS, Tarbell NJ, Kun LE. *Pediatric Radiation Oncology.* 2nd ed. New York: Raven Press; 1994.

117. Freeman CR, Krischer J, Sanford RA, et al. Hyperfractionated radiotherapy in brain stem tumors: results of a Pediatric Oncology Group study. *Int J Radiat Oncol Biol Phys* 1988;15:311–318.

118. Freeman CR, Krischer J, Sanford RA, et al. Hyperfractionated radiation therapy in brain stem tumors: results of treatment at the 7020 cGy dose level of Pediatric Oncology Group #8495. *Cancer* 1991;68:474–481.

119. Packer RJ, Littman PA, Sposto RM, et al. Results of a Pilot study of hyperfractionated radiation therapy for children with brain stem gliomas. *Int J Radiat Oncol Biol Phys* 1987;13:1647–1651.

120. Hyperfractionated radiation therapy (72 Gy) for children with brain stem gliomas: a Children's Cancer Group phase I/II trial. *Cancer* 1993;72:1414–1421.

121. Stea B. Acute Nonlymphocytic leukemia. In: Cassady JR, ed. *Radiation Therapy in Pediatric Oncology.* New York: Springer-Verlag; 1994.

122. Halperin EC. Impact of radiation technique upon the outcome of treatments for medulloblastoma. *Int J Radiat Oncol Biol Phys* 1996;36:233–239.

123. Dunbar SF, Barnes PD, Tarbell NJ. Radiologic determination of the caudal border of the spinal field in craniospinal irradiation. *Int J Radiat Oncol Biol Phys* 1993; 26:669.

124. Bentel GC, Halperin EC. High-dose areas are unintentionally created as a result of gap shifts when the prescribed dose in the two adjacent areas are different. *Med Dosim* 1990;15:179–183.

125. Twining EW. Radiology of the third and fourth ventricles: Part II. *Br J Radiol* 1939;12:569.

126. Goldwein JW, Zimmerman R, Corn BW. Easy method for defining intracranial target volumes on orthogonal simulation films using magnetic resonance images. *Radiat Oncol Invest.* 1997;5:38–42.

127. Tobias CA, Roberts JE, Lawrence JH, et al. Irradiation hypophysectomy and related studies using 340-MeV protons and 190-MeV deuterons. *Peaceful Uses of Energy* 1956;10:95–106.

128. Archambeau JO, Slater JD, Slater JM, Tangeman R. Role for proton beam irradiation in treatment of pediatric CNS malignancies. *Int J Radiat Oncol Biol Phys* 1992;22: 287–294.

129. Wambersie A, Gregroire V, Brucher JM. Potential clinical gain of proton (and heavy ion) beams for brain tumors in children. *Int J Radiat Oncol Biol Phys* 1992;22:275–286.

130. Schuchter LM. Guidelines for the administration of amifostine. *Semin Oncol* 1996;23(4 Suppl 8):40–43.

131. Hall EJ. *Radiobiology for the Radiologist.* 4th ed. Philadelphia: JB Lippincott; 1994.

132. Wasserman TH, Chapman JD, Coleman CN, Kligerman MM. Chemical modifiers of radiation. In: Perez CA, Brady LW, eds. *Principles and Practice of Radiation Oncology.* 3rd ed. Philadelphia: Lippincott-Raven Publishers; 1997.

133. NIH Consensus Conference. Adjuvant therapy for patients with colon and rectal cancer. *JAMA* 1990;264: 1444–1450.

Chapter 9

Stereotactic Radiosurgery

Douglas Kondziolka, L. Dade Lunsford, and John C. Flickinger

Stereotactic radiosurgery is an effective and widely used treatment technique for the management of carefully selected brain tumors and vascular malformations in children.[1-4] Ongoing analysis of results has led to refinements in technique, a better understanding of target dose response as well as that for normal tissue, and an evolution in patient selection. These analyses have led to improved results. Radiosurgery is a minimally invasive technique, but it is not risk-free. Because long-term survival can be expected for most patients with benign disorders of the brain, both the short- and long-term outcomes of radiosurgery must be rigorously evaluated and available for review. In this chapter, we will present data from the first 12 years' experience in the treatment of childhood brain tumors at the University of Pittsburgh, as part of an overall series of more than 3300 radiosurgery cases (Table 9–1).

TABLE 9–1 Radiosurgery for Brain Tumors in Children, University of Pittsburgh, 1987–1997

Diagnosis	No. of Cases
Pilocytic astrocytoma	15
Astrocytoma	4
Anaplastic astrocytoma	6
Glioblastoma multiforme	3
Ependymoma	11
Pituitary adenoma	8
Craniopharyngioma	8
Acoustic schwannoma	6
Meningioma	3
Primitive neuroectodermal tumor	4
Pineocytoma	2
Metastasis	2
Germinoma	1
Chondrosarcoma	1
Pineoblastoma	1
Chordoma	1
Embryonal cell carcinoma	1
Total = 77	

THE RADIOBIOLOGY OF RADIOSURGERY

In the early 1950s radiation oncologists learned the importance of fractionation in the use of external-beam radiotherapy to treat malignant tumors. Fractionation preferentially reduced radiation effects for late-reacting normal tissue, compared with the more rapid and early response of malignant cells. This concept improved the therapeutic window of treatment so that the rates of tumor control versus risk of complications remained favorable. The lessons learned regarding fractionation, combined with economic incentives to increase fractionation, have led many radiation oncologists to use fractionation in most situations. *However, when both the target tissue and the surrounding normal brain have more similar types of response (both may be late-responding tissues), then nothing significant is likely to be gained by extended fractionation schemes.* Such a situation is relevant in functional radiosurgery where the target *is* normal brain, probably in the treatment of vascular malformations, and possibly for most benign tumors of the brain, cranial nerves, or meninges. The actual $\alpha:\beta$ ratio for most of these lesions is not well characterized.

The radiobiologic power of single-fraction delivery is the basis for radiosurgery.[5, 6] Conformal radiosurgery allows radiation of only a small volume of surrounding normal tissue in the region of radiation dose fall-off. *The opportunity to deliver a high single-session dose to a properly defined target allows effective doses to be delivered to solid neoplasms or vascular malformations that do not contain normal brain.*[7] It is likely that some of the effects of radiosurgery are observed through both indirect vascular effects as well as direct cytotoxic effects. Dose prescription formulas assist in selection of the dose depending on imaging and clinical factors.[8, 9] It may soon be possible for molecular biologic analyses to identify tumors with low $\alpha:\beta$ ratios so that specific therapies, such as radiosurgery, or limited fractionation regimens can be selected. Adjuvant radiosurgery can also be of value in early-responding malignant tumors, such as brain metastasis or glial neoplasms, likely due to the enhanced radiobiologic effectiveness of the single-fraction dose.[10]

CHILDREN AND RADIATION THERAPY

The brain is more tolerant of radiation than most other organs in the body, particularly in adults. The effects of radiation are of greater concern in the developing brain of children, who appear more likely to respond adversely than adults given similar doses. *Because of this risk to subsequent brain development, exposure to potential radiation injury may be unacceptable if other treatment strategies exist.*

The risks of conventional fractionated therapy to the brain of children have been well described in the literature. They can be classified as acute, early-delayed, or late. Acute effects of fractionated radiotherapy include mild fatigue, skin redness, and hair loss. The main subacute or early-delayed effect is a somnolence syndrome that was observed in children under 10 years following low-dose prophylactic whole-brain radiotherapy for leukemia or higher dose focal irradiation for childhood brain tumors. Somnolence typically occurs 1 to 2 months after radiotherapy and lasts 1 to 6 weeks. Late sequelae of radiotherapy are location-, volume-, dose-, and age-dependent. The list of possible late effects of therapeutic radiation includes impaired mental development, interference in bone growth resulting in an abnormally shaped face or skull, hypopituitarism, radiation necrosis, rare vascular sequelae such as moyamoya disease, and delayed oncogenesis.[11, 12]

BOX 9–1
Side Effects of Radiotherapy

- **Acute: mild fatigue, skin redness, hair loss**
- **Early-delayed: somnolence syndrome (occurs 1 to 2 months after treatment, lasts 1 to 6 weeks)**
- **Late: impaired mental development, bone growth abnormalities, endocrine disturbances, radiation necrosis, vascular changes (e.g., moyamoya), secondary tumors**

TECHNIQUE OF RADIOSURGERY IN CHILDREN

Application of the Leksell Model G stereotactic coordinate frame is applied using general anesthesia in children younger than 14 years. For older children, local anesthesia is supplemented with mild sedation. In some children, continuous infusion of propofol anesthesia without intubation provides deep and adequate anesthesia. This approach has mainly been used in children between the ages of 8 and 12. Once the stereotactic frame is applied, a stereotactic magnetic resonance imaging (MRI) scan is performed with intravenous paramagnetic contrast enhancement. High-resolution 1-mm slice thickness volume acquisition images using a 512×252 matrix provide exclusive anatomical detail in most cases. The images are transferred via ethernet to the computer workstation of the gamma knife. Using the current version of GammaPlan (Elekta Instruments, Atlanta, GA), the axial images can be used to create stereotactically accurate coronal and sagittal high-resolution images for planning (Fig. 9–1). The 201-source cobalt 60 gamma knife (Elekta Instruments) is used for radiosurgery after completion of volumetric dose planning with a high-speed computer workstation.

At our center, dose planning is performed by the neurosurgeon in conjunction with the radiation oncologist and med-

ical physicist. Our goal is precise, conformal, three-dimensional irradiation of the tumor target. In most patients, this requires conforming to the enhancing margin of the tumor on MRI. For tumors without enhancement, we can form the plan to the imaging changes identified on the long TR images. *Dose selection is based on tumor location, histology, volume, patient age, and an estimated risk of delayed radiation injury of less than 3%* based on volume (integrated logistic formula).[8] The dose is reduced if the patient received prior radiation therapy. After radiosurgery, the patient receives a weight-adjusted dose of intravenous methylprednisolone. He or she is sent to an observation unit or back to the neurosurgical ward and discharged home the next morning. After stereotactic frame removal, occasional use of acetaminophen may be necessary for headache, which usually clears within several hours.

RESULTS

Pilocytic Astrocytomas

Pilocytic astrocytoma is a distinct histologic subtype of astrocytoma that is most often diagnosed in children and young adults.[2] Pilocytic astrocytomas are usually well circumscribed on contrast-enhanced imaging. Many tumors have an indolent course and long-term survival (and even cure) following complete surgical resection. However, in some patients tumor recurrence or progression occurs after subtotal resection of tumors in a high-risk brain location. The effectiveness of fractionated external-beam radiation therapy has been questioned. *We anticipated that single-fraction, high-dose volumetric irradiation of these often well-circumscribed tumors might provide a superior alternative to other therapies.*[13]

To date, 15 children with pilocytic astrocytoma have had stereotactic radiosurgery at our center. Mean patient age was 9 years (range 4 to 17). The mean duration of symptoms prior to radiosurgery was 2 years. Eleven patients had undergone prior resection (6 had residual tumors and 5 had recurrent tumors). Ten of 15 patients had a neurologic deficit at the time of radiosurgery. One patient was treated for tumor progression after prior fractionated radiation therapy. Tumor locations included the cerebellum ($n = 6$), thalamus ($n = 2$), pons/midbrain ($n = 5$), frontal lobe ($n = 1$), and temporal lobe ($n = 1$). Mean tumor volume at radiosurgery was 1.9 mL (range, 0.06 to 7.1). Mean dose delivered to the tumor margin was 15.4 Gy (range 13 to 20) and mean maximal dose 29.6 Gy (range 21.4 to 40). After radiosurgery, all patients had stabilization in their tumor volume. In a detailed review of the first 9 patients who were evaluated for up to 4 years, five tumors had decreased in size and four showed no further growth.[13] In patients whose tumors regressed, reduction in tumor volume after radiosurgery varied from 72 to 99% (Fig. 9–2). No morbidity or mortality was associated with radiosurgery. No patient developed a new or progressive neurologic deficit from tumor growth. Six patients had improvement in their preoperative neurologic deficit; and in the first 9 patients, school performance and intellectual/emotional development were judged by family members to be unchanged after radiosurgery.[13]

Radiosurgery may be especially valuable for pilocytic astrocytomas because these tumors are often well circumscribed histologically. Radiosurgery likely leads to tumor growth

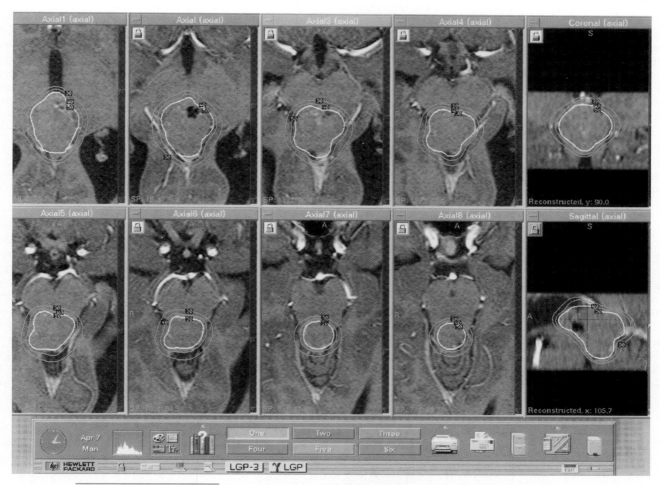

Figure 9–1 Dose planning using the gamma knife. In this patient with a germinoma, axial images and the isodose configuration are displayed, with simultaneous display of stereotactically accurate coronal and sagittal images. (See also Fig. 9–6.)

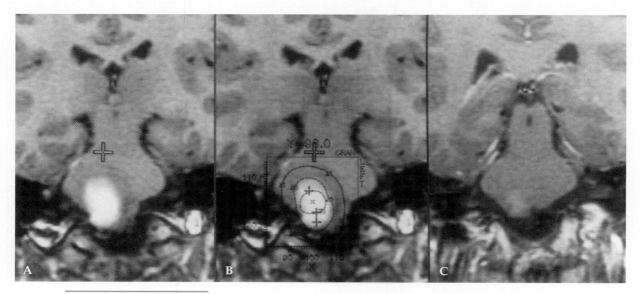

Figure 9–2 Pilocytic astrocytoma in a child after prior subtotal resection (A). The radiosurgery plan is shown on the coronal magnetic resonance image (B). Eleven months later, the tumor was barely identified (C). The child remains with a normal MRI result 6 years after radiosurgery.

arrest by preventing further cellular division coupled with delayed intratumoral vascular obliteration. Many pilocytic astrocytomas (even after resection) remain clinically and biologically dormant without any other intervention. *However, children with progressive, well-circumscribed tumors that are located in critical or deep areas are potential candidates for radiosurgery.* Larger tumors (greater than 3.5 cm in diameter) should again be considered for resection. Fortunately, many brain stem pilocytic astrocytomas are small and therefore suitable for radiosurgery. A tumor margin dose of 13 to 15 Gy can be effective for these patients.[14] Additional long-term follow-up will be required to confirm that radiosurgery provides tumor control for localized and progressive pilocytic astrocytoma.

Astrocytoma

Patients with nonpilocytic, nonanaplastic astrocytomas may be candidates for stereotactic radiosurgery. To date, four patients were treated at our institution at a mean age of 10 years (range 3 to 17). One patient had prior external-beam radiation therapy. Subtotal resection had been performed in two patients. Brain locations included frontal lobe ($n = 1$), intraventricular ($n = 1$), thalamus ($n = 1$), and brain stem ($n = 1$). The mean tumor volume was 1.4 mL and the mean tumor margin dose 15.8 Gy. Upon follow-up (2 to 11 years, one patient's tumor had disappeared on

imaging, and other patients experienced no tumor growth. *For an astrocytoma to be suitable for radiosurgical targeting, it should be small (less than 2.5 cm diameter) and in a location where larger field fractionated radiation should be avoided.*[2] For well-circumscribed proven astrocytomas, radiosurgery should be considered as potentially less toxic and of more therapeutic benefit than fractionated radiotherapy. Other centers have used radiosurgery for children with astrocytomas and report small series.[4]

Anaplastic Astrocytoma and Glioblastoma Multiforme

Patients with malignant glial tumors are suitable for radiosurgery as a boost to their fractionated radiation therapy regimen or in addition to other adjuvant treatments, such as chemotherapy.[2, 10] We treated six patients with anaplastic astrocytoma and three with glioblastoma in our first 10 years of experience. The mean dose for anaplastic astrocytoma was 9 years (range, 4 to 16) and for glioblastoma, 6 years. Four of six patients with anaplastic astrocytoma had prior radiation therapy (41 to 60 Gy) and all three with glioblastoma had XRT. Two patients with glioblastoma continue to be followed up to 60 months after treatment, and one patient died. Of the anaplastic astrocytoma patients, one patient remains tumor-free on imaging 9 years after radiosurgery (Fig. 9–3). One patient with a mid-

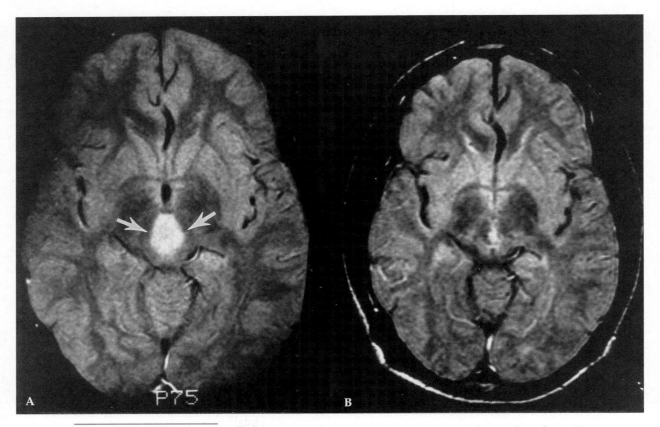

Figure 9–3 (A) Anaplastic astrocytoma of the midbrain tectum in an adolescent boy (long-TR magnetic resonance image). Two years after radiosurgery and radiation therapy, no tumor was identified (B). The patient remains well with no imaging evidence of tumor 10 years after treatment.

brain anaplastic astrocytoma with long term follow-up (10 years) had a Parinaud's syndrome 1 year after radiosurgery and radiation therapy that subsequently resolved. Only one of six patients died during the mean follow-up period of 3 years.

Ependymoma

Radiosurgery has been used as an adjuvant management approach to recurrent or residual ependymomas after microsurgical resection.[4, 15] Eleven children had radiosurgery (mean age 8 years) at our center. Nine patients (82%) had undergone prior external-beam radiation therapy before radiosurgery. Ten of 11 patients had undergone prior resection (maximum four resections). Tumor locations included fourth ventricle and brain stem ($n = 6$), cerebellum ($n = 2$), and middle fossa skull base ($n = 2$). Mean tumor volume was 2.9 mL (range 0.8 to 11.8 mL). Mean dose delivered to the tumor margin was 14 Gy (range 11 to 17 Gy) and the mean maximum dose 28.5 Gy. Impressive local tumor responses were noted in many patients. Those with anaplastic ependymomas often had distant recurrences, even when initial regression was noted. *Radiosurgical treatment for ependymoma continues to be evaluated. When the biologic behavior of the tumor enters a phase of rapid progression, radiosurgery can be an effective palliation for circumscribed small-volume tumors, but the tendency for these tumors to recur outside their imaging-defined borders remains problematical.* Effective therapy may await the development of potent tumor-specific radiation sensitizers or brain protectant agents that permit a higher radiosurgical dose.

Pituitary Tumors

Radiosurgery of pituitary adenomas offers potentially higher response rates over shorter time intervals than fractionated radiotherapy, with a greater chance of preserving normal pituitary function.[16] Radiosurgery of hormone-secreting or non–hormone-secreting tumors must achieve long-term tumor growth control with low morbidity. For hormone-secreting tumors, the additional goal of hormone suppression is required. *Tumors are suitable for radiosurgery only if they can be well localized on imaging and are located at least 2 mm from the optic chiasm.* Custom beam blocking can allow the delivery of a satisfactory radiation dose to the tumor and still limit the optic chiasm dose to less than 8 Gy.[17] Older charged-particle irradiation series utilized poor, nonstereotactic tumor targeting.

In a series involving more than 100 pituitary tumors, we used radiotherapy to treat eight children with pituitary adenomas. The mean patient age was 14 years (range 9 to 17 years). One patient had received prior radiation therapy, one a gross total resection, and seven a subtotal resection. Three patients had prolactin-secreting adenomas, one a mixed growth hormone/prolactin–secreting tumor, two Cushing's disease, and one Nelson's syndrome. The cavernous sinus space was involved in two patients. After radiosurgery, tumor mass was controlled in seven of eight patients (Fig. 9–4). One developed a posterior fossa metastasis of an adrenocorticotropic hormone–secreting tumor requiring resection.

In an attempt to improve results with hormone-secreting tumors, we aim to deliver as high a dose as possible to the tumor while preserving the safety of the optic nerve and chiasm.[7] Using conformal planning and selective beam blocking, we aimed to deliver an optic chiasm nerve dose of less than 8 Gy and deliver as much to the tumor as possible based on that limitation.[18] Thus, for this tumor, the mean maximum dose was 44.4 Gy (range, 30 to 60 Gy) and the mean margin dose was 22 Gy—significantly higher than that delivered to acoustic tumors or meningiomas. In children, radiosurgery should be used as an adjuvant management strategy for treatment of recurrent or residual tumors following resection where larger field fractionated radiation therapy is not desired.

The minimal rate of short-or long-term pituitary insufficiency after radiosurgery provides another compelling reason to select radiosurgery over radiation therapy. We believe that radiosurgery will have an increasing role in the management of small-volume pituitary tumors within the sella or cavernous sinus.

Craniopharyngiomas

As for other sellar and suprasellar tumors, radiosurgery can be used to treat craniopharyngiomas provided that the tumor can be identified on imaging and does not distort the optic apparatus. *We believe that radiosurgery is best suited for treatment of solid tumors rather than cystic ones.*[19] Intracavitary irradiation may be a more effective and radiobiologically powerful technique for the treatment of monocystic craniopharyngiomas.[20] For mixed tumors, a combination of therapies can be effective. Surgical resection often must first be considered in patients with large solid tumors.

Eight children with craniopharyngiomas had radiosurgery at the University of Pittsburgh. The mean patient age was 11 years (9 to 17). Three patients had undergone "gross total" resection and another three subtotal resection. Six patients had pituitary insufficiency and six a fixed neurologic deficit associated with prior tumor treatment. The mean tumor margin dose was 17 Gy (range 14 to 22.5) and the mean maximum dose 32.5 Gy. For the most part, craniopharyngiomas represented small-tumor residuals after prior resection and thus the mean tumor-volume was small at 0.47 mL. Seven of eight patients have had stabilization of their tumor on imaging (mean follow-up, 43 months; range, 12 to 110 months). One patient developed cystic enlargement of an initially solid tumor that required additional resection.

Indications for radiosurgery in these patents are similar to those for patients with nonsecreting pituitary tumors. The optic chiasm should remain at a distance of 2 mm or so from the tumor margin to allow the delivery of an adequate tumor dose that is safe to vision.

Acoustic Neuromas

Radiosurgery has been established as a useful alternative to surgical resection in the management of acoustic tumors.[21–26] The application of conventional radiation therapy to these tumors was questioned or ignored by surgeons due to the lack of satisfactory results observed. It is only since the late 1980s, when increasing numbers of patients were treated and results reported, that acoustic neuroma radiosurgery

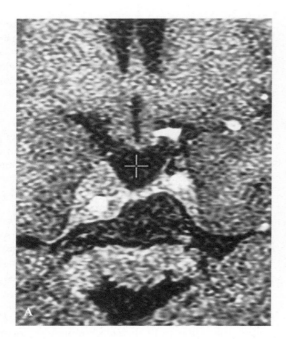

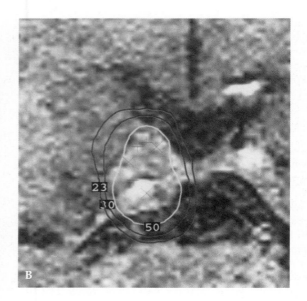

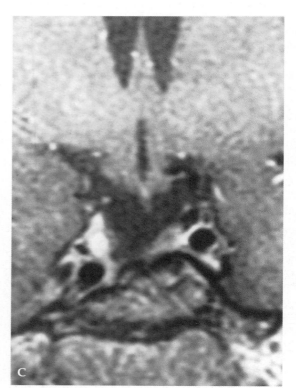

Figure 9–4 (A) Coronal magnetic resonance image showing a pituitary tumor involving the right cavernous sinus in a 15-year-old boy who presented with acromegaly following two transsphenoidal resections. He had a growth hormone– and prolactin-secreting tumor, and was later found to have a pheochromocytoma. (B) The radiosurgery dose plan is shown (tumor margin recieved 18 Gy to the 50% isodose) with the optic chiasm kept below the 20% isodose line. Six months after radiosurgery (C), the tumor had regressed.

has been embraced. Most series report tumor control rates with radiosurgery that exceed 90%.[21, 27] There is variation in the reported risks of radiation injury to facial, trigeminal, and auditory nerves based on differences in tumor size and technique.[28] These risks have decreased with time.[21, 29] Radiobiological studies confirm the histologic effects of this technique.[25]

Long-term follow-up in adults (5 to 10 years) substantiates the role of radiosurgery for acoustic tumor. Children, who most often have neurofibromatosis type 2 (NF-2), pose additional challenges. To date, six acoustic tumors in children (all with NF-2) were managed with radiosurgery. Two patients had radiosurgery for bilateral tumors, staged at 6 and 12 months, respectively. Five of six tumors were controlled after irradiation, at maximum follow-up of 8 years. There was no major morbidity after radiosurgery. Initially, we attempted to use radiosurgery with the goal of preserving the hearing of patients with these difficult tumors.

However, all patients treated prior to 1992 lost useful hearing.[30] Since then, radiosurgical technique involving the use of multiple small isocenters and a reduced radiation dose has been associated with hearing preservation in some patients.[31] *At present, we recommend radiosurgery or surgery only for growing tumors on serial imaging studies, or when documented hearing loss or clinical progression has occurred with a stable tumor on imaging.*

Meningiomas

Radiosurgery is an exciting development in the management of brain meningiomas. Because these tumors are often well circumscribed, easily defined on imaging, and rarely invade the brain, they can be targeted using conformal radiosurgical techniques.[32] *The utility of radiosurgery for cranial base meningiomas has been proven effective for the treatment of tumors in critical brain locations adjacent to cranial nerves or the brain stem.*[33, 34] Radiosurgery can be used as a second-stage approach after prior microsurgical resection to treat residual tumor, for the management of recurrent tumors after prior gross total resection, or as a primary method for the treatment of smaller meningiomas (Fig. 9–5).

Meningiomas are uncommon tumors in children. We have used radiosurgery as an adjuvant strategy for patients with recurrent tumors after resection.[17, 18, 35] To date, three patients were treated (mean age, 14 years).[2, 3, 10, 27, 36] Tumor locations included two that were intraventricular and one that was suprasellar; the latter occurred following radiation therapy. All tumors were successfully treated without subsequent growth at average follow-up of 37 months (range 20 to 50 months).

The roles of radiosurgery alone (for small tumors), surgical resection plus radiosurgery (for larger tumors), and the utility of fractionated radiation therapy for meningiomas are currently being defined. Long-term follow-up is mandatory to evaluate the optimum roles of different treatments for intracranial meningiomas.

Pineal Region Tumors

Malignant and benign tumors that arise from the pineal gland present difficult management challenges because of the tumor itself, associated neurologic deficits, and hydrocephalus.[37] For tumors such as germinoma (germinomatous germ cell tumor), excellent results have been reported after fractionated radiation therapy.[38] More recently, both intravenous chemotherapy regimens and radiosurgery have been considered in an effort to avoid craniospinal irradiation for younger patients. To date, we managed three patients with germinomatous germ cell tumors using radiosurgery followed by chemotherapy. Total tumor regression was noted within 4 months in all three (Fig. 9–6). Another patient with a pineoblastoma and hydrocephalus in the setting of the trilateral syndrome had prompt resolution of both the pineoblastoma and a pituitary stalk tumor within a month of radiosurgery (Fig. 9–7). Hydrocephalus resolved promptly without the need for a shunt. This patient died 1.5 years after radiosurgery when diffuse subarachnoid tumor spread developed. We have observed that tumors with rapid cellular division rates respond quickly to radiosurgery. The treatment of recurrent embryonal carcinoma was less satisfactory in the one patient treated so far. Two

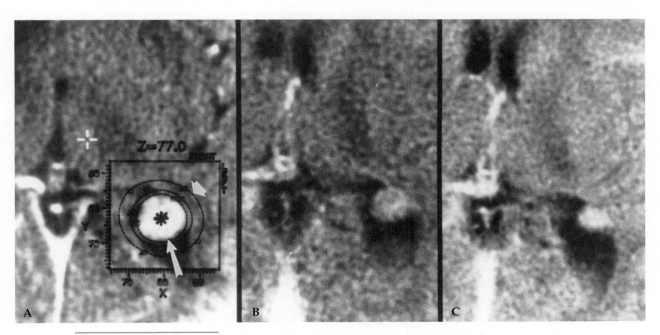

Figure 9–5   CT imaging in a 14-year-old boy during radiosurgical treatment for a recurrent intraventricular meningioma (A). The radiosurgery plan is shown: large arrow represents an 80% isodose (25 Gy) and small arrow a 20% isodose. Four months (B) and 8 months (C) after radiosurgery, the tumor has regressed. The patient is now 22 years old.

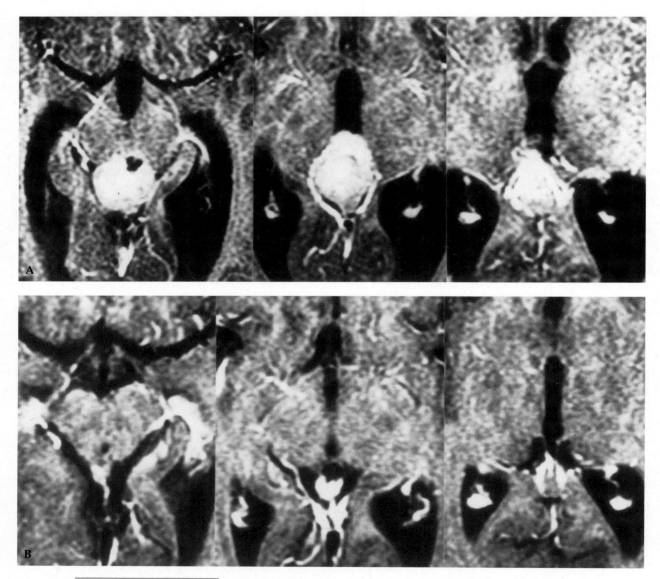

Figure 9–6 (A) Serial axial magnetic resonance images in a 15-year-old boy with a pineal germinoma. Radiosurgery was performed with 13 Gy to the 50% isodose (see Fig. 9–1). (B) Three months after radiosurgery no tumor was identified.

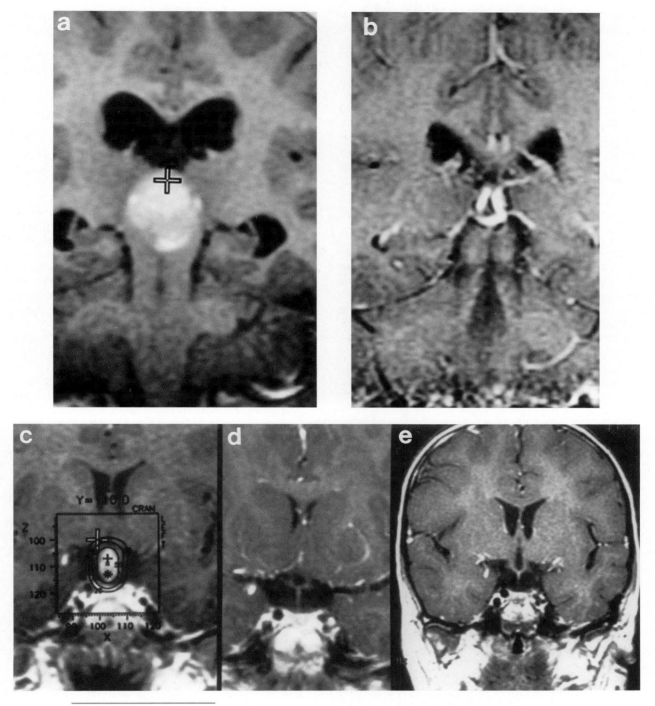

Figure 9–7   (A) Coronal magnetic resonance image in a 3-year-old girl with pineoblastoma and bilateral retinoblastomas. One month after radiosurgery, no tumor was identified and her ventricular size had decreased (B). For a newly identified pituitary stalk tumor found during the scan at (B), radiosurgery was performed (C). (D) One month later that tumor could not be found; she remained without hormonal deficits (E) 4 months later.

patients with pineocytomas have had tumor growth arrest after radiosurgery in early follow-up.

Other Tumors

Radiosurgery is used to treat patients with other benign brain tumors including trigeminal and jugular foramen schwannomas),[39] hemangioblastomas,[40] glomus tumors, and hemangiopericytomas.[41] Occasionally, children with NF-2, von Hippel–Lindau disease, or other genetic disorders present with these neoplasms and are considered for radiosurgery. Other malignant tumors managed in this way include chordoma and chondrosarcoma.[36]

SUMMARY

When the tumor can be clearly identified on imaging, when the risks of other therapies seem excessive, and when an effective radiosurgery dose can be administered, stereotactic radiosurgery can be a valuable treatment option for patients. The opportunity to use radiation as a biologic treatment for cerebral neoplasms without the concomitant risks of large-volume brain irradiation will ensure the increasing use of stereotactic radiosurgery for children with brain tumors.

REFERENCES

1. Baumann G, Wara W, Larson D, et al. Gamma knife radiosurgery in children. *Pediatr Neurosurg* 1996;24:193–201.
2. Grabb P, Lunsford LD, Albright AL, et al. Stereotactic radiosurgery for glial neoplasms of childhood. *Neurosurgery* 1996;38:696–702.
3. Kondziolka D, Lunsford LD, Flickinger JC. Stereotactic radiosurgery in children and adolescents. *Pediatr Neurosurg* 1992;16:219–221.
4. Loeffler JS, Rossitch E, Siddon R, et al. Role of stereotactic radiosurgery with a linear accelerator in treatment of intracranial arteriovenous malformations and tumors in children. *Pediatrics* 1990;85:774–782.
5. Larsson B, Leksell L, Rexed B, et al. The high-energy proton beam as a neurosurgical tool. *Nature* 1958;182:1222–1223.
6. Leksell L. The stereotaxic method and radiosurgery of the brain. *Acta Chir Scand* 1951;102:316–319.
7. Witt TC, Kondziolka D, Flickinger JC, et al. Stereotactic radiosurgery for pituitary tumors. *Radiosurgery* 1996;1:55–65.
8. Flickinger JC. An integrated logistic formula for prediction of complications from radiosurgery. *Int J Radiat Oncol Biol Phys* 1989;17:879–885.
9. Flickinger JC, Lunsford LD, Kondziolka D. Dose prescription and dose volume effects in radiosurgery. *Neurosurg Clin North America* 1992;3:51–59.
10. Kondziolka D, Somaza S, Comey C, et al. Radiosurgery and radiation therapy: comparison of different techniques in an in vivo rat glioma model. *J Neurosurg* 1996;84:1033–1038.
11. Painter MJ, Chutorian A, Hilal A. Cerebrovasculopathy following irradiation in childhood. *Neurology* 1975;25:189–194.
12. Wara W, Richards G, Grumbach M, et al. Hypopituitarism after irradiation in children. *Int J Radiat Oncol Biol Phys* 1977;2:549–552.
13. Somaza S, Kondziolka D, Lunsford LD, et al. Early outcomes after stereotactic radiosurgery for growing pilocytic astrocytomas in children. *Pediatr Neurosurg* 25:109–115, 1996.
14. Kondziolka D, Lunsford LD. Intraparenchymal brainstem radiosurgery. *Neurosurg Clin North Am* 1993;4:469–479.
15. Kondziolka D, Lunsford LD. Current concepts in gamma knife radiosurgery. *Neurosurg Q* 1993;3:253–271.
16. Pollock BE, Kondziolka D, Lunsford LD, et al. Stereotactic radiosurgery for pituitary adenomas: imaging, visual, and endocrine results. *Acta Neurochir* 1994;62(Suppl):33–38.
17. Flickinger JC, Maitz A, Kalend A, et al. Treatment volume shaping with selective beam blocking using the Leksell gamma unit. *Int J Radiat Oncol Biol Phys* 1990;19:783–789.
18. Tishler RB, Loeffler JS, Lunsford LD, et al. Tolerance of the cranial nerves of the cavernous sinus to radiosurgery. *Int J Radiat Oncol Biol Phys* 1993;27:215–221.
19. Lunsford LD, Pollock B, Kondziolka D, et al. Stereotactic options in the management of craniopharyngioma. *Pediatr Neurosurg* 1994;21(Suppl 1):90–97.
20. Pollock BE, Lunsford LD, Kondziolka D, et al. Phosphorus-32 intracavitary irradiation of cystic craniopharyngiomas: current technique and long-term results. *Int J Radiat Oncol Biol Phys* 1996;35:437–446.
21. Flickinger JC, Kondziolka D, Pollock BE, et al. Evolution of technique for vestibular schwannoma radiosurgery and effect on outcome. *Int J Radiat Oncol Biol Phys* 1996;36:275–280.
22. Flickinger JC, Lunsford LD, Coffey RJ, et al. Radiosurgery of acoustic neurinomas. *Cancer* 1991;67:345–353.
23. Flickinger JC, Lunsford LD, Linskey ME, et al. Gamma knife radiosurgery for acoustic tumors: multivariate analysis of four-year results. *Radiother Oncol* 1993;27:91–98.
24. Linskey ME, Lunsford LD, Flickinger JC, et al. Stereotactic radiosurgery for acoustic tumors. *Neurosurg Clin North Am* 1992;3:191–205.
25. Linskey ME, Martinez AJ, Kondziolka D, et al. The radiobiology of human acoustic schwannoma xenografts after stereotactic radiosurgery evaluated in the subrenal capsule of athymic mice. *J Neurosurg* 1993;78:645–653.
26. Linskey ME, Flickinger JC, Lunsford LD. Cranial nerve length predicts the risk of delayed facial and trigeminal neuropathies after acoustic tumor stereotactic radiosurgery. *Int J Radiat Oncol Biol Phys* 1993;25:227–233.
27. Foote RL, Coffey RJ, Swanson JW, et al. Stereotactic radiosurgery using the gamma knife for acoustic neuromas. *Int J Radiat Oncol Biol Phys* 1995;32:1153–1160.
28. Flickinger JC, Kondziolka D, Lunsford LD. Dose and diameter relationships for facial, trigeminal, and acoustic neuropathies following acoustic neuroma radiosurgery. *Radiother Oncol* 1996;41:215–219.
29. Ogunrinde OK, Lunsford LD, Flickinger JC, et al. Stereotactic radiosurgery for acoustic nerve tumors in patients

with useful preoperative hearing: results at two-year follow-up examination. *J Neurosurg* 1994;80:1011–1017.

30. Linskey ME, Lunsford LD, Flickinger JC. Tumor control after stereotactic radiosurgery in neurofibromatosis patients with bilateral acoustic tumors. *Neurosurgery* 1992;31:829–839.
31. Subach BR, Kondziolka D, Lunsford LE, et al. Stereotactic radiosurgery in the management of acoustic neuromas associated with neurofibromatosis type 2. *J Neurosurg* 1999; 90:815–822.
32. Kondziolka D, Lunsford LD, Coffey RJ, et al. Stereotactic radiosurgery of meningiomas. *J Neurosurg* 1991;74:552–559.
33. Kondziolka D, Lunsford LD. Radiosurgery of meningiomas. *Neurosurg Clin North Am* 1992;3:219–230.
34. Lunsford LD, Witt T, Kondziolka D, et al. Stereotactic radiosurgery for anterior skull base tumors. *Clin Neurosurg* 1994;42:99–118.
35. Duma CM, Lunsford LD, Kondziolka D, et al. Stereotactic radiosurgery of cavernous sinus meningiomas as an addition or alternative to microsurgery. *Neurosurgery* 1993;32:699–705.
36. Kondziolka D, Lunsford LD, Flickinger JC. The role of radiosurgery in the management of chordoma and chondrosarcoma of the cranial base. *Neurosurgery* 1991;29:38–46.
37. Dempsey PK, Kondziolka D, Lunsford LD. Stereotactic diagnosis and treatment of pineal region tumors and vascular malformations. *Acta Neurochir* 1992;116:14–22.
38. Casentini L, Colombo F, Pozza F, et al. Combined radiosurgery and external radiotherapy of intracranial germinomas. *Surg Neurol* 1990;34:79–86.
39. Pollock BE, Kondziolka D, Lunsford LD, et al. Preservation of cranial nerve function after radiosurgery for nonacoustic schwannomas. *Neurosurgery* 1993;33:597–601.
40. Patrice S, Sneed P, Flickinger JC, et al. Radiosurgery for hemangioblastoma: results of a multi-institutional experience. *Int J Radiat Oncol Biol Phys* 1996;35:493–499.
41. Coffey RJ, Cascino TL, Shaw EG. Radiosurgical treatment of recurrent hemangiopericytoma of the meninges: preliminary results. *J Neurosurg* 1993;78:903–908.

Chapter 10

Chemotherapy

H. Stacy Nicholson and Roger J. Packer

The combination of surgery, radiotherapy, and chemotherapy in the treatment of primary central nervous system (CNS) tumors of childhood has resulted in slowly improving survival rates over the past two decades. Until the late 1970s and early 1980s, treatment for children with both benign and malignant brain tumors primarily consisted of surgery with or without radiation therapy. Chemotherapy was rarely used, except for children with recurrent malignant brain tumors. However, clinical trials completed since the mid-1970s have demonstrated the efficacy of chemotherapy for children with recurrent and newly diagnosed malignant and benign primary CNS tumors. For some childhood brain tumors, chemotherapy at diagnosis, when added to radiation therapy, increases the likelihood of survival.[1-3] Chemotherapy is clearly beneficial for medulloblastoma, and high-grade gliomas also appear to benefit. Furthermore, for some children without metastatic disease, chemotherapy may replace some of the radiation.[4] The use of chemotherapy to delay radiotherapy in infants and very young children with malignant brain tumors is now extensive;[5] in fact, some children have had such an excellent response to chemotherapy that radiotherapy was not needed. The specific role of chemotherapy in the management of childhood brain tumors is still being defined through clinical trials.

GENERAL CONSIDERATIONS

Many factors must be considered in designing chemotherapy for children with CNS tumors, some of which are unique to these tumors. First, childhood primary CNS tumors are composed of a heterogeneous group of lesions, each with their own biologic characteristics, mitotic activity, and responsiveness to chemotherapy. Therefore, it is difficult to generalize about brain tumors as a class, and each tumor type must be considered separately.[6, 7] Second, for chemotherapeutic agents to be effective the tumor must be sensitive to the agent employed. The selection of a drug or drug regimen for a given type of tumor has primarily been based on clinical studies investigating the response of the tumor to treatment (i.e., Phase II trials).[8] However, with the development of laboratory methods to ascertain the therapeutic profile of a given tumor, a more rational choice of chemotherapeutic agents can be made. Agents with possible activity are first tested by in vitro methods. Those agents that show promise are then studied in animal models, such as a xenograft model in which human tumors are grown in immune-deprived (nude) mice.

Thus, potentially active new compounds must show considerable promise before human clinical trials are undertaken. Also, agents that are unlikely to benefit patients are often discarded prior to reaching human clinical trials.

TYPES OF CLINICAL TRIALS

Most drugs presently used for pediatric CNS tumors were chosen initially on the basis of their efficacy against other forms of cancer and subsequent results in clinical trials in adults and children with brain tumor (see Table 10–1). In general, human clinical trials can be separated into three major categories, which are described in greater detail in Chapter 37. Phase I trials are designed to determine the maximum tolerated dose (MTD) of a drug, to identify its toxicities, and to obtain pharmacokinetic data. These studies are usually performed in children with recurrent disease who have exhausted all proven means of therapy. In pediatrics, most drugs that enter Phase I testing have already been shown to be active in adults with primary CNS tumors.

When the MTD and schedule of a drug have been defined in the Phase I study, a Phase II trial is carried out to determine the activity of a drug against a specific tumor. Such a trial measures the response rate of a tumor type (or types) to the drug. A 50% reduction in tumor size on neuroradiographic studies is a partial response, and a complete disappearance of the tumor is a complete response. Most trials require that a response persist for at least 4 weeks. Phase II trials are most often performed in children with recurrent disease; however, for some tumor types, especially those that are highly resistant to any known form of treatment, preirradiation chemotherapeutic Phase II trials (also known as Phase II window trials or neoadjuvant trials) have been performed. The rationale for utilizing preirradiation Phase II trials includes improved tolerance to the drug or drug combination and the potential that a chemotherapy-naive tumor may be less resistant to chemotherapy. Thus, trials in newly diagnosed patients may more accurately reflect the true activity of the drug or drug combination under study.

The final step in establishing the efficacy of a chemotherapeutic agent or combination is a randomized comparison to the standard therapy for the disease being studied. Because pediatric CNS tumors are rare, Phase III studies usually must be done in a multi-institutional setting. Generally, in the United States, these trials have only been possible through the pediatric cooperative groups sponsored by the National Cancer Institute.

TABLE 10–1   Chemotherapeutic Agents Commonly Used for Childhood Brain Tumors

Drug	Route	Tumor Type	Common Toxicities
Alkylating Agents			
Cyclophosphamide	IV	Medulloblastoma, germ cell tumor	Myelosuppression, hemorrhagic cystitis
Ifosfamide	IV	Medulloblastoma	Hemorrhagic cystitis
Melphalan	IV (SCR)	Medulloblastoma, high-grade glioma	Myelosuppression, gastrointestinal
Thiotepa	IV (SCR)	Medulloblastoma, high-grade glioma	Myelosuppression,
CCNU (BCNU)	PO (IV)	Medulloblastoma; high-grade glioma; oligodendroglioma	Myelosuppression, gastrointestinal, pulmonary
Cisplatin	IV	Medulloblastoma, ependymoma, germ cell tumors	Ototoxity, nephrotoxicity, myelosuppression, peripheral neuropathy, nausea and vomiting
Carboplatin	IV	Low-grade glioma, medulloblastoma; ependymoma, germ cell tumors	Peripheral neuropathy, nausea and vomiting, myelosuppression
Procarbazine	PO	High-grade glioma, low-grade glioma; oligodendroglioma	Myelosuppression, nausea, vomiting
Temozolomide	PO	High-grade glioma	Myelosuppression, hepatotoxicity
Antimetabolites			
Methotrexate	PO, IV	Medulloblastoma, high-grade glioma	Myelosuppression; gastrointestinal, hepatotoxicity
Cytarabine	IV	Medulloblastoma	Gastrointestinal, hepatic
Plant Alkaloids			
Vincristine	IV	Medulloblastoma, low-grade glioma, high-grade glioma	Peripheral and autonomic neuropathy
Etoposide (VP-16)	IV or PO	Medulloblastoma, high-grade glioma, low-grade glioma, germ cell tumor	Myelosuppression

IV, intravenous; SCR, stem cell rescue (either autologous bone marrow rescue or peripheral blood hernatopoietic stem cell rescue); PO, orally; CCNU, lomustine; BCNU, carmustine.

DETERMINANTS OF DRUG EFFICACY/RESISTANCE

In addition to the sensitivity of the tumor to a chemotherapeutic agent, other characteristics of the drug, such as its pharmacokinetics, its ability to cross the blood-brain barrier (BBB) in high enough concentrations to affect tumor growth, the ability of the tumor cells to accumulate and retain the drug, and the ability of the tumor cells to repair drug-induced damage,[9, 10] also affect its efficacy as a chemotherapeutic agent. A great deal of emphasis has been placed on the delivery of the drug, or drugs, to the tumor, but increasing information suggests that just as important are the cellular mechanisms within the tumor that are responsible for drug resistance.

BOX 10–1
Determinants of Drug Efficacy

- **Sensitivity of the tumor to the drug**
- **Pharmacokinetics of the drug**
- **Drug's ability to cross the BBB**
- **Ability of the tumor cells to accumulate and retain the drug**
- **Ability of the tumor cells to repair damage caused by the drug**

The BBB has been identified as a major cause of ineffectiveness of certain chemotherapeutic agents.[11–13] In some pediatric brain tumors, such as medulloblastoma, which often has a robust blood supply, the significance of the BBB is questionable. In contrast, for infiltrating gliomas, drug delivery is a more important issue as it is often difficult to deliver adequate concentrations of drugs to the periphery of the tumor.[11–13] Several methods of enhanced drug delivery have been tested, including the use of higher doses of chemotherapy, the use of osmotic agents to disrupt the BBB, and the coupling of chemotherapeutic agents with other drugs that selectively and transiently open the BBB.[11–16] Other methods, such as intra-arterial therapy, intracavitary therapy, intraoperative use of biodegradable polymers impregnated with a chemotherapeutic agent allowing a slow local release of a chemotherapeutic agent (wafer therapy), and direct intraparenchymal infusional therapy, also attempt to increase local delivery of chemotherapy to the tumor.[17–23] Although these are potentially useful techniques, their efficacy has yet to be proven in adults or children with CNS tumors. One concern with the modification of the BBB and delivery of drugs at higher concentrations to the normal surrounding brain is the potential for increased neurotoxicity.

The mechanisms of drug resistance in primary CNS tumors are important topics for basic research.[24] *Resistance to a given therapy may be an intrinsic property of the tumor or may be acquired during treatment. Tumors may acquire resistance by the loss of normal properties or by the amplification of existing cellular mechanisms.* In addition, tumors may become cross-resistant to multiple agents by a similar mechanism.

Mechanisms of drug resistance include alterations in cell transport, expression or amplification of genes such as the multi-drug resistance gene (*MDR1*), and elevated intracellular levels of enzymes that interfere with the antitumor activity of a drug. For the alkylator agents, which constitute the most widely used class of drugs enployed against CNS tumors, elevated levels of intracellular aldehyde dehydrogenase and glutathione (or glutathione S-transferase), decrease drug efficacy.[24–28] Similarly, intrinsic or acquired resistance to the nitrosoureas may be attributable to increased repair of DNA mediated by the O^6-alkyl guanine DNA alkyl transferase protein or by elevated levels of thiol or glutathione S-transferases.[24–28] Attempts to overcome drug resistance, including saturation of enzymes by alternative substrates and the use of drugs that inactivate cell resistance mechanisms, have not yet shown clear clinical efficacy.

In 1979, Goldie and Coldman proposed a mathematical model that related curability of malignancy to the appearance of resistant cell lines.[29, 30] They proposed that control of the neoplasm was a function of various factors favoring resistance, including the tumor's spontaneous mutation rate. *The major contribution of the Goldie-Coldman hypothesis is the recognition that a tumor is less likely to be resistant to multiple agents administered simultaneously than it is to individual agents because cells are not given an opportunity to mutate and develop pleotropic multiple drug resistance.* In fact, multiagent chemotherapy has become the standard of care for most childhood cancers. In addition, if multiple drugs are given over a relatively short time, myelosuppression should be less because damage to hematopoietic precursor cells is partially dependent on the duration of exposure. Most ongoing chemotherapeutic trials involving childhood brain tumors

utilize a combination of drugs rather than single agents in attempts to improve efficacy.

The use of chemotherapy at higher doses to both overcome drug resistance and allow delivery of higher, more effective concentrations of drugs to the periphery of the tumor has also been utilized.[31, 32] The primary toxicity of such high-dose chemotherapy is hematopoietic toxicity, although other organs can be injured by high doses of chemotherapeutic agents. High-dose chemotherapy trials in children with recurrent brain tumors with hematopoietic support provided by hematopoietic growth factors, autologous bone marrow rescue, and/or peripheral blood hematopoietic stem cell rescue have been done.[31] Although the toxicity of these therapies is considerable, including mortality rates as high as 15 to 20% in some autologous bone marrow rescue trials, preliminary results show promise for subgroups of patients with recurrent malignant brain tumors and, possibly, for infants with malignant brain tumors.

In pediatric neuro-oncology, the use of chemotherapy has not been limited to trials seeking to improve survival. Given the long-term toxicities of radiation, especially that associated with whole-brain and/or neuraxis irradiation, chemotherapy has also been implemented to reduce the amount of radiation required for disease control. In rare patients, the need for radiotherapy has been eliminated by the use of chemotherapy.[4, 5] Chemotherapy is now widely utilized for infants and young children with malignant brain tumors and for selected patients with low-grade tumors that are not surgically resectable without prohibitive morbidity.

SPECIFIC TUMOR TYPES AND CHEMOTHERAPY
Medulloblastoma

Of all the major childhood primary CNS tumors, the most experience with chemotherapy has been in the treatment of medulloblastoma. Prospective randomized trials have shown that children with medulloblastoma can be broadly separated into two risk groups.[1, 7, 33] Children with disseminated disease at diagnosis and those whose tumors are not amenable to total resection have a relatively poor prognosis, with an overall survival rate of approximately 40% at 5 years after radiation therapy alone (poor-risk patients). *In contrast, medulloblastoma patients without metastatic disease at diagnosis and whose tumors can be completely resected have approximately a 50 to 60% survival rate at 5 years with radiotherapy alone (average-risk patients).* Younger patients also have a less favorable survival rate, although the reasons for this are not well understood. The benefit of chemotherapy in poor-risk pediatric patients has been clearly demonstrated, and although improved survival has not been demonstrated for those children with average-risk disease in randomized chemotherapy clinical trials,[1, 33] most investigators consider the benefit of chemotherapy in patients with average-risk disease to be substantial enough to warrant trials using reduced-dose radiotherapy combined with chemotherapy.

These principles led to a generation of studies of children with poor-risk medulloblastoma that utilized more aggressive chemotherapy in an attempt to improve survival. In these same studies, patients with average-risk disease were treated with protocols primarily directed at reducing the amount of radiotherapy given as a way of potentially decreasing the late effects of treatment. However, more recently, the concept that children with average-risk disease do not benefit from chemotherapy has been questioned. Because radiotherapy has been implicated as a primary cause of cognitive and endocrinologic sequelae, especially in young children, there has been significant interest in utilizing chemotherapy as adjuvant therapy as a way of reducing the amount of radiation administered to children with average-risk medulloblastoma. Similarly, there has been a strong rationale for using chemotherapy as primary therapy for some children with medulloblastoma (especially very young children) to allow deferral and, occasionally, total avoidance of radiotherapy.

Treatment of Recurrent Disease

The initial reports of responses to chemotherapy pertained to patients with recurrent disease. Activity in recurrent medulloblastoma has been documented in studies of numerous agents, including cisplatin, carboplatin, cyclophosphamide, and etoposide, both singly and in combination.[34–41] However, despite response rates as high as 80% in some studies, long-term survival has rarely been documented after conventional doses of chemotherapy in children with recurrent medulloblastoma following surgery and craniospinal radiotherapy. Subsequently, high-dose chemotherapy supplemented by autologous bone marrow rescue has been used in children with recurrent medulloblastoma.[42–45] Excellent response rates have been documented in such studies; however, a high rate of treatment-related morbidity is also seen. For example, the combination of high-dose thiotepa, etoposide, and carboplatin was utilized in 23 patients with recurrent medulloblastoma.[42] Three patients (13%) in this series died of treatment-related toxicity. However, three patients survived without evidence of progression at a median of 36 months from treatment (range 10 to 63 months). The patients who fared best after high-dose chemotherapy were those who had minimal residual disease prior to the use of chemotherapy and no evidence of leptomeningeal dissemination. Other centers, using other high-dose chemotherapeutic regimens, have not reported as many patients with long-term disease control.[43, 44, 46] If the effectiveness of high-dose chemotherapeutic regimens is confirmed in children with recurrent medulloblastoma, autologous bone marrow rescue will likely be replaced by peripheral blood hematopoietic stem cell rescue.

Newly Diagnosed Disease

Because many agents are active in children with recurrent medulloblastoma, postsurgical trials have been undertaken to evaluate the efficacy of chemotherapy, in combination with radiotherapy, for children with newly diagnosed disease (Table 10–2).[1, 33, 47–49, 53–55] Two large, prospective randomized

TABLE 10–2 Selected Adjuvant Chemotherapy Trials for Children with Medulloblastoma

Study (No. Patients)	Type of Trial	Dose CSRT	Drugs Utilized	Outcome
McIntosh (21)	Single-arm; all risk	WB 3925 Spinal 3300	VCR, CPM	PFS 5 y: 81%
Levin (47)	Single-arm; all risk	WB 3300 Spinal 2500	PCZ, HU	PFS 5 y: 55%
Kretschmar (21)	Single-arm; high risk	WB 3060 Spinal 2550	CDDP, VCR, mustard	PFS 35 mo: 71%
Bloom (38)	Single-arm; all-risk	Variable	CCNU, VCR	Survival 5 y: 65%
Evans (179)	Randomized; all-risk	WB 3600 Spinal 3600	CCNU/VCR, prednisone vs RT alone	PFS 5 y: 60%, with chemo (high risk: 46% with chemo vs 0% RT alone)
Tait (251)	Randomized; all-risk	WB 3500–4500 Spinal 3000–3500	CCNU, VCR vs RT alone	PFS 5 y: 53%
Krishner (71)	Randomized; all-risk	WB 3500 Spinal 3000 (reduced in younger)	MOPP	PFS 5 y: 68 ± 9%
Packer (63)	Single-arm; high-risk	WB 3600 Spinal 3600	CCNU, VCR, CDDP	PFS 5 y: 85 ± 6%
Packer (65)	Single-arm; low-risk	WB 2400 Spinal 2400	CCNU, VCR, CDDP	PFS 3 y: 82 ± 7%

CSRT, craniospinal radiotherapy; WB, whole brain; VCR, vincristine; CPM, cyclophosphamide; PCZ, procarbazine; HU, hydroxyurea; CCNU, lomustine; CDDP, cisplatin; RT, radiotherapy; MOPP, mechlorethamine, vincristine, prednisone, procarbazine; PFS, progression-free survival.

trials were performed independently by the Children's Cancer Group and the International Society of Paediatric Oncology.[1, 33] In both studies, patients were randomized to receive either radiation therapy alone (3600 cGy craniospinal irradiation plus local tumor boost to a total dose of 5400 to 5600 cGy) or identical radiation therapy plus vincristine during the radiation and postradiation therapy cycles of lomustine (CCNU) and vincristine. For children on the Children's Cancer Group trial, the postradiation chemotherapy regimen also included prednisone. These trials demonstrated a statistical benefit for the addition of chemotherapy for children with poor-risk posterior fossa medulloblastoma. In the Children's Cancer Group trial, the estimated 5-year progression-free survival was 59% for children treated with radiation and chemotherapy and 50% for those treated with radiation alone. However, in patients with metastatic disease at diagnosis, event-free survival was 48% for those receiving chemotherapy, as compared with 0% for those treated with radiation alone.

While these prospective randomized trials were being performed, other single- or limited-institution trials were also being completed. McIntosh reported that 81% of 21 children treated with postirradiation therapy cyclophosphamide and vincristine were alive and free of disease at a median of 6 years after diagnosis.[47] Also, Packer and co-workers reported a trial evaluating 63 children with medulloblastomas that used CCNU, cisplatin, and vincristine. The progression-free survival at 5 years was 85 ± 6%.[48, 49] For eligibility in the latter study, children had to be at least 3 years old and must have had either subtotal resection, evidence of metastatic disease at the time of diagnosis, or brain stem involvement. Patients with metastatic disease at diagnosis had a 5-year progression-free survival of 67 ± 15%, compared with 90 ± 6% for those with localized disease.

After demonstrating that chemotherapy improved survival in patients with poor-risk medulloblastoma, the Children's Cancer Group completed a prospectively randomized clinical trial that compared two chemotherapy regimens. One group was treated with craniospinal and local-boost radiotherapy and concomitant vincristine followed by eight 6-week cycles of postirradiation CCNU, vincristine, and prednisone. The other group received the 8-drugs-in-1-day regimen for two cycles prior to irradiation, followed by craniospinal and local boost radiation and then eight postirradiation therapy cycles of 8-in-1.[50, 51] The 3-year event-free survival for the group as a whole was 57%. However, those children who received the control arm of CCNU and vincristine had a statistically higher 5-year event-free survival than those who received pre- and postirradiation 8-in-1-day therapy (3-year progression-free survival 62 ± 8% vs 48 ± 8%). Also, a multicenter randomized trial performed by the International Society of Paediatric Oncology, which involved 364 children with biopsy-proven medulloblastoma, failed to demonstrate a benefit for the use of a preirradiation chemotherapy regimen consisting of methotrexate, procarbazine, and vincristine.[52] The Paediatric Oncology Group utilized postirradiation mechlorethamine, vincristine [Oncovin], prednisone, and procarbazine (MOPP) as adjuvant therapy in another randomized trial, compared with craniospinal irradiation alone.[53] The 5-year event-free survival for the group receiving radiotherapy and chemotherapy was 68%,

compared with 57% for those receiving irradiation alone; however, given the small number of patients in the study, this difference was not statistically significant.

These studies show that adjuvant chemotherapy is of benefit for children with medulloblastoma. Randomized trials have clearly demonstrated this improvement in survival only for children with poor-risk disease who have received chemotherapy during and after radiation therapy. Preirradiation chemotherapy has shown no advantage over postirradiation chemotherapy, and in some trials survival disadvantages were demonstrated, possibly due to the delayed radiotherapy. The benefit of chemotherapy in children with average-risk medulloblastoma has not been shown in a prospective randomized trial comparing chemotherapy with radiotherapy alone. *However, it is paradoxical that children with average-risk disease treated with radiation therapy alone have the same or poorer survival than children with poor-risk disease treated with radiation plus chemotherapy.* This suggests that although chemotherapy should be of benefit for those with low-risk disease, the most effective regimen was not used in the earlier clinical trials.

Another potential use of chemotherapy for children with medulloblastoma is in reducing the amount of radiation needed, especially in younger children. Early reports of randomized trials that attempted to reduce the dose of radiation without the addition of chemotherapy in children with nondisseminated medulloblastoma suggested a higher rate of relapse outside the primary site and an overall poorer disease-free survival rate in patients treated with reduced-dose radiotherapy.[54] However, an update of the randomized trial performed in collaboration by the Children's Cancer Group and the Pediatric Oncology Group showed that the difference in survival between the reduced-dose radiotherapy group (2400 cGy) and the group that received 3600 cGy of craniospinal irradiation was no longer be statistically significant ($p = 0.058$). Moreover, in a prospective randomized trial performed by SIOP, survival was similar in patients receiving full-dose (3600 cGy) or reduced-dose (2400 cGy) craniospinal radiotherapy.[52]

Chemotherapy has also been used in conjunction with reduced-dose radiotherapy for children with medulloblastoma. In one trial utilizing procarbazine following surgery and hydroxyurea during radiation therapy, and a dose of 2500 cGy to the brain and spine for children with nondisseminated disease, the estimated 5-year progression-free survival and overall survival was 63% and 68%, respectively.[55] Of the 17 patients with nondisseminated disease at diagnosis who relapsed in the series, only 1 had an initial recurrence outside the primary site. The Children's Cancer Group has recently completed a study utilizing vincristine, CCNU, and cisplatin following irradiation in children with nondisseminated medulloblastoma coupled with 2400 cGy of craniospinal irradiation (with concomitant vincristine).[4] In this trial of 65 evaluable patients, the overall progression-free survival at 3 years was 82 ± 7%. These studies suggest that reducing the dose of radiation therapy for children with nondisseminated medulloblastoma may be a reasonable approach when chemotherapy is added. However, the optimal chemotherapeutic regimen to be used in combination with reduced-dose radiotherapy has not been defined, although prospective randomized trials are ongoing. As chemotherapy improves, the use of radiation may be further reduced.

Infants with Medulloblastoma

Another subset of children with medulloblastoma who have been extensively treated with chemotherapy are infants.[5, 56, 57] Most studies have shown a poorer prognosis for children diagnosed in the first 3 to 4 years of life than older children, independent of whether they were treated with radiation alone or with radiation plus chemotherapy. Because cranial irradiation in young children is associated with potentially severe adverse delayed toxicities, including intellectual deterioration and endocrinologic (especially growth-related) sequelae, there have been multiple studies, dating back to the 1970s, that utilized postsurgical chemotherapy, with delayed or no radiotherapy, for infants with medulloblastoma. In an early study, MOPP chemotherapy was used in 13 children with medulloblastoma who were younger than 36 months, resulting in a progression-free survival of 55%.[58] The largest experience has been that of the Pediatric Oncology Group, which utilized a four-drug regimen of vincristine, cyclophosphamide, cisplatin, and etoposide until 36 months of age or for at least 12 months in children with medulloblastoma who were younger than 3 years.[5] In this protocol, delayed irradiation was given upon completion of chemotherapy, and the median time of relapse in patients with medulloblastoma was 9 months; 34% of patients remained progression-free a median of 2 years from diagnosis. No patient relapsed beyond 26 months of diagnosis, raising the issue of the necessity of irradiation in those with complete response. The Children's Cancer Group has utilized the 8-in-1-day chemotherapy regimen for children younger than 18 months with newly diagnosed medulloblastoma.[56] In this study, radiation therapy was not routinely employed in children who showed a complete response, and the 3-year progression-free survival was 22%. The German Cooperative Group has utilized four cycles of an aggressive regimen of ifosfamide, methotrexate, cisplatin, vincristine, and intravenous cytosine arabinoside for infants with medulloblastoma.[59] Treatment of patients with localized disease at diagnosis resulted in a 92% 2-year disease-free survival rate without radiotherapy. In contrast, all patients with disseminated disease ultimately progressed.

An even more aggressive approach has been used by investigators at Memorial Sloan Kettering and participating institutions. This protocol included children younger than 3 years with localized medulloblastoma and children between 3 and 6 years with disseminated medulloblastoma. Treatment included five cycles of induction chemotherapy (cisplatin high-dose cyclophosphamide, etoposide, and vincristine) followed by a consolidation cycle of myeloablative chemotherapy (thiotepa, etoposide, and carboplatin) supported by autologous bone marrow rescue.[60] In 13 patients, the 2-year event-free and overall survival was 51% and 61%, respectively.

These studies suggest that chemotherapy alone may be an appropriate approach for some young children with medulloblastoma. Although most of these studies have used age 36 months or younger as an eligibility criterion, it is not yet clear to what age such an approach could be extended and what type of therapy would best consolidate an initial good response to chemotherapy. An important issue is whether, in those patients with a complete response, irradiation (either local or craniospinal) or high-dose chemotherapy is required to sus-

tain disease control. Some patients without residual disease after induction chemotherapy may do just as well with maintenance chemotherapy alone. Only a prospective randomized trial can address this issue. However, all of the completed studies show that most infants and young children with metastatic medulloblastoma at diagnosis respond only transiently to chemotherapy. For these children, more effective initial treatments are needed.

Other Primitive Neuroectodermal Tumors

Chemotherapy trials for children with primitive neuroectodermal tumors (PNETs) arising outside the posterior fossa, including pineoblastomas, have been similar to those for children with medulloblastomas. *Children with supratentorial PNETs have a poorer prognosis than those with medulloblastoma, possibly because of younger age at the time of diagnosis or because such tumors (especially pineoblastomas) are frequently disseminated at diagnosis or disseminate early in the course of illness.*[61, 62] Although not proven, nonposterior fossa PNETs may be biologically different from medulloblastomas.

The role of adjuvant chemotherapy for children with supratentorial PNETs has not been clearly established,[61, 62] partially due to the small numbers of patients available for study. Children with both pineal PNETs and other supratentorial PNETs were treated in the Children's Cancer Group trial that compared preirradiation and postirradiation chemotherapy with the 8-in-1-day regimen to radiation therapy plus CCNU, vincristine, and prednisone. For those with supratentorial PNETs, the progression-free survival at 5 years in 44 patients was 45 ± 8%. Twenty-five children with pineal PNETs were also treated. Eight were younger than 18 months and were nonrandomly treated with the 8-in-1-day chemotherapy regimen. The remaining 17 patients were randomized between the two treatments. All infants in this study developed progressive disease at a median of 4 months from the start of treatment. Of the 17 older patients, the overall 3-year progression-free survival was 61 ± 13%. The numbers in this study are too small to compare the two adjuvant chemotherapy regimens. However, given the poor outcome of children with pineal and other supratentorial PNETs, most investigators are using some form of chemotherapy in addition to radiation therapy.

Glioma
High-Grade Gliomas

The role of chemotherapy for malignant gliomas in childhood and adolescence remains less clear.[3] *It has been postulated, but not proven, that the biology of malignant gliomas in children differs from that in adults.*[63] Although the molecular alterations in both childhood and adult malignant gliomas are still being studied, preliminary evidence suggests that malignant astrocytic tumors arising in childhood are more likely to have *p53* gene mutations and, thus, a different genetic composition than those occurring during adulthood, which are believed to undergo a cascade of genetic changes as they progress from low-grade to high-grade malignancies.[64] This may partially explain differences between the sensitivity of adult and pediatric malignant gliomas to therapy.

Recurrent Disease

At recurrence, malignant gliomas may transiently respond to chemotherapeutic agents. Interpretation of chemotherapy trials is difficult, especially in adult series, as many trials combine patients showing an objective neuroradiographic response with those who have disease stabilization, considering both groups as "responders."[65–67] The nitrosoureas, singly or in combination with other drugs, such as procarbazine and vincristine, have been the most extensively studied drugs in adult Phase II trials; overall objective response rates usually have ranged between 10% and 20% (although some report transient benefit in as many as 75% of patients). Median time to progression in most series, which may be a better marker of efficacy, is usually less than 6 months. Studies in pediatric patients with recurrent malignant gliomas have been undertaken less commonly. Drugs that have been evaluated include vincristine, procarbazine, intravenous etoposide, oral etoposide, BCNU, PCNU, cisplatin, cyclophosphamide, carboplatin, and thiotepa as single agents or in combination with other agents, such as ifosfamide or high-dose cytosine arabinoside.[68–86] These studies have shown objective response rates ranging between 0% and 50%, with most studies reporting tumor shrinkage in 10% of patients or less. As in adult trials, even in series reporting a higher rate of response, median time to progression has been well less than a year and, usually, less than 6 months.

There has been increasing interest in the use of higher dose chemotherapy for children with malignant gliomas, supplemented by either autologous bone marrow rescue or peripheral blood hematopoietic stem cell rescue.[87–92] Thiotepa and etoposide have been administered at high dose in children with malignant gliomas. Objective responses to therapy were noted in 6 of the first 10 patients treated. Later studies combining high-dose BCNU with thiotepa and etoposide or high-dose carboplatin with thiotepa and etoposide had a similar overall response rate in a larger group of patients. Encouragingly, these studies also disclosed a small subgroup of children with prolonged survival, including those with anaplastic gliomas and glioblastoma multiforme. Enthusiasm for this approach is tempered by a toxic mortality rate of nearly 20% in some studies. Other investigators, using different chemotherapeutic agents, such as busulfan and thiotepa, or melphalan-based regimens, have shown less activity.[87–94] The reasons for these disparities in studies are unclear. *However, patients with minimal residual disease prior to treatment with high-dose chemotherapy (i.e., those with tumors that could be resected prior to chemotherapy) seem to have been the most likely to benefit from treatment with high-dose chemotherapy.*

Newly Diagnosed Disease

Chemotherapy for adults with malignant gliomas, when given as an adjuvant with or after radiotherapy, produces a modest prolongation in median survival but has not clearly improved the likelihood of long-term survival.[95–100] A meta-analysis of major adjuvant chemotherapy trials in adults concluded that there was a 10% increase in survival at 1 year and an 8.6% survival advantage at 2 years for adults with glioblastoma treated with chemotherapy and radiotherapy, compared with those treated with irradiation alone.[101, 102]

Chemotherapy has shown somewhat more promise in children (Table 10–3).[3, 103] The study that has provided the strongest evidence that adjuvant chemotherapy is of benefit for children with high-grade gliomas was completed by the Children's Cancer Group in 1982.[3] In this trial, the addition of CCNU, vincristine, and prednisone during and after radiotherapy was compared with treatment with radiation alone. Forty-six percent of children who received radiotherapy and adjuvant chemotherapy were alive and free of disease 5 years following treatment, compared with 18% of those treated with postsurgical radiotherapy alone. The benefit of chemotherapy was statistically significant for children with glioblastoma multiforme.

In a follow-up study, the Children's Cancer Group compared preirradiation chemotherapy and postirradiation chemotherapy with the 8-drugs-in-1-day regimen to the standard therapy with irradiation and chemotherapy with CCNU, vincristine, and prednisone.[103] No survival advantage was shown for those children treated with pre- and postirradiation 8-in-1-day therapy, compared with adjuvant CCNU and vincristine. Overall, the survival rates for children with anaplastic gliomas and glioblastomas were lower in the most recent Children's Cancer Group trial, but approximately 30% of children with anaplastic gliomas and 20% of children with glioblastoma were alive and free of disease 5 years after treatment. A statistical comparison of these two trials showed no difference in overall survival between the trials.[104] A more recent review of this information suggested that some of the children considered to have high-grade gliomas in the first Children's Cancer Group trial may have had low-grade gliomas. However, even when pathologic materials were re-reviewed, the statistical benefit for the addition of CCNU and vincristine for children with glioblastoma multiforme remained.

Studies are ongoing utilizing high-dose chemotherapy either prior to or following radiation therapy for children with both anaplastic gliomas (primarily subtotally resected tumors) and glioblastoma multiforme. Trials are also under

TABLE 10–3 Randomized Adjuvant Chemotherapy Trials for Children with High-Grade Astrocytoma

Study (No. Patients)	Dose RT	Drugs Utilized	Outcome
Sposto (58)	5250 cGy	CCNU, VCR, Prednisone vs no chemotherapy	PFS 5 y: chemo + RT = 46% RT only = 18%
Finlay (172)	5400 cGy	CCNU, VCR, prednisone vs."8-in-1"	PFS 5 y: 33%—no difference by type of chemotherapy

CCNU, lomustine; VCR, vincristine; RT, radiotherapy; PFS, progression-free survival; Chemo, chemotherapy.

5. Duffner PK, Horowitz ME, Krischer JP, et al. Postoperative chemotherapy and delayed radiation in children less than three years of age with malignant brain tumors. *N Engl J Med* 1993;328:1725–1731.

6. Kleihues P, Burger PC, Scheithauer BW, et al. *World Health Organization International Classification of Tumors, Histological Typing of Tumors of the Central Nervous System.* Berlin: Springer-Verlag; 1993.

7. Packer RJ. Chemotherapy for medulloblastoma/primitive neuroectodermal tumors of the posterior fossa. *Ann Neurol* 1990;28:823–828.

8. Friedman HS, Schold SC. Rational approaches to the chemotherapy of medulloblastoma. *Neurol Clin* North Am 1985;3:843–853.

9. Kornblith P, Walker M. Chemotherapy for malignant gliomas. *J Neurosurg* 1988;68:1–17.

10. Groothius DP, Blasberg RG. Rational brain tumor chemotherapy: the interaction of drug and tumor. *Neurol Clin North Am* 1985;3:801–816.

11. Sipos EP, Brem H. New delivery systems for brain tumor therapy. *Neurol Clin North Am* 1995;13:813–822.

12. Neuwelt EA, Howieson J, Frenkel EP, et al. Therapeutic efficacy of multiagent chemotherapy with drug delivery enhancement by blood-brain barrier modification in glioblastoma. *Neurosurgery* 1986;19:573–582.

13. Tamargo RJ, Brem H. Drug delivery to the central nervous system: a review. *Neurosurg Q* 1992;2:259–279.

14. Black KL, Chio CC. Increased opening of blood-tumour barrier by leukotriene C4 is dependent on size of molecules. *Neurol Res* 1992;14:402–404.

15. Pardridge WM, Boado RJ, Black KL, et al. Blood-brain barrier and new approaches to brain drug delivery. *West J Med* 1992;156:281–286.

16. Dahlborg SA, Petrillo A, Crossen JR, et al. The potential for complete and durable response in nonglial primary brain tumors in children and young adults with enhanced chemotherapy delivery. *Cancer J Sci Am*;110–124.

17. Bullard DE, Bigner SH, Bigner DD. Comparison of intravenous versus intracarotid therapy with 1,3-bis(2-chloroethyl)-1-nitrosourea in a rat brain tumor model. *Cancer Res* 1985;45:5240–5245.

18. Brem H, Mahaley MSJ, Vick NA, et al. Interstitial chemotherapy with drug polymer implants for the treatment of recurrent gliomas. *J Neurosurg* 1991;74:441–446.

19. Brem H, Piantadosi S, Burger PC, et al. Intraoperative controlled delivery of chemotherapy by biodegradable polymers: safety and effectiveness of recurrent gliomas evaluated by a prospective, multi-institutional placebo-controlled clinical trial. *Lancet* 1995;345:1008–1012.

20. Brem H, Tamargo RJ, Olivi A, et al. Biodegradable polymers for controlled delivery of chemotherapy with and without radiation therapy in the monkey brain. *J Neurosurg* 1994;80:283–290.

21. Harbaugh RE, Saunders RL, Reeder RF. Use of implantable pumps for central nervous system drug infusions to treat neurological disease. *Neurosurgery* 1988;23:693–698.

22. Cahan MA, Walter KA, Colvin OM, et al. Cytotoxicity of taxol in vitro against human and rat malignant brain tumors. *Cancer Chemother Pharmacol* 1994;33:441–444.

23. Bobo RH, Laske DW, Akbasak A, et al. Convection-enhanced delivery of macromolecules in the brain. *Proc Natl Acad Sci U S A* 1994;91:2076–2080.

24. Phillips PC. Antineoplastic drug resistance in brain tumors. *Neurol Clin North Am* 1991;9:383–404.

25. Ali-Osman F, Caughlan J, Gray GS. Decreased DNA interstrand cross-linking and cytotoxicity induced in human brain tumor cells by 1,3-bis(2-chloroethyl)-1-nitrosourea after in vitro reaction with glutathione. *Cancer Res* 1989;49:5954–5958.

26. Buller AL, Clapper ML, Tew KD. Glutathione S-transferases in nitrogen mustard-resistant and -sensitive cell lines. Molec Pharmacol 1987;31:575–578.

27. Friedman HS, Skapek SX, Colvin OM, et al. Melphalan transport, glutathione levels and glutathione-S-transferase activity in human medulloblastoma. *Cancer Res* 1988;48:5397–5402.

28. Schold SC, Brent TP, von Hofe E, et al. O^6-alkylguanine-DNA-alkyltransferase and sensitivity to procarbazine in human brain-tumor xenografts. *J Neurosurg* 1989;80:573–577.

29. Goldie JH, Coldman AJ. A mathematical model for relating the drug sensitivity of tumors to their spontaneous mutation rate. *Cancer Treat Rev* 1979;63:1727–1733.

30. Goldie JH, Coldman AJ. Application of theoretical models to chemotherapy protocol design. *Cancer Treat Rev* 1986;70:127–132.

31. Finlay J, August C, Packer R, et al. High-dose multi-agent chemotherapy followed by bone marrow "rescue" for malignant astrocytomas of childhood and adolescence. *J Neuro-oncol* 1990;9:239–248.

32. Graham ML, Herndon JE II, Casey JR, et al. High-dose chemotherapy with autologous stem-cell rescue in patients with recurrent and high-risk pediatric brain tumors. *J Clin Oncol* 1997;15:1814–1823.

33. Tait DM, Thorton-Jones H, Bloom HJG, et al. Adjuvant chemotherapy for medulloblastoma: the first multi-centre control trial of the International Society of Paediatric Oncology (SIOP I). *Eur J Cancer* 1990;26:464–469.

34. Bertolone SJ, Baum ES, Kirvit W, et al. A phase II study of cisplatin therapy in recurrent childhood brain tumors: a Children's Cancer Group phase II trial. *J Neuro-oncol* 1989;7:5–11.

35. Walker RW, Allen JC. Cisplatin in the treatment of recurrent childhood primary brain tumors. *J Clin Oncol* 1988;6:62–66.

36. Gaynon PS, Ettinger LJ, Baum ES, et al. Carboplatin in childhood brain tumors: a Children's Cancer Group phase II trial. *Cancer* 1990;66:2465–2469.

37. Friedman HS, Krischer JP, Burger P, et al. Treatment of children with progressive or recurrent brain tumors with carboplatin or iproplatin: a Pediatric Oncology Group randomized phase II trial. *J Clin Oncol* 1992;10:249–256.

38. Allen JC, Walker RW, Luks E, et al. Carboplatin and recurrent childhood brain tumors. *J Clin Oncol* 1987;5:459–463.

39. Mograbi A, Fuchs H, Brown M, et al. Cyclophosphamide in combination with sagramostim in the treatment of recurrent medulloblastoma. *Med Pediatr Oncol* 1995;25:190–196.

40. Boor R, Huber A, Gutjahr P. Etoposide treatment in recurrent medulloblastoma. *Neuropediatrics* 1994;25:39–41.

41. Ashley DM, Meier L, Kerby T, et al. Response of recurrent medulloblastoma to low-dose oral etoposide. *J Clin Oncol* 1996;14:1922–1927.

42. Dunkel IJ, Boyett JM, Yates A, et al. High-dose carboplatin, thiotepa, and etoposide with autologous stem-cell rescue for patients with recurrent medulloblastoma: Children's Cancer Group. *J Clin Oncol* 1998;16:222–228.

43. Kalifa C, Hartmann O, Vassal G, et al. High-dose busulfan and thiotepa with autologous bone marrow transplantation in childhood malignant brain tumors: a phase II study. *Bone Marrow Transplant* 1992;9:227–233.

44. Mahoney DH Jr, Strother D, Camitta B, et al. High-dose melphalan and cyclophosphamide with autologous bone marrow rescue for recurrent/progressive malignant brain tumors in children: a pilot Pediatric Oncology Group study. *J Clin Oncol* 1996;14:382–388.

45. Finlay J, Grovas A, Garvin J, et al. The "head start" regimen for children less than six years of age with newly-diagnosed malignant brain tumors. International Society of Paediatric Oncology (SIOP) XXVIIth Meeting, Montevideo, Uruguay 1995.

46. Dupuis-Girod S, Hartmann O, Benhamou E, et al. Will high-dose chemotherapy followed by autologous bone marrow transplantation supplant cranio-spinal irradiation in young children treated for medulloblastoma? *J Neuro-oncol* 1996;27:87–98.

47. McIntosh S, Chen M, Sartain PA, et al. Adjuvant chemotherapy for medulloblastoma. *Cancer* 1985;56:1316–1319.

48. Packer RJ, Siegel KR, Sutton LN, et al. Efficacy of adjuvant chemotherapy for patients with poor-risk medulloblastoma: a preliminary report. *Ann Neurol* 1988;24:503–508.

49. Packer RJ, Sutton LN, Elterman R, et al. Outcome for children with medulloblastoma treated with radiation and cisiplatin, CCNU and vincristine chemotherapy. *J Neurosurg* 1994;81:690–698.

50. Zelzer P, Boyett J, Finlay JL, et al. Tumor staging at diagnosis and therapy type for PNET determine survival. Report from the Childrens Cancer Group CCG–921. *Med Pediatr Oncol* 1995;25:238.

51. Packer RJ: Brain tumor studies of the Childrens Cancer Group (CCG): an update. *J Neuro-Oncal* 1996;28:48.

52. Bailey CC, Gnekow A, Wellek S, et al. Prospective randomized trial of chemotherapy given before radiotherapy in childhood medulloblastoma. International Society of Paediatric Oncology (SIOP) and the (German) Society of Paediatric Oncology (GPO): SIOP II. *Med Pediatr Oncol* 1995;25:166–178.

53. Krischer JP, Ragab AH, Kun L, et al. Nitrogen mustard, vincristine, procarbazine, and prednisone as adjuvant chemotherapy in the treatment of medulloblastoma. *J Neurosurg* 1991;74:905–909.

54. Deutsch M, Thomas PRM, Krishner J, et al. Results of a prospective randomized trial comparing standard dose neuroaxis irradiation (3600 cGy/20) with reduced neuroaxis irradiation (2340 cGy/13) in patients with low stage medulloblastoma: a combined Children's Cancer Group/Pediatric Oncology Group study. *Pediatr Neurosurg* 1996;24:167–177.

55. Levin VA, Rodriguez LA, Edwards MSB, et al. Treatment of medulloblastoma with procarbazine, hydroxyurea, and reduced radiation doses to whole brain and spine. *J Neurosurg* 1988;68:383–387.

56. Geyer JR, Zelzer PM, Boyett JM, et al. Survival of infants with primitive neuroectodermal tumors or malignant ependymomas of the CNS treated with eight drugs in one day: a report from the Children's Cancer Group. *J Clin Oncol* 1994;12:1607–1615.

57. White L, Johnston H, Jones R, et al. Postoperative chemotherapy without irradiation in young children with malignant non-astrocytic brain tumors: a report from the Australia and New Zealand Childhood Cancer Study Group. *Cancer Chemother Pharmacol* 1993;32:403–406.

58. van Eys J, Cangir A, Coody D, et al. MOPP regimen as primary chemotherapy for brain tumors in infants. *J Neuro-oncol* 1985;3:237–243.

59. Kuhl J, Gnekow A, Havers W, et al. Primary chemotherapy after surgery and delayed irradiation in children under three years of age with medulloblastoma: pilot trial of the German Pediatric Brain Tumor Study Group. *Med Pediatr Oncol* 1992;20:387.

60. Finlay JL. The "head start" regimen for children less than six years of age newly diagnosed with malignant brain tumors. *J Neuro-oncol* 1996;23:68.

61. Jakacki RI, Zeltzer PM, Boyett JM, et al. Survival and prognostic factors following radiation and/or chemotherapy for primitive neuroectodermal tumors of the pineal region in infants and children: a report of the Children's Cancer Group. *J Clin Oncol* 1995;13:1377–1383.

62. Cohen BH, Zeltzer PM, Boyett JM, et al. Prognostic factors and treatment results for supratentorial primitive neuroectodermal tumors in children using radiation and chemotherapy: a Children's Cancer Group randomized trial. *J Clin Oncol* 1995;13:1687–1696.

63. Collins VP: Genetic alterations in gliomas. *J Neuro-Oncol* 1995;24:37–38.

64. Rasheed BKA, McLendon RD, Herndon JE, et al. Alterations of the TP53 gene in human gliomas. *Cancer Res* 1994;54:1324–1330.

65. Mahaley JR MS: Neuro-oncology index and review (adult primary brain tumors). *J Neuro-oncol* 1991;11:85–147.

66. Yung WKA, Levin VA. Chemotherapy: current and future role and expectations. In: Apuzzo ML, ed. *Malignant Cerebral Gliomas: Neurosurgical Topics*. Park Ridge, IL: American Association of Neurologic Surgeons, 1990;207–216.

67. Conrad C, Milosauljevic VP, Yung WKA. Advances in chemotherapy for brain tumors. *Neurol Clin North Am* 1995;13:795–812.

68. Ward H: Central nervous system tumors of childhood treated with CCNU, vincristine, and radiation. *Med Pediatr Oncol* 1978;4:315–320.

69. Rosenstock J, Evans A and Schut L: Response to vincristine of recurrent brain tumors in children. *J Neurosurg* 1976;45:135–140.

70. Kumar A, Renaudin J, Wilson C, et al. Procarbazine hydrochloride in the treatment of brain tumors. *J Neurosurg* 1974;40:365–371.

71. Rosen G, Ghavimi F, Nirenberg A. High dose methotrexate with citrovorum factor rescue for the treatment of central nervous system tumors in children. *Cancer Treat Rep* 1977;6:681–690.

72. Walker R , Allen J. Cisplatin in the treatment of recurrent childhood primary brain tumors. *J Clin Oncol* 1988;6: 62–66.

73. Bertolone S, Baum E, Krivit W, et al. A phase II study of cisplatin therapy in recurrent childhood brain tumors: a report from the Children's Cancer Group. *J Neuro-oncol* 1989;7:5–11.

74. Allen JC, Walker R, Lucks E, et al. Carboplatin and recurrent childhood brain tumors. *J Clin Oncol* 1987;5:459–463.

75. Gaynon PS, Ettinger LJ Baum ES, et al. Carboplatin in childhood brain tumors: a Children's Cancer Study Group phase II trial. *Cancer* 1990;66:2465–2469.

76. Allen JC Helson L. High-dose cyclophosphamide chemotherapy for recurrent CNS tumors in children. *J Neurosurg* 1981;55:749–756.

77. Abrahamsen T, Lange B, Packer R, et al. A phase I and II trial of dose intensified cyclophosphamide and GM-CSF in pediatric malignant brain tumors. *J Pediatr Hematol Oncol* 1995;17:134–139.

78. Heideman RL, Packer RJ, Reaman GH, et al. A phase II evaluation of thiotepa in pediatric central nervous system malignancies. *Cancer* 1993;762:271–275.

79. Bouffet E, Mottolese C, Biron P, et al. High-dose thiotepa and etoposide followed by bone marrow rescue for malignant gliomas: a single institution experience. Houston, TX: Sixth International Symposium on Pediatric Neuro-oncology 67, 1994.

80. Kobrinski N, Packer R, Boyett J, et al. Etoposide with or without mannitol for the treatment of recurrent brain tumors: a Children's Cancer Group Study, CCG-9881 *J Neuro-oncol* 1999;45:47–54.

81. Miser J, Krailo M, Smithson W, et al. Treatment of children with recurrent brain tumors with ifosfamide, etoposide and MESNA. *Proc Am Soc Clin Oncol* 1989;8:328.

82. Castgello M, Clerico A, Giovanni D, et al. High-dose carboplatin in combination with etoposide(JEt Regimen) for childhood brain tumors. *Am J Pediatr Hematol Oncol* 1990; 2:297–300.

83. Corden B, Strauss L, Killmond T, et al. Cisplatin, ara-C and etoposide (PAE) in the treatment of recurrent childhood brain tumors. *J Neuro-oncol* 1991;11:57–63.

84. Allen J, Walker R, Rosen G. Preradiation high-dose intravenous methotrexate with leucovorin rescue for untreated primary childhood brain tumors. *J Clin Oncol* 1988;6:649–653.

85. Pendergrass T, Milstein J, Geyer J, et al. Eight-drugs-in-one day chemotherapy for brain tumors: experience with 107 children and rationale for pre-radiation chemotherapy. *J Clin Oncol* 1987;5:1221–1231.

86. Allen JC, Hancock C, Walker R, et al. PCNU and recurrent childhood brain tumors. *J Neuro-oncol* 1987;5:241–244.

87. Goldman S, Wong M, Garvin J, et al. High dose thiotepa and etoposide with autologous marrow rescue (ABMR) for children and young adults with recurrent central nervous system (CNS) tumors. Sixth International Symposium on Pediatric Neuro-oncology 157, 1994.

88. Papadakis V, Malkin M, Thompson S, et al. High-dose thiotepa, etoposide and BCNU with autologous bone marrow rescue in patients with malignant brain tumors. Houston, TX: Sixth International Symposium on Pediatric Neuro-oncology 65, 1994.

89. Foreman N, Pamphilon D, Cornish J, et al. Dose escalation study of cyclophosphamide in high dose with peripheral stem cell rescue. Houston, TX: Sixth International Symposium on Pediatric Neuro-oncology 50, 1994.

90. Heideman R, Douglass E, Krance A, et al. High-dose chemotherapy and autologous bone marrow rescue followed by interstitial and external-beam radiotherapy in newly diagnosed pediatric malignant gliomas. *J Clin Oncol* 1993;11:1458–1465.

91. Shen V, Bennetts G, Renna G, et al. The safety and efficacy of repetitive peripheral stem cell support in children with brain tumors receiving dose-intensified chemotherapy. Houston, TX: Sixth International Symposium on Pediatric Neuro-oncology 52, 1994.

92. Finlay J. High-dose chemotherapy and autologous marrow rescue for malignant brain tumors. Houston, TX: Sixth International Symposium on Pediatric Neuro-oncology 31, 1994.

93. Bouffet E, Mottolese C Jouvet A, et al. Etoposide and thiotepa followed by ABMT (autologous bone marrow transplantation) in children and young adults with high-grade gliomas. *Eur J Cancer* 1997;33:91–5.

94. Bouffet E, Khelfaoui F, Philip I, et al. High-dose carmustine for high-grade gliomas in childhood. *Cancer Chemother Pharmacol* 1997;39:376–9.

95. Levin VA, Wara WM, Davis RL, et al. NCOG protocol 6G91: seven-drug chemotherapy and irradiation for patients with glioblastoma multiforme. *Cancer Treat Rep* 1986;70:739–744.

96. Walker MD, Alexander E, Hunt WE, et al. Evaluation of BCNU and/or radiotherapy in the treatment of anaplastic gliomas. *J Neurosurg* 1978;49:333–343.

97. Walker MD, Green SB, Byar DP, et al. Randomized comparisons of radiotherapy and nitrosoureas for the treatment of malignant gliomas after surgery. *N Engl J Med* 1980;303:1323–1329.

98. Walker MD, Hurwitz BS. BCNU (1,3-bis(2-chloroethyl)-1 nitrosourea: NSC-409962) in the treatment of malignant brain tumor—a preliminary report. *Cancer Chemother Rep* 1970;54:263–271.

99. Levin VA, Silver P, Hannigan J, et al. Superiority of postradiotherapy adjuvant chemotherapy with CCNU, procarbazine, and vincristine (PCV) over BCNU for anaplastic gliomas: NCOG 6G61 final report. *Int J Radiat Oncol Biol Phys* 1990;18:321–324.

100. Levin VA, Wara WM, Davis Rlm, et al. Phase III comparison of BCNU and the combination of procarbazine, CCNU, and vincristine administered after radiation therapy with hydroxyurea to patients with malignant gliomas. *J Neurosurg* 1985;61:1063–1068.

101. Fine HA, Dear KBH, Loeffler JS, et al. Meta-analysis of radiation therapy with and without adjuvant chemotherapy for malignant gliomas in adults. *Cancer* 1993;71:2585–2597.

102. Fine HA. The basis for current treatment recommendations for malignant gliomas. *J Neuro-oncol* 1994;20:111–120.

103. Finlay JL, Boyett JM, Yates AJ, et al. Randomized phase III trial in childhood high-grade astrocytoma comparing vincristine, lomustine, and prednisone with the eight-drugs-in-1-day regimen. *J Clin Oncol* 1995;13:112–123.

104. Packer RJ, Sposto R, Finlay J, et al. Survival of children with high-grade gliomas (HGG): a comparison of two sequential randomized Children's Cancer Group (CCG) trials. *Ann Neurol* 1995;38:343.

105. Chamberlain MC. Recurrent brainstem gliomas treated with oral VP-16. *J Neuro-oncol* 1993;15:133–139.

106. Rodriguez LA, Prados M, Fulton D, et al. Treatment of recurrent brain stem gliomas and other central nervous system tumors with 5-fluorouracil, CCNU, hydroxyurea, and 6-mercaptopurine. *Neurosurgery* 1988;22:691–693.

107. Doz F, Bouffet E, Tron P. Clinical trial of carboplatin before and during irradiation for malignant brain stem tumor: a study by the Societé Française d'Oncologie Pédiatrique. *Proceedings of the Sixth International Symposium on Pediatric Neuro-oncology* 77, 1994.

108. Kalifa C, Hartman O Vassal G, et al. High-dose busulfan and thiotepa following radiation therapy in childhood malignant brain stem glioma. Houston, TX: Sixth International Symposium on Pediatric Neuro-oncology 78, 1994.

109. Dunkel I, Garvin J, Goldman S, et al. High-dose chemotherapy with autologous bone marrow rescue does not cure children with brain stem tumors. Sixth International Symposium of Pediatric Neuro-oncology: 78, 1994.

110. Jenkin DT, Boesel C, Ertel I, et al. Brain stem tumors in childhood: a prospective randomized trial of irradiation with and without adjuvant CCNU, VCR, and prednisone: a report of the Children's Cancer Group. *J Neurosurg* 1987;66:227–233.

111. Kretschmar CS, Tarbell NJ, Barnes PD, et al. Pre-irradiation chemotherapy and hyperfractionated radiation therapy 66 Gy for children with brain stem tumors: a phase II study of the Pediatric Oncology Group, protocol 8833. *Cancer* 1993;72:1404–1413.

112. Allen J, Packer R, Bleger A, et al. Recombinant beta-interferon (Betaseron): a phase I–II trial in children with recurrent brain tumors. *J Clin Oncol* 1991;9:783–788.

113. Nagai M, Arai T. Interferon therapy for malignant brain tumours: present and future. *No Shinkei Geka* 1982;10:463–476.

114. Packer RJ, Prados M, Phillips P, et al. Treatment of children with newly diagnosed brain stem gliomas with intravenous recombinant beta-interferon and hyperfractionated radiation therapy: a Children's Cancer Group phase I/II study. *Cancer* 1996;77:2150–2156.

115. Wakabayashi T, Yoshida J, Mizuno M, et al. Effectiveness of interferon-β, ACNU, and radiation therapy in pediatric patients with brainstem glioma. *Neurol Med Chir (Tokyo)* 1992;32:942–946.

116. Garvey M, Packer RJ. An integrated approach to the treatment of chiasmatic-hypothalamic gliomas. *J Neuro-oncol* 1996;28:167–183.

117. Rosenstock JG, Packer RJ, Bilaniuk L, et al. Chiasmatic optic gliomas treated with chemotherapy. *J Neurosurg* 1985;63:862–866.

118. Lefkowitz IB, Packer RJ, Sutton LN, et al. Results of the treatment of children with recurrent gliomas with lomustine and vincristine. *Cancer* 1988;61:896–902.

119. Pons M, Finlay JL, Walker RW, et al. Chemotherapy with vincristine (VCR) and etoposide (VP-16) in children with low grade astrocytoma. *J Neuro-oncol* 1992;14:151–158.

120. Friedman HS, Krischner JP, Burger P, et al. Treatment of children with progressive of recurrent brain tumors with carboplatin or iproplatin: a pediatric oncology group randomized phase II study. *J Clin Oncol* 1992;10:249–256.

121. Packer RJ, Ater J, Allen J, et al. Carboplatin and vincristine chemotherapy for children with newly diagnosed low-grade gliomas of childhood. *J Neurosurg* 1997;86:747–754.

122. Chamberlain M, Grafe MR. Recurrent chiasmatic-hypothalamic glioma treated with oral etoposide. *J Clin Oncol* 1996;13:2072–2076.

123. Packer RJ, Sutton LN, Bilaniuk LT, et al. Treatment of chiasmatic/hypothalamic gliomas of childhood with chemotherapy: an update. *Ann Neurol* 1988;23:79–85.

124. Prados M, Edwards MS, Rabbitt J, et al. Treatment of pediatric low-grade gliomas with a nitrosourea-based multiagent chemotherapy regimen. *J Neuro-oncol* 1997;32:235–241.

125. Cairncross G, Macdonald D, Ludwin S, et al. Chemotherapy for anaplastic oligodendroglioma. *J Clin Oncol* 1994;12:2013–2021.

126. Friedman H Oakes W. The chemotherapy of posterior fossa tumors in childhood. *J Neuro-oncol* 1987;5:217–229.

127. Goldwein JW, Glauser T, Packer RJ, et al. Recurrent intracranial ependymoma: treatment, survival and prognosis. *Cancer* 1990;66:557–563.

128. Evans AE, Anderson JR, Lefkowitz-Bourdreaux IB, Finlay JL. Adjuvant chemotherapy of childhood posterior fossa ependymoma: cranio-spinal irradiation with or without adjuvant CCNU, vincristine, and prednisone: a Children's Cancer Group study. *Med Pediatr oncol* 1996;27:8–14.

129. Robertson PL, Zeltzer PM, Boyett JM, et al. Survival and prognostic factors following radiation therapy and chemotherapy for ependymomas in children: a report of the Children's Cancer Group. *J Neurosurg* 1998;88:695–703.

130. Needle M, Goldwein J, Grass J, et al. Adjuvant chemotherapy for the treatment of intracranial ependymoma of childhood. *Cancer* 1997;80:341–347.

131. Grill J, Kalifa C, Doz F, et al. A high-dose busulfan-thiotepa combination followed by autologous bone marrow transplantation in childhood recurrent ependymoma: a phase II study. *Pediatr Neurosurg* 1996;25:7–12.

132. Gosl GJ, Geller NL, Bajorin DSP, et al. A randomized trial of etoposide and cisplatin versus vinblastin + bleomycin + cisplatinum + cyclophosphamide + dactinomycin in patients with good prognosis germ-call tumors. *J Clin Oncol* 1988;6:1231–1238.

133. Einhorn LH, Williams SD, Loehrer PJ, et al. Evaluation of optimal combination of chemotherapy in favorable prognosis disseminated germ-cell tumors: a Southeastern Cancer Study Group protocol. *J Clin Oncol* 1989;7:387–391.

134. Allen JC, Gosl G, Walker R. Chemotherapy trials in recurrent primary intracranial germ-cell tumors. *J Neuro-oncol* 1985;3:147–152.
135. Allen JC, DaRosso RC, Donahue B, Nirenberg A. A phase II trial of preirradiation carboplatin in newly diagnosed germinoma of the central nervous system. *Cancer* 1994;74(3):940–944.
136. Allen JC, Kim JH, Packer RJ. Neoadjuvant chemotherapy for newly-diagnosed germ-cell tumors of the CNS. *J Neurosurg* 1987;67:65–70.
137. Allen JC, Bruce J, Kun LE and Langford LA: Pineal region tumors. In: Levin VA, ed. *Cancer in the Nervous System*. New York: Churchill Livingstone; 1995:171–186.
138. Yoshida J, Sugita K, Kobayashi T, et al. Prognosis of intracranial germ-cell tumors: effectiveness of chemotherapy with cisplatin and etoposide (CDDP and VP-16). *Acta Neurochirurg* 1993;120:111–117.
139. Balmaceda C, Heller G, Rosenblu M, et al. Chemotherapy without irradiation: a novel approach for newly diagnosed central nervous system (CNS) germ-cell tumors (GCT): results of an international cooperative trial. *J Clin Oncol* 1996;14:2908–2915.
140. Duffner PK, Kun LE, Burger PC, et al. Postoperative chemotherapy and delayed radiation in infants and very young children with choroid plexus carcinomas. *Pediatr Neurosurg* 1995;22:189–196.
141. Cangir A, van Eys J, Hvizdala E, et al. Combination chemotherapy with MOPP in children with recurrent brain tumors. *Med Pediatr Oncol* 1978;4:253–261.
142. Horowitz M, Mulhern R, Kun L, et al. Brain tumors in the very young child: postoperative chemotherapy in combined modality treatment. *Cancer* 1988;61:428–434.
143. Ater J, van Eys J, Woo SY, et al. MOPP chemotherapy without irradiation as primary postsurgical therapy for brain tumors in infants and young children. *J Neuro-oncol* 1997;32:243–252.
144. Geyer J, Finlay J, Boyett J, et al. Survival of infants with malignant astrocytomas: a report from the Children's Cancer Group. *Cancer* 1995;75:1045–1050.
145. Duffner PK, Krischer JP, Burger PC, et al. Treatment of infants with malignant gliomas: the Pediatric Oncology Group experience. *J Neuro-oncol* 1996;28:245–256.

Chapter 11

Gene Therapy

Andrew T. Parsa, David W. Pincus, Neil A. Feldstein, and Jeffrey N. Bruce

In recent years, advances in chemotherapy and radiation therapy have increased survival rates for children with a variety of pediatric brain tumors. Despite this encouraging progress, there remains an impetus to use less toxic and more specific means of preventing tumor progression and recurrence. Minimizing the side effects associated with chemotherapy and radiation is an especially important consideration in the pediatric patient population. A better understanding of the molecular events leading to tumor development has provided an opportunity to intervene with experimental modalities, such as gene therapy and immunotherapy. These modalities may provide more efficacious treatment by targeting specific molecular characteristics, such as pathogenic gene expression and tumor antigens.

FROM BENCHTOP TO BEDSIDE

For children with brain tumors, gene therapy offers the hope of replacing defective genes, amplifying the immune response to cancer, and sensitizing tumor cells to systemic therapies. The simplest paradigm of gene therapy in a somatic cell is the replacement of a mutated protein with a genetically engineered, functional protein. In this scenario the pathologic phenotype of the cell is reversed once its genotype is restored. Gene therapy starts in the laboratory with the identification of a defect that can be corrected. A delivery method is selected for the gene and the hypothesis of restoring function is tested. Once confirmed in the laboratory, there are several methods of delivery (ex vivo or in vivo) that can be used to restore function in a patient. Such pediatric diseases as severe combined immunodeficiency (SCID),[1] cystic fibrosis,[2] and various inborn errors of metabolism[3] are being treated with gene therapy in this manner.

The malignant phenotype of a brain tumor results from a series of mutations, including genetic deletions.[4] Therefore, the simple paradigm of replacing a defective protein does not typically apply to children with brain tumors. However, the problems faced by early investigators using gene therapy to treat diseases such as SCID remain challenges for clinicians using gene therapy to treat children with brain tumors today.

ASHANTI DESILVA: THE SEVERE COMBINED IMMUNODEFICIENCY STORY

In 1990, a 4-year-old girl by the name of Ashanti Desilva became the first person to be treated in a federally approved gene therapy protocol.[5, 6] She suffered from a rare form of SCID, a disease caused by a dysfunctional immune system. Children with this disease have a defect in the protein adenosine deaminase (ADA) and if untreated usually sustain fatal complications of infection 1 to 2 years following diagnosis. ADA is an enzyme vital to the purine salvage pathway. Absence or dysfunction of ADA results in an accumulation of deoxyadenosine, which is cytotoxic to T cells and B cells. The only treatments for children with this type of SCID prior to 1990 were allogenic bone marrow transplantation and injection of bovine ADA conjugated to polyethylene glycol.[1]

The first step toward gene therapy of ADA-SCID children came with the identification, characterization, and cloning of the human genetic sequence that codes for the ADA protein.[7] Subsequent expression of the human protein in mammals, first in mice and later in monkeys, paved the way for human trials.[1] Before treating Ashanti Desilva and other children in the trial, investigators were faced with the questions of how and where to deliver the normal ADA genetic sequence. The term "vector" is used to describe the genetic vehicle that delivers the therapeutic gene of interest. Investigators had a number of different vectors to choose from at the time of the ADA-SCID trial, and there are even more today. Vectors come from the genomic sequence of a bacterium or virus.

Plasmid vectors are circular pieces of DNA derived from bacteria that can be genetically engineered to contain an antibiotic resistance gene as well as the therapeutic gene of interest. The antibiotic resistance gene permits large-scale preparation of the plasmid. Bacteria are transformed with the plasmid after insertion of the therapeutic gene and grown in broth containing the antibiotic. Subsequently, cultures are harvested by a method that allows for easy separation of the small circular plasmid from the larger circular bacterial genome.[8] After purification the plasmid can be used to transfect human cells by a number of different techniques, resulting in expression of the therapeutic protein.[9, 10]

Viral vectors consist of a viral genome stripped of its harmful pathogenic genes. The genome of these vectors is usually linear, typically larger than that of a plasmid, and can be engineered to contain an antibiotic resistance gene, a marker gene, a therapeutic gene, or a combination thereof.[11] Unlike the plasmid vector, viral vectors require eukaryotic cells (usually mammalian) in which to grow, prior to purification and transfection of human cells. For the ADA-SCID trial, investigators used a vector derived from the Moloney murine leukemia virus. This vector had been successfully used in vitro to transfer the ADA gene into T cells derived from SCID patients, thus restoring ADA function to the T cells.[12]

Transfer of genetic material from a vector to a target cell can be accomplished in vivo or ex vivo. The treatment of Ashanti Desilva involved harvesting autologous T cells, transfecting the Moloney murine leukemia virus containing ADA into the T cells, and transfusing the genetically engineered cells back into the children. As of the last published report, all patients in the initial ADA-SCID gene therapy trial tolerated the ex vivo therapy without complications.[1] Currently, the children in the study require significantly less exogenous ADA for maintenance of normal immune responses.[1A]

GENE REGULATION: SEVERAL POSSIBLE POINTS OF INTERVENTION FOR GENE THERAPY

The synthesis of a protein and subsequent biologic action of that protein is the end point of a series of events referred to as the central dogma (i.e., DNA is transcribed into RNA, which is translated into protein).[13, 14] The starting point for protein synthesis is genomic DNA, which is organized into chromosomes containing a set number of genes. The majority of DNA found in the genome does not code for proteins; instead, this noncoding DNA has important regulatory and structural functions. Each gene has a discrete organization that includes genetic sequences designated for transcription into RNA and regulatory elements that facilitate initiation of transcription (Fig. 11–1).

Regulatory elements can be found upstream or downstream of the genetic sequence where RNA synthesis begins, also known as the transcriptional start site. *Those elements found proximal to the start site are referred to as promoter elements, and can include basic sequences such as the TATA box as well as more specific elements such as the* interferon stimulatory response element (ISRE).[15–17] *More distal regulatory elements are referred to as enhancers and can be found several kilobases away from the transcriptional start site.*[18] Transcription of a gene into RNA begins with specific DNA/protein interactions occurring at and around promoter elements. Specific proteins, called transcription factors, bind to basic promoter sequences

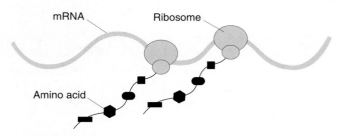

Figure 11–1 The translation of RNA sequence into amino acid sequence of protein is facilitated by ribosomes.

to stabilize the RNA polymerase complex and facilitate the initiation of transcription.[19, 20]

DNA sequence downstream of the transcriptional start site can be divided into exons and introns (Fig. 11–2). Exons contain sequences that ultimately make it into the final messenger RNA (mRNA) molecule, whereas introns contain the intervening sequences that are spliced out.[21] Once transcription begins, a rough draft of the final mRNA is made with both transcribed exon and intron sequences. The introns are subsequently spliced out as part of natural processing, bringing the exon sequences together in order.[22] The enzymatic addition of a methylated guanosine triphosphate to the 5′ end[23] and a polyadenylated tail to the 3′ end[24] of the final mRNA molecule completes the processing.

Protein synthesis occurs after mRNA molecules move from the nucleus into the cytoplasm. Translation refers to the process that converts the information encoded by nucleic acid sequence into an amino acid sequence constituting a protein (Fig. 11–3).[25] An adaptor molecule, referred to as a transfer RNA (tRNA), acts as the translator by matching an amino acid with a 3-bp anticodon. A multimeric protein complex called a ribosome moves along the RNA strand, providing a docking station for the tRNA. As the ribosome moves along the template, a new tRNA matches up with the appropriate RNA codon, and the peptide chain grows longer with the addition of another amino acid. The process of translation starts at a specific codon, called the translation initiation site (AUG, which codes for the amino acid methionine). There are three termination signals that stop translation when recognized by the ribosome complex (UAA, UAG, and UGA).[26] Because the codons come in triplets, every RNA molecule has the potential to contain three separate reading frames; however, usually only one of these acts as the reading frame, resulting in a complete protein. A consensus sequence around the AUG start site has been described that makes it

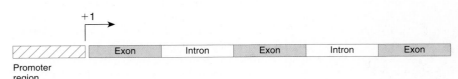

+1

| Promoter region | Exon | Intron | Exon | Intron | Exon |

Figure 11–2 Each gene has a discrete organization that includes genetic sequences designated for transcription into RNA. Intron sequences are spliced out during RNA processing, allowing exon sequences to be joined in contiguity to form mRNA. The rate of transcription and gene activation can be modulated by the promoter element located 5′ to the transcriptional start site (designated as +1).

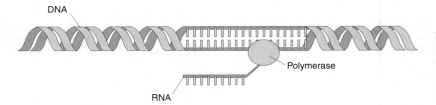

Figure 11–3 A multisubunit RNA polymerase facilitates the transcription of the double-stranded DNA template into the single-stranded RNA template used for protein synthesis.

more likely to serve as a start codon than AUG codons without the consensus sequence.[25] In addition, there is increasing evidence that certain cellular signals can change the rate of translation.[27–29]

In the flow of genetic information from DNA to protein, RNA is the least stable molecule, with a half-life that can range from seconds to minutes.[30] The relative instability of RNA makes it the rate-limiting molecule in the events that lead up to the synthesis of most proteins.[31, 32] The sum total of a specific mRNA is a function of both the rate at which it is synthesized and the rate at which it degrades. When a gene becomes activated the rate of its transcription increases significantly over basal levels, resulting in a transient but significant rise in the sum total of a specific mRNA, which in turn results in more protein.[16] Similarly, in some biological states, specific mRNA molecules become more stable (degrade at a slower rate), also resulting in a rise in the sum total of a specific mRNA.[33]

Several possible points of intervention for gene therapy exist along the pathways of transcription and translation (Fig. 11–4). The simplest intervention can occur toward the end by replacing the missing or mutated protein with exogenous protein, as in the case of SCID children treated with ADA conjugated to polyethylene glycol. In the case of Ashanti Desilva, the missing or mutated protein was replaced by a cloned version inserted into the genome of a host cell. The complementary DNA (cDNA) molecule encoding the wild-type protein is a double-stranded DNA version of the single-stranded mRNA (i.e., no introns). Once inserted into the genome the cDNA is transcribed and translated just like an endogenous gene, resulting in expression of the wild-type protein. Other strategies for genetic intervention include targeting events prior to protein synthesis (i.e., antisense RNA molecules[34] and promoter decoy molecules[35]). Regardless of the target, successful gene therapy is dependent on delivery of a therapeu-

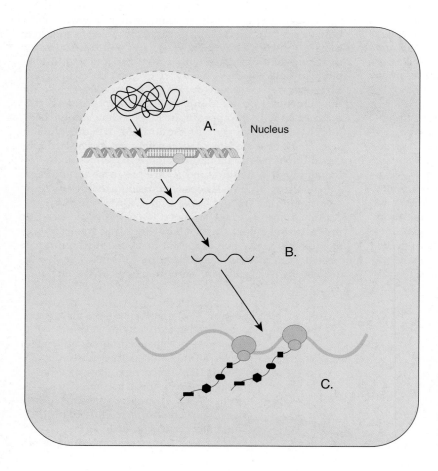

Figure 11–4 Several possible points of intervention for gene therapy exist along the pathway of transcription and translation. Some of these are illustrated in this figure. Direct insertion of therapeutic genetic sequences into the genome can occur in the nucleus (A). RNA molecules or oligonucleotides encoding antisense sequences can be introduced to block translation of RNA in the cytoplasm (B). A missing or mutated protein can be directly replaced by synthetic protein introduced into the cell (C).

tic molecule into the cell. Several vectors to achieve this task exist, each with unique advantages and disadvantages.

VECTORS: VIRAL AND NONVIRAL
Retrovirus-Based Vectors

The retrovirus derives its name from its genome comprising RNA. Each virus encodes a protein referred to as reverse transcriptase, which performs the opposite task of RNA polymerase (it copies an RNA molecule into a DNA molecule). The mature retrovirus contains an inner-core icosahedral protein shell surrounded by a phospholipid envelope derived from the previous host's cell membrane. The inner core, also referred to as a capsid, acts to protect the RNA genome found within. There are three subfamilies in the family *Retroviridae*, which are divided into categories based on pathogenesis. These include the *Spumavirinae*, *Lentivirinae* (i.e., HIV types 1 and 2), and *Oncovirinae*, which is further subdivided into five categories based on morphology.[36] The murine C type of oncovirus from the *Oncovirinae* class has been used most extensively to derive retroviral vectors for human gene therapy protocols.[37]

The life cycle of a retrovirus starts with the attachment of envelope proteins to a surface receptor on the target cell. Subsequent membrane fusion permits release of the viral core into the cytoplasm of the target cell. The RNA genome is then converted to double-stranded DNA, transported to the nucleus, and randomly integrated into the host's genome. After integration into the host, virus-specific promoters in the upstream region of the integrated sequence initiate transcription. Subsequently, viral proteins are synthesized with the use of the host's own transcriptional and translational machinery. The life cycle is completed when the viral particles are reassembled and new viral particles bud from the cell surface, utilizing part of the host cell's membrane to form its envelope.[36]

Most human gene therapy protocols require retroviral vectors that are replication-defective. This term implies an ability to infect the cell and integrate the viral genome but a deficiency in subsequent steps of replication (i.e., packaging and budding). A retrovirus is genetically engineered to be replication-defective by removing the genes responsible for packaging and budding (genes designated *gag, pol*, and *env*).[37] Besides the reverse transcriptase gene, other sequences that are absolutely necessary for a retroviral vector to function include (1) a packaging signal sequence, denoted "Psi" in murine viruses and "E" in avian viruses, that allows the RNA genome to be attached to the protein core; (2) the primer binding site for the tRNA primer of reverse transcriptase; and (3) repetitive sequences found at the ends of the vector, denoted "long terminal repeats (LTRs)," which include adjacent sequences necessary for priming of DNA synthesis and integration.[38] Up to 8 kb of exogenous DNA encoding marker genes, therapeutic genes, or antibiotic resistance genes can be inserted into a retroviral vector following removal of the *gag, pol*, and *env* sequences.

Once a retroviral vector has been engineered, a packaging cell line is required to provide the proteins that have been deleted from the vector. These cell lines have been altered to contain special versions of the *gag, pol*, and *env* genes. After a retroviral vector is transfected into a packaging cell line it undergoes the typical life cycle of a retrovirus, including packaging and budding. However, because the *gag, pol*, and *env* sequences in the packaging cell line have been designed to lack a packaging signal sequence, they do not leave the cell line. Thus, the retrovirus produced is missing the genes necessary for subsequent infection once integrated into the host's genome (i.e., is replication-defective).[37]

The obvious disadvantage associated with retroviral vectors in gene therapy is the necessity of placing a packaging cell line in proximity to the target cell. For in vivo gene therapy, this requires the injection of packaging cells that have been transfected with the retroviral vector into a patient. The main advantage of the retroviral gene therapy approach is the highly stable, long-term expression of the therapeutic gene. Another consideration is that retroviruses preferentially infect rapidly divided cells.[36] In the brain tumor patient this provides an important and advantageous level of specificity.

BOX 11–1
Retroviral Vectors

- **Advantages**
  - **Stable, long-term expression of gene product**
  - **Preferentially infect rapidly dividing cells**
- **Disadvantage: packaging cell line must be in proximity to the target cell**

Herpesvirus-Based Vectors

Herpesviruses contain *double-stranded DNA genomes* ranging in size from 100 kb to 250 kb. They constitute a diverse group of viruses with distinct genomic organization, genetic content, and pathogenesis.[39] Unlike the retrovirus, herpesviruses do not require integration for replication; rather, their genome can exist as a separate episome (i.e., exogenous chromosome) that remains stable, allowing the virus to establish a latent infection without harming the host cell.[40] Herpesviruses are divided into three subfamilies: alpha, beta, and gamma—which can be distinguished based on their ability to establish latent infections. *Gammaherpesviruses, such as Epstein-Barr virus, can establish latent infections in dividing cells, whereas alphaherpesviruses, such as the herpes simplex virus (HSV), cannot.*[41] *Betaherpesviruses, such as cytomegaloviruses, can vary with respect to establishing a latent infection depending on cell type.* Although other herpesviruses are being investigated as potential gene therapy vectors, applications with HSV from the alpha subfamily have shown the most promise. This is partly because of the association of gammaherpesviruses with lymphoproliferative disease and the paucity of information on the details of latent infections with the beta herpesviruses.[42]

Natural infection of humans with HSV has been well described and involves initial infection of epithelial cells on the skin or mucosa.[43] Subsequently, a cytolytic phase of infection results in production of more virus, which finds its way in rapid retrograde fashion to the neuronal cell bodies connected to sensory nerve endings. The virus then may either continue along the productive cytolytic pathway of infection or establish a latent infection. During a natural infection it is not known what environmental cues cause the switch from cytolytic to latent infection. However, with the full sequence and characterization of all HSV genes, it has been easy to identify the gene products necessary for cytolytic infection.

The genome of HSV includes 70 genes that can be divided into three sections based on the order in which they are expressed during a cytolytic infection (immediate early, early, and late).[39] Immediate early genes encode proteins necessary for initiation of a cytolytic cycle; early genes encode proteins required for DNA synthesis; and late genes encode viral structural proteins. Deletion of some of these genes renders a virus replication-defective and fosters the establishment of a latent infection. HSV mutant stocks are viruses that lack the ability to establish a productive infection because specific immediate early, early, or late genes have been deleted. As with the replication-deficient retroviruses, these mutants require helper cell lines that can provide some of the missing gene products for the initial transfection. Since the HSV, as opposed to the retrovirus, is very stable, large stocks of a given HSV construct can be purified from helper cell lines and stored until needed. This increased stability of HSV allows investigators to avoid the cumbersome task of injecting helper cells proximal to the target cell for gene therapy.[39]

The main advantages of HSV mutants as gene therapy vectors include their ability to transfect large pieces of foreign DNA (up to 30 kb) and the potential for establishing latent infections in nondividing cells.[11] The possible reversion of an HSV mutant to its wild-type form is a concern. Many current studies with HSV mutant vectors are aimed at reducing the rate of reversion to wild-type while increasing transfection efficiency.[44]

BOX 11–2
Herpesvirus-Based Vectors

- **Advantages**
  - **Double-stranded genome does not require integration for replication**
  - **Able to transfect large pieces of foreign DNA and establish latent infection in nondividing cells**
- **Disadvantage: possible reversion of a herpes simplex virus mutant to its wild type**

Adenovirus Vectors

Adenoviruses belong to the family *Adenoviridae*, with the human version of these viruses belonging to the class *Mastadenovirus*. There are 47 serotypes of human adenovirus grouped in categories A–F.[45] Wild-type human adenoviruses are ubiquitous and commonly infect epithelial cells in the upper respiratory tract, gastrointestinal tract, and urinary tract. The adenovirus is made up of an icosahedral-shaped capsid containing a double-stranded DNA genome that averages 36 kb in length. The structure is maintained by proteins on the outer coat of the capsid that interact with target cells. Other viral proteins hold the capsid together and stabilize the genome by directly binding DNA. When infecting a cell, proteins projecting from the capsid interact with receptors on the target cell to facilitate viral entry and subsequent migration of the viral DNA to the cell nucleus.

The adenovirus genome, like that of HSV, can be divided into sets of genes based on when they are activated after infection. Early genes code for several different proteins, including those involved in DNA synthesis and DNA binding, whereas late genes code for structural proteins found in the capsid. As with the other viral vectors, an adenovirus can be rendered replication-defective by deletion of certain genes. *After infection these replication-defective adenoviral vectors exist in the host cell nucleus without integrating into the host's genome.*[46]

Adenoviruses can infect both dividing and nondividing cells. Because they are very stable viruses, it is possible to purify large amounts of adenoviral particles from helper cell lines after infection with a replication-defective virus.[47] Once purified, these adenoviral particles can be used to infect target cells in vivo or ex vivo. The stability of the adenoviral particle circumvents the problems associated with in vivo gene therapy, exemplified by retroviral vectors that require the helper cell line to be proximal to the target cell.[11] Other advantages of adenoviral vectors include their relative safety and long-term expression in cells as a nonreplicating extra chromosome. A major drawback is that upon cell division the adenoviral vector is lost, as it neither segregates nor replicates.[47] In addition, humans can attenuate the effect of gene therapy by mounting a significant immune response to adenoviral vectors.[48]

BOX 11–3
Adenovirus Vectors

- **Advantages**
  - **Can infect both dividing and nondividing cells**
  - **Very stable**
  - **Relatively safe**
  - **Long-term expression**
- **Disadvantages**
  - **Adenoviral vector lost when the cell divides**
  - **Effect possibly attenuated by significant immune response**

Nonviral Approaches

Plasmid vectors derived from bacteria represent an alternative to virus-based vectors. The circular DNA of a plasmid can be engineered to contain a strong eukaryotic promoter (one that will function in the target cell) to direct the transcription of a therapeutic gene. Large amounts of plasmid can be easily purified and transfected into target cells in vivo or ex vivo by different methods.[8–10] *The main obstacle in using a nonviral approach is in finding a method that will efficiently deliver the vector without harming the plasmid or the target cell.*

Particle bombardment has been described as an efficient method for transferring plasmid DNA to mammalian cells.[49] In this method, the plasmid is conjugated to the surface of gold beads with a 1 to 3-μn diameter. The particles are then "fired" at the tissue or cell using an electric discharge device (referred to as a "gene gun") and the plasmid DNA is carried through the cell membrane with the gold particle. Once inside the cytoplasm the plasmid can dissociate from the gold particle and undergo transcription and translation. The utility of this technique is limited in vivo by the lack of specificity and the possibility of causing trauma to nontumorigenic cells. In addition, the transfection efficiency falls off dramatically as a cell lies further from the surface. It is unlikely that the gene gun will be used commonly for in vivo gene therapy. However, the gene gun has been used successfully in some in vitro and ex vivo gene therapy protocols.[50]

Currently, the preferred method for transferring plasmid vectors into cells utilizes a biochemically engineered molecule referred to as a "cationic lipid."[49] Many different versions of this type of molecule are commercially available, with all having a common basic structure consisting of two parts: (1) a head group containing single or multiple positive charge(s) at physiologic pH and (2) a lipophilic tail made up of a lipid moiety.[51] Plasmid DNA, which is negatively charged at physiologic pH, is bound by the positively charged head of the cationic lipid. Multiple cationic lipids interact with the plasmid DNA until a microsphere is formed with the charged head group in the middle and the lipophilic tails on the outside. When the plasmid/cationic lipid hybrid is stable, it can easily traverse the lipid bilayer of the cell membrane, delivering the plasmid vector to the cell.

The foremost advantage of nonviral vectors is the elimination of potentially pathogenic properties associated with reversion of viral vectors to wild-type strains. The availability of cationic lipid reagents and the simplicity of the technique make it an attractive modality for many investigators who lack a background in virology.[10] As with other vectors that do not replicate or integrate, the nonviral approach is limited by the transient nature of the plasmid DNA. Once inside the cell the plasmid does not replicate or segregate when the cell divides. Although its promoter may foster incessant expression of the therapeutic protein, this expression is eventually limited by the viability and doubling time of the target cell.[49]

BOX 11–4
Nonviral Vectors

- **Advantages**
  - **Avoids potentially pathogenic reversion of viral vectors to wild-type strains**
  - **No replication inside cell**
- **Disadvantages**
  - **Transient nature of plasmid DNA (unstable)**
  - **Finding efficient means of delivery**
  - **Incessant expression of protein**

Progenitor Cells as Vectors for Gene Therapy

Neural stem cells are multipotential progenitors of neurons and glia capable of mitosis. The isolation of neural stem cells from human specimens has led to possible clinical application in cell replacement therapy and gene therapy.[1, 2] Stable transfection of stem cells with a therapeutic construct would be an elegant means of circumventing the limitations associated with more conventional gene therapy vectors. *Because of*

their inherent mitotic activity, stem cells offer the advantage of continuously producing a therapeutic protein with each cell division. The migratory characteristics of stem cells could be an additional advantage by facilitating production of a therapeutic protein distal to the site of stereotactic injection.

A progenitor cell gene therapy approach has been tested with success in a murine model of the type VII mucopolysaccharidosis (MPS), also known as Sly's syndrome.[3] In this lysosomal storage disorder, a deficiency in the enzyme β-glucoronidase causes an accumulation of glycosaminoglycan in lysosomes, resulting in a progressively fatal neurodegenerative disorder. Snyder and colleagues treated mice with type VII MPS by engrafting them as neonates with intraventricular injection of progenitor cells genetically engineered to express β-glucoronidase. After the mice had matured into adulthood, the brains receiving the stem cell injection revealed diffuse migration of grafted cells and ubiquitous expression of β-glucoronidase. Long-term engrafted animals appeared behaviorally and neurologically normal, whereas the untreated control animals died prematurely.

VECTOR DELIVERY METHODS

There are several anatomical and physiologic factors that hinder the delivery of gene therapy vectors to target cells in patients with brain tumors.[52] The blood-brain barrier (BBB) prevents transcellular transport of molecules and can be naturally disrupted by factors secreted by the tumor, as demonstrated by enhancement on contrast computed tomography (CT). However, in these cases high interstitial fluid pressure within the tumor often precludes delivery of a gene therapy vector.[53] Other obstacles to vector delivery include heterogeneity of target cells, microvasculature, and hemodynamics within the tumor.[54] The eloquence of brain tissue surrounding the tumor is also an important consideration.

BOX 11–5
Obstacles to Vector Delivery

- **Blood-brain barrier**
- **Target cell heterogeneity**
- **Microvasculature**
- **Tumor hemodynamics**

Methods for delivering vectors to CNS targets can be divided into intraparenchymal and intravascular strategies. *Intraparenchymal methods rely on direct injection, infusion, or passive diffusion after a vector is placed within the brain. Intravascular methods require transient disruption or compromise of the BBB for delivery of the vector.*

Intraparenchymal Delivery

Direct stereotactic injection of vectors into target tissue has been accomplished in a number of animal trials as well as some human trials.[55–57] *This method allows precise localization of the target and subsequent vector delivery to specified locations.* Once injected, the bolus of vector can diffuse along a concentration gradient that is dependent in part on the number of target cells it encounters along the gradient. Diffusion of a vector in the brain is not like a model of diffusion in which a solute dissolves and spreads through a liquid media, eventually achieving a state of equilibrium with a uniform concentration. *The diffusion of a vector in the brain is hindered by interaction of the vector with target cells.*[58] As a vector encounters the target cell it can interact with its receptor and become internalized.[56] This interaction has been hypothesized to be the cause of limited distribution after direct inoculation.[58]

Convection-enhanced delivery (also referred to as intracerebral clysis) was devised as a means of overcoming the limitations of passive diffusion.[59] This method utilizes a pressure gradient during infusion to augment distribution. *Stereotactic localization allows precise placement of the infusion catheter to optimize the distribution of vector to target tissue.* Several studies have shown that intracerebral clysis is a superior method for delivery in comparison with passive diffusion after direct inoculation.[60, 61]

BOX 11–6
Means of Intraparenchymal Vector Delivery

- **Direct stereotactic injection (passive diffusion)**
- **Convection-enhanced delivery (pressure gradient)**

Intravascular Delivery

The vascular endothelial cells, tight junctions, and astrocytic foot processes combine to form a relatively impermeable structure. *Transient disruption of the BBB for vector delivery is dependent on compromising the function of one of these key components.* Osmotic disruption of the BBB can be achieved by reducing the intracellular volume of endothelial cells and subsequently separating tight junctions.[62] The agent associated with the most successful outcome is mannitol. When mannitol is injected into a vessel the osmolarity of the intravascular solution is increased, establishing an osmotic gradient that draws solution out of endothelial cells. As a result, the endothelial cell shrinks, pulling components of the tight junction apart. When the mannitol solution washes out the osmotic equilibrium is reestablished, the endothelial cells return to their normal size, and the tight junctions reform to complete the BBB. The transient disruption of the BBB with mannitol has been effective at delivering HSV and adenovirus in several animal models.[63, 64]

Vasoactive peptides have also been used to disrupt the BBB. These peptides interact with specific endothelial cell receptors on the systemic side of the BBB. The end result is an increase in the level of intracellular calcium, which in turn activates various signal transduction pathways that foster transient permeability of the BBB. Leukotrienes and vasoactive peptides, such as bradykinin, have been studied for their ability to increase vector delivery in animal models.[64] Reports on a bradykinin analogue, denoted RMP-7, have shown encouraging results, with significant uptake of gene therapy vectors in animal models.[65] As with the osmotic disruption of the BBB, the use of vasoactive peptides is limited by the rate of clearance (wash-out) from the intravascular volume.

A significant disadvantage of intravascular approaches is the lack of localization in comparison with the stereotactic intraparenchymal techniques. Another disadvantage is the potential for vectors to interact with endothelial cells and astrocytes on their way to the target tissue. These interactions could potentially attenuate the dose of vector being delivered, requiring higher concentrations to a achieve a therapeutic effect and thus increasing the likelihood systemic and intracranial side effects will develop.

BOX 11–7
Intravascular Delivery

- **Advantage: disruption of the blood-brain barrier (mannitol, vasoactive peptides, leukotrienes)**
- **Disadvantages**
  - **Lack of localization**
  - **Possible interaction with endothelial cells (nontarget cells)**

GENE THERAPY STRATEGIES FOR BRAIN TUMOR PATIENTS

The rapid pace of advancements in gene therapy precludes a complete summary of current protocols. There are some basic strategies, however, that are being adapted in different ways for patients with brain tumors.[11, 66–68] The majority of these protocols are being applied to the adult patient population exclusively. As more information is gathered on safety and efficacy, it is likely that these protocols will be applied to the pediatric patient population as well.

Prodrug Activation

In prodrug activation, also referred to as "suicide gene therapy," a vector is designed to carry a gene that codes for a protein that sensitizes cells to a specific drug. The most widely applied version of this therapy is the herpes simplex virus thymidine kinase ganciclovir (HSVTK-GCV) protocol.[69–73] In this protocol, patients with recurrent tumor are stereotactically injected with a mouse fibroblast packaging cell line near the site of glioma recurrence. A retrovirus containing the *HSVTK* gene is shed from the packaging cell line and taken up preferentially by nearby glioma cells. Once inside the cell the virus integrates into the genome and expresses TK. Subsequently, patients are administered GCV, which is converted by the TK protein to a toxic metabolite, thus killing the tumor cell. The specificity of this protocol is dependent on the localization provided by the stereotactic injection, as well as the biologic restriction of the retrovirus, which only infects rapidly dividing cells.

The HSVTK-GCV protocol has had limited success in clinical trials in part because of the poor transfection efficiency of the retrovirus. Several studies have shown less than 10% transfection efficiency after treatment.[74] In addition, some laboratory and clinical observations have suggested that this therapy kills tumor cells by more than one mechanism. The bystander effect describes the in vitro and in vivo observation that tumor cells that have not been infected by the HSVTK retrovirus respond to the therapy.[75] Three mechanisms for this have been proposed: (1) coinfection of endothelial cells that are proliferating at the time of treatment, resulting in devascularization and tumor infarction[76]; (2) gap junction–facilitated transfer of toxic metabolites from cells infected with the HSVTK construct to those that have not been infected[77]; and (3) a generalized immune response fostered by the presence of foreign cells (i.e., the murine fibroblasts).[78]

The future application of prodrug therapy will be dependent on increasing the transfection efficiency of the virus. More efficient vectors, such as adenovirus, are being investigated as alternatives to the cumbersome retroviral packaging cell line approach used initially.[79] There are several other proteins being evaluated as alternative prodrug activators, including guanine phosphoribosyltransferase,[80] cytosine deaminase,[81] cytochrome $P450_{2B1}$,[82] and deoxycytidine kinase.[83] Ongoing studies with these proteins and their respective prodrugs might provide more potent combinations for prodrug activation gene therapy in the future.

Antisense Gene Therapy

The goal of antisense gene therapy is to prevent the expression of proteins that facilitate tumor progression.[84, 85] Knowledge of the target gene sequence makes it possible to design a vector that will produce a molecule with the complementary sequence (i.e., antisense). Once the vector is taken up by the target cell, the antisense gene is expressed and the single-stranded RNA synthesized by the vector can bind to the mRNA of the target gene. The antisense binding sterically hinders the ribosome apparatus and prevents translation of the mRNA; the end result is a decrease in the synthesis of the pathogenic protein. Antisense inhibition can also be achieved by directly transfecting short sequences of nucleic acid molecules referred to as "oligonucleotides."[86] These oligonucleotides can be designed to match the complement sequence of a target transcript proximal to the translation initiation site (the AUG with the consensus sequence). Once the oligonucleotide binds to this key area of the mRNA, translation is inhibited.

Several genes have been inhibited with the antisense method in an attempt to prevent glioma progression in animal models. Studies evaluating the inhibition of the K-*ras* oncogene,[87] insulin-like growth factor receptor,[88] and transforming growth factor β[89] have shown effects ranging from complete regression of the tumor to decreases in growth rate. Many of these animal studies are confounded by the use of allogenic cell lines.[90] This raises the possibility that experimental observations are attributable to a graft host rejection phenomenon, as opposed to treatment-induced tumor regression. Studies evaluating antisense protocols in syngenic systems will provide a better estimate of possible therapeutic efficacy.

The potential application of antisense therapy to brain tumor patients has several advantages over the prodrug activation protocol. The use of adenoviral and oligonucleotide protocols would circumvent the problem of low transfection efficiency rates found with retroviruses in the HSVTK-GCV protocol. In addition, multiple pathogenic genes could be inhibited by using a variety of oligonucleotides or adenoviral vectors during one treatment. A distinct disadvantage of the antisense approach is the relative instability of the therapeutic molecule (the single stranded antisense nucleic acid). Current efforts in the field are aimed at biochemically altering the therapeutic oligonucleotides to make them more stable and therefore theoretically more efficacious.[34, 91]

Tumor Suppressor Gene Therapy

Several genes have been implicated in the progression of familial and sporadic tumors. These can be loosely grouped into proto-oncogenes and tumor suppressor genes.[92] *Proto-oncogenes become oncogenic when overexpressed or amplified as a result of genetic mutation or translocation.*[93, 94] These genes can also become oncogenic when mutations in the coding sequence of the gene result in constitutive activation of the protein. Proto-oncogenes typically code for proteins that promote cell growth (i.e., the epidermal growth factor receptor).[95] *In contrast, tumor suppressor genes can code for proteins that inhibit cell growth.* A number of tumor suppressor genes have been implicated in the progression of primary central nervous system tumors.[92, 96, 97] The purpose of tumor suppressor gene therapy is to replace the missing or mutated tumor suppressor protein and thus restore the normal nonpathologic cellular phenotype.

The p53 tumor suppressor gene has been termed the "guardian of the genome" because of its role in preventing the propagation of cells with genetic mutations. Loss of *p53* is an early event in many adult malignant glial neoplasms.[98, 99] Several studies have successfully induced cell growth arrest and apoptosis (programmed cell death) in cell lines derived from tumors with *p53* deletions or mutations. This has been achieved by transfecting cells with vector constructs containing a wild-type *p53* gene.[100, 101] Although animal studies have been promising, the heterogeneity of tumors in vivo is a significant obstacle to applying *p53* gene therapy to patients.[102, 103] Glioma cells within a defined region of tumor tissue can have different molecular profiles, with several different genes contributing to the malignant phenotype.[104] Furthermore, mutations of the *p53* tumor suppressor gene are common in astrocytomas that occur in adults but are rarely found in astrocytomas or medulloblastomas of children.[105] This difference highlights another disadvantage of a *p53* gene therapy protocol in the treatment of children with brain tumors.

A more recently identified tumor suppressor gene implicated in brain tumors is the cellular phosphatase gene known as PTEN (*also known as* MMAC *and* TEP1).[106–108] This gene is located at 10q23.3 in the human genome and is frequently mutated or deleted in a number of solid tumors. Phosphatases act by turning off signaling pathways that are dependent on phosphorylation, many of which result in cellular proliferation.[109] When phosphatase activity is lost, signaling pathways become activated constitutively, resulting in aberrant proliferation. Several reports have demonstrated the feasibility of using gene therapy to rescue cells containing *PTEN* mutations. In 1997, Furnari and colleagues demonstrated that transferring wild-type *PTEN* into glioma cell lines with *PTEN* mutations resulted in growth suppression.[110] In this study, transfer of *PTEN* with a mutated phosphatase domain did not suppress growth, underscoring the importance of the *PTEN* phosphatase activity. More recently, Tamura and colleagues have shown that overexpression of *PTEN* inhibits cell migration, whereas antisense *PTEN* enhances migration. Integrin-mediated cell spreading and the formation of focal adhesions were shown to be decreased by wild-type *PTEN* but not by *PTEN* with an inactive phosphatase domain.[111]

The potential of gene therapy rescue with *PTEN* in vivo has also been confirmed. Using a replication-defective adenovirus containing the wild-type *PTEN*, Cheney and colleagues markedly decreased the growth rate and neoplastic characteristics of the human glioma cell line U87MG in nude mice.[112] As with the *p53* gene therapy strategy, any application of *PTEN* gene therapy to patients will be hindered by the molecular heterogeneity of the tumor.[107, 108]

Promoter Down-regulation with Decoy Oligonucleotides

Gene transcription is dependent on stabilization of RNA polymerase and its associated proteins at specific regions within the promoter. This stabilization process is one of dynamic equilibrium whereby forces can increase or decrease the stability of RNA polymerase.[16] Transcription factors are cellular proteins that interact with specific sequences in the promoter and as a result, increase the stability of the RNA polymerase and subsequent transcription of the gene.[20] Activation of a transcription factor is often the end point of a signal transduction process that starts at the cell surface and results in the up-regulation of a specific set of genes.[113]

In the late 1980s, Darnell and colleagues discovered a signaling pathway that rapidly activates a specific subset of responsive genes.[114] This pathway begins with the interaction of an interferon molecule with its specific cell surface receptor. After interferon binding, a cytoplasmic tyrosine kinase associated with the receptor is activated and phosphorylates a specific subset of proteins, referred to as signal transducers and activators of transcription, or STAT proteins.[17] These STAT proteins form multimeric complexes and migrate to the nucleus. Once in the nucleus they bind to specific DNA sequences in the promoter region [i.e., interferon stimulatory response elements (ISREs), or gamma interferon-γ activation sequences.] The binding of the STAT proteins to the regulatory elements stabilizes the RNA polymerase apparatus and facilitates an increase in transcription. The pathway allows interferons to up-regulate specific cellular genes, which in turn code for proteins that manifest the various antiproliferative, immunomodulatory, and antiviral effects of interferons.[114]

The STAT pathway is used by a number of other ligands, including growth factors, and is an excellent model for the potential of decoy gene therapy. The STAT proteins, like other transcription factors, will bind double-stranded DNA oligonucleotides (DS-oligos) that are designed to contain the exact sequence of the regulatory elements found in the promoter of a gene. These DS-oligos can vary in length depending on the target sequence. Once transfected inside the cell the DS-oligos competitively inhibit binding to the regulatory sequence of the gene being targeted. In the interferon

pathway described above, transfecting the cell with multiple copies of a DS-oligo ISRE could significantly reduce the rate of transcription for some interferon-responsive genes. The promoter decoy strategy has been applied successfully to the inhibition of smooth-muscle proliferation in vivo and in vitro.[35]

The effective application of promoter decoy gene therapy to patients with brain tumors remains to be seen. Theoretically this strategy could be used to inhibit transcription of specific genes implicated in tumor progression. Use of multiple decoy molecules would allow for a wide range of inhibition. A potential disadvantage of the therapy is that not all pathogenic genes manifest their effects as a result of an increase in transcription. However, this strategy offers an exciting possibility for disrupting the effects of certain genes known to be transcriptionally up-regulated in brain tumors.

FUTURE OUTLOOK

The application of gene therapy to children with brain tumors will depend on several factors, including (1) further characterization of genetic mutations in pediatric brain tumors, (2) development of more efficient and safer gene therapy vectors, (3) development of more efficient delivery methods, (4) evaluation of novel forms of combined therapy that use gene therapy as a means of augmentation, (5) evaluation of antiangiogenic gene therapy, and (6) completion of ongoing clinical trials in adult patients being treated with gene therapy protocols.

The discovery of genes such as *PTEN* is a good example of recent progress in defining genetic mutations in brain tumors. Techniques that identify subtle differences between tumor cells and normal cells, such as differential display polymerase chain reaction,[115] will undoubtedly contribute to the list of genetic mutations found in pediatric brain tumors. Current studies using newly developed gene therapy vectors, such as adeno-associated viruses,[68] HSV amplicons,[116] and replication-competent adenovirus and HSV[44] will also play a role in future application of gene therapy in children with brain tumors. Some of these experimental vectors are now being used to augment chemotherapy,[117] immunotherapy,[118] and radiotherapy[119, 120] in adult patients. Gene therapy augmentation of these therapies in children would be a logical step after completion of clinical trials in adults. The possibility of inhibiting angiogenesis in tumors is currently being investigating with gene therapy.[121] Antiangiogenic gene therapy could augment aspects of antiproliferative gene therapy in patients with brain tumors.

The future of gene therapy in the treatment of children with brain tumors is hopeful. As with the initial treatment of children suffering from SCID, a multidisciplinary approach involving clinicians and scientists will be necessary to achieve the goal of effective treatment.

SUMMARY

The experimental modality of gene therapy may provide effective treatments for preventing tumor progression and recurrence in children with brain tumors. Physicians and researchers hope therapeutic genes may be utilized to increase the immune response to cancer, sensitize tumor cells to systemic therapies, or replace defective genes. Gene therapy offers the potential for reducing the toxic side effects of radiation therapy and chemotherapy, which is an important consideration in the pediatric patient population.

REFERENCES

1. Hooger brugge P, et al. Gene therapy for adenosine deaminase deficiency. *BMJ*, 1995;51(1):72–81.

1A. Parkman R, et al. Gene therapy for adenosine deaminase deficiency. *Ann Rev Med* 2000;51:33–47.

2. Rosenecker J, et al. Towards gene therapy of cystic fibrosis. *Eur J Med Res* 1998;3(3):149–156.

3. Grossman M, et al. Successful ex vivo gene therapy directed to liver in a patient with familial hypercholesterolemia. *Nat Genet* 1994;6:335–341.

4. Sehgal A. Molecular changes during the genesis of human gliomas. *Semin Surg Oncol* 1998;14(1):3–12.

5. Anderson WF. GeneTherapy. *Sci Am* 1995;273:124–128.

6. Maria BL, et al. Gene therapy for neurologic disease: benchtop discoveries to bedside applications. 2. The bedside. *J Child Neurol* 1997;12(2):77–84.

7. Valerio D, et al. Cloning of human adenosine deaminase cDNA and expression in mouse cells. *Gene* 1984.31: 147–153.

8. Edwardson PA, et al. A new rapid procedure for the preparation of plasmid DNA. *Anal Biochem* 1986;152(2): 215–20.

9. Goldman CK, et al. In vitro and in vivo gene delivery mediated by a synthetic polycationic amino polymer. *Nat Biotechnol* 1997;15(5):462–466.

10. Verma RS, et al. Increased efficiency of liposome-mediated transfection by volume reduction and centrifugation. *Biotechniques* 1998;25(1):46–9.

11. Spear MA, et al. Targeting gene therapy vectors to CNS malignancies. *J Neurovirol* 1998;4(2):133–47.

12. Kantoff PW, et al. Correction of adenosine deaminase deficiency in cultured human T and B cells by retro-virus mediated gene transfer. *Proc Natl Acad Sci USA* 1986;83: 6563–6567.

13. Cooper S. The central dogma of cell biology. *Cell Biol Int Rep* 1981;5(6):539–49.

14. Sollner-Webb B. *RNA* editing. *Curr Opin Cell Biol* 1991; 3(6):1056–1061.

15. Burley SK. *The TATA* box binding protein. *Curr Opin Struct Biol* 1996;6(1):69–75.

16. Tjian R. The biochemistry of transcription in eukaryotes: a paradigm for multisubunit regulatory complexes. *Philos Trans R Soc Lond B Biol Sci* 1996;351(1339):491–499.

17. Darnell JE. Jr. *STATs* and gene regulation. *Science* 1997; 277(5332):1630–1635.

18. Blackwood EM, Kadonaga JT. Going the distance: a current view of enhancer action. *Science* 1998;281(5373):61–63.

19. Latchman DS. Eukaryotic transcription factors. *Biochem J* 1990;270(2):281–289.

20. van der Vliet PC, Verrijzer CP. Bending of DNA by transcription factors. *Bioessays* 1993;15(1):25–32.

21. Long M, de Souza SJ. Gilbert, W. Evolution of the intron-exon structure of eukaryotic genes. *Curr Opin Genet Dev* 1995;5(6):774–778.

22. Zaphiropoulos PG. Mechanisms of pre-mRNA splicing: classical versus non-classical pathways. *Histol Histopathol* 1998;13(2):585–589.

23. Varani G. A cap for all occasions. *Structure* 1997;5(7): 855–858.

24. Wahle E, Keller, W. The biochemistry of polyadenylation. *Trends Biochem Sci* 1996;21(7):247–250.

25. Kozak M. Regulation of translation in eukaryotic systems. *Annu Rev Cell Biol* 1992;8:197–225.

26. Kisselev LL, Frolova, L. Termination of translation in eukaryotes. *Biochem Cell Biol* 1995;73(11–12):1079–1086.

27. Altmann M, Trachsel, H. Regulation of translation initiation and modulation of cellular physiology. *Trends Biochem Sci* 1993;18(11):429–432.

28. Brostrom CO, Brostrom, MA. Regulation of translational initiation during cellular responses to stress. *Prog Nucleic Acid Res Mol Biol* 1998;58:79–125.

29. Kleijn M, et al. Regulation of translation initiation factors by signal transduction. *Eur J Biochem* 1998;253(3):531–544.

30. Wickens M, Anderson P. Jackson, R.J. Life and death in the cytoplasm: messages from the 3' end. *Curr Opin Genet Dev* 1997;7(2):220–232.

31. Liebhaber SA. mRNA stability and the control of gene expression. *Nucleic Acids Symp Ser* 1997;36:29–32.

32. Day DA, Tuite, M.F. Post-transcriptional gene regulatory mechanisms in eukaryotes: an overview. *J Endocrinol* 1998;157(3):361–371.

33. Ross J. Control of messenger RNA stability in higher eukaryotes. *Trends Genet* 1996;12(5):171–175.

34. Weiss B, Davidkova G, Zhang, SP. Antisense strategies in neurobiology. *Neurochem Int* 1997;31(3):321–348.

35. Morishita R, et al. A gene therapy strategy using a transcription factor decoy of the E2F binding site inhibits smooth muscle proliferation in vivo. *Proc Natl Acad Sci USA* 1995;92(13):5855–5859.

36. Varmus HE. Retroviruses. *Science* 1988;240:1427–1435.

37. Miller AD. Retroviral vectors. *Curr Top Microbiol Immunol* 1992;158:1–24.

38. Vile RG, Russell, SJ. Retroviruses as vectors. *Br Med Bull* 1995;51(1):12–30.

39. Efstathiou S, Minson, AC. Herpes virus-based vectors. *Br Med Bull* 1995;51(1):45–55.

40. Goins WF, et al. Herpes simplex virus vectors for gene transfer to the nervous system. *J Neurovirol*, 1997;3 (Suppl 1): S80–S88.

41. McGeoch DJ, Barnett BC. Maclean, CA. Emerging functions of alpha-herpes virus genes. *Semin Virol* 1993;4:125–134.

42. Geller A.I. Herpesviruses: expression of genes in postmitotic brain cells. *Curr Opin Genet Dev* 1993;3(1):81–85.

43. Kennedy PG. Potential use of herpes simplex virus (HSV) vectors for gene therapy of neurological disorders. *Brain* 1997;120(Pt 7):1245–1259.

44. Mineta T, et al. Attenuated multi-mutated herpes simplex virus–1 for the treatment of malignant gliomas. *Nature Med* 1995;1(9):938–943.

45. Ginsberg HS, et al. A proposed terminology for the adenovirus antigens and virion morphology. *Virology* 1966; 28:782–783.

46. Kovesdi I, et al. Adenoviral vectors for gene transfer. *Curr Opin Biotechnol* 1997;8(5):583–589.

47. Kremer EJ, Perricaudet, M. Adenovirus and adeno-associated virus mediated gene transfer. *Br Med Bull* 1995; 51(1):31–44.

48. Maria BL, Friedman, T. Gene therapy for pediatric brain tumors. *Semin Pediatr Neurol* 1997;4(4):333–339.

49. Schofield JP, Caskey, C.T. Non-viral approaches to gene therapy. *Br Med Bull* 1995;51(1):56–71.

50. Yang N-S, et al. In vivo and in vitro gene transfer to mammalian somatic cells by particle bombardment. *Proc Natl Acad Sci USA* 1991;88:2726–2730.

51. Balasubramaniam RP, et al. Structural and functional analysis of cationic transfection lipids: the hydrophobic domain. *Gene Ther* 1996;3(2):163–172.

52. Chung RY, Chiocca EA. Gene therapy for tumors of the central nervous system. *Surg Oncol Clin North Am* 1998; 7(3):589–602.

53. Jain RK. Barriers to drug delivery in solid tumors. *Sci Am* 1994;271:58–64.

54. Torres-Filho IP, et al. Noninvasive measurement of microvascular and interstitial oxygen profiles in a human tumor in SCID mice. *Proc Natl Acad Sci USA* 1994;91: 2081–2085.

55. Badie B, et al. Stereotactic delivery of a recombinant adenovirus into a C6 glioma cell line in a rat brain tumor model. *Neurosurgery* 1994;35(5):910–915;discussion 915–916.

56. Kun LE, et al. Stereotactic injection of herpes simplex thymidine kinase vector producer cells (PA317-G1Tk1SvNa.7) and intravenous ganciclovir for the treatment of progressive or recurrent primary supratentorial pediatric malignant brain tumors. *Hum Gene Ther* 1995; 6(9):1231–1255.

57. Maron A, et al. Gene therapy of rat C6 glioma using adenovirus-mediated transfer of the herpes simplex virus thymidine kinase gene: long-term follow-up by magnetic resonance imaging. *Gene Ther* 1996;3(4):315–322.

58. Boviatsis, EJ, et al. Gene transfer into experimental brain tumors mediated by adenovirus, herpes simplex virus, and retrovirus vectors. *Hum Gene Ther* 1994;5(2):183–191.

59. Bobo RH, et al. Convection-enhanced delivery of macromolecules in the brain. *Proc Natl Acad Sci USA* 1994;91: 2076–2080.

60. Muldoon LL, Nilaver G, Kroll RA. Comparison of intracerebral inoculation and osmotic blood brain barrier disruption for delivery of adenovirus, herpes virus, and iron oxide nanoparticles to normal rat brain. *Am J Pathol* 1995; 147:1840–1851.

61. Zhu J, et al. A continuous intracerebral gene delivery system for in vivo liposome-mediated gene therapy. *Gene Ther* 1996;3(6):472–476.

62. Rapoport SI, et al. Quantitative aspects of reversible osmotic opening of the blood-brain barrier. *Am J Physiol* 1980; 238:421–431.

63. Nilaver G, et al. Delivery of herpesvirus and adenovirus to nude rat intracerebral tumors after osmotic blood-brain barrier disruption. *Proc Natl Acad Sci USA* 1995; 92(21):9829–9833.

64. Kroll RA, Neuwelt EA. Outwitting the blood-brain barrier for therapeutic purposes: osmotic opening and other means [In Process Citation]. *Neurosurgery* 1998;42(5): 1083–1099; discussion 1099–1100.

65. LeMay DR, et al. Intravenous RMP-7 increases delivery of ganciclovir into rat brain tumors and enhances the

effects of herpes simplex virus thymidine kinase gene therapy [In Process Citation]. *Hum Gene Ther* 1998;9(7): 989–995.

66. Kramm CM, et al. Gene therapy for brain tumors. *Brain Pathol*, 1995;5(4):345–381.

67. Zlokovic BV, Apuzzo ML. Cellular and molecular neurosurgery: pathways from concept to reality—part I: target disorders and concept approaches to gene therapy of the central nervous system. *Neurosurgery* 1997;40(4):789–803; discussion 803–804.

68. Zlokovic BV, Apuzzo ML. Cellular and molecular neurosurgery: pathways from concept to reality—part II: vector systems and delivery methodologies for gene therapy of the central nervous system. *Neurosurgery* 1997;40(4): 805–812; discussion 812–813.

69. Short MP, et al. Gene delivery to glioma cells in rat brain by grafting of a retrovirus packaging cell line. *J Neurosci Res* 1990;27(3):427–439.

70. Ezzeddine ZD, et al. Selective killing of glioma cells in culture and in vivo by retrovirus transfer of the herpes simplex virus thymidine kinase gene. *New Biol* 1991;3(6): 608–614.

71. Takamiya Y, et al. Gene therapy of malignant brain tumors: a rat glioma line bearing the herpes simplex virus type 1—thymidine kinase gene and wild type retrovirus kills other tumor cells. *J Neurosci Res* 1992;33(3):493–503.

72. Ram Z, et al, Toxicity studies of retroviral-mediated gene transfer for the treatment of brain tumors. *J Neurosurg* 1993; 79(3):400–407.

73. Izquierdo M, et al. Human malignant brain tumor response to herpes simplex thymidine kinase (HSVtk)/ganciclovir gene therapy. *Gene Ther* 1996;3(6):491–495.

74. Viola JJ, Martuza RL. Gene therapies for glioblastomas. *Baillieres Clin Neurol* 1996;5(2):413–424.

75. Wu JK, et al. Bystander tumoricidal effect in the treatment of experimental brain tumors. *Neurosurgery* 1994;35(6): 1094–1102; discussion 1102–1103.

76. Ram Z, et al. The effect of thymidine kinase transduction and ganciclovir therapy on tumor vasculature and growth of 9L gliomas in rats. *J Neurosurg* 1994;81(2):256–260.

77. Dilber MS, et al. Gap junctions promote the bystander effect of herpes simplex virus thymidine kinase in vivo. *Cancer Res* 1997;57(8):1523–1528.

78. Vrionis FD, et al. A more potent bystander cytocidal effect elicited by tumor cells expressing the herpes simplex virus-thymidine kinase gene than by fibroblast virus-producer cells in vitro. *J Neurosurg* 1995;83(4):698–704.

79. Sterman DH, et al. Adenovirus-mediated herpes simplex virus thymidine kinase/ganciclovir gene therapy in patients with localized malignancy: results of a phase I clinical trial in malignant mesothelioma [In Process Citation]. *Hum Gene Ther* 1998;9(7):1083–1092.

80. Ono Y, et al. Regression of experimental brain tumors with 6–thioxanthine and Escherichia coli gpt gene therapy. *Hum Gene Ther* 1997;8(17):2043–2055.

81. Ge K, et al. Transduction of cytosine deaminase gene makes rat glioma cells highly sensitive to 5-fluorocytosine. *Int J Cancer* 1997;71(4):675–679.

82. Rainov NG, et al. New prodrug activation gene therapy for cancer using cytochrome P450 4B1 and 2-aminoanthracene/4-ipomeanol [In Process Citation]. *Hum Gene Ther* 1998; 9(9):1261–1273.

83. Manome Y, et al. Viral vector transduction of the human deoxycytidine kinase cDNA sensitizes glioma cells to the cytotoxic effects of cytosine arabinoside in vitro and in vivo. *Nat Med* 1996;2(5):567–573.

84. Yung WK. New approaches in brain tumor therapy using gene transfer and antisense oligonucleotides. *Curr Opin Oncol* 1994;6(3):235–239.

85. Alama A, et al. Antisense oligonucleotides as therapeutic agents. *Pharmacol Res* 1997;36(3):171–178.

86. Hall WA, Flores EP, Low WC. Antisense oligonucleotides for central nervous system tumors. *Neurosurgery* 1996;38(2):376–383.

87. Aoki K, et al. Liposome-mediated in vivo gene transfer of antisense K-ras construct inhibits pancreatic tumor dissemination in the murine peritoneal cavity. *Cancer Res* 1995;55(17):3810–3816.

88. Burfeind P, et al. Antisense RNA to the type I insulin-like growth factor receptor suppresses tumor growth and prevents invasion by rat prostate cancer cells in vivo. *Proc Natl Acad Sci USA* 1996;93(14):7263–7268.

89. Fakhrai H, et al. Eradication of established intracranial rat gliomas by transforming growth factor beta antisense gene therapy. *Proc Natl Acad Sci USA* 1996;93(7):2909–2914.

90. Saleh M, Stacker SA, Wilks AF. Inhibition of growth of C6 glioma cells in vivo by expression of antisense vascular endothelial growth factor sequence. *Cancer Res* 1996;56(2):393–401.

91. Chavany C, Connell Y, Neckers L. Contribution of sequence and phosphorothioate content to inhibition of cell growth and adhesion caused by c-myc antisense oligomers. *Mol Pharmacol* 1995;48(4):738–746.

92. von Deimling A, Louis DN, Wiestler OD. Molecular pathways in the formation of gliomas. *Glia* 1995;15(3):328–338.

93. Akbasak A, Sunar-Akbasak B. Oncogenes: cause or consequence in the development of glial tumors. *J Neurol Sci* 1992;111(2):119–133.

94. Collins VP. Amplified genes in human gliomas. *Semin Cancer Biol* 1993;4(1):27–32.

95. Hurtt MR, et al. Amplification of epidermal growth factor receptor gene in gliomas: histopathology and prognosis. *J Neuropathol Exp Neurol* 1992;51(1):84–90.

96. Godbout R, et al. Lack of expression of tumor-suppressor genes in human malignant glioma cell lines. *Oncogene* 1992;7(9):1879–1884.

97. Cogen PH, McDonald JD. Tumor suppressor genes and medulloblastoma. *J Neurooncol* 1996;29(1):103–112.

98. del Arco A, et al. Timing of p53 mutations during astrocytoma tumorigenesis. *Hum Mol Genet* 1993;2(10):1687–1690.

99. Bogler O, et al. *The* p53 gene and its role in human brain tumors. *Glia* 1995;15(3):308–327.

100. Hsiao M, et al. Intracavitary liposome-mediated p53 gene transfer into glioblastoma with endogenous wild-type p53 in vivo results in tumor suppression and long-term survival. *Biochem Biophys Res Commun* 1997;233(2):359–364.

101. Kokunai T, Kawamura A, Tamaki N. Induction of differentiation by wild-type p53 gene in a human glioma cell line. *J Neurooncol* 1997;32(2):125–133.

102. Koga H, et al. Analysis of p53 gene mutations in low- and high-grade astrocytomas by polymerase chain reaction-assisted single-strand conformation polymorphism and immunohistochemistry. *Acta Neuropathol* 1994;87(3):225–232.

103. Kock H, et al. Adenovirus-mediated p53 gene transfer suppresses growth of human glioblastoma cells in vitro and in vivo. *Int J Cancer* 1996;67(6):808–815.

104. Li Y, et al. p53 mutations in malignant gliomas. *Cancer Epidemiol Biomarkers Prev* 1998;7(4):303–308.

105. Litofsky NS, Hinton D, Raffel C. The lack of a role for p53 in astrocytomas in pediatric patients. *Neurosurgery* 1994;34(6): 967–972; discussion 972–973.

106. Li J, et al. PTEN, a putative protein tyrosine phosphatase gene mutated in human brain, breast, and prostate cancer [see comments]. *Science* 1997;275(5308):1943–1947.

107. Rasheed BK, et al. PTEN gene mutations are seen in high-grade but not in low-grade gliomas. *Cancer Res* 1997;57(19):4187–4190.

108. Wang SI, et al. Somatic mutations of PTEN in glioblastoma multiforme. *Cancer Res* 1997;57(19):4183–4186.

109. Parsons R. Phosphatases and tumorigenesis. *Curr Opin Oncol* 1998;10(1):88–91.

110. Furnari FB, et al. Growth suppression of glioma cells by PTEN requires a functional phosphatase catalytic domain. *Proc Natl Acad Sci USA* 1997;94(23):12479–12484.

111. Tamura M, et al. Inhibition of cell migration, spreading, and focal adhesions by tumor suppressor PTEN. *Science* 1998;280(5369):1614–1617.

112. Cheney IW, et al. Suppression of tumorigenicity of glioblastoma cells by adenovirus-mediated MMAC1/PTEN gene transfer. *Cancer Res* 1998;58(11):2331–2334.

113. Wagner S, Green MR. DNA-binding domains: targets for viral and cellular regulators. *Curr Opin Cell Biol* 1994;6(3):410–414.

114. Darnell JE, Jr. Studies of IFN-induced transcriptional activation uncover the Jak-Stat pathway [In Process Citation]. *J Interferon Cytokine Res* 1998;18(8):549–554.

115. Sehgal A, et al. Application of the differential hybridization of Atlas human expression arrays technique in the identification of differentially expressed genes in human glioblastoma multiforme tumor tissue. *J Surg Oncol* 1998;67(4):234–241.

116. Geller AI, et al. Helper virus-free herpes simplex virus-1 plasmid vectors for gene therapy of Parkinson's disease and other neurological disorders. *Exp Neurol* 1997;144(1):98–102.

117. Trepel M, et al. Chemosensitivity of human malignant glioma: modulation by p53 gene transfer [In Process Citation]. *J Neurooncol* 1998;39(1):19–32.

118. Jean WC, et al. Interleukin-12-based immunotherapy against rat 9L glioma. *Neurosurgery* 1998;42(4):850–856; discussion 856–857.

119. Geng L, et al. Transfection of a vector expressing wild-type p53 into cells of two human glioma cell lines enhances radiation toxicity. *Radiat Res* 1998;150(1):31–37.

120. Lang FF, et al. Enhancement of radiosensitivity of wild-type p53 human glioma cells by adenovirus-mediated delivery of the p53 gene [In Process Citation]. *J Neurosurg* 1998;89(1): 125–132.

121. Tanaka T, et al. Viral vector-targeted antiangiogenic gene therapy utilizing an angiostatin complementary DNA. *Cancer Res* 1998;58(15):3362–3369.

Intracranial Tumors

Chapter 12

Infratentorial Astrocytoma

Michael D. Medlock

HISTORY

Found predominantly in children, cerebellar astrocytomas account for 12% to 18% of pediatric intracranial tumors.[1, 2] In 1931, Harvey Cushing was the first to report extensively and specifically on these tumors in an article that appeared in the journal, *Surgery, Gynecology and Obstetrics*.[3] Since that time, many major series of studies of cerebellar astrocytomas have been published,[4-21] such as those by Ilgren and Stiller, in which the authors summarize 2916 cases reported between 1926 and 1984.[22-25]

EPIDEMIOLOGY

Increases in the incidence of pediatric astrocytomas over the past several decades have been reported in Australia,[26] Sweden,[27] England,[28] Italy,[29] Delaware,[30] and Minnesota.[31] The Delaware study reported that the overall incidence of childhood central nervous system (CNS) tumors, including the subgroup of gliomas, increased 2.7% per year from 1970 to 1989. The Swedish study found that the incidence of astrocytomas increased 3% per year from 1973 to 1992.[27] The Swedish scientists found that malignant brain tumors as a group increased at an average annual rate of 2.6%, although they were unable to identify any spatial or temporal clustering that might warrant further investigation. The reason for this trend of increasing incidence remains unclear, although in several counties in California and Washington state,[32] paternal employment in the chemical and electrical industries has been associated with an increased risk of astrocytomas.

GENETICS

Reproducible genetic markers have not yet been identified for the low-grade astrocytomas of childhood.[33] Malignant pediatric astrocytomas have abnormalities similar to those seen in adult tumors, for example, polyploidy, loss of alleles on l7p13 and TP53 mutations, trisomy 7, and loss of chromosomes 10 and 22.[33, 34] It has been proposed in the literature that early dysfunction of p53 protein expression may be the first step in malignant degeneration of pilocytic astrocytomas.[35]

PRESENTATION

Approximately 70% of cerebellar astrocytomas occur in children, and most patients with these tumors present before 7 years of age.[22] Congenital cerebellar astrocytomas have been diagnosed as early as 29 weeks of estimated gestational age.[36, 37] When these tumors occur in adults, they exhibit biological behavior similar to those seen in children.[38] Patients having tectal and cerebellar astrocytomas most often present with symptoms similar to those that occur with other posterior fossa masses, namely insidious onset of hydrocephalus, lethargy, nausea, vomiting, ataxia, and dysmetria. Isolated and intermittent cranial neuropathies, nystagmus, precocious puberty, and hemorrhage also have been reported as presenting symptoms.[39-43] In addition, patients may present with benign symptoms such as positional vertigo or deterioration in handwriting.[44, 45]

Some described symptoms of cerebellar astrocytomas are atypical for lesions in the posterior fossa and for brain stem dysfunction. For example, hallucinations are atypical among presenting symptoms, with surgical tumor removal resulting in their cessation.[46] In addition, invasion of superficial soft tissues[47] or transmission of increased pressure to the upper cervical spinal cord, which may cause syringomyelia,[48] can be seen among the symptoms of patients with cerebellar astrocytomas.

BOX 12–1
Clinical Presentation

- **Hydrocephalus**
- **Lethargy**
- **Nausea and vomiting**
- **Ataxia**
- **Dysmetria**
- **Central nervous dysfunction**
- **Precocious puberty**

Associations

Neurofibromatosis predisposes children to neoplasms throughout the central and peripheral nervous systems. *A history of neurofibromatosis and a cerebellar astrocytoma should prompt the clinician to look closely for other CNS tumors, such as optic pathway astrocytomas*.[49] Cerebellar astrocytomas have been reported in association with multiple hereditary exostoses of the thoracic spine.[50] Cranial arachnoid seeding is not uncommon, and spinal cord seeding has also been reported.[51]

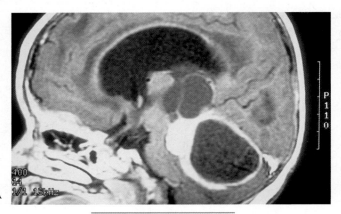 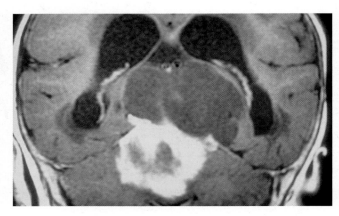

Figure 12–1 This 12-year-old boy presented with headache secondary to his hydrocephalus. (A) Sagittal MRI (T1-weighted) with gadolinium enhancement of large multicystic infratentorial juvenile pilocytic astrocytoma. Note the characteristic enhancement of the tumor capsule as well as anterior solid component. (B) Coronal MRI (T1-weighted) demonstrating gadolinium enhancement of the solid tumor component in the infratentorial compartment. As seen on the sagittal view as well, this patient has a significant supratentorial cystic extension into the posterior third ventricle.

IMAGING CHARACTERISTICS

It is difficult to predict the histological diagnosis with certainty based on imaging studies. Other common and uncommon tumors of the posterior fossa in children, such as medulloblastoma, ependymoma, astrocytoma, choroid plexus papilloma, epidermoid, meningioma, and neurofibroma have significant overlap in their appearance on magnetic resonance (MR) imaging (Fig. 12–1) and on computed tomography (CT) (Fig. 12–2). Cerebellar astrocytomas can present as a homogeneously enhancing mass, a ring enhancing cyst, or a cystic cavity with an enhancing mural nodule.[52] Nevertheless, some distinguishing features can assist with making a presumptive preoperative diagnosis.

Computed Tomography Imaging

The extension of tumor into the cerebellopontine angle from within the fourth ventricle or hemorrhage within the tumor are characteristic features of an ependymoma. Medulloblastomas rarely form cysts, although the necrotic core of a malignant tumor may be indistinguishable on MR imaging from the high protein cyst fluid found in benign tumors such as pilocytic astrocytomas. Epidermoid tumors tend to be homogeneous, nonenhancing masses that have imaging characteristics similar to cerebral spinal fluid (CSF). Calcification can be seen in up to 20%, and cysts in 70%, of posterior fossa astrocytomas.[53, 54]

Magnetic Resonance Imaging

On MR imaging, astrocytomas are typically hypointense or isointense to the surrounding brain on T1-weighted images (Fig. 12–3), and hyperintense on T2-weighted images (Fig. 12–2).[52] The MR images in Figures 12–1 and 12–3 show many of these typical features. Astrocytomas may extend into the cervical spinal canal, mimicking a characteristic feature of ependymomas.[55] During the past 10 years taking an MR scan within the first 2 days following surgery has been routine to determine the extent of residual tumor. The surgeon's estimate of whether a gross total resection was achieved may be inaccurate in up to one third of cases,[56, 57] although recent evidence suggests that false positives and false negatives based on MR imaging studies may be more common than previously thought.[58] Postsurgical areas may enhance, and residual tumor may not enhance.

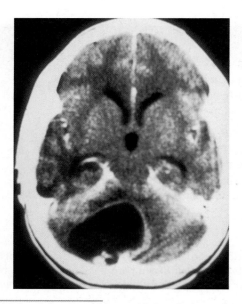

Figure 12–2 A 9-year-old boy with headache and vomiting seen to have a cystic mass in the posterior fossa with contrast enhancement of the capsule. A low-grade astrocytoma was responsible for his hydrocephalus.

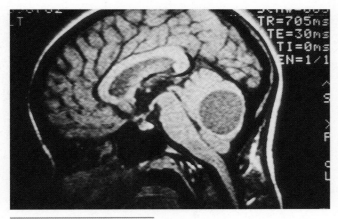

Figure 12–3 Sagittal MRI of a 13-year-old girl with a history of ataxia and intermittent nausea and vomiting. There was minimal enhancement with gadolinium and this tumor was characterized as a low-grade glioma.

BOX 12–2
Imaging Features

- **CT**
  - **Enhancing cysts**
  - **Calcifications (20%)**
- **MRI**
  - **T1-weighted images: hypo- to isointense**
  - **T2-weighted images: hyperintense**

SURGERY

Surgery is the primary mode of treatment for both diagnostic and therapeutic purposes, and the goal of surgical treatment is gross total resection. Hoffman describes a gross physical distinction between cyst walls that are neoplastic and those that are composed of reactive gliosis: neoplastic cyst walls have shaggy borders, whereas gliotic cyst walls have smooth borders.[59] Resection of a cyst wall is not required for gross total resection if the wall is thin and shows gliosis without neoplasia.

More than 90% of astrocytomas are completely resectable, and surgical resection should be tailored to minimize acute morbidity.[4] Because of the proximity to cranial nerves and important brainstem structures controlling heart rate and respiration, surgery in the posterior fossa carries a higher morbidity than supratentorial surgery.

Positioning

Most posterior fossa tumors are approached using one of three basic positions: prone, supine, or sitting. Intra-operative frameless stereotactic navigation is rarely helpful in the posterior fossa as conventional anatomical landmarks are usually sufficient. Ultrasound may be helpful in determining the amount of residual tumor attached to the floor of the fourth ventricle.

The most commonly used position for midline tumors is the prone position; for lateral tumors, the supine position. Tumors in the lateral portion of the hemisphere may be approached using a supine position with a shoulder roll under the ipsilateral shoulder and the head turned to the contralateral side. The sitting position is less commonly used because of the risks of hypotension and air embolism. Air embolism to the lungs is a problem associated with surgical positions in which the surgical field is elevated above the heart. In the sitting position venous channels such as the dural venous sinuses, cortical veins, and bone can entrain air.

Approach

Cushing often used a "T" incision to expose the entire subocciput.[3] Today, the more commonly used incision is a longitudinally oriented linear skin incision made over the axis of the surgical approach. The dura may be opened in a stellate fashion, or in a U-shape with the base toward the sigmoid sinus. Dural sinus laceration can result in life-threatening hemorrhage, and prior to surgery at least 1 blood volume equivalent should be cross matched. Dural venous sinuses that may be injured include the transverse sinus, sigmoid sinus, sinus cerebelli, and circular sinus. The transverse sinus and confluens of sinuses (torcula of Hirophilus) may lie low on the occiput, and the midsagittal MR image must be examined closely prior to placing the first burr hole.

Several of the dural venous channels in the posterior fossa undergo involution during childhood. The circular sinus, a dural venous sinus at the foramen magnum that encircles the cervicomedullary junction, can be large with high venous blood flow, particularly in the first year of life. It can transmit blood in volumes equivalent to the sigmoid sinuses, and opening this sinus can be life-threatening. Likewise, the midline sinus cerebelli is a potential site of large volume blood loss. Lastly, the posterior fossa dura frequently contains venous lakes that may, in addition to bipolar cautery, require suture ligature or metal (vascular) clip closure.

Cerebellar mutism is a disorder sometimes seen following partial or complete resection of the cerebellar vermis, and it may be accompanied by personality changes, bradykinesia, hypotonia, reduced oral intake, urinary retention, and long-tract signs.[60] The syndrome has been reported in up to 13% of patients undergoing surgery for tumors in, or around, the cerebellar vermis.[61] Edema in the brachium pontis has been associated with the development of this syndrome.[61]

BOX 12–3
Cerebellar Mutism

- **Personality changes**
- **Bradykinesia**
- **Hypotonia**
- **Decreased oral intake**
- **Decreased verbal output**

Piatt suggests a surgical approach to the fourth ventricle that precludes sectioning of the vermis. This approach involves elevation of the cerebellar tonsils with, and sectioning of, the tela choroidea, thus avoiding incision of the vermis or traction on the dentate nuclei and allowing visualization from one foramen of Luschka to the other.[62] In the literature, Piatt describes eleven cases in which surgical section of the vermis would have been performed but was avoided. Following the resection of fourth ventricle tumors through the use of the above-described technique, none of the patients developed post-operative mutism.

Brain stem injury may result from over-aggressive tumor resection, and the scope of potential injuries is broad, ranging from isolated cranial nerve or tract injury to death and coma. For example, pontine tegmental injury can result in a "one-and-a-half" syndrome.[63] This syndrome affects the ipsilateral paramedian pontine reticular formation or abducens nerve nucleus and the internuclear fibers crossing the midline to the contralateral abducens nerve nucleus. Palatal myoclonus may result from injury to the deep cerebellar nuclei.[64] Injury to the lower cranial nerves, that is, the glossopharyngeal, vagus, spinal accessory, and hypoglossal nerves, confers a high cost to the patient because such injury can result in compromised airway protection and swallowing, requiring tracheostomy and gastrostomy.

Late complications of surgical resection of astrocytomas include superficial siderosis and hydrocephalus.[65] Closure of the dura is essential as the incidence of postoperative hydrocephalus has been reported near 20% for cases in which the dura is not closed.[66]

HISTOLOGICAL SPECTRUM

Cerebellar astrocytomas can be classified histologically using specific and nonspecific grading systems. The cerebellum-specific two-tiered classification system proposed by Winston and Gilles is based on histological criteria, and its authors have found that it correlates with outcome (Table 12–1). Other standards for histological classification not specific to the cerebellum include those of Russell and Rubenstein and the World Health Organization.[67, 68] The widely used St. Anne-Mayo astrocytoma grading system focuses on atypia, mitosis, endothelial proliferation, and necrosis (Table 12–2).

TABLE 12–1 Winston and Gilles Classification of 132 Cerebellar Gliomas

Type A	Type B
Microcyst	Perivascular pseudorosette
Leptomeningeal deposit	High cell density
Rosenthal fiber	Necrosis
Oligodendroglial focus	Mitosis
	Calcification

To qualify for each type, the tumor must have ≥1 of the characteristics in that column.
From Winston K, et al. Cerebellar gliomas in children. *J Natl Cancer Inst* 1977;58:833–838.

TABLE 12–2 St. Anne-Mayo Astrocytoma Grading System

Grade	Number of features
1	0
2	1
3	2
4	3–4

Features are atypia, mitosis, endothelial proliferation, and necrosis.
From Daumas-Duport C, et al. Grading of astrocytomas: a simple and reproducible method. *Cancer* 1988;62:2152–2165.

Malignant histological characteristics, such as vascular proliferation and necrosis, may be found in benign tumors such as pilocytic astrocytomas and pleomorphic xanthoastrocytomas.[69] Histologically malignant astrocytomas are far less common: less than 30 glioblastomas of the cerebellum in childhood have been reported.[70, 71] *The MIB-1 labeling index may be a useful means of predicting biological activity in pediatric anaplastic astrocytomas.*[72] Ho and his colleagues at the Veteran's General Hospital in Taipei studied 101 pediatric non-pilocytic astrocytomas, and they found that children who had anaplastic astrocytomas with a MIB-1 labeling index ≤ 11 had survival rates similar to those of children with low grade astrocytomas. Those children who had anaplastic astrocytomas and a MIB-1 labeling index > 11 had survival rates similar to those of children with glioblastomas.

Gjerris and Klinken reported a series on the cases of 44 children with cerebellar astrocytomas who were operated on between 1935 and 1959. The histologic diagnoses were divided into juvenile (pilocytic) and diffuse type tumors. The 25-year cumulative survival was 94% for the juvenile type and 38% for the diffuse type.[11] But the importance of this histological distinction has not gone without challenge—the ability to achieve a gross total resection may be more important than the presence or absence of certain histological characteristics.[17]

Accordingly, local leptomeningeal dissemination is not necessarily a poor prognostic sign, and it may occur in up to 70% of benign astrocytomas.[73–75] More diffuse leptomeningeal metastases from CSF seeding may occur in up to 4% of pediatric astrocytomas, and in particular, in those that are adjacent to ventricular or subarachnoid spaces at presentation.[76–80] Peritoneal seeding of benign astrocytomas through a ventriculoperitoneal shunt has been reported.[76]

RADIATION THERAPY

Radiation therapy is not recommended in the initial management of benign cerebellar astrocytomas because exposure to radiation risks developmental delay, endocrine failure, and malignant degeneration of the tumor.[81] However, progression of unresectable tumor on follow-up may offer no alternative to radiation therapy,[81–85] and in the case of resection of malignant astrocytomas radiation therapy is frequently recommended as a second line agent immediately following surgery.[86]

Degeneration of the astrocytoma into a more histologically malignant astrocytoma may occur as many as 28 years after initial treatment[82, 85, 87–89] whether or not the patient underwent radiation therapy. Radiation therapy may play a causative role in the induction of benign and malignant tumors of the temporal bone and dura,[90] and according to the study of the long-term follow-up of patients irradiated for other tumors, such as medulloblastoma,[91] it has been shown to be associated with a risk of malignant astrocytomas.

CHEMOTHERAPY

If leptomeningeal dissemination is symptomatic, high-dose cyclophosphamide has been reported to be effective in some patients.[92] Despite intensive chemotherapy among 172 children with high grade astrocytomas, surgery was the only factor that affected outcome in a recent prospective study.[93]

PROGNOSTIC FACTORS

The long-term outcome of cerebellar astrocytornas is favorable,[9–12, 23, 94] and long-term survival is possible despite obvious residual tumor.[2, 16, 97] However, residual tumor may progress, remain stable, or regress.[56] Progression free survival is much lower in patients with residual tumor, approximately 70% to 80% at 10 years and 40% to 50% at 20 years. Pathologically proven astrocytomas may involute for unclear reasons[96] and unresectable brainstem involvement confers a poorer prognosis.[8, 17, 19, 22, 95] Median survival among patients with high grade astrocytomas of the cerebellum may be less than 12 months despite aggressive chemotherapy and radiation therapy.[52]

In the literature, five year survival rates among patients who have had gross total resections are 100%, in some series,[7] and ten year survival rates of greater than 90% are common. Several more current series have noted up to 100% survival at 20 years,[4, 13, 21] and in one study of children with Grade I tumors a 94% 25-year survival rate has been noted.[11]

Recurrent disease in patients who have undergone a gross total resection can be as high as 10%[52] and given this low rate of recurrence radiation therapy is not justified. Even when low grade astrocytomas recur, there is no clear evidence in the form of controlled trials that radiation therapy improves the quality of, or prolongs, life.

The slow growth of these tumors accounts for late recurrences, and patients must be evaluated periodically throughout childhood.[6] Recurrences of benign tumors have been reported as long as 36 and 48 years after initial gross-total resection[6, 98, 99] and cerebellar astrocytomas with benign histology and malignant progression have also been reported.[100, 101] Malignant conversion has been reported as long as 48 years after initial resection of a benign lesion.[83, 88, 102, 103]

Although cerebellar astrocytomas are apparently distant from neocortex, more than half of children with these tumors have neuropsychological problems independent of radiation therapy.[97]

SUMMARY

Cerebellar astrocytomas are tumors found predominantly in children. They generally carry a good prognosis, with surgical removal being the primary mode of treatment.

REFERENCES

1. Larson, DA, Wara WM, Edwards MS. Management of childhood cerebellar astrocytoma. *Int J Radiat Oncol* 1990;18:971–973.
2. Pollack, IF. Brain tumors in children. *N Engl J Med* 1994;331:1500–1507.
3. Cushing H. Experiences with the cerebellar astrocytomas. *Surg Gyn Obs* 1931;52:129–205.
4. Abdollahzadeh M, et al. Benign cerebellar astrocytoma in childhood: experience at the Hospital for Sick Children 1980–1992. *Childs Nerv Syst* 1994;10:380–383.
5. Akyol FH, et al. Results of post-operative or exclusive radiotherapy in grade I and grade Il cerebellar astrocytoma patients. *Radiotherapy Onc* 1992;23:245–248.
6. Austin EJ, Alvord ECY. Recurrences of cerebellar astrocytomas: a violation of Collins' Law. *J Neurosurg* 1988;68:41–47.
7. Conway PD, et al. Importance of histologic condition and treatment of pediatric cerebellar astrocytoma. *Cancer* 1991;67:2772–2775.
8. Ferbert A, Gullotta FY. Remarks on the follow-up of cerebellar astrocytomas. *J Neurol* 1985;232:134–136.
9. Garcia DM, et al. Astrocytomas of the cerebellum in children. *J Neurosurg* 1989;71:661–664.
10. Garcia DM, et al. Childhood cerebellar astrocytomas: is there a role for postoperative irradiation? *Int J Radiat Oncol* 1990;18:815–818.
11. Gjerris F, Klinken L. Long-term prognosis in children with benign cerebellar astrocytoma. *J Neurosurg* 1978;49:179–184.
12. Hayostek CJ, et al. Astrocytomas of the cerebellum: a comparative clinicopathologic study of pilocytic and diffuse astrocytomas. *Cancer* 1993;72:856–869.
13. Heiskanen O, Lehtosalo J. Surgery of cerebellar astrocytomas, ependymomas and medulloblastomas in children. *Acta Neurochir* 1985;78:1–3.
14. Kehler U, Arnold H, Muller HY. Long-term follow-up of infratentorial pilocytic astrocytomas. *Neurosurg Rev* 1990;13:315–320.
15. Laws ER, Jr, Bergstralh EJ, Taylor WF. Cerebellar astrocytoma in children. *Prog Exp Tumor Res* 1987;30:122–127.
16. Mandigers CMPW, et al. Astrocytoma in childhood: survival and performance. *Ped Hemat Onc* 1990;7:121–128.
17. Palma L, Russo A, Celli P. Prognosis of the so-called "diffuse" cerebellar astrocytoma. *Neurosurgery* 1984;15:315–317.
18. Slavcf I, Salchegger C, Hauer C. Follow-up and quality of survival of 67 consecutive children with CNS tumors. *Child's Nerv Syst* 1994;10:433–443.
19. Undjian S, Marinov M, Georgiev KY. Long-term follow-up after surgical treatment of cerebellar astrocytomas in 100 children. *Child's Nerv Syst* 1989;5:99–101.

20. Wallner KE, et al. Treatment results of juvenile pilocytic astrocytoma. *J Neurosurg* 1988;69:171–176.
21. Winston K, et al. Cerebellar gliomas in children. *J Natl Cancer Inst* 1977;58:833–838.
22. Ilgren EB, Stiller CA. Cerebellar astrocytomas: clinical characteristics and prognostic indices. *J Neurooncol* 1987;4:293–308.
23. Ilgren EB, Stiller CA. Cerebellar astrocytomas: therapeutic management. *Acta Neurochir* 1986;81:11–26.
24. Ilgren EB, Stiller CA. Cerebellar astrocytomas, I: macroscopic and microscopic features. *Clin Neuropathol* 1987; 6:185–200.
25. Ilgren EB, Stiller CA. Cerebellar astrocytomas, II: pathologic features indicative of malignancy. *Clin Neuropathol* 1987;6:201–214.
26. McWhirter WR, Dobson C, Ring I. Childhood cancer incidence in Australia, 1982–1991. *Int J Cancer* 1996;65:34–38.
27. Hjalmars U, et al. Increased incidence rates but no space-time clustering of childhood astrocytoma in Sweden, 1973–1992: a population-based study of pediatric brain tumors. *Cancer* 1999;85:2077–2090.
28. McKinney PA, et al. Epidemiology of childhood brain tumours in Yorkshire, UK, 1974–1995: geographical distribution and changing patterns of occurrence. *Br J Cancer* 1998;78:974–979.
29. Farinotti M, et al. Incidence and survival of childhood CNS tumours in the region of Lombardy, Italy. *Brain* 1998;121:1429–1436.
30. Bunin GR, et al. Increasing incidence of childhood cancer. *JUL* 1996;10(3):319–338.
31. Swensen AR, Bushhouse SA. Childhood cancer incidence and trends in Minnesota, 1988–1994. *Minn Med* 1998;81: 27–32.
32. McKean-Cowdin R, et al. Parental occupation and childhood brain tumors: astroglial and primitive neuroectodermal tumors. *J Occup Environ Med* 1998;40:332–340.
33. Biegel JA. Genetics of pediatric central nervous system tumors. *J Pediatr Hematol Oncol* 1997;19:492–501.
34. Bigner SH, et al. Chromosomal characteristics of childhood brain tumors. *Cancer Genet Cytogenet* 1997;97:125–134.
35. Bodey B, et al. Immunohistochemical detection of p53 protein expression in various childhood astrocytoma subtypes: significance in tumor progression. *Anticancer Res* 1997;17:1187–1194.
36. Doren M, et al. Prenatal diagnosis of a highly undifferentiated brain tumour: a case report and review of the literature. *Prenat Diagn* 1997;17:967–971.
37. Podskalny GD, et al. Report of congenital anaplastic astrocytoma discovered in a newborn. *J Child Neurol* 1993;8:389–394.
38. Hassounah M, et al. Cerebellar astrocytoma: report of 13 cases aged over 20 years and review of the literature. *Br J Neurosurg* 1996;10:365–371.
39. Chopra K, et al. Precocious puberty—unusual manifestation of cerebellar astrocytoma. *Indian Pediatr* 1977;14:321–323.
40. Astle WF, Miller SJ. Bilateral fluctuating trochlear nerve palsy secondary to cerebellar astrocytoma. *Can J Ophthalmol* 1994;29:34–38.
41. Fogelson MH, Oppenheim RE, McLaurin RL. Childhood cerebellar astrocytoma presenting with hemorrhage. *Neurology* 1980;30:669–670.
42. Traccis S, et al. Upbeat nystagmus as an early sign of cerebellar astrocytoma. *J Neurol* 1989;236:359–360.
43. Vincent FM, Bartone JR, Jones MZ. Cerebellar astrocytoma presenting as a cerebellar hemorrhage in a child. *Neurology* 1980;30:91–93.
44. Gregorius FK, Crandall PH, Baloh PW. Positional vertigo with cerebellar astrocytoma. *Surg Neurol* 1976;6:283–286.
45. Harel S, et al. Cerebellar astrocytoma presenting as deterioration of handwriting in a child. *Eur J Pediatr* 1985; 143:235–237.
46. Nadvi SS, Ramdial PK. Transient peduncular hallucinations secondary to brain stem compression by a cerebellar pilocytic astrocytoma. *Br J Neurosurg* 1998;12:579–581.
47. Kepes JJ, Lewis RC, Vergara GG. Cerebellar astrocytoma invading the musculature and soft tissues of the neck. Case report. *J Neurosurg* 1980;52:414–418.
48. Kumar C, et al. Cerebellar astrocytoma presenting as a syringomyelic syndrome. *Surg Neurol* 1987;27:187–190.
49. Miller NR. Optic nerve glioma and cerebellar astrocytoma in a patient with von Recklinghausen's neurofibromatosis. *Am J Ophthalmol* 1975;79:582–588.
50. Decker RE, Wei WC. Thoracic cord compression from multiple hereditary exostoses associated with cerebellar astrocytoma. Case report. *J Neurosurg* 1969;30:310–312.
51. Shapiro K, Shulman K. Spinal cord seeding from cerebellar astrocytoma. *Child's Brain* 1976;2:177–186.
52. Campbell JW, Pollack IF. Cerebellar astrocytomas in children. *J Neuro-Oncol* 1996;28:223–231.
53. Chang T, Teng MMH, Lirng JF. Posterior cranial fossa tumours in childhood. *Neuroradiology* 1993;35:274–278.
54. Lee Y, et al. Juvenile pilocytic astrocytomas. *AJR* 1989;52: 1263–1270.
55. Leproux F, et al. Extension of a cerebellar cystic astrocytoma into the cervical canal, demonstrated by magnetic resonance imaging. *Can Assoc Radiol J* 1993;44:460–462.
56. Dirven CM, Mooij JJ, Molenaar WM. Cerebellar pilocytic astrocytoma: a treatment protocol based upon analysis of 73 cases and a review of the literature. *Child's Nerv Syst* 1997;13:17–23.
57. Smoots DW, et al. Predicting disease progression in childhood cerebellar astrocytoma. *Child's Nerv Syst* 1998;14: 636–648.
58. Rollins NK, Nisen P, Shapiro KN. The use of early postoperative MR in detecting residual juvenile cerebellar pilocytic astrocytoma. *Am J Neuroradiol* 1998;19:151–156.
59. Hoffman HJ. Cerebellar astrocytomas. In Apuzzo M, ed., *Brain Surgery: Complication Avoidance and Management.* New York: Churchill Livingston; 1993:1813–1824.
60. van Dongen HR, Catsman-Berrevoets CE, van Mourik M. The syndrome of "cerebellar" mutism and subsequent dysarthria. Comments. *Neurology* 1994;44:2040–2046.
61. Pollack IF, et al. Mutism and pseudobulbar symptoms after resection of posterior fossa tumors in children: incidence and pathophysiology. Comments. *Neurosurgery* 1995;37:885–893.
62. Kellogg JX, Piatt JH Jr. Resection of fourth ventricle tumors without splitting the vermis: the cerebellomedullary fissure approach. Comments. *Pediatr Neurosurg* 1997;27:28–33.
63. Newton HB, Miner ME. "One-and-a-half" syndrome after a resection of a midline cerebellar astrocytoma: case

report and discussion of the literature. *Neurosurgery* 1991;29:768–772.

64. Nishigaya K, et al. Palatal myoclonus induced by extirpation of a cerebellar astrocytoma. Case report. *J Neurosurg* 1998;88:1107–1110.

65. Anderson NE, Sheffield S, Hope JK. Superficial siderosis of the central nervous system: a late complication of cerebellar tumors. *Neurology* 1999;52:163–169.

66. Stein BM, Tenner MS, Fraser RA. Hydrocephalus following removal of cerebellar astrocytomas in children. *J Neurosurg* 1972;36:763–768.

67. Russell D, Rubinstein L. *Pathology of Tumours of the - Nervous System.* Baltimore: Williams & Wilkins; 1977:183.

68. Kleihaus P, et al. World Health Organization histological typing of tumours of the central nervous system. 1993.

69. Giannini C, Scheithauer BW. Classification and grading of low-grade astrocytic tumors in children. *Brain Pathol* 1997;7:785–798.

70. Bristo R, et al. Malignant cerebellar astrocytomas in childhood: experience with four cases. *Child's Nerv Syst* 1998; 14:532–536.

71. Katz DS, et al. A rare case of cerebellar glioblastoma multiforme in childhood: MR imaging. *Clin Imaging* 1995;19: 162–164.

72. Ho DM, et al. MIB-1 labeling index in nonpilocytic astrocytoma of childhood: a study of 101 cases. *Cancer* 1998; 82:2459–2466.

73. Medlock MD, Scott RM. Optic chiasm astrocytomas of childhood, II: surgical management. *Pediatr Neurosurg* 1997;27:129–136.

74. Mishima K, et al. Leptomeningeal dissemination of cerebellar pilocytic astrocytoma. Case report. *J Neurosurg* 1992;77:788–791.

75. Morikawa M, et al. Cerebellar pilocytic astrocytoma with leptomeningeal dissemination. Case report. *Surg Neurol* 1997;48:49–51;(discussion)51–52.

76. Pollack IF, et al. Dissemination of low grade intracranial astrocytomas in children. *Cancer* 1994;73:2869–2878.

77. Packer RJ, et al. Leptomeningeal dissemination of primary central nervous system tumors of childhood. *Ann Neurol* 1985;18:217–221.

78. McLaughlin JE. Juvenile astrocytomas with subarachnoid spread. *J Pathol* 1976;118:101–107.

79. Kocks W, et al. Spinal metastasis of pilocytic astrocytoma of the chiasma opticum. *Child's Nerv Syst* 1989;5: 118–120.

80. Civitello LA, et al. Leptomeningeal dissemination of low-grade gliomas in childhood. *Neurology* 1988;38: 562–565.

81. Sgouros S, Fineron PW, Hockley AD. Cerebellar astrocytoma of childhood: long-term follow-up. *Child's Nerv Syst* 1995;11:89–96.

82. Casadei GP, et al. Late malignant recurrence of childhood cerebellar astrocytoma. *Clin Neuropathol* 1990;9: 295–298.

83. Schwartz AM, Ghatak NR. Malignant transformation of benign cerebellar astrocytoma. *Cancer* 1990;65:333–336.

84. Danoff BF, et al. Assessment of the long-term effects of primary radiation therapy for brain tumors in children. *Cancer* 1982;49:1580–1586.

85. Budka H. Partially resected and irradiated cerebellar astrocytoma of childhood: malignant evolution after 28 years. *Acta Neurochir* 1975;32:139–146.

86. Salazar OM. Primary malignant cerebellar astrocytomas in children: a signal for postoperative craniospinal irradiation. *Int J Rad Oncol Biol Phys* 1981;7:1661–1665.

87. Alpers CE, Davis RL, Wilson CB. Persistence and late malignant transformation of childhood cerebellar astrocytoma. Case report. *J Neurosurg* 1982;57:548–551.

88. Scott RM, Ballantine HT Jr. Cerebellar astrocytoma: malignant recurrence after prolonged postoperative survival. Case report. *J Neurosurg* 1973;39:777–779.

89. Kleriga E, et al. Development of cerebellar malignant astrocytoma at site of a medulloblastoma treated 11 years earlier. Case report. *J Neurosurg* 1978;49:445–449.

90. Casentini L, et al. Osteogenic osteosarcoma of the calvaria following radiotherapy for cerebellar astrocytoma: report of a case in childhood. *Tumori* 1985;71:391–396.

91. Furuta T, et al. Malignant cerebellar astrocytoma developing 15 years after radiation therapy for a medulloblastoma. *Clin Neurol Neurosurg* 1998;100:56–59.

92. McCowage G, et al. Successful treatment of childhood pilocytic astrocytomas metastatic to the leptomeninges with high-dose cyclophosphamide. *Med Pediatr Oncol* 1996;27:32–39.

93. Wisoff JH, et al. Current neurosurgical management and the impact of the extent of resection in the treatment of malignant gliomas of childhood: a report of the Children's Cancer Group trial no. CCG-945. *J Neurosurg* 1998;89:52–59.

94. Fulchiero A, et al. Secular trends of cerebellar gliomas in children. *J Natl Cancer Inst* 1977;58:839–843.

95. Pencalet P, et al. Benign cerebellar astrocytomas in children. *J Neurosurg* 1999;90:265–273.

96. Kernan JC, et al. Spontaneous involution of a diencephalic astrocytoma. *Pediatr Neurosurg* 1998;29:149–253.

97. LeBaron S, et al. Assessment of quality of survival in children with medulloblastoma and cerebellar astrocytoma. *Cancer* 1988;62:1215–1222.

98. Yoshizumi MO. Neuro-ophthalmologic signs in a recurrent cerebellar astrocytoma after 48 years. *Ann Ophthalmol* 1979;11:1714–1719.

99. Pagni CA, Giordana MT, Canavero S. Benign recurrence of a pilocytic cerebellar astrocytoma 36 years after radical removal. Case report. *Neurosurgery* 1991;28:606–609.

100. Auer RN, et al. Cerebellar astrocytoma with benign histology and malignant clinical course. Case report. *J Neurosurg* 1981;5:128–132.

101. Sioutos PJ, et al. Unusual early recurrence of a cerebellar pilocytic astrocytoma following complete surgical resection: case report and review of the literature. *J Neurooncol* 1996;30:47–54.

102. Kleinman GM, et al. Malignant transformation in benign cerebellar astrocytoma. Case report. *J Neurosurg,* 1978;49: 111–118.

103. Ushio Y, et al. Malignant recurrence of childhood cerebellar astrocytoma. Case report. *Neurosurgery* 1987;21: 251–255.

104. Daumas-Duport C, et al. Grading of astrocytomas: a simple and reproducible method. *Cancer* 1988;62:2152–2165.

Chapter 13

Brain Stem Tumors

Keith S. Blum and James Tait Goodrich

Intrinsic brain stem tumors are relatively common in children, comprising approximately 10 to 25% of all pediatric brain tumors[1–9] and 25–30% of posterior fossa tumors in children.[5, 7, 8, 10] The majority of patients present before the age of 16 years, with a peak tumor prevalence observed at 6 to 10 years of age.[11–14] There is no sex predilection or geographical distribution.

The majority of these tumors are diffuse, infiltrating, aggressive lesions that typically occur most frequently in the pons, invade the surrounding brain stem, and are not amenable to surgical resection.[2, 10, 12, 15–19] Most patents die within 2 years after diagnosis; however, 20–35% of patients with brain stem tumors are reported to survive for several years with a relatively good prognosis.[10, 13] Less common lesions, such as focal intrinsic lesions of the midbrain,[4, 20] tumors of the cervicomedullary junction,[4, 21, 22] and dorsally exophytic tumors arising from the floor of the fourth ventricle,[23–25] are primarily slow growing, histologically benign lesions. In some instances, radical surgery alone has provided adequate long-term disease control.

Limited diagnostic and radiologic techniques in the past have accounted for brain stem lesions being regarded as an homogeneous group of tumors which are uniformly malignant and viewed with a sense of hopelessness. The risk of operating on the brain stem in the past, together with the failure of surgery to alter prognosis, led to treatment recommendations consisting of radiotherapy and supportive measures alone.

In 1968, Pool[26] reported useful long-term survival following surgical and X-ray treatment for verified brain stem gliomas in three cases of confirmed astrocytoma. Patient survival was 10, 20, and 23 years without clinical progression. All patients were operated on via a suboccipital approach. Two cases consisted of "partial removal" and in one case biopsy of the tumor led to bleeding, so further removal was not attempted. Pool suggests that if a brain stem tumor is suspected, an exploratory craniotomy is generally advisable; otherwise a benign lesion may be overlooked that could readily have been removed and the patient cured.

The advent of magnetic resonance imaging (MRI) has simplified the diagnosis of brain stem tumors and has helped in their further classification based on their location and imaging characteristics. The location of a tumor within the brain stem has been found to greatly influence not only the histologic outcome but also whether surgical excision can be accomplished with acceptable morbidity and mortality.[2, 21, 27, 28]

Wide variations in clinical and radiologic features exist that relate to the site and behavior of these brain stem tumors and so influence their surgical management.[4, 25] Over the course of the last few decades, several authors have identified certain categories of brain stem tumors that are associated with a better prognosis.[21, 23, 28, 29] In 1971, Lassiter et al[29] reported long-term survivors in five patients who had largely cystic brain stem masses with mural nodules. Surgery included uncapping of the tumor, biopsy of the nodule, and postoperative radiotherapy. In 1980, Hoffman et al[23] reported their experience with dorsally exophytic brain stem gliomas. They found that this distinct subgroup of brain stem gliomas behaved in a significantly different fashion than the typical infiltrating brain stem glioma and could be treated successfully by subtotal resection. In 1986, Epstein and McCleary[21] presented their experience with radical excision of intrinsic nonexophytic brain stem gliomas in 34 pediatric patients. They classified intrinsic brain stem neoplasms as diffuse, focal, and cervicomedullary. All diffuse tumors and one focal tumor were malignant astrocytomas (grade III or IV), and all of the cervicomedullary tumors were low-grade astrocytomas (grade I or II). No patient with a malignant tumor benefited from surgery, whereas patients with benign neoplasms either were stabilized or improved with surgery. The authors conclude that although surgery may be accomplished within the substance of the brain stem with acceptable morbidity and mortality, it is not indicated for malignant astrocytomas of the brain stem.

More recent approaches to brain stem tumors recognize that there are clearly defined subgroups of pediatric brain stem tumors with markedly differing clinicopathologic features and dramatically different prognoses. The treatment of each must be tailored appropriately.[4, 12, 16, 21, 30, 31] Although the patient's history and neurologic examination will always remain important aspects of the diagnostic process, the advent of MRI has made it possible to accurately diagnose the nature of a specific lesion. In 1993, Epstein and Farmer[28] classified brain stem tumors according to growth patterns that were obvious on MRI appearance. They helped clarify why cervicomedullary, dorsally exophytic, and focal tumors have a better prognosis and helped establish a selection criteria for the surgical treatment of specific brain stem lesions.

Advancements in imaging and neurosurgical techniques have led to an improvement in the surgical management of children with brain stem tumors. Many children with brain stem tumors previously considered "inoperable" can now benefit from surgery. New theories concerning the natural history, growth pattern, classification, and optimal management of brain stem tumors continue to evolve with increased experience.

NATURAL HISTORY AND CLINICAL FEATURES

The clinical syndrome at the time of presentation is determined by the anatomical site of origin of the tumor and its rate of growth. Appearance on imaging studies as well as clinical manifestations are useful in categorizing brain stem tumors and formulating a therapeutic plan.

Diffuse Tumors

Diffuse intrinsic brain stem gliomas compose 60 to 80% of brain stem tumors.[1, 21, 32, 33] They almost always involve the pons, with or without infiltration rostral to the midbrain or caudal extension to the medulla.[5, 30, 32] Earlier reports based on computed tomography (CT) studies showed a lower incidence of this type of tumor. MRI has provided increased resolution, and some tumors that appear on CT as focal may in fact extensively involve the brain stem with MRI. Diffuse brain stem tumors occur most frequently in children between the ages of 6 and 10 years and in the majority of cases are malignant in both histologic type and clinical behavior. The majority of children present with a brief clinical history of 6 weeks or less and imaging consistent with a diffuse tumor expanding the pons. Few children survive longer than 18 months.[2, 30, 34] The short duration of symptoms reflects the invasive and destructive nature of these lesions.[1, 16, 17, 35] These tumors have remained highly resistant to treatment despite many intensive clinical efforts.[11, 21, 33, 36, 37]

Bilateral cranial nerve involvement, gait instability, ataxia, mild motor weakness, and hyperreflexia are common clinical findings. The sixth and seventh cranial nerves are most commonly involved.[11] Symptoms usually reflect the involvement of more than one level of the brain stem. Signs of increased intracranial pressure (ICP) and hydrocephalus are late findings with diffuse intrinsic tumors.[2, 25] Death within 18 months is the usual course of the disease in patients with diffuse symptomatology reflecting involvement of more than one level of the brain stem.[35]

BOX 13–1
Clinical Features of Diffuse Tumors

- **Brief clinical history with bilateral cranial nerve involvement and long-tract signs.**
- **Gait instability, ataxia, mild motor weakness, and hyperreflexia are common.**

Focal Tumors

A focal brain stem tumor is a circumscribed mass usually less than 2 cm in diameter without associated edema.[21] These tumors can arise anywhere in the brain stem. Whether solid or cystic patients present with symptoms related to the part of the brain stem where the tumor originated.

Patients with focal tumors usually have an atypical history associated with a paucity of neurologic signs and slow clinical progression. Symptoms are usually referable to a sin-gle focus in the brain stem that is unilateral, often single cranial nerve dysfunction, and contralateral hemiparesis.[21, 34]

Focal intrinsic tumors of the midbrain are generally slow-growing, histologically benign lesions.[15] They typically occur within the cerebral peduncle or the tectal plate and are usually low-grade astrocytomas.[5] Previous reports of tectal and periaqueductal tumors have shown an overall poor prognosis, with few patients surviving longer than 18 months after diagnosis.[38] These lesions were often diagnosed on postmortem examination, supporting the statement of Kernohan and Sayre that these are "in all probability the smallest tumors in the human body that lead to the death of the patient."[39]

In 1982, Sanford et al[38] described two patients with "pencil" gliomas of the aqueduct of Sylvius diagnosed at autopsy. They reviewed the 12 cases reported in the literature at that time and confirmed the poor prognosis of patients with periaqueductal and tectal tumors. In only two cases reported in the literature then was the diagnosis made while the patient was alive, although at that time none of the cases reported in the literature had been evaluated with CT or MRI. In the two cases reported, the tumors were so small that enhancement in the region of the aqueduct was not recognized using ordinary contrast techniques with CT.

More recently, a subset of indolent gliomas arising in relationship to the midbrain tectum has come into sharper focus.[40–43] These tumors arise in a remarkably circumscribed locus centered on the quadrigeminal plate and have long been recognized as a potential cause of late-onset aqueductal stenosis.[23, 26, 38, 39, 42–46] The most striking feature of these tumors is that they behave as extremely indolent masses, suggesting a congenital origin and limited growth potential.[40]

The clinical presentation of raised ICP secondary to hydrocephalus in the absence of brain stem signs is well known.[15, 45, 47] Patients usually exhibit either signs and symptoms of raised ICP caused by obstructive hydrocephalus or signs and symptoms caused by pressure on the tegmentum and cerebral peduncles.[20] Typical signs of increased ICP include headache, vomiting, and papilledema, which are common.

Chapman et al,[40] in a series of eight patients with dorsal midbrain masses, found that all patients presented with hydrocephalus. In each case the clinical course was remarkable for its chronicity, extending over years, with evidence of having its onset in infancy or early childhood. The progression of brain stem, cerebellar, and long-tract signs typically associated with intrinsic brain stem tumors was notably absent in this group of tumors. The appearance of focal signs was related to formation or expansion of a cystic component of the tumor.

Tumors of the tectal plate can range from 50% to 67% of focal midbrain tumors.[20, 41] The majority of these tumors present with obstructive hydrocephalus at the level of the sylvian aqueduct.[39, 42] In contrast to the majority of brain stem gliomas, which are inherently invasive and produce progressive cranial nerve deficits and long-tract signs in the absence of hydrocephalus, intrinsic tectal tumors almost always present with clinical findings of increased ICP from severe hydrocephalus, often without associated brain stem signs.[15, 42] Parinaud's syndrome (paralysis of conjugate upward gaze) is surprisingly uncommon at presentation, despite the anatomical location of the tumor within the dorsal midbrain.[40, 42, 43] Headache, vomiting, and papilledema are common findings on presentation.

In a series of 89 patients treated at the Hospital for Sick Children between 1976 and 1991,[41] 18 patients (20.22%) were diagnosed with focal midbrain tumors. Sixty-seven percent of all tumors occurred predominantly in the tectal region, giving rise to obstructive hydrocephalus in 92%. The most common presenting symptoms were headache, vomiting, diplopia, and loss of motor function (usually a hemiparesis).

Tumors of the tegmentum usually present with motor deficits, resulting from involvement of the cerebral peduncle or cranial nerve deficits due to pressure on the nuclei of oculomotor nerves or their connecting pathways with or without associated long-tract findings.[41] Hemiparesis is common if the tumor involves the cerebral peduncle.[20, 41]

BOX 13–2
Clinical Features of Focal Tumors

- **Atypical history associated with a paucity of neurologic signs and slow clinical progression.**
- **Symptoms are usually referable to a single focus in the brain stem that is unilateral, often single cranial nerve dysfunction and contralateral hemiparesis if cerebral peduncle involved.**
- **Brain stem signs are typically absent.**
- **Focal tectal tumors present with signs of increased intracranial pressure secondary to hydrocephalus: headaches, vomiting, papilledema, often without associated brain stem signs.**
- **Clinical course for focal tectal tumors is remarkable for its chronicity, extending over years, usually with evidence of having its onset in infancy or early childhood.**
- **Patients with tegmental tumors usually present with cranial nerve deficits, which may occur due to pressure on the nuclei of oculomotor nerves or their connecting pathways with or without associated long-tract findings.**
- **Hemiparesis is common in tegmental tumors that involve the cerebral peduncle.**

Dorsally Exophytic Tumors

Dorsally exophytic brain stem tumors represent a distinct group of atypical brain stem tumors that behave in a significantly different fashion from the typical infiltrating brain stem glioma.[23, 24] They may account for up to 22% of newly diagnosed brain stem tumors.[23–25] These children have been shown to survive substantially longer than children with the usual diffuse intrinsic tumors.[23, 25] Dorsally exophytic tumors grow from the subependymal surface of the brain stem posteriorly into the fourth ventricle and cause relatively early obstruction of the ventricular system, leading to hydrocephalus.[34] They do not extend deeply into the brain stem but instead are exophytic into the fourth ventricle, often filling it with tumor.[5]

Epstein et al[28] have hypothesized the growth pattern of the dorsally exophytic tumor. They feel that it grows initially within the substance of the brain stem as a focal tumor. The low malignant nature of the lesion causes focal swelling of the medulla. Transverse fiber tracts of the pontomedullary and cervicomedullary junction limit growth in the rostral and caudal directions. Because of these rostral and caudal barriers the mass expands in the direction of least resistance, which results in the floor of the fourth ventricle becoming a dorsally exophytic mass.

Dorsally exophytic tumors may present with signs of increased ICP if the tumor has a large exophytic component that blocks the outlets of the fourth ventricle or the aqueduct. Growth is usually slow with these tumors, and the clinical course develops gradually. Children typically present with a longer history of symptoms in comparison with the more malignant intrinsic type. Long-tract signs are uncommon; however, in cases of diffuse brain stem gliomas these are prevalent.[25]

Because symptoms are often insidiously progressive, many children are symptomatic for extended periods of time before diagnosis. Hydrocephalus is common and may result in increased ICP and an isolated sixth-nerve palsy. Mass effect or involvement of the peduncles may cause ataxia or motor weakness. Cranial nerve deficits are rare despite the tumor's close relationship with the floor of the fourth ventricle. Vomiting is common as tumors frequently arise from the floor of the fourth ventricle in the region of the area postrema. Very young patients commonly present with failure to thrive, whereas older patients tend to present with headache, vomiting, and ataxia.[4, 23, 24]

Pollack et al[24] reported a series of 18 patients with dorsally exophytic tumors. All patients who developed symptoms before the age of 1 year manifested failure to thrive as a result of chronic vomiting. Papilledema, ataxia, and torticollis were also common. None of the children had long-tract signs, whereas 15 of 18 patients (83%) presented with varying degrees of obstructive hydrocephalus on imaging. Five children required a ventriculoperitoneal shunt as a stabilizing measure prior to tumor resection.

BOX 13–3
Clinical Features of Dorsally Exophytic Tumors

- **Clinical history is gradual.**
- **Signs of increased intracranial pressure occur if the tumor has a large exophytic component blocking the outlets of the fourth ventricle.**
- **Proximity to the peduncles frequently may cause ataxia, and long-tract signs are uncommon.**
- **Cranial nerve deficits are rare despite their close approximation to the floor of the fourth ventricle.**
- **Vomiting is common as tumors frequently arise from the floor of the fourth ventricle in the region of the area postrema.**
- **Very young patients commonly present with failure to thrive, whereas older patients tend to present with a combination of headache, vomiting, and ataxia.**
- **Papilledema, ataxia, and torticollis are also common.**

Cervicomedullary Tumors

In the past, radical surgery for intra-axial tumors of the cervicomedullary junction was not employed with any regularity because it was generally assumed that dissection in this eloquent area resulted in unacceptable morbidity and mortality. Because of this, radiation therapy (with or without biopsy) was considered the treatment of choice, and this usually resulted in transient remission of symptoms; however, progressive disability and death were considered inevitable.[22]

Epstein et al[22] in their initial experience with intrinsic tumors of the spinal cord and brain stem noted that in eight cases the neoplasm extended from the medulla to the cervical spinal cord. Preoperative clinical states were improved or stabilized following radical surgical excision. Five neoplasms were low-grade astrocytomas and three were gangliogliomas. The authors suggested, based on this experience, that cervicomedullary neoplasms were often benign and that an aggressive surgical approach can result in neurologic recovery and long-term survival with acceptable levels of morbidity and mortality. More recently, subtotal or even radical removal of cervicomedullary tumors has been shown to significantly improve the prognosis for long-term survival with a relatively good quality of life.[5, 21, 22, 34]

Cervicomedullary lesions typically involve the lower two-thirds of the medulla and the rostral segments of the spinal cord.[21] These cervicomedullary lesions commonly have an indolent clinical course, reflecting either medullary or cervical spinal cord dysfunction, and tend to arise in the upper cervical cord growing into the medulla in a posterior exophytic fashion.[22] *A subtype of the cervicomedullary tumor group has recently been identified that originates in the medulla and may infiltrate dorsally into the fourth ventricle and down to the cervical cord. This "medullary-cervical" subset of cervicomedullary tumors has a more malignant nature and behaves more like the intrinsic diffuse brain stem tumor.*[48]

Primary clinical manifestations are those that present with cranial nerve dysfunction or spinal cord dysfunction.[22, 34] Both groups have a particularly indolent course. Motor weakness and lower cranial nerve dysfunction, such as difficulty in swallowing, nasal speech, or chronic nausea, may be the first presenting signs of this tumor. Occasionally, intractable neck pain and torticollis are the only complaints. Symptoms are usually present for months to years prior to definitive diagnosis, reflecting the low-grade nature of these lesions. Hydrocephalus may occur if the rostral pole of the tumor obstructs the outlet of the fourth ventricle.

Epstein and Wisoff[22] identified a correlation between the primary clinical symptoms and the primary location of the neoplasm. Patients with lower cranial nerve dysfunction invariably had a noncystic medullary component of the neoplasm. In other patients with early spinal cord symptoms and/or neck pain, the solid part of the neoplasm was in the high cervical cord and was associated with an apparently nonneoplastic cyst, which "capped" the neoplasm and extended into the medulla.

NEURORADIOLOGIC FEATURES

MRI is the diagnostic study of choice for the evaluation of brain stem tumors. Tumors should be assessed for location, signal intensity, focality, extent of infiltration, degree of brain stem enlargement, presence or absence of a cyst, necrosis, hemorrhage, or exophytic components.[11] The density and enhancement characteristics can be diagnostic of the various tumor types.[4] Categorizing the tumor as focal, diffuse, cervicomedullary, or dorsally exophytic based on the MRI results when correlated with the clinical history is helpful in determining the prognosis and formulating a treatment plan.

MRI is more sensitive than CT at detecting more benign subgroups of brain stem tumors.[49] Frequently, MRI reveals brain stem gliomas to be more extensive than they appear to be on CT scans, and they often may be reclassified as diffuse tumors.[34, 50, 51] Epstein et al[28] retrospectively correlated the pathologic findings and MRI appearance of 88 brain stem gliomas. They propose that the growth of more benign gliomas of the brain stem is guided by secondary structures, such as the pia, fiber tracts, and the ependyma. This leads to stereotypical growth patterns that are clearly identified on magnetic resonance images and help clarify why cervicomedullary, dorsally exophytic, and focal tumors have a more favorable prognosis.[28]

Signal abnormalities in the brain stem are common in patients with neurofibromatosis, type 1 (NF-1). These lesions have a particularly indolent course and exhibit little if any tumor growth over time.[52, 53] Patients with such lesions require a more conservative approach to intervention than those without NF-1.[1, 54]

Diffuse Tumors

More recently with MRI a higher incidence of diffuse intrinsic brain stem tumors has been reported as compared with earlier

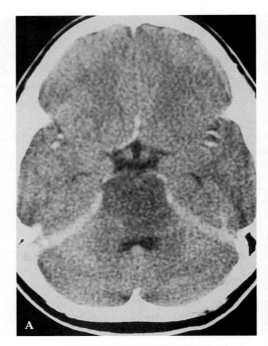
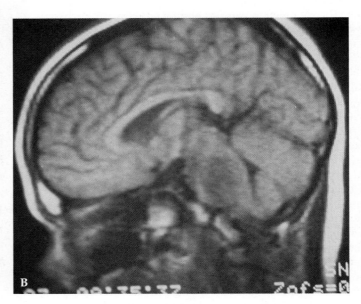

Figure 13–1 A diffuse intrinsic glioma involving the pons. (A) Unenhanced computed tomography (CT) scan showing a hypodense intrinsic brain stem tumor. (B) Sagittal T1-weighted magnetic resonance image showing a diffuse intrinsic mass expanding the pons with low signal intensity. The lesion showed irregular enhancement following the administration of gadolinium.

studies using CT.[49] Albright et al[33] found that 76% of their patients had tumors that were considered diffuse on MRI. Earlier reports using CT scans showed these tumors to compromise 14 to 36% of brain stem gliomas.[32] These tumors typically invade the surrounding brain stem extending up to the midbrain or down to the medulla and classically cause diffuse enlargement with ill-defined margins on imaging studies (Fig. 13–1). The surface of the brain stem may become irregu-

lar, and exophytic nodules may penetrate the pia and can encase or displace the basilar artery to one side (Fig. 13–2).[2, 55]

Despite anaplastic tendencies, they are usually hypodense on nonenhanced CT, rarely enhance with contrast, and show diffuse enlargement of the brain stem. Most diffuse brain stem gliomas have low signal intensity on T1-weighted images and high signal on T2-weighted sequences. The increased signal on T2-weighted sequences has been shown to represent infiltrating malignant tumor rather than edema.[16] Enhancement is variable and exophytic components are more likely to do so.[11] Regardless of treatment these patients do poorly and death ensues usually within 12 to 18 months. Thus, treatment for these patients is palliative.[4, 21, 33, 34]

Figure 13–2 Sagittal T1-weighted magnetic resonance image showing a diffuse intrinsic mass expanding the pons with mixed signal intensity. The surface of the brain stem is irregular, and exophytic nodules have penetrated the pia.

BOX 13–5
Neuroradiologic Features
of Diffuse Tumors

- Almost always involve the pons, with or without infiltration rostral to the midbrain or caudal extension to the medulla.
- CT shows diffuse enlargement of the brain stem, which is hypodense on nonenhanced study and rarely enhances with contrast.
- MRI characteristics are low signal intensity on T1-weighted images and high signal on T2-weighted sequence with variable enhancement of exophytic components.

Focal Tumors

Focal tumors of the brain stem can occur in the midbrain, pons, or medulla. They are usually solid but can be cystic. These tumors are usually hypodense on CT and will enhance with contrast administration. Occasionally, they may be isodense and show no enhancement. Cystic tumors usually have a contrast-enhancing cyst wall, rarely with a mural nodule component.[2] The T1- and T2-weighted images closely resemble each other in size, and the edges of the tumor are well defined. These tumors are usually low-grade astrocytomas and occasionally gangliogliomas.

Lesions involving the tectal plate or the tegmentum may extend upward to the thalamus or downward to the pons, displacing rather than infiltrating these structures.[20, 41] The majority of tumors in this area have a solid consistency with intense regular enhancement after intravenous contrast (Fig. 13–3). Cystic tumors may have intense rim enhancement after intravenous contrast.[41] In a series of 12 focal midbrain tumors, all of the tectal tumors were solid with intense regular enhancement, whereas 3 of the 6 tegmental tumors were cystic with intense rim enhancement after intravenous contrast.[20]

Tumors involving the tectal region commonly give rise to obstructive hydrocephalus. In a series of six patients, May et al[42] found that in six patients with tectal tumors, all had ventriculomegaly at the time of diagnosis, together with tectal distortion by a focal tectal mass, focal calcification, persistently abnormal MRI, and lack of growth of lesions over time. Increase in T2-weighted signal was seen in five cases involving the tectum and periaqueductal region, and the tectum alone in one case.

In the past, tectal gliomas have tended to be grouped with tumors that occur at closely adjacent sites such pineal, mid-

brain tegmentum, and rostral cerebellum.[40] This has occurred due to limitations in radiographic studies such as ventriculography, angiography, and even CT to provide adequate anatomical resolution.[47] Prior to MRI these lesions were not observed well on CT and were commonly labeled as late aqueductal stenosis. On CT it is not uncommon to find a central tectal calcification.[41, 42] The calcium usually produces reduction or loss of signal on both T1- and T2-weighted sequences, although the characteristics of its T1-weighted signal may be variable. Typical appearance of these lesions on MRI is a globular tectal mass that is isointense or hypointense in comparison with the surrounding brain on T1-weighted images, hyperintense on T2-weighted images, and devoid of enhancement.[15] The periaqueductal region commonly appears hyperintense on T2-weighted images (Fig. 13–4).[41] Tectal thickening may be caused by suprapineal recess enlargement associated with hydrocephalus alone, as well as by intrinsic mass lesions.[56, 57] Serial radiologic examinations reveal that small focal masses in the dorsal tectum do not progress in size in the majority of patients.[41, 42] Enhancement of benign tectal masses is uncommon and, if present, becomes less prominent over time as these lesions become progressively more calcified.[41, 42]

Differentiating benign from tumoral aqueductal stenosis by MRI can be difficult. The concept of distortion of the tectum by suprapineal recess enlargement in patients with benign aqueductal narrowing should be understood. In general, tectal gliomas are bulbous masses that can obstruct the aqueduct at any location. In contrast to benign aqueductal stenosis, the location of the obstruction is usually more specific.[57] Barkovich et al[57] found that among six patients with neoplastic stenosis of the aqueduct, all exhibited a bulbously enlarged tectum and

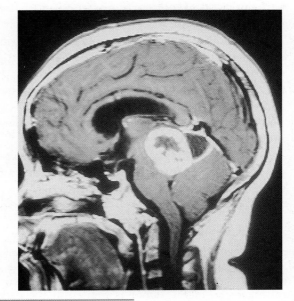

Figure 13–3 Magnetic resonance imaging (MRI) appearance of a large tectal glioma. Sagittal T1-weighted magnetic resonance image with gadolinium shows an enhancing tectal mass with a cystic component that is occluding the aqueduct of Sylvius.

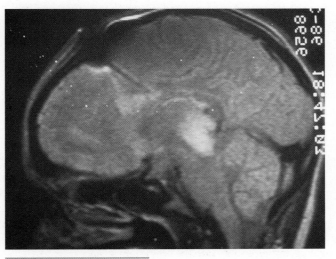

Figure 13–4 Sagittal magnetic resonance image showing a hyperintense mass involving the tectal and tegmental region.

prolonged T2 relaxation time as compared with normal brain tissue, whereas in 17 patients with benign aqueductal stenosis the location of the obstruction was more limited and the tectum, though sometimes appearing thickened, was never bulbous. Increased T2 signal occurred in only four patients with benign aqueductal stenosis, which was thought to possibly represent gliosis from previous infection or interstitial edema from transependymal cerebrospinal fluid (CSF) flow.

BOX 13–6
Neuroradiologic Features
of Focal Tumors

- A focal brain stem tumor is a circumscribed mass usually less than 2 cm in diameter without associated edema.
- Tumors can occur anywhere in the brain stem and may be solid or cystic.
- Solid tumors usually will be hypodense on CT and will contrast-enhance.
- Occasionally, solid tumors may be isodense and show no enhancement.
- Focal cystic tumors usually will have a contrast-enhancing cyst wall, rarely with a mural nodule component.
- The T1- and T2-weighted images on MRI closely resemble each other in size, and the edges of the tumor are well defined.
- On CT, tectal tumors may commonly have a central tectal calcification.
- Cystic tegmental tumors may have intense rim enhancement after intravenous contrast.
- Typical appearance of tectal tumors on MR images is a globular tectal mass that is isointense or hypointense in comparison to the surrounding brain on T1, with the tectal plate and periaqueductal region having hyperintensity on T2-weighted images usually devoid of enhancement.

Dorsally Exophytic Tumors

Dorsally exophytic tumors grow from the subependymal surface of the brain stem posteriorly into the fourth ventricle, causing relatively early obstruction of the ventricular system and symptomatic hydrocephalus.[25, 28] On CT these lesions are isodense or slightly hypodense and enhance brightly with contrast agent.[23–25] The tumor often largely obliterates the fourth ventricle on sagittal MRI, a cap of CSF is sometimes seen dorsally or at the rostral and caudal poles of the tumor. Ventrally the tumor blends imperceptibly into the brain stem surface (Fig. 13–5).[24]

The tumor will be hypointense on T1, hyperintense on T2, and will enhance. Sagittal MRI is helpful in establishing the exophytic nature of these tumors and the rostral and caudal extents of the mass. Exophytic tumors that grow in an anterolateral or posterolateral direction may have more malignant potential.[34]

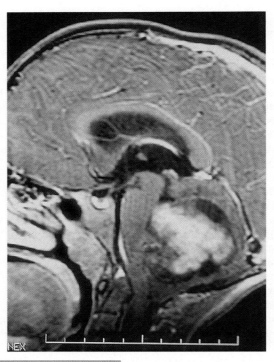

Figure 13–5   An enhancing dorsally exophytic tumor that fills the fourth ventricle. Note the lack of infiltration into the brain stem.

BOX 13–7
Neuroradiologic Features
of Dorsally Exophytic Tumors

- Grow from the subependymal surface of the brain stem posteriorly into the fourth ventricle and cause relatively early obstruction of the ventricular system.
- These tumors do not extend deeply into the brain stem; instead, they are exophytic into the fourth ventricle, often filling it with tumor.
- On CT they are isodense or slightly hypodense and enhance brightly with contrast agent.
- The tumor will be hypointense on T1 and hyperintense on T2 and will enhance.
- Sagittal MRI is helpful in establishing the exophytic nature of these tumors and identifying the rostral and caudal extents of the mass.

Cervicomedullary Tumors

Preoperative investigation of cervicomedullary tumors requires MRI. Sagittal images delineate the rostrocaudal boundaries of the mass and assess for associated cysts at those boundaries. Rostral extension of the tumor is limited at the cervicomedullary junction by decussating fibers.[28] The low-grade nature of these tumors results in displacement rather than infiltration of fiber tracts. This causes a posterior bulge at the level of the obex and results in some tumors erupting into the fourth ventricle, possibly causing hydrocephalus.[28]

Tumors may have mixed low or intermediate signal intensities within the solid component of the tumor and may enhance homogeneously or heterogeneously when intravenous gadolinium contrast is administered. The medullary component of the lesion may consist of a nonneoplastic cyst or may be noncystic. Epstein et al[22] found that in a series of 22 patients with cervicomedullary tumors, 8 patients had a medullary component of the lesion that consisted of a nonneoplastic cyst that extended from the rostral pole of the tumor. In 11 patients the medullary component of the neoplasm was noncystic or contained a small intratumoral cyst.

> ## BOX 13–8
> ## Neuroradiologic Features
> ## of Cervicomedullary Tumors
>
> - Typically involve the lower two-thirds of the medulla and the rostral segments of the spinal cord.
> - MRI typically show mixed low or intermediate signal intensities within the solid component of the tumor, which may enhance homogeneously or heterogenously when intravenous gadolinium contrast is administered.

SURGERY

The role of surgical intervention for brain stem gliomas is controversial but is becoming clearer with time. In the past, empirical treatment with steroids and irradiation were recommended for most brain stem tumors.[58, 59] Presently a more aggressive surgical approach has been shown to be of more benefit for the treatment of benign focal tumors, whereas palliative therapy is recommended for the treatment for diffuse intrinsic tumors.

With better imaging modalities and increased surgical experience with these tumors over the years, several authors have attempted to devise preoperative clinical and radiologic criteria to identify children that are likely to benefit from surgery.[4, 12, 21, 23, 34] Clinical correlates, such as duration of the disease, severity of neurologic deficits, in addition to MRI characteristics, are helpful in assessing the histologic grade of a brain stem lesion, categorizing the tumor and ultimately in establishing the therapeutic plan.[28]

Surgery for intrinsic brain stem tumors is only potentially beneficial for "benign" neoplasms.[14, 21, 34, 54] Surgery, if offered at all, should be done only when neurologic signs and symptoms and MRI results support the diagnosis of a focal and potentially benign tumor.[14, 32–34, 37, 60, 61] Pierre-Kahn et al[14] demonstrated the benefit of aggressive surgical removal in benign brain stem tumors.[14] Among his patients the 3-year actuarial survival rate increased from 52% after partial removal to 94% after total or subtotal removal. This 94% survival rate was much higher than the best reported rates of 58% at 5 years obtained by irradiation of low-grade gliomas.[62] Epstein and McCleary[21] presented their results of radical surgical excision of 34 intrinsic nonexophytic brain stem gliomas. While surgery was relatively well tolerated, it was apparent retrospectively that this therapy did not have a favorable impact on malignant tumors. Although transiently improved, all patients with malignant tumors succumbed to tumor progression within 6 to 9 months of surgery. Radical removal of benign neoplasms resulted in significant neurologic improvement and long-term clinical remission.

Some authors have advocated the importance of performing routine open or stereotactic biopsy of brain stem tumors to obtain an accurate pathologic diagnosis and to provide prognostic information before making treatment recommendations.[10, 16, 63, 64] This was especially common before the availability of MRI. Sampling error can be a significant factor, and when biopsy results show a low-grade neoplasm, the small amount of biopsy specimen obtained may not represent other areas of the neoplasm with more malignant histology.[21, 33] Thus treatment recommendations based on low-grade histologic biopsy specimens in patients with classic diffuse intrinsic brain stem tumors are not useful and do not alter the poor prognosis. The diagnostic specificity of MR scans when combined with the clinical history and examination identifies the diffuse intrinsic brain stem tumor and predicts a poor prognosis; biopsy should be deferred.

Advances in mapping and monitoring techniques have facilitated systematic approaches to surgery of the brain stem. Monitoring brain stem evoked potentials is valuable because the electrical activity becomes relatively disorganized as more normal neural tissue is approached.[22, 34] Motor nuclei can usually be located relative to specific anatomical landmarks on the ventricular floor; however, these landmarks are not evident in most patients because of the distorting effects of the tumor.[65]

In 1993, Strauss et al[66] introduced a method of neurophysiologic mapping of the facial colliculus and the nucleus of cranial nerve XII in patients with a variety of brain stem and cerebellar lesions. The method was performed successfully in 10 patients during surgery for brain stem lesions and the facial colliculus and the trigone of the hypoglossal nerve were reliably identified. Electrophysiologic identification of the facial colliculus guided the surgical approach into the brain stem in all cases. In three cases, instead of placing an incision at the level of maximum bulging, a different site was chosen because the facial colliculus was located at the maximum bulging site. In no case were complications observed relating to the seventh and underlying sixth nerve resulting from incision into the brain stem. More recent brain stem mapping techniques have been used to intraoperatively locate the facial colliculus and the motor nuclei of cranial nerves IX/X and XII on the floor of the fourth ventricle.[65–67]

Nuclear and infranuclear palsies are well-known complications of posterior fossa surgery in children. Cushing relates these injuries to contusions of cranial nerve nuclei on the floor of the fourth ventricle, which may occur during operative manipulation.[68] The region of the calamus scriptorius and facial colliculi is especially susceptible to cauterization, and injury to this area may result in bulbar cranial nerve dysfunction and ataxia.[69] Wisoff and Epstein[69] describe delayed onset of supranuclear cranial nerve palsies associated with emotional incontinence and lability that resolved over several weeks to months in seven patients. They feel retractor pressure on the medial cerebellum, and splitting of the vermis was the operative insult responsible for edema that subsequently tracked along fiber pathways in the middle and superior cerebellar peduncle into the upper pons and midbrain, causing delayed onset of pseudobulbar palsy. To avoid this complication, they recommend performing a limited resection of the medial 1 to 1.5 cm of cerebellar hemisphere overhanging the vermis to provide adequate exposure of large, deep midline vermian/fourth ventricular tumors and thereby eliminating the need for retraction.

Resection of brain stem tumors involving incision of the floor of the fourth ventricle may result in significant morbidity.[24, 34] The stria medullares forms the border between the rostral and caudal ventricular floors.[65] Areas above and below the facial colliculus in the rostral portion of the fourth ventricular floor above the stria medullares are areas that may be incised to provide passage to the upper brain stem.[70] Injury to areas below the stria medullares is associated with significant morbidity.[65] Mapping can help the surgeon understand the way in which the tumor distorts the brain stem anatomy. This information can help locate cranial nerve nuclei and determine the entry area before tumor resection, potentially avoiding unnecessary injury.[65]

Adequate exposure is essential to visualize surrounding structures that will help with orientation during resection. Tumor margins may not be clear, and changes in tissue characteristics may be subtle. Intraoperative ultrasonography is sometimes useful in delineating rostral and caudal boundaries of the tumor and presence or absence of associated cysts. Gentle packing and hemostatic agents should be used to control bleeding in the tumor cavity whenever possible rather than cautery to avoid unnecessary injury. Use of an ultrasonic surgical aspirator decreases excessive mobilization of normal brain during tumor removal and may decrease the intraoperative morbidity associated with brain stem surgery.[14, 71] All tissue removed with the ultrasonic aspirator may be collected and sent for histologic examination.

The availability of surgical adjuncts, such as the operating microscope, ultrasonic aspirators, frameless stereotactic guidance, intraoperative evoked potentials, and motor nuclei mapping, has made extensive removal of subsets of brain stem gliomas safer and more feasible.

Diffuse Tumors

Recent literature suggests that diffuse intrinsic brain stem tumors should not be biopsied and that extensive removal is not indicated.[21, 34, 72] Biopsy results are prone to sampling error and may fail to identify the malignant component of the tumor. Stereotactic biopsy is unreliable in determining the nature of the tumor or its prognosis.[2] Imaging characteristics on CT and MRI, along with the clinical course, are uniformly diagnostic of this dreadful tumor and obviate the need to operate on these sick children.[2, 34, 73] Attempts at radical removal are futile, and most patients die within 18 months of diagnosis.[5, 51]

BOX 13–9
Treatment/Outcome of Diffuse Tumors

- **Palliative therapy consisting of radiation therapy with or without chemotherapy.**
- **Biopsy should be deferred if clinical course and imaging are consistent with a diffuse intrinsic tumor.**
- **Current treatment for diffuse pontine glioma is ineffective, and death usually occurs within 2 years in 90 to 100% of patients.**

Focal Tumors

Children with focal low-grade tumors appear to benefit from extensive tumor removal.[16, 34] These focal tumors have an indolent course spanning many months to years, a focal neurologic exam, imaging consistent with a focal tumor, and no evidence of diffuse infiltration. A focal tumor with a limited clinical history, paucity of neurologic signs, and imaging that supports the diagnosis may be regarded as potentially benign and considered amenable to surgery. Surgery should be questioned and approached with caution in any patient with a short clinical history, bilateral cranial nerve dysfunction, and long-tract signs despite imaging that suggests a focal tumor.[4, 16, 21] Surgical procedures may be considered for patients with focal tumors, with or without associated cysts. Cystic astrocytomas of the brain stem with mural enhancing nodules and nonenhancing cyst walls are amenable to surgical resection and carry a good prognosis.[34] Several authors have reported on the successful outcome of cyst aspiration in patients with cystic tumors in the brain stem,[29, 64, 74] whereas an enhancing cyst wall may be more consistent with malignant glioma and a worse outcome.[34]

Stroink et al[4] in a series of 49 patients with brain stem tumors had 4 patients with cystic tumors of the brain stem with enhancing cyst walls. All patients presented with cranial nerve deficits and long-tract signs. All patients underwent surgical therapy for biopsy and drainage of the cyst. All patients did poorly, 2 of 4 patients had high-grade gliomas, 3 patients died, and 1 was doing poorly 8 months following surgery. Although patients with focal cystic brain stem tumors are amenable to cyst aspiration and surgical biopsy, patients with enhancing cyst wall usually have a poor outcome.

Tectal mass lesions manifest with a paucity of neurologic findings. Imaging exhibits a characteristic appearance and demonstrates indolent-growth characteristics. Therefore, biopsy of tectal mass lesions and radiotherapy are often deferred until there is clear-cut evidence of disease progression.[5, 41, 42] These patients are managed expectantly with CSF shunting or third ventriculostomy, and close follow-up monitoring.[2, 15, 42, 47] Wait-and-watch is a good rationale for these types of tumors.

Tumors of the cerebral peduncles are commonly low-grade astrocytomas.[5] They may be cystic or solid, but an attempt at removal is justified when the patient has progressive symptomatology from a mostly solid lesion.[5] Some have advocated stereotactic cyst aspiration for cystic lesions.[29, 76]

Laterally projecting tumors of the mid- and upper midbrain, cystic midbrain tumors, and intrinsic lesions of the tegmentum can be approached subtemporally.[34, 41, 54] Cystic cavities can be marsupialized to the subarachnoid space.[34] The tentorium can be incised to provide more exposure of the lateral midbrain if necessary. This approach provides excellent access to the tegmentum and cerebral peduncle.[41] Certain intrinsic lesions in the cerebellar peduncles are surgically resectable with acceptable morbidity and mortality.[75] Tomita[75] divides the cerebellar peduncle into three portions: brain stem, ventricular, and cerebellar. He describes a midline posterior fossa approach for lesions involving the ventricular or cerebellar portion of the cerebellar peduncle in four patients with no mortality and minimal morbidity. Tumors within the brainstem portion of the cerebellar peduncle are considered brain stem tumors.

The supracerebellar infratentorial approach is ideal for large tumors in the tectum that extend inferiorly to the posterior fossa, whereas an occipital transtentorial approach is useful for large tumors that extend posteriorly above the level of the tentorium. Limited tumor debulking or drainage of cystic components in patients with radiographic progressive disease can be performed using an infratentorial/supracerebellar approach or via transfrontal stereotactic biopsy, respectively.[76] In some patients a combination of the above approaches is used.

BOX 13–10
Treatment/Outcome of Focal Tumors

- **Benefited by extensive tumor removal. Focal solid tumors are treated by resection alone.**
- **Cystic astrocytomas of the brain stem with mural enhancing nodules and nonenhancing cyst walls are amenable to surgical resection and carry a good prognosis.**
- **Several authors have reported on the success of cyst aspiration in patients with cystic tumors the brain stem.**
- **Cystic tumors with enhancing cyst walls may have more malignant potential and require adjuvant therapy if malignant histology is found.**
- **Focal tectal tumors are managed expectantly with CSF shunting or third ventriculostomy, and close follow-up monitoring.**
- **Focal tectal tumors have a particularly indolent course and good long-term outcome.**
- **Adjuvant therapy is reserved for progressive or recurrent tectal tumors.**

Dorsally Exophytic Tumors

Dorsally exophytic brain stem tumors originate just below the ependymal surface of the floor of the fourth ventricle and penetrate into the brain stem minimally. As the tumor grows and fills the fourth ventricle, proximal hydrocephalus ensues. There is general agreement that these tumors are usually low grade and lend themselves to surgical treatment. Removal of the exophytic portion without aggressively entering the pons appears to be the appropriate therapy.

Dorsally exophytic brain stem tumors are approached via a midline suboccipital craniotomy. Occasionally, a C1 laminectomy is required to expose the lower pole of the tumor. The exophytic portion of the tumor typically splays apart the cerebellar tonsils; if possible, they are elevated to expose the rostral portion of the tumor. Otherwise, the vermis is split accordingly. It is helpful to identify the rostral and caudal extent of the tumor and floor of the fourth ventricle. Often there may be a cystic component at the rostral or caudal extents. The area of attachment of the exophytic component to the brain stem can then be identified. The tumor is aggressively debulked and then shaved to the level of the floor. No attempt is made to pursue it into the brain stem, thus avoiding potential injury to cranial nerve nuclei and fiber tracts.

Cervicomedullary Tumors

Because of the benign nature of lesions in this location, radical surgical resection is considered the primary treatment.[22, 34, 61, 77]

BOX 13–11
Treatment/Outcome of Dorsally Exophytic Tumors

- **Surgical treatment is warranted.**
- **Simply shaving off the exophytic portion without being aggressive with going into the pons appears to be the appropriate therapy.**
- **A second surgical procedure should be considered in cases of recurrence.**
- **Radiotherapy in general should be reserved for as long as possible. However, in cases where the pathology is malignant, radiotherapy is required.**
- **These tumors usually remain stable over time, and some may actually involute following surgical resection.**

Intraoperative monitoring of sensory evoked potentials and motor evoked potentials is an important adjunct to successful surgery.[65] Placement of a recording electrode on the rostral floor of the fourth ventricle allows for much faster updating of the averaged signals.[32] Epidural electrodes can be placed caudal to the tumor to pick up potentials evoked by transcranial stimulation of the motor cortex during surgery.[32, 65]

Surgery is carried out with the patient in the prone position. Surgical exposure is through a midline-incision, upper cervical laminectomy with or without a small suboccipital craniotomy. Transdural ultrasonography is helpful in identifying the rostrocaudal limits of the neoplasm and the presence or absence of associated cysts.[78] After the dura has been opened, a midline myelotomy is carried out over the entire length of the solid component of the neoplasm.[22] A cyst, if present, should be completely drained as it may contribute to the symptomatology.[34] The ultrasonic aspirator and surgical laser are helpful for central debulking. Ultrasonography can be used throughout the procedure to follow the extent of the resection and residual tumor.

BOX 13–12
Treatment/Outcome of Cervicomedullary Tumors

- **Early surgical intervention is warranted in cervicomedullary tumors prior to neurological, deterioration.**
- **Tumors arising at the cervicomedullary junction represent a more diverse array of pathology.**
- **The majority of tumors are benign and are amenable to surgical extrication with good results.**

NEUROPATHOLOGY

Diffuse intrinsic brain stem gliomas are the most common brain stem tumors in children. The differential diagnosis of lesions in the brain stem include more benign masses, such as low-grade astrocytomas and gangliogliomas, as well as nonglial tumors, such as ependymomas and primitive neuroectodermal tumors (PNETs), or even nontumoral lesions such as inflammation and hamartomas. Brain stem masses in patients with NF-1 tend to behave in a more benign fashion.[52] The classical history of brief clinical onset, multiple cranial nerve deficits, long-tract signs with MRI showing a diffuse mass enlarging the brain stem and increased signal on T2 surrounding the tumor is almost pathognomonic of a highly malignant diffuse brain stem glioma. The prognosis still remains poor despite the availability of multiple therapies. Autopsy reports confirm that the majority of diffuse intrinsic tumors of the pons are malignant, regardless of their histology on biopsy, and thus are reflected in their extremely poor survival rate.[41, 59] Histologic specimens of malignant brain stem tumors are often heterogeneous and often have areas of low-grade tumors adjacent to regions of glioblastoma. Specimens obtained by biopsy, whether open or stereotactic, are usually very small and may not be representative of the malignant component of the tumor. Unfortunately, the clinical course is essentially the same even if the histology is low-grade and is in most cases universally fatal. Epstein and McCleary[21] reported that 22 of 34 patients with intrinsic brain stem tumors had diffuse gliomas. All 22 patients had malignant gliomas grade III or IV on histologic examination and poor outcome. Other clinical series have reported similar findings that support this as well.[4, 12, 21, 34]

BOX 13–13
Differential Diagnosis of Brain Stem Lesions

- **Low-grade astrocytoma**
- **Ganglioglioma**
- **Ependymoma**
- **PNET**
- **Hamartoma**

In contrast to diffuse brain stem tumors, the majority of focal brain stem tumors are low grade in nature. In a total of 30 patients in two series with focal midbrain tumors the authors found that all focal tumors were fibrillary low-grade astrocytomas.[20, 41] Most small, intrinsic tectal tumors are of an astroglial origin, usually low-grade astrocytoma. These tumors typically have a particularly indolent course and remain stable in size over several years.[15, 40, 42, 43] Tumors of the cerebral peduncle frequently are low-grade astrocytomas and can often be surgically removed. It is not uncommon to find a large cyst associated with the lesion: drainage of the cyst and removal of the surrounding tumor tissue often gives relief of symptoms and long-term stability before further tumor growth occurs.[5]

Dorsally exophytic tumors are usually low-grade astrocytomas or gangliogliomas. In a series of 121 brain stem tumors, 10 patients were admitted with dorsally exophytic tumors, 8 had low-grade fibrillary astrocytomas, and 2 had benign gangliogliomas.[23] The low malignant potential of these lesions is illustrated by the low invasiveness of the tumor and the tendency to grow into the fourth ventricle.[28] Other series have also supported the benign histology in the majority of these lesions.[4, 23, 24]

Tumors at the cervicomedullary junction are usually histologically benign, and typically are low-grade astrocytomas, but do represent a wider spectrum of pathology. In a series presented by Epstein and Wisoff, it was found that 80% of cervicomedullary tumors were low-grade astrocytomas or gangliogliomas and were favorably affected by radical surgical excision. There were five grade I astro-

cytomas, six grade II astrocytomas, three gangliogliomas, two ependymomas, and four anaplastic tumors.[22] In another series, it was found that of 34 pediatric patients with brain stem tumors, 8 pa-tients were found to have cervicomedullary tumors, all of which were found to be low-grade astrocytomas.[21] Results of various series suggest that intrinsic tumors arising at the cervicomedullary junction represent a diverse array of pathology; the majority of such tumors are benign and amenable to surgical resection with good results.

ADJUNCTIVE THERAPY

Of all childhood tumors, diffuse intrinsic brain stem tumor remains one of the most resistant to therapy.[11, 21, 36] Despite this finding, the hallmark of treatment of diffuse intrinsic pontine gliomas remains radiation therapy. Despite a transient response to radiotherapy, most patients with diffuse tumors relapse, and death occurs within 2 years in 90 to 100% of patients after diagnosis.[5, 19, 72] Standard treatment for a diffuse tumor uses a total dose of 5400 cGy delivered in 30 fractions of 180 cGy. Higher total doses are limited by the tolerance of the normal surrounding brain.

In the past, radiotherapy was used routinely for most low-grade gliomas. Presently, subgroups of brain stem tumors, such as focal tumors of the midbrain and tectum, have been shown to have a particularly indolent and slow-growing course. In these instances, after subtotal removal or CSF diversion procedures alone, an expectant approach is taken and is often associated with a good long-term outcome.[20] Radiotherapy should be reserved for patients with progressive enlargement of residual tumor or tumors with histologic signs of malignancy.

In present-day management, it is recommended that dorsally exophytic tumors should undergo aggressive subtotal resection of the lesion. These patients do not require any further adjunctive therapy and have been known to survive for extended periods of time without evidence of tumor recurrence or progression. Radiotherapy should be limited to those patients with histologic signs of malignancy or those who develop recurrence of the tumor and for whom a second surgical procedure is not an option.[4, 24] Reoperation without any further adjunctive therapy is an option in patients with recurrence if the tumor regrowth took place over several years.[2, 24] Exophytic tumors that grow in an anterolateral or posterolateral direction may show more malignant potential and require adjunctive therapy if histologic signs of malignancy are found.[34]

Factors that play a role in biologic response to radiation include total dose, size, number of individual treatment fractions, overall treatment time, and volume irradiated.[79–81] *Radiation-induced tissue injury is a dose-related phenomenon.* The estimated incidence of radiation-induced tissue injury is below 5% for a dose of 5500 cGy at 180 to 200 cGy per fraction. The probability of radionecrosis increases with higher doses (more than 5500 cGy). Fraction size appears to be the dominant factor in influencing the frequency of posttreatment necrosis. The acceptable daily dose is considered to be 170 to 200 cGy. Tolerance of the brain to radiation therapy is also effected by age. In children younger than 2 years, brain tolerance is 10 to 20% lower.[82–86] The risk of radiation-induced tissue damage in the brain is less over the age of 2 with standard fractional dosage, but is increased by augmentation techniques of interstitial brachytherapy as well as chemotherapy.

Attempts to improve the results of external-beam radiotherapy include altered fractionation schedules, concomitant chemotherapy, and radiation sensitizers. *Hyperfractionation is the delivery of larger numbers of smaller fractions of radiotherapy over an equivalent period of time as standard treatment.* A typical hyperfractionation schedule employs a total dose of 7200 cGy delivered in 100-cGy doses twice a day.[18, 19] Preliminary data suggested that hyperfractionation would allow increased dose delivery without increased damage to surrounding brain tissue.[18, 19, 87] Unfortunately, phase III trials conducted by the Pediatric Oncology Group have shown no additional benefit.[88]

Angiogenesis inhibitors, radiation sensitizers, and concomitant high-dose chemotherapy remain interesting adjuncts to possibly improving the survival in these patients.[89–91] However, radiation therapy continues to be the primary modality of treatment for the majority of children with brain stem glioma, and there are no data to support the routine use of hyperfractionated radiotherapy.[92, 93] Stereotactic radiosurgery techniques and temporary and permanent brain implants (I-125, Ir-192, and Au-198) are being employed with moderate success in pediatric and adult populations.[73, 94–96]

Chemotherapy has become an integral part of the treatment in many forms of childhood brain cancer. Phase II trials using single agents and preradiotherapy chemotherapy have produced low response rates in the range of 15 to 20%.[97] High-dose chemotherapy with stem cell support has also met with disappointment.[97] One phase III trial conducted by the Children's Cancer Study Group[98] comparing radiotherapy with radiotherapy plus chemotherapy (CCNU, vincristine, and prednisone) failed to establish a benefit to multimodality therapy as compared with radiation alone. The overall 5-year survival rate was 20% and was not improved by adjuvant chemotherapy.[98] High-dose chemotherapy followed by autologous bone marrow infusion and involved field hyperfractionated radiation therapy also has not been shown to have any better survival than conventional therapy alone.[99]

Current studies include the use of radiosensitizing chemotherapy (carboplatin, estramustine, and cisplatin) and more intensive neoadjuvant chemotherapy trials.[97] Major advances in patient treatment await further insight into the molecular vulnerability of high-grade gliomas and new chemotherapeutic drugs with an improved spectrum of activity and diminished acute or chronic toxicity. At present, the effectiveness of chemotherapy in the treatment of brain stem gliomas in children is discouraging.

OUTCOME

Diffuse intrinsic tumors of the brain stem continue to carry a poor prognosis,[23, 24] *though up to 30% of patients with brain stem neoplasms continue to survive many years after diagnosis following radiotherapy.*[10, 12, 16, 58] The current treatment for diffuse pontine glioma is ineffective, and death usually occurs within 2 years in 90 to 100% of patients.[1, 72] Many patients have an initial period of radiologic and clinical improvement during and soon after radiotherapy. Follow-up MRI 4 to 6 weeks after treatment has shown dramatic regression in some cases.[87, 88] The incidence of central nervous system dissemination is 15 to 23% and is usually found on postmortem examination.[100] Packer and Allen et al. diagnosed meningeal gliomatosis ante mortem in 5 of 15 (33%) brain stem glioma patients. These patients developed an antemortem clinical syndrome of meningeal gliomatosis that manifested as local or radiating back pain, segmental weakness, paresthesias, and incontinence.[101]

True focal medullary tumors have little tendency to infiltrate; thus, incomplete resection is possible, with acceptable morbidity and mortality, and often leads to a marked clinical improvement and prolonged progression-free survival. In some cases, residual tumor has been reported to involute after surgery and cannot be demonstrated on follow-up imaging.[41] In one series of 12 focal midbrain tumors, Vandertop et al[20] reported that surgery was well tolerated, with no surgical mortality and minimal morbidity. All tumors were nonpilocytic, low-grade astrocytomas. Mean follow-up was 2.5 years, and all patients were alive and doing well.

The natural history of tumors of the tectal plate and their long-term potential for clinical and radiographic progression is becoming clearer. Hoffman et al[41] found that all patients with small, intrinsic tectal mass lesions treated with CSF diversion as the only treatment had no evidence of progression during a follow-up period of up to 18 years, suggesting that this group of lesions is truly benign. Pollack et al[15] reviewed their experience with 16 children diagnosed with late-onset aqueductal stenosis and intrinsic tectal tumors. All patients underwent CSF diversion initially, with conservative management of the tectal lesion and close long-term follow-up monitoring. Four children ultimately demonstrated clinical signs of progressive tumor growth with the onset of Parinaud's syndrome, despite the presence of a functioning shunt. Symptom progression had a median interval of 7.8 years from the time of shunt insertion and 11.5 years from the onset of initial symptoms and signs of hydrocephalus. All four patients with clinical evidence of disease progression were treated with conventional radiotherapy. One patient with an anaplastic astrocytoma received local stereotactic radiosurgery. These patients subsequently remained stable, with three showing tumor regression and one showing stable disease on serial MRI (median follow-up period from time of tumor progression was 4.25 years). May et al[42] found in a series of six patients with tectal tumors that all patients presented with raised intracranial pressure as a result of hydrocephalus due to obstruction of the sylvian aqueduct. Shunt placement was the only surgical procedure performed in all patients. No patient underwent radiotherapy, and there has been no evidence of progression in the follow-up period ranging from 8 months to 17 years. Five patients had normal intellectual development.

The vast majority of dorsally exophytic tumors are low-grade astrocytomas and gangliogliomas. These tumors remain stable over time, and some tumors may actually involute following surgical resection.[2] Pollack et al[24] reviewed their long-term results in 18 patients with dorsally exophytic brain stem gliomas. All patients underwent surgical intervention. There were no perioperative deaths; morbidity was generally limited to transient exacerbation of preoperative ataxia, dysmetria, nystagmus, and cranial nerve deficits (particularly sixth- and seventh-nerve paresis). Seventeen patients were alive at a mean follow-up time of 110 months (range 33 to 212 months). One child died of a shunt malfunction at another hospital. Two patients received postoperative radiotherapy and had had no evidence of residual disease on follow-up imaging 61 and 135 months after surgery. At the conclusion of the study, 15 children had follow-up radiographic evaluation; of there, 3 had complete disappearance of the residual tumor, 8 had stable residual disease, and 4 had obvious tumor regrowth (mean time to recurrence was 41 months after surgery). A second operation was performed in all patients with recurrent tumor and was well tolerated. Hoffman et al[23] found that subtotal resection of dorsally exophytic brain stem tumors was extremely successful; the longest surviving patient was still alive 15 years after treatment. Two patients were alive and well 7 and 8 years after operation and radiotherapy. Five patients who did not receive radiotherapy have been followed for 1 to 5 years; none have had clinical or radiographic evidence of tumor growth. Other series support similar findings that subtotal surgical resection provides most patients with excellent outcome, and in some cases the residual tumor may involute on follow-up imaging.[4] Tumors that demonstrate recurrence are amenable to a second attempt at radical tumor excision. Radiotherapy should be deferred for as long as possible.

Epstein and Wisoff[22] operated on 20 patients with cervicomedullary tumors. There were no surgical mortalities, but the following morbidity was reported: one patient had a sleep apnea syndrome, three had impaired position sense in the upper extremities, and six had transient weakness and spasticity in the lower extremities postoperatively. One patient was moderately disabled preoperatively and became quadriplegic postoperatively. They found that postoperative neurologic recovery was directly related to the preoperative neurologic status and that an aggressive surgical approach offers potential for both neurologic recovery and long-term survival. In a series of 17 children who underwent surgical resection of intra-axial cervicomedullary tumors, surgery was well tolerated, and the 4-year progression-free and total survival rates for patients who had surgery for cervicomedullary tumors as initial therapy were 70% and 100%, respectively.[102] In another series, Weiner et al[103] found that the overall 5-year progression-free and total survivals were 60% and 89%, respectively. They also noted a trend for preoperative neurologic grade to predict functional neurologic outcome at follow-up. Early surgical intervention is warranted in cervicomedullary tumors prior to neurologic deterioration. Medullary-cervical tumors represent a subset of cervicomedullary tumors that originate in the medulla and may infiltrate dorsally into the fourth ventricle and down to the cervical cord. These tumors behave in a manner similar to that of diffuse intrinsic brain stem tumors.[48]

SUMMARY

Diffuse brain stem gliomas are a relatively common form of childhood tumor that remain highly resistant to therapy. The development of MRI has mode possible detailed visualization of tumors within the brain stem. Imaging information combined with the clinical history and neurologic examination allows for a more refined subcategorization of such tumors and delineation of children who might benefit from surgery. Surgical candidates include children with long clinical histories and focal neurologic deficits. Imaging should be consistent with focal, solid or cystic, dorsally exophytic, or cervicomedullary tumors. The majority of these tumors are amenable to surgical treatment and carry a good prognosis.

Serial studies show a poor prognosis for diffuse pontine gliomas, with better outcomes for dorsally exophytic tumors, most focal midbrain tumors, and cervicomedullary tumors. Routine biopsy of the "classic" diffuse intrinsic brain stem tumor should be considered a thing of the past. The optimal management of children with brain tumors remains a multidisciplinary approach. Improved outlook for children with brain stem gliomas will require further research in tumor neurobiology and new therapeutic modalities.

REFERENCES

1. Shuper A, Kornreich L, Loven D, et al. Diffuse brain stem gliomas. are we improving outcome? *Child's Nerv Syst* 1998;14:578–581.
2. Hoffman HJ, Goumnerova L. Pediatric brain stem gliomas. In: Wilkins RH, Rengachary SS, eds. *Neurosurgery.* 2nd ed. New York: McGraw-Hill; 1996:1183–1194.
3. Bruno L, Schut L. Survey of pediatric brain tumors. In: American Association of Neurological Surgeons, ed. *Pediatric Neurosurgery: Surgery of the Developing Nervous System.* New York: Grune and Stratton; 1982:361–365.
4. Stroink AR, Hoffman HJ, Hendrick EB, et al. Diagnosis and management of pediatric brain-stem gliomas. *J Neurosurg* 1986;65:745–750.
5. Walker ML, Emadian SM, Honeycutt JH Jr. Diagnosis and management of primary pediatric brain tumors. In: Grossman RG, Loftus CM, ed. *Principals of Neurosurgery.* 2nd ed. Philadelphia: Lippincott-Raven Publishers; 1999: 33–46.
6. Panitch HS, Berg BO. Brainstem tumors of childhood and adolescence. *Am J Dis Child* 1970;119:465–472.
7. Schoenberg BS, Schoenberg DG, Christine BW, et al. The epidemiology of primary intracranial neoplasms of childhood: a population based study. *Mayo Clin Proc* 1976;51:51–56.
8. Farwell JR, Dohrmann GJ, Flannery JT. Central nervous system tumors in children. *Cancer* 1977;40:3123–3132.
9. Koos WT, Miller MH. *Intracranial Tumors of Infants and Children.* St Louis: CV Mosby; 1971:346–350.
10. Albright AL, Price RA, Guthkelch AN. Brainstem gliomas of children: a clinicopathological study. *Cancer* 1983;52: 2313–2319.
11. Packer RJ, Nicholson SH, Vezina LG, et al. Brainstem gliomas. *Neurosurg Clin North Am* 1992;3:863–879.
12. Berger MS, Edwards MS, LeMasters D, et al. Pediatric brain stem tumors: radiographic, pathological and clinical correlations. *Neurosurgery* 1983;12:298–302.
13. Littman P, Jarrett P, Bilaniuk LT, et al. Pediatric brainstem gliomas. *Cancer* 1980;45:2787–2792.
14. Pierre-Kahn A, Hirsch JF, Vinchon M, et al. Surgical management of brain-stem tumors in children: results and statistical analysis of 75 cases. *J Neurosurg* 1993;79:845–852.
15. Pollack IF, Dachling P, Albright AL. The long-term outcome in children with late-onset aqueductal stenosis resulting from benign intrinsic tectal tumors. *J Neurosurg* 1994;80:681–688.
16. Albright AL, Guthkelch AN, Packer RJ, et al. Prognostic factors in pediatric brain-stem gliomas. *J Neurosurg* 1986;65:751–755.
17. Cohen M, Duffner P, Heffner R, et al. Prognostic factors in brainstem gliomas. *Neurology* 1986;36:602–605.
18. Edwards MSB, Wara WM, Urtansun RC, et al. Hyperfractionated radiation therapy for brain-stem glioma: a phase I-II trial. *J Neurosurg* 1989;70:691–700.
19. Packer RJ, Allen JC, Goldwein JL, et al. Hyperfractionated radiotherapy for children with brain stem gliomas: a pilot study using 7,200 cGy. *Ann Neurol* 1990;27:167–173.
20. Vandertop WP, Hoffman HJ, Drake JM, et al. Focal midbrain tumors in children. *Neurosurgery* 1992;31:186–194.
21. Epstein F, McCleary EL. Intrinsic brain-stem tumors of childhood: surgical indications. *J Neurosurg* 1986;64:11–15.
22. Epstein F, Wisoff J. Intra-axial tumors of the cervicomedullary junction. *J Neurosurg* 1987;67:483–487.
23. Hoffman HJ, Becker L, Craven MA. A clinically and pathologically distinct group of benign brain stem gliomas. *Neurosurgery* 1980;7:243–248.

24. Pollack IF, Hoffman HJ, Humphreys RP, et al. The long-term outcome after surgical treatment of dorsally exophytic brain-stem gliomas. *J Neurosurg* 1993;78:859–863.
25. Stroink AR, Hoffman HJ, Hendrick EB, et al. Transependymal benign dorsally exophytic brain stem gliomas in childhood: diagnosis and treatment recommendations. *Neurosurgery* 1987;20:439–444.
26. Pool JL. Gliomas in the region of the brain stem. *J Neurosurg* 1968;29:164–167.
27. Tomita T, Radkowski M, Cheddia A. Brain stem tumors in childhood. *Concepts Pediatr Neurosurg* 1990;10:78–96.
28. Epstein FJ, Farmer JP. Brain-stem glioma growth patterns. *J Neurosurg* 1993;78:408–412.
29. Lassiter KRL, Alexander E Jr, Davis CH Jr, et al. Surgical treatment of brainstem gliomas. *J Neurosurg* 1971;34:719–725.
30. Grigsby PW, Thomas PRM, Schwartz HG, et al. Irradiation of primary thalamic and brain stem tumors in a pediatric population: a 33-year experience. *Cancer* 1987;60:2901–2906.
31. Hoffman HJ, Stroink AR, Davidson G, et al. Pediatric brain stem gliomas: evaluation of biopsy. *Concepts Pediatr Neurosurg* 1987;7:105–116.
32. Abbott R, Ragheb J, Epstein FJ. Brainstem tumors: surgical indications. In: Cheek WR, ed. *Pediatric Neurosurgery: Surgery of the Developing Nervous System*. 3rd ed. Philadelphia: WB Saunders; 1994:374–382.
33. Albright AL, Packer RJ, Zimmerman R, et al. Magnetic resonance scans should replace biopsies for the diagnosis of diffuse brain stem gliomas: a report from the Children's Cancer Group. *Neurosurgery* 1993;33:1026–1030.
34. Epstein F, Wisoff JH. Surgical management of brainstem tumors of childhood and adolescence. *Neurosurg Clin North Am* 1990;1:111–121.
35. Sanford RA, Freeman CR, Burger P, et al. Prognostic criteria for experimental protocols in pediatric brainstem gliomas. *Surg Neurol* 1988;30:276–280.
36. Barkovich AJ, Krischner J, Kun LE, et al. The characteristics of brainstem gliomas: correlation with survival statistics in a three-center study. *Pediatr Neurosurg* 1991;16:73–83.
37. Packer RJ, Nicholson HS, Johnson DL, et al. Dilemmas in the management of childhood brain tumors: brainstem glioma. *Pediatr Neurosurg* 1991–92;17:37–43.
38. Sanford RA, Bebin J, Smith RW. Pencil gliomas of the aqueduct of Sylvius: report of two cases. *J Neurosurg* 1982;57:690–696.
39. Kernohan WJ, Sayre GS. *Tumors of the Central Nervous System. Atlas of Tumor Pathology*. Section 10, Fascicle 35. Washington, DC: Armed Forces Institute of Pathology; 1952:19–42.
40. Chapman PH. Indolent gliomas of the midbrain tectum. *Concepts Pediatr Neurosurg* 1990;10:97–107.
41. Hoffman HJ, Vandertoop WP. Tumors of the midbrain. *Neurosurg Clin North Am* 1993;4:537–542.
42. May PL, Blaser SI, Hoffman HJ, et al. Benign intrinsic tectal "tumors" in children. *J Neurosurg* 1991;74:867–871.
43. Boydston WR, Sanford RA, Muhlbauer MS, et al. Gliomas of the tectum and periaqueductal region of the mesencephalon. *Pediatr Neurosurg* 1991–1992;17:234–238.
44. Sheldon WD, Parker HL, Kernohan JW. Occlusion of the aqueduct of sylvius. *Arch Neurol Psychiatry* 1930;23:1183–1202.
45. Steinbok P, Boyd CM. Periaqueductal tumor as a cause of late-onset aqueductal stenosis. *Childs Nerv Syst* 1987;3:170–174.
46. Stookey B, Scarff JE. Occlusion of the aqueduct of Sylvius by neoplastic and non-neoplastic processes with a ratio-nal surgical treatment for relief of resultant obstructive hydrocephalus. *Bull Neurol Inst NY* 1936;5:348–377.
47. Raffel C, Hudgins R, Edwards MSB. Symptomatic hydrocephalus: initial findings in brainstem gliomas not detected on computer tomography scans. *Pediatrics* 1988;82:733–737.
48. Squires LA, Constantini S, Miller DC, et al. Diffuse infiltrating astrocytoma of the cervicomedullary region: clinicopathologic entity. *Pediatr Neurosurg* 1997;27:153–159.
49. Smith RR, Zimmerman RA, Packer RJ, et al. Pediatric brainstem glioma: post-radiation clinical and radiographic follow-up. *Neuroradiology* 1990;32:265–271.
50. Packer RJ, Zimmerman RA, Luerssen TG, et al. Brain stem gliomas of childhood: magnetic resonance imaging. *Neurology* 1985;35:397–401.
51. Epstein F, Wisoff JH. Intrinsic brain stem tumors in childhood: surgical indications. *J Neuro-oncol* 1988;6:309–317.
52. Millstein JM, Geyer JR, Berger MS, et al. Favorable prognosis for brainstem gliomas in neurofibromatosis. *J Neuro-oncol* 1989;7:367–371.
53. Raffel C, McComb G, Bodner S, et al. Benign brain stem lesions in pediatric patients with neurofibromatosis: case reports. *Neurosurgery* 1989;25:959–964.
54. Abbott R, Goh KYC. Brain stem gliomas. In: Albright AL, Pollack IF, Adelson DP, ed. *Principles and Practices of Pediatric Neurosurgery*. New York: Thieme Medical Publishers; 1999:629–640.
55. Mantravardi RVP, Phatak R, Bellur S, et al. Brainstem glioma: an autopsy study of 25 cases. *Cancer* 1982;49: 1294–1296.
56. Sherman JL, Citrin CM, Barkovich AJ, et al. MR imaging of the mesencephalic tectum: normal and pathologic variations. *Am J Neuroradiol* 1987;8:59–64.
57. Barkovich AJ, Newton TH. MR of aqueductal stenosis: evidence of a broad spectrum of tectal distortion. *Am J Neuroradiol* 1989;10:471–476.
58. Tokuriki Y, Handa H, Yamoshita J, et al. Brainstem glioma: an analysis of 85 cases. *Acta Neurochir (Wein)* 1986; 79:67–73.
59. Tomita T, McClone DG, Nadich TP. Brain stem gliomas in childhood: rational approach and treatment. *J Neuro-oncol* 1981;2:117–122.
60. Albright AL. Brain stem gliomas. In: Youmans JR, ed. *Neurological Surgery: A Comprehensive Reference Guide to the Diagnosis and Management of Neurosurgical Problems*. 4th ed. Vol. 4. Philadelphia: WB Saunders; 1996: 2603–2611.
61. Epstein F, Constantini S. Practical decisions in the treatment of pediatric brain stem tumors. *Pediatr Neurosurg* 1996;24:24–34.
62. Mundinger F, Braus DF, Krauss JK, et al. Long-term outcome of 89 low-grade brain-stem gliomas after interstitial radiation therapy. *J Neurosurg* 1991;75:740–746.
63. Hood TW, Gebarski SS, McKeever PE, et al. Stereotactic biopsy of intrinsic lesions of the brain stem. *J Neurosurg* 1986;65:172–176.
64. Reigel DH, Scarff TB, Woodford JE. Biopsy of pediatric brain stem tumors. *Child's Brain* 1979;5:329–340.
65. Morota N, Deletis V, Epstein FJ, et al. Brain stem mapping: neurophysiological localization of motor nuclei on the floor of the fourth ventricle. *Neurosurgery* 1995;37: 922–930.
66. Strauss C, Romstöck J, Nimsky C, et al. Intraoperative identification of motor areas of the rhomboid fossa using direct stimulation. *J Neurosurg* 1993;79:393–399.
67. Bricolo A, Turazzi S. Surgery for gliomas and other mass lesions. In: Symon L, ed. *Advances and Technical Standards in Neurosurgery*, Vol. 22. New York: Springer-Verlag; 1995:261–342.

68. Cushing H. The intracranial tumors of preadolescence. *Am J Dis Child* 1927;33:551–584.

69. Wisoff JH, Epstein FJ. Pseudobulbar palsy after posterior fossa operation in children. *Neurosurgery* 1984;15:707–709.

70. Kyoshima K, Kobayashi S, Gibo H, et al. A study of safe entry zones via the floor of the fourth ventricle for brain-stem lesions: report of three cases. *J Neurosurg* 1993;78: 987–993.

71. Albright AL, Sclabassi RJ. Use of the cavitron ultrasonic surgical aspirator and evoked potentials for the treatment of thalamic and brain stem tumors in children. *Neurosurgery* 1985;17:564–568.

72. Chuba PJ, Zamarano L, Hamre M, et al. Permanent I-125 brain stem implants in children. *Child's Nerv Syst* 1998; 14:570–577.

73. Steck J, Friedman WA. Stereotactic biopsy of brainstem mass lesions. *Surg Neurol* 1995;43:563–568.

74. Kruyff E, Munn JD. Posterior fossa tumors in infants and children. *AJR Am J Roentgenol* 1963;89:951–965.

75. Tomita T. Surgical management of cerebellar peduncle lesions in children. *Neurosurgery* 1986;18:568–575.

76. Coffey RJ, Lunsford LD. Stereotactic surgery for mass lesions of the midbrain and pons. *Neurosurgery* 1985; 17:12–18.

77. Abbott R. Tumors of the medulla. *Neurosurg Clin North Am* 1993;4:519–528.

78. Epstein F, Wisoff J. Spinal cord astrocytomas of childhood: surgical considerations. In: Long DM, ed. *Current Therapy in Neurological Surgery*. Philadelphia: BC Decker; 1984:159–161.

79. Gttoothuis DR, Vick NA. Radionecrosis of the central nervous system: the perspective of the clinical neurologist and neuropathologist. In: Gilbert HA, Kagen AR, eds. *Radiation Damage to the Nervous System*. New York: Raven Press; 1980:83–106.

80. Safdari H, Fluentes JM, Dubois JB, et al. Radiation necrosis of the brain: time of onset and incidence related to total dose and fractionation of radiation. *Neuroradiology* 1985;27:44–47.

81. Kaufman M, Swartz BE, Mandelkern M, et al. Diagnosis of delayed cerebral radiation necrosis following proton beam therapy. *Arch Neurol* 1990;47:474–476.

82. Yamashita J, Handa H, Yumitori K, et al. Reversible delayed radiation effect on the brain after radiotherapy of malignant astrocytoma. *Surg Neurol* 1980;13:413–417.

83. Woo E, Lam K, Lee PW, et al. Cerebral radionecrosis: is surgery necessary? *J Neurol Neurosurg Psychiaty* 1987;50: 1407–1414.

84. Safdari H, Bouluix B, Gros C. Multifocal brain radionecrosis masquerading as tumor dissemination. *Surg Neurol* 1984;21:35–41.

85. Leibel SA, Sheline GE. Radiation therapy for the neoplasms of the brain. *J Neurosurg* 1987;66:1–22.

86. Sheline GE. Irradiation injury of the human brain: a review of clinical experience. In: Gilbert HA, Kagen AR, eds. *Radiation Damage to the Human Nervous System*. New York: Raven Press; 1980:39–58.

87. Freeman CR, Krischer, Sanford RA, et al. Hyperfractionated radiotherapy in brain stem tumors: results of a Pediatric Oncology Group study. *Int J Radiat Oncol Biol Phys* 1988;15:311–318.

88. Mandell L, Kadota R, Douglass EC, et al. Is it time to rethink the role of hyperfractionated radiotherapy in the management of children with newly diagnosed brainstem glioma? Results of a pediatric oncology group phase III trial comparing conventional vs hyperfractionated radiotherapy. Proceedings of the 39th Annual ASTRO Meeting, Orlando, FL, 19–23 October 1997. *Int J Radiat Oncol Biol Phys* 1997;39:143.

89. Wesseling P, Ruiter DJ, Burger PC. Angiogenesis in brain tumors: pathobiological and clinical aspects. *J Neuro-oncol* 1997;32:253–265.

90. Graham ML, Herndon JE II, Casey JR, et al. High-dose chemotherapy with autologous stem-cell rescue in patients with recurrent and high-risk pediatric brain tumors. *J Clin Oncol* 1997;15:1814–1823.

91. Dutton SC, Pomeroy SL, Billett AL, et al. A phase I trial of etanidazole and hyperfractionated radiotherapy in children with diffuse brain stem glioma. Proceedings of the 39th Annual ASTRO Meeting, Orlando, Florida, 19-23 October 1997. *Int J Radiat Oncol Biol Phys* 1997;39:333.

92. Fallai C, Olmi P. Hyperfractionated and accelerated radiation therapy in central nervous system tumors (malignant gliomas, pediatric tumors, and brain metastases). *Radiother Oncol* 1997;43:235–246.

93. Botturi M, Fariselli L. Clinical results of unconventional fractionation radiotherapy in central nervous system tumors. *Tumori* 1998;84:176–187.

94. Gutin PH, Edwards MSB, Wara WM, et al. Preliminary experience with 125-I brachytherapy of pediatric brain tumors. *Concepts Pediatr Neurosurg* 1985;5:187–206.

95. Gutin PH, Leibel SA, Wara WM, et al. Recurrent malignant glioma: survival following interstitial brachytherapy with high activity iodine-125 sources. *J Neurosurg* 1987;67:864–873.

96. Leibel SA, Gutin PH, Wara WM. Survival and quality of life after interstitial implantation of removable high-activity iodine-125 sources for the treatment of patients with recurrent malignant gliomas. *Int J Radiat Oncol* 1990;17:1129–1139.

97. Allen JC, Siffert J. Contemporary chemotherapy issues for children with brain stem gliomas. *Pediatr Neurosurg* 1996;24:98–102.

98. Derek R, Jenkin MB, Boesel L, et al. Brain-stem tumors in childhood: a prospective randomized trial of irradiation with and without adjuvant CCNU, VCR, and prednisone. A report of the Children's Cancer Study Group. *J Neurosurg* 1987;66:227–233.

99. Kedar A, Maria BL, Graham-Pole J, Ringdahl DM, et al. High-dose chemotherapy with marrow reinfusion and hyperfractionated irradiation for children with high-risk brain tumors. *Med Pediatr Oncol* 1994;23: 428–436.

100. Yung WA, Horten BC, Shapiro WR. Meningeal gliomatosis: a review of 12 cases. *Ann Neurol* 1980;8:605–608.

101. Packer RJ, Allen J, Nielsen S, et al. Brainstem glioma: clinical manifestations of meningeal gliomatosis. *Ann Neurol* 1983;14:177–182.

102. Robertson PL, Allen JC, Abbott IR, et al. Cervico-medullary tumors in children: a distinct subset of brain stem gliomas. *Neurology* 1994;44:1798–1803.

103. Weiner HL, Freed D, Woo HH, et al. Intra-axial tumors of the cervicomedullary junction: surgical results and long-term outcome. *Pediatr Neurosurg* 1997;27:12–18.

Chapter 14

Supratentorial Astrocytoma

Philip V. Theodosopoulos and Mitchel S. Berger

Primary brain tumors are the most common pediatric solid tumors and, second to the leukemias, the most common form of cancer occurring in children.[1, 2] The annual incidence of primary pediatric brain tumors is 2.4 in every 100,000 children. Thirty percent of these tumors are supratentorial, and the number increases to 55% in children younger than 2 years. Approximately 60 to 75% of all pediatric brain tumors are of glial origin.[2] Supratentorial astrocytomas account for 35% of all pediatric primary brain tumors. Unlike the distribution of astrocytoma subtypes in the adult population, low-grade astrocytomas are more common among children than high-grade astrocytomas.[1] Only 11% of pediatric brain tumors are high-grade supratentorial astrocytomas.

Supratentorial astrocytomas usually present with headache, seizures, and papilledema and occasionally with weakness.[3–6] When they involve the optic pathway and diencephalon, visual changes and endocrinologic dysfunction account for the majority of presenting symptoms.[7] Strabismus, proptosis, and nystagmus are common. Spasms nutans and diencephalic syndrome, with failure to thrive despite adequate intake, euphoria, and hyperactivity, are characteristic of lesions of the optic chiasm and the diencephalon.[5]

BOX 14–1
Presenting Signs and Symptoms

- **Headaches**
- **Seizures**
- **Papilledema**
- **Weakness**
- **Visual changes**
- **Endocrine dysfunction**
- **Failure to thrive**

HISTOPATHOLOGIC CLASSIFICATION

The different subtypes of tumors of astrocytic origin are classified according to their histologic, macroscopic, and clinical characteristics. Several different grading systems for astrocytomas exist. According to the most recent recommendations of the World Health Organization (WHO), there are four grades of astrocytoma malignancy, with differentiation depending on indicators of anaplasia, including nuclear atypia, mitotic activity, presence of necrosis, and vascular proliferation[8] (Table 14–1).

TABLE 14–1   WHO and St. Anne-Mayo Astrocytic Tumor Grading System

WHO grade	WHO designation	St. Anne-Mayo designation	St. Anne-Mayo criteria
1	Pilocytic astrocytoma	—	—
2	Astrocytoma (low-grade diffuse)	Astrocyloma grade 1 Astrocytoma grade 2	Zero criterion One criterion, usually nuclear atypia
3	Anaplastic astrocytoma	Astrocytoma grade 3	Two criteria, usually nuclear atypia and mitotic activity
4	Glioblastoma multiforme	Astrocytoma grade 4	Three criteria, usually nuclear atypia, mitoses, endothelial proliferation and/or necrosis

Data from Kleihues P, Cavenee, KW, eds. *Pathology and Genetics: Tumours of the Nervous System.* Lyon: International Agency for Research on Cancer; 1997:2.

The authors thank Richard Davis, M.D. and Nancy Fishbein, M.D. for their generous assistance with chapter figures.

BOX 14–2
Indications of Anaplasia

- **Nuclear atypia**
- **Mitotic activity**
- **Necrosis**
- **Vascular proliferation**

Diffuse Astrocytoma

Diffuse astrocytomas are the most common of all astrocytic tumors. They may arise anywhere in the central nervous system and can be highly infiltrative. These tumors have a propensity to undergo malignant transformation. According to the WHO grading system, they are classified as low grade, anaplastic, or glioblastoma multiforme.

Low-grade diffuse astrocytomas appear macroscopically to be infiltrative, with some blurring of the gross anatomical boundaries and usually little mass effect. Their histologic characteristics include the presence of few reactive astrocytes, a mild increase in cellularity, and monotonous nuclei (Fig. 14–1). *Subtypes include fibrillary astrocytomas, which most often have scant cytoplasm and mucin-filled microcysts, and gemistocytic astrocytomas, which have a predominance of astrocytes with eosinophilic cytoplasm positioned in the middle of a coarse fibrillary network.*

Macroscopically, anaplastic astrocytomas are not substantially different from low-grade astrocytomas. However, histologically they present with increased cellularity, increased nuclear atypia, presence of mitoses, increased number of gemistocytes, and, in some cases, a proliferation of tumor blood vessels (Fig. 14–2).

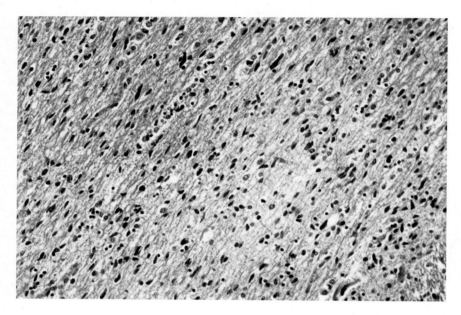

Figure 14–1 Infiltrating grade 2 astrocytoma in white-matter tracts. There is little nuclear pleomorphism, but mainly an increase in cellularity of the elongated nuclei. Original magnification × 10.

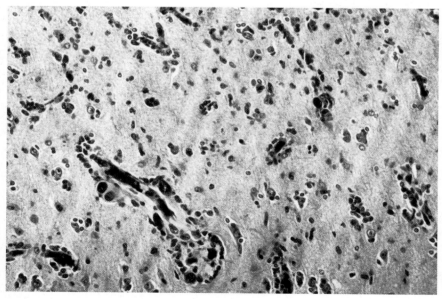

Figure 14–2 Infiltrating grade 3 astrocytoma in cortex. There is neuronal neoplastic satellitosis and cuffing of small blood vessels by pleomorphic tumor cells. Original magnification × 10.

Glioblastomas multiforme have obvious macroscopic invasion of neighboring structures and frequently have extension to both hemispheres. Histologically there is markedly increased cellularity, regional heterogeneity, vascular proliferation, and necrosis. Hallmarks also include multinucleated giant cells and perivascular cuffing.

Pilocytic Astrocytoma

Pilocytic astrocytomas are low-grade tumors that usually arise in the optic pathway, hypothalamus, basal ganglia, or cerebral hemispheres. Macroscopically they are well circumscribed.[4] Histologically they have a characteristic biphasic pattern of compact areas that stain for glial fibrillary acidic protein (GFAP) and microcystic areas that do not. They have uniform cell types, Rosenthal fibers, and characteristic eosinophilic granular bodies (Fig. 14–3).

BOX 14–3
Common Locations
of Pilocytic Astrocytoma

- Optic pathway
- Hypothalamus
- Basal ganglia
- Cerebral hemispheres

Pleomorphic Xanthoastrocytoma

Pleomorphic xanthoastrocytoma was only recently identified as an individual subtype of astrocytoma. Between 1979 and 1994, 79 cases of pleomorphic xanthoastrocytoma were reported.[9] These tumors usually present during a child's second decade of life after a long, symptomatic course,

most often characterized by seizures. Macroscopically they are firm, rubbery, well-circumscribed masses located superficially and associated with cysts containing xanthochromic fluid. Often they have meningeal involvement. Histologically they have cellular and nuclear pleomorphism, prominent infiltration into the subarachnoid space, intracellular accumulations of lipids (hence the designation xanthoastrocytoma), a mix of spindle cells with multinucleated cells, a high density of reticulin fibers usually surrounding clusters of tumor cells, occasional mitoses, and, rarely, areas of necrosis (Fig. 14–4). These tumors are frequently surrounded by regions of gliosis with Rosenthal fibers and occasionally have features of diffuse low-grade astorocytoma.

Desmoplastic Cerebral Astrocytoma

Desmoplastic cerebral astrocytomas are low-grade tumors involving the cortex and meninges. They usually develop in infants and invariably are supratentorial. Macroscopically they have multiloculated cysts with clear or xanthochromic fluid. Histologically they are densely cellular, having spindle and pleomorphic cells in a characteristic desmoplastic stroma with scattered clusters of gemistocytes and aggregates of poorly differentiated neuroepithelial cells, uncommon mitoses, and positive GFAP and vimentin staining[10] (Fig. 14–5).

Subependymal Giant Cell Astrocytoma

Otherwise known as spongioblastoma or neurinoma, subependymal giant cell astrocytomas arise from the walls of the lateral ventricles. There is a very clear association of this tumor subtype with tuberous sclerosis (TS), and although only 3 to 14% of all patients with TS harbor such tumors, they are almost never found in patients who are not afflicted with that disease. On histologic examination the lesion consists of

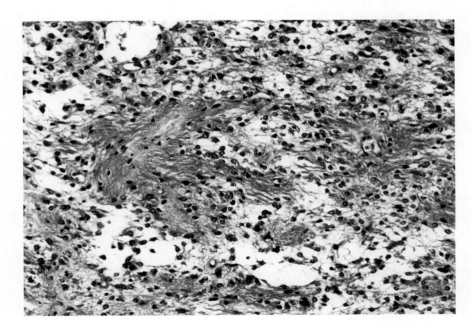

Figure 14–3 Juvenile pilocytic astrocytoma with alternating loose and compact areas, the former with microcysts. Original magnification × 10.

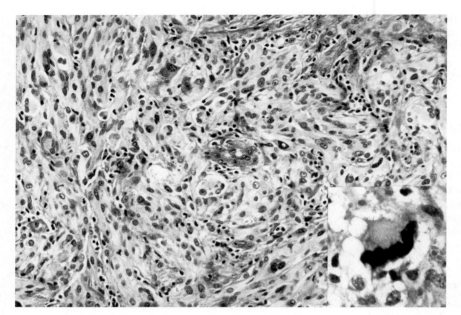

Figure 14–4 Pleomorphic xanthoastrocytoma with sheets of variably sized cells and nuclei, the latter also with different shapes. Endothelial proliferation is present, and some multinucleated cells have finely vacuolated cytoplasm (inset). Original magnification × 10, inset magnification × 25.

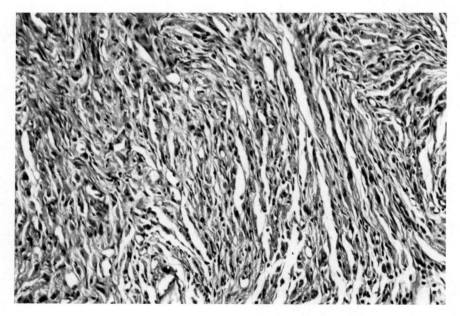

Figure 14–5 Desmoplastic astrocytoma showing parallel bundles of spindle-shaped tumor cells. GFAP and vimentin stains show positivity in elongated pattern paralleling elongated nuclei.

heterogeneous astrocytes with giant pyramidal processes, nuclear polymorphism, and multinucleated cells that show variable expression of GFAP, S100, and neuronal immunohistochemical markers[11] (Fig. 14–6).

MOLECULAR BIOLOGY OF PEDIATRIC ASTROCYTOMAS

Extensive molecular biologic and cytogenetic studies of adult astrocytic tumors have been reported. Mutations of chromosome 17p, which are considered an early event in the development of an astrocytic tumor, are present in 40% of diffuse and anaplastic astrocytomas and in 30% of glioblastomas. Loss of homogeneity of chromosomes 9p and 19p has also been linked to the progression from anaplastic astrocytoma to glioblastoma, and loss of homogeneity of chromosome 10q has been linked to the de novo development of glioblastoma. In addition, mutations of the tumor suppressor gene *p53* associated with 17p deletions have also been linked to the development of astrocytic tumors.

Molecular biologic and cytogenetic results of primary brain tumors differ in the pediatric population. In children, astrocytomas of any grade show only a 15% association with 17p mutations, and *p53* mutations are rarely seen, even when there is a 17p mutation.[12] Low-grade astrocytic tumors most often are karyotypically normal.[13] Still, a review of cytoge-

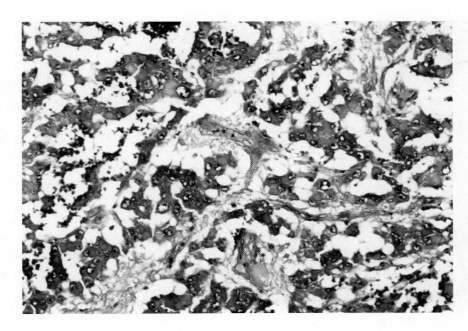

Figure 14–6 Subependymal giant cell astrocytoma from lateral ventricle. Numerous large astrocytes with round to oval nuclei are present. These are much larger than gemistocytes. Original magnification × 10.

netically abnormal pediatric brain tumors has shown an association with mutations in chromosomes X, 7, 9, and 10, with loss of homogeneity for chromosome 10 in 33% of glioblastomas and in 23% of anaplastic astrocytomas.[13] Although these results are preliminary, they are strongly suggestive of some association of specific karyotypic abnormalities with the development of aggressive astrocytic tumors in children.

A promising new histologic marker with prognostic value as a predictor of outcome for malignant gliomas is MIB1, a labeling index that binds to a nuclear antigen specific for the growth phase of the cell cycle. In a study of 31 high-grade gliomas not involving the brain stem, Pollack and colleagues[14] showed a statistically significant correlation of MIB1 and outcome, with progression-free survival and overall survival of more than 48 months for patients with MIB1 less than 12 and a progression-free survival of 6 months and overall survival of 16 months for patients with MIB1 higher than 12.

Familial Tumor Syndromes

Several well-characterized familial syndromes have been linked to an increased incidence of pediatric brain tumors.

Neurofibromatosis Type 1 or Von Recklinghausen's Disease

Neurofibromatosis type 1 (NF-1) is a neurocutaneous disease associated with a mutation at the gene for neurofibrin on 17q12, a protein that is thought to be a tumor suppressor by inactivating Ras, a protein involved in growth factor–mediated cell proliferation.[12] The incidence of von Recklinghausen's disease is 1 in every 4000 children. The disease is transmitted in an autosomal dominant fashion. In addition, a very high incidence of spontaneous mutations has been documented as being responsible for nearly 50% of the new cases. Patients with von Recklinghausen's disease often develop neurofibromas but are also susceptible to developing gliomas, most frequently pilocytic optic pathway astrocytomas[7] and, next most frequently, diffuse astrocytomas of all grades.

Tuberous Sclerosis

Tuberous sclerosis, another neurocutaneous disease, is characterized by the development of hamartomas that involve many organs, including benign lesions in the brain, cutaneous angiofibromas, cardiac rhabdomyomas, and subungual fibromas. The incidence is 1 in every 5000 to 10,000 children, and the disease is transmitted in an autosomal dominant fashion with high penetrance. Clinically patients present with seizures, mental retardation, and sebaceous adenomas. In addition to brain hamartomas, there is a clear association of TS with subependymal giant cell astrocytomas, which rarely occur in patients who do not have TS.[5, 11]

Li-Fraumeni Syndrome

The autosomal dominant syndrome known as Li-Fraumini is caused by a *p53* germline mutation. Children with this syndrome have multiple primary neoplasms, including soft-tissue sarcomas, osteosarcomas, brain tumors, breast cancer, and leukemia. Of the brain tumors, 77% are astrocytic in origin.[5]

DIAGNOSTIC IMAGING

Hemispheric astrocytomas often present on computed tomography (CT) as a mass that is isodense to hypodense and that enhances after administration of a contrast agent. Cystic areas are not uncommon and are often accompanied by a mural nodule. Magnetic resonance imaging (MRI) of the brain is more helpful than CT in differentiating the grade of the tumor. Low-grade astrocytomas are usually homogeneous and often lack enhancement with the contrast agent gadolinium. High-grade tumors, in contrast, are inhomogeneous, with areas of necrosis and hemorrhage, and they frequently enhance after the administration of gadolinium (Fig. 14–7).

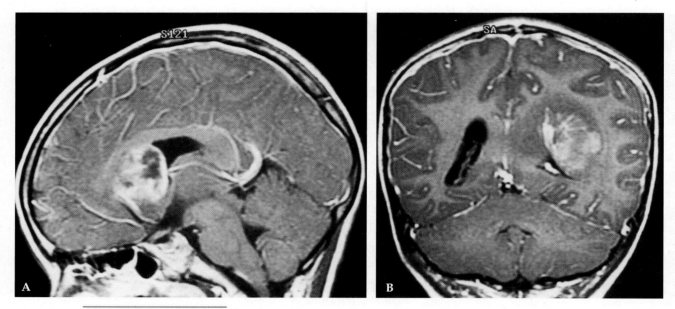

Figure 14–7 Glioblastoma multiforme. Sagittal (A) and coronal (B) views of T1-weighted gadolinium enhanced image showing variable enhancement and surrounding edema.

Thalamic gliomas often present with mass effect to adjacent structures, and they can cause obstruction of the ventricular system and possibly entrapment of one lateral ventricle secondary to unilateral compression of the foramen of Monro[15] (Fig. 14–8). The presence of a cyst is usually an indication of a juvenile pilocytic astrocytoma, whereas contrast enhancement seen after the administration of gadolinium is correlated with a higher grade tumor (Fig. 14–9). It is important when treating such tumors to examine the radiographic studies for possible tumor extension into the ventricular ependymal surface and the corpus callosum.

Subependymal giant cell astrocytomas often present with multifocal disease at the time of diagnosis. On CT, they appear well circumscribed, isodense or hypodense, and close to the foramen of Monro. Partial calcifications are often present. MRI often reveals low signal on T1 and T2 signal prolongation, and uniform contrast enhancement[14] (Fig. 14–10).

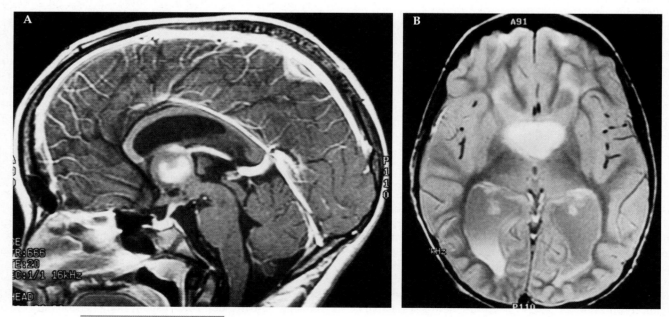

Figure 14–8 Hypothalamic juvenile pilocytic astrocytoma. Sagittal (A) T1-weighted and axial (B) T2-weighted postgadolinium image showing a partially enhancing mass in the hypothalamus. This mass appears hyperintense in the proton intensity image.

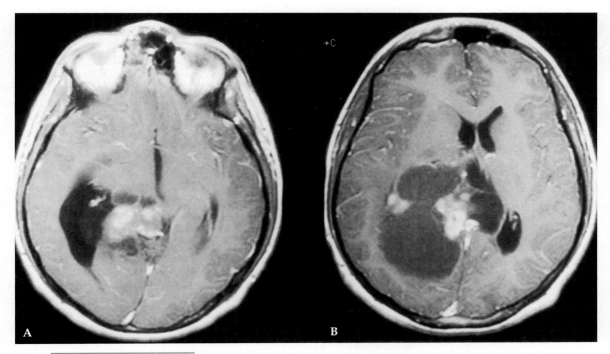

Figure 14–9 Juvenile pilocytic astrocytoma. Axial T1-weighted, postgadolinium images showing a cystic mass with prominent nodular enhancement at the level of the third ventricle (A) and above the foramen of Monro (B).

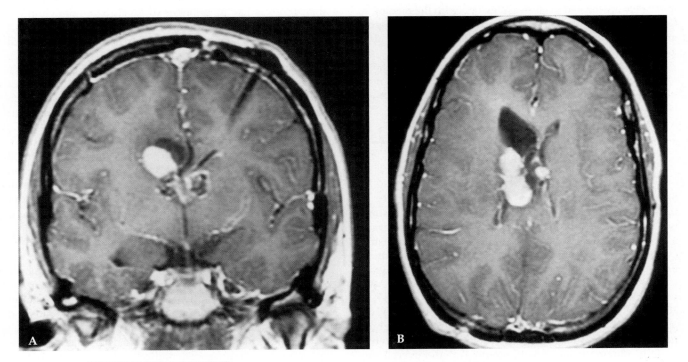

Figure 14–10 Subependymal giant cell astrocytoma. Coronal (A) and axial (B) T1-weighted post-gadolinium images reveal a uniformly enhancing mass based at the inferolateral aspect of the right lateral ventricle extending to the foramen of Monro.

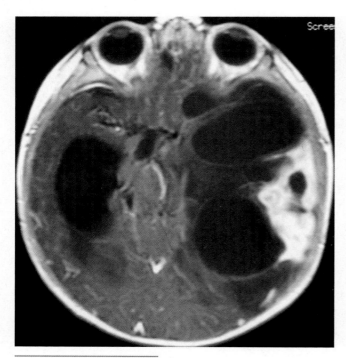

Figure 14–11 Desmoplastic infantile ganglioglioma. Axial T1-weighted postgadolinium image showing nodular enhancement and a large multiloculated cyst.

Pleomorphic xanthoastrocytomas usually present as a large cystic mass with a mural nodule that enhances following administration of contrast agent for CT.[16, 17] They almost invariably are located in close association with the meninges. On MRI, they commonly exhibit prolongation of T2 signal and uniform enhancement of the solid component after gadolinium administration.

Desmoplastic cerebral astrocytomas present on MRI as a hypointense cystic mass, with enhancement of the solid nodule and, on occasion, the periphery after gadolinium administration (Fig. 14–11).

TREATMENT
Surgery

Supratentorial astrocytomas include a wide variety of tumors, some promptly amenable to treatment and some with a less favorable prognosis. Patients with low-grade astrocytomas, including WHO grade I and II diffuse astrocytomas, xanthoastrocytomas, pilocytic astrocytomas, desmoplastic astrocytomas, and giant cell subependymal astrocytomas, have overall survival rates of 82 to 94% at 5 years after diagnosis,[2, 18, 19, 20] 79% at 10 years,[17] and 76% at 20 years.[18] Most studies show a progression-free survival after surgery of 70 to 95% at 5 years. In contrast, high-grade tumors have significantly shorter progression-free survival periods, ranging from 10 to 18 months[21, 22] and overall survival ranging from 18 to 42 months.[2, 21–24]

The mainstay of treatment for pediatric supratentorial astrocytomas is surgical resection. Several studies have assessed the prognostic value of the patient's age, tumor location, extent of resection, histologic characteristics, and a variety of other factors. *Extent of resection has been shown in many studies to be the only reliable independent prognostic factor for both low-grade and high-grade astrocytomas.* Pollack and colleagues[18] showed that for low-grade astrocytomas gross total resection was associated with 100% progression-free and overall survival at 10 years of follow-up evaluation. Campbell and colleagues[21] showed a similar effect of resection on high-grade gliomas, reporting disease-free survival at 84 months for patients who underwent gross total resection. In contrast, patients undergoing subtotal resection had a median overall survival of 25 months and a progression-free period of 11 months, and those undergoing less than a subtotal resection had an overall survival of 10.5 months with a progression-free period of 5.5 months. Heideman and colleagues[25] also found a significant difference in progression-free survival of patients with high-grade astrocytomas who underwent gross total resection, achieving 60% survival at 3 years, as compared with survival 4% of patients with any lesser degree of resection.

Histologic differentiation of the tumor beyond the distinction between low-grade and high-grade lesions has been found to be of predictive value only in cases of partial resection, in which glioblastoma multiforme has a worse prognosis than anaplastic astrocytoma.[21] In studying high-grade gliomas, Heideman[25] and Al-Mefty[24] and their colleagues showed no difference in prognosis between patients with anaplastic astrocytoma and those with glioblastoma multiforme.

The patient's age at diagnosis is a more controversial prognostic factor. Several studies have emphasized younger age as a good prognostic factor.[22, 26–28] Phuphanich and colleagues[22] showed that age at diagnosis was the only statistically significant prognostic factor, with children younger than 10 years having a longer survival than older children. Packer and colleagues[28] found that in patients younger than 5 years who have newly diagnosed low-grade gliomas treated with chemotherapy, there is a 74 ± 7% rate of positive response, as compared with a response rate of 39 ± 21% among patients older than 5 years. These findings are in accordance with those of Rosenblum and colleagues,[27] which showed age-dependent in vitro sensitivity of malignant glioma cells to carmustine.

In contrast, Heideman and colleagues[25] showed that progression of tumor development and survival from malignant gliomas is not associated with the patient's age. Moreover, Gajjar and colleagues[29] showed that younger children with low-grade gliomas have a worse prognosis than have older children, with patients younger than 5 years having a progression-free survival of 53% at 4 years, and patients older than 5 years having a progression-free survival of 77%. Nonetheless, overall survival for the two groups was the same. Al-Mefty and colleagues[24] showed that, among children with malignant gliomas, those in the 5- to 10-year age bracket have a significantly worse prognosis, with a 6-month survival rate of 50% as compared with a 62-month survival rate of 50% for the rest of the pediatric population.

Therefore, it appears that the degree of resection is the single most reliable prognostic indicator. It is not unusual for supratentorial gliomas to have ill-defined borders or to be located adjacent to or within functional cortical and subcortical areas. In such situations, it is imperative to use such adjuvant techniques as frameless stereotaxy and functional brain mapping to localize the tumor accurately and make resection safer and more complete.

Frameless navigational systems calibrate fiducial markers that are attached to the patient's scalp so that the area under surgical consideration can be visualized relative to reconstructed three-dimensional preoperative magnetic resonance images. The tip of a probe is then used intraoperatively for localizing areas of interest, including functional regions of brain. Functional mapping is achieved by electrical stimulation of the cortex using a unipolar or bipolar stimulating electrode. Motor or sensory responses are monitored to identify functional areas of the motor and somatosensory cortex. Alternatively, somatosensory evoked potentials (SSEPs) may be used to identify the central sulcus. SSEPs are especially useful in treating children younger than 5 years, whose cortex is still electrically inexcitable.[30] Mapping of the cortical regions governing speech is essential in operations on tumors located in the dominant frontotemporal hemisphere. Speech mapping can be achieved either by placement of a subdural grid or, in older children who can tolerate such a procedure, through a craniotomy performed with the child awake.

Surgery has also been shown to be an effective treatment for seizures associated with the presence of a supratentorial astrocytoma. In children with low-grade gliomas and seizures, Packer[31] showed complete seizure control postoperatively in 75% (45 of 60) of the patients, with 2 of the remaining 15 patients having significant reduction in seizure frequency. In a study of seizure control after resection of childhood hemispheric low-grade gliomas with the use of intraoperative electrocorticography, Berger and colleagues[32] demonstrated 93% of the patients to be free of seizures while off anticonvulsant medications, or on tapering doses, at least 1 year postoperatively.

Radiation Therapy

Several studies have shown the usefulness of irradiation in the treatment of adult high-grade gliomas.[33] For children, radiation therapy is beneficial in the treatment of recurrent tumors[3] and even as the primary treatment for unresectable tumors of the thalamus, hypothalamus, and optic pathways. Tao and colleagues[34] showed that children with chiasmatic gliomas treated with radiation therapy alone have a 10-year progression-free survival of 89% and an overall survival of 100%, with a median time to the onset of radiographic response of 62 months. In a study of radiation therapy given after the subtotal removal or biopsy of chiasmatic childhood gliomas, Erkal and colleagues[35] demonstrated an overall survival rate of 93 ± 5% at 5 years and 79 ± 10% at 10 years, with a progression-free survival rate of 82 ± 8% at 5 years and 77 ± 10% at 10 years. Vision improved in 50% of those patients and stabilized in the rest of them.

The utility of radiation therapy in treating children is tempered by its effects on the developing brain. It has been shown that long-term complications of radiation therapy in children include necrosis of the central nervous system, myelopathy, leukoencephalopathy, vascular injury, neuropsychological deficits, hormonal imbalances, bone and teeth abnormalities, ocular toxicity, and ototoxicity. In addition, any of a number of secondary malignancies may arise

after treatment, including meningiomas, gliomas, and sarcomas.[36] In a study of the treatment of low-grade astrocytomas of the cerebral hemispheres, Pollack and colleagues[18] found that all patients who had malignant progression of their gliomas had undergone irradiation. Similarly, in a series of 56 children who had optic pathway and thalamic low-grade tumors, Dirks and colleagues[37] found that all six children who developed anaplastic changes had been treated with radiation therapy and that the location new tumor was within the irradiated field. *Given the toxic effect of radiation and the very low risk of recurrence after gross total resection, radiation therapy is not indicated for the treatment of low-grade astrocytomas, including diffuse, pilocytic, desmoplastic, and xanthoastrocytoma lesions.*

BOX 14–4
Potential Complications of Radiation Therapy

- Necrosis
- Myelopathy
- Leukoencephalopathy
- Vascular injury
- Neuropsychiatric deficits
- Hormonal imbalance
- Bone/tooth abnormalities
- Ocular toxicity
- Ototoxicity
- Secondary malignancy

Despite the great success of stereotactic radiosurgery in the treatment of adults with brain tumors, its use in children is still novel. In a study by Grabb and colleagues[38] of children with unresectable low-grade or high-grade gliomas who were treated with stereotactic radiosurgery, all patients with low-grade gliomas and four of five patients with high-grade gliomas were alive at a median of 21 months after treatment. In this study, toxicity was mild, including nausea, vomiting, and transient paresis that resolved promptly with steroid treatment in all cases.

Chemotherapy

Chemotherapy has proved to be an important treatment modality for astrocytomas of childhood. In a randomized study, Sposto and colleagues[39] showed significantly prolonged overall survival and progression-free survival in children with new diagnoses of high-grade astrocytoma who were treated with radiation therapy and chemotherapy rather than radiation therapy alone. The chemotherapy regimen used in this study consisted of vincristine, lomustine, and prednisone. Overall survival for the group undergoing chemotherapy and radiation therapy was 43% at 5 years, as compared to 18% at 5 years for the group receiving radiation therapy alone.[39] Packer and colleagues[28] studied the effect of carboplatin and vincristine for newly diagnosed and nonresectable low-grade gliomas and demonstrated a response rate of 56%. Progression-free survival in this study was 75 ± 6% at 2 years and 68 ± 7% at 3 years after completion of the chemotherapy regimen.

A study by Duffner and colleagues[40] assessed the efficacy of postoperative chemotherapy and delayed irradiation in patients younger than 3 years who had malignant brain tumors. Vincristine, cyclophosphamide, cisplatin, and etoposide were used for 24 months for patients younger than 24 months and for 12 months for children older than 24 months, followed by traditional radiation therapy. Overall survival for patients with malignant gliomas was 83 ± 9% at 1 year and 65 ± 13% at 2 years, with a progression-free survival of 54 ± 12% at 1 year and 54 ± 18% at 2 years from initiation of therapy.

Another randomized study by Lyden and colleagues[41] compared a course of radiation therapy followed by conventional chemotherapy with a regimen of radiation therapy followed by the 8-in-1-day chemotherapy regimen consisting of lomustine, cisplatin, cyclophosphamide, cytosine arabinoside, hydroxyurea, methylprednisone, procarbazine, and vincristine, all given in one day. No statistically significant difference in outcome was observed, but toxicity of the 8-in-1 regimen was observed to be substantially higher. The Children's Cancer Group studied the effect of the intensive eight-drug chemotherapy regimen on malignant astrocytoma of infants younger than 24 months. They showed an overall survival of 51 ± 8% at 3 years, with a progression-free survival of 36 ± 8%, and progression-free survival for children with cerebral hemispheric astrocytomas of 50%.[42]

More recently, high-dose chemotherapy administered with autologous bone marrow reconstitution has been considered for the treatment of high-grade gliomas. In a pilot study, Finlay and colleagues[43] treated children who had high-grade recurrent gliomas with high-dose thiotepa and etoposide, along with autologous bone marrow reconstruction, and found an overall response rate of 23%. In the group with high-grade gliomas, he observed a median progression-free survival of 9.6 months, with a median overall survival of 12.7 months. Of all patients, 29% were free of disease at a median follow-up interval of 49 months after autologous bone marrow reconstruction. The usefulness of this form of treatment remains to be established, especially considering the high degree of toxicity, which in this study accounted for a 16% mortality rate.[43]

SUMMARY

Supratentorial astrocytoma is a very common childhood tumor. Most lesions are low-grade and amenable to treatment with a high rate of cure. The extent of surgical resection is the only statistically significant prognostic factor for recurrence and survival. For low-grade lesions gross total resection is very likely to be curative, whereas in high-grade gliomas adjuvant therapy may be required. Given the toxicity of radiation to the developing nervous system, radiation therapy is reserved for recurrent, unresectable, and high-grade tumors. Chemotherapy is a proven alternative as a postoperative adjuvant treatment for effective control of disease progression and for delaying irradiation. Advances in intraoperative localization, functional mapping, stereotactic radiosurgery, and chemotherapeutic regimens define the future in the treatment of supratentorial gliomas of childhood.

REFERENCES

1. Bruce DA, Shut L, Sutton LN. Supratentorial brain tumors of children. In: Youmans JR, ed. *Neurological Surgery.* 3rd. ed. Philadelphia: WB Saunders; 1990.
2. Butler D, Jose B, Summe R, et al. Pediatric astrocytomas: the Louisville experience, 1978–1988. *Am J Clin Oncol* 1994;17:475–479.
3. Hirsch J-F, Sainte Rose C, Pierre-Kahn A, et al. Benign astrocytic and oligodendrocytic tumors of the cerebral hemispheres in children. *J Neurosurg* 1989;70:568–572.
4. Palma L, Guidetti B. Cystic pilocytic astrocytomas of the cerebral hemispheres. *J Neurosurg* 1985;62:811–815.
5. Packer RJ, Vezina G, Chadduck WM. Brain tumors of glial and neuronal origin in infants and children: clinical features and natural history. In: Tindall GT, Cooper PR, Barrow DL, eds. *The Practice of Neurosurgery.* Baltimore: Williams & Wilkins, 1996;780–798.
6. Clark GB, Henry JM, McKeever PE. Cerebral pilocytic astrocytoma. *Cancer* 1985;56:1128–1133.
7. Garvey M, Packer RJ. An integrated approach to the treatment of chiasmatic hypothalamic gliomas, *J Neuro-oncol* 1996;28:167–183.
8. Kleihues P, Cavenee, KW, eds. *Pathology and Genetics: Tumours of the Nervous System.* Lyon: International Agency for Research on Cancer, 1997:2.
9. Rostomily RC, Rostomily RC, Hoyt JW, et al. Pleomorphic xanthoastrocytoma, DNA flow cytometry and outcome analysis of 12 patients. *Cancer* 1997;80:2141–2150.
10. Aydin F, Ghatak BR, Salvant J, Muizelaar P. Desmoplastic cerebral astrocytoma of infancy. *Acta Neuropathol* 1993;86:666–680.
11. Sinson G, Sutton LN, Yachnis AT, et al. Subependymal giant cell astrocytomas in children. *Pediatr Neurosurg* 1994;20:233–239.
12. Raffel C. Molecular biology of pediatric gliomas. *J Neuro-oncol* 1996;28:121–128.
13. Bhattacharjee MB, Armstrong DD, Vogel H, Cooley LD. Cytogenetic analysis of 120 primary pediatric brain tumors and literature review. *Cancer Genet Cytogenet* 1997;97:39–53.
14. Pollack IF, Campbell JW, Hamilton RL, et al. Proliferation index as a predictor of prognosis in malignant gliomas of childhood. *Cancer* 1997;79:849–859.
15. Souweidane MM, Hoffman HJ. Current treatment of thalamic gliomas in children. *J Neuro-oncol* 1996;28:157–166.
16. Pahapill PA, Ramsay DA, Del Maestro RF. Pleomorphic xanthoastrocytoma: case report and analysis of the literature concerning the efficacy of resection and significance of necrosis. *Neurosurgery* 1996;38:822–827.
17. Kawano N. Pleomorphic xathoastrocytoma: some new observations. *Clin Neuropathol* 1992;11:323–328.

18. Pollack IF, Claassen D, Al-Shboul Q, et al. Low grade gliomas of the cerebral hemispheres in children: an analysis of 71 cases. *J Neurosurg* 1995;82:536–547.
19. Mercuri S, Russo A, Palma L. Hemispheric supratentorial astrocytomas in children. *J Neurosurg* 1981;55:170–173.
20. Gajjar A, Sanford RA, Heideman R, et al. Low grade astrocytoma: a decade of experience at St Jude Children's Research Hospital. *J Clin Oncol* 1997;15:2792–2799.
21. Campbell JW, Pollack IF, Martinez AJ, Shultz B. High grade astrocytomas in children: radiologically complete resection is associated with an excellent long-term prognosis. *Neurosurgery* 1996;38:258–264.
22. Phuphanich S, Edwards MSB, Levin VA, et al. Supratentorial malignant gliomas of childhood: results of treatment with radiation therapy and chemotherapy. *J Neurosurg* 1984;60:495–499.
23. Duffner PK, Kirscher JP, Burger PC, et al. Treatment of infants with malignant gliomas: the Pediatric Oncology Group experience. *J Neuro-oncol*, 1996;28:245–256.
24. Al-Mefty O, Al-Rodan NRF, Phillips RL, et al. Factors affecting survival of children with malignant gliomas. *Neurosurgery* 1987;20:416–420.
25. Heideman RL, Kuttesch J, Gajjar AJ, et al. Supratentorial malignant gliomas in childhood. *Cancer* 1997;80:479–504.
26. Gold EB, Gordis L. Determinants of survival in children with brain tumors. *Ann Neurol* 1979;5:569–574.
27. Rosenblum ML, Gerosa M, Dougherty DV, et al. Age-related chemosensitivity of stem cells from human malignant brain tumor. *Lancet* 1982; 1 (April 17):885–887.
28. Packer RJ, Ater J, Allen J, et al. Carboplatin and vincristine chemotherapy for children with newly diagnosed progressive low-grade gliomas. *J Neurosurg* 1997;86:747–754.
29. Gajjar A, Heideman RL, Kovnar EH, et al. Response of pediatric low grade gliomas to chemotherapy. *Pediatr Neurosurg* 1993;19:113–120.
30. Berger MS. The impact of technical adjuncts to the surgical management of cerebral hemispheric low-grade gliomas of childhood. *J Neuro-oncol* 1996;28:129–155.
31. Packer RJ, Sutton LN, Patel KM, et al. Seizure control following tumor surgery for childhood cortical low-grade gliomas. *J Neurosurg* 1994;80:998–1003.
32. Berger MS, Ghatan S, Geyer JR, et al. Seizure outcome in children with hemispheric tumors and associated intractable epilepsy: the role of tumor removal combined with seizure foci resection. *Pediatr Neurosurg* 1991–92;17:185–191.
33. Berger MS, Geyer JR. Management of brain tumors of glial and neuronal origin in infants and children. In: Tindall GT, Cooper PR, Barrow DL, eds. *The Practice of Neurosurgery*. Baltimore: Williams & Wilkins; 1996;797–819.
34. Tao ML, Bames PD, Billett AL, et al. Childhood optic chiasm gliomas: radiographic response following radiotherapy and long-term clinical outcome. *Int J Radiat Oncol Biol Phys* 1997;39:579–587.
35. Erkal HS, Serin M, Cakmak A. Management of optic pathway and chiasmatic-hypothalamic gliomas in children with radiation therapy. *Radiother Oncol* 1997;45:11–15.
36. Donahue B. Short and long-term complications of radiation therapy for pediatric brain tumors. *Pediatr Neurosurg* 1992;18:207–217.
37. Dirks PB, Jay V, Becker LE, Drake JM, et al. Development of anaplastic changes in low grade astrocytomas of childhood. *Neurosurgery* 1994;34:68–77.
38. Grabb PA, Lunsford LD, Albright AL, et al. Stereotactic radiosurgery for glial neoplasms of childhood. *Neurosurgery* 1996;38:696–702.
39. Sposto R, Ertel IJ, Jenkin RDT, et al. The effectiveness of chemotherapy for the treatment of high grade astrocytoma in children: results of a randomized study. *J Neuro-oncol* 1989;7:165–177.
40. Duffner PK, Horowitz ME, Krischer JP, et al. Post-operative chemotherapy and delayed radiation in children less than three years of age with malignant brain tumors. *N Engl J Med* 1993;328:1725–1731.
41. Lyden DC, Mason WP, Finlay JL. The expanding role of chemotherapy for pediatric supratentorial malignant gliomas. *J Neuro-oncol* 1996;28:185–191.
42. Geyer JR, Finlay JL, Boyett JM, et al. Survival of infants with malignant astrocytomas: a report of the Children's Cancer Group. *Cancer* 1995;75:1045–1050.
43. Finlay JL, Goldman S, Wong MC, et al. Children's Cancer Group. Pilot study of high-dose thiotepa and etoposide with autologous bone marrow rescue in children and young adults with recurrent central nervous system tumors. *J Clin Oncol* 1996;14:2495–2503.

Chapter 15

Infratentorial Ependymoma

David M. Weitman and Philip H. Cogen

Tumors of ependymal cell origin occur throughout the neural axis; on occasion, they are found outside the central nervous system (CNS) in the parasacral soft tissues.

EPIDEMIOLOGY

Ependymoma is the third most common pediatric brain tumor, following astrocytoma and medulloblastoma, accounting for approximately 10% of childhood intracranial neoplasms.[1] In children, 90% of ependymomas are intracranial, with the remainder located in the spinal canal. Approximately 50% of pediatric ependymomas are identified in children younger than 5 years. Ependymal tumors of the posterior fossa predominate in this younger population. Infratentorial lesions represent approximately two thirds of the total number of reported cases,[2,3] with a greater proportion of tumors seen in the posterior fossa in children younger than 3 years.[4] Approximately 25% of posterior fossa ependymomas arise in the cerebellopontine angle and/or lateral cerebellum, with the remainder originating in the midline structures.[5,6]

PRESENTATION

The presenting signs and symptoms of infratentorial ependymoma are dependent on the age of the patient and the location of the tumor. The earliest symptoms include behavioral changes such as lethargy, irritability, and decreased social interaction. These symptoms and signs are then often followed by headache, most pronounced upon awakening, and vomiting, particularly in the absence of nausea. Tumors located in the midline of the cerebellum may result in truncal and gait ataxia, whereas lesions in the cerebellar hemispheres cause ipsilateral dysmetria. Ependymomas that exit the foramen of Luschka from the cerebellopontine angle may present with cranial neuropathies. Hydrocephalus secondary to cerebrospinal fluid (CSF) obstruction at the level of the cerebral aqueduct or fourth ventricle is common (Fig. 15–1). Papilledema due to intracranial hypertension is one of the most common signs and has been reported in as many as 90% of patients in some series. Sudden death due to obstructive hydrocephalus has been reported in two children with ependymomas.[7] Acquired torticollis may be a manifestation of cerebellar tonsillar herniation, and children with the new onset of a head tilt should be considered suspect for a posterior fossa tumor. In very young children, increasing head circumference may be the only presenting feature of the tumor.

Rapid, sudden deterioration in the neurologic status of a child with an infratentorial ependymoma may be due to hemorrhage into either the tumor[8] or the subarachnoid space.[9] Primary presentation with spinal cord or radicular symptoms secondary to drop metastasis is extremely rare in ependymoma.[10] As emesis is one of the earliest and most common manifestations of posterior fossa tumors, it is not unusual for children to undergo an extensive gastrointestinal workup for several weeks or months prior to the diagnosis of the tumor.[11] With the more frequent use of neuroimaging studies, this problem has become less common.

The signs and symptoms described for infratentorial ependymoma are not pathognomonic for this tumor type and may result from other posterior fossa tumors and/or nonneoplastic processes in this location.

BOX 15–1
Clinical Presentation

- **Headache**
- **Vomiting**
- **Lethargy**
- **Irritability**
- **Ataxia/dysmetria**
- **Cranial neuropathies**
- **Papilledema**
- **Torticollis**

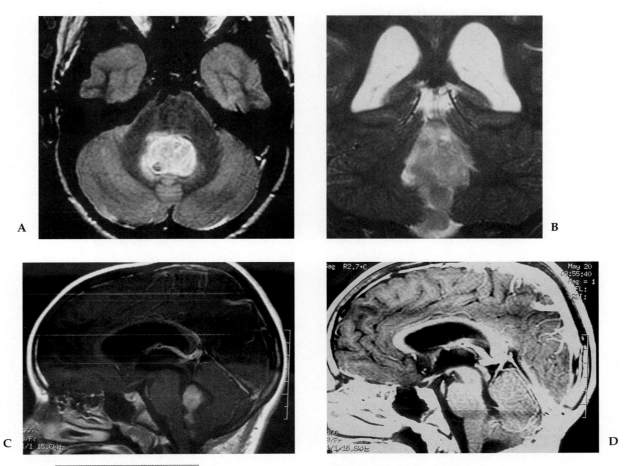

Figure 15–1 Infratentorial ependymoma in a 10-year-old girl with a history of headache and vomiting. (A) T2-weighted axial MRI showing fourth ventricular location. (B) T2-weighted coronal MRI image showing associated hydrocephalus. The ventricles returned to normal size following tumor resection without the need for a shunt. (C, D) T1-weighted gadolinium–enhanced MRI scans showing the lesion before and after total resection. MRI of the spine revealed no metastases, and the cerebrospinal fluid cytology was negative for tumor cells. The child received focal irradiation after the resection.

DIAGNOSTIC STUDIES

For patients who present with acute symptoms, computed tomography (CT) will identify the tumor mass and is useful in identifying hydrocephalus, brain stem compression, and cerebral edema. However, magnetic resonance imaging (MRI), with and without contrast administration, is the imaging modality of choice for surgical planning, due to its greater soft-tissue detail and multiplanar imaging capacity. On precontrast CT scans, most ependymomas are homogeneous, with approximately 75% of tumors iso- to hyperdense to gray matter, which is evidence of high cellularity.[4] Fifty percent of tumors show calcifications. The vast majority strongly enhance with contrast administration. These imaging characteristics are shared by all intracranial ependymomas irrespective of their location[12] (Fig. 15–2A).

> **BOX 15–2**
> **CT Features**
>
> - **Homogeneous**
> - **Iso-/hypodense**
> - **50% Ca^{2+}**
> - **Enhancement with contrast**

On precontrast T1-weighted magnetic resonance images (Figs. 15–1, 15–2, and 15–3) more than 85% of these tumors have signal intensity iso- to hypointense to gray matter, with only a small proportion of tumors exhibiting high signal intensity. Almost all tumors have high signal intensity on T2-weighted images. As with CT scans, almost all tumors show

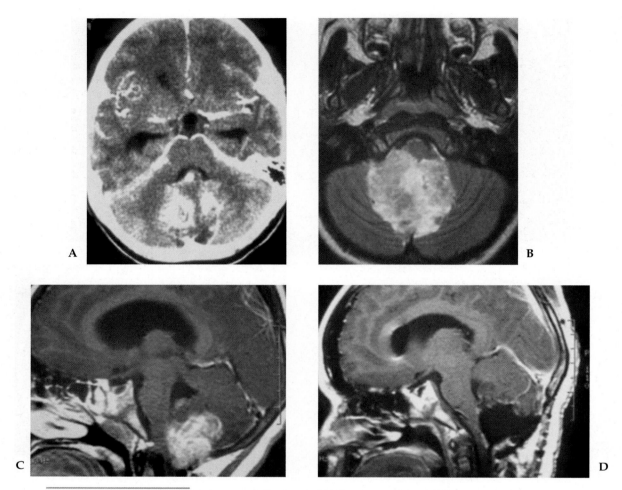

Figure 15–2   Large posterior fossa ependymoma. (A) Contrast-enhanced CT scan of an 11-year-old girl with headaches and gait ataxia. Note the irregular enhancement of the lesion. There is important hydrocephalus. (B) T2-weighted axial MRI scan. The lesion compresses the brain stem, and a clear plane is difficult to discern. (C) Sagittal T1-weighted gadolinium-enhanced MRI showing extension of the lesion below the foramen magnum into the cerebellar tonsil. This is a common pattern for ependymomas. (D) Postoperative T1-weighted gadolinium-enhanced sagittal MRI. Note the minimal area of contrast enhancement on the brain stem representing an area of unresectable tumor. This child received a combined focal irradiation/chemotherapy protocol because of the presence of residual disease.

enhancement on MRI following the administration of gadolinium-diethylenetriaminepentaacetic acid (DPTA) (Fig. 15–2). Radiologic features less commonly identified in infratentorial ependymomas include cystic change and dural involvement.[4, 12, 13]

BOX 15–3
MRI Features

- **T1-weighted images: iso-/hypointense**
- **T2-weighted images: hyperintense**
- **Enhancement with contrast**

These radiologic features are not totally specific for ependymoma. The radiographic differential diagnosis includes medulloblastoma, choroid plexus papilloma, and dorsally exophytic brain stem glioma. *MR spectroscopy has recently been investigated as a means of differentiating among these pathologic entities.*[14] By comparing the signal intensities generated by choline containing compounds N-acetylaspartate, creatine/phosphocreatine, and lactate, spectroscopic signatures of various tumors can be generated. However, in one study this technique had only a 0.75 sensitivity and a 0.60 positive predictive value for identification of ependymoma.[14] By adding clinical data, such as patient age, sex, tumor size and other radiographic information, algorithms can be generated that identify tumor type with up to 95% accuracy.[13]

Chapter 16

Supratentorial Ependymoma

Charles L. Rosen and Robert F. Keating

In the pediatric population, supratentorial ependymomas are an uncommon but not altogether rare neoplasm. It is inappropriate to treat them like any other "glioma." The constellation of neoplasms known as ependymoma have a distinct biology unto themselves, and the treatment plan for supratentorial ependymomas differs from that for supratentorial gliomas, as well as for infratentorial ependymoma. This chapter will focus on high- and low-grade ependymomas in the supratentorial compartment and will also review data from previously published studies. We have purposely excluded subependymoma and ependymoblastoma from the bulk of our analysis as these are clearly very different neoplasms (discussed further in the section on pathology).

HISTORY

Virchow[1] first described ependymoma in 1864, and Bailey[2] further classified it as a distinct neoplasm in 1924. Bailey found a total of five cases in the literature that seemed authentic. To these five cases he added six more from Dr. Cushing's clinic. Ten cases were localized to the posterior fossa and one to the sacral region,[3] but no supratentorial lesions were described in this early series. Initially ependymoblastoma was recognized as representing a distinct entity. Ependymomas differ in that "they are polygonal and have no tails ... but show characteristic blepharoplasten."[3] Though described as a separate entity, until recently ependymoblastoma was often considered a more malignant form of ependymoma. Thus many series of "ependymomas" include ependymoblastoma.

EPIDEMIOLOGY

Incidence

Following pilocytic astrocytoma and medulloblastoma, ependymoma is the most common tumor of childhood.[4–6] In the classic series of Bailey et al, ependymomas represented 7% of the intracranial neoplasms[7]; similarly, Cuneo and Rand found an incidence of 7.3%.[8] In more recent studies, 6 to 12% of intracranial tumors are ependymomas.[8–10] In one of the few large studies that quantified supratentorial ependymomas, out of 4054 primary intracranial tumors, 1.2% were ependymoma, and 0.35% were supratentorial ependymomas (age not specified).[12]

Location

In contrast to infratentorial ependymomas, supratentorial ependymomas are encountered in the cerebral substance, not the ventricular system.[13] As many as 85% of tumors are away from the ventricular surface.[14] In fact, few cases of supratentorial ependymomas are restricted to the ventricular lumen.[14–16] Tumors have even been identified adjacent to the cortical surface.[17] The explanation for how ependymal-based tumors occur in the parenchyma has been well described. Ependymal cells have been identified deep in the cerebral hemispheres, far removed from the ventricles, thought to be extensions or inclusions where the primitive ventricular walls have fused.[18–21] It is these cellular rests that are believed to develop into supratentorial ependymomas.

Ependymomas are located in the supratentorial region, as opposed to the infratentorial region, in 20 to 49% of patients.[9, 11–13, 22–33] Significant difficulty exists with the interpretation of published data on supratentorial ependymomas, as many studies group supratentorial and infratentorial ependymomas together.[13, 26–28, 31, 34, 35] However, some authors have specifically examined supratentorial ependymomas (though many do not limit themselves to the pediatric population).[18, 22, 28, 31, 36–39] In Table 16–1, the total number of patients and percentage of lesions located in the supratentorial region are tabulated. Children have a lower proportion of supratentorial ependymomas (35%) than their adult counterparts (40%). The fact that some studies have demonstrated equal numbers of supratentorial and infratentorial ependymomas,[10] (even up to 55.6% supratentorial lesions[39]) is most likely due to selection bias. Another explanation may be that more malignant tumors, or tumors in the older child, have an increased propensity to grow in the supratentorial region, with nearly 65% of anaplastic ependymomas being supratentorial.[12, 31, 36, 39, 40] Spinal seeding from supratentorial ependymomas has been reported only occasionally.[24, 41–45]

TABLE 16–1   Incidence of Supratentorial Ependymoma in Adults and Children[a]

Series	No. of patients	% Supratentorial	% Supratentorial in children
Cushing[101]	25	24.0	
List[102]	81	34.6	
Ringertz and Reymond[13]	54	38.9	
Svien et al[21]	126	40.5	38.9
Phillips et al[46]	42	45.2	
Kricheff et al[28, 37]	59	24.0	
Fokes and Earle[23]		25.0	
Shuman et al[33]	74		24.0
Liu et al[59]	31		42.0
Dohrmann et al[40]	44		40.0
Coulon and Till[9]	43		30.2
Mork and Loken[12]	48	28.0	24.2
Marks and Adler[38]	36		44.0
Pierre-Kahn et al[30]	47		31.9
Read[35]	25		28.0
Shaw et al[32]	33		33.0
Ernestus et al[36]	134	38.8	55.8
Undjian and Marinov[63b]	60		38.3
Total	962	40.3	35.1

[a] The reported incidence of supratentorial ependymomas in several large series. Where possible, pediatric tumors are distinguished from adult lesions.
[b] Includes children with ependymoblastoma.

Age/Sex

The demographics of age are complex with respect to supratentorial ependymomas. In studies not confined to a particular age group, children represented 20 to 70% of the patient population (table 16–2). The mean age for presentation in studies not limited to the pediatric population ranged from 17 to 25 years,[12, 28, 31, 46] whereas in studies that focused on the pediatric population the mean age of presentation ranged from 4.2 to 4.9 years. Overall, supratentorial ependymomas appear to affect a slightly older population than infratentorial ependymomas.

TABLE 16–2   Patients with Supratentorial Ependymoma in Childhood[a]

Series	% Pediatric
Fokes and Earle[23]	20.0
Svien at al[21]	41.2
Ringertz and Reymond[13]	39.0
Rawlings et al[31]	35.5
Hahn et al[14]	70.0
Minauf et al[103]	68.9
Mork and Loken[12]	57.0

[a] Several reports provide direct data for the percentage of patients with supratentorial ependymomas who are children. Studies that report a particular age usually use the term "pediatric" to imply persons 16 years of age or younger.

The majority of studies showed a male predominance for supratentorial ependymomas, with a male/female ratio of 1.2–2.25:1.[9, 14, 28, 39, 40] Two studies showed a slight female predominance with a male/female ratio of 0.82–0.88:1.[26, 47]

PRESENTATION

The signs and symptoms of supratentorial ependymomas are more often related to a large mass lesion causing increased intracranial pressure. Focal signs and seizures are less common. Table 16–3 tabulates the data from four separate series. Clearly, papilledema is the most common sign and headache the most common symptom in patients with supratentorial ependymomas. Patients also frequently experience mental status changes, lethargy, cranial nerve palsies (especially dysconjugate gaze), nausea, and vomiting.

BOX 16–1
Clinical Presentation
of Supratentorial Ependymomas

- **Papilledema**
- **Headache**
- **Mental status changes**
- **Lethargy**
- **Cranial nerve palsies**
- **Nausea and vomiting**

TABLE 16–3 Signs and Symptoms of Supratentorial Ependymoma[a]

Sign/Symptom	Dohrmann et al (n = 24)[40]	Rawlings et al (n = 22)[31]	Coulon and Till (n = 13)[9]	Hahn et al (n = 20)[14]	Mean (%)
Papilledema	13	19	10	6	60.8
Ataxia	14	1	3	4	27.8
Lethargy/change in mental status	12	8	7		45.8
Cranial nerve palsy	11	14	2		45.8
Focal paresis	9	4	7		33.9
Enlarged fontanel	6		3		24.3
Headache	12	14	5	12	54.4
Nausea and vomiting	15	1	8	11	44.3
Seizures	6	2		3	16.7

[a] The presenting signs and symptoms of patients with supratentorial ependymomas were reported in these four series. Means are calculated only for those values reported.

RADIOGRAPHIC CHARACTERISTICS

Plain Films

Plain skull X rays are not routinely recommended for evaluation of children with supratentorial ependymomas. However, a number of findings have been documented in older series. Hahn et al in a study of 19 children found abnormal skull X rays in 63% of patients with supratentorial ependymomas, which included separation of sutures in 50%, erosion of dorsum sella in 17%, and calcification in 25%.[14] Similarly, Coulon and Till in a study of 13 children found suture diastasis in 77%, general vault thinning in 23%, focal vault thinning in 31%, sella changes in 23%, calcification in 23%, and increased digital markings in 8% of the study population.[9]

Computed Tomography

Two detailed studies of computed tomography (CT) scan characteristics have been reported. In a study by Centeno et al, all patients exhibited a hyperdense lesion, with *calcification* in 80%. Mild edema was present in 40% and marked edema in 30% of patients. *Contrast enhancement* was uniformly present, ranging from moderate to markedly enhanced.[18] No correlation was seen between CT scan characteristics and the grade of the ependymomas.

In a similar report by Armington et al, the CT Scans of 17 patients with tissue-proven diagnosis of supratentorial ependymoma (mean age 9.4 years) were characterized. Lesions were intraventricular in 23.5%, periventricular in 29.4%, parenchymal in 41.2%, and extra-axial in 5.9% of patients. Tumor size varied widely, with 5.9% less than 1 cm, 11.8% about 1 to 4 cm, and 82.4% greater than 4 cm. The tumors were further characterized as solid 29.4%, solid with lucency 23.5%, and cystic 47.1%. In contrast to the report of Centeno et al, no enhancement was present in 5.9% of lesions. Slight enhancement was present in 5.9% of lesions, whereas 41% had moderate enhancement and 35.3% had intense enhancement. Edema was present in 47.1% of patients and calcification in 29.4%.[15]

Thus, a differential diagnosis based on CT scan includes astrocytoma, primitive neuroectodermal tumor, choroid plexus papilloma, and giant cell subependymal astrocytoma.[15] Though CT scanning may be helpful, magnetic resonance imaging (MRI) remains superior for the diagnosis and definition of tumor and adjacent structure anatomy.

Magnetic Resonance Imaging

Presently, MRI is the imaging modality of choice (Fig. 16–1). However, due to the relative rarity of supratentorial ependymomas and recent development of MRI, there are few studies demonstrating the magnetic resonance characteristics of these lesions. One of the few existing MRI studies has only six patients after excluding patients over the age of 20 and those with subependymomas. The imaging characteristics were as follows: four lesions were cystic, two had evidence of calcium, and three enhanced (Fig. 16–2). They had an average size of 4.2 cm. MRI signal characteristics are outlined in Table 16–4.[48] Tominaga et al found similar characteristics in their three patients.[49]

PATHOLOGY

In terms of gross pathology, supratentorial ependymomas are often characterized as large, firm, cystic, lobulated, partially encapsulated, vascular, reddish gray tumors that can be found at a distance from the ventricular system.[8, 50] When cystic fluid is present, it is yellow to deep amber, often cloudy, and contains red blood cells. Supratentorial ependymoma is the commonest hemispheric tumor to show calcification. It frequently manifests numerous areas of hemorrhage and necrosis.[11]

Histology

Bailey was the first to describe the histologic criteria of ependymal tumors. Such tumors were characterized by ependymal cells forming rosettes and pseudorosettes (Fig. 16–3).[2, 21, 27, 51] In addition, Bailey described "blepharoplasts, the basal bodies of cilia that can best be demonstrated with

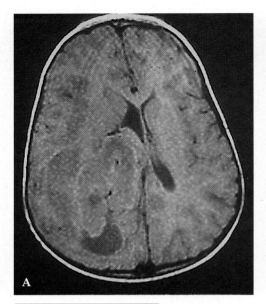
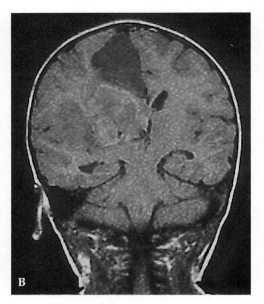

Figure 16–1 (A) A 13–year-old-boy presenting with headaches and seizures, demonstrating on a non–contrast-enhanced T1-weighted magnetic resonance image a mass in the right posterior periventricular region with effacement of the lateral ventricle. This lesion was seen to be an epithelial type of ependymoma. (B) Same patient with a coronal view of his ependymoma with a cystic component above the body of the tumor.

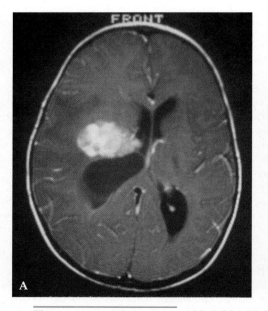
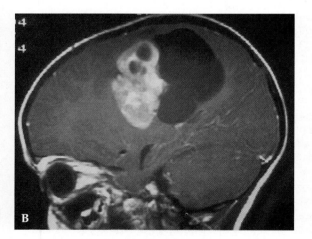

Figure 16–2 (A) An 8-year-old child with headache, vomiting, and recent difficulty running. A gadolinium-enhancing mass is seen in a periventricular area with multiple cysts also present. At the time of surgical excision, this lesion was diagnosed as an ependymoma. (B) Sagittal view of the same patient demonstrating significant mass effect due to the tumor as well as cyst.

phosphotungstic acid–hematoxylin staining, as characteristic of ependymomas, but often difficult to find."[2, 50, 51]

As a result of these early descriptions, subependymoma and ependymoblastoma were grouped with ependymomas as two ends of a continuous spectrum of ependymal lesions. Subependymoma is currently classified as a low-grade neoplasm (WHO grade 1). It is considered a hamartomatous lesion of the periventricular space, mostly limited to patients with tuberous sclerosis. This lesion usually causes symptoms by obstructive hydrocephalus, is slow growing, and even partial removal may yield a cure. As such, many believe that subependymomas should not be grouped with ependymomas. Inclusion of these lesions in any series may falsely elevate treatment efficacy.

On the opposite end of the spectrum, ependymoblastoma is considered a primitive neuroectodermal tumor. It is a highly malignant lesion that is similar in both appearance and

TABLE 16–4   MRI Characteristics of Supratentorial Ependymoma (%)[a]

Signal	Isointense	Heterogeneous	Increased	Decreased
T1-weighted	50.0	33.3	0	16.7
T2-weighted	16.7	50.0	33.3	0

[a] Two studies on MRI characteristics were combined to yield this table of data concerning the MRI characteristics of supratentorial ependymomas.

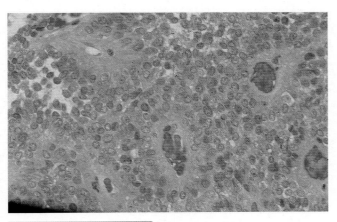

Figure 16–3   A hemotoxylin and eosin–stained ependymoma demonstrating characteristic perivascular pseudorosette formation with cuboidal cells.

biology to other primitive neuroectodermal tumors, such as medulloblastoma, retinoblastoma, pinealoblastoma, and so forth, as opposed to ependymoma, with which it has little in common. Inclusion of ependymoblastoma in the patient populations under study will severely skew the data toward the "malignant" end of the spectrum. Thus, treatments with possible benefits to patients with ependymoma will appear as worthless if no effect is seen on the more malignant entity of ependymoblastoma.

Significant difficulty exists in the interpretation of data from papers published with respect to ependymoblastoma and subependymoma. In many series, these tumors were included with ependymoma[15, 36, 40, 48, 52–63] despite the fact that the grading systems separated these entities. The two predominant grading systems will be described below; a corresponding summary of the clinical series with respect to these grading systems will also be given.

Kernohan Classification

In Kernohan's first description, four subtypes of ependymomas were defined:

(1) The *cellular* group, characterized by compact masses of ependymal cells. There is frequent mingling of the myxopapillary and epithelial types and a tendency to form pseudorosettes and especially perivascular pseudorosettes; (2) the *epithelial* group, a type of cell which

gives the general impression of true rosette formation (as well as pseudorosettes) and always contains "blepharoplasten" (minute granules) in the cytoplasm; (3) the *myxopapillary* group, which occurs anywhere along the cerebrospinal axis but is most frequently found in the sacral region of the spinal cord. The cells are high cuboidal with a heavy process attached to the core of a papilla; and (4) the *papilloma choroideum* group, a tumor composed of a special secreting type of cell which lines the choroid plexus. These types tend to be mixed, except for the papilloma group.[64]

This system evolved over time with many modifications. The classifications based on Kernohan by Mabon et al and later Svien et al were the most commonly used.[21, 65]

BOX 16–2
Kernohan's Grading System

- **Grade 1: Cells appear similar to normal ependymal cells. Pseudorosettes, true rosettes, and papilla are well formed. No pleomorphism, hyperchromatism, or mitotic figures are present.**
- **Grade 2: The architectural pattern is less distinct than grade 1 lesions, but still present. A few cells show moderate pleomorphism and hyperchromatism, though the majority of cells appear like normal ependymal cells.**
- **Grade 3: Architectural pattern more severely disrupted. Only about half the cells appear like normal ependymal cells. There are many cells with pleomorphism of the cytoplasm and nuclei, hyperchromatism, and mitotic figures are present.**
- **Grade 4: Only a few at best "normal ependymal cells." Architecture is nearly fully disrupted. Only a few remnants of ependymal structures. Cells have marked pleomorphism and hyperchromatism, and mitotic figures are abundant.**

World Health Organization Classification[66]

The current WHO classification simply divides ependymomas into (1) *classic ependymoma*, including variants (cellular, papillary, and clear cell), WHO grade 2; (2) *anaplastic ependymoma*, WHO grade 3; (3) *myxopapillary ependymoma* (found principally in the cauda equina) and (4) *subependymoma* (often associated with tuberous sclerosis), WHO grade 1.

In terms of grading the different classifications, the cellular criteria are different from those used for gliomas.

BOX 16–3
WHO Grading System

- **Grade 1: devoid of mitotic activity, hamartomatous lesion**
- **Grade 2: mitotic figures present but no endothelial proliferation or necrosis**
- **Grade 3: mitotic figures, plus endothelial proliferation or necrosis or both**
- **Grade 4: basic features similar to those of primitive neuroectodermal tumor but with evidence of ependymal differentiation (these highly cellular tumors contained numerous mitotic figures and usually had endothelial proliferation as well as necrosis). Grade 4 ependymoma is not equal to glioblastoma multiforme.[32, 105]**

Literature Review with Respect to Pathologic Features

A grading system must accomplish two very significant goals. It should demonstrate an accurate separation of tumors into meaningful and reproducible classes as well as provide pertinent clinical relevance. With these features in mind, the WHO grading system has merit with respect to identification of lesions as well as prognosis for given pathology.

Some authors have reported very high levels of grade 3/4 lesions in their series. Pierre-Kahn et al report that 86% of supratentorial ependymomas in children were malignant, but they include an unspecified number of ependymoblastomas.[30] Other authors have also stated that "many supratentorial ependymomas are malignant."[13, 21, 32, 40, 59, 67–69] This may be secondary to the tendency for the grade of a tumor to increase as the distance from the ventricular system increases.[36] In addition, supratentorial ependymomas, in contrast to infratentorial ependymomas and spinal ependymomas, have increased cell density and microcystic change, perhaps demonstrating a more malignant appearance to supratentorial ependymomas than infratentorial ependymomas.[31]

In other studies, the proportion of high-grade to low-grade lesions is reversed. Hahn et al found that 63.2% of the lesions in their study were benign.[14] In another study presented by Perilongo et al,[47] 32 patients with supratentorial ependymomas had benign lesions 69% of the time.

Ernestus et al reported 73 supratentorial ependymomas with 4.1% identified as subependymomas, 56.2% as grade 2 ependymomas, and 39.7% grade 3 ependymomas.[36] Anaplastic or malignant lesions were characterized by pleomorphism, including multinucleation and giant cells, mitotic figures, vascular changes, and necrosis. With this criteria, only 35.7% of 14 lesions were anaplastic.[12] We conclude that classic ependymoma is slightly more common than anaplastic ependymoma, but the ratio seen at any one hospital can vary tremendously based on physician referral patterns.

Regardless of the incidence of the various grades of ependymoma, the question remains whether any correlation may be made between prognosis and tumor grade. Svien et al reported the average age, sex, and mean survival for their cohort of patients with supratentorial ependymomas as they related to pathologic grade. They found after using a four level grading system that patients with low-grade lesions had improved survival (Table 16–5). Their study was not limited to pediatric cases and the data do not allow for strict extrapolation to pediatric outcome.[21]

Schiffer et al had similar results, showing that a high number of mitoses and high cell density were negative prognostic factors in supratentorial ependymomas in 72 patients (half of patients were older than 16 years).[70] Hypervascularity, endothelial proliferation, mitosis, and calcification have been shown to negatively affect prognosis in other reports.[67, 71, 72] Median survival of supratentorial ependymomas with vascular proliferation was 3.7 years versus 20.1 years in those patients with ependymomas that did not have vascular proliferation.[31] Ernestus et al[73] had very convincing results, with a median survival time without recurrence of 15.5 years with grade 2 lesions and 1.5 years with grade 3 lesions. At 5 years, grade 2 lesions were associated with a 75% survival, whereas grade 3 lesions were associated with a 31% survival. At 15 years, both curves remained at 31% survival, and no spinal seeding was seen in any patient. Conversely, some authors have found no prognostic significance to histologic grading systems in ependymomas.[12, 27, 28, 60] This may be due to the limited number of patients in many studies. Nevertheless, using the current WHO criteria, grade 3 ependymomas are likely to have a poorer outcome than grade 2 lesions with respect to 5-year survival. Convergence of the survival curves as seen in the study by Ernestus et al[73] is also expected.

TABLE 16–5 Patient Survival Based on Pathology Grade[a]

Grade	No. of Patients	M/F	Avg. age (y)	Postop survival (mo)
1	17	3:2	27.2	95.0
2	8	2:1	27.8	22.7
3	16	3:5	23.3	18.6
4	10	3:4	32.1	3.9

[a]These data, first presented by Svien et al,[21] show a correlation between outcome and tumor pathology.

SURGICAL TREATMENT

Olivecrona was one of the first surgeons to consider total surgical extirpation for supratentorial ependymomas to be sufficient therapy. In a series of patients (both adults and children), he reported that 8 of 25 patients who had gross total resection and received no radiotherapy were alive and well more than 10 years later. Olivecrona's series included a total of 30 patients with supratentorial ependymomas, with an operative mortality of 16.6%. Their 5-year survival was 16.1%, as opposed to his experience with infratentorial ependymomas, which had a 5-year survival of 35%.[74]

Fokes and Earle[23] reported similar results. They demonstrated 5-year survival rates for supratentorial and infratentorial ependymomas of 16.1% and 53.2%, respectively. Matson believed that surgical excision of a benign lesion was sufficient therapy. He reported that 8 patients with benign ependymomas with gross total resection (there were 24 patients in the series), no radiotherapy, were alive and well more than 10 years later.[11] All of these studies showed increased morbidity and mortality for supratentorial ependymomas versus infratentorial ependymomas.

Ten years later, Salazar reported results wherein supratentorial ependymomas had a 5-year survival similar to that of infratentorial ependymomas (approximately 37%), though 25% of their patients were older than 12 years.[43] This ratio then reversed in other reports at about the same time as well as more recently. Patients with supratentorial ependymomas had a mean survival of 53 months, versus 15 months for patients with infratentorial ependymomas in the series reported by Dohrman et al. The 1, 2, and 5-year survival rates for supratentorial ependymomas were 62%, 61%, and 32%, respectively.[40] In the series reported by Rawlings et al, patients with supratentorial ependymoma had a much better outcome than patients with infratentorial ependymoma: 1-year survival of 85% versus 71%, and 5-year survival of 49% versus 23%.[31] This reversal of outcome may in part be due to use of steroids, as well as improved operative techniques and earlier diagnosis.

In a recent study of supratentorial ependymomas in children 20 years or younger, Palma et al reported a mean age of 13.2 at diagnosis. They were able to obtain a gross total resection in 89.9% of patients. They had an operative mortality rate of 11.1%. Patients had a mean survival of 8.9 years, with 22.2% of them being cured as per Collins' law. In five of the six patients who survived for less than 5 years (range 7 to 54 months), the diagnosis was malignant ependymoma. With respect to the patients without malignant ependymoma, two died postoperatively, one died at 54 months, and the total survival of patients surviving postoperatively was 12 years and counting.[39] Similar results were obtained by Perilongo et al. Of 32 patients with supratentorial ependymomas, 56% had a gross total resection. This resulted in a 10-year progression-free survival of 37.7% and an overall 10-year survival of 66.8%.[47]

Radical surgery without adjuvant therapy is being revisited as treatment of choice for ependymoma. In 1996, Awaad et al published their results with 10 children who had supratentorial ependymomas. The average age of the children was 8.3 years, the male/female ratio was 2:1, and all patients had an attempt at gross total excision of low-grade ependymoma.

Postoperative MRI showed complete resection in five patients; two patients had small blood clots that prevented accurate assessment. The two patients with blood clots had recurrences at 3 and 11 months and underwent repeat resection. The five patients with negative MRI had a progression-free survival of 42 months at the end of the study. The whole group had a total survival of 39.5 months and no deaths. It is important to note that this was a highly selected group of patients, drawn from a population of 52 ependymomas, 19 of which were supratentorial.[75, 76]

In addition to the change in outcome of infratentorial lesions versus supratentorial lesions, operative and perioperative mortality changed drastically with the use of corticosteroids. Perioperative mortality dropped precipitously, from 40% to 17%,[30, 40] with operative mortality being demonstrated to be lower with supratentorial ependymomas versus infratentorial ependymomas.[9, 12, 28–30, 33, 37, 43, 46, 77, 78] In Table 16–6 the operative mortality rate, 5-year survival, and median survival are summarized from several major series.

Ependymomas are known for their ability to seed the neuraxis via the subarachnoid space. This is less common in patients with supratentorial ependymomas, in contrast to infratentorial ependymomas. Reports of metastasis range from 5%[38] to 20%.[41] In studies with 10 or more patients with supratentorial ependymomas, the average incidence of metastasis was 8%.[79] In a large pediatric study by Pierre-Kahn et al, only three (9%) instances of metastasis were seen and no lesions metastasized to below the tentorium.[30] Extraneural metastases are very rare. The most common site for metastatic spread is to the lungs and lymph nodes, with a slightly higher representation of supratentorial ependymomas versus infratentorial ependymomas as a source.[80]

RADIATION THERAPY

The use of radiotherapy for supratentorial ependymoma remains controversial. Several surgeons, as previously discussed, believe that radiotherapy is not indicated when a gross total resection of classic ependymoma is achieved, assuming that no evidence of metastatic disease exists. Furthermore, given that the correlation of tumor grade with outcome is unclear, complete resection of even anaplastic ependymoma may qualify as sufficient treatment. Nevertheless, there is much previous experience with radiotherapy as an adjunctive treatment for supratentorial ependymomas.

Experience with radiotherapy includes patients with low-grade and high-grade tumors, even after gross total resection. Several variables have been explored, including dosage, schedule, and fields treated. The enthusiasm for radiotherapy must also be tempered by an appreciation of the real costs of radiotherapy, including but not limited to the risk of oncogenesis[35, 60, 81, 82] and mental retardation.[43, 83, 84]

Given the potential destructive nature of radiotherapy, it is considered prudent to use lower radiation doses for younger patients. Salazaar et al have previously published a set of guidelines for reduced whole-brain radiotherapy based on the age of the patient.[90] Their guidelines are summarized in Table 16–7. Regions to be irradiated are also open to review. Many physicians recommend treatment for the

TABLE 16–6   Mortality Rate and Survival after Surgery for Supratentorial Ependymoma

Series	No. of patients	Operative mortality rate (%)	5-Year survival (%)	Median survival (mo)
Cushing[101]	6	33.3		
Ringertz and Reymond[13]	21	22.0	15.0	< 24.0
Kricheff et al[28, 37]	18	33.3	14.0–33.0	33.6
Phillips et al[46]	21	33.3	31.0	
Olivecrona[74]	30	16.6	15.0	
Fokes and Earl[23]			16.1	15.1
Shuman et al[33]	18	5.6		
Hahn et al[14]	14			38.7
Dohrman et al[40]			25.0	50.0
Mork and Loken[12]	28	16.6	18.0	
Goutelle[104]	102	34.3		
Coulon and Till[9]	13	15.4	10.0	22.2
Pierre-Kahn et al[30]		6.0	39.0	
Undjian and Marinov[63a]	23	17.4	26.1	
Goldwein et al[25]	18		35.0	
Palma et al[39]		11.1		106.0

[a] Operative mortality rate (includes 1 month postoperative), 5-year survival, and median survival for supratentorial ependymomas.
[b] includes children with ependymoblastoma.

TABLE 16–7   Proposed Radiotherapy Schedule (rads)[90]

Age (y)	WB radiotherapy	Target boost	Daily fraction
≤3	3600	4400	150
4–12	4500	5500	150
>12	4500	5500	180

The age of the patient is thought to play a large role in the risk of radiotherapy. This table is one recommendation for tailoring the radiotherapy to the patient's age.

TABLE 16–8   Radiotherapeutic Guidelines for Treatment (Gy)[88a]

Lesion	Supratentorial low-grade	Supratentorial high-grade
Whole brain	40.00	40.00
Primary tumor	54.40	54.40
Spinal cord	–	35.20

[a] This proposed radiotherapy is for children older than 3 years. In this algorithm, radiotherapy is changed according to the pathologic features of the lesion.

tumor bed and the whole brain regardless of tumor grade.[85] Others recommend that the whole craniospinal axis be radiated for all malignant lesions.[30, 43, 78, 86, 87] Silverman et al published their recommendations for supratentorial ependymomas based on the histologic grading of the lesion (Table 16–8). Their algorithm does not take into consideration the extent of resection.[88]

Some studies have shown an improvement in 5-year survival with 45 Gy or more to the primary site.[12, 23, 87] Dohrman et al showed a large improvement in survival with radiotherapy: 19 months with surgery versus 53 months with surgery plus radiotherapy. They also demonstrated significant improvement in short-term but not long-term, survival (Table 16–9).[40] Phillips et al also demonstrated improved survival with radiotherapy, though their data encompass adult patients as well as infratentorial lesions.[46]

A comparison of patient outcome with low-dose radiotherapy (less than 45 Gy) and high-dose radiotherapy (45 to 55 Gy) has shown a change in improved survival from 10 to 30% after the lower dose of radiation to 35 to 60% with the higher dose of radiation.[37, 89, 90]

Using high-dose radiotherapy, Ernestus et al in a study not limited to the pediatric population exhibited demonstrable benefit from radiotherapy (Table 16–10). In their experience, the use of radiotherapy correlated with an improved outcome. Gross total resection and lower grade lesions were also associated with improved outcomes in their study.[36] For all ependymomas, Mork and Loken saw the 50% survival time increase by 2 years with radiotherapy, but the survival curves converged at 9 years. Thus there appeared to be a short-term benefit with radiotherapy, but no long-term improvement.[12]

Conversely, Perilongo et al reported 32 patients with supratentorial ependymomas who had a doubling of survival with gross total resection but no increase in survival with radiotherapy.[47] In addition, excellent results without recurrence have been demonstrated with gross total

TABLE 16–9 Radiotherapy Improves Short-Term Survival[40a]

Treatment	No. of cases	Median survival (mo)	% Survival 1 y	2 y	5 y
Operation	6	19	50	50	50
Op + radiotherapy	4	53	100	100	60

[a] Radiotherapy had a large effect on short-term outcome and a minimal effect on long-term outcome.

TABLE 16–10 Radiotherapy and Surgery Improves Survival[36a]

Procedure	5-Year survival rate without recurrence (%)	Median survival time without recurrence (mo)
Grade 2 ependymoma	57.4	83
Resection only	40.7	38
Resection plus radiotherapy	80.0	185
Grade 3 ependymoma	24.1	18
Resection only	11.1	16
Resection plus radiotherapy	30.0	21
Resection:		
Gross Total	48.7	54
Partial	40.5	30
Resection	17.6	9
Resection plus radiotherapy	60.0	108

[a] Quality of resection has an important role in patient survival. In this study, radiotherapy had a major role in patient outcome.

resection and no adjuvant therapy in patients with low-grade ependymomas.[75, 76]

CHEMOTHERAPY

Prior studies on the efficacy of chemotherapy are limited by the lack of patients who meet strict categorical criteria. These studies lump together not only different grades of ependymoma but also different pathologic entities, including gliomas and primitive neuroectodermal tumors (i.e., medulloblastomas and ependymoblastomas). In addition, patients have had various degrees of surgical resection as well as tumor burden. In several studies, the few patients with supratentorial ependymomas did not benefit from chemotherapy.[91–93]

Although minimal responses to nitrosoureas and vincristine have been reported,[94–96] there are other studies whereby diaziquone and cisplatin have demonstrated a large reduction in tumor volume by CT criteria, but only in a minority of cases.[97, 98] Supratentorial ependymomas treated with PCV (procarbazine, CCNU, vincristine) and CVM (CCNU, vincristine, methotrexate) have also had poor response rates.[99, 100] At this point, the data are insufficient to support the use of chemotherapeutic agents except as an experimental protocol after surgery and radiotherapy have failed to control the tumor.

SUMMARY AND FUTURE DIRECTION

Supratentorial ependymomas continue to present as a challenging clinical entity and confront the clinician on many levels. The lower grade lesions are often situated in the midline, intimately involved with vital anatomical structures that are sensitive to surgical manipulation. Lesions at a distance from the midline, in less eloquent brain, are frequently high grade or anaplastic, having a tendency to recur despite surgical extirpation. The use of radiotherapy may permit some improvement in outcome, especially when a gross total excision is not achieved, but chemotherapy has yet to be proven useful.

Avoiding radiotherapy in children who may not benefit directly should also be a therapeutic goal. Long-term survival leading to mental retardation or the development of another malignancy is a poor trade-off. Furthermore, irradiating the spinal cord without having objective clinical evidence of cord involvement should also be avoided. Unlike anaplastic and low-grade gliomas, the data presented here clearly argue for radical resection. Biopsy followed by radiation strategies has not proven useful in the treatment of supratentorial ependymomas.

Future research in this arena should address the long-term outcome of children with low-grade ependymoma with gross total resection who are not treated with radiotherapy. At what point does disease-free progression truly constitute a cure? In addition, the use of stereotactic guided resection is likely to have a vital role in the achievement of gross total resection. Furthermore, treatment of these tumors may also eventually include genetic manipulation. Nevertheless, if an adequate understanding of an effective treatment armamentarium is to be obtained, it will be necessary to investigate these tumors within their respective pathologic categories and exclude subependymomas and ependymoblastomas from subsequent outcome studies.

REFERENCES

1. Virchow R. Die Krankhaften Geschülste Band II. Berlin 1864–1865.
2. Bailey P. A study of tumors arising from ependymal cells. *Arch Neurol Psychiatry* 1924;11:1–27.
3. Bailey P, Cushing H. A classification of the tumors of the glioma group on a histogenetic basis with a correlated study of prognosis. Philadelphia: Lippincott; 1926;66–69.
4. Flores LE, Williams DL, Bell BA, et al. Delay in the diagnosis of pediatric brain tumors. *Am J Dis Child* 1986;140:684–686.
5. Hooper R. Intracranial tumours in childhood. *Child's Brain* 1975;1:136–140.
6. West CR, Bruce DA, Duffner PK. Ependymomas: factors in clinical and diagnostic staging. *Cancer* 1985;56:1812–1816.
7. Bailey P, Buchanan D, Bucy P. Intracranial tumors of infancy and childhood. Chicago; 1939:13–40.
8. Cuneo H, Rand C. Ependynoma. In: *Brain Tumors of Childhood*. Springfield: Charles C Thomas; 1952;58–69.
9. Coulon RA, Till K. Intracranial ependymomas in children: a review of 43 cases. *Child's Brain* 1977;3:154–168.
10. Koos W, Miller M. Intracranial tumors in infants and children. Stuttgart; 1971.
11. Matson DD. Gliomas of the cerebral hemispheres. In: *Neurosurgery of Infancy and Childhood*. Springfield; 1969:502–504.
12. Mork SJ, Loken AC. Ependymoma: a follow-up study of 101 cases. *Cancer* 1977;40:907–915.
13. Ringertz N, Reymond A. Ependymomas and choroid plexus papollomas. *J Neuropathol Exp Neurol* 1949;8:355–380.
14. Hahn F, Schapiro R, Okawara S-H. Supratentorial ependymoma. *Neuroradiology* 1975;10:5–13.
15. Armington WG, Osborn AG, Cubberley DA, Harnsberger HR, Boyer R, Naidich TP, Sherry RG. Supratentorial ependymoma: CT appearance. *Radiology* 1985;157:367–372.
16. Swartz JD, Zimmerman RA, Bilaniuk LT. Computed tomography of intracranial ependymomas. *Radiology* 1982;143:97–101.
17. Vernet O, Farmer JP, Meagher VK, Montes JL. Supratentorial ectopic ependymoma. *Can J Neurol Sci* 1995;22:316–319.
18. Centeno RS, Lee AA, Winter J, Barba D. Supratentorial ependymomas: neuroimaging and clinicopathological correlation. *J Neurosurg* 1986;64:209–215.
19. Hanchey RE, Stears JC, Lehman RA, Norenberg MD. Interhemispheric ependymoma mimicking falx meningioma: case report. *J Neurosurg* 1976;45:108–112.
20. Kernohan J, Sayre G. *Tumors of the Central Nervous System.* Sec. X, Fasc. 35. Washington DC: Armed Forces Institute of Pathology; 1952.
21. Svien H, Mabon R, Kernohan J, McK Craig W. Ependymoma of the brain: pathological aspects. *Neurology* 1953;3:1–15.
22. Barone BM, Elvidge AR. Ependymomas: a clinical survey. *J Neurosurg* 1970;33:428–438.
23. Fokes EJ, Earle KM. Ependymomas: clinical and pathological aspects. *J Neurosurg* 1969;30:585–594.
24. Garrett PG, Simpson WJ. Ependymomas: results of radiation treatment. *Int J Radiat Oncol Biol Phys* 1983;9:1121–1124.
25. Goldwein JW, Leahy JM, Packer RJ, et al. Intracranial ependymomas in children [see comments]. *Int J Radiat Oncol Biol Phys* 1990;19:1497–1502.
26. Ilgren EB, Stiller CA, Hughes JT, et al. Ependymomas: a clinical and pathologic study. Part I. Biologic features. *Clin Neuropathol* 1984;3:113–121.
27. Ilgren EB, Stiller CA, Hughes JT, et al. Ependymomas: a clinical and pathologic study. Part II. Survival features. *Clin Neuropathol* 1984;3:122–127.
28. Kricheff I, Becker M, Schneck S, Taveras J. Intracranial ependymomas: factors influencing prognosis. *J Neurosurg* 1964;21:7–14.
29. Namer I, Pamir M, Benli K, and Erbengi, A. Les épendymomes intracrâniens: etude de 81 cas et comparaison avec la littérature. *Neurochirugie* 1984;30.
30. Pierre-Kahn A, Hirsch JF, Roux FX, et al. Intracranial ependymomas in childhood: survival and functional results of 47 cases. *Child's Brain* 1983;10:145–156.
31. Rawlings CD, Giangaspero F, Burger PC, Bullard DE. Ependymomas: a clinicopathologic study. *Surg Neurol* 1988;29:271–281.
32. Shaw EG, Evans RG, Scheithauer BW, et al. Postoperative radiotherapy of intracranial ependymoma in pediatric and adult patients. *Int J Radiat Oncol Biol Phys* 1987;13:1457–1462.
33. Shuman RM, Alvord EJ, Leech RW. The biology of childhood ependymomas. *Arch Neurol* 1975;32:731–739.
34. Kim YH, Fayos JV. Intracranial ependymomas. *Radiology* 1977;124:805–808.
35. Read G. The treatment of ependymoma of the brain or spinal canal by radiotherapy: a report of 79 cases. *Clin Radiol* 1984;35:163–166.
36. Ernestus RI, Wilcke O, Schroder R. Intracranial ependymomas: prognostic aspects. *Neurosurg Rev* 1989;12:157–163.
37. Kricheff I, Becker M, Schneck S, Taveras J. Intracranial Ependymomas: a study of survival in 65 cases treated by surgery and irridiation. *Am J Roentgenol* 1964;91:7–14.
38. Marks JE, Adler SJ. A comparative study of ependymomas by site of origin. *Int J Radiat Oncol Biol Phys* 1982;8:37–43.
39. Palma L, Celli P, Cantore G. Supratentorial ependymomas of the first two decades of life: long-term follow–up of 20 cases (including two subependymomas). *Neurosurgery* 1993;32:169–175.
40. Dohrmann GJ, Farwell JR, Flannery JT. Ependymomas and ependymoblastomas in children. *J Neurosurg* 1976;45:273–283.
41. Renaudin JW, DiTullio MV, Brown WJ. Seeding of intracranial ependymomas in children. *Child's Brain* 1979;5:408–412.

42. Sagerman R, Bagshaw M, Hanbery J. Considerations in the treatment of ependymoma. *Radiology* 1965;84:401–408.

43. Salazar OM, Castro VH, VanHoutte P, et al. Improved survival in cases of intracranial ependymoma after radiation therapy: late report and recommendations. *J Neurosurg* 1983;59:652–659.

44. Tarlov I, Davidoff L. Subarchnoid and ventricular implants in ependymal and other gliomas. *J Neuropathol Exp Neurol* 1946;5:213–224.

45. Wentworth P, Birdsell DC. Intracranial ependymoma with extracranial metastases. *J Neurosurg* 1966;25:648–651.

46. Phillips T, Sheline G, Boldrey E. Therapeutic considerations in tumors affecting the central nervous system: ependymomas. *Radiology* 1964;83:98–105.

47. Perilongo G, Massimino M, Sotti G, et al. Analyses of prognostic factors in a retrospective review of 92 children with ependymoma: Italian Pediatric Neuro-oncology Group. *Med Pediatr Oncol* 1977;29:79–85.

48. Furie DM, Provenzale JM. Supratentorial ependymomas and subependymomas: CT and MR appearance. *J Comput Assist Tomogr* 1995;19:518–526.

49. Tominaga T, Kayama T, Kumabe T, et al. Anaplastic ependymomas: clinical features and tumour suppressor gene *p53* analysis. *Acta Neurochir (Wien)* 1995;135:163–170.

50. Ford FR. *Diseases of the Nervous System.* Springfield: Charles C Thomas; 881–883, 1945.

51. Russel D, Rubinstein L. *Pathology of Tumors of the Nervous System.* London: Williams & Wilkins; 1989.

52. Casentini L, Gullotta F, Mohrer U. Clinical and morphological investigations on ependymomas and their tissue cultures. *Neurochirurgia (Stuttgart)* 1981;24:51–56.

53. Chin HW, Hazel JJ, Kim TH, Freeman C, Maruyama Y. Intracranial ependymomas and ependymoblastomas. *Strahlentherapie* 1984;160:191–194

54. Chin HW, Maruyama Y, Markesbery W, Young AB. Intracranial ependymoma: results of radiotherapy at the University of Kentucky. *Cancer* 1982;49:2276–2280.

55. Ernestus RI, Schroder R, Stutzer H, Klug N. Prognostic relevance of localization and grading in intracranial ependymomas of childhood. *Child's Nerv Syst* 1996;12:522–526.

56. Kudo H, Oi S, Tamaki N, et al. Ependymoma diagnosed in the first year of life in Japan in collaboration with the International Society for Pediatric Neurosurgery. *Child's Nerv Syst* 1990;6:375–378.

57. Levin VA, Clancy TP, Ausman JI, Rall DP. Uptake and distribution of ^{3}H-methotrexate by the murine ependymoblastoma. *J Natl Cancer Inst* 1972;48:875–883.

58. Levin VA, Freeman DM, Maroten CE. Dianhydrogalactitol (NSC-132313): pharmacokinetics in normal and tumor–bearing rat brain and antitumor activity against three intracerebral rodent tumors. *J Natl Cancer Inst* 1976;56:535–539.

59. Liu HM, Boogs J, Kidd J. Ependymomas of childhood. I. Histological survey and clinicopathological correlation. *Child's Brain* 1976;2:92–110.

60. Ross GW, Rubinstein LJ. Lack of histopathological correlation of malignant ependymomas with postoperative survival. *J Neurosurg* 1989;70:31–36.

61. Rubinstein LJ. Embryonal central neuroepithelial tumors and their differentiating potential: a cytogenetic view of a complex neuro-oncological problem. *J Neurosurg* 1985;62:795–805.

62. Schiffer D, Chio A, Giordana MT. Histologic prognostic factors in ependymoma. *Child's Nerv Syst* 1991;7:177–182.

63. Undjian S, Marinov M. Intracranial ependymomas in children. *Child's Nerv Syst* 1990;6:131–134.

64. Kernohan J, Fletcher-Kernohan E. The ependymomas, a study of 109 cases. *Proc Res Nerv Ment Dis* 1935;16:182.

65. Mabon R, Svien H, Kernohan J, Craig WM. Ependymomas. *Proc Staff Meet Mayo Clin* 1949;24:65.

66. Kleihues P, Burger P, Scheithauer B. Histological typing of tumors of the central nervous system. In: *World Health Organization International Histological Classification of Tumors.* Berlin: Springer-Verlag; 1993:17–18.

67. Gilles FH, Leviton A, Hedley WT, Jasnow M. Childhood brain tumor update. *Hum Pathol* 1983;14:834–845.

68. Kernohan J. Ependymomas. In: Minckler J ed. *Pathology of the Nervous System.* New York: McGraw-Hill; 1968: 1976–1993.

69. Zulch K. *Brain Tumors: Their Biology and Pathology.* New York: Springer; 1986.

70. Schiffer D, Chio A, Cravioto H, et al. Ependymoma: internal correlations among pathological signs: the anaplastic variant. *Neurosurgery* 1991;29:206–210.

71. Kitahara M, Katakura R, Kanno M, et al. Results of intracranial ependymoma combined with radiochemotherapy. *Neurol Surg* 1987;15:495–501.

72. Rorke LB. Relationship of morphology of ependymoma in children to prognosis. *Prog Exp Tumor Res* 1987;30:170–174.

73. Ernestus RI, Wilcke O, Schroder R. Supratentorial ependymomas in childhood: clinicopathological findings and prognosis. *Acta Neurochir (Wien)* 1991;111:96–102.

74. Olivecrona H. The surgical treatment of intracranial tumors. In: Olivecrona H, Tonnis W, eds: *Handbuch der Neurochirugie.* Berlin: Springer-Verlag 1967;1–301.

75. Awaad YM, Allen JC, Miller DC, Schneider SJ, Wisoff J, Epstein FJ. Deferring adjuvant therapy for totally resected intracranial ependymoma. *Pediatr Neurol* 1996;14:216–219.

76. Hukin J, Epstein F, Lefton D, Allen J. Treatment of intracranial ependymoma by surgery alone. *Pediatr Neurosurg* 1998;29:40–45.

77. Bloom H, Walsssh L. Tumors of the central nervous system. In: Bloom, Lemerle, Neidhardt, and Voute, eds. *Cancer in Children: Clinical Management.* Berlin: Springer-Verlag; 1975:93.

78. Pierre-Kahn A, Hirsch J, Renier D, et al. Les épendymomes intrâcraniens de l'enfant: pronostic et perspectives thérapeutiques. *Arch Fr Pediatr* 1983;40:5–9.

79. Cohen M, Duffner P. *Brain Tumors of Childhood: Principles of Diagnosis and Treatment.* New York; 1994.

80. Cohen ME, Duffner PK. Current therapy in childhood brain tumors. *Neurol Clin* 1985;3:147–164.

81. Palma L, Vagnozzi R, Annino L, et al. Postradiation glioma in a child: case report and review of the literature. *Child's Nerv Syst* 1988;4:296–301.

82. Shapiro S, Mealey JJ, Sartorius C. Radiation induced intracranial malignant gliomas. *J Neurosurg* 1989;71:77–82.

83. Jacobi G, Kornhuber B. Malignant brain tumors in children. In Jellinger K, ed. *Therapy of Malignant Brain Tumors.* Wien: Springer-Verlag; 1987.

84. Oi S, Raimondi A. Ependymoma. In: *Pediatric Neurosurgery*. New York: Grune and Stratton; 1982;419–427.

85. McLaughlin MP, Marcus RB Jr, Buatti JM, et al. Ependymoma: results, prognostic factors and treatment recommendations. *Int J Radiat Oncol Biol Phys* 1998;40:845–850.

86. Bloom H. Recent concepts in the conservative treatment of intracranial tumors in children. *Acta Neurochir* 1979;50:103–116.

87. Wallner KE, Wara WM, Sheline GE, Davis RL. Intracranial ependymomas: results of treatment with partial or whole brain irradiation without spinal irradiation. *Int J Radiat Oncol Biol Phys* 1986;12:1937–1941.

88. Silverman C, Thomas P, Cox W. Ependymomas. In: Deutsch M, ed. *Management of Childhood Brain Tumors*. Boston: Kluwer Academic; 1990:369–382.

89. Kim T, Chin H, Pollan S, et al. Radiotherapy of primary brainstem tumors. *Int J Radiat Oncol Biol Phys* 1980;6:51–57.

90. Salazar OM, Rubin P, Bassano D, Marcial VA. Improved survival of patients with intracranial ependymomas by irradiation: dose selection and field extension. *Cancer* 1975;35:1563–1573.

91. Carrie C, Bouffet E, Brunat-Mentigny M, Philip T, Lacroze M. Les tumeurs cerebrales primitives de l'enfant. Partie II: Etude topographique et traitment. *Bull Cancer* 1989;76: 255–272.

92. Kun LE, Kovnar EH, Sanford RA. Ependymomas in children. *Pediatr Neurosci* 1988;14:57–63.

93. Marsh WR, Laws EJ. Intracranial ependymomas. *Prog Exp Tumor Res* 1987;30:175–180.

94. Friedman H, Oakes W. The chemotherapy of posterior fossa tumors in childhood. *J Neuro-oncol* 1987;5:217–229.

95. Levin VA. Chemotherapy of primary brain tumors. *Neurol Clin* 1985;3:855–866.

96. Wilson C, Cutin P, Baldrey E, et al. Single-agent chemotherapy of brain tumors. *Arch Neurol* 1976;33:739–744.

97. Khan A, D'Souza B, Wharam M, et al. Cisplatin therapy in recurrent childhood brain tumors. *Cancer Treat Rep* 1982;66:2013–2020.

98. Sexauer CL, Khan A, Burger PC, et al. Cisplatin in recurrent pediatric brain tumors: a POG Phase II study. A Pediatric Oncology Group Study. *Cancer* 1985;56: 1497–1501.

99. Gutin P, Wilson C, Kumar A, et al. Phase II study of procarbazine, CCNU, and vincristine in the treatment of malignant brain tumors. *Cancer* 1975;35:1398–1404.

100. Hildebrand J, Brihaye J, Wagenknecht J, et al. Combination chemotherapy with 1-(2-chloroethyl-3-cyclohexyl-1-nitrosurea)(CCNU), vincristine, and methotrexate in primary and metastatic brain tumor: a preliminary report. *Eur J Cancer Clin Oncol* 1973;9:627–634.

101. Cushing H. *Intracranial Tumours: Notes Upon a Series of 2000 Verified Cases with Surgical Mortality Percentages Thereto*. Springfield; 1932.

102. List C. Intracranial ependymomas: a preliminary report. *Univ Hosp Bull Ann Arbor* 1936;2:27.

103. Minauf M, Jellinger K, Grunert V. [Frequency and morphology of supratentorial ependymomas in adults]. *Acta Neurochir (Wien)* 1970;22:181–193.

104. Goutelle A. Les ependymomes intra-craniens sustentoriels. *Neurochirugie* 1977;23(Suppl):1977;53–109.

105. Zülch K. Histological typing of tumours of the central nervous system. Geneva; 1979.

106. Zülch K, Kleinsasser O. Ortsgebundene Abweichungen in der Histologie und im biologischen Verhalten der Ependymome. *Zentralbl Allg Pathol Pathol Anat* 1957; 97:59–66.

Chapter 17

Infratentorial Primitive Neuroectodermal Tumors

Ian F. Pollack

Medulloblastoma is the most common posterior fossa tumor of childhood and one of the most common pediatric solid tumors. The term "medulloblastoma" is a misnomer, reflecting the belief of Bailey and Cushing that these small-cell neoplasms were derived from a multipotential medulloblast.[1] These lesions were subsequently classified by Rorke et al[2] with other primitive neuroectodermal tumors (PNETs),[3] and the terms "medulloblastoma" and "infratentorial PNET" are now used interchangeably. These lesions have a characteristic mode of presentation, with rapidly progressive headache, nausea, and vomiting from obstructive hydrocephalus and brain stem compression, and show a high frequency of dissemination at the time of diagnosis. Current treatment approaches for medulloblastoma address both of these clinical factors: surgery plays an essential role in immediately reducing the tumor burden and opening the ventricular system, whereas intensive adjuvant therapy is employed postoperatively to treat what is in reality an invasive, potentially multicentric disease process. *During the last 25 years, advances in the surgical and adjuvant management have led to substantial improvements in outcome for children harboring these tumors, increasing the 5-year progression-free survival from less than 20% to more than 70%, making this one of the real "success stories" of pediatric neuro-oncology.* Ongoing studies are directed at further improving the survival rate of children with these tumors while minimizing treatment-induced morbidity.

EPIDEMIOLOGY

Medulloblastomas account for approximately 20% of pediatric brain tumors and 30% of posterior fossa tumors.[4] Approximately 300 new cases are diagnosed in the United States each year, which corresponds to approximately 5 cases per million children per year.[5, 6] A 2:1 male predominance has been noted in most large series.[7–9] The median age at diagnosis is 5 to 7 years, and more than 75% of cases are diagnosed in the first 15 years of life.[10] Approximately 20% of lesions arise in adults, where they are often located within the cerebellar hemispheres and are histologically desmoplastic.[11–13]

Exhaustive studies of risk factors have failed to identify a single environmental factor that had a clear relationship to the development of these tumors. Similarly, various maternal dietary factors, such as folate, multivitamin, and iron supplements, have been associated with a slightly lower risk of having a child with medulloblastoma,[14, 15] but no factor that predisposes to the development of medulloblastoma has been identified.

In contrast, children with several genetically transmissible syndromes, such as nevoid basal cell carcinoma (Gorlin's) syndrome, Turcot's syndrome, and Li-Fraumeni syndrome, are known to be at significantly increased risk for developing medulloblastoma. Gorlin's syndrome is characterized by multiple nevoid basal cell carcinomas, jaw cysts, skeletal abnormalities, pits on the palms and soles, dural calcifications, hydrocephalus, and mental retardation. Approximately 3 to 5% of affected children develop medulloblastomas,[16, 17] which are frequently desmoplastic in appearance. These lesions have been attributed to inactivation of a tumor suppressor gene at chromosome 9q.[18] Patients with Turcot's syndrome exhibit multiple colonic polyposis in association with central nervous system tumors, such as malignant gliomas and medulloblastomas.[19, 20] This disorder has been linked to mutations in the *APC* gene on chromosome 5q and in various DNA mismatch repair genes,[20] but these regions have not been convincingly linked to the development of sporadic medulloblastomas.[19, 21] Patients with Li-Fraumeni syndrome, which results from germline mutations of the *p53* gene, exhibit an increased risk of a variety of carcinomas, sarcomas, and other tumor types, including PNETs.[22] Interestingly, *p53* mutations have been reported to be rare in sporadic medulloblastomas.[23]

BOX 17–1
Genetic Syndromes Associated with Medulloblastoma

- **Gorlin's syndrome**
- **Turcot's syndrome**
- **Li-Fraumeni syndrome**

PATHOLOGY AND MOLECULAR PATHOGENESIS
Nosology

The histopathologic characterization of these tumors has been controversial since their initial description by Bailey and Cushing as "spongioblastoma cerebelli."[24] These authors soon realized that a similar term had been used for malignant

This work was supported in part by NIH grant 1KO8-NS01810.

supratentorial tumors and modified the name to "medulloblastoma"[1] to reflect their belief that these lesions arose from medulloblasts, which were thought to be one of the five cell types populating the primitive neural tube. In reality, the medulloblast has never been conclusively identified and, instead, these tumors have been considered by many to arise from undifferentiated cells of the fetal external granular cell layer.[25, 26] This belief is by no means uniformly held, and others have suggested that these tumors may arise from undifferentiated subependymal cells of the medullary velum or the internal granular cell layer.[27]

Even more controversial is the relation of these tumors to other PNETs, such as neuroblastoma, pineoblastoma, retinoblastoma, and peripheral PNETs. Rorke[2] suggested that these tumors all be grouped together because their appearance is similar regardless of their site of origin in the nervous system. She hypothesized that undifferentiated neuroepithelial cells at a variety of sites in the nervous system could develop into PNETs. Conversely, Rubinstein felt that despite the histologic similarity of the above tumor types, the different lesions arose from malignant transformation along the pathway of differentiation of resident cells in different areas of the brain and that the various tumor types should be categorized separately.[28] With advances in the molecular characterization of the above lesions, it has become clear that at least some of these lesions are indeed pathogenetically distinct entities, such as retinoblastomas and peripheral PNETs, which result from consistent patterns of genomic alterations (i.e., Rb gene deletions and chromosome 11/22 translocations, respectively) that are not typically present in intracranial PNETs. It remains to be determined whether cerebral, pineal, and infratentorial PNETs arise from common or distinct genomic insults. However, the fact that these lesions differ significantly in terms of their response to therapy[29, 30] suggests that they may in reality be distinct entities. In view of the uncertainty regarding the appropriate nomenclature of these lesions, most investigators use the terms "medulloblastoma" and "infratentorial PNET" interchangeably or in combination (e.g., PNET-MB).

Cellular Pathology

Medulloblastomas are soft, friable, purplish gray tumors that usually arise in the cerebellar vermis and displace the surrounding structures. Although these lesions appear in places to be well circumscribed, they are generally invasive on a microscopic level, which precludes a truly complete resection. Desmoplastic medulloblastomas tend to be firmer and well circumscribed but are nonetheless invasive of the surrounding structures. Histologically, these tumors are characterized by their high cellularity comprising small oval to round cells with a high nuclear/cytoplasmic ratio (Fig. 17–1A) that exhibit foci of clustering into Homer Wright rosettes. Differentiation of cells along glial or neuronal lines has been noted in up to 50% of tumors,[31–34] but the relationship between this feature and outcome has been unclear.[31–37] Similarly, the relationship between desmoplasia (Fig. 17–1B) and prognosis has been uncertain.[38, 39]

Molecular Pathogenesis

On a genomic level, abnormalities in several chromosomes have been observed consistently in medulloblastomas, particularly loss of the short arm of chromosome 17 (17p), which

has been noted in about half of these tumors.[40, 41] Although a common site of deletions occurs near 17p13, which is the locus of the p53 gene, this gene is rarely mutated in medulloblastomas;[23, 42, 43] a nearby, heretofore uncharacterized, tumor suppressor gene distal to p53 (at 17p13.3) is likely to be involved.[44] Other sites of DNA sequence loss in medulloblastomas include chromosomes 6q, 16q, and 22q,[40, 45] although a common site of deletions on these chromosomes has yet to be identified conclusively.

Although amplification of a number of oncogenes and activation of various growth factor pathways have been noted anecdotally in sporadic medulloblastomas, no consistent pattern of abnormalities has been apparent.[46] A possible explanation for this observation is that the defining signaling abnormality in these tumors may be a loss or impairment of a normal mitogenic cascade that permits neural differentiation, such as a neurotrophin receptor–mediated pathway, rather than excessive stimulation of an aberrant pathway. This view is supported by the observation in neuroblastoma that tumors expressing high levels of the nerve growth factor (NGF) receptor (TrkA) have a more favorable prognosis than those without this feature, which is presumed to reflect the capacity of tumors with high TrkA expression to differentiate along normal lines, if an appropriate stimulus is provided. Although a role for NGF/TrkA has not been confirmed in medulloblastoma,[47] compelling evidence has recently been provided that high levels of expression of TrkC, the receptor for neurotrophin-3, may correlate with a favorable prognosis.[48] The contribution of other growth factor pathways to medulloblastoma growth and differentiation remains uncertain.

SYMPTOMS AND SIGNS

Medulloblastoma is the prototypical posterior fossa tumor of childhood, producing headache, nausea, and vomiting from obstructive hydrocephalus that characteristically occur early in the morning and remit shortly thereafter. Symptoms are usually present for 1 to 2 months before a diagnosis is made and become progressively more severe during that time. Not uncommonly, children exhibit head tilt or neck pain by the time of presentation from chronic tonsillar herniation. If the diagnosis is delayed significantly, children may manifest with progressive lethargy from a combination of hydrocephalus, dehydration, and brain stem compression by the tumor. Rarely, patients present with symptoms of spinal dissemination, such as back and leg pain or paraparesis, or with evidence of rapid neurologic deterioration from intratumoral hemorrhage.[49, 50] In comparison with older children, the mode of presentation in infants is often more insidious, with gradually progressive macrocephaly, irritability, failure to thrive, and loss of developmental milestones.[51]

On examination, most children exhibit papilledema. Sixthnerve palsies resulting from intracranial hypertension and ataxia from a combination of cerebellar compression and hydrocephalus are also common. Multiple cranial neuropathies and long-tract signs are uncommon and suggest major brain stem invasion by the tumor.

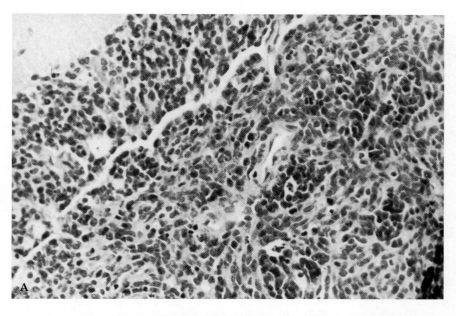

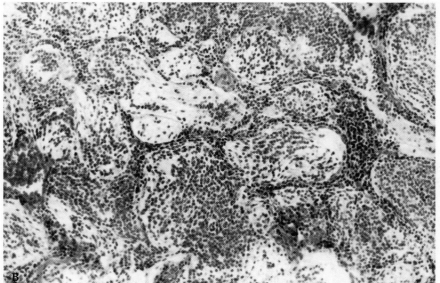

Figure 17–1   (A) Typical histologic appearance of a medulloblastoma showing a hypercellular neoplasm composed of small round to oval cells. (B) Desmoplastic medulloblastoma is characterized by delicate reticulin bands with hypocellular areas encompassing hypercellular areas, composed of cells with dense, round nuclei and scant cytoplasm.

BOX 17–2
Signs and Symptoms

- **Headache**
- **Nausea and vomiting**
- **Head tilt**
- **Neck pain**
- **Cranial nerve palsies**
- **Lethargy**
- **Irritability**
- **Spinal dissemination (including back pain, leg pain, neurologic deterioration)**
- **Gait abnormalities**
- **Ataxia**

DIAGNOSTIC EVALUATION

Computed tomography (CT) or magnetic resonance imaging (MRI) can each be used to establish the diagnosis of a posterior fossa tumor. Although no single feature is pathognomonic of a medulloblastoma, certain typical imaging characteristics are commonly noted. On CT, medulloblastomas are generally hyperdense, homogeneously enhancing vermian lesions that fill the fourth ventricle (Fig. 17–2). Calcifications and small cystic areas are also commonly observed.[52] On MRI, these lesions are often isointense or hypointense to brain on T1-weighted images, hyperintense on T2-weighted images, and intensely enhancing (Fig. 17–3). Mixed signal characteristics, indicative of foci of cyst formation, calcification, or hemorrhage, are observed in the majority of medulloblastomas.[53, 54] *In lesions that are thought to be*

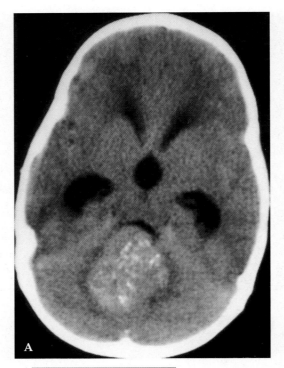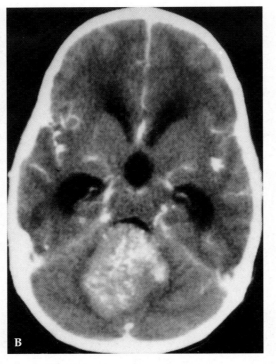

Figure 17–2 (A) Typical CT appearance of a medulloblastoma, showing a hyperdense fourth ventricular mass. Foci of calcification, noted in this image, are commonly observed. (B) Following administration of contrast, enhancement may be uniform or, as shown here, irregular.

medulloblastomas or ependymomas based on initial cranial imaging, we routinely obtain spinal MRI preoperatively, if this can be conveniently accomplished, because both lesion types show a significant incidence of cerebrospinal fluid (CSF) dissemination. Although such studies can also be obtained after surgery, artifacts from blood and high protein complicate interpretation of the images during the first few postoperative weeks, which may delay efforts to appropriately stage the patient's disease in preparation for adjuvant therapy. Needless to say, lumbar puncture for cytologic examination of CSF is contraindicated preoperatively in a child with a posterior fossa mass; such studies are performed after tumor resection has been completed.

BOX 17–3
Imaging Features

- **CT**
  - **Hyperdense**
  - **Homogeneous vermin lesions**
  - **Calcifications**
  - **Cystic areas**
- **MRI**
  - **T1: iso-/hypodense**
  - **T2: hyperintense, mixed signal**

SURGERY

Preresection Management

Most children who present with posterior fossa tumors can be stabilized with the administration of steroids (e.g., dexamethasone 1 to 6 mg q6h, depending on the weight of the patient) so that surgery can be performed electively on the next available operating day. Because of the known risk of perioperative stress ulceration in these patients, we generally administer an H_2 blocker in conjunction with the steroids, although we recognize that a benefit of this approach has not been proven.

Rarely, patients present *in extremis* and urgent intervention is required. Although significant symptomatic improvement can often be obtained by CSF diversion, we generally do not wait to see if the patient "wakes up" after this maneuver, but instead proceed directly with tumor removal. Although in the past, CSF shunting was advocated as a temporizing measure before resection of a midline posterior fossa tumor with associated hydrocephalus,[55–59] it is clear that the majority of such patients do not require long-term CSF diversion and thus can be spared the potential morbidity of shunting.

Anesthetic Considerations and Operative Positioning

The anesthetic technique generally consists of a mixture of fentanyl, vecuronium, nitrous oxide, and isoflurane, with the

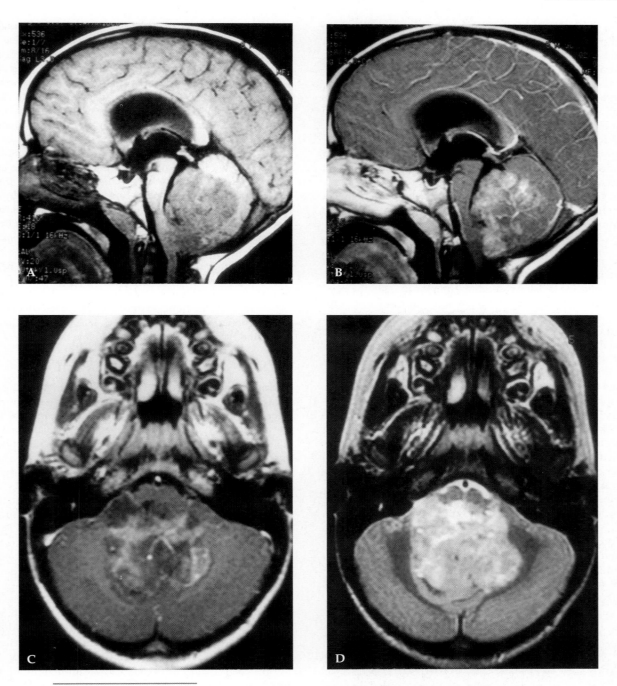

Figure 17–3 (A) T1-weighted sagittal magnetic resonance image of a medulloblastoma showing a vermian mass obstructing the fourth ventricle with apparent infiltration of the brain stem caudally. (B) Following administration of gadolinium, enhancement may be uniform or, as shown here, irregular. (C, D) These axial T1- and T2-weighted images reveal extensive brain stem infiltration and growth of the tumor through the foramen of Luschka.

doses adjusted to facilitate monitoring of somatosensory and brain stem auditory evoked potentials and lower cranial nerve electromyography. *We routinely monitor sixth- and seventh-nerve function and, depending on the predominant direction of tumor growth, may incorporate monitoring of the third, fourth, tenth, and twelfth cranial nerves because the sites of origin*

of these nerves within the brain stem are often involved by the tumor.[60] Achieving reliable monitoring while keeping the patient appropriately anesthetized requires that the anesthesiologist be made aware of the surgeon's plans preoperatively. Other common features of the surgical preparation include insertion of a urinary drainage catheter, arterial line, and, in most cases, a central line, and placement of sizable peripheral intravenous lines to facilitate blood replacement, if needed. Prophylactic antibiotics are administered during skin preparation and every 6 to 8 hours during the procedure. Steroids are also continued intraoperatively.

Under ideal circumstances, an external ventricular drain is placed immediately before the tumor removal and then clamped to avoid the risk of upward herniation[61-63] from rapid decompression of the ventricular system in the setting of a large posterior fossa mass. The patient is then placed in a modified prone (Concorde) position[62] using pin fixation of the head in children older than 3 years and a horseshoe head-rest in younger children. Care must be taken to pad points of dependency and avoid excessive flexion of the neck, which can compromise jugular venous return.

Tumor Resection

Following skin preparation, most lesions are approached using a midline incision extending from the inion to the spinous process of C2. A posterior fossa craniectomy or craniotomy (my preference) is then performed. Removal of the arch of C1 is also required for tumors with significant growth below the foramen magnum.

At this point, I usually ask the anesthesiologist to let off 10 to 20 mL of CSF if the dura is tense. The dura is then opened in a Y-shaped fashion beginning over the cerebellar hemispheres and extending toward the midline at the occipitocervical junction. Large venous sinuses at the foramen magnum region should be anticipated and occluded using either clips or sutures to avoid major bleeding. The incision is then extended inferiorly in the midline to the top of C1 or to the caudal pole of the tumor, whichever is lower. Then the cisterna magna is opened and the cerebellar tonsils are gently elevated using self-retaining retractors. In many cases, the tumor is immediately apparent within the cisterna magna (Fig. 17–4); if not, it is usually readily exposed by coagulation and incision of the inferior pole of the vermis. The vermian incision is then extended upward approximately 1 to 2 cm to provide a corridor for resection of the tumor. A frozen section is obtained and the central component of the tumor is debulked with the ultrasonic aspirator.

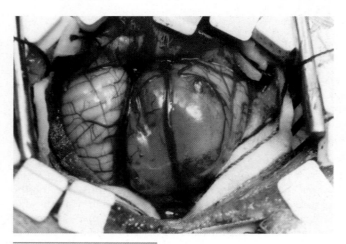

Figure 17–4 This large medulloblastoma fills the cisterna magna.

Although a tumor capsule is never present, a clear demarcation between tumor and normal brain is often apparent, particularly in the cerebellum. After coring out the center of the lesion, I usually follow the plane between the tumor and the cerebellum rostrally until the tongue of tumor extending into the roof of the fourth ventricle is identified. This typically yields a burst of CSF from the aqueduct, which is visualized and covered with a small cottonoid patty to prevent inflow of blood and tumor cells, and exposes the rostral fourth ventricular floor well beneath the residual tumor. With this landmark exposed, I debulk additional tumor in a rostral to caudal direction until the region where the tumor extends through the foramen of Magendie has been reached. Areas in which the tumor has clearly invaded the cerebellar peduncles and brain stem, which are encountered in the majority of tumors,[61, 64] are left for last. To minimize the risk of postoperative neurologic impairment, I generally resect the tumor flush with these surfaces without violating them because microscopic residual disease does not appear to adversely affect prognosis. Hemostasis in then achieved and the dura is closed in a "water-tight" fashion, usually with some form of graft material. The bone is replaced (if a craniotomy has been performed) and the wound closed in layers.

Postoperative Management

Patients are generally observed at least overnight in the intensive care unit and, if stable, are then transferred to the neurosurgical ward. In children who fail to awaken promptly after the anesthetics and muscle relaxants have worn off, an urgent CT scan should be obtained to rule out intracranial hemorrhage or infarction. Otherwise, a postoperative MRI is performed electively during the first 24 hours after surgery to determine the extent of residual disease.

The drip chamber of the external ventricular drain is kept at a height of 5 cm for the first 2 days to facilitate drainage of bloody CSF and then raised over the next 3 to 5 days. Steroids are tapered concurrently. Patients who do not tolerate weaning of the ventriculostomy, as evidenced by continued high CSF outputs at chamber heights above 30 cm, the development of a large pseudomeningocele, or the onset of progressive lethargy, may undergo an additional course of external drainage or, alternatively, a third ventriculostomy, but most such patients will ultimately require CSF diversion. Although there has long been concern that CSF shunting increases the patient's risk of extraneural seeding of tumor,[59] this point has never been proven.[65, 66] Because the addition of millipore filters to the shunt system to prevent dissemination[59, 64] has been associated with a prohibitive rate of shunt failure,[67] this strategy is not routinely used.

Surgical Morbidity

Neurologic complications, which may range from minor to severe, have been reported in approximately 25 to 40% of patients, even when the most up-to-date surgical techniques were utilized.[62, 68] An uncommon but potentially serious problem that mandates special attention is lower cranial nerve and brain stem dysfunction. Such patients may require a prolonged period of intubation and possibly tracheostomy and gastrostomy to facilitate adequate nutrition and airway protection. *Mutism and pseudobulbar dysfunction are seen in at* least 10% of children[61, 69-71] and encompass a spectrum of deficits, which range from impaired initiation of speech and oropharyngeal movements to a global impairment in the initiation of voluntary activities. These impairments usually manifest 24 to 72 hours after surgery, often after a period of relatively normal functioning. Although this syndrome is presumed to result from injury to the dentatorubrothalamic connections to the supplementary motor cortex,[72] this mechanism remains conjectural. Although symptoms often begin to resolve within several weeks after operation, some deficits persist for months.

Another syndrome of delayed onset is aseptic meningitis, which is characterized by fever, photophobia, and nuchal rigidity, usually occurring 5 to 7 days after operation.[67] This syndrome must be distinguished from bacterial meningitis by examination of the CSF Gram stain and culture. Whereas aseptic meningitis is treated using corticosteroids, bacterial meningitis requires appropriately selected antibiotics, which may be instituted empirically until the culture results are reported.

BOX 17–4
Morbidity

- **Cranial nerve deficits**
- **Brain stem dysfunction**
- **Mutism**
- **Pseudobulbar dysfunction**
- **Dysconjugate gaze**
- **Aseptic meningitis**

Postoperative Staging and Prognostic Factors

It has long been recognized that patients with large, incompletely resected medulloblastomas and those with disease dissemination had a worse prognosis after surgery than those with small, extensively resected, non-disseminated lesions. This observation has provided an impetus for various attempts at developing staging systems that facilitate risk stratification and therapeutic decision making. The Chang system represented an early attempt to solidify staging criteria, which were based on tumor size and extent as assessed by the surgeon's impression (T-stage) and the presence and location of metastases (M-stage).[73] In more recent studies, the presence of metastases has consistently been shown to be an adverse prognostic factor.[74, 75] However, the preoperative extent of disease at the primary site (T-stage) has been shown to be a less reliable predictor of outcome than the postoperative tumor volume (as assessed objectively by neuroimaging).[74-79] Evidence suggesting that the extent of residual disease correlates with outcome has been provided by several single- and multi-institutional studies.[74-79] For example, Jenkin et al reported a 5-year progression-free survival of 93% in patients undergoing "total" resection versus 45% in those undergoing incomplete resection.[76] In a study of the International Society of Paediatric Oncology (SIOP), 5-year survival was 52% after gross total or subtotal resections versus 33% after partial (less than 50%) resections ($p < 0.05$).[77] In larger studies, the benefit of extensive resection has not unexpectedly

been most apparent in children without evidence of disease dissemination. A recent Children's Cancer Group (CCG) study (CCG-921) demonstrated a clear relationship between extent of resection and outcome in the subset of patients with no evidence of tumor dissemination, but only a nonsignificant trend toward better outcomes after extensive resections in patients with evidence of tumor seeding.[75]

In view of the strong relationship between the extent of residual disease and outcome, contemporary staging guidelines depend on the following evaluations (Fig. 17–5): (1) a postoperative cranial CT or MRI, preferably within 48 hours of operation, to determine the volume of residual tumor; (2) spinal MRI, performed either preoperatively or two weeks postoperatively, or postoperative CT/myelography, to identify drop metastases; and (3) CSF cytology from the lumbar thecal space, which can be obtained either immediately after the craniotomy or several weeks later, to rule out dissemination in the absence of radiologically apparent spread. To facilitate rapid initiation of postoperative treatment, we favor obtaining preoperative spinal MRI and intraoperative cytologies, if possible, because the interpretation of these studies during the first 2 weeks after operation is complicated by the presence of blood and operative debris.[80] Because extraneural dissemination is rarely observed at initial diagnosis, a systemic staging evaluation is not routinely performed.

Apart from the prognostic significance of disease extent, recent studies have indicated that age younger than 3 or 4 years is also an unfavorable feature.[74-76] This in part reflects the fact that young children are more likely to present with advanced disease that is less amenable to radical resection or with disease dissemination[74] and that these patients often receive reduced doses of radiotherapy.[74, 76] However, it is conceivable that heretofore uncharacterized biologic factors may also contribute to the unfavorable prognosis of young children.

Based on the results of the aforementioned studies, patients are categorized as "standard-risk" or "low-stage" if they are older than 3 years, have less than 1.5 cm^2 of residual tumor after operation, and have no evidence of dissemination. Patients with any adverse factor are considered to be "poor-risk" or "high-stage." These two risk categories have formed the basis for current approaches to treatment stratification in children with medulloblastoma (Fig. 17–5). Implicit in these criteria is that a radiologically complete resection does not confer any measurable benefit over a nearly complete resection that leaves a small amount of tumor attached to the brain stem, which probably reflects that even with a gross total resection, truly complete removal of these inherently invasive tumors is not feasible. Accordingly, although we strongly advocate extensive tumor removal, there appears to be no indication for proceeding with potentially dangerous efforts to resect small amounts of tumor within the brain stem if this is the only site of residual disease.

BOX 17–5
Adverse Prognostic Factors

- **Significant residual disease**
- **Disseminated leptomeningeal spread**
- **Age less than 3 to 4 years**

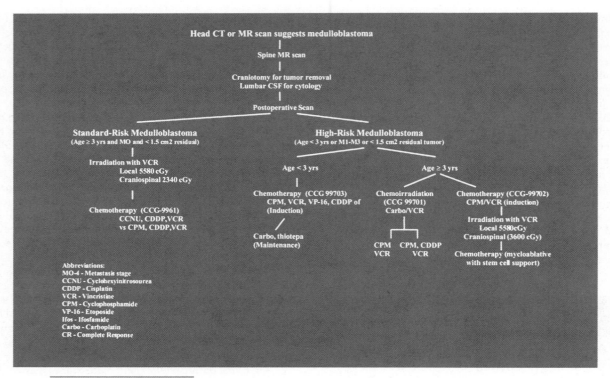

Figure 17–5   Management schema for medulloblastomas (based on open Children's Cancer Group studies).

ADJUVANT THERAPY
Radiation Therapy

It has long been recognized that surgical resection alone is insufficient to cure a medulloblastoma.[81] Early on, radiotherapy was administered in the hopes of improving outcome. Initial results using inadequate doses (less than 5000 cGy) and local treatment fields were generally disappointing.[82] The benefit of adequate doses of craniospinal axis irradiation (5000 to 6000 cGy to the posterior fossa and 3500 cGy to the rest of the neuraxis) was demonstrated in the landmark report of Patterson and Farr,[83] which effectively increased survival from 20% to almost 50%. The importance of using posterior fossa doses greater than 5000 cGy has been confirmed by other groups.[84]

Although the widespread use of craniospinal irradiation for these tumors has had a major impact on overall survival, this approach is far from optimal in terms of ensuring functional long-term outcome. First, less than 30% of patients with poor-risk disease enjoy long-term survival with craniospinal irradiation alone. Second, even among patients with standard-risk disease, approximately 30 to 40% ultimately die of tumor progression. Finally, the morbidity of high doses of craniospinal irradiation is substantial. Unfortunately, attempts to lower the doses of neuraxis irradiation for standard-risk patients from 3600 to 2340 cGy in a cooperative CCG/Pediatric Oncology Group (POG) study conducted between 1986 and 1990 led to a significant increase in the frequency of relapses outside the primary site and a slightly worse overall progression-free survival (52% vs. 60%).[85, 86] Taken together, these factors have formed an impetus for combining radiotherapy

with chemotherapy both to improve disease control in patients with standard- and poor-risk disease and to allow reduction in the dose of craniospinal radiotherapy in patients with standard-risk disease to reduce radiotherapy-induced morbidity (Fig. 17–5).

Chemotherapy

The efficacy of chemotherapy against medulloblastoma has been demonstrated in several studies and has convincingly been shown to improve long-term outcome in patients with poor-risk disease. In CCG-942, patients with evidence of tumor dissemination and brainstem invasion at presentation had a 5-year survival rate of 0% with craniospinal radiotherapy alone but had a significantly better outcome when chemotherapy, using a combination of prednisone, CCNU [lomustine], and vincristine (PCV), was added to the treatment regimen (46% 5-year survival),[74] which approaches the outcome of standard-risk patients who receive radiotherapy alone. A POG study also confirmed the beneficial effect of chemotherapy with MOPP (mechlorethamine, oncovin [vincristine], procarbazine, and prednisone); children receiving chemotherapy had a 5-year survival of 74% versus 56% in those receiving radiotherapy alone ($p = 0.06$).[79] Attempts to improve survival further using the more complex "8-drugs-in-1-day" regimen (which combined multiple agents, some with uncertain efficacy against medulloblastoma, at relatively low dose intensity) have not yielded a convincing benefit over the results achieved with either PCV or MOPP.[87, 88] Accordingly, protocol design in more recent studies has focused on incorporating agents known to be active against medulloblastoma and administering them at adequate dose intensity.

In this context, recent studies by Packer et al have reported particularly encouraging results in poor-risk patients (those with disseminated disease, brain stem invasion, or less than 90% resection) using a combination of cisplatin, which is independently active against medulloblastoma, with CCNU and vincristine.[89, 90] The 5-year disease-free survival rate of more than 70% exceeded the results in standard-risk patients treated with radiotherapy alone.[90] An extension of this study to two other centers achieved a 5-year progression-free survival of 85%, even including patients younger than 5 years, who received reduced doses of craniospinal radiation.[91] The 5-year survival among patients with metastatic disease was 67% versus 90% for those with localized disease at diagnosis.

The favorable results with adjuvant chemotherapy have provided a rationale for efforts to reduce neuraxis irradiation doses in order to minimize toxicity. Several studies have shown that neuraxis doses of 2400 cGy, if supplemented with chemotherapy, yielded 5-year survival rates in standard-risk patients of approximately 70%, comparable to the results achieved with conventional radiotherapy doses without chemotherapy.[92–94] In a recent CCG study, Packer's protocol yielded a 3-year progression-free survival in standard-risk patients of 80% ± 9% with the use of only 2400 cGy to the neuraxis.[95] A subsequent CCG/POG study (A9961) is comparing in a randomized format the efficacy and toxicity of two adjuvant regimens (CCNU, cisplatin, vincristine vs. cyclophosphamide, cisplatin, vincristine) and reduced-dose craniospinal radiotherapy in the management of these standard-risk patients.

The apparent chemosensitivity of medulloblastoma has also provided a rationale for efforts to defer radiotherapy in young patients using neoadjuvant (preirradiation) chemotherapy,[87, 88, 92] with the thought that a delay of irradiation for 1 to 2 years, if feasible, would be beneficial in improving long-term functional outcome. In a POG study of patients younger than 3 years who were treated with chemotherapy alone to defer administration of radiotherapy, 34% remained progression-free 2 years after diagnosis.[96] In some institutions, radiotherapy is now avoided altogether in young patients who have a complete response to chemotherapy unless they develop recurrent disease. Preirradiation chemotherapy has also been shown to produce objective disease regression in a high percentage of older children with poor-risk PNETs.[97] Accordingly, a recent CCG study (CCG-9931) evaluated the efficacy of intensive neoadjuvant chemotherapy as a means for reducing disease burden prior to high-dose hyperfractionated craniospinal radiotherapy in patients with poor-risk medulloblastomas. Studies of further dose intensification and chemo-irradiation are also in progress (Fig. 17–5).

DIAGNOSIS AND MANAGEMENT OF RECURRENT DISEASE
Diagnosis

Although the overall outlook for patients with medulloblastoma has improved dramatically during the last 20 years, as many as 30 to 50% of patients in most series die from tumor "recurrence," which in reality represents progression of residual disease. The majority of recurrences occur at the primary site.[8, 74, 98] However, many patients will manifest CSF dissemination either alone or in combination with local recurrences; systemic dissemination is detected in a small percentage of children.[74, 86, 98] Extraneural metastases seem to be more common in children who have not received postoperative chemotherapy,[99] particularly if reduced neuraxis irradiation doses have been administered.[86]

The utility of routine surveillance imaging as a means for identifying disease recurrence or progression at an early stage has become increasingly controversial during the last few years.[100–102] Torres et al[100] reported that there was little benefit to surveillance scans, both because most patients in their series had symptomatic recurrences that became apparent between scheduled scans and because the outlook was almost uniformly poor in their patients with recurrent disease (even if the lesions were detected at a presymptomatic stage). Subsequently, other groups have noted that children in whom recurrences are detected at a presymptomatic stage may enjoy longer postrecurrence survival than those with symptomatic recurrences.[101, 102] However, this may simply reflect a lead-time bias in that the asymptomatic recurrences were detected earlier in their growth process and thus would be expected to be associated with longer survival.

At present, the efficacy of surveillance scanning for prolonging survival must be viewed as unproven; however, in view of the hope that earlier detection of the recurrent disease will increase the chances for a cure as new therapeutic approaches are implemented (see below), this practice is maintained at most centers, including our own. In general, we obtain scans of the head (and spine in patients with disease dissemination at presentation) every 3 months for a year, every 6 months for 2 years, and annually thereafter for an additional 2 years. Subsequent scans are obtained approximately 7 and 10 years after diagnosis. It is generally assumed that medulloblastoma, as an embryonal tumor, follows Collins' law;[8] patients without evidence of recurrence for a duration equal to their age at diagnosis plus 9 months are presumed to be "cured." In reality, there are numerous reports in which this "law" has been violated in medulloblastoma.[98, 103, 104] Alternatively, it has been observed that medulloblastomas rarely recur more than 8 years after diagnosis,[98] although we have observed an exception to this rule as well. *Accordingly, the duration for which a patient must be followed before the disease can be referred to as cured remains problematic.*

Treatment

The treatment of patients with recurrent disease remains a major therapeutic challenge. Although disease regression has been achieved with a variety of conventional chemotherapeutic regimens, both alone and in combination with repeat radiotherapy, long-term disease control is uncommon.[105–107] Similarly, radiosurgery has shown some efficacy in shrinking small, focal recurrences, but such patients generally die of disease dissemination.[108] In recent years, the use of highly intensive chemotherapy coupled with bone marrow or peripheral blood stem cell reconstitution has shown some promise in the control of progressive disease.[109, 110] Dunkel and Finlay[110] reported that 6 of 17 patients with recurrent medulloblastoma survived event-free for a median of 33 months after treatment of their recurrent disease with marrow-ablative doses of carboplatin, thiotepa, and etoposide. Patients whose gross recurrent disease could be eliminated using reoperation or conventional chemotherapy had a particularly favorable response, with 5 of 11 becoming long-term survivors.

SEQUELAE OF TREATMENT

With improvements in the overall survival of children with medulloblastoma, increasing emphasis has been placed on evaluating functional outcome in these patients. Although the majority of treatment-related sequelae (e.g., chemotherapy-induced myelotoxicity, ototoxicity, and nephrotoxicity) are acute, a significant component of the treatment-induced morbidity manifests several years after diagnosis, mandating long-term multidisciplinary follow-up of the childhood brain tumor patient. Radiotherapy is known to induce leukoencephalopathy, vasculopathy, and, at higher doses, necrosis, which may translate to profound cognitive deficits.[111–118] Sequential measurements of IQ in children younger than 7 years who received whole-brain radiotherapy have demonstrated a progressive deterioration in intelligence during the first 2 years after irradiation.[114, 115, 117] In the series of Radcliffe et al, children younger than 7 years lost an average of 27 IQ points and all required special education; in addition, 50% of children older than 7 years also were receiving supplemental educational services.[115] Ellenberg et al reported a drop of 20 IQ points in children younger than 6 years, 10 points in children between 6 and 8 years, and no consistent change in children 9 years and older.[114] In a comparative study, Hirsch et al[119] noted that IQ scores were below 90 in almost 90% of medulloblastoma survivors who had received craniospinal irradiation, versus less than 40% of children with cerebellar astrocytomas who had not received radiotherapy. Cognitive and behavioral problems have been noted in the majority of medulloblastoma survivors, and these deficits appear to become increasingly severe over time.[111, 115, 118, 120] Although young children are clearly at higher risk for these impairments, older patients frequently exhibit at least some cognitive deterioration from treatment.[115, 118]

Endocrinopathies are also extremely common in children who have received adjuvant therapy for brain tumors. Growth hormone deficiency is seen in the vast majority of children who have received whole-brain irradiation.[121–123] Growth may be further impaired by spinal irradiation, which directly interferes with spinal bone growth.[124, 125] Spinal irradiation and chemotherapy may also contribute to the development of primary endocrine deficiencies. Livesey et al noted primary thyroid dysfunction in 23% of patients treated with craniospinal irradiation and in 69% of those receiving craniospinal irradiation and chemotherapy.[123] Primary ovarian or testicular dysfunction was seen in 60% and 20% of girls and boys, respectively, who received craniospinal radiotherapy and chemotherapy. In another series, testicular dysfunction was seen almost uniformly in boys who had received chemotherapy in combination with radiotherapy;[126] alkylating agents appear to be particularly deleterious in this regard.

Secondary neoplasms are an additional concern in children with a brain tumor, even in the absence of a genetic syndrome. The incidence of secondary malignancies ranges from 1% to 5%.[111, 127, 128] The majority of secondary tumors are malignant gliomas, meningiomas, and meningeal and skull sarcomas that occur within radiotherapy treatment fields 10 to 20 years after irradiation. The combination of radiotherapy and chemotherapy appears to increase risk over that seen with radiotherapy alone.[129]

SUMMARY

Infratentorial PNET, or medulloblastoma, is the most common tumor of childhood. Its pathogenesis remains elusive despite great advances in diagnosis and treatment. During the last 25 years, such significant advances have been made that 5-year progression-free survival has increased from less than 20% to 70%, making this one of the real "success stories" in pediatric neurosurgery. The goal of current studies is to decrease treatment-induced morbidity while improving the survival rate of children with these tumors.

REFERENCES

1. Cushing H. Experiences with cerebellar medulloblastomas: critical review. *Acta Pathol Microbiol Scand* 1930; 1:1–86.
2. Rorke LB. The cerebellar medulloblastoma and its relationship to primitive neuroectodermal tumors. *J Neuropathol Exp Neurol* 1983;42:1–15.
3. Hart MN, Earle KM. Primitive neuroectodermal tumors of the brain in children. *Cancer* 1973;32:890–897.
4 Pollack IF. Brain tumors in children. *N Engl J Med* 1994; 331:1500–1507.
5. Young JL, Miller RW. Incidence of malignant tumors in U.S. children. *J Pediatr* 1974;86:254–258.
6. Schoenberg BS, Schoenberg DG, Christine BW, et al. The epidemiology of primary intracranial neoplasms of childhood: a population study. *Mayo Clin Proc* 1976;51:51–56.
7. Farwell JR, Dohrmann GJ, Flannery JT. Medulloblastoma in childhood: an epidemiological study. *J Neurosurg* 1984; 61:657–664.
8. Hershatter BW, Halperin EC, Cox EB. Medulloblastoma: the Duke University Medical Center experience. *Int J Radiat Oncol Biol Phys* 1986;12:1771–1777.
9. Finlay JL. Natural history and epidemiology of medulloblastoma. In: Zeltzer PM, Pochedly C, eds. *Medulloblastomas in Children: New Concepts in Tumor Biology, Diagnosis, and Treatment.* 1986; 22–36.
10. Roberts RO, Lynch CF, Jones MP, et al. Medulloblastoma: a population-based study of 532 cases. *J Neuropathol Exp Neurol* 1991;50:134–144.
11. Maleci A, Cervoni L, Delfini R. Medulloblastoma in children and adults: a comparative study. *Acta Neurochir* 1992; 119:62–67.

Chapter 18

Supratentorial Primitive Neuroectodermal Tumors

Ian F. Pollack

The term "primitive neuroectodermal tumor" (PNET) was first used by Hart and Earle[1] to describe a cerebral hemispheric tumor composed of primitive neuroepithelial cells with evidence of differentiation along glial, neuronal, ependymal, or mesenchymal lines. Rorke later proposed that such tumors were the supratentorial counterparts of medulloblastoma and that such tumors should be grouped with similar lesions in other locations, such as pineoblastoma and retinoblastoma, based on their comparable appearances and their presumed common origin from pluripotential neuroepithelial cells.[2] Cerebral neuroblastomas and pineoblastomas were thus viewed as supratentorial PNETs and medulloblastomas as infratentorial PNETs. An opposing opinion, espoused by Rubinstein, is that these lesions are distinct entities arising from progenitor cells unique to the tumor's site of origin.[3] Despite the obvious similarities between cerebral, pineal, and infratentorial PNETs in terms of their microscopic appearance and tendency to disseminate, these lesions differ significantly in terms of their prognosis after therapy and, thus, are evaluated separately in most therapeutic studies. This chapter focuses primarily on the diagnosis, treatment, and outcome of cerebral and pineal PNETs; medulloblastomas are discussed in more detail in Chapter 17.

EPIDEMIOLOGY

Cerebral and pineal PNETs occur most commonly in early childhood: more than 60% of cerebral cases are detected before the age of 5 years and 80% before 10 years[4–9] and more than 60% of pineal lesions are detected within the first decade.[10] No sex predilection is apparent for cerebral lesions,[4] but a slight male predominance has been noted for pineal PNETs,[10] similar to the situation with medulloblastomas.[11] Cerebral and pineal PNETs are each only one-tenth as common as medulloblastomas.[12] In the recent Children's Cancer Group (CCG) study (CCG-921), which included 255 children with PNETs, 27 had supratentorial PNETs and 17 had pineal PNETs.[4] These lesions account for about 5% of cerebral hemispheric tumors,[13, 14] approximately 15% of pineal region tumors, and about 3% of all brain tumors in children.[14] The vast majority of cases occur sporadically without a known genetic or environmental predisposition.[15] However, patients with bilateral retinoblastoma secondary to loss of the retinoblastoma susceptibility gene are at increased risk for the development of a pineal PNET, so-called trilateral retinoblastoma.[16, 17]

PATHOLOGY

Cerebral PNETs are presumed to arise from multipotential cells of the subpial granular layer of the cerebral hemispheres,[18] although this has yet to be confirmed. Similarly, pineal PNETs are thought to originate from pineal progenitor cells, which are capable of differentiating along retinal, ganglionic, or astrocytic lines.

On gross inspection, PNETs are soft, friable, gelatinous, highly vascular, purplish gray tumors that widely infiltrate the surrounding structures. Foci of hemorrhage are commonly observed.[10] Although these lesions appear in places to be well circumscribed, they are generally invasive on a microscopic level, which precludes a truly complete resection. Histologically, these tumors are characterized by their high cellularity, composed of small round to oval cells with a high nuclear/cytoplasmic ratio that exhibit foci of clustering into Homer Wright rosettes and numerous mitotic figures (Fig. 18–1). Some tumors exhibit varying degrees of connective tissue proliferation, resembling desmoplastic medulloblastoma. About half of pineal PNETs exhibit some evidence of differentiation, which may occur along retinal, ganglionic, astrocytic, or ependymal lines.[19] Immunoreactivity for retinal S-antigen[20–22] is observed in a significant percentage of tumors. In addition, foci of differentiation to pineocytoma are also commonly observed. Differentiation of cerebral PNETs along glial, neuronal, ependymal, or oligodendroglial lines has been noted in approximately 40% of tumors,[6,10,23] but even in such cases, the majority of the tumor is undifferentiated.[6,13,24] Medulloepitheliomas, which make up a morphologically distinct subset of PNETs, typically exhibit differentiation along primitive lines, with the formation of neural tube–like structures, often in association with areas of astrocytic or ganglionic morphology.[25] The relationship between differentiation in PNETs and outcome has been unclear; although it has been suggested that differentiated tumors may be associated with a more favorable outcome,[13] a number of studies have failed to confirm this observation.[7, 10, 25–27] Interestingly, transformation of these tumors into ganglioneuromas has been observed anecdotally.[28] Similarly, the relationship between desmoplasia and prognosis is uncertain.[9]

This work was supported in part by NIH grant 1KO8–NS01810.

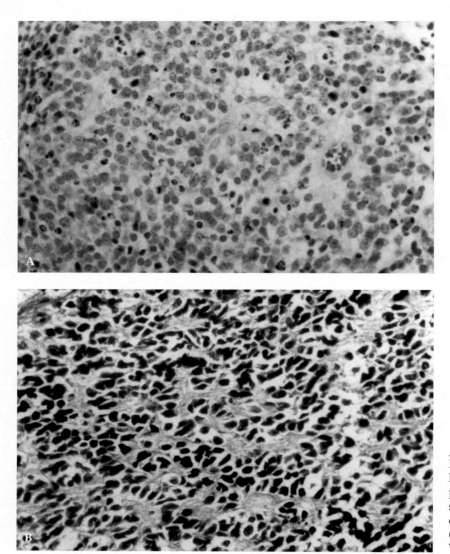

Figure 18–1 (A) The characteristic histologic appearance of a cerebral primitive neuroectodermal tumor (H&E), showing closely packed small cells with dense nuclei and scant cytoplasm. (B) Focal clustering of cells in Homer Wright rosettes is often apparent.

On a cytogenetic level, pineal lesions have anecdotally been observed to have isochromosome 17q, similar to the characteristic finding in medulloblastomas.[29] This abnormality has not been consistently noted in cerebral lesions. However, because cytogenetic and molecular genetic analyses of only a limited number of pineal PNETs and even fewer cerebral PNETs have been reported, it is not possible to determine conclusively whether these tumors are similar to or distinct from medulloblastomas on a genetic level.

From a diagnostic standpoint, it is essential to distinguish cerebral PNETs from central neurocytoma, which is a benign lesion with neuronal differentiation that morphologically shows greater resemblance to oligodendroglioma than medulloblastoma[30–33] and is associated with a much more favorable prognosis, even in the absence of adjuvant therapy. In the past, these lesions were often included with supratentorial PNETs as cerebral neuroblastomas. However, because these tumors tend to occur in an intraventricular location in older patients[7, 9] and are morphologically distinct from typical PNETs, the separation of these two entities is now generally straightforward. *Another lesion that must be distinguished is the desmoplastic infantile ganglioglioma,[34] which is a meningeal-based lesion of infancy with astrocytic and ganglionic differentiation in association with a profound desmoplastic response.* These lesions also have a relatively favorable prognosis. Pineal PNETs with pineocytic differentiation must be distinguished from pineocytomas because the latter lesions generally have a much more indolent course and often respond well to surgery and local radiotherapy or to radiosurgery.

PRESENTING SYMPTOMS AND SIGNS

Because these lesions generally grow rapidly, the duration of symptoms before diagnosis is correspondingly brief, rarely exceeding 3 months.[6] Patients often present with nonspecific symptoms of increased intracranial pressure, such as headache, nausea, vomiting, and lethargy.[6] Children with hemispheric lesions may exhibit seizures,[8, 35] whereas those with pineal lesions may manifest with Parinaud's syndrome. Occasionally, patients present with a rapid decline in neurologic function as a result of hemorrhage into the tumor. Frequently, these lesions are large at the time of diagnosis.[4, 8]

DIAGNOSTIC EVALUATION

Supratentorial PNETs appear isodense or, more commonly, hyperdense to the surrounding brain on computed tomography (CT) (Fig. 18–2) and exhibit variable signal characteristics on magnetic resonance imaging (MRI)[36] (Figs. 18–3 and 18–4). Cerebral lesions are located most commonly in the frontal and parietal lobes.[4] Enhancement after administration of intravenous contrast is heterogeneous. Intratumoral cysts, hemorrhage, and calcification are common,[6, 37, 38] and some lesions exhibit a sizable cystic component.[7, 39] These lesions characteristically have a deceptively distinct border with the surrounding brain,[4] which belies their inherently invasive properties. *Because no single imaging feature is absolutely diag-nostic of these tumors, it is difficult to conclusively establish the diagnosis of a PNET preoperatively.* Other lesions that can mimic PNETs in the cerebral hemispheres include malignant glioma, choroid plexus carcinoma, and ependymoma. In the pineal region, germ cell tumors may occasionally be indistinguishable from PNETs.

Because 20 to 40% of these lesions exhibit evidence of intracranial or leptomeningeal dissemination at presentation,[4, 6] a staging evaluation of the neuraxis is an essential component of the diagnostic evaluation (Table 18–1). This can be accomplished with MRI or, if unavailable, CT/myelography (if intracranial mass effect has been reduced by tumor resection).

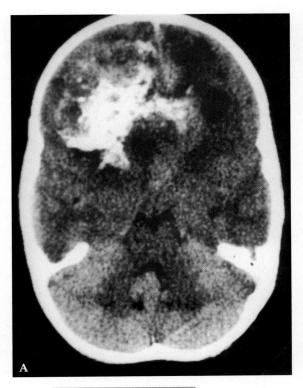
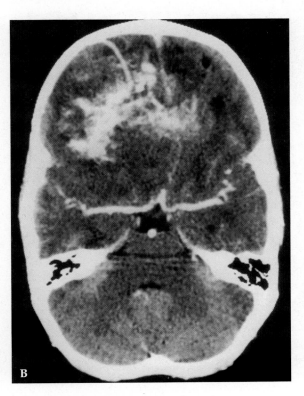

Figure 18–2 (A) The characteristic CT appearance of a cerebral primitive neuroectodermal tumor on an unenhanced scan, showing a hyperdense hemispheric mass. (B) The lesion enhanced irregularly with intravenous contrast.

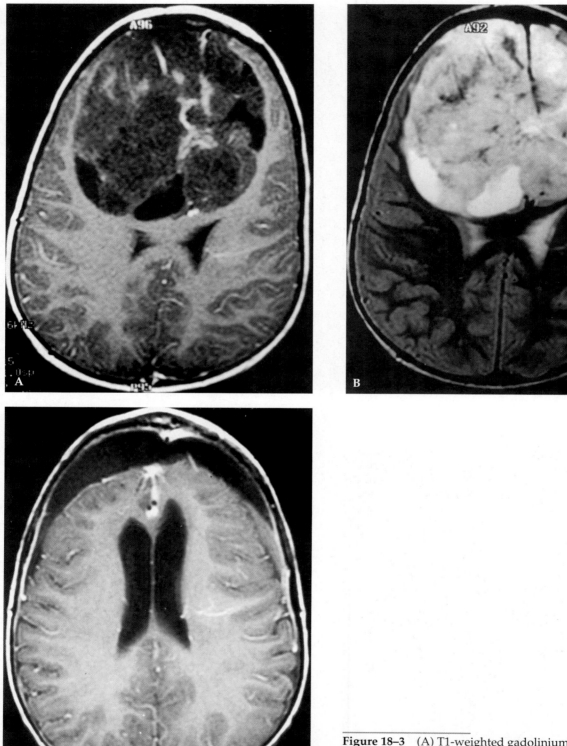

Figure 18–3 (A) T1-weighted gadolinium-enhanced magnetic resonance image of the above tumor, showing a hypointense, seemingly well-circumscribed bifrontal mass. (B) T2-weighted image of the same tumor. (C) Postoperative image of the same tumor.

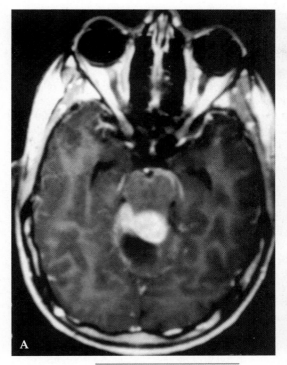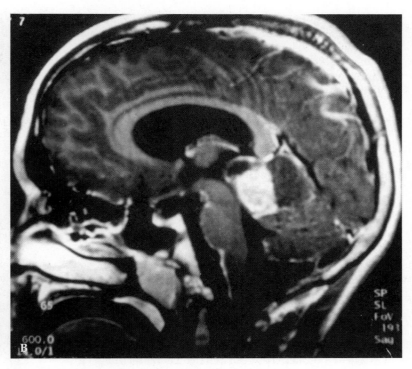

Figure 18–4   Gadolinium-enhanced axial (A) and sagittal (B) T1-weighted gadolinium-enhanced magnetic resonance image of a pineal primitive neuroectodermal tumor. Leptomeningeal dissemination was apparent within the basal cisterns.

A postoperative cytologic examination of the cerebrospinal fluid (CSF) is also indicated to rule out occult seeding of the neuraxis. Lesions are graded as M0 if there is no evidence of seeding, M1 if the cytology is positive without radiologically detectable spread, M2 if there is intracranial spread alone, and M3 if there is spinal dissemination. Because systemic (M4) dissemination is rarely present at the time of diagnosis, a systemic staging evaluation is not routinely pursued.

Table 18–1 Staging of Supratentorial PNET

Stage	Description
M0	No evidence of seeding
M1	Positive cytology, no radiographic evidence of spread
M2	Intracranial spread only
M3	Spinal dissemination
M4	Systemic dissemination

SURGICAL TREATMENT
Operative Preparation

Patients are begun on steroids (e.g., dexamethasone 1 to 6 mg q6h, depending on the weight of the patient) preoperatively. Anticonvulsants are administered to patients with hemi-spheric lesions. Both medications are continued during the perioperative period; steroids are weaned during the first few postoperative days if an extensive resection has been achieved, and the anticonvulsant is stopped after a week if the patient has been seizure-free. Because of the known risk of perioperative stress ulceration in these patients, we generally administer an H_2 blocker in conjunction with the steroids, although we recognize that a benefit of this approach has not been conclusively proven.

If the child is alert and neurologically intact, the operative procedure is scheduled for the next available day. Surgery is performed on a more urgent basis if the patient is lethargic at the time of diagnosis. *The operative goals are to establish a diagnosis, to open occluded CSF pathways, and to remove as much tumor as is safely feasible.* At our institution, pineal lesions are often biopsied stereotactically before open resection is attempted. This is useful for excluding lesions that may not require resection, such as germinomas.[40] The biopsy is performed using a low-frontal entry site (at the hairline) near the midpupillary line to pass anteriorly and inferiorly to the great veins in the vicinity of the tumor. Stereotactic biopsy is rarely used for cerebral PNETs, which generally are large lesions that require major debulking to relieve the significant associated mass effect.

In patients with ventricular obstruction from the tumor, which is particularly common for pineal lesions, placement of an external ventricular drain and/or endoscopic third ventriculostomy is often performed after the stereotactic biopsy or immediately before the tumor resection, which facilitates the operative approach to the tumor by relieving intracranial hypertension. If the tumor resection unblocks the CSF pathways, then the ventriculostomy can generally be weaned within several days of operation. Patients with persistence of symptomatic hydrocephalus postoperatively require insertion of a ventriculoperitoneal shunt.

An important caveat before embarking on the open resection of any of these large, highly vascular cerebral and pineal lesions is to have adequate intravenous access to facilitate blood replacement, if needed, as well as central venous and arterial lines. A urinary drainage catheter is also routinely inserted. Prophylactic antibiotics are administered during skin preparation and every 6 to 8 hours during the procedure. Steroids and anticonvulsants are also continued intraoperatively.

Operative Procedure

Cerebral hemispheric lesions are approached using a standard craniotomy situated over the site of the lesion. For subcortical lesions, stereotactic guidance may be employed to minimize the risk of injury to surrounding normal structures. Because intracranial pressure is often significantly elevated in association with large cerebral PNETs, even after CSF drainage (if indicated) has been initiated, mannitol (0.5 g/kg) is often administered before opening of the dura. For large superficial cerebral PNETs, the dura is then opened over the lesion and the central component of the mass debulked expeditiously to prevent herniation of the brain through the opening. After the initial debulking, the dural opening is extended to facilitate wide visualization of the mass. For smaller or deep-seated lesions, a more standard one-step opening is performed as determined by the location of the mass and the approach being employed.

Pineal PNETs (Fig. 18–4) are approached using either a supracerebellar or an occipital transtentorial exposure, depending on whether the predominant direction of tumor growth is below or above the tentorium. At our institution, these procedures are performed using a modified prone (Concorde) position, although others use a sitting position. We favor the prone position for pineal region lesions because it minimizes (but does not eliminate entirely) the risk of air embolism and because it avoids the arm fatigue that can accompany prolonged sitting. For a supracerebellar approach, the head is flexed laterally 20 degrees away from the surgeon. The skin incision extends from just above the inion to the spinous process of C2. A craniotomy or craniectomy is then made that extends about 3 cm on either side of the midline, exposes the transverse sinuses superiorly, and courses just above the foramen magnum inferiorly. Approximately 10 to 20 mL of CSF is usually drained from the ventriculostomy at this point to ensure that the dura is "slack" prior to opening. The dura is then opened in a V-shaped fashion, based superiorly. The cerebellum is gently retracted inferiorly as bridging veins between the cerebellum and the tentorium are coagulated and divided. Near the tentorial hiatus, a dense arachnoidal covering is encountered extending upward from the rostral cerebellum. Coagulation and sharp division of this structure exposes the precentral cerebellar vein, which is also coagulated and divided. The tumor is generally apparent at this point.

For an occipital transtentorial approach, the head is both flexed laterally 20 degrees away from the surgeon and rotated 20 degrees toward the surgeon to allow gravity to retract the occipital lobe on the operative (usually right) side away from the falx. An inverted U-shaped skin incision is used, which extends from the midline at the level of the inion over the occipital convexity and down toward the mastoid region. The craniotomy exposes both the sagittal and transverse sinuses. After drainage of CSF, if needed, the dura is opened in an inverted U, based medially and inferiorly, with a relaxing incision directed to the junction of the sagittal and transverse sinuses. The occipital lobe is then gently retracted laterally, and the tentorium is coagulated and incised just lateral to its attachment to the falx. The precentral cerebellar vein is exposed and divided as noted above, which exposes the tumor extending both above and below the tentorium.

After the lesion has been made visible, the outer pole of the tumor is coagulated and the tumor centrally debulked using the ultrasonic aspirator. Although a tumor capsule is never present, a clear demarcation between tumor and normal brain is often apparent. After coring out the center of the lesion, I usually follow the plane between the tumor and the surrounding brain, if such a plane is present. *It is usually possible to resect the majority of cerebral lesions in a piecemeal fashion from the inside out, but because these lesions are inherently invasive, there is no indication for "chasing" the tumor into the surrounding cortex if a functionally significant area of the brain is involved.* With pineal lesions, the plane between tumor and third ventricular ependyma is often preserved rostrally. Removing this component of the tumor typically yields a burst of CSF from the anterior third ventricle and exposes the fornices. More posterior tumor that is adherent to the wall of the third ventricle and great vessels is removed bit by bit, with care taken not to damage these structures. After the resection has been completed, hemostasis is achieved and the dura is closed in a "water-tight" fashion.

Because of the large size, dense vascularity, and invasive characteristics of supratentorial PNETs, gross total resection is achieved in a minority of tumors, particularly in the pineal region.[4, 6] Nonetheless, near-total resection is often an attainable goal (Fig. 18–3C); in a recent CCG study, 56% of children with cerebral PNETs had less than 1.5 cm^2 of residual disease after resection. In that study, there was a correlation between preoperative tumor size and postoperative residual disease; not surprisingly, patients with large tumors were more likely to have more than 1.5 cm^2 of residual disease after resection.[4]

Although an unequivocal benefit of resection extent on outcome has not been established because of the small numbers of patients included in previous studies, a trend toward better results among patients with more extensive resections has been noted. In CCG-921, 4-year survival was 40% in children with less than 1.5 cm^2 of residual tumor, compared with only 13% in patients with more residual disease.[4] Similarly, Dirks et al[6] noted a more favorable prognosis among patients who underwent gross total resections ($p = 0.08$). Cystic lesions, which are inherently more amenable to radical resection, seem to carry a particularly favorable prognosis with extensive tumor removal.[7, 41] Accordingly, there is at least a theoretical rationale for attempting to aggressively resect these lesions, if feasible.

PROGNOSTIC FACTORS AND ADJUVANT THERAPY

In general, patients with supratentorial PNETs are treated with craniospinal radiotherapy in addition to surgery (Fig. 18–5) because these lesions show a high propensity for dissemination. Radiotherapy doses to the primary site of 5000 to 6000 cGy are associated with the best chance for local control;[42] these have typically been combined with craniospinal doses of 3600 cGy. Despite these high doses of radiation, the prognosis for children with supratentorial PNETs has been less favorable than for children with medulloblastoma.[4, 6, 9, 13, 26, 27, 37, 42–47] Kosnik et al[37] in 1978 reported a 1-year survival of only 10% in children with cerebral PNETs. In the experience at the Hospital for Sick Children, reported by Dirks et al,[6] 5-year survival for patients with these tumors was only 12%. Similarly, overall 5-year survival for cerebral PNETs in CCG-921 was only 34%.[4] Adverse prognostic factors for children with cerebral PNETs include (1) age younger than 3 years ($p < 0.02$ in Ref. 4; $p = 0.006$ in Ref. 6), possibly reflecting the fact that patients younger than 3 years typically receive reduced doses of craniospinal radiation, and (2) disease dissemination.[4, 43] Age younger than 3 years and disease dissemination have also been observed to be unfavorable prognostic factors in patients with pineal PNETs.[44, 46–48]

BOX 18–3
Adverse Prognostic Factors

- Age <3 years
- Metastases
- Residual tumor (?)

Although in some studies patients with pineal PNETs (Fig. 18–4) have fared slightly better than those with cerebral PNETs,[6, 46, 49] this has not been observed uniformly. Dirks et al[6] reported a 5-year survival of 30% for children with pineal PNETs, which was more than twice that of patients with cerebral lesions. Similarly, in CCG-921, 3-year survival for pineal PNETs was 74%, which was substantially better than the results obtained for cerebral tumors.[43, 46] However, Mena et al[50] observed a median survival of only 24 months in seven patients with pineal PNETs, and Duffner et al[47] noted that all 11 children in the infant Pediatric Oncology Group (POG) study with pineal lesions had progressive disease within 1 year of diagnosis. Thus, at best, the results in children with cerebral and pineal PNETs are in keeping with those in children with poor-risk medulloblastomas,[51] which has formed the basis for grouping these lesions together as "poor-risk PNETs" in ongoing therapeutic studies (Fig. 18–5).

In view of the generally discouraging results in children with supratentorial PNETs who have been treated with surgery and radiotherapy alone, there has been considerable interest during the last decade in examining the effect of chemotherapy in these tumors. A number of regimens have shown efficacy against these lesions. Ashley et al reported partial responses to high-dose cyclophosphamide in three of six patients with newly diagnosed PNETs and stable disease in the other three patients.[52] Responses have also been observed with ifosfamide,[53] melphalan,[54] and carboplatin.[55] The combination of cisplatin, vinblastine, and bleomycin has also been effective in inducing disease regression prior to irradiation.[56] Using a neoadjuvant regimen of cisplatin, etoposide, and vincristine, Ghim et al[57] achieved disease-free survival for more than 2 years in two of three patients. The combination of cisplatin and etoposide has also been reported by Kovnar et al[58] to have efficacy against high-risk PNETs, with preirradiation responses in 10 of 11 patients, including

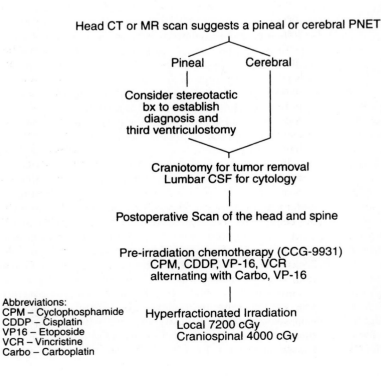

Figure 18–5 Recent management schema for supratentorial primitive neuroectodermal tumors. Current CCG protocols are illustrated in Figure 17–5. (Adapted from Children's Cancer Group "High-Risk" PNET Protocol, CCG-9931.)

both children with pineoblastoma.[58] Halperin et al[59] reported long-term progression-free survival in four of five patients treated with maximal resection, hyperfractionated irradiation, and chemotherapy, using cyclophosphamide, vincristine, and cisplatin. An intensive neoadjuvant regimen of cyclophosphamide and vincristine alternating with cisplatin and etoposide, administered in the infant POG study, achieved a 3-year progression-free survival of 55% in children with cerebral PNETs but failed to have a significant effect on pineal PNETs.[44, 47] After two cycles of treatment, only 1 of 11 children had objective disease regression and all patients progressed within 2 to 11 months of starting treatment. All children ultimately died despite the use of subsequent craniospinal irradiation. Similarly discouraging results in infants with pineal PNETs were noted by Jakacki et al using neoadjuvant 8-in-1 chemotherapy.[46]

Because a variety of regimens have been used in different studies, which have each included small numbers of patients, it has been difficult to prove that chemotherapy truly prolongs survival in children with these tumors.[60–62] In some studies, no benefit of chemotherapy has been confirmed and, as noted above, a variety of regimens have been largely ineffective.[46, 47] However, in a large single-institution study, Dirks et al[6] noted a trend toward longer survival for children who received adjuvant chemotherapy in addition to radiotherapy than for those who received irradiation alone ($p = 0.07$). Despite the uncertain benefits of chemotherapy, the otherwise poor prognosis of supratentorial PNETs treated with surgery and radiotherapy alone has provided some rationale to continue with efforts to optimize adjuvant therapy. A recent CCG study (CCG-9931) (Fig. 18–5) examined the effect on disease control of intensive neoadjuvant therapy followed by high-dose hyperfractionated craniospinal irradiation (7200 cGy to the primary site and up to 5000 cGy to the neuraxis with boosts to areas of metastatic disease). Ongoing studies are examining further dose intensification and chemo-irradiation for high-risk medulloblastomas (see Chapter 17).

DIAGNOSIS AND MANAGEMENT OF PROGRESSIVE DISEASE

Although there are no clear guidelines regarding the frequency of postoperative surveillance imaging, we generally follow the same schema as that used for medulloblastomas, recognizing that, even for these lesions, the utility of surveillance scanning remains controversial.[63, 64] It is our hope that early detection of progressive disease will increase the chances for a cure as new therapeutic approaches are implemented. In general, we obtain scans of the head (and spine in patients with disease dissemination at presentation) every 3 months for a year, every 6 months for 2 years, and annually thereafter for 2 additional years. Subsequent scans are obtained approximately 7 and 10 years after diagnosis.

In general, recurrences are thought to follow Collins' law, occurring within an interval after diagnosis equal to the patient's age plus 9 months, although exceptions for posterior fossa PNETs have been reported.[65] Although most recurrences are local, a significant percentage of patients exhibit radiologic or cytologic evidence of disease dissemination.[8] In addition, extraneural

dissemination has been reported[10] and, in some cases, has been attributed to tumor seeding through the shunt.[66, 67]

Management of progressive disease remains a major therapeutic challenge. Although transient disease regression has been achieved with a variety of conventional chemotherapeutic regimens and repeat radiotherapy, long-term disease control is rare. Similarly, we have found radiosurgery to be effective in shrinking small, focal recurrences, but such patients generally die of disease dissemination. In recent years, the use of highly intensive chemotherapy (e.g., with marrow-ablative doses of carboplatin, thiotepa, and etoposide), coupled with bone marrow or peripheral blood stem cell reconstitution, has shown some promise in controlling progressive disease in patients with recurrent PNETs.[68] This approach appears to have the highest likelihood of success in patients whose gross disease can be eliminated using reoperation or conventional chemotherapy.[68]

SEQUELAE OF TREATMENT

Because the treatment approaches that are employed for supratentorial PNETs carry the potential for long-term morbidity, patients must be monitored periodically in a multidisciplinary setting for several years after diagnosis, even if they have no evidence of tumor recurrence. Radiotherapy is known to induce leukoencephalopathy, vasculopathy, and, at higher doses, necrosis, which may translate to profound cognitive deficits.[69–74] Sequential measurements of IQ in children younger than 7 years who received whole-brain radiotherapy have demonstrated a progressive deterioration in intelligence during the first 2 years after irradiation.[71, 72, 74] In the series of Radcliffe et al, children younger than 7 years lost an average of 27 IQ points and all required special education; in addition, 50% of children older than 7 years also were receiving supplemental educational services.[72] Ellenberg et al reported a drop of 20 IQ points in children younger than 6, 10 points in children between 6 and 8, and no consistent change in children 9 years and older.[71] Cognitive and behavioral problems appear to increase in severity over time.[72] Although young children are clearly at higher risk for these impairments, older patients frequently exhibit at least some cognitive deterioration as a result of treatment.[72]

Endocrinopathies are also extremely common in children who have received adjuvant therapy for brain tumors. Growth hormone deficiency is seen in the vast majority of children who have received whole-brain irradiation.[75–77] Growth may be further impaired by spinal irradiation, which directly interferes with spinal bone growth. Spinal irradiation and chemotherapy can also contribute to the development of primary endocrine deficiencies. Livesey et al noted primary thyroid dysfunction in 23% of patients treated with craniospinal irradiation and in 69% of those receiving craniospinal irradiation and chemotherapy.[77] Primary ovarian or testicular dysfunction was seen in 60% and 20% of girls and boys, respectively, who received craniospinal radiotherapy and chemotherapy. In another series, testicular dysfunction was seen almost uniformly in boys who had received chemotherapy in combination with radiotherapy;[78] alkylating agents appear to be particularly deleterious in this regard.

Secondary neoplasms are an additional concern in children with a brain tumor, even in the absence of a genetic syndrome. The incidence of secondary malignancies ranges from 1% to 5%.[79, 80] The majority of second tumors are malignant gliomas, meningiomas, and meningeal and skull sarcomas that occur within radiotherapy treatment fields 10 to 20 years after irradiation. The combination of radiotherapy and chemotherapy appears to increase risk over that seen with radiotherapy alone.[81]

SUMMARY

Occurring most frequently in early childhood, cerebral and pineal PNETs present a diagnostic and therapeutic challenge to the neurosurgeon. It is imperative that these tumors be distinguished from other more benign lesions that may have similar symptomatology and imaging characteristics. Because PNETs are invasive, thay usually cannot be completely resected. Therefore, adjuvant treatment, including radiotherapy and/or chemotherapy, and long-term follow-up are crucial for improving outcome.

REFERENCES

1. Hart MN, Earle KM. Primitive neuroectodermal tumors of the brain in children. *Cancer* 1973;32:890–897.
2. Rorke LB. The cerebellar medulloblastoma and its relationship to primitive neuroectodermal tumors. *J Neuropathol Exp Neurol* 1983;42:1–15.
3. Rubinstein LJ. Embryonal central neuroepithelial tumors and their differentiating potential: a cytogenetic view of a complex neuro-oncological problem. *J Neurosurg* 1985;62:795–805.
4. Albright AL, Wisoff JH, Zeltzer P, et al. Prognostic factors in children with supratentorial (nonpineal) primitive neuroectodermal tumors. *Pediatr Neurosurg* 1995;22:1–7.
5. Pendergrass TW, Milstein JM, Geyer JR, et al. Eight drugs in one day chemotherapy for brain tumors: experience in 107 children and rationale for preradiation chemotherapy. *J Clin Oncol* 1987;5:1221–1231.
6. Dirks PB, Harris L, Hoffman HJ, et al. Supratentorial primitive neuroectodermal tumors in children. *J Neuro-oncol* 1996;29:75–84.
7. Berger MS, Edwards MSB, Wara WM, et al. Primary cerebral neuroblastoma: long-term follow-up review and therapeutic guidelines. *J Neurosurg* 1983;59:418–423.
8. Horten BC, Rubinstein LJ. Primary cerebral neuroblastoma: a clinicopathological study of 35 cases. *Brain* 1976; 99:735–756.
9. Bennett JP, Rubinstein JL. The biological behavior of primary cerebral neuroblastoma: a reappraisal of the clinical course in a series of 70 cases. *Ann Neurol* 1984;16:21–27.
10. Russell DS, Rubinstein LJ. In: *Pathology of Tumours of the Nervous System.* 5th ed. Baltimore: Williams & Wilkins; 1989:279–289, 383–387.
11. Farwell JR, Dohrmann GJ, Flannery JT. Medulloblastoma in childhood: an epidemiological study. *J Neurosurg* 1984; 61:657–664.

12. Park TS, Hoffman HJ, Hendrick EB, et al. Medulloblastoma: clinical presentation and management—experience at the Hospital for Sick Children, Toronto, 1950–1980. *J Neurosurg* 1983;58:543–552.
13. Gaffney CC, Sloane JP, Bradley NH, et al. Primitive neuroectodermal tumours of the cerebrum. *J Neuro-oncol* 1985;3:23–33.
14. Pollack IF. Brain tumors in children. *N Engl J Med* 1994; 331:1500–1507.
15. Bunin GR, Buckley JD, Boessel CP, et al. Risk factors for astrocytic glioma and primitive neuroectodermal tumor of the brain in young children: a report from the Children's Cancer Group. *Cancer Epidemiol, Biomarkers Prev* 1994;3:197–204.
16. Bader JL, Meadows AT, Zimmerman LE, et al. Bilateral retinoblastoma with ectopic intracranial retinoblastoma: trilateral retinoblastoma. *Cancer Genet Cytogenet* 1982;5:203–213.
17. Kingston JE, Plowman PN, Hungerford JL. Ectopic intracranial retinoblastoma in childhood. *Br J Ophthalmol* 1985;69:742.
18. Brun A. The subpial granular layer of the foetal cerebral cortex in man: its ontogeny and significance in congenital cortical malformations. *Acta Patholog Microbiol Scand* 1965; 179(suppl):3–98.
19. Herrick MK, Rubinstein LJ. The cytological differentiating potential of pineal parenchymal neoplasms (true pinealomas): a clinicopathological study of 28 tumours. *Brain* 1979;102:289–320.
20. Numoto RT. Pineal parenchymal tumors: cell differentiation and prognosis. *J Cancer Res Clin Oncol* 1994;120:683–690.
21. Perentes E, Rubinstein LJ, Herman MM, et al. S-Antigen immunoreactivity in human pineal glands and pineal parenchymal tumors: a monoclonal antibody study. *Acta Neuropathologica* 1986;71:224.
22. Lopes MB, Gonzalez-Fernandez F, Scheithauer MB, et al. Differential expression of retinal proteins in a pineal parenchymal tumor. *J Neuropathol Exp Neurol* 1993;52:516–524.
23. Zeltzer PM, Bodey B, Marlin A, et al. Immunophenotype profile of childhood medulloblastomas and supratentorial primitive neuroectodermal tumors using 16 monoclonal antibodies. *Cancer* 1990;66:273–283.
24. Sarkar C, Roy S, Tandon PN. Primitive neuroectodermal tumours of the central nervous system—an electron microscopic and immunohistochemical study. *India J Med Res* 1989;90:91–102.
25. Molloy PT, Yachnis AT, Rorke LB, et al. Central nervous system medulloepithelioma: a series of eight cases including two arising in the pons. *J Neurosurg* 1996;84:430–436.
26. Grant JW, Steart PV, Gallagher PJ. Primitive neuroectodermal tumors of the cerebrum: a histological and immunohistochemical study of 10 cases. *Clin Neuropathol* 1988;7:229–233.
27. Tomita T, McLone DG, Yasue M. Cerebral primitive neuroectodermal tumors in childhood. *J Neuro-oncol* 1988;6:233–243.
28. Torres LF, Grant N, Harding BN, et al. Intracerebral neuroblastoma: report of a case with neuronal maturation and long survival. *Acta Neuropathol* 1985;68:110.
29. Kees UR, Biegel JA, Ford J, et al. Enhanced MYCN expression and isochromosome 17q in pineoblastoma cell lines. *Genes Chrom Cancer* 1994;9:129–135.

30. Laidlaw JD, McLean CA, Sui K, et al. Intraventricular neurocytoma, a recently recognized pathological entity: report of two cases and review of the literature. *Br J Neurosurg* 1991;5:371–378.

31. Pearl GS, Takei Y, Bakai RAE, et al. Intraventricular primary cerebral neuroblastomas in adults: report of three cases. *Neurosurgery* 1985;16:847–849.

32. Nishio S, Tashima T, Takeshita I, et al. Intraventricular neurocytoma: clinicopathological features of six cases. *J Neurosurg* 1988;68:665–670.

33. Townsend JJ, Seaman JP. Central neurocytoma—a rare benign intraventricular tumor. *Acta Neuropathol* 1986;71: 167–170.

34. VandenBerg SR, May EE, Rubinstein LJ, et al. Desmoplastic supratentorial neuroepithelial tumors of infancy with divergent differentiation potential ("desmoplastic infantile gangliogliomas"). Report on 11 cases of a distinctive embryonal tumor with a favorable prognosis. *J Neurosurg* 1987;66:58–71.

35. Pigott TJD, Punt JAG, Lowe JS, et al. The clinical, radiological and histopathological features of cerebral primitive neuroectodermal tumors. *Br J Neurosurg* 1990;4: 287–298.

36. Chiechi MV, Smirniotopoulos JG, Mena H. Pineal parenchymal tumors: CT and MR features. *J Comp Asst Tomogr* 1995;19:509–517.

37. Kosnik EJ, Boesel CP, Bay J, et al. Primitive neuroectodermal tumors of the central nervous system in children. *J Neurosurg* 1978;48:741–746.

38. Chambers EF, Turski PA, Sobel D, et al. Radiological characteristics of primary cerebral neuroblastomas. *Radiology* 1981;139:101–104.

39. Davis PC, Wichman RD, Takei Y, et al. Primary cerebral neuroblastoma: CT and MR findings in 12 cases. *Am J Neuroradiol* 1990;11:115–120.

40. Regis J, Bouillot P, Rouby-Volot F, et al. Pineal region tumors and the role of stereotactic biopsy: review of mortality, morbidity, and diagnostic results in 370 cases. *Neurosurgery* 1996;39:907–914.

41. Cangemi M, Maiuri F, Fiorillo A, et al. Primary cerebral neuroblastomas. *Neurochirurgic* 1987;30:48–52.

42. Schild SE, Scheithauer BW, Schomberg PJ, et al. Pineal parenchymal tumors: clinical, pathologic, and therapeutic aspects. *Cancer* 1993;72:870–880.

43. Cohen BH, Zeltzer PM, Boyett JM, et al. Prognostic factors and treatment results for supratentorial primitive neuroectodermal tumors in children using radiation and chemotherapy: a Children's Cancer Group randomized trial. *J Clin Oncol* 1995;13:1687–1696.

44. Duffner PK, Horowitz ME, Krischer JP, et al. Postoperative chemotherapy and delayed radiation in children less than three years of age with malignant brain tumors. *N Engl J Med* 1993;24:1725–1731.

45. Geyer JR, Zeltzer PM, Boyett JM, et al. Survival of infants with primitive neuroectodermal tumors or malignant ependymomas of the CNS treated with eight drugs in one day. *J Clin Oncol* 1994;12:1607–1615.

46. Jakacki RI, Zeltzer PM, Boyett JM, et al. Survival and prognostic factors following radiation and/or chemotherapy for primitive neuroectodermal tumors of the pineal region in infants and children: a report of the Children's Cancer Group. *J Clin Oncol* 1995;13:1377–1383.

47. Duffner PK, Cohen ME, Sanford RA, et al. Lack of efficacy of postoperative chemotherapy and delayed radiation in very young children with pineoblastoma: Pediatric Oncology Group. *Med Pediatr Oncol* 1995;25:38–44.

48. Chang SM, Lillis-Hearne PK, Larson DA, et al. Pineoblastoma in adults. *Neurosurgery* 1995;37:383–390.

49. Goldwein JW, Phillips PC, Sutton LN, et al. Primitive neuroectodermal tumors of the pineal gland (pineoblastoma): patterns of presentation and relapse, survival and treatment recommendations. Proceedings from the 6th International Symposium on Pediatric Neuro-oncology. *Pediatr Neurosurg* 1993:321.

50. Mena H, Rushing EJ, Ribas JL, et al. Tumors of pineal parenchymal cells: a correlation of histological features, including nucleolar organizer regions, with survival in 35 cases. *Hum Pathol* 1995;26:20–30.

51. Evans AE, Jenkin DT, Sposto R, et al. The treatment of medulloblastoma: results of a prospective randomized trial of radiation therapy with and without CCNU, vincristine, and prednisone. *J Neurosurg* 1990;72:572–582.

52. Ashley DM, Longee D, Tien R, et al. Treatment of patients with pineoblastoma with high dose cyclophosphamide. *Med Pediatr Oncol* 1996;26:387–392.

53. Heideman RL, Douglass EC, Langston JA, et al. A phase II study of every other day high-dose ifosfamide in pediatric brain tumors: a Pediatric Oncology Group Study. *J Neuro-oncol* 1995;25:77–84.

54. Friedman HS, Schold SC Jr, Mahaley MS Jr et al. Phase II treatment of medulloblastoma and pineoblastoma with melphalan: clinical therapy based on experimental models of human medulloblastoma. *J Clin Oncol* 1989;7: 904–911.

55. Allen JC, Walker R, Luks E, et al. Carboplatin and recurrent childhood brain tumors. *J Clin Oncol* 1987;5:459–463.

56. Kurisaka M, Arisawa M, Morika A, et al. Successful combination chemotherapy (cisplatin, vinblastine, and bleomycin) with small-dose irradiation in the treatment of pineoblastoma metastasized into spinal cord: case report. *Surg Neurol* 1993;39:152–157.

57. Ghim TT, Davis P, Seo JJ, et al. Response to neoadjuvant chemotherapy in children with pineoblastoma. *Cancer* 1993;72:1795–1800.

58. Kovnar EH, Kellie SJ, Horowitz ME, et al. Preirradiation cisplatin and etoposide in the treatment of high-risk medulloblastoma and other malignant embryonal tumors of the central nervous system: a phase II study. *J Clin Oncol* 1990;8:330–336.

59. Halperin EC, Friedman HS, Schold SC, et al. Surgery, hyperfractionated craniospinal irradiation and adjuvant chemotherapy in the management of supratentorial embryonal neuroepithelial neoplasms in children. *Surg Neurol* 1993;40:278–283.

60. Zeltzer P, Boyett J, Finlay J, et al. Prognostic factors for survival differ in high-risk infra- and supratentorial primitive neuroectodermal tumors. *Pediatr Neurosurg* 1993;19:333.

61. Ashwal S, Hinshaw DB, Bedros A. CNS primitive neuroectodermal tumors of childhood. *Med Pediatr Oncol* 1984;12:180–188.

62. Zeltzer PM, Gaskil SJ, Marlin AE. Supratentorial primitive neuroectodermal tumors. In: Deutsch M, ed. *Management of Childhood Brain Tumors*. Boston: Kluwer Academic; 1990.

63. Torres CF, Rebsamen S, Silber JH, et al. Surveillance scanning of children with medulloblastoma. *N Engl J Med* 1994;330:892–895.

64. Steinbok P, Hentschel S, Cochrane DD, et al. Value of postoperative surveillance imaging in the management of children with some common brain tumors. *J Neurosurg* 1996;84:726–732.

65. Brown WD, Tavare CJ, Sobel EL et al. The applicability of Collins' law to childhood brain tumors and its usefulness as a predictor of survival. *Neurosurgery* 1995;36:1093–1096.

66. Cranston PE, Hatten MT, Smith EE. Metastatic pineoblastoma via a ventriculoperitoneal shunt: CT demonstration. *Comp Med Imaging Graphics* 1992;16:349–351.

67. Gururangen S, Heideman RL, Kovnar EH, et al. Peritoneal metastases in two patients with pineoblastoma and ventriculo-peritoneal shunts. *Med Pediatr Oncol* 1994;22:417–420.

68. Dunkel IJ, Finlay JL. High dose chemotherapy with autologous stem cell rescue for patients with medulloblastoma. *J Neuro-oncol* 1996;29:69–74.

69. Donahue B. Short- and long-term complications of radiation therapy for pediatric brain tumors. *Pediatr Neurosurg* 1992;18:207–217.

70. Duffner PK, Cohen ME, Thomas PRM, et al. The long-term effects of cranial irradiation on the central nervous system. *Cancer* 1985;56:1841–1846.

71. Ellenberg L, McComb JG, Siegel S, et al. Factors affecting intellectual outcome in pediatric brain tumor patients. *Neurosurgery* 1987;21:638–644.

72. Radcliffe J, Packer RJ, Atkins TE, et al. Three- and four-year cognitive outcome in children with noncortical brain tumors treated with whole-brain radiotherapy. *Ann Neurol* 1992;32:551–554.

73. Packer RJ, Sutton LN, Atkins TE, et al. A prospective study of cognitive function in children receiving whole-brain radiotherapy and chemotherapy: two-year results. *J Neurosurg* 1989;70:703–713.

74. Mulhern RK, Kun LE. Neuropsychologic function in children with brain tumor: interval changes in the six months following treatment. *Med Pediatr Oncol* 1985;13:318–324.

75. Kanev PM, Lefebvre JF, Mauseth RS, et al. Growth hormone deficiency following radiation therapy of primary brain tumors in children. *J Neurosurg* 1991;74:743–748.

76. Duffner PK, Cohen ME, Voorhess ML, et al. Long-term effects of cranial irradiation on endocrine function in children with brain tumors: a prospective study. *Cancer* 1985; 56:2189–2193.

77. Livesey EA, Hindmarsh PC, Brook CGD, et al. Endocrine disorders following treatment of childhood brain tumours. *Br J Cancer* 1990;61:622–625.

78. Clayton PE, Shalet SM, Price DA, et al. Testicular damage after chemotherapy for childhood brain tumors. *J Pediatr* 1988;112:922–926.

79. Hawkins MM, Draper GJ, Kingston JE. Incidence of second primary tumors among childhood cancer survivors. *Br J Cancer* 1987;56:339–347.

80. Farwell J, Flannery JT. Second primaries in children with central nervous system tumors. *J Neuro-oncol* 1984;2:371–375.

81. De Vathaire F, Francois P, Hill C, et al. Role of radiotherapy and chemotherapy in the risk of second malignant neoplasms after cancer in childhood. *Br J Cancer* 1989; 59:792–796.

Chapter 19

Craniopharyngioma

Jeffrey H. Wisoff

Craniopharyngiomas constitute approximately 3% of all intracranial neoplasms.[1,2] They are the most common nonglial tumor of childhood, accounting for 6 to 9% of pediatric brain tumors.[3–5] Cushing graphically described craniopharyngiomas as "the kaleidoscopic tumors, solid and cystic, which take their origin from epithelial rests ascribable to an imperfect closure of the hypophyseal or craniopharyngeal duct" and whose management is "one of the most baffling problems to the neurosurgeon."[6] The benign histologic features of these tumors are often in marked contrast to their malignant clinical course in children. The location of craniopharyngiomas, with their intimate association with the visual pathways, hypothalamus, and limbic system, predisposes patients with these tumors to severe visual, endocrine, and cognitive deficits, both at presentation and as a result of treatment. Although most children can compensate for neurologic deficits and endocrinologic deficiencies, the cognitive and psychosocial squelae may be functionally devastating, interfering with education, limiting independence, and adversely affecting the quality of life as these children approach adulthood.[7]

EPIDEMIOLOGY

Although craniopharyngiomas compose a significant proportion of pediatric brain tumors, on a population basis they are rare. Based on an analysis of three population-based cancer registries, the incidence of craniopharyngioma in the United States is between 0.13 and 0.18 per 100,000 person years.[8] A bimodal distribution by age has been noted, with peak incidence rates in children and older adults. Incidence is lowest in late adolescence and early adulthood (age 15 to 34 years). Among children, the incidence is greatest at 6 to 10 years, followed by 11 to 15 years.[8,9] Although previous studies have reported that the majority of craniopharyngiomas occurred in children,[4,10–14] the population-based registry data suggest that only 33 to 35% of all craniopharyngiomas occur in childhood.[8] Based on these assumptions, approximately 338 cases of craniopharyngioma are expected to be diagnosed annually in the United States, with 96 occurring in children from 0 to 14 years of age.

Although there does not appear to be any racial or ethnic predilection for craniopharyngiomas, the influence of sex is unclear. Bunin et al describe an incidence that is nearly identical: 0.13 males and 0.12 females per 100,000 per year.[8] There is also no sex difference in a population-based study from

Finland.[13] In contrast, clinical series have shown a mixed picture. A large hospital-based series of cases from the United Kingdom showed a ratio of 1.3 (107 males and 66 females),[15] whereas in case series of craniopharyngiomas in children the male/female ratios varied from 0.9 (42 tumors),[16] to 1.2 (80 tumos),[9] to 1.6 (105 tumors).[17] Considering all of the data, craniopharyngiomas may occur slightly more often in boys.

Stiller and Nectoux[18] have reported that the proportion of brain tumors that are craniopharyngiomas varied substantially among different global regions: 1.5% in Australia, 4.7 to 7.9% in Europe, 3.9% in Japan, 2.7% in U.S. whites, 4.9% in U.S. blacks, and 11.6% in Africa. Although this international variation in occurrence has led to speculation regarding environmental influences, the data must be interpreted with caution. Since socioeconomic conditions preclude population-based reporting of all brain tumors in developing countries, variation in incidence is not a reliable statistic. Although percentages of reported tumor are more useful in comparing international rates because they will be less prejudiced by incomplete reporting, they are influenced by the proportions of other types of tumors, including those with nonspecific diagnosis, such as brain tumor or malignant brain tumor. Although the incidence of craniopharyngioma appears increased in Africa and decreased in Australia, this conclusion is specious and not supported by clear data.[8]

PATHOLOGY

Craniopharyngiomas develop from epithelial nests that are embryonic remnants of Rathke's pouch, located along an axis extending from the sella turcica along the pituitary stalk to the hypothalamus and the floor of the third ventricle.[2,19] Craniopharyngiomas gradually enlarge as partially calcified solid and cystic masses predominantly in the suprasellar region; the cystic component can reach several centimeters in size. Purely cystic tumors are uncommon in childhood. They extend along the path of least resistance into the basal cisterns or can invaginate into the third ventricle. With continued growth superiorly into the third ventricle, hydrocephalus may develop.

Craniopharyngiomas have two basic patterns of cellular growth: adamantinomatous and papillary.[1,2,10,14,20,21] Mixed tumors with both adamantinomatous and squamous papillary components or combinations of craniopharyngioma and Rathke's cleft cysts can occur.[1,2,10,14,20–22]

The adamantinomatous tumors are the most common variant, occurring at all ages. They resemble the epithelium of tooth-forming tumors containing three distinct components: a basal layer of small cells; an intermediate layer of variable thickness with loose, stellate cells; and a top layer facing the cyst lumen where the cells are abruptly enlarged, flattened, and keratinized. At the cyst surface, desquamated epithelial cells are present either singly or in characteristic stacked clusters (keratin nodules). These nodules may undergo mineralization with accumulation of calcium salts, which in rare instances progress to metaplastic bone formation. The cysts in adamantinomatous craniopharyngiomas usually contain an oily liquid composed of desquamated epithelium rich in cholesterol, keratin, and, occasionally, calcium.

Squamous papillary craniopharyngiomas occur nearly exclusively in adults and have a predilection to involve the third ventricle.[23] They consist of solid epithelium, without loose stellate zones, in a papillary architecture that resembles metaplastic respiratory epithelium.[2, 3, 10, 20] They are predominantly solid and rarely undergo mineralization. When cysts occur, the fluid is less oily and dark than adamantinomatous tumors. As a result of the absence of calcification and minimal cyst formation, complete curative surgical resection may be obtained more often than with adamantinomatous or mixed craniopharyngiomas.[9, 10, 22] Histology does not affect the risk of recurrence after subtotal resection or the response to radiation therapy.

Microscopic islets, or "fingers," of adamantinomatous tumor embedded in densely gliotic parenchyma are frequently seen when the tumor arises in the region of the tuber cinereum, hypothalamus, and floor of the third ventricle.[20, 22, 24–28] The gliotic reaction of Rosenthal fibers and fibrillary astrocytes, varying between several hundred micrometers to millimeters in thickness,[26] effectively separates tumor from brain, thus providing a safe plane for surgical dissection.[12, 22, 28, 29] The presence of this gliotic tissue on surgical pathologic examination is associated with a decreased risk of recurrence following a gross total tumor resection.[22]

RADIOLOGY

The role of neuroimaging is to establish a preoperative diagnosis and then define the location and extent of the cystic, solid, and calcified portions of the tumor and its relationship to the distorted normal anatomy. Radiographic evaluation includes computed tomography (CT), magnetic resonance imaging (MRI), magnetic resonance angiography (MRA), and, where available, magnetic resonance spectroscopy (MRS).[30–32] Vascular anatomy can be well demonstrated by MRI and MRA, obviating the need for invasive cerebral angiography.[30]

CT and MRI have complementary roles in the diagnosis of craniopharyngioma[30, 32, 33] (Fig. 19–1). CT is superior in

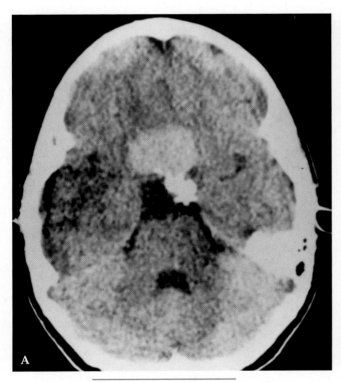
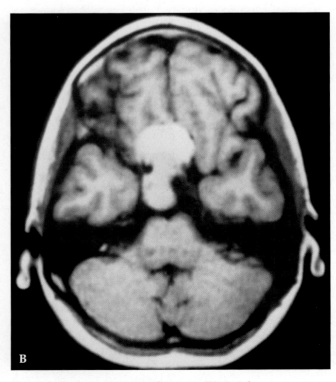

Figure 19–1 (A) Noncontrast CT scan demonstrating calcified component of tumor. (B) Axial T1-weighted gadolinium-enhanced magnetic resonance image demonstrating solid and cystic tumor. Note how the image does not delineate the calcified portion as well as the CT scan.

the detection of the varied and complex calcifications. The non–contrast-enhanced CT scan usually demonstrates a suprasellar and often intrasellar mass with calcifications as well as hypodense solid and cyst components. The low density is usually greater than the attenuation of cerebrospinal fluid (CSF). A small percentage of craniopharyngiomas may be of high density.[32] CT may show secondary changes in the skull base, such as enlargement of the sella turcica and/or erosion of the dorsum sella.

BOX 19–1
CT Appearance

- **Calcifications**
- **Hypodense solid and cystic components**
- **Erosion of sella**

MRI and MRA provide valuable information about the relationships of the tumor to surrounding structures, delineating the involvement or displacement of the visual pathways, hypothalamus, ventricles, and vessels of the circle of Willis. Non–contrast-enhanced sagittal T1-weighted images may show the normal pituitary, leading to the correct diagnosis.[33] Fine calcifications may not be visible, may demonstrate a paradoxical increased signal on T1-weighted imaging, or, if more substantial, may exhibit characteristic signal voids. Craniopharyngioma cysts are uniformly bright on T2-weighted sequences; however, on T1-weighted sequences the signal intensity of the fluid may range from hypointense to hyperintense,[30, 32, 34] reflecting the heterogeneous contents. The correlation between MRI and the biochemical composition of cyst fluid is complex, with protein, lipid, and iron concentrations having a major influence on cyst signals.[30, 35] Cyst capsule and solid tumor vividly enhance with contrast.

BOX 19–2
MRI Appearance

- **Variable solid tumor**
- **Cysts**
  - **Bright on T2**
  - **Hypo- to hyperdense on T1**

Noncalcified solid craniopharyngiomas may have CT and MRI characteristics that are indistinguishable from those of other pediatric suprasellar neoplasms, including chiasmatic hypothalamic gliomas, germinomas, and pituitary adenomas. Proton MRS demonstrates unique spectroscopic profiles that differentiate these tumors.[31] Craniopharyngiomas show a dominant peak consistent with lactate or lipids and only trace amount of other metabolites. In contrast, gliomas demonstrate choline, N-acetylaspartate, and creatine, with an increased ratio of choline to N-acetylaspartate compared with normal brain. Pituitary adenomas show either choline peaks or no metabolites at all.

The surgeon's impression of extent of tumor resection must be confirmed by neuroimaging. Postoperative imaging with both enhanced MRI and CT is best done within 48 hours to avoid the artifacts of surgical trauma.[30] Residual tumor should be graded according to the method of Hoffman:[29] grade 1—no residual timor or calcification; grade 2—tiny (<1 min) fleck of calcification without evidence of enhancement or mass; grade 3—small "calcific chunk" without enhancement or mass effect; grade 4—small contrast-enhancing lesion without significant mass effect, and grade 5—contrast-enhancing mass.

BOX 19–3
Hoffman's Grading System

- **Grade 1: no residual tumor or calcification**
- **Grade 2: less than 1 mm calcification, no enhancement or mass effect**
- **Grade 3: small calcification without enhancement or mass effect**
- **Grade 4: small enhancing lesion without mass effect**
- **Grade 5: enhancing mass**

CLINICAL PRESENTATION

In children, the slow growth of a craniopharyngioma often results in a delay between onset of symptoms and diagnosis, with a typical prodrome of 1 to 2 years.[36, 37] The main presenting signs and symptoms of craniopharyngioma are related to pressure on adjacent neural structures.[4, 22, 25, 36, 38–45] Headache from increased intracranial pressure is the most common complaint, occurring in 60 to 75% of cases. Visual symptoms are noted in approximately half of these children. Progressive visual loss is often well tolerated by children and not diagnosed until they are noted to be sitting progressively closer to the television. Evidence of hormonal insufficiency, including growth failure, delayed sexual maturation, excessive weight gain, and diabetes insipidus (DI), is present in 20 to 50% of the children at diagnosis but is rarely the symptom that brings the child to medical attention. With progressive growth into frontal lobes, hypothalamus, and/or the onset of hydrocephalus, psychomotor slowing, apathy, and short-term memory deficits may also occur with a decline in academic performance.

Formal preoperative neuro-ophthalmologic, endocrinologic, and neuropsychological evaluations are mandatory. Seventy to eighty percent of patients will demonstrate abnormal visual acuity or field on preoperative testing.[22, 25, 36, 38, 45, 46] The specific ophthalmologic deficits reflect the direction of growth of the tumor and its compression of various portions of the visual apparatus: prechiasmatic extension will compress optic nerves with loss of visual acuity, whereas posterior tumors cause chiasmatic compression with complex visual field defects. Frank papilledema is present in approximately 20% of patients.[37]

The essential preoperative endocrine testing includes an evaluation of adrenal function, thyroid function, and salt and water balance before initiation of steroid therapy; measurement of gonadotropin and growth hormone (GH) levels is also routinely performed. Failure to preoperatively recognize and correct adrenocorticotropic hormone (ACTH) or thyroid hormone deficiency or appropriately manage DI can result in severe morbidity or death.

Less than 30% of children are endocrinologically normal at diagnosis.[43, 47, 48] GH deficiency is the most common finding, present in up to 75% of pediatric patients. Gonadotropin deficiency is observed in up to 60% of children, and thyroid or adrenal dysfunction in approximately 30%. DI is relatively uncommon, occurring in only 9 to 17% of patients.

SURGERY

Most pediatric neurosurgeons in North America and Europe favor complete microsurgical resection as the treatment of choice for newly diagnosed craniopharyngiomas.[12, 22, 36, 40, 45, 49, 50] The feasibility and success of radical resection are dependent on the availability of surgical expertise and postoperative endocrinologic support, understanding the size and extent of the tumor, whether the tumor is primary or recurrent, the clinical condition of the patient, and the societal resources for coping with potential postoperative deficits. If the socioeconomic conditions applicable to an individual patient do not provide appropriate long-term endocrinologic support and neurologic care, functional morbidity or even death may overshadow the merits of curative resection.

Operative Planning

Categorization of the pattern and extent of growth assists in evaluating treatment options, determining potential surgical approach, and predicting outcome. Several different clinicoradiologic classification systems have been proposed;[29, 36, 37, 49, 51] all attempt to describe the degree of vertical and horizontal extension, displacement of the optic nerves and chiasm, number of anatomical regions involved by tumor, and overall tumor size. The tumors may be entirely within the sella or intra- and extrasellar infradiaphragmatic (Yasargil type a and b, Samii grade I–II, Hoffman sellar group, Choux group A), suprasellar supradiaphragmatic extending anteriorly to displace the optic nerves and chiasm posteriorly (Yasargil type c, Samii grade III–V, Hoffman prechiasmatic, Choux group B), suprasellar supradiaphragmatic with tumor extending posterior to the chiasm, displacing chiasm and optic nerves forward and invaginating into the hypothalamus, mamillary bodies, basilar artery, third ventricle, and brain stem (Yasargil type d and e, Samii grade III–V, Hoffman retrochiasmatic, Choux group B and ABC), and purely intraventricular (Yasargil type e, Choux group C).

The size is graded as small (2 cm), moderate (2 to 4 cm), large (4 to 6 cm), and giant (greater than 6 cm).[45] Giant tumors may extend into multiple or all compartments, extending from the medulla to the foramen of Monro (Figs. 19–2) to 19–4). In children, small tumors compose 4 to 10%,

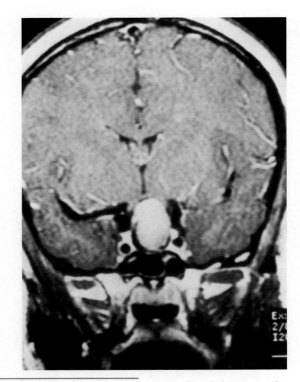

Figure 19–2 Coronal T1-weighted gadolinium-enhanced magnetic resonance image demonstrating a small craniopharyngioma.

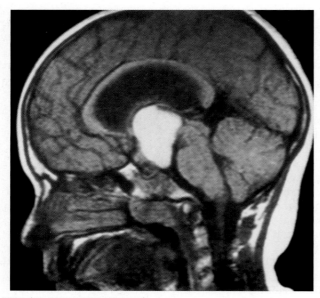

Figure 19–3 Sagittal T1-weighted gadolinium-enhanced magnetic resonance image demonstrating a large craniopharyngioma.

moderate tumors 29 to 51%, and tumors greater than 4 cm approximately 50%, with 5 to 10% classified as giant.[9, 22, 36, 52, 53]

Operative Technique—Craniotomy

A variety of operative approaches have been described and championed by different surgeons, including the subfrontal,[4, 12, 28, 54] pterional,[49, 55, 56] bifrontal interhemispheric,[57, 58] subtemporal,[59] transcallosal,[9] and transsphenoidal approaches.[56, 60–63] All intracranial surgery is performed with the operating microscope, usually under moderate to high magnification. Surgical adjuncts, including the ultrasonic aspirator, frameless stereotaxy, and rigid and flexible neuroendoscopes, should be available and utilized when appropriate.

The author has utilized the pterional craniotomy as advocated by Yasargil et al[45] in 76 of 79 consecutive operations for craniopharyngioma. This approach offers the shortest and most direct route to the suprasellar region and, with splitting of the sylvian fissure, minimizes or eliminates retraction of normal brain. Tumors extending from the pontomedullary junction (Fig. 19–4) to above the foramen of Monro can be removed through the pterional approach. In no patient is a cortical resection[64] or sacrifice of the olfactory nerve[28] necessary.

Dexamethasone (0.1 mg/kg), phenytoin (15 mg/kg), and cephalexin (25 mg/kg) are administered after induction and intubation. Mannitol (0.25 g/kg) is given at the time of skin incision to help maximize brain relaxation. The diuretic effect is maximal within the first hour of surgery, long before manipulation of the pituitary stalk and hypothalamus may produce DI, which complicates fluid and electrolyte management. A 7-cm frontotemporal craniotomy is performed with removal of the sphenoid wing; when necessary, the orbital rim can be removed with the craniotomy flap to obtain a wider operative corridor and shorter distance to the tumor. Prior to opening the dura either intraopetative ultrasonography or frameless stereotaxy is used to determine the location and extent of the tumor and its relationship to the operative exposure.

Throughout the surgery retraction of the brain is minimized. Mannitol, hyperventilation, and gradual drainage of CSF through the opened sylvian fissure and basal cisterns will usually provide excellent relaxation, even in the presence

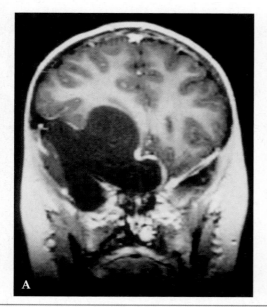
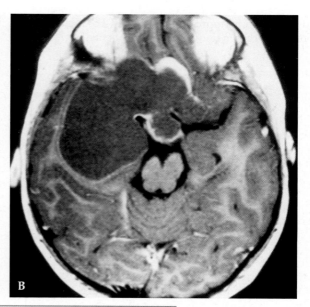

Figure 19–4 (A) Axial and (B) coronal T1-weighted gadolinium-enhanced magnetic resonance image demonstrating a giant craniopharyngioma.

of moderate degrees of hydrocephalus. Ventricular drainage is reserved for cases refractory to these maneuvers or when the use of an intraventricular endoscope is anticipated (vide infra). Although hydrocephalus is present in 15 to 66% of patients,[12, 22, 36, 42, 45, 52, 55, 57] preoperative shunting is reserved for patients with severe symptoms of increased intracranial pressure that is unresponsive to medical management.

As these tumors often extend diffusely throughout the suprasellar cisterns, displacing and distorting normal structures, identification of the vascular anatomy provides essential landmarks. Starting laterally, the sylvian fissure is widely split and the distal branches of the middle cerebral artery are identified. Bipolar cauterization is limited to avoid fusing arachnoid planes. The arachnoidal dissection proceeds medially to the main trunk of the middle cerebral artery, which is followed proximally to the ipsilateral carotid bifurcation, anterior cerebral artery, and internal carotid artery. As the carotid is followed proximally to the clinoid, the optic nerve, chiasm, and tracts are identified in relation to the tumor.

Premature decompression of craniopharyngiomas, especially cystic tumors, causes the tumor capsule and arachnoid to become redundant, thus obscuring the planes of dissection. Working in the prechiasmatic, opticocarotid, and carotidotentorial triangles, one may develop and maintain an arachnoidal plane between the intact tumor and the branches of the ipsilateral carotid artery and vessels of the circle of Willis, preserving all vessels and their perforating branches. This plane is developed posteriorly until the basilar artery is identified. In primary tumors, the membrane of Lillequist invariably separates the tumor from the basilar artery.

Once the vascular anatomy has been identified and separated from the tumor, the cyst is aspirated and the solid internal component debulked. Care is taken to preserve the capsule of the tumor. Again working in the parachiasmal spaces and maintaining arachnoidal planes, the tumor is progressively dissected free from the optic nerves, the contralateral carotid and its branches, and the inferior aspect of the optic chiasm. Manipulation of the optic nerves, chiasm, and tracts should be minimized. The optic nerves, as they exit the optic canal, are susceptible to injury by traction over the sharp, fixed edge of the dura proprium. Both the optic nerves and/or the chiasm may be pinched between the anterior cerebral artery above and the tumor below. Optic tract injury can occur with relatively little retraction.

An attempt is always made to identify and preserve the pituitary stalk; this can be accomplished in 30% of patients. When the stalk cannot be separated from the tumor, it is sectioned as distally as possible to prevent undo traction on the hypothalamus. After the tumor is dissected free from the entire circle of Willis, the pituitary stalk, and the optic apparatus, the capsule is grasped and, with continuous traction and blunt dissection, the gliotic plane is developed, which allows the tumor to be delivered from its attachment to the hypothalamus in the region of the tuber cinereum. After the tumor has been removed, the entire bed must be inspected for residual disease. A micromirror or angle endoscope is used to view the undersurface of the chiasm and hypothalamus to confirm a complete resection.

If the tumor extends into the third ventricle or has a significant retrochiasmatic component, the lamina terminalis is fenestrated. The lamina terminalis is easily distinguished from the chiasm as it appears pale, avascular, and often is distended by tumor. As retrochiasmatic tumor is removed, the prechiasmatic space may widen, providing an additional avenue for dissection.

Third ventricular tumor is delivered through the lamina terminalis as well as from below the chiasm. Placement of a 2.3-mm neuroendoscope into the lateral or third ventricle assists in monitoring the delivery of the intraventricular component of the tumor. With the endoscope, simultaneous or sequential transcallosal exposure of the intraventricular tumor[9] is usually not obligatory.

When the tumor extends into the sella turcica, removal of the posterior planum sphenoidale and tuberculum sellae may be required to gain adequate intrasellar exposure.[54] After removal of tumor, any defects communicating with the sphenoid sinus must be obliterated with fat and pericranial grafts.

Operative Technique—Transsphenoidal Surgery

Although most craniopharyngiomas of childhood arise in the region of the tuber cinereum, a small percentage originate from more caudal craniopharyngeal duct cells resting in the sella turcica.[63] As these tumors grow, the diaphragma sellae stretches over the dorsal aspect, separating it from suprasellar structures and preventing tumor adherence to the optic apparatus, hypothalamus, and vessels of the circle of Willis. This feature of the pathologic anatomy allows radical removal of infradiaphragmatic intrasellar tumors by a transsphenoidal approach.[9, 56, 62, 63, 65] In pediatric craniopharyngiomas, between 3 and 15% of the tumors may be amenable to transsphenoidal resection.[36, 66]

Transsphenoidal surgery in young children may present anatomical difficulties related to the small size of the bony structures and to the lack of a pneumatized sphenoid sinus. The presence of a conchal or prepneumatized sphenoid sinus is not a contraindication to transsphenoidal surgery; however, the bone must be meticulously drilled or chiseled under fluoroscopic control to obtain wide access to the sella turcica.[63] Other than the bony exposure, the technical aspects of the operation do not differ significantly from similar surgery in adults, particularly with regard to the overall approach and tumor resection.[55, 56, 60, 63, 67] However, the rarity of these tumors suggests that this approach be utilized only by surgical teams with adequate experience.[68]

After a wide dural opening, the normal ventrally displaced pituitary gland is encountered. The gland must be incised in the midline and then gently pushed laterally to obtain exposure of the dorsally located craniopharyngioma. Once an initial plane of cleavage between the tumor and the sella wall is established, the capsule is opened, resulting in drainage of cyst fluid and debulking of solid neoplasm. Following this internal decompression, the capsule is dissected from the walls of the cavernous sinuses and pituitary gland to complete mobilization of the intrasellar tumor. When the superior capsule is adherent to the diaphragma, it must be incised and resected. As the superior craniopharyngioma is delivered, the remaining attachment of tumor to the pituitary stalk is made visible and detached with bipolar coagulation and sharp dissection to achieve a gross total resection. Resection of the diaphragma invariably produces an intraoperative CSF leak. Obliteration of the sella and sphenoid sinus with a free fat graft is mandatory. Several days of postoperative lumbar drainage is recommended.[56]

Extent of resection is confirmed with postoperative MRI and CT. Accessible tumor that was inadvertently left unresected during primary surgery should be removed. A second operation within several weeks of a primary surgery is not associated with significant added risk or technical difficulty.

OUTCOME
Craniotomy

Radiographically confirmed total resection can be accomplished in 80 to 100% of primary tumors in children.[9, 12, 22, 36, 49, 50, 57] Perioperative mortality following radical surgery has decreased substantially in the last decade from 6–11% to 0–4%.[9, 12, 22, 28, 36, 49, 52, 55, 56, 69–72] The philosophy[25] and experience of the surgeon[22, 52, 53] significantly affects the likelihood of achieving a curative total resection with low mortality or disabling morbidity. Centers performing fewer than two operations for radical resection per year had a good outcome in only 52% of cases, compared with 87% for institutions that performed radical surgery more often.[53] In addition, age of patient, size and location of tumor, severity of preoperative deficits, and presence of hydrocephalus all impact on postoperative morbidity.[9, 52]

BOX 19–5
Postoperative Morbidity
Following Craniotomy

- **Hormonal changes**
- **Visual deterioration**
- **Vascular injury (carotid)**
- **Neuropsychological defects**

Endocrine disturbances are common after radical resection as a result of hypothalamic manipulation and pituitary stalk sectioning.[5, 9, 36, 49, 73, 74] Endocrine morbidity may be more severe when tumor resection involves bilateral manipulation of the hypothalamus.[9] Although a significant percentage of deaths in earlier series were attributable to pituitary insufficiency,[74, 75] this is uncommon today provided adequate endocrinologic expertise and socioeconomic resources are available.

Hormonal replacement therapy is required in approximately 80% of pediatric patients.[22, 43, 47, 48, 76, 77] Thyroid and cortisol replacement therapy is administered as necessary.

DI is universally present immediately following surgery. Over the course of the first week, DI may alternate with the syndrome of inappropriate antidiuretic hormone (SIADH). Meticulous attention to fluid balance and electrolyte status is essential to avoid severe fluctuations from hypernatremia to hyponatremia. Permanent DI will develop in approximately 75% of children.[22, 45, 78] Replacement with synthetic vasopressin (DDAVP) provides excellent control of DI in children with an intact thirst mechanism. However, the rare combination of ADH insufficiency and an impaired sense of thirst following aggressive surgery with severe hypothalamic injury remains one of the most complex management problems.[73]

Weight gain without overt hyperphagia may occur in half of all children undergoing radical surgery, although morbid obesity with lack of satiety is far less common.[8, 36, 43, 76, 79, 80] Bilateral hypothalamic damage, particularly in larger tumors, may result in an insensitivity to endogenous leptin and a disturbed feedback mechanism from the hypothalamic leptin receptors to the adipose tissue.[80] Preoperative weight gain and MRI evidence of extensive involvement of the hypothalamus may help identify patients most at risk for severe postoperative obesity.[79]

Excess weight is often the overriding concern during long-term follow-up. As Hoffman et al[12] noted, "in a society where fitness and slim bodies are praised, obesity has led to problems with peers." Many children may become distraught over the alteration in habitus and body image[5]: four of our early patients required individual or family counseling to address these psychological and emotional issues. We now routinely advise families and older children preoperatively that they may experience a 10 to 15% permanent weight gain.

Although most children with craniopharyngiomas are GH-deficient, some will maintain a normal or even accelerated growth rate after surgery, often associated with hyperphagia and obesity.[47, 48] Normal or accelerated growth following surgery does not indicate the presence of normal GH secretion nor does it ensure continued growth. A complex series of metabolic events, including activation of insulin-like growth factor 1 by hypothalamic hyperphagia/obesity–induced hyperinsulinemia may explain this growth pattern.[43, 81] Many children later fail to maintain this growth and, if GH treatment is not instituted, adult height is compromised.[47] GH treatment may be recommended in these children for long-term improved growth velocity, adult height, and other GH-dependent metabolic processes.[82] Even when GH replacement may not affect growth, it may help decrease body mass index.[83]

Total removal of the tumor offers the optimal ophthalmologic recovery and outcome.[36] Some degree of deterioration in visual function is present in approximately 20% of children after surgery.[36] Maximum improvement in visual acuity and fields is noted within the first postoperative month.[46] Extent and duration of preoperative deficits but not age are associated with a worse outcome.[22, 36, 45, 70] Visual outcome from the author's experience and current literature is summarized in Table 19–1.

Fusiform dilatation of the carotid artery on postoperative MRI has been noted in 10 to 29% of children following radical

TABLE 19–1   Visual Function after Radical Resection

	Hoffman[12] (50 children— all primary)	Yasargil[45] (67 children— 51 primary/ 16 recurrent)	Tomita[49] (27 children— all primary)	Wisoff (2001)* (66 children— 45 primary/ 21 recurrent)
Visual field:				
Improved	39	63	62	53
Stable	20	32	19	20
Worse	41	5	19	27
Visual acuity:				
Improved	55	60	59	60
Stable	15	25	30	27
Worse	30	15	11	13

*Author's series, this volume.

surgery.[84, 85] Retraction of the vessels and dissection of tumor capsule from the adventitia may damage the vasovasorum, weakening the muscular wall and causing progressive diffuse expansion of the artery. The natural history appears to be benign: there have been no anecdotal or published reports of hemorrhage or stroke attributable to these lesions to date. Observation with serial MRI/MRA appears to be the appropriate management. When additional surgery for craniopharyngioma is required, approaching the tumor from the side opposite to the fusiform dilatation has been recommended.[85] It is uncertain whether there is any benefit to wrapping the dilatation with muslin gauze; attempts at arterial reconstruction are not warranted.

The impact of extent of resection on neuropsychological functioning is controversial.[7, 12, 22, 72, 86–90] Evidence of preoperative hypothalamic dysfunction and size of tumor may predict those children at risk for postoperative intellectual and behavioral difficulties.[52] Isolated results on neuropsychological testing may not predict psychosocial or academic performance. Mild deficits in recent memory may not impair normal educational advancement if intelligence is adequate.[12]

Many of the reports describing a poor neuropsychological outcome are from institutions with either limited experience with radical microsurgical resection or multiple surgeons caring for a relatively small number of patients.[7, 42, 52, 53] In contrast, among centers with a large volume of radical surgeries and a dedicated neurosurgeon, a good outcome with normal psychosocial integration and age-appropriate academic performance is reported in over 70% of children[12, 22, 43, 49, 53] and was seen in 87% of the author's 45 patients with primary tumors radically resected since 1985. Memory disturbances are seen in half of children on psychometric testing; however, this impairment does not interfere with schooling when intelligence is normal.[12] Some of the deficits associated with impairment of frontal lobe function following radical subfrontal resections[87] may be avoided by the pterional approach, which inherently has less retraction on the frontal lobe. Giant tumors, retrochiasmatic location, and severe preoperative hydrocephalus all impact negatively on psychosocial outcome.

Following radiographically confirmed total resection, no adjuvant therapy is administered. Recurrence rates following total resection range from 0 to 20% (Table 19–2).[9, 12, 22, 36, 49, 53] Most recurrences in children occur within 2 to 3 years.[9, 12, 22, 36, 49, 72, 91, 92] Hoffman et al reported that 70% of recurrences became evident within 3 years (mean 2.46 years);

TABLE 19–2   Recurrence Following Total Resection

Study	Total no. children	Radical surgery (no.)	Recurrence (%)	Mortality (%)
Choux (1991)[36]	454	251	19	4
Fahlbusch (1997)[55]	30	13	17	0
Hoffman (1992)[12]	50	45	29	2
Tomita (1993)[49]	27	23	5	0
Wisoff (2001)*	45	43	12	2
Yasargil (1995)[9]	61	61	10	2

*Author's series, this volume.

however, some recurrences took place as late as 7 years after primary surgery.[25] With a mean follow-up of more than 6 years, 12% of our 43 totally resected primary tumors have recurred, all within 2 years of initial surgery. Rarely, tumor may recur distant from the primary site as a result of implantation at the time of initial resection.[49, 93, 94] Reoperation can be curative, especially with solid tumors; however, scarring from previous surgery may increase the technical difficulty of surgery (vide infra). The morbidity following reoperation is high, with only 30 to 60% having a good outcome.[45, 92]

Transsphenoidal Resection

Total resection can be accomplished in 60 to 90% of primary infradiaphragmatic itrasellar craniopharyngiomas; however, the rate of success drops to 10 to 60% for recurrent tumors.[55, 56, 60, 61, 66, 67] In experienced hands, operative mortality ranges from 0 to 4% and nonendocrine morbidity in 15 to 25% of the patients, with children tending to have a better outcome than adults.[55, 56, 60, 63, 66] The incidence of new DI but not other endocrine deficiencies appears to be less than with transcranial surgery.[9, 55, 56, 67] Impairment of psychosocial function is uncommon.[55, 56] Recurrence after total resection of primary tumors occurs in 0 to 43% of patients, with the incidence of recurrence substantially less in the most experienced centers.[55, 56, 61, 66, 67]

IRRADIATION

When total resection cannot be achieved, either for technical or socioeconomic reasons, additional adjuvant therapy is required to control tumor growth: 90% of these tumors will have radiographic and symptomatic progression within 5 years.[84, 95] In an era of prohibitive morbidity and mortality following aggressive surgery for craniopharyngioma, Kramer et al first described the efficacy of combining limited surgery with irradiation in the early 1960s.[96, 97] Subsequent reports showed that irradiation added to surgery resulted in a 50 to 90% 5-year and 10-year disease-free survival.[7, 22, 39, 42, 88, 95, 98–103] Neuropsychological outcome and quality of life are excellent, especially when treating smaller tumors.[7, 42, 87] Endocrine replacement is required; however, few patients will develop DI.

Stereotactic radiosurgery has been employed for small solid tumors (under 2.5 cm), often in conjunction with intracystic irradiation.[104–106] Long-term results in 88 patients demonstrated disease control with a good quality of life in 63% and tumor-related mortality in 16%.[105] Radiation injury to the optic nerve was present in 10% of patients. At least 3 to 5 mm must separate the target volume from the optic pathways to limit the dose to less than 1000 cGy and thus avoid this complication.[106]

Radiation injury occurs in a predictable manner depending on dose, volume, and fractionation.[107] Doses of 5000 to 5500 cGy delivered in 180-cGy fractions are required to obtain tumor control with minimal toxicity.[51, 98, 102, 103] Current conformal technology minimizes radiation damage to adjacent neural

structures; however, panhypopituitarism occurs almost universally. Stereotactic radiotherapy, the application of stereotactic radiosurgical technique to conventional fractionation, provides tighter isodose curves around the tumor, further limiting collateral irradiation to the mesial temporal lobes, hypothalamus, and skull base.[107] The technique is limited to small volumes. With large tumors, significant portions of the temporal and frontal lobes will be included in the radiation portals. Long-term sequelae of irradiation include secondary tumors, optic neuropathy, and vascular injury accompanied by the development of moyamoya disease.[7, 12, 42, 92, 103, 108]

INTRACAVITARY THERAPY

Indications for intracavitary therapy and choice of agents (radionuclide or bleomycin) are still in evolution. Both tumor and patient characteristics should be considered when considering intracystic therapy. Intracavitary therapy is most effective and often curative in primary monocystic tumors with relatively thin walls, although significant control of the cystic components of recurrent tumors can be achieved as well.[105, 106, 109–113, 132]

Aspiration

Simple stereotactic aspiration of tumor cysts or placement of an Ommaya reservoir in the cyst for serial aspirations is never indicated as primary therapy in children and should be reserved for palliation when all other treatment modalities have failed.[92, 106, 114] Frequent aspirations tend to stimulate cyst fluid production, leading to progressively shorter symptom-free intervals. Solid tumor growth is unimpeded and may extend into areas of decompressed cysts. Aspiration may be required to control cyst volume while awaiting the therapeutic effect of intracavitary irradiation (vide infra).

Intracavitary Irradiation

Local treatment of cystic craniopharyngioma with intracavitary β irradiation was first described 45 years ago by Leksell and Liden.[115] The ideal agents are colloidal suspensions of β-emitting radionuclides that evenly distribute along the walls of cystic tumors, have tissue half-lives that achieve adequate but not excessive dosage, and have a rapid fall-off in tissue penetrance to avoid corollary radiation injury to adjacent neural tissue.

Four radioisotopes have been evaluated over the past five decades: ^{32}P, ^{90}Y, ^{193}Au, and ^{186}Re.[36, 106, 111, 113, 116, 117] Clinical experience has established an ideal dose of 200 to 250 Gy to the cyst wall.[106,111,112,116] Use of ^{186}Re and ^{193}Au has been largely abandoned: both of these radioisotopes have inadequate β-emission penetration of the cyst wall, produce undesirable γ rays, and have yielded disappointing clinical results.[111, 113] There has been controversy over the relative efficacy and safety of ^{90}Y compared with ^{32}P.[105, 106, 111–113, 116] This resulted in part from the fact that access to ^{90}Y was limited to patients in Great Britain, Europe, and Japan. Early studies also questioned whether the slightly lower ^{32}P β-particle energy adequately penetrated and treated the cyst wall.[113, 116] Contemporary reports show similar cyst response rates to both of these radionuclides, with diminution or obliteration of cysts reported in 74 to 100%.[105, 106, 112, 113, 118–120] ^{32}P is currently the preferred agent because its shorter tissue penetration and longer half-life offer the possibility of diminished injury to adjacent structures, especially the visual pathways and hypothalamus.[106, 112, 113]

Radionuclide is administered by stereotactic cannulation of the cyst, usually through a precoronal trajectory utilizing a fine needle. Use of an indwelling catheter connected to an Ommaya reservoir has been abandoned by most centers because the catheters have distal holes that may be located outside of the cyst.[106, 113] Leakage of radionuclide has been reported in 10 to 22% of patients although clinical sequelae have been rare.[106, 112, 113, 117–121]

Cyst regression after intracavitary irradiation occurs gradually over several months. Large symptomatic cysts often require subsequent puncture and drainage during this period of involution. Durable control is seen in 80 to 96% of the treated cysts with 12 to 45% having a complete response with permanent obliteration of the cyst.[105, 106, 112, 113] Intracystic irradiation does not control solid tumor growth or prevent the development of new cysts.

Treatment-related mortality is low (less than 2%); however, morbidity varies in different series from 6 to 58%.[106, 111, 113, 120–123] Preoperative optic atrophy, intimate contact of the cyst wall with the optic nerves, previous or concurrent external-beam irradiation, and the use of ^{90}Y, with its greater tissue half value, are risk factors for visual deterioration.[106, 113, 120] New endocrine deficiencies occur in approximately 10% of the patients; however, treatment-related DI is uncommon.[112, 113] Other neurologic complications and delayed cognitive deficits are rare.

Intracavitary Bleomycin

The cell cycle kinetics and spatial distribution of S-phase proliferative cells in the squamous epithelium of craniopharyngioma cysts provide a rationale for the use of antineoplastic agents.[124] Bleomycin is an antineoplastic antibiotic that interferes with DNA production and has demonstrated clinical efficacy in squamous cell carcinomas.[125] Clinical use of intracavitary bleomycin in craniopharyngiomas was first reported by Takahashi et al.[126] Long-term control was demonstrated in 3 of 7 children treated by minimal tumor excision followed by postoperative adjuvant injection of bleomycin into the remaining cystic tumor. Although the total number of patients treated remains small, subsequent published[36, 109, 110, 127, 128] and anecdotal reports (personal communication Choux, 1996; Sainte-Rose and Pierre-Kahn, 1997; Hoffman, 1998) have established general treatment guidelines, response rates, and pattern of complications.

An Ommaya catheter is placed into the cyst either stereotactically or at craniotomy. Several days after catheter place-

ment a contrast injection and CT are perfomed to verify that there has been no leakage of cyst contents. Bleomycin 1.5 to 10 mg is injected at 1- to 2-day intervals depending on the cyst volume. Repeat injections are performed over a 10- to 21-day period for an average total dose of 60 to 80 mg.[110, 128] Although most centers have measured cyst fluid lactate dehydrogenase, no consistent pattern has emerged to guide therapy.[109] The major risk is leakage of bleomycin into the subarachnoid space or ventricles with ensuing ventriculitis, meningitis, or vasospasm. To date, this has only been reported anecdotally (personal communication, Sainte-Rose, 1997). Visual deterioration and new hearing deficits have been noted in individual patients.[109, 128]

Similar to intracystic irradiation, involution of cysts occurs slowly over several months. Reduction in cyst volume is seen in almost all patients, with up to 50% of patients showing, complete disappearance of the cyst and indefinite remission.[36, 109, 110, 127, 128] Bleomycin may also be used as a surgical adjunct to decrease the technical difficulty of subsequent surgical resection, particularly in patients with mixed solid and cystic craniopharyngiomas. Intracavitary therapy produces a thick, tough cyst wall, resistant to tearing, that is easier to maintain intact, dissect, and remove en masse than the more common fragile, diaphanous cyst tissue. In contrast to other treatment modalities, bleomycin chemotherapy does not induce arachnoidal scarring or damage the gliotic plane between tumor and normal hypothalamus that is crucial for safe resection.

RECURRENCE

The most common complication of all treatment modalities is tumor recurrence. As discussed in previous sections, extent of surgical resection and postoperative adjuvant irradiation are the most significant factors limiting the likelihood of recurrence. In an international multicenter report of 474 children with craniopharyngiomas,[36] the overall recurrence rate was 29.7%: 19.1% following total resection, 29.6% after subtotal resection plus adjuvant irradiation, and 56.6% with subtotal resection alone. Tumors in younger children recurred more frequently: 36.6% of tumors in children younger than 5 years recurred.

Although considered "slow growing," craniopharyngiomas tend to recur early, often as a result of rapid regrowth of tumor cysts. *Most series report recurrences occurring within 2 to 5 years after primary treatment,*[12, 36, 45, 49, 72, 91, 129] *although recurrences as late as 30 years after surgery have been described.*[69] The average time to recurrence in the international series was 33 months.[36]

Surgical resection should be considered for recurrent craniopharyngioma; however, age of the patient, location of the tumor, nature of previous therapy, and severity of symptoms and signs must be thoroughly assessed prior to embarking on any treatment. Although neither prior surgery nor irradiation precludes the possibility of a curative operation in recurrent tumors, many surgeons have reported increased morbidity, mortality, and failure to obtain a total removal compared with surgery in primary tumors.[9, 12, 84, 92, 130]

Most pediatric neurosurgeons are supportive of reoperation following a less extensive primary procedure; however, all caution that previous radical surgery may render further resection hazardous or even impossible.[9, 12, 84, 92, 130, 131] When radical surgery is contemplated, the pterional approach with a wide sylvian dissection allows the start of a clean plane of dissection free from arachnoidal scarring and adhesions, particularly in patients who have had a previous subfrontal resection. Because both tumor and cicatrix from previous surgery may extend diffusely throughout the suprasellar cisterns, displacing and distorting normal structures, identification of normal vascular anatomy provides essential landmarks. In recurrent tumors that have not had a previous radical resection, the membrane of Lillequist usually separates the tumor from the basilar artery. The violation of arachnoidal planes during an aggressive primary resection may promote a dense mesenchymal reaction from the arterial adventitia to recurrent tumor, precluding development of a safe plane of dissection and total removal. Calcific tumor is particularly likely to adhere to major vessels. Previous surgery can damage the vasovasorum and weaken the arterial wall.[84, 85] Excessive imprudent manipulation may cause carotid or basilar laceration, resulting in significant morbidity or death.[49, 64, 130] The single death in the author's series of 24 operations for recurrent tumor was a consequence of carotid laceration.

The gliotic reaction that forms a natural cleavage plane between the craniopharyngioma and hypothalamus may be destroyed at the primary surgery. Unlike primary tumors where gentle traction will establish a plane,[12, 131] careful blunt dissection must be utilized to separate recurrent tumor from the chiasm, hypothalamus, or cortex. Dissection must remain on the capsule surface and not penetrate the parenchyma. The increased incidence of visual, neurologic, and neuropsychological deficits accompanying surgery for recurrence may be partially related to direct hypothalamic and optic pathway injury due to the lack of this glial barrier.

Recurrent tumor limited to the sella turcica is best removed through a transsphenoidal approach.[63] Careful consideration of anatomical features, meticulous surgical technique, and extensive experience with transsphenoidal surgery are essential for success. Significant suprasellar tumor is a relative contraindication to this approach; however, cyst drainage for palliation may occasionally be appropriate.

Recurrent craniopharyngiomas are radiosensitive tumors. Excellent long-term tumor control can be achieved with external-beam irradiation in previously nonirradiated children.[103] The author strongly recommends that no radiation be administered following radiographically confirmed total resection of a recurrent craniopharyngioma. Even a small fleck of calcium without enhancing tumor (Hoffman grade II) should probably be treated as a total resection.[29, 92] The one child in our series who developed a radiation-induced glioblastoma had a small fleck of residual calcium on the anterior communicating artery after undergoing resection of a recurrent 5-cm tumor (Fig. 19–5). Clearly, adjuvant irradiation for that patient would not be recommended today.

Children who have previously received maximum tolerance doses of radiation are not candidates for further conventional external-beam irradiation. If their tumors are not resectable they can be considered for intracystic therapy and/or stereotactic radiosurgery. Intracavitary therapy with either radionuclide or bleomycin will obliterate the cystic component but will not affect solid tumor growth. Simple stereotactic aspiration of tumor cysts or placement of an Ommaya reservoir into the cyst for serial may provide palliation when all other treatment modalities have failed.

In the author's series of 26 patients who had surgery for recurrence, 68% had a gross total resection. There was 1 operative death, 2 late treatment–related deaths, and 2 deaths from tumor progression, for a case mortality of 20%. The multicenter international study reported a 3.7% surgical mortality for primary surgery, increasing to 13% after secondary radical surgery.[36] Tomita and McClone[49] reported total resection in 55% of recurrent tumors versus 79% in primary operations. Most of these patients had a second recurrence that required further surgery and irradiation for tumor control. Hoffman et al[12] operated on 16 of 17 recurrent tumors, achieving a radical resection in only 5 patients; 47% of the 17 patients experienced a second recurrence.

Yasargil et al[45] reported 32 radical resections (19 children and 13 adult) for recurrent tumor; total resection was obtained in 56.3%. He did not experience an increase in operative mortality; however, the long-term survival was 59.4% after secondary microsurgery, compared with 90% for primary tumors. Both children and adults with recurrent craniopharyngiomas faired poorly, with a case mortality of 42.1% and 38.5%, respectively. Yasargil et al comment that the difference in outcome could "largely be attributed to the difficulty in dissection at second or subsequent operation."[45]

SUMMARY

In experienced centers with appropriate surgical expertise, endocrinologic support, and socioeconomic resources, curative resection of craniopharyngiomas can be achieved in 70 to 90% of children, with maintenance of a good quality of life in more than 90% of those cured. Although uncommon in the pediatric group, small intrasellar tumors are best treated by a transsphenoidal route. Intracystic therapy may be appropriate for monocystic tumors without a solid component. Irradiation is effective in controlling craniopharyngioma growth and is appropriate as initial treatment when the criteria for total surgical resection cannot be met. Recurrent tumors are problematical: a multimodality approach should be considered, often utilizing a combination of surgery, irradiation, and intracystic therapy to salvage the majority of these patients.

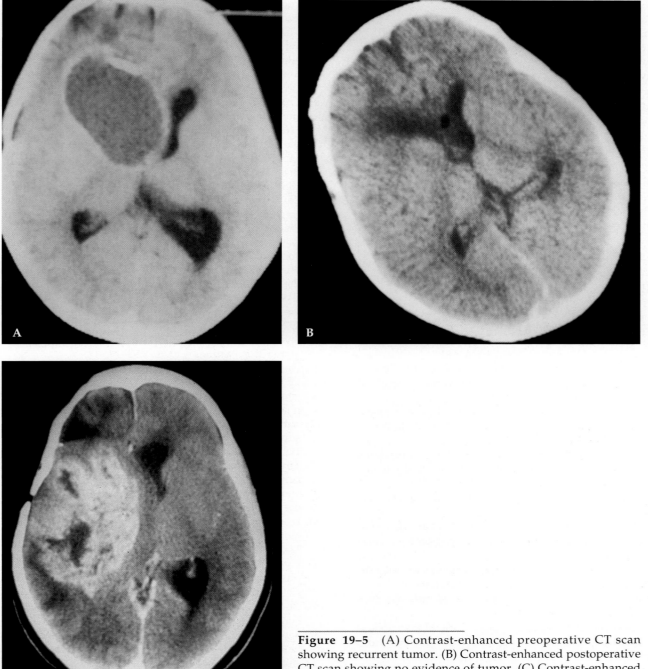

Figure 19–5   (A) Contrast-enhanced preoperative CT scan showing recurrent tumor. (B) Contrast-enhanced postoperative CT scan showing no evidence of tumor. (C) Contrast-enhanced CT scan 5 years after irradiation showing radiation-induced glioblastoma.

REFERENCES

1. Burger PC, Scheithauer BW, Vogel FS. *Surgical Pathology of the Nervous System and Its Coverings*. New York: John Wiley and Sons; 1991.
2. Russell DS, Rubinstein L. *Pathology of Tumours of the Nervous System*. 6th ed. Baltimore: Williams & Wilkins; 1999: 629–640.
3. Hoffman HJ, Hendrick EB, Humphreys RP, et al. Management of craniopharyngioma in children. *J Neurosurg* 1977;47:218–227.
4. Matson DD, Crigler JF Jr. Management of craniopharyngioma in childhood. *J Neurosurg* 1969;30:377–390.
5. Shiminski-Maher T, Rosenberg M. Late effects associated with treatment of craniopharyngiomas in childhood. *J Neurosci Nurs* 1990;22:220–226.
6. Cushing H. The craniopharyngiomas. In: *Intracranial Tumors—Notes upon a Series of Two Thousand Verified Cases with Surgical Mortality Percentages Thereto*. Springfield, IL: Charles C Thomas, 1932.
7. Fischer EG, Welch K, Shillito J Jr, et al. Craniopharyngiomas in children: long-term effects of conservative surgical procedures combined with radiation therapy [see comments]. *J Neurosurg* 1990;73:534–540.
8. Bunin GR, Surawicz TS, Witman PA, et al. The descriptive epidemiology of craniopharyngioma. *J Neurosurg* 1998;89:547–551.
9. Yasargil M. Craniopharyngiomas. In: *Microneurosurgery IVB: Microneurosurgery of CNS Tumors*. New York: Thieme Medical Publishers; 1996:205–216.
10. Adamson TE, Wiestler OD, Kleihues P, et al. Correlation of clinical and pathological features in surgically treated craniopharyngiomas. *J Neurosarg* 1990;73:12–17.
11. Banna M. Craniopharyngioma: based on 160 cases. *Br J Radiol* 1976;49:206–223.
12. Hoffman H, DeSilva M. Humphreys R, et al. Aggressive surgical management of craniopharyngiomas in childhood. *J Neurosurg* 1992;76:47–52.
13. Sorva R, Heiskanen O. Craniopharyngioma in Finland: a study of 123 cases. *Acta Neurochir* 1986;81:85–89.
14. Zulch K. *Brain Tumors: Their Biology and Pathology*. New York: Springer-Verlag; 1986.
15. Rajan B, Ashley S, Gorman C, et al. Craniopharyngioma—a long-term results following limited surgery and radiotherapy. *Radiother Oncol* 1993;26:1–10.
16. Farwell JR, Dohrmann GJ, Flannery JT. Central nervous system tumors in children. *Cancer* 1977;40:3123–3132.
17. Stewart AM, Lennox EL, Sanders BM. Group characteristics of children with cerebral and spinal cord tumors. *Br J Cancer* 1973;28:568–574.
18. Stiller CA, Nectoux J. International incidence of childhood brain and spinal tumors. *Int J Epidemiol* 1994;23: 458–464.
19. Erdheim J. Über Hypophysengangsysgeschwulste und Hirncholesteatome. *Sitzungsb Akad Wissensch* 1904;113:537.
20. Miller D. Pathology of craniopharyngiomas: clinical importance of pathological findings. *Pediatr Neurosurg* 1994;21 (Suppl):11–17.

21. Petito CK, DeGirolami U, Earle KM. Craniopharyngiomas: a clinical and pathological review. *Cancer* 1976; 37:1944–1952.
22. Weiner H, Wisoff J, Rosenberg M, et al. Craniopharyngiomas: a clinicopatliological analysis of factors predictive of recurrence and functional outcome. *Neurosurgery* 1994;35:1001–1011.
23. Crotty TB, Scheithauer BW, Young WF, Jr, et al. Papillary craniopharyngioma: a clinicopathological study of 48 cases. *J Neurosurg* 1995;83:206–214.
24. Bartlett J. Craniopharyngiomas: an analysis of some aspects of symptomatology, radiology, and histology. *Brain* 1971;94:725.
25. Hoffman H, Raffel C. Craniopharyngiomas. In: McLaurin RL, Schut L, Venes JL, Epstein F, eds. *Pediatric Neurosurgery: Surgery of the Developing Nervous System*. 2nd ed. Philadelphia: WB Saunders; 1989:399–408.
26. Kobayashi T, Kageyama N, Yoshida J, et al. Pathological and clinical basis of the indications for treatment of craniopharyngiomas. *Neurol Med Chir (Tokyo)* 1981;21:39–47.
27. Pertuiset B. Craniopharyngiomas. In: Vinken PJ, Broyen GW, eds. *Handbook of Clinical Neurology, vol 18. Tumours of the Brain and Skull, Part III*. Amsterdam: North Holland; 1975:531–572.
28. Sweet WH. Radical surgical treatment of craniopharyngioma. *Clin Neurosurg* 1976;23:52–79.
29. Hoffman HJ. Craniopharyngiomas. *Can J Neurol Sci* 1985; 12:348–352.
30. Harwood-Nash DC. Neuroimaging of childhood craniopharyngioma. *Pediatr Neurosurg* 1994;21:2–10.
31. Sutton L, Wang Z, Wehrli S, et al. Proton spectroscopy of suprasellar tumors in pediatric patients. *Neurosurgery* 1997;41:388–394.
32. Zimmerman R. Imaging of intrasellar, suprasellar, and parasellar tumors. *Semin Roentgenol* 1990;25:174–197.
33. Tsuda M, Takahashi S, Higano S, et al. CT and MR imaging of craniopharyngioma. *Eur Radiol* 1997;7:464–469.
34. Freeman MP, Kessler RM, Allen JH, et al. Craniopharyngioma: CT and MR imaging in nine cases. *J Comput Assist Tomogr* 1987;11:810–814.
35. Pigeau I, Sigal R, Halimi P, et al. MRI features of craniopharyngiomas at 1.5 Tesla: a series of 13 cases. *J Neuroradiol* 1988;15:276–287.
36. Choux M, Lena G, Genitori L. Le craniopharyngiome de l'enfant. *Neurochirurgie* 1991;37:1–174.
37. Samii M, Tatagiba M. Craniopharyngioma. In: Kaye A, Laws E, eds. *Brain Tumors*. New York: Churchill Livingstone; 1995:873–894.
38. Abrams LS, Repka MX. Visual outcome of craniopharyngioma in children. *J Pediatr Ophthalmol Strabismus* 1997;34: 223–228.
39. Baskin DS, Wilson CB. Surgical management of craniopharyngiomas: a review of 74 cases. *J Neurosurg* 1986;65: 22–27.
40. Carmel PW, Antunes JL, Chang CH. Craniopharyngiomas in children. *Neurosurgery* 1982;11:382–389.
41. Pang D. Surgical management of craniopharyngioma. In: Sekhar L, Janecka I, eds, *Surgery of Cranial Base Tumors*. New York: Raven Press; 1993:787–807.
42. Scott RM, Hetelekidis S, Barnes PD, et al. Surgery, radiation, and combination therapy in the treatment of child-

hood craniopharyngioma—a 20-year experience. *Pediatr Neurosurg* 1994;21:75–81.
43. Sklar CA. Craniopharyngioma: endocrine sequelae of treatment. *Pediatr Neurosurg* 1994;21:120–123.
44. Sorva R. Children with craniopharyngioma: early growth failure and rapid postoperative weight gain. *Acta Paediatr Scand* 1988;77:587–592.
45. Yasargil MG, Curcic M, Kis M, et al. Total removal of craniopharyngiomas: approaches and long-term results in 144 patients. *J Neurosurg* 1990;73:3–11.
46. Repka MX, Miller NR, Miller M. Visual outcome after surgical removal of craniopharyngiomas [see comments]. *Ophthalmology* 1989;96:195–199.
47. Blethen SL. Growth in children with a craniopharyngioma. *Pediatrician* 1987;14:242–245.
48. Stahnke N, Grubel G, Lagenstein I, et al. Long-term follow-up of children with craniopharyngioma. *Eur J Pediatr* 1984;142:179–185.
49. Tomita T, McClone D. Radical resections of childhood craniopharyngiomas. *Pediatr Neurosurg* 1993;19:6–14.
50. Villani RM, Tomei G, Bello L, et al. Long-term results of treatment for craniopharyngioma in children. *Child's Nerv Syst* 1997;13:397–405.
51. Rougerie J, Fardeau M. *Les cranio-pharyngeomes.* Paris: Masson; 1962.
52. De Vile CJ, Grant DB, Kendall BE, et al. Management of chilhood craniopharyngioma: can the morbidity of radical surgery be predicted? *J Neurosurg* 1996;85:73–81.
53. Sanford RA. Craniopharyngioma: results of survey of the American Society of Pediatric Neurosurgery. *Pediatr Neurosurg* 1994;21:39–43.
54. Patterson RH Jr, Danylevich A. Surgical removal of craniopharyngiomas by the transcranial approach through the lamina terminalis and sphenoid sinus. *Neurosurgery* 1980;7:111–117.
55. Fahlbusch R, Honegger J, Paulus W, et al. Surgical treatment of craniopharyngiomas. Part I. Experience with 168 patients. *Neurosurg Focus* 1997;3:Article 2.
56. Maira G, Anile C, Rossi G, et al. Surgical treatment of craniopharyngiomas: an evaluation of the transsphenoidal and pterional approaches. *Neurosurgery* 1995;36:715–724.
57. Samii M, Bini W. Surgical treatment of craniopharyngiomas. *Zentralbl Neurochir* 1991;52:17–23.
58. Suzuki J, Katakura R, Mori T. Interhemispheric approach through the lamina terminalis to tumors of the anterior part of the third ventricle. *Surg Neurol* 1984;22:157–163.
59. Symon L, Pell MF, Habib AH. Radical excision of craniopharyngioma by the temporal route: a review of 50 patients. *Br J Neurosurg* 1991;5:539–549.
60. Honegger J, Buchfelder M, Fahlbusch R. et al. Transsphenoidal microsurgery, for craniopharyngioma. *Surg Neurol* 1992;37:189–196.
61. Landolt A, Zachman M. Results of transsphenoidal extirpation of craniopharyngiomas and Rathke's cysts. *Neurosurgery* 1991;28:410–415.
62. Laws ER, Craniopharyngiomas in children and young adults. *Prog Exp Tumor Res* 1987;30:335–340.
63. Laws ER Jr. Transsphenoidal removal of craniopharyngioma. *Pediatr Neurosurg* 1994;21:57–63.
64. Symon L, Sprich W. Radical excision of craniopharyngioma. Results in 20 patients. *J Neurosurg* 1985;62:174–181.
65. Laws ER Jr. Transsphenoidal microsurgery in the management of craniopharyngioma. *J Neurosurg* 1980;52:661–666.
66. Nicola G, Lasio G, Valentini L, et al. Role of the transphenoidal approach in the surgical management of craniopharyngiomas. In: Broggi G, ed. *Craniopharyngioma: Surgical Treatment.* Milan: Springer-Verlag; 1995:97–103.
67. Laws E. Craniopharyngiomas: transphenoidal surgery. In: Apuzzo M, ed. *Brain Surgery: Complication Avoidance and Management.* New York: Churchill Livingstone; 1993:357–362.
68. Ciric IS, Cozzens JW. Craniopharyngiomas: transsphenoidal method of approach—for the virtuoso only? *Clin Neurosurg* 1980;27:169–187.
69. Kahn EA, Gosch HH, Seeger JF, et al. Forty-five years experience with the craniopharyngiomas. *Surg Neurol* 1973;1:5–12.
70. Pierre-Kahn A, Brauner R, Renier D, et al. Treatment of craniopharyngiomas in children: retrospective analysis of 50 cases. *Arch Fr Pediatr* 1988;45:163–167.
71. Sanford RA, Muhlbauer MS. Craniopharyngioma in children. *Neurol Clin* 1991;9:453–465.
72. Shapiro K, Till K, Grant DN. Craniopharyngiomas in childhood: a rational approach to treatment. *J Neurosurg* 1979;50:617–623.
73. De Vile CJ, Grant DB, Hayward RD, et al. Growth and endocrine sequelae of craniopharyngioma. *Arch Dis Child* 1996;75:108–114.
74. Lyen K, Grant D. Endocrine function, morbidity, and mortality after surgery for craniopharyngioma. *Arch Dis Child* 1982;57:837–841.
75. Katz EL. Late results of radical excision of craniopharyngiomas in children. *J Neurosurg* 1975;42:86–93.
76. Sorva R, Heiskanen O, Perheentupa J. Craniopharyngioma surgery in children: endocrine and visual outcome. *Child's Nerv Syst* 1988;4:97–99.
77. Thomsett M, Conte F, Kaplan S, et al. Endocrine and neurologic outcome in childhood craniopharyngioma: review of effect of treatment in 42 patients. *J Pediatr* 1980;97:728–735.
78. Hetelekidis S, Barnes PD, Tao ML, et al. Twenty-year experience in childhood craniopharyngioma [see comments]. *Int J Radiat Oncol Biol Phys* 1993;27:189–195.
79. De Vile CJ, Grant DB, Hayward RD, et al. Obesity in childhood craniopharyngioma: relation to post-operative hypothalamic damage shown by magnetic resonance imaging. *J Clin Endocrinol Metab* 1996;81:2734–2737.
80. Roth C, Wilken B, Hanefeld F, et al. Hyperphagia in children with craniopharyngioma is associated with hyperleptinaemia and a failure in the downregulation of appetite. *Eur J Endocrinol* 1998;138:89–91.
81. Blethen SL, Weldon VV. Outcome in children with normal growth following removal of a craniopharyngioma. *Am J Med Sci* 1986;292:21–24.
82. Price DA, Jonsson P. Effect of growth hormone treatment in children with craniopharyngioma with reference to the KIGS (Kabi International Growth Study) database. *Acta Paediatr Suppl* 1996;417:83–85.
83. Schoenle EJ, Zapf J, Prader A, et al. Replacement of growth hormone (GH) in normally growing GH-deficient patients operated for craniopharyngioma. *J Clin Endocrinol Metab* 1995;80:374–378.

84. Carmel P. Craniopharyngioma: transcranial approaches. In: Apuzzo M, ed. *Brain Surgery: Complication Avoidance- and Management*. New York: Churchill Livingstone, 1993; 339–357.

85. Sutton LN. Vascular complications of surgery for craniopharyngioma and hypothalamic glioma. *Pediatr Neurosurg* 1994;21:124–128.

86. Anderson CA, Wilkening GN, Filley CM, et al. Neurobehavioral outcome in pediatric craniopharyngioma. *Pediatr Neurosurg* 1997;26:255–260.

87. Cavazzuti V, Fischer EG, Welch K, et al. Neurological and psychophysiological sequelae following different treatments of craniopharyngioma in children. *J Neurosurg* 1983;59:409–417.

88. Colangelo M, Ambrosio A, Ambrosio C. Neurological and behavioral sequelae following different approaches to craniopharyngioma. Long-term follow-up review and therapeutic guidelines. *Child's Nerv Syst* 1990;6:379–382.

89. Galatzer A, Nofar E, Beit-Halachmi N, et al. Intellectual and psychosocial functions of children, adolescents and young adults before and after operation for craniopharyngioma. *Child Care Health Dev* 1981;7:307–316.

90. Stelling MW, McKay SE, Carr WA, et al. Frontal lobe lesions and cognitive function in craniopharyngioma survivors. *Am J Dis Child* 1986;140:710–714.

91. Hoff JT, Patterson RH Jr. Craniopharyngiomas in children and adults. *J Neurosurg* 1972;36:299–302.

92. Wisoff J. Surgical management of recurrent craniopharyngiomas. *Pediatr Neurosurg* 1994; 21 (Suppl):108–113.

93. Barloon TJ, Yuh WT, Sato Y, et al. Frontal lobe implantation of craniopharyngioma by repeated needle aspirations. *Am J Neuroradiol* 1988;9:406–407.

94. Ragoowansi A, Piepgras D. Postoperative ectopic craniopharyngioma: case report. *J Neurosurg* 1991;74:653–655.

95. Amacher AL. Craniopharyngioma: the controversy regarding radiotherapy. *Child's Brain* 1980;6:57–64.

96. Kramer S, Southard M, Mansfield C. Radiotherapy in the management of craniopharyngiomas: further experience and late results. *Am J Roentgenol* 1868;103:44–52.

97. Kramer S, McKissock W, Concannon J. Treatment by surgery and radiation therapy. *J Neurosurg* 1961;18: 217–226.

98. Flickinger JC, Lunsford LD, Singer J, et al. Megavoltage external beam irradiation of craniopharyngiomas: analysis of tumor control and morbidity. *Int J Radiat Oncol Biol Phys* 1990;19:117–122.

99. Manaka S, Teramoto A, Takakura K. The efficacy of radiotherapy for craniopharyngioma. *J Neurosurg* 1985; 62:648–656.

100. Richmond IL, Wara WM, Wilson CB. Role of radiation therapy in the management of craniopharyngiomas in children. *Neurosurgery* 1980;6:513–517.

101. Thompson IL, Griffin TW, Parker RG, et al. Craniopharyngioma: the role of radiation therapy. *Int J Radiat Oncol Biol Phys* 1978;4:1059–1063.

102. Wara WM, Sneed PK, Larson DA. The role of radiation therapy in the treatment of craniopharyngioma. *Pediatr Neurosurg* 1994;21:98–100.

103. Weiss M, Sutton L, Marcial V, et al. The role of radiation therapy in the management of childhood craniopharyngioma. *Int J Radiat Oncol Biol Phys* 1989:17:1313–1321.

104. Backlund EO. Studies on craniopharyngiomas. IV. Stereotaxic treatment with radiosurgery. *Acta Chir Scand* 1973;139:344–351.

105. Backlund EO, Axelsson B, Bergstrand CG, et al. Treatment of craniopharyngiomas—the stereotactic approach in a ten to twenty-three years' perspective. I. Surgical, radiological and ophthalmological aspects. *Acta Neurochir* 1989;99:11–19.

106. Lunsford LD, Pollock BE, Kondziolka DS, et al. Stereotactic options in the management of craniopharyngioma. *Pediatr Neurosurg* 1994;21:90–97.

107. Tarbell N, Barnes P, Scott R, et al. Advances in radiation therapy for craniopharyngiomas. *Pediatr Neurosurg* 1994;21(Suppl):101–107.

108. Ushio Y, Arita N, Yoshimine T, et al. Glioblastoma after radiotherapy for craniopharyngioma: case report. *Neurosurgery* 1987;21:33–38.

109. Broggi G, Giorgi C, Franzini A, et al. Therapeutic role of intracavitary bleomycin administration in cystic craniopharyngioma. In: Broggi G, ed. *Craniopharyngioma: Surgical Treatment*. Milan: Springer-Verlag; 1995:113–119.

110. Cavalheiro S, Sparapani FV, Franco JO, et al. Use of bleomycin in intratumoral chemotherapy for cystic craniopharyngioma: case report [see comments]. *J Neurosurg* 1996;84:124–126.

111. Kobayashi T, Kageyama N, Ohara K. Internal irradiation for cystic craniopharyngioma. *J Neurosurg* 1981;55:896–903.

112. Pollock B, Lunsford L, Kondziolka D, et al. Phosphorus-32 intracavitary irradiation of cystic craniopharyngiomas: current technique and long-term results. *Int J Radiat Oncol Biol Phys* 1995;33:437–446.

113. Voges J, Sturm V, Lehrke R. et al. Cystic craniopharyngioma: long-term results after intracavitary irradiation with stereotactically applied colloidal beta-emitting radioactive sources. *Neurosurgery* 1997;40:263–269; discussion 269–270.

114. Gutin PH, Klemme WM, Lagger RL, et al. Management of the unresectable cystic craniopharyngioma by aspiration through an Ommaya reservoir drainage system. *J Neurosurg* 1980;52:36–40.

115. Leksell L, Liden K. A therapeutic trial with radioactive isotopes in cystic brain tumor. In: *Radioisotope Techniques, Vol 1, Medical and Physiological Applications*. London: Her Majesty's Stationery Office; 1953:76–78.

116. Backlund EO. Studies on craniopharyngiomas. 3. Stereotaxic treatment with intracystic yttrium-90. *Acta Chir Scand* 1973;139:237–247.

117. Munari C, Landre E, Musolino A, et al. Long term results of stereotactic endocavitary beta irradiation of craniopharyngioma cysts. *J Neurosurg Sci* 1989;33:99–105.

118. Julow J, Lanyi F, Hajda M, et al. Further experiences in the treatment of cystic craniopharyngiomas with yttrium-90 silicate colloid. *Acta Neurochir (Wien)* 1988;42 (Suppl):113–119.

119. Pan D, Lee L, Huang C, et al. Stereotactic internal irradiation for cystic craniopharyngiomas: a 6-year experience. *Stereotact Funct Neurosurg* 1990;54–55:525–530.

120. Van den Berge J, Blaauw G, Breeman W, et al. Intracavitary brachytherapy of cystic craniopharyngioma. *J Neurosurg* 1992;77:545–550.

121. Backlund EO, Johansson L, Sarby B. Studies on craniopharyngiomas. II. Treatment by stereotaxis and radiosurgery. *Acta Chir Scand* 1972;138:749–759.

122. Anderson DR, Trobe JD, Taren JA, et al. Visual outcome in cystic craniopharyngiomas treated with intracavitary phosphorus-32. *Ophthalmology* 1989;96: 1786–1792.

123. Guevara JA, Bunge HJ, Heinrich JJ, et al. Cystic craniopharyngioma treated by [90]yttrium silicate colloid. *Acta Neurochir* 1988; Suppl 42:109–112.

124. Broggi G, Franzini A, Cajola L, et al. Cell kinetic investigations in craniopharyngioma: preliminary results and considerations. *Pediatr Neurosurg* 1994;21:21–23.

125. Umezawa H, Maeda K, Takeuchi T, et al. New antibiotics, bleomycin A and B. *J Antibiot (A)* 1966;19:200–209.

126. Takahashi H, Nakazawa S, Shimura T. Evaluation of postoperative intratumoral injection of bleomycin for craniopharyngioma in children. *J Neurosurg* 1985;62: 120–127.

127. Broggi G, Giorgi C, Franzini A, et al. Preliminary results of intracavitary treatment of craniopharyngioma with bleomycin. *J Neurosurg Sci* 1989;33:145–148.

128. Mottolese C, Guyotat J, Bret P, et al. Treatment of craniopharyngiomas with local intracystic chemotherapy with bleomycin: our experience (abstract). *J Neurosurg* 1996;84:343A.

129. Sung D, Chang C, Harisiadis L, et al. Treatment results of craniopharyngiomas. *Cancer* 1981;47:847–852.

130. Sweet WH. Recurrent craniopharyngiomas: therapeutic alternatives. *Clin Neurosurg* 1980;27:206–229.

131. Sweet W. Craniopharyngiomas (With a note on Rathke's cleft or epithelial cysts and on suprasellar cysts). In: Schmidek H, Sweet W, eds. *Operative Neurosurgical Techniques: Indications, Methods, and Results*. Orlando, FL: Grune & Stratton; 1988;349–379.

132. Kumar PP, Good RR, Skultety FM, et al. Retreatment of recurrent cystic craniopharyngioma with chromic phosphorus P 32. *J Natl Med Assoc* 1986;78:542–543, 547–549.

Chapter 20

Pituitary Tumors

Marc S. Arginteanu and Kalmon D. Post

The proper functioning pituitary gland is an integral component of the normal growth and sexual maturation of a child. The pituitary gland must orchestrate the hormonal milieu through the drastic changes that occur between childhood and adolescence, then again during the transition to young adulthood. This is a complex and poorly understood process, and its upset may lead to an arrest of growth or prevention of sexual maturation. Pituitary dysfunction during childhood may be caused by radiation damage, craniopharyngiomas, or other tumorous lesions involving the pituitary gland or hypothalamus.[1, 2]

Tumors affecting the pituitary gland of children and adolescents are uncommon. Most authors who have gathered large series of patients with pituitary adenomas have found only 2.0 to 3.5% of those harboring these lesions to be children,[3-6] although one group has reported 6% of patients with pituitary tumors to be children.[7]

The adenohypophysis contains several populations of cells, most of which produce distinct hormones. Each type of cell is capable of neoplastic degeneration.[1] Tumors of the pituitary gland in children are invariably adenomas, as pituitary carcinoma is virtually unheard of in this age group.[8, 9] The patient's clinical presentation, the diagnostic tests required, and the proper treatment will vary depending on the type of cell from which the tumor originated.

COMPARISON WITH ADULT POPULATION

A relative incidence of each type of pituitary adenoma in the adult population was gleaned by reviewing two large series of cases[3, 7] encompassing more than 4300 patients. Prolactinomas were found to be the most common type of pituitary adenoma, accounting for 33% of the total. About 29% of adult patients harbor adenomas that do not produce endocrinologic symptoms. Cushing's disease is present in 14% of adults with pituitary tumors. Acromegaly is present in another 14% of these patients. Both prolactin and growth hormone are secreted by 5% of pituitary tumors. The remaining 5% of tumors manifest a clinical syndrome from secretion of one of the gonadotropic hormones, thyrotropin, or are plurihormonal with a hormone combination other than growth hormone and prolactin.

Several series, with a combined total of 330 patients, were reviewed to determine the relative incidence of various adenoma types in the pediatric population.[3-7] The differences are striking (Fig. 20–1). As in adults, the most common type of pituitary tumor is prolactinoma, accounting for 48% of lesions. Corticotropic adenomas represent 37% of pediatric pituitary tumors. Growth hormone is secreted by 7% of tumors.

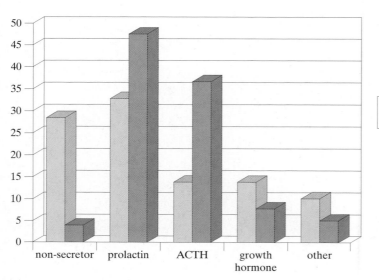

Figure 20–1 Percentage of various types of pituitary adenomas in adults and children, segregated by type of hormone secretion (ACTH = adrenocorticotropic hormone).

Only 3% of tumors in the pediatric population are nonsecretory. About 2% of pediatric pituitary adenomas secrete both prolactin and growth hormone, and another 2% of patients have a clinical syndrome consistent that a plurihormonal tumor that secretes a different combination of hormones. Gonadotropin-secreting tumors account for less than 1% of the total. Most of the reported series of children with pituitary tumors show no cases of thyrotropin-secreting adenomas.[3-7] Thyrotropin-secreting pituitary adenomas are rare, being described in only a handful of case reports.[7, 10]

In both adults and children, the percentage of plurihormonal tumors may be underestimated by the tendency of some authors to classify them according to the predominant endocrine symptoms.[7] In fact, based on the preoperative clinical and biochemical evaluation, most patients who harbor a plurihormonal tumor will have been thought to have a tumor that secretes only one hormone.[6] Using immunohistochemical staining of the pathologic specimen, up to 29% of pediatric pituitary tumors may be classified as plurihormonal.[7] The majority of plurihormonal tumors have been noted to be macroadenomas.[6] If a plurihormonal tumor manifests clinically as a plurihormonal endocrinopathy, the most common syndrome seen will result from a combination of the effects of growth hormone and prolactin.[6]

Pituitary adenomas account for a smaller percentage of brain tumors in children than in adults. Pituitary adenomas represent 1.2% of all intracranial tumors, and 2.7% of all supratentorial tumors in children.[6, 7] In adults, pituitary tumors account for about 15% of intracranial tumors.[8]

Some authors believe pituitary adenomas in children and adolescents to be more aggressive than those in adults.[4, 11] They have argued that pediatric pituitary tumors are more likely to have late recurrences when followed over the long term and are more likely to be invasive. Others argue that pituitary tumors in children are probably no more aggressive than those in adults.[3, 6] Both groups agree that the difference between tumors found in childhood and those found in adulthood lies in the fact that more children harbor macroadenomas at the time of diagnosis than adults, and these are more difficult to cure than microadenomas. The reason for the larger size of tumors in children is at the heart of the dispute. The first group would claim that childhood tumors are more biologically aggressive. Others would argue that the problem is one of diagnosis and not tumor biology.[12] Endocrinologic symptoms are more difficult to detect in prepubertal children. Furthermore, children will tolerate neurologic symptoms, such as visual field deficits, without complaint for a longer time than will adults.

CLINICAL PRESENTATION

The clinical presentation of a pituitary adenoma is usually precipitated by one or more of the following factors:

1. The effects of a hormone secreted by the tumor may cause a discrete clinical syndrome.
2. The tumor may cause a focal neurologic deficit by mass effect on, or invasion into, the parasellar structures, such as the optic apparatus or cranial nerves of the cavernous sinus (Fig. 20-2).

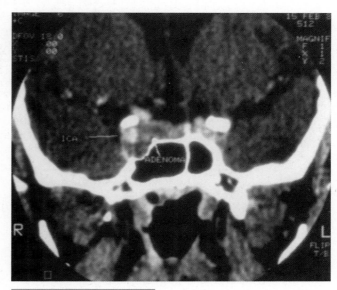

Figure 20–2 Coronal CT scan with contrast enhancement demonstrating a pituitary tumor with invasion of the right cavernous sinus.

3. The tumor may impair pituitary glandular function, most commonly from mass effect within the sella. This usually results in growth retardation and impairment of sexual maturation.

There are also several less common ways in which pediatric pituitary adenomas present:

1. A pituitary adenoma may cause diabetes insipidus (DI). This development is extremely rare. Most large pediatric series noted no patients presenting with DI.[4, 5, 7, 13-15] One group noted DI in 5% of patients.[3]
2. Apoplexy is the impetus for clinical presentation only on rare occasions. Apoplexy is seen significantly less often in children than in adults.[16] When apoplexy is encountered it is heralded by sudden severe headache and acute decrease in visual acuity. A change in mental status and extraocular muscle palsies also may be present.
3. On rare occasions, a macroadenoma attains a sufficient size to obstruct the third ventricle. The patient may then present with signs and symptoms of acute hydrocephalus.

> **BOX 20–1**
> **Clinical Presentation**
>
> - **Common**
>   - **Growth arrest**
>   - **Pubertal delay**
>   - **Focal neurologic deficit**
>   - **Endocrinopathy**
> - **Rare**
>   - **Apoplexy**
>   - **Hydrocephalus**
>   - **Diabetes insipidus**

TABLE 20–1   Common Signs and Symptoms in Pediatric Pituitary Adenomas

Tumor type	Signs and symptoms
Prolactinoma	Galactorrhea, amenorrhea, gynecomastia, pubertal delay, weight gain, growth delay, neurologic deficit
Cushing's disease	Weight gain, growth delay, pubertal delay, hypertension, acne, buffalo hump, amenorrhea, psychiatric disturbance
Growth hormone	Gigantism, acromegaly, neurologic deficit
Nonsecreting adenoma	Growth delay, pubertal delay, neurologic deficit

Almost 66% of pediatric pituitary tumors occur during puberty.[7] This may be because puberty is a time of life when the pituitary gland undergoes rapid growth. Another explanation is that a long existing tumor is first noted in puberty when a parent becomes concerned about failure of sexual maturation or absence of a "growth spurt."

The remainder of this section is dedicated to examining the clinical manifestations of various adenomas. Some characteristics associated with pituitary adenomas are listed in Table 20–1.

Prolactinoma

Patients harboring prolactinoma often present with symptoms due to effects of endocrinopathy. Hypersecretion of prolactin causes galactorrhea in 30 to 60% of patients.[5, 7, 14] Boys may present with gynecomastia or pubertal delay.[4, 17] Pubertal delay and amenorrhea are due to feedback inhibition of the secretion of hypothalamic gonadotropin-releasing hormones by prolactin.[1] Girls present with primary or secondary amenorrhea in up to 76% of cases.[5, 14] Weight gain is sometimes noted in children harboring prolactinomas.[6, 7, 14] Growth delay is noted in 10 to 40% of patients[6, 7, 14] and is probably evidence of hypopituitarism. The mean age at presentation is 15 years.[4–6, 14] Prolactinomas affect girls more commonly than boys (3.5:1).[4–6, 14]

Mass effect causing headache and focal neurologic deficit is often noted, with visual changes found in up to 44% of cases.[4] Macroadenomas outnumber microadenomas 1.5:1.[3–5] Larger tumors are more commonly found in boys.[5, 7] This is probably because the endocrinologic consequences of hyperprolactinemia are not as readily noticed in boys, allowing them to grow to a larger size before presentation.

> # BOX 20–2
> ## Signs and Symptoms of Prolactinoma
>
> - **Galactorrhea**
> - **Gynecomastia**
> - **Amenorrhea**
> - **Pubertal delay**
> - **Weight gain**
> - **Growth delay**
> - **Neurologic deficit (visual change, hydrocephalus)**

Cushing's Disease

The clinical state resulting from a chronic excess of cortisol is known as Cushing's syndrome. The etiology of Cushing's syndrome is varied. Ectopic production of adrenocorticotropic hormone (ACTH) or corticotropin-releasing hormone (CRH) from extrapituitary or extra-adrenal tumors is a possible cause of Cushing's syndrome. However, in children ectopic sources of CRH or ACTH secretion cause less than 5% of cases of Cushing's syndrome.[15] Certain psychiatric illnesses or alcohol abuse may cause a clinical syndrome that mimics Cushing's syndrome. "Pseudo-Cushing's" syndrome, caused by alcohol abuse or depression, is less common in children than in adults as a cause of Cushing's syndrome.[11] Long-term administration of a supraphysiologic dose of corticosteriods will cause iatrogenic Cushing's syndrome. Inordinate cortisol production directly from the adrenal glands or from an adrenal tumor is another possible cause of Cushing's syndrome.[18] ACTH overproduction by a pituitary adenoma accounts for 50 to 80% of cases of Cushing's syndrome[19, 20] and has been given the eponym "Cushing's disease," which is the focus of our discussion.

Children with Cushing's disease often present for evaluation with growth retardation, which is seen in up to 80% of patients, and increase in weight, seen in up to 90% of patients.[5, 13] Other common clinical manifestations are hypertension, hirsutism, acne, buffalo hump, menstrual irregularities, and psychiatric disturbances.[5–7, 13, 19] Diabetes mellitus is a much less common manifestation of Cushing's disease in children than in adults.[21] The mean age at presentation is 12.9 years.[5–7, 15] The age at presentation for children with Cushing's disease has been noted to be significantly younger than that for children with prolactinomas.[7] Girls suffering from Cushing's disease outnumber boys 1.3:1.[4–7, 15] The pediatric ratio differs from the adult ratio of 3:1, which is considerably more skewed to women.[15]

It is uncommon for children with Cushing's disease to harbor a macroadenoma. One group found ACTH-secreting adenomas to be significantly smaller on presentation than other types of pituitary tumors.[7] Thus, it is unusual for an ACTH-secreting tumor to cause focal neurologic deficit from mass effect.

Growth Hormone–Secreting Pituitary Adenomas

The endocrinopathy caused by a growth hormone–secreting pituitary tumor is what usually leads a patient to a doctor. A patient who is a prepubertal child when affected by this type of

---

BOX 20–3
Signs and Symptoms of Cushing's Disease

- **Growth delay**
- **Pubertal delay**
- **Weight gain**
- **Hypertension**
- **Hirsutism**
- **Acne**
- **Buffalo hump**
- **Menstrual irregularity**
- **Psychiatric disturbances**

---

tumor will experience an abnormally brisk rate and an abnormally large extent of somatic growth. Excess growth hormone causes gigantism indirectly, by the stimulation of other growth factors.[1] If the patient is postpubertal when affected by such a tumor, the epiphyses of his or her long bones will already have been fused. The clinical syndrome caused by the tumor in these cases is acromegaly.[1] The abnormal somatic growth will be limited to hands, feet, face, and soft tissues, giving the patient the typical acromegalic appearance. Aside from cosmetic considerations, an enlarging tongue may cause sleep apnea. Arthritis and diabetes are common in these patients. The effects of acromegaly on visceral structures, such as the heart and lungs, are the most debilitating aspect of the disease.[1] Untreated acromegalics develop hypertension and congestive heart failure, which is ultimately deadly.

BOX 20–4
Signs and Symptoms of Growth Hormone Abnormalities

- **Gigantism**
- **Acromegaly**
  - **Arthritis**
  - **Diabetes**
  - **Hypertension**
  - **Congestive heart failure**

Growth hormone–secreting tumors in children have been noted to be significantly larger upon presentation, on average, than prolactinomas.[7] *Despite this finding, it is much more common for children and adolescents to present with gigantism or acromegaly than focal neurologic deficits due to mass effect.*[4, 6, 7]

Other Pituitary Adenomas

Thyrotropin–secreting adenomas have been reported to manifest clinically as an unusual cause of hyperthyroidism, which proves difficult to control by anti-thyroid drugs.[10] Pediatric gonadotropin secretion (either follicle-stimulating hormone or leuteinizing hormone) by pituitary tumors has been noted to cause precocious puberty.[3]

Pituitary tumors that do not secrete endocrinologically active hormones most often manifest due to mass effect in the sella and on parasellar areas. *Nonsecretory pituitary adenomas have been reported to be significantly larger than any other type of pituitary adenoma upon presentation.*[7] Most children present with visual field deficits, although other focal deficits have been noted.[4, 6, 7] In addition, intrasellar compression often causes hypopituitarism.[4, 6, 7] Usually hypopituitarism causes growth arrest or delay in sexual development, but panhypopituitarism with adrenal failure may occur. A macroadenoma may cause obstructive hydrocephalus, which can result in an acute change in mental status.

BOX 20–5
Signs and Symptoms of Nonsecreting Adenoma

- **Pubertal delay**
- **Precocious puberty**
- **Hyperthyroidism**
- **Visual field deficits**
- **Hydrocephalus**

DIAGNOSIS
Laboratory

Blood studies are usually the first confirmatory tests the practitioner obtains when clinical suspicion of a pituitary tumor in a child arises. Each individual tumor is capable of producing a distinctive biochemical profile.

Prolactinoma

The normal serum prolactin in a male and nonpregnant, nonnursing female is less than 20 and 25 (ng/mL), respectively.[5] In the normal resting state the hypothalamus secretes dopamine, and possibly other factors, which inhibit pituitary prolactin secretion.[1] The most common cause for an elevated prolactin level is pregnancy, with a peak level usually less than 200 ng/mL.[1] A mild hyperprolactinemia may also be seen in end-stage renal failure, primary hypothyroidism, ingestion of antidopaminergic drugs (e.g., phenothiazines), and with any mass lesion that impinges on the pituitary stalk.[1] Increased prolactin level from the so-called stalk effect is due to blockade of hypothalamic prolactin inhibitory factors. In a nonpregnant patient, a serum prolactin level of greater than 150 ng/mL is almost always caused by a prolactinoma.[1, 22]

Cushing's Disease

Diagnosing Cushing's disease based on laboratory studies is quite complex. Serum cortisol normally shows a circadian rythm, with levels highest in the morning and lowest in the evening. Cushing's syndrome of any etiology causes an elevation of serum and urine cortisol as well as loss of the normal diurnal variation in serum cortisol levels.[5, 7, 13] Elevation in serum cortisol normally inhibits the pituitary release of ACTH through a feedback loop, causing the cortisol level to fall. Administration of decadron in a low dose (i.e., 30 μg/kg per day)[13] causes an inhibition of pituitary function and a decrease in serum cortisol in patients with pseudo-Cushing's but not in patients with Cushing's disease, ACTH secretion from an ectopic tumor, or cortisol secretion from hyperplastic or tumorous adrenals. Decadron does not interfere with the laboratory assay for cortisol. Administration of decadron in a high dose (i.e., 120 μg/kg per day)[13] usually suppresses the cortisol level in patients with Cushing's disease, but not in those with ectopic secretion of ACTH or secretion of cortisol from adrenal hyperplasia or tumors. Thus, the low- and high-dose suppression tests are usually performed to investigate the causes of Cushing's syndrome. *Patients with Cushing's disease will have suppression of cortisol on high-dose but not low-dose suppression tests in 86% of cases.*[13]

CRH recently became available for clinical use. A CRH stimulation test has been found by some authors[13] to be more convenient and less costly than a dexamethasone suppression test. In this test, CRH is administerred with follow-up serum checks of ACTH and cortisol levels. Of patients with ACTH-secreting pituitary adenomas, 75% have an increase in ACTH after the test and 80% have an increase in cortisol. This may be compared to none of the patients with ectopic production of corticotropin or cortisol having an increase in corticotropin after administration of CRH and only 16% having an increase in cortisol.

Inferior petrosal sinus sampling (IPSS) can be helpful in confirming a pituitary source of ACTH hypersecretion if a suspected adenoma is poorly visualized on CT and MRI.[5, 23] In this procedure bilateral femoral veins are catheterized. Under flouroscopic guidance the catheters are then guided into the inferior petrosal sinuses (Fig. 20–3). The physician thus may sample the effluent from the cavernous sinuses. The ACTH level of this blood is compared to that in blood drawn at a peripheral site. A central-to-peripheral ACTH ratio of greater than 2:1 is 86 to 90% sensitive and almost 100% specific for Cushing's disease.[13, 24] The accuracy of this test has been improved by adding CRH stimulation to the testing protocol.[25, 26] Administration of CRH, with a central-to-peripheral corticotropin ratio of greater than 3:1, improves the sensitivity to more than 95% and retains excellent specificity.[13] The advanced imaging studies currently available, used in conjunction with IPSS, have reduced the incidence of sellar explorations for an ectopic source of ACTH production.[24]

IPSS has also been used to aid in localizing the side of the pituitary gland in which a tumor is located. IPSS has been reported to give correct lateralization in 54 to 76% of patients.[13, 15, 27] This test might help guide the surgeon intraoperatively. If no discrete tumor is found during operative exploration, it may suggest which side of the gland to remove. One caveat is that false lateralization has been reported in 8 to 31%[15, 24] and no lateralization in 15%.[8]

Despite the test's utility in the situations outlined above, the physician should not order IPSS indiscriminately. It will not be indicated or helpful unless Cushing's syndrome has been documented. IPSS has been referred to as an invasive and expensive test that most children find quite disturbing.[15] *Nevertheless, if Cushing's syndrome has been diagnosed and imaging studies are normal, this study must be performed to confirm a pituitary cause.*

Other Tumor Types

The biochemical diagnosis of a growth hormone–secreting tumor is based on the measurement of serum growth hormone levels 60 to 120 minutes after oral ingestion of 100 g of glucose. In a normal individual, the growth hormone level will be suppressed to less than 2 to 5 ng/mL. In the presence of a growth hormone–secreting pituitary adenoma the serum growth hormone level remains above 5 to 10 ng/mL, and often increases in response to ingestion of a glucose bolus.[1]

Children with nonsecreting pituitary adenomas have normal or low hormonal levels, with the possible exception of prolactin.[7] There may be a mild prolactinemia present due to compression of the pituitary stalk by a nonsecreting macroadenoma.

The biochemical diagnosis of a gonadotropin-secreting adenoma is clear when an elevated gonadotropin level is found along with a radiologically evident tumor. Diagnostic difficulty arises when an elevated gonadotropin level is found with no radiologically demonstrable tumor. In these cases, the differential diagnosis includes ectopic gonadotropin production and primary hypogonadism.[1] The differentiation of these entities requires provocative endocrinologic testing beyond the scope of this chapter.[1]

Imaging

Currently available imaging studies, such as computed tomography (CT) and, especially, contrast-enhanced magnetic resonance imaging (MRI), have allowed the identification of an increasing number of pituitary microadenomas and virtually all macroadenomas.[17] For example, growth hormone–secreting tumors and prolactinomas, which are likely to be macroadenomas, may be localized on CT or MRI in 72 to 86% of cases.[4, 6] On the other hand, ACTH-secreting tumors, which are microadenomas in 96% of cases,[13] are diagnosed on CT or MRI in only 29 to 52% of cases.[4, 6, 13] In addition, the need for angiography, with its attendant risks, to delineate

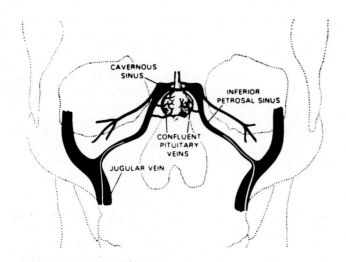

Figure 20–3 Catheters in position for sampling effluent from inferior petrosal sinuses bilaterally.

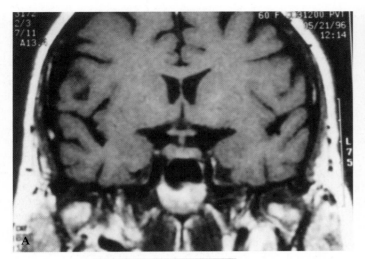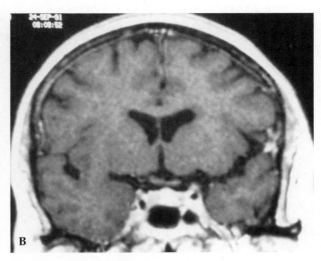

Figure 20–4   Coronal magnetic resonance image without (A) and with (B) intravenous contrast demonstrating bilateral pituitary adenomas, which do not enhance as brightly as the surrounding normal gland. The left-sided microadenoma was proven pathologically to be the cause of this patient's Cushing's disease, whereas the right sided tumor proved to be an incidental nonsecreting tumor.

tumor vascularity or the position of the carotid arteries has been virtually eliminated by MRI (Fig. 20–4).

Despite recent advances in neuroimaging, one must be cautious about their interpretation. Perceived abnormalities on imaging studies may not represent the position of an adenoma. Incorrect lateralization of microadenomas by CT has been reported to be up to 14% and also has been reported with MRI.[15, 28] Incidental pituitary tumors may be the cause of some of these errors (Fig. 20–5). Pituitary tumors have been found in up to 27% of nonselected patients studied at autopsy.[23] In one study of 100 normal volunteers, contrast-enhanced MRI was performed to search for sellar lesions, which could be suggestive of adenoma. Of these asymptomatic patients, 10% harbored focal pituitary lesions measuring 3 to 6 mm in greatest diameter.[29] Not surprisingly, previous operation or radiation renders CT less useful. In one series looking at such patients, microadenoma localization by CT was only 9%.[30]

CT and MRI are indispensable for evaluation of structures contiguous to the pituitary gland. Invasion of the cavernous sinus or parasellar tissues by tumor may be noted (Fig. 20–2). This changes the operative plan, as will be discussed later. The anatomy of the sphenoid sinus should be evaluated carefully (Fig. 20–6). An incompletely pneumatized sphenoid sinus is sometimes seen, which makes a transsphenoidal approach to the sella more difficult. Septations of the sphenoid sinus should also be noted. They may fortuitously act as a guide to a radiographically visible tumor. Conversely, if the location of intraoperative dissection relative to a sphenoid septation is not carefully noted, the patient's midline may be misinterpreted. One cell of a septated sinus may remain unentered. This could result in opening the anterior wall of the sella in a far lateral position, thus endangering the cavernous sinus, cranial nerves, and carotid artery. Alternatively, in this situation, the contralateral portion of the sella may remain unexplored, and a small macroadenoma may be missed (a special concern in Cushing's disease).[30]

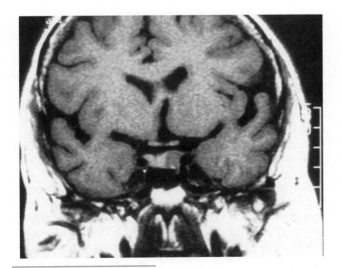

Figure 20–5   Coronal magnetic resonance image showing a pituitary tumor abutting the left carotid artery. The position of the carotid arteries can usually be well demonstrated on MRI, obviating the need for angiogram in preoperative planning.

TREATMENT

Transsphenoidal selective adenomectomy offers the best chance at cure with the best chance of allowing normal development to proceed in all types of symptomatic pediatric pituitary tumors except prolactinomas. Successful selective removal of tumor may enable "catch-up" growth, or a resumption of normal growth, in up to 73% of patients.[13, 31] Eighty-six percent of patients resume normal menses after transsphenoidal resection of

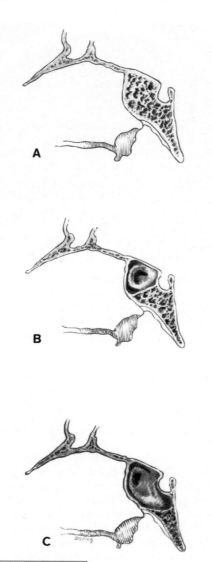

Figure 20–6 Pneumatization of the sphenoid sinus: (A) conchal; (B) partially pneumatized; (C) fully pneumatized.

pituitary tumors, and many have demonstrated normal fertility.[6] Primary surgical treatment of pituitary tumors results in panhypopituitarism in 9% of cases and partial hypopituitarism in 29% of cases.[6]

Kane et al use the transsphenoidal approach for selective adenomectomy as primary treatment for most pediatric pituitary adenomas.[3] In their series on microadenomas (excluding Cushing's disease), they report a 70% immediate cure rate, with a 25% recurrence rate. When treating macroadenomas (again excluding Cushing's disease) they report a 33% cure rate. This immediate cure rate increases to 55% with adjuvant treatment, with a 33% recurrence. Recurrences are treated by this group with radiation or reoperation.

In most cases it is possible to perform the standard sublabial transsphenoidal approach to the pituitary gland with the aim of selective tumor removal with sparing of the normal gland.[4] The further normal development of facial structures is not disturbed by this type of procedure.[6] One difficulty that

arises in children much more commonly than in adults is an incompletely pneumatized or conchal-type sphenoid sinus (Fig. 20–6). This has been reported in 6 to 18% of cases of pediatric pituitary tumors.[4, 6, 15] Several strategies have been used with success access the sella through an incompletely pneumatized sphenoid sinus. Most authors suggest drilling out the sphenoid under fluoroscopic guidance.[4, 6] A diamond drill may be used for the deepest portion until both cavernous sinuses are clearly delineated.[15] Some have suggested using a chisel to broach the anterior wall of the sphenoid. The medullary center of the bone is sharply curetted to reach the inner surface, which is removed with use of a chisel.[32] Regardless of the means by which the sella is exposed through an incompletely pneumatized sphenoid, care must be taken to avoid the carotid arteries.[12] In the fully pneumatized sphenoid sinus the carotid arteries form a visible indentation in the superior posterior lateral walls. In the incompletely pneumatized sphenoid, the carotid position is not as clear.

Pituitary irradiation is the chief modality of adjuvant therapy used to achieve remission when pituitary tumors do not respond to surgical therapy alone. The cure rate for pediatric pituitary adenomas using conventional radiotherapy has been reported at 80% after 18 months.[19] Maximal effects of radiotherapy may not be seen for 5 to 10 years.[33] The chief concern in administration of radiotherapy to children is delayed, often insidious occurrence of pituitary insufficiency. Although normal sexual maturation and fertility have been demonstrated in many patients after pituitary irradiation,[19] 66% of patients in one series[2] had postirradiation growth retardation, and 100% had hormonal abnormalities. The introduction of stereotactic radiotherapy has increased the efficacy and safety of this treatment. Using the gamma knife, one group has reported an 88% remission rate.[21] A radiation dose of 50 to 70 G was directed at the sella, with less than 10% of the isodose reaching the optic tracts. Although panhypopituitarism was not often seen in this cohort, 100% of the children needed some form of hormonal replacement after the treatment. Recurrence of tumor 5 years after apparent radiotherapy cure has been reported.[34]

Prolactinoma

The first-line of therapy for the treatment of prolactinomas in children, as in adults, is medical. Treatment with bromocriptine leads to resolution of the endocrinopathy, as well as resolution of laboratory and radiologic abnormalities in most patients.[5, 14, 17] Pretreatment visual deficits related to macroprolactinomas significantly regress in 90% of patients.[17] The mechanism of action of bromocriptine is activation of dopamine receptors on lactotrophs leading to inhibition of prolactin secretion.[14] It has also been suggested that bromocriptine has a direct tumoricidal effect.[14] In most cases, return of normal menses and fertility is seen during treatment of prolactinomas with bromocriptine.[17] Smaller tumors have a more rapid and complete response to medical treatment.[17]

After clinical and radiologic regression of the tumor, the patient may be weaned from bromocriptine.[5, 14, 17] *A slow taper of dopamine agonists with close follow-up is needed because sudden termination has been reported to result in rapid increase in tumor size.*[14] Some patients remain cured after the cessation of therapy, whereas others require continued medical therapy for an indefinite period of time.[17]

Some macroprolactinomas compress the surrounding normal gland and cause hypopituitarism. Despite shrinkage or regression of a prolactinoma on bromocriptine therapy, some children suffer from continued hypopituitarism, requiring growth hormone, testosterone, and/or thyroxine.[14, 17]

Failure of tumor response to bromocriptine, or a continued or worsening neurologic deficit while taking bromocriptine, are indications for surgical therapy.[5, 17] Intolerance of the side effects of bromocriptine had previously been another surgical indication[5]; however, newer dopamine agonists, such as pergolide, are now available, and cabergoline will soon be available.[22] Adolescent girls with prolactinomas who are receiving medical treatment may become pregnant. Continued medical treatment during pregnancy is successful in more than 95% of patients with microprolactinomas and 65 to 85% of those with macroprolactinomas.[1] Symptomatic tumor enlargement during pregnancy may occur in the remainder of patients and should be addressed surgically.

BOX 20–6
Surgical Indications
for Prolactinoma

- **Continued/worsening neurodeficits (i.e., vision)**
- **Failure to respond to bromocriptine**
- **Intolerance of side effects**

The surgical curability of a prolactinoma is related to its size, with larger tumors less likely to be cured surgically.[7] One group has reported an immediate surgical cure rate in microprolactinomas to be 70% with a 29% recurrence rate, compared with macroprolactinomas, which had a 35% immediate surgical cure rate with 38% recurrence.[3] Others have reported similarly disappointing results after surgery for macroprolactinomas.[5] Serum prolactin level has been found to increase directly with tumor size and also gives some indication of surgical curability.[7] Some authors use a cutoff prolactin level of 200 ng/mL.[3, 4] Surgical cure is extremely unlikely in patients found to have prolactin levels greater than that. Dyer et al were able to acheive postoperative normalization of prolactin in 86% of patients with a preoperative serum prolactin level less than 200 ng/mL, compared with 9% of patients who had a preoperative prolactin level greater than 200 ng/mL.[4]

Some have recommended transsphenoidal adenomectomy as a first-line therapy for children with prolactin-secreting microadenomas.[3] Their argument is that this will provide a high likelihood of cure, with minimal morbidity and mortality, sparing the patient from long-term dependance on bromocriptine.

Radiotherapy should be used in the treatment of children with prolactinomas only if clinical and radiographic remission cannot be induced by medical or surgical treatment.[5]

Cushing's Disease

Selective removal of an ACTH-secreting adenoma is the treatment of choice for pediatric Cushing's disease, whenever possible. Magiakou et al reviewed their experience in treating childhood Cushing's disease at the National Institutes of Health

between 1982 and 1992. Remission of hypercortisolism was attained in 48 of the 49 patients who underwent transsphenoidal surgery.[13] Knapp et al, recently reported their experience with a series of 55 pediatric patients with Cushing's disease.[15] The patients ranged in age from 4 to 19 years. The primary modality of therapy used by this group is selective surgical extirpation of the tumor. They identified and removed discrete adenomas in 88% of their patients and tumorous tissue in another 10%. They failed to find tumor upon initial exploration in only one patient. They subsequently brought this child back to surgery for reexploration and successfully removed a tumor. This group believes in early surgical reexploration for persistent hypercortisolism. Practicing this strategy they report a remarkable 96% rate of remission of hypercortisolism, with 100% remission when early reexploration is included. Haddad et al achieved control of hypercortisolism in all five cases of pediatric Cushing's disease treated by their group.[5] The admirable rates of control of hypercortisolism compare favorably to those of most large series of adult patients with Cushing's disease. Postoperative remission of hypercortisolism in adult patients with Cushing's disease has been reported in 70 to 86% of patients.[24, 31, 35–40] One group thinks that the discrepancy in remission rates suggests that ACTH–secreting adenomas in children are more often noninvasive and well localized than those in adults.[5]

IPSS is routinely used after a histologically negative exploration of the gland with persistent hypercortisolism (if it was not performed preoperatively) to reassure the physician that a pituitary source for hypercortisolism exists.[15, 23]

Recurrence of hypercortisolism has been reported in range 0 to 32% of children.[5–7, 11, 13, 15, 21] Many tumors recurred after 7 years.[11, 21] If possible, a recurrent tumor should be selectively removed. If it is localizable to one part of the gland but a discrete adenoma is not encountered, a partial hypophysectomy may also be performed. If remission of hypercortisolism is not induced by partial hypophysectomy, consideration should be given to administering radiation therapy. *Complete hypophysectomy in a child or young woman of childbearing age should be avoided.*

Radiation therapy is usually reserved for cases in which cure by surgery alone had not been possible.[5, 6, 11, 13, 15, 21] *For example, radiation is used in conjunction with surgery for treatment of invasive tumors. In addition, radiation may be used for surgical failures, after multiple attempts at surgical cure.* On the other hand, there are some proponents of radiation therapy as primary treatment for pediatric Cushing's disease. An initial success rate of 80% has been reported.[13] Use of stereotactic radiosurgical techniques may increase the remission rate to 88%.[7] Delayed onset of hypopituitarism (especially diminished growth hormone) and late recurrences have dampened enthusiasm for the procedure.[6, 7, 15, 19]

Medical treatment of hypercortisolism with ketoconazole has been reported.[41] This type of treatment will not suffice as the sole therapy for Cushing's disease. However, ketoconazole may be used while the patient is awaiting surgery or awaiting the effects of radiotherapy. Patients must remain on adrenostatic medication after pituitary irradiation for months, sometimes years, until the effects of radiotherapy are seen.[15]

Bilateral adrenalectomy should only be only used in the treatment of Cushing's disease when all other measures have failed.[15, 24] There is a reported operative mortality of 4% for the procedure. Nelson's syndrome has a reported incidence of 10% to 26% and has been noted to be a more common sequela of bilateral adrenalectomy in children than adults.[15, 21, 24] Nelson's syndrome has been characterized by continued growth of a pituitary adenoma after bilateral adrenalectomy, with progressive sellar enlargement and extreme elevations in ACTH.[19] Patients with Nelson's syndrome have been noted to have worsening headaches, visual field deficits, oculomotor palsies, and hyperpigmentation.[19, 21] Even after this procedure, Cushing's syndrome may recur from growth of adrenal rests or remnants.[33]

Chronic hypercortisolism affects the nontumorous portion of the pituitary gland, decreasing the ability of the corticotropic cells to secrete ACTH. Postoperative hypocortisolism has been noted by many authors and serves to reassure the surgeon that a remission of the disease has been achieved.[4, 13] Supplemental corticosteroids should be provided for the patient to avert addisonian crisis. These should be tapered gradually over a 6- to 8-month period as the patient's hypocortisolism gradually returns to eucortisolemic levels.[4, 13]

Gigantism and Acromegaly

Surgical extirpation of the offending adenoma remains the first-line therapy for growth hormone–secreting pituitary tumors in children. However, the surgical cure rate in children falls short of the reported rate of 60 to 88% demonstrated in adults.[4] One group was able to cure only 13% of patients with surgery alone.[4] This discrepancy in cure rate may be explained by a higher rate of children harboring tumors with suprasellar extension than adults.[4]

Medical treatment is indicated for those patients who are not cured by surgery alone. A somatostatin analog is the most effective agent currently available in the treatment of growth hormone–secreting tumors. Somatostatin has been found to reduce serum growth hormone level and control symptoms in 66% of patients and to induce partial tumor regression in 20 to 50% of patients.[1] Currently, in the United States the only available form of the medication is expensive and must be administered in a subcutaneous regimen three times a day. A longer lasting formulation should soon become available, making medical treatment cheaper and more convenient, and allowing for much less frequent administration.

If surgery and medical therapy fail, radiation therapy should be provided. Somatostatin should be provided to control the endocrinopathy while awaiting the effects of pituitary irradiation.[42]

Other Adenoma Types

It is reasonable to attempt surgical resection of nonsecreting pituitary tumors, or to debulk the adenoma, for relief of neurologic deficit. However, as noted earlier, these tumors are most frequently the largest type of pituitary adenoma upon presentation, which renders their surgical cure difficult. Adjuvant radiotherapy is required in their treatment more commonly than in the treatment of the other tumors.[7]

General comments made about the treatment of thyrotropin-secreting tumors in children are of limited value due to their rarity. Difficulty in medically controlling clinical hyperthyroidism in these cases has been reported.[10] *Surgery with complete removal of the adenoma is the best hope for cure.* If attempts at surgical extirpation fail to cure the affected individual, radiosurgical treatment should be offered.

SUMMARY

Several aspects of pediatric pituitary tumors distinguish them from pituitary tumors in adults: Pituitary adenomas account for a smaller percentage of intracranial tumors in children than adults. The distribution of adenoma type in children is distinct from that of adults. Many children with pituitary tumors come to clinical attention because of growth retardation or pubertal delay. There is some debate as to whether pituitary tumors in children are more biologically aggressive than those in adults.

Diagnosis of pituitary adenomas has been facilitated by advances in imaging techniques and biochemical testing. Synthetic hormones and hormonal assays render biochemical definition of endocrinopathy possible. The use of MRI has allowed accurate localization of many pituitary tumors. IPSS has been useful in cases of Cushing's syndrome for confirming the pituitary etiology of ACTH hypersecretion.

The primary treatment of pituitary adenomas in children is surgical, with the exception of prolactinomas. The primary treatment of prolactinomas should be with a dopamine agonist. If surgical treatment is not curative, medical and/or radiation treatment should be administered, depending on adenoma type.

REFERENCES

1. Daniels G, Martin J. Neuroendocrine regulation and diseases of the anterior pituitary and hypothalamus. In: Wilson JD, ed. *Harrison's Principals of Internal Medicine.* New York: McGraw-Hill; 1991:1655–1668.
2. Wara WM, Richards GE, Grumbach MM, et al. Hypopituitarism after irradiation in children. *Int J Radiat Oncol Biol Phys.* 1977;2(5–6):549–552.
3. Kane LA, Leinung MC, Scheithauer BW, et al. Pituitary adenomas in childhood and adolescence. *J Clin Endocrinol Metab.* 1994;79(4):1135–1140.
4. Dyer EH, Civit T, Visot A, et al. Transsphenoidal surgery for pituitary adenomas in children. *Neurosurgery.* 1994; 34(2):207–212.
5. Haddad SF, VanGilder JC, Menezes AH. Pediatric pituitary tumors. *Neurosurgery* 1991;29(4):509–514.
6. Partington MD, Davis DH, Laws ER Jr, Scheithauer BW. Pituitary adenomas in childhood and adolescence. Results of transsphenoidal surgery. *J Neurosurg.* 1994; 80(2):209–216.
7. Mindermann T, Wilson CB. Pediatric pituitary adenomas. *Neurosurgery.* 1995;36(2):259–268.
8. Jamjoom A, Moss T, Coakham H, et al. Cervical lymph nodes metastases from a pituitary carcinoma. *Br J Neurosurg.* 1994;8(1):87–92.
9. Gollard R, Kosty M, Cheney C, et al. Prolactin secreting pituitary carcinoma with implants in the cheek pouch and metastases to the ovaries. *Cancer* 1995;76:1814–1820.
10. Avramides A, Karapiperis A, Triantafyllidou E, et al. TSH-secreting pituitary macroadenoma in an 11-year-old girl. *Acta Paediatr.* 1992;81(12):1058–1060.

11. Laws ER. Comments on: Knapp UJ, Ludecke DK, Transnasal microsurgery in children and adolescents with Cushing's disease. *Neurosurgery.* 1996;39:484–493.

12. Landolt AM. Comments on: Haddad SF, VanGilder JC, Menezes AH. Pediatric pituitary tumors. *Neurosurgery.* 1991;29(4):509–514.

13. Magiakou MA, Mastorakos G, Oldfield EH, et al. Cushing's syndrome in children and adolescents. Presentation, diagnosis, and therapy. *N Engl J Med.* 1994;331(10):629–636.

14. Oberfield SE, Nino M, Riddick L, et al. Combined bromocriptine and growth hormone (GH) treatment in GH-deficient children with macroprolactinoma in situ. *J Clin Endocrinol Metab.* 1992;75(1):87–90.

15. Knapp UJ, Ludecke DK. Transnasal microsurgery in children and adolescents with Cushing's disease. *Neurosurgery* 1996;39:484–493.

16. Sugita S, Hirohata M, Tokutomi T, et al. A case of pituitary apoplexy in a child. *Surg Neurol.* 1995;43(2):154–157.

17. Tyson D, Reggiardo D, Sklar C, David R. Prolactin-secreting macroadenomas in adolescents. Response to bromocriptine therapy. *Am J Dis Child.* 1993;147(10):1057–1061.

18. Laws ER. Comments on: Nakane T, Kuwayama A, Watanabe M, et al. Long term results of transsphenoidal adenomectomy in patients with Cushing's disease. *Neurosurgery.* 1987;21(2):218–222.

19. Jennings AS, Liddle GW, Orth DN. Results of treating childhood Cushing's disease with pituitary irradiation. *N Engl J Med.* 1977;297(18):957–962.

20. Hardy J. Presidential address: XVII Canadian Congress of Neurological Sciences. Cushing's disease: 50 years later. *Can J Neurol Sci.* 1982;9(4):375–380.

21. Thoren M, Rahn T, Hallengren B, et al. Treatment of Cushing's disease in childhood and adolescence by stereotactic pituitary irradiation. *Acta Paediatr Scand.* 1986;75(3):388–395.

22. Ciccarelli E, Camanni F. Diagnosis and drug therapy of prolactinoma. *Drugs.* 1996;51(6):954–965.

23. Post KD, Habas J. Cushing's disease: results of operative treatment. In: Cooper PR, ed. *Neurosurgical Topics: Contemporary Diagnosis and Management of Pituitary Adenomas.* Park Ridge, IL: AANS; 1991.

24. Mampalam TJ, Tyrrell JB, Wilson CB. Transsphenoidal microsurgery for Cushing disease. A report of 216 cases. *Ann Intern Med.* 1988;109(6):487–493.

25. Zarrilli L, Colao A, Merola B, et al. Corticotropin-releasing hormone test: improvement of the diagnostic accuracy of simultaneous and bilateral inferior petrosal sinus sampling in patients with Cushing syndrome. *World J Surg.* 1995;19(1):150–153.

26. Freda PU, Wardlaw SL, Bruce JN, et al. Differential diagnosis in cushing syndrome. Use of corticotropin-releasing hormone. *Med Baltimore.* 1995;74(2):74–82.

27. Landolt AM, Schubiger O, Maurer R, Girard J. The value of inferior petrosal sinus sampling in diagnosis and treatment of Cushing's disease. *Clin Endocrinol Oxf.* 1994;40(4):485–492.

28. Peck WW, Dillon WP, Norman D, et al. High-resolution MR imaging of pituitary microadenomas at 1.5 T: experience with Cushing disease. *Am J Roentgenol.* 1989;152(1):145–151.

29. Hall WA, Luciano MG, Doppman JL, et al. Pituitary magnetic resonance imaging in normal human volunteers: occult adenomas in the general population. *Ann Intern Med.* 1994;120(10):817–820.

30. Friedman RB, Oldfield EH, Nieman LK, et al. Repeat transsphenoidal surgery for Cushing's disease. *J Neurosurg.* 1989;71(4):520–527.

31. Fahlbusch R, Buchfelder M, Muller OA. Transsphenoidal surgery for Cushing's disease. *J R Soc Med.* 1986;79(5):262–269.

32. Laws ER. Comments on: Dyer EH, Civit T, Visot A, et al. Transsphenoidal surgery for pituitary adenomas in children. *Neurosurgery.* 1994;34(2):207–212.

33. Yanovski JA, Cutler GB. Cushing's disease: medical treatment. In: Cooper PR, ed. *Neurosurgical Topics: Contemporary Diagnosis and Management of Pituitary Adenomas.* Park Ridge, IL: AANS; 1991.

34. Cappa M, Stoner E, DiMartino Nardi J, et al. Recurrence of Cushing's disease in childhood after radiotherapy-induced remission. *Am J Dis Child.* 1987;141(7):736–740.

35. Tindall GT, Herring CJ, Clark RV, et al. Cushing's disease: results of transsphenoidal microsurgery with emphasis on surgical failures. *J Neurosurg.* 1990;72(3):363–369.

36. Carpenter PC. Cushing's syndrome: update of diagnosis and management. *Mayo Clin Proc.* 1986;61(1):49–58.

37. Chandler WF, Schteingart DE, Lloyd RV, et al. Surgical treatment of Cushing's disease. *J Neurosurg.* 1987;66(2):204–212.

38. Guilhaume B, Bertagna X, Thomsen M, et al. Transsphenoidal pituitary surgery for the treatment of Cushing's disease: results in 64 patients and long term follow-up studies. *J Clin Endocrinol Metab.* 1988;66(5):1056–1064.

39. Ram Z, Nieman LK, Cutler GB Jr, et al. Early repeat surgery for persistent Cushing's disease. *J Neurosurg.* 1994;80(1):37–45.

40. Nakane T, Kuwayama A, Watanabe M, et al. Long term results of transsphenoidal adenomectomy in patients with Cushing's disease. *Neurosurgery.* 1987;21(2):218–222.

41. Sonino N, Boscaro M, Merola G, Mantero F. Prolonged treatment of Cushing's disease by ketoconazole. *J Clin Endocrinol Metab.* 1985;61(4):718–722.

42. Gelber SJ, Heffez DS, Donohoue PA. Pituitary gigantism caused by growth hormone excess from infancy. *J Pediatr.* 1992;120(6):931–934.

Chapter 21

Optic Nerve Glioma

Harold J. Hoffman and Robin P. Humphreys

Optic nerve gliomas in childhood have long been known to follow a highly unpredictable course. Some remain static for many years, whereas others increase in size and can lead to significant morbidity and even death. This extreme variability has led to what Oxenhandler and Sayers described as a dilemma in the management of these tumors,[1] a dilemma that still exists today. Observation only or treatment by radiotherapy, chemotherapy, and surgical resection have all been proposed, individually or in combination. The advocates of each approach have stressed the benefits of the therapy they espouse and the danger of other forms. Consequently, there is no uniform method for management of these tumors, which in childhood are generally recognized as low-grade astrocytomas.

LOCATION OF OPTIC NERVE GLIOMAS

Optic nerve gliomas can arise anywhere in the optic system from just behind the globe, through the chiasm and hypothalamus, to the geniculate body. They can also originate in the walls of the third ventricle and infiltrate the optic pathways anteriorly and laterally, or can arise in the chiasm and infiltrate the hypothalamus posteriorly. For this reason, tumors that are located primarily in the hypothalamus or in the optic chiasm are often labeled "optic pathway gliomas" because it is difficult to distinguish these neoplasms clinically or radiologically. About 10% of optic pathway tumors are located in one optic nerve. One-third of the tumors involve both optic nerves and chiasm, another third involve predominantly the chiasm itself, and one-fourth are predominantly in the hypothalamus.

INCIDENCE AND NATURAL HISTORY

Optic pathway gliomas are not common. In Cushing's series of 2000 brain tumors, only 1% were gliomas involving the optic pathways.[2] However, 75% of these tumors occur during the first decade of life, and so the series reported from major pediatric neurosurgical centers reflect the significantly higher incidence in children. Optic gliomas composed 4% of the brain tumors seen at the Children's Hospital National Medical Center in Washington, DC,[3] 3.6% from the Children's Hospital in Boston,[4] 4% from the Columbus Children's Hospital in Ohio,[5] and 6% from the Hospital for Sick Children in Toronto.[6]

Optic and chiasmatic gliomas can be large tumors with unpredictable growth rates. Literature exists with respect to reports that these tumors are congenital, nonneoplastic, and self-limiting.[7, 8] Although it is true that some of these gliomas remain quiescent for several years, behaving as hamartomas, others unquestionably grow slowly and cause progressive visual decline, neurologic deficits, and even death in 20 to 30% of patients.[8] *In general, most reports have shown that although optic and chiasmatic gliomas are histologically low-grade astrocytomas, those arising in the chiasm and hypothalamus are more aggressive and invasive than those confined to the optic nerve. There are no clinical, histologic, or neuroimaging features that differentiate between aggressive and indolent tumors.[9]*

The effect of age on the clinical behavior of these tumors is noteworthy. Generally, the optic system gliomas are more aggressive, with an increased tendency to recur, and a higher mortality rate in patients younger than 5 years than in those between 5 and 20 years. This is especially the case when the tumor occurs in the infant. Whether this represents an intrinsic growth advantage of these tumors in this vulnerable age group or reflects the results of the reluctance to use radiation therapy in infants is uncertain.[1, 10–12] Optic glioma is strongly associated with neurofibromatosis type 1 (NF-1). Among patients with NF-1, 14 to 40% are at risk of developing this tumor; or, virtually all patients with the glioma restricted to the optic nerve will have NF-1.[13]

A peculiar feature of the optic glioma, albeit rare, is its tendency to disseminate along the neuraxis.[14, 15] Gajjar et al[16] reported a 5% rate of central nervous system dissemination in a series of 150 consecutive accrued patients with low-grade glioma. Interestingly, half of those patients with metastases had optic glioma. This tumor spreads through the cerebrospinal fluid (CSF) pathways, in particular the ventricule, gaining access to different sites along the neuraxis.

CLINICAL PRESENTATION

If the tumor is confined to one optic nerve the patient presents with unilateral visual loss, often accompanied by proptosis and associated with optic atrophy. (Fig. 21–1)

BOX 21–1
Presentation of Unilateral Optic Nerve Glioma

- **Visual loss**
- **Proptosis**
- **Optic atrophy**

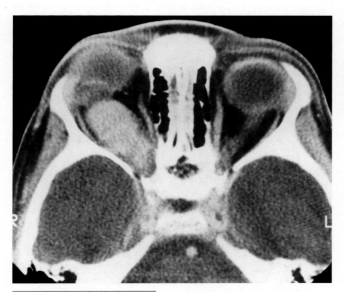

Figure 21–1   A 5 year-old girl with neurofibromatosis type 1 has proptosis and severe visual loss in the right eye. Enhanced CT scan shows an intraorbital glioma that was resected.

Patients with tumors involving the optic chiasm present with visual loss, manifested in the infant as poor visual fixation and, occasionally, see-saw nystagmus (Fig. 21–2). Thus neuro-ophthalmologic assessment should include accurate measurements of visual acuity and formal tests of the visual fields with perimetry techniques.

Furthermore, tumors in the chiasm can fill the third ventricle, thus producing hydrocephalus and raising intracranial pressure, resulting in headaches, vomiting, and papilledema

(Fig. 21–3). Rarely, chiasmal tumors can extend laterally to involve motor tracts and produce a hemiparesis (Fig. 21–4).

BOX 21–2
Presentation of Optic Nerve Glioma in the Optic Chiasm

- **Visual loss (bitemporal)**
- **See-saw nystagmus**
- **Hydrocephalus**
- **Hemiparesis**
- **Seizures**

DIAGNOSTIC AND IMAGING FEATURES

When the tumor involves the optic nerve there is usually a fusiform enlargement of the nerve that can continue through the optic foramen to involve the intracranial portion of the nerve. The lesion can then extend posteriorly into the chiasm (Fig. 21–3). Tumors of the chiasm present as suprasellar masses that are particularly large in infancy. The tumor can fill the third ventricle, blocking the foramina of Monro and producing hydrocephalus. It can also spread posteriorly along the optic tracts to involve the geniculate body. The glioma that involves the chiasm and the hypothalamus can become enormous, particularly in infants.

Magnetic resonance imaging (MRI) shows the optic glioma to be wholly solid, cystic, or of mixed signal intensity. Typically, there is marked gadolinium enhancement. When the tumor involves only the optic nerve, there is usually a

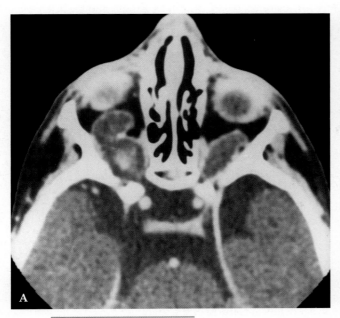
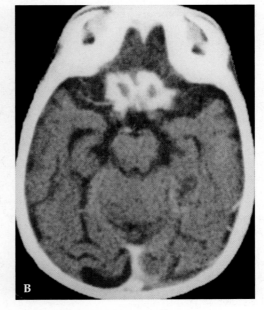

Figure 21–2   (A) Bilateral optic nerve tumors in an infant with severe visual loss. (B) Chiasmatic extension of the tumor.

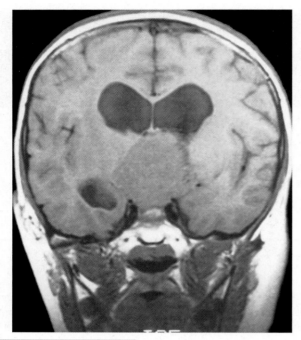

Figure 21–3 Coronal magnetic resonance image of large chiasmatic tumor extending into the third ventricle and producing obstructive hydrocephalus.

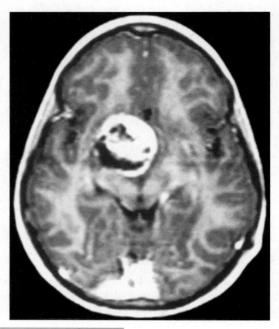

Figure 21–4 Axial magnetic resonance image outlining partially cystic chiasmatic-hypothalamic tumor that extends lateral and posterior to impact on the cerebral peduncle.

fusiform enlargement of the nerve that can continue through the optic foramen to involve the intracranial portion of the nerve and perhaps also the chiasm. *Patients with NF-1 frequently demonstrate involvement of both optic nerves.* From this point, a common pathway for the tumor's continuing growth is posterosuperiorly as the tumor courses toward the brain stem and invaginates superiorly into the third ventricle. Lateral growth may also be appreciated, and the vessels of the circle of Willis can become circumferentially engulfed by tumor. These major arteries may demonstrate marked narrowing on the magnetic resonance angiography component of the study.

BOX 21–3
MRI Appearance

- **Solid/cystic**
- **Gadolinium enhancement**

PATHOLOGY OF OPTIC PATHWAY GLIOMAS

Optic pathway gliomas occurring in childhood are low-grade astrocytomas and, rarely, gangliogliomas. Only in adults may these gliomas present as malignant tumors that cause early loss of vision and lead to death.[17]

The low-grade astrocytomas in childhood involving the optic pathways have a highly unpredictable course. Some remain static

and quiescent for many years. This fact no doubt led Hoyt and his colleagues to regard them as hamartomas.[8, 14, 18] However, some of these low-grade astrocytomas can adopt an aggressive course, increasing rapidly in size and perhaps leading to death. Despite this marked difference in behavior these tumors are histologically similar. Childhood optic pathway gliomas are pilocytic astrocytomas (60%), fibrillary astrocytomas (40%), or, rarely, gangliogliomas. *Despite the benign nature of juvenile pilocytic astrocytoma, children who have these tumors within optic pathways do not fare nearly as well as patients with fibrillary astrocytomas.* Patients with pilocytic astrocytomas have a significantly increased risk of tumor recurrence and tumor progression.[13]

BOX 21–4
Types of Optic Pathway Gliomas

- **Pilocytic astrocytoma (60%)**
- **Fibrillary astrocytoma (40%)**
- **Ganglioglioma (rare)**

MANAGEMENT STRATEGIES

Management of the optic pathway glioma is truly a challenge for the clinician. Is one to be more influenced by the glioma's clinical features or the changing tumor architecture noted on contemporary imaging studies? It is inappropriate to construct a treatment algorithm that would be applied to each and every patient with an optic nerve glioma. However, one should acknowledge the following principles:

- Patients with NF-1 associated with optic pathway tumors seem to have a better prognosis than patients without NF-1. About one-half of patients with optic pathway gliomas and NF-1 seen at our hospital have required no treatment for their tumors, which have remained quiescent.[6]

- A skilled neuro-ophthalmologist is the individual best able to assess the clinical impact of this particular tumor. Changes in visual acuity or field, characteristics of the optic fundus, and ocular motility or protuberance are highly objective hallmarks of disease progression.

- The emergence of superior imaging techniques has allowed neurosurgeons to monitor the course of these lesions as well as to assess the effects of therapy. Most patients with childhood optic pathway gliomas survive for many years. With contemporary neuroimaging, neurosurgeons can see what happens to these tumors with time—whether they shrink, remain the same, expand, or even disappear.

The therapeutic choices for patients with gliomas of the visual system are to a large degree arbitrary and uncertain. Treatment recommendations for such patients range from expectant observation to operative exploration and biopsy or nerve and tumor resection, to chemotherapy and irradiation adjunctive therapy, or to any combination of these. Much effort has thus been devoted to analyzing the specific treatment goals for these patients, so that the techniques of optic nerve tumor surgery and its complications have received less emphasis.[19]

Thus, patients with optic pathway tumors who do not have NF-1 should undergo tissue sampling. A limited biopsy is less desirable because substantial resection of a glioma may lead to regression of some of these tumors.[13] Furthermore, chiasmatic tumors must be distinguished from suprasellar germinomas and occasionally from craniopharyngiomas. In addition, one should be aware that a limited biopsy may lead to confusion between an optic pathway glioma and a germinoma.[12]

OPERATIVE TREATMENT

Whether the patient has NF-1 or not, a tumor that is located anteriorly within the orbit requires treatment if it produces proptosis, particularly if vision also is significantly compromised.

Computed tomography (CT) and MRI studies, in addition to detailing the features of the optic nerve and tumor, will also show the optic canal and its size, the relationship of the extraocular muscle cone to the tumor, the size and position of the ethmoid air cells, and the cavernous sinus.

The neurosurgical approach to the optic nerve tumor is via a frontal craniotomy ipsilateral to the tumor and a subfrontal extradural and intradural exposure of the orbital roof, the optic canal, and the optochiasmatic junction and adjacent carotid artery. The goal is to resect tumor-bearing nerve from the globe to the chiasm. Some surgeons may choose to include the supraorbital rim in the craniotomy as well.

As the target of the procedure lies within the orbital cavity, it is tempting to expose the orbital roof by dissecting across it in the extradural plane. Sooner or later the dura covering the undersurface of the frontal lobe must be opened to expose the intradural portion of the optic nerve and the anterior clinoid process and superior margin of the optic foramen. *The surgeon is advised to inspect the optic nerve and chiasm intradurally prior to orbital exploration.* The "lie" of the nerve and the course of the optic canal are determined, and if tumor is evident, the nerve may be sectioned adjacent to the chiasm (6 mm or more beyond the optochiasmatic junction in order to preserve the looping Willbrand knee fibers). If the intradural, intracranial nerve appears normal, the orbital roof and optic canal are approached extradurally. The goal is not to remove the entire orbital roof but rather to remove just that part covering the optic canal even if it is expanded.

From this point on, the somewhat complex normal anatomical configuration of the orbital contents, blurred as it is through the periorbital tissue and orbital fat, tends to be even more confusing due to distortion from the optic nerve mass. Muscle bundles are flattened, blanched, and pushed up or aside. Branches of cranial nerves are thinned and may be deviated; the surgeon's aim is to identify the frontalis nerve, which is a relatively broad band running about parallel to the optic nerve and on top of the levator palpebrae superioris and superior rectus muscles. In order to maintain continuity through the optic canal and foramen, the annulus of Zinn must be opened; this act risks sacrificing the trochlear nerve.

Microdissectors and retractors are used to withdraw the muscle bellies and develop a plane to the tumor sheath and optic nerve. The tumor can be further delineated with blunt dissection, and the surgeon should expect its outline to be irregular though smooth. As the exploration proceeds around the girth of the optic nerve tumor, a blunt microhook assists in ventral dissection and confirms the site of the union of the nerve and tumor with the globe. Once identified, the junction can be coagulated with bipolar forceps and the nerve sectioned. Branches of the ophthalmic artery that serve the nerve can be traced to it and divided after coagulation.

If the tumor is so large and irregular that it cannot be easily removed, the mass can be reduced by laser vaporization or ultrasonic aspiration. The tumor and nerve can then be removed as far back as the optochiasmatic junction, either en bloc or as two separate portions, depending on whether the annulus has been opened. At the end, the surgeon must make a decision about reconstruction of the bony defect in the orbital roof to prevent visible globe pulsation with proptosis. As microscopic techniques increasingly permit a much more conservative removal of the glioma through the roof of the optic canal, roof reconstruction will not be required in many circumstances.

If the tumor extends into the chiasm and upward into the third ventricle, it may be necessary to open the lamina terminalis. At this juncture the tumor characteristically has a different appearance from that of normal optic fibers, thereby assisting with the bulk removal of the lesion without impairing the patient's vision or creating an endocrinologic deficit. In this circumstance, one is advised to beware of the major arteries—anterior and middle cerebral—that may be engulfed by tumor. Not only may their exact position be unclear, but they can be subject to reactive vasospasm with even minor manipulations. In a few circumstances the biologic effect of diminishing the tumor bulk can result in its stabilization and even regression.[13]

HYDROCEPHALUS

As previously indicated, patients with NF-1 presenting with an optic pathway tumor and stable vision may be treated expectantly. However, some of these patients, as well as those who do not have NF-1, may present with hydrocephalus because of obstruction of the third ventricle by upward growth of the tumor (Fig. 21–3). In such cases, only a ventriculoperitoneal shunt is needed. On occasion, when such a shunt is performed ascites develops.[20] Presumably, this results from the shunting of proteinaceous fluid to the peritoneal cavity.

CHEMOTHERAPY

In large part because of the adverse effects of radiation therapy on the developing brain and the therapeutic frustration that is experienced when a child younger than 3 years shows disease progression from an optic glioma, some groups have reported on chemotherapy for this tumor.[15, 21–23] Although the efficacy for chemotherapy for low-grade gliomas remains uncertain, Packer and colleagues have described their experience treating 24 patients with chiasmatic or hypothalamic tumors using actinomycin D and vincristine.[15] In nine patients the tumors responded to chemotherapy, and this delayed the necessity for radiation therapy until the children were older. Petronio et al have reported good results with combination chemotherapy in 19 patients.[21] In both groups there have been no deaths. Vision was stabilized in 85% of patients and the tumors shrank or were stable in more than 90%.

RADIATION TREATMENT

External-beam irradiation has reduced or controlled tumor bulk when it occupies the optic nerves and chiasm.[3, 24–26] A dose of 5200 to 5600 cGy has been recommended. However, this is not universally true, and radiotherapy does produce significant sequelae. In general, radiation therapy can be very detrimental to the developing brain, and children with optic gliomas who are younger than 3 years can be neurologically harmed by this technique.[27] In our own series, we have also become concerned about four patients who developed malignant astrocytomas in the field of their irradiation[6] (Fig. 21–5). In addition, five children who received radiation therapy developed the moyamoya phenomenon following the irradiation.[9, 10, 28] However, in patients older than 5 years who do not respond to resection alone or to chemotherapy, and in whom the tumor is leading to significant visual compromise, radiotherapy may be the only option available.

There is also some experience reported with the use of stereotactic radiosurgery whose application appears to have considerable advantages and appeal over conventional irradiation techniques.[29] However, the long-term efficacy of this strategy for patients with optic and chiasmatic gliomas

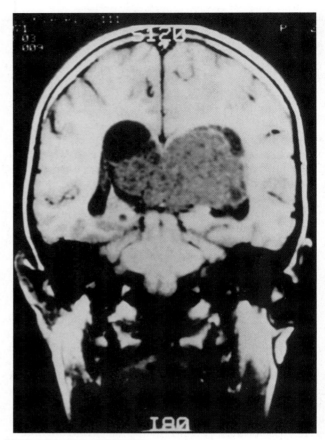

Figure 21–5 Coronal magnetic resonance image of a child 10 years after irradiation for a low-grade optic glioma. A large anaplastic tumor occupies the ventricular cavities.

remains to be determined. The same might also be said about the proposed use of conformal irradiation techniques.

SUMMARY

Optic pathway gliomas have been considered benign and self-limiting. However, most series report significant morbidity and mortality, especially with the more extensive, posteriorly placed tumors. The emergence of modern imaging techniques allows one to monitor the course of the disease and the effects of therapy. Most patients with these tumors survive for many years with a varying clinical course. In their report on this tumor, Oxenhandler and Sayers stressed that individualization is necessary when the neurosurgeon is confronted with a rare tumor of indeterminate natural history and a potential of multidecade duration.[1] This principle still holds true. The current policy at our center is to resect anteriorly located tumors that are restricted to one orbit and are causing unsightly proptosis and significant visual loss. Patients with NF-1 and posteriorly located tumors that are not interfering significantly with vision are treated symptomatically, namely, CSF shunting for hydrocephalus and medical therapy for endocrinologic dysfunction, if required. Patients with posteriorly located tumors without NF-1, as well as those with NF-1 who show deteriorating vision or progressive neurologic deficits, are treated by operation. After resection, patients with significantly compromised vision and patients who show progression of their disease on neuroimaging or on clinical evaluation receive chemotherapy. If chemotherapy proves ineffective, then radiotherapy is used. Patients who are stable clinically and have vision that is not compromised receive no therapy and are followed with neuroimaging.

REFERENCES

1. Oxenhandler DC, Sayers MP. The dilemma of childhood optic gliomas. *J Neurosurg* 1978;48:34–41.
2. Martin P, Cushing H. Primary gliomas of the chiasm and optic nerves in their intracranial portion. *Arch Ophthalmol* 1923;52:209.
3. McCullough DC, Johnson DL. Optic nerve gliomas and other tumors involving the optic nerve and chiasm. In: McLaurin RL, ed. *Pediatric Neurosurgery.* Philadelphia: WB Saunders; 1989;391–397.
4. Matson DD. *Neurosurgery of Infancy and Childhood.* Springfield, IL: Charles C Thomas; 1969;436–448.
5. Sayers MP. Optic nerve gliomas. In: McLaurin RL, ed. *Pediatric Neurosurgery.* New York: Grune & Stratton; 1982;513–522.
6. Hoffman HJ. Optic pathway gliomas. In: Amador LD, ed. *Brain Tumors in the Young.* Springfied, IL: Charles C Thomas; 1983:622–633.
7. Wong JYM, Uhl V, Wara WM, et al. Optic glioma reanalysis of the University of California, San Francisco experience. *Cancer* 1987;60:1847–1855.
8. Imes RK, Hoyt WF. Childhood chiasmal gliomas: update on the fate of patients in the 1969 San Francisco study. *Br J Ophthalmol* 1986;70:179–182.
9. Servo A, Puranen M. Moyamoya syndrome as a complication of radiation therapy: case report. *J Neurosurg* 1978;48:1026–1029.
10. Kestle JRW, Hoffman HJ, Mock AR. Moyamoya phenomenon after radiation for optic glioma. *J Neurosurg* 1993;79:32–35.
11. Pierce SM, Barnes PD, Loeffler JS, et al. Definitive radiation therapy in the management of symptomatic patients with optic glioma: survival and long-term effects. *Cancer* 1990;65:45–52.
12. Cohen DH, Steinberg M, Buchwald R. Suprasellar germinoma diagnostic confusion with optic gliomas: case report. *J Neurosurg* 1974;41:490–493.
13. Hoffman HJ, Soloniuk DS, Humphreys RP, et al. Management and outcome of low-grade astrocytomas of the midline in childhood. *Neurosurgery* 1993;33:964–977.
14. Glaser JS, Hoyt WF, Corbett J. Visual morbidity with chiasmal glioma: long-term studies of visual fields in untreated and irradiated cases. *Arch Ophthalmol* 1971;85:3–12.
15. Packer RJ, Sutton LN, Bilaniuk LT, et al. Treatment of chiasmatic/hypothalamic gliomas of childhood with chemotherapy: an update. *Ann Neurol* 1988;23:79–85.
16. Gajjar A, Bhargava R, Jenkins JJ, et al. Low grade astrocytoma with neuraxis dissemination at diagnosis. *J Neurosurg* 1995;83:67–71.
17. Taphoorn MJB, de Vries-Knoppert AEJ, Ponssen H, et al. Malignant optic gliomas in adults. *J Neurosurg* 1989;70:277–279.
18. Hoyt WF, Baghdassarian SA. Optic gliomas of childhood: natural history and rationale for conservative management. *Br J Ophthalmol* 1969;53:793–798.
19. Humphreys RP: Optic gliomas. In: Apuzzo MLJ ed. *Brain Surgery: Complication Avoidance and Management.* New York: Churchill Livingstone; 1993:643–652.
20. Weidmann MJ. Ascites from a ventriculoperitoneal shunt: case report. *J Neurosurg* 1975;43:233.
21. Petronio J, Edwards MSB, Prados M, et al. Management of chiasmal and hypothalamic gliomas of infants and childhood with chemotherapy. *J Neurosurg* 1992;74:701–708.
22. Weiss L, Sagerman RH, King GA, Chung CT, Dubowy RL. Controversy in the management of optic nerve gliomas cancer. *Cancer* 1987;59:1000–1004.
23. Wisoff JH, Abbott R, Epstein F. Surgical management exophytic chiasmatic-hypothalamic tumors of childhood. *J Neurosurg* 1990;73:661–667.
24. Gold RJ, Hilal SK, Chutorian AM. Efficacy of radiotherapy in optic gliomas. *Pediatr Neurol* 1987;3:29–32.
25. Packer RJ, Savino PJ, Bilaniuk LT, et al. Chiasmatic gliomas of childhood: a reappraisal of natural history and effectiveness of cranial irradiation. *Child's Brain* 1983;10:393–403.
26. Taveras JM, Mount LA, Wood EH. The value of radiation therapy in the management of glioma of the optic nerves and chiasm. *Radiology* 1956;66:518–528.
27. Richards GE. Effects of irradiation on the hypothalamic and pituitary regions. In: Gilbert HA, Kogan AR, eds. *Radiation Damage to the Nervous System.* New York: Raven Press; 1980:175–180.
28. Rajakulasingam K, Cerullo LJ, Raimondi AJ. Childhood moyamoya syndrome: postradiation pathogenesis. *Child's Brain* 1979;5:467–475.
29. Bakardjiev AI, Barnes PD, Goumernova LC, et al. Magnetic resonance imaging changes after stereotactic radiation therapy for childhood low grade astrocytoma. *Cancer* 1996;76:864–874.

Chapter 22

Pineal Region Tumors

Andrew T. Parsa, David W. Pincus, Neil A. Feldstein, Casilda M. Balmaceda, Michael R. Fetell, and Jeffrey N. Bruce

In the early part of this century, pineal region surgery had a poor outcome, with operative mortality approaching 90%.[1-3] From Horsley's initial attempt at removing a pineal mass in 1910 through the development of the lateral transventricular approach in 1931 by Van Wagenan, primitive anesthetic technique and the lack of an operating microscope hindered pineal region surgery.[4, 5] In 1948, Torkildsen argued for abandoning aggressive surgical resection in favor of cerebrospinal fluid (CSF) diversion followed by empirical radiotherapy.[6] If the patient did not respond to radiation, a surgical procedure to remove radioresistant tumor was performed. The algorithm of CSF diversion, radiation, and observation was sometimes successful; however, patients with benign lesions were exposed to unnecessary and ineffective radiation. Modification of this treatment strategy gave rise to the "radiation test" heralded by Japanese clinicians managing an inordinately high percentage of radiosensitive germinomas in their patient populations. In this protocol, patients were given small doses of radiation and followed radiologically. If the pineal tumor decreased in size it was presumed to be radiosensitive and a full course of radiation was instituted. Patients not responding to radiotherapy underwent surgical exploration. Despite the low dose of radiation initially used there remained significant potential morbidity associated with this strategy, particularly in children.[7, 8]

The advent of microsurgical techniques and stereotactic procedures in the latter part of the twentieth century has obviated the need for empirical radiotherapy without tissue diagnosis. Therapeutic decision making is now based on tumor histology rather than radiation responsiveness. Currently, initial surgical management for tissue diagnosis and possible resection is the standard of care for most children with pineal region tumors.

CLINICAL PRESENTATION

The clinical syndromes associated with pineal region tumors relate directly to normal pineal anatomy as well as tumor histology. The pineal gland develops during the second month of gestation as a diverticulum in the diencephalic roof of the third ventricle. It is flanked by the posterior and habenular commissures in the rostral portion of the midbrain directly below the splenium of the corpus collosum. The velum interpositum is found rostral and dorsal to the pineal gland and contains the internal cerebral veins, which join to form the vein of Galen.[9, 10] The principal cell of the pineal gland is the pineal parenchymal cell, or pineocyte. This cell is a specialized neuron related to retinal rods and cones. The pineocyte is surrounded by a stroma of fibrillary astrocytes that interact with adjoining blood vessels to form part of the blood-pial barrier.

The pineal gland is richly innervated with sympathetic noradrenergic input via a pathway originating in the retina and coursing through the suprachiasmatic nucleus of the hypothalamus and the superior cervical ganglion.[9] Upon stimulation, the pineal gland converts sympathetic input to hormonal output by producing melatonin, which in turn has regulatory effects on hormones such as leuteinizing hormone and follicle-stimulating hormone.[11] *The pineal gland can be considered a neuroendocrine transducer that synchronizes hormonal release with phases of the light-dark cycle by means of its sympathetic input.* However, the exact relationship between the pineal gland and human circadian rhythm remains unclear and is an active area of investigation.

In their 1954 pineal tumor study, Ringertz and colleagues defined the pineal region as being bound by the splenium of the corpus collosum and telachoroidea dorsally, the quadrigeminal plate and midbrain tectum ventrally, the posterior aspect of the third ventricle rostrally, and the cerebellar vermis caudally.[12] Mass lesions that compress these adjacent structures result in typical clinical syndromes. One of the most common presentations is headache, nausea, and vomiting caused by aqueductal compression and resultant obstructive hydrocephalus.[13] Left untreated, hydrocephalus may progressively lead to lethargy, obtundation, and death. Compromise of the superior colliculus through direct compression or tumor invasion results in a syndrome of vertical gaze palsy that can be associated with pupillary or oculomotor nerve paresis. This eponymic syndrome was first described by the French ophthalmologist Henri Parinaud in the late 1800s and has become virtually pathognomonic for lesions involving the quadrigeminal plate. Further compression of the periaqueductal gray region may cause mydriasis, convergence spasm, pupillary inequality, and convergence or retractory nystagmus. Impairment of downgaze becomes more pronounced in children with tumor involving the ventral midbrain.[14] Children can also present with motor impairment, such as ataxia and dysmetria, resulting from compromise of cerebellar efferent fibers in the superior cerebellar peduncle.[13]

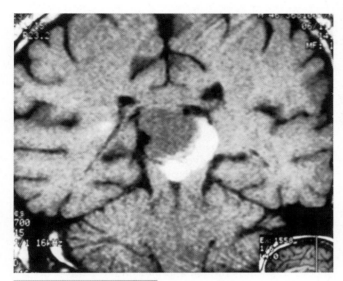

Figure 22–1 Coronal magnetic resonance image of a pineo-cytoma demonstrating areas of increased signal due to hemorrhage. This patient presented with apoplectic symptoms and acute hydrocephalus.

Endocrine malfunction in children with pineal region tumors can present with diabetes insipidus secondary to hydrocephalus or concurrent suprasellar tumor.[13, 15] More specific endocrine syndromes can arise from secretion of hormones by germ cell tumors. Pseudoprecocious puberty caused by β–human chorionic gonadotropin (β-hCG) can be observed with germ cell tumors in either the pineal or suprasellar region.[16, 17] In a large series of germ cell tumor patients with suprasellar involvement, 93% of girls older than 12 years had secondary amenorrhea, whereas 33% of patients younger than 15 years had growth arrest.[18]

Pineal apoplexy has been described as a rare presenting feature of pineal region tumors[19, 20] (Fig. 22–1). Hemorrhage into a vascular rich-pineal tumor can occur pre-operatively and is a well-described post-operative complication.[21]

DIAGNOSTIC CONSIDERATIONS

The symptoms of pineal region tumors can be as varied as their diverse histology, with prodromal periods lasting from weeks to years. A rigorous and uniform preoperative workup is therefore requisite for all children suspected of harboring a pineal region tumor. Any endocrine abnormalities revealed during medical evaluation should be investigated prior to surgery. Children presenting with signs and symptoms of raised intracranial pressure must undergo head computed tomography (CT) or magnetic resonance imaging (MRI) to assess the need for emergency management. Subsequent nonemergency workup of a child with a pineal region tumor can be divided into radiologic and laboratory studies.

Radiologic Diagnosis

High-resolution MRI with gadolinium is necessary in the evaluation of pineal region lesions. Tumor characteristics such as size, vascularity, and homogeneity can be assessed, as can the anatomical relationship with surrounding structures.[22] Irregular tumor borders can be suggestive of tumor invasiveness and associated histologic malignancy. Although the type of tumor cannot be reliably determined from the radiographic characteristics alone, some radiographic patterns are associated with specific tumors (Table 22–1).

Non–germ cell tumors consist of tumor derived from pineal parenchymal cells as well as surrounding tissue. Pineocytomas and pineoblastomas are typically hypointense to isointense on T1-weighted images with increased signal on T2-weighted images and demonstrate homogeneous enhancement. Pineoblastomas can be distinguished by their irregular shape and large size (i.e., some greater than 4 cm).[23] Astrocytomas that arise from the glial stroma of the gland and surrounding tissue are also hypointense on T1- and hyperintense on T2-weighted images. Astrocytomas have variable enhancement patterns. Calcium may be present in either pineal cell tumors or astrocytomas. Meningiomas typically enhance homogeneously with smooth borders. Tentorial meningiomas can have a dural tail of enhancement and are anatomically distinguished by their dorsal location relative to the deep venous system.

Germ cell tumors arise from the neoplastic transformation of residual primordial tissue derived from ectoderm, mesoderm, or endoderm. Each tumor subtype represents the malignant correlate of a distinct stage of embryonic development. In some cases, the stage of tissue development can have distinct radiographic features.

Germinomas are isointense on T1-weighted images and slightly hyperintense on T2-weighted images with strong

TABLE 22–1   Radiologic Features

| Tumor | Pattern | | Enhancement Pattern |
	T1	T2	
Pineocytoma/blastoma	Hypo/isointense	Increased signal	Homogeneous enhancement
Astrocytoma	Hypo/isointense	Increased signal	Variable enhancement
Germinoma	Isointense	Slightly hyperintense Cysts may be visible	Homogeneous enhancement
Teratoma	Heterogeneous	Multilocular	Irregular enhancement

homogeneous enhancement.[22, 24] Calcification surrounds the pineal gland as the germinoma grows, as opposed to the intratumoral calcium within a pineocytoma.[25] Intratumoral cysts can exist as well.[26] In contrast to germinomas, teratomas can contain tissue from all three germinal layers, resulting in a heterogeneous signal. They are well-circumscribed benign tumors characterized by their heterogeneity, multilocularity, and irregular enhancement. Contrast enhancement of teratomas can also be ring enhancing. In some cases, a well-circumscribed teratoma can have areas of low attenuation that correlate with adipose tissue, which serves to further distinguish it from other pineal region tumors.[27] Malignant nongerminomatous germ cell tumors can also have a heterogeneous appearance due to a mixture of benign and malignant germ cell components[22, 24] (Fig. 22–2). Areas of intratumoral hemorrhage may distinguish specific subtypes, such as choriocarcinoma.[28]

In addition to MRI, angiography is sometimes used in cases of suspected vascular anomalies. However, the anatomical and vascular information provided by MRI has largely circumvented the need for routine angiography in the evaluation of pineal region neoplasms.

Laboratory Diagnosis

Measurements of serum and CSF tumor markers are a valuable component of the preoperative evaluation.[29] As with radiographic studies they can be suggestive of tumor type but are seldom diagnostic.[30] Markers have been most helpful in the workup of children with germ cell tumors. In addition to their histologic characteristics, germ cell tumors retain molecular characteristics of their primordial lineage. As a result, the expression of embryonic proteins such as α-fetoprotein

(AFP) and β-hCG are indicative of malignant germ cell elements (Table 22–2).[31, 32] Serum and CSF measurements can be used for diagnostic purposes or for monitoring a response to therapy.[33, 34] In general, CSF measurements are more sensitive than serum measurements, and a CSF/serum gradient may be consistent with an intracranial lesion. However, there is still active debate in the literature regarding the diagnostic value of CSF and serum measurements.[35]

Other biologic markers for germ cell tumors include lactate dehydrogenase isoenzymes and placental alkaline phosphatase.[15, 36, 37] AFP is a glycoproytein produced by fetal yolk sac elements and has been implicated in a wide range of cancers, including gastric, liver, and colon adenocarcinoma, as well as extracranial germ cell tumors.[30] Serum levels of AFP are greatest in the newborn and decline thereafter. The biologic half-life of AFP is approximately 5 days, and levels should always be normalized to known age standards to prevent false-positive results. AFP is markedly elevated with endodermal sinus tumors and elevated to a lesser degree

TABLE 22–2   CSF Markers

Tumor	Marker AFP	BHCG
Endodermal sinus	+++	+/−
Embryonal cell carcinoma	++	+/−
Teratoma	+/−	+/++
Choriocarcinoma	+/−	+++

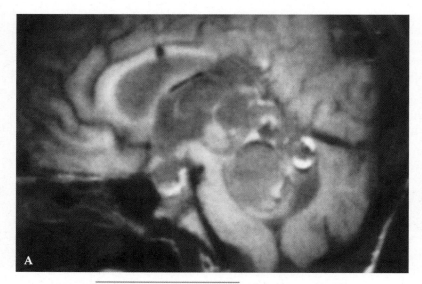
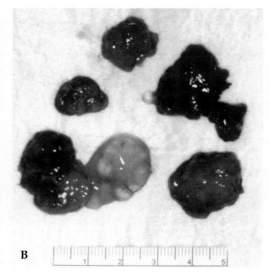

Figure 22–2   (A) Sagittal magnetic resonance image showing multiloculated mixed germ cell tumor extending superiorly with significant heterogeneity. (B) The gross specimens obtained upon resection of the tumor also reflect this heterogeneity.

with embryonal cell carcinomas.[30–33, 38, 39] Although teratomas do not secrete AFP, the less differentiated immature teratomas can produce detectable amounts.[40]

β-hCG is a glycoprotein with a half-life of 15–20 hours and is normally produced by placental trophoblastic cells.[30] Choriocarcinomas secrete large amounts of β-hCG, whereas lesser elevations can occur in patients with embryonal cell carcinomas.[18, 31–33, 41] The presence of syncytiotrophoblastic giant cells in mixed germinomas may result in detectable levels of β-hCG; however, the majority of germinomas are non-secretory.[39, 42] *There is significant variability in expression of tumor markers such that the absence of AFP or β-hCG does not rule out a mixed germ cell tumor.* Although recent studies suggest a less favorable prognosis for patients with germinomas secreting β-hCG, there is no established prognostic significance of tumor markers.[43] Determination of AFP and β-hCG levels prior to surgical resection is extremely important as it provides a reference point, allowing follow-up measurements to assess recurrence.

Pineal parenchymal cell tumor markers are less well characterized than their germ cell counterparts and include melatonin and the S antigen.[9] Neither of these proteins has proven valuable in the diagnosis of pineal parenchymal cell tumors. However, some authors report the use of melatonin levels in the follow-up of patients with pineocytoma after surgical treatment.[44]

PATHOLOGIC FEATURES

The diversity of tumors in the pediatric age group is exemplified by Edward's series of 36 patients under the age of 18 years with pineal region masses.[7] Tumors of the pineal region have varied histology, which can be generally divided into germ cell and non–germ cell derivatives. Most tumors are a result of displaced embryonic tissue, malignant transformation of pineal parenchymal cells, or transformation of surrounding astroglia. Pineal region tumors make up 0.4 to 1.0% of intracranial tumors in adults and 3.0 to 8.0% of brain tumors in children.[26] Most children present between 10 and 20 years of age, with an average age of presentation of 13 years.[7, 45]

Germ Cell Tumors

Germ cell tumors are the most prevalent neoplasm of the pineal region and are histologically indistinguishable from tumors found at extracranial locations, including the mediastinum and gonads.[46] These extracranial locations are most commonly midline. Pineal germ cell tumors are more commonly found in male children, whereas suprasellar germinomas have no sex-specific prevalence.[47, 48] Germ cell tumors can compress the aqueduct and distort the quadrigeminal plate, resulting in headaches, mental status changes, and gaze palsies. In addition, a less common but classic presentation is pseudoprecocious puberty.[49, 50] Approximately half of children presenting with pineal germ cell tumors have suprasellar extension of the tumor.[47] As a result, diabetes insipidus, visual loss, and hypopituitarism may be added to the list of clinical presenting signs. Diabetes insipidus is a common initial symptom for suprasellar germinomas.[40]

BOX 22–1
Germ Cell Tumors

- **Most prevalent tumor**
- **Pineal, suprasellar, and extracranial (midline) locations**
- **Hydrocephalus**
- **Precocious puberty**
- **Gaze palsies**
- **Diabetes insipidus**
- **Visual changes**
- **Hypopituitarism**

Intracranial germ cell tumors can be divided into two categories: (1) germinomas and (2) tumors derived from totipotential germ cells.[46, 51] Germinomas make up 60% to 70% of all pediatric germ cell tumors.[46] Nongerminomatous germ cell tumors fall along a spectrum of differentiation. Least differentiated is the embryonal cell carcinoma, with further differentiation being described as either embryonic or extraembryonic. Immature and mature teratomas result from maturation along embryonic cell lines, whereas endodermal sinus tumor or yolk sac tumor and choriocarcinoma are the result of extraembryonic differentiation.[52–54] Description and classification of a given lesion are sometimes confounded when more than one type of germ cell component is found in a surgical specimen. Mixed germ cell tumors are a result of simultaneous differentiation along more than one pathway such that at presentation two or more well-characterized components are recognized.[55] An example of this is the teratocarcinoma, which is an embryonal carcinoma containing elements of an immature teratoma.[56]

Germinoma is most likely to occur in pure form and is characterized histologically by large round tumor cells interspersed with lymphocytes and septae of fibrous tissue.[57] At low-power magnification with hematoxylin and eosin staining, the contrast between the smaller darkly staining lymphocytes and larger pale staining cytoplasm of neoplastic cells is virtually pathognomonic (Fig. 22–3). At higher magnification, germinoma cells are characterized by a nucleus with an open chromatin structure and prominent nucleoli. The cytoplasm is glycogen rich, making these cells periodic acid–Schiff (PAS)–positive and diastase-labile. Characteristic cytoarchitecture of these cells includes cellular junctions in the form of simplified desmosomes and focal microvilli within intercellular lumina. The presence of microvilli is one of the few histologic characteristics that distinguishes the intracranial lesion from its extracranial correlate.[51]

BOX 22–2
Pathologic Features of Germinoma

- **Large round cells interspersed with lymphocytes and fibrous tissue**
- **PAS-positive**
- **Focal microvilli**

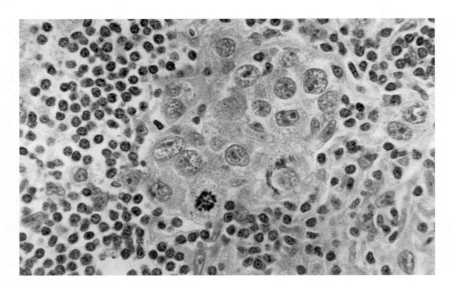

Figure 22–3 Typical two-cell population in a germinoma with lymphocytes interspersed with larger tumor cells.

The pathologic diagnosis of a germinoma can be confounded when the specimen examined contains an infiltrating portion of the tumor or tumor amid significant inflammation. Infiltrating germinomas can elicit atypical gliosis, which may be confused with malignant glial neoplasm. This is particularly true of specimens on the periphery of the germinoma containing a paucity of true germinoma cells. Another example of peripheral change is the noncaseating granulomatous inflammation with multinucleated giant cells seen with some germinomas.[46] An important consideration is that the degree of inflammation can vary significantly among specimens, thus underscoring the need to obtain an adequate amount of diagnostic tissue during surgical intervention.

Nongerminomatous germ cell tumors are more likely to arise in the pineal region than the suprasellar region.[58–60] Embryonal cell carcinoma is a tumor consisting of cuboidal to columnar cells arranged in sheets and cords with large nuclei, prominent irregular nucleoli, and significant mitotic activity (Fig. 22–4). Unlike germinomas, there is little or no lymphocytic infiltrate. Signs of differentiation of embryonal cell carcinomas are seen in cases of mixed germ cell tumors and can proceed along embry-

onal cell lineage toward teratoid cells, or along extraembryonic cell lineage toward yolk sac or placental elements.[51]

**BOX 22–3
Pathologic Features
of Embryonal Cell Carcinoma**

- **Cuboidal-columnar cells in sheets and cords**
- **Large nuclei and prominent nucleoli**
- **Little or no lymphocytic infiltrate**

Teratomas can be composed of a mixture of tissues derived from all three germinal layers with varying degrees of differentiation.[54] Structured variants of teratomas may resemble adult tissue histologically, whereas unstructured examples do not recapitulate known tissue. Hosoi first used the term "teratoid" in 1930 to describe less structured tumors in which derivatives of all three germinal layers could not easily be identified.[61] Current description of teratomas divides these tumors

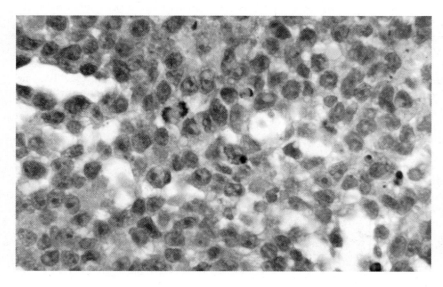

Figure 22–4 Embryonal cell carcinoma consisting of sheets of primitive cells with frequent mitoses.

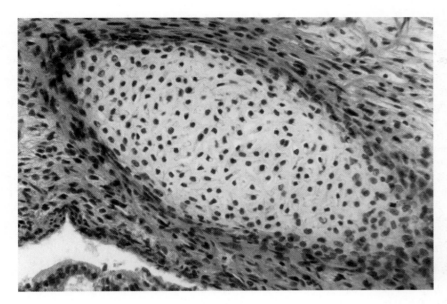

Figure 22–5 Cartilaginous tissue within a teratoma.

into mature teratomas containing fully differentiated ectodermal, mesodermal, and endodermal elements and immature teratomas containing more primitive elements closely resembling embryonic histology.[54] The spectrum of differentiation that exists within the teratoma lineage precludes definitive descriptions of immature versus mature lesions. There are, however, some general microscopic characteristics that can help guide the diagnosis.[46] Mature lesions often contain solid or cystic foci of squamous epithelium, cartilage, or glandular elements embedded in tubular structures lined with mucin-secreting columnar epithelium (Fig. 22–5). Mesenchymal stroma consisting of smooth muscle can be seen interspersed among these well-differentiated tissue elements. Immature teratomas are usually composed of primitive cells derived from one of the three germinal layers. These small round cells, when viewed at lower magnification, can resemble the hypercellularity of a medulloblastoma. Lesions containing primitive cells from all three germinal layers have also been described.

> ## BOX 22–4
> ## Pathologic Features of Teratoma
>
> - **All three germ cell layers**
> - **Varying degrees of differentiation**
> - **Solid or cystic foci of squamous epithelium cartilage, or glandular elements**

Extraembryonic differentiation of embryonal cell carcinoma results in either an endodermal sinus tumor or a choriocarcinoma.[47, 62–65] These two entities represent differentiation toward the yolk sac and trophoblast, respectively, and, as with the teratomas, these tumors may exist admixed with germinomas. The yolk sac carcinoma is derived from the endoderm and therefore contains endodermal sinuses or Schiller-Duval bodies[46, 66] (Fig. 22–6). These pathognomonic

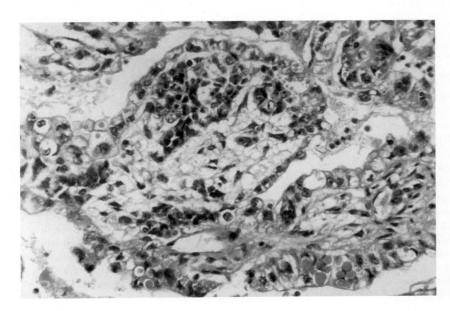

Figure 22–6 Schiller-Duval body within an endodermal sinus tumor.

glomeruloid structures contain a tumor cell–lined space with an invaginated vascular pedicle covered by a single layer of tumor cells. Other characteristic cytoarchitecture includes perivascular endodermal cells and thin-walled cystic spaces. At higher magnification, globules of PAS-positive and diastase-resistant proteins can be easily seen within endodermal sinus cells and the surrounding extracellular stromal matrix. These globules of protein correlate with the presence of AFP in the CSF and blood, a marker associated with endodermal sinus tumors.[53] Trophoblastic differentiation can result in isolated syncytiotrophoblasts expressing gonadotropins or bilaminar arrangements of syncytiotrophoblasts and cytotrophoblasts typified by the choriocarcinoma.[67]

BOX 22–5
Pathologic Features
of Endoderm Sinus Tumor

- **Differentiation (yolk sac)**
- **Pathognomonic glomeruloid structures (Schiller-Duval bodies)**
- **Invaginated vascular pedicle lined by single layer of tumor cells**

Unlike other nongerminomatous germ cell tumors, the choriocarcinoma very rarely appears as an isolated lesion. At low magnification, the bilaminar cytotrophoblastic and syncytiotrophoblastic cells can be identified surrounding blood. Intratumoral hemorrhage is common in choriocarcinoma and correlates with these blood-filled sinuses.[68]

BOX 22–6
Pathologic Features
of Choriocarcinoma

- **Differentiation (trophoblast)**
- **Bilaminar cytotrophoblasts/syncytiotrophoblasts**
- **Intratumoral hemorrhage common**

Non–Germ Cell Tumors

Non–germ cell tumors of the pineal region arise from the pineal gland or its surrounding tissue. The rarity of pineal cell lesions and the lack of an extracranial correlate have complicated the classification of these tumors. Currently, pineal parenchymal tumors are divided into high- and low-grade variants based on the extent of differentiation. The primitive pineoblastoma and the differentiated pineocytoma exist at opposite ends of the spectrum with intermediate-grade variants in between. Russell and Rubinstein have described a more specific classification such that pineoblastomas include types without differentiation, types with pineocytic differentiation, and types with neuronal, glial, or retinoblastic differentiation.[46] Similarly, pineocytomas have been divided into types without further differentiation, types with neuronal differentiation only, types with astrocytic differentiation only,

and types with divergent neuronal and astrocytic differentiation (i.e., the ganglioglioma).[46]

BOX 22–7
Non–Germ Cell Tumors

- **Pineoblastoma**
  - **No differentiation**
  - **Glial**
  - **Pineocytic neuronal**
  - **Retinoblastic**
- **Pineocytoma**
  - **No differentiation**
  - **Neuronal**
  - **Astrocytic**
  - **Ganglioglioma**

Pineoblastomas consist of dense populations of small primitive cells that can form neuroblastic rosettes or Homer Wright rosettes[69] (Fig. 22–7). Less common examples of pineoblastoma cytoarchitecture are the Flexner-Wintersteiner rosettes, which have a ciliary 9 + 0 configuration similar to that of the retinal photoreceptor.[70, 71] Further differentiation of the pineoblastoma can be seen in some cases of familial bilateral retinoblastoma in which a pineoblastoma with retinoblastic features is found. This rare syndrome has been referred to as "trilateral retinoblastoma."[72–74] *The pineoblastoma is an aggressive tumor that resembles the medulloblastoma with respect to age of presentation and its propensity to seed the subarachnoid space.*[42, 47] The pineocytoma is significantly less aggressive than the pineoblastoma. It usually presents during adolescence and rarely seeds the subarachnoid space. Pineocytomas consist of rosette-forming small cells similar to those of the pineoblastoma; however, they appear more spread out and more lobular, and are further distinguished by large hypocellular zones containing fibrillary stroma[23, 75] (Fig. 22–8). At the ultrastructural level these fibrils contain microtubules and dense-core granules.[71] The normal pineal gland tissue contains lobular cells of uniform size with an easily identified astroglial stroma, two features that can be used to distinguish normal gland from pineocytoma.[9]

Glial cell–derived neoplasms occur second most frequently in children with pineal region tumors, exceeded only by germinomas in two large series that include children with pineal region tumors.[7, 76] The histologic and macroscopic appearances are similar to those of malignant glial neoplasms found in other areas of the CNS.[46] Glial-derived neoplasms in the pineal region can include low-grade and high-grade lesions.[47]

Nonneoplastic Lesions

Benign cysts of the pineal gland are being diagnosed more frequently with the increased use of MRI for standard workups unrelated to pineal region pathology.[77, 78] These incidental lesions appear radiographically as cystic structures with peripheral calcification and rimlike contrast enhancement.[79] They are normal variants of pineal gland anatomy and once documented require no treatment unless they

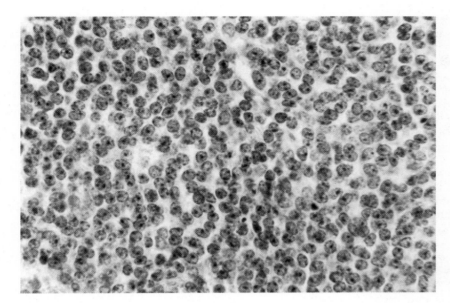

Figure 22–7 Pineoblastoma consisting of small, densely packed primitive cells.

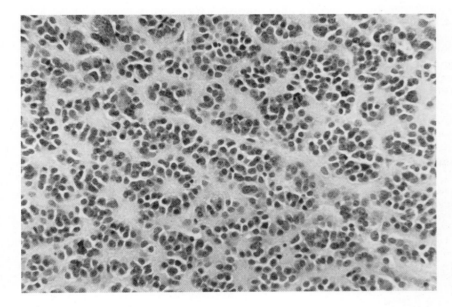

Figure 22–8 Rosettes formed within a pineocytoma.

grow.[80] Pineal cysts may be difficult to distinguish from low-grade cystic astrocytomas based exclusively on radiographic criteria. Any doubts of diagnosis should be addressed by carefully following the patient with serial MRI scanning to ensure that the lesion is not growing.[81, 82]

BOX 22–8
Benign Pineal Lesions

- **Peripheral calcification**
- **Rim contrast enhancement**
- **No growth**

TREATMENT CONSIDERATIONS

Management of children with pineal region tumors should be directed at treating hydrocephalus and establishing a diagnosis. Preoperative evaluation should include the following: (1) high-resolution MRI scan of the head with gadolinium; (2) measurement of serum and CSF markers; (3) cytologic examination of CSF; (4) evaluation of pituitary function if endocrine abnormalities are suspected; and (5) visual field examination if suprasellar extension of tumor is noted on MRI. The ultimate management goal should be to refine adjuvant therapy based on tumor pathology.[29, 39]

BOX 22–9
Preoperative Evaluation

- **MRI (with and without contrast)**
- **Serum and CSF markers**
- **CSF cytology**
- **Pituitary function**
- **Visual fields (for suprasellar lesions)**

The treatment of hydrocephalus can be effectively accomplished temporarily with the placement of an external ventricular drain, or permanently with ventriculoperitoneal shunt placement or third ventriculostomy. For symptomatic patients with hydrocephalus, preoperative third ventriculostomy is extremely effective and often eliminates the need for shunt placement.[83] Successful resection of the lesion may remove the obstruction and allow free flow from the third ventricle, obviating the need for any form of CSF diversion.[84, 85]

Patients presenting with hydrocephalus and radiographic evidence of a malignant pineal region tumor may have their hydrocephalus treated with third ventriculostomy or vetriculoperitoneal shunt prior to biopsy or resection. The staged procedure allows for definitive control of the hydrocephalus prior to surgical resection of lesions suspected as malignant. A similar strategy may be employed for patients with marked, symptomatic hydrocephalus and benign-appearing lesions. The timing of the second procedure can vary according to the surgeon's preference. Peritoneal seeding with shunting is a rare but well documented complication in these patients.[86–91] However, the use of a filter to decrease the incidence of seeding has been associated with frequent shunt malfunctions and is generally not recommended, particularly because third ventriculostomy is a better option.[92]

Improved endoscopic techniques have made third ventriculostomy an easy and reliable method to divert CSF.[84, 85, 93] Third ventriculostomy is performed free-hand or stereotactically with an endoscope passed via a burrhole into the right lateral ventricle and through the foramen of Monro (Fig. 22–9). The floor of the third ventricle is then fenestrated to provide an alternate route for CSF flow and subsequent absorption. As with all CSF diversion procedures, CSF may be obtained and sent for cytologic and biochemical analysis during the procedure. Third ventriculostomy has the added advantage of potentially allowing for a biopsy during the procedure by endoscopic guidance. This provides the opportunity to make an intraoperative diagnosis with subsequent tailoring of further additional therapy.

The decision to perform biopsy versus an open procedure has been debated extensively in the pineal region tumor literature.[29, 39, 94–96] While the ultimate choice of procedure will be based to some extent on the surgeon's personal bias and experience, there are some distinct advantages and disadvantages to each of these procedures. Stereotactic biopsy has been described as the procedure of choice for obtaining a tissue diagnosis in certain situations, such as when a patient has widely disseminated disease, clearly invasive malignant tumor, or multiple medical problems. Early experience with stereotactic biopsies encountered morbidity and mortality specifically related to the targeting of periventricular structures adjacent to the deep venous system. However, more recent studies however have shown stereotactic biopsy to be a safe and efficient means of obtaining a tissue diagnosis. In their 1996 series, Regis and colleagues revealed a mortality rate of 1.3% and a less than 1.0% morbidity rate in 370 stereotactic biopsies of pineal region tumor patients.[76] The study included data from 15 French neurosurgical centers and documented statistical homogeneity among the different centers. In a similar study, Kreth and colleagues retrospectively evaluated the risk profile, diagnostic accuracy, and therapeutic relevance of the stereotactic approach in 106 patients.[97] They showed a morbidity rate of 2 in 106, a mortality rate of 9 in 106, and a definitive tissue diagnostic rate of 103 in 106 patients. Although stereotactic biopsy can be performed safely and effectively at centers familiar with the technique, it falls short of one main operative goal that may be advantageous to some patients, namely, the complete or nearly complete resection of tumor.

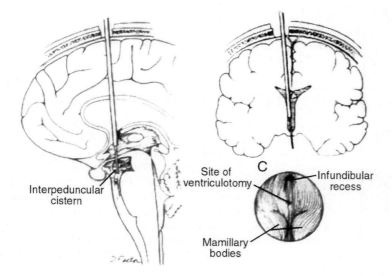

Interpeduncular cistern

Site of ventriculotomy

C

Infundibular recess

Mamillary bodies

Figure 22–9 Stereotactically guided endoscopic third ventriculostomy is the optimal method for treating most patients with hydrocephalus secondary to a pineal region mass. Under stereotactic guidance, an endoscope is advanced into the third ventricle through the foramen of Monro. The ventriculostomy is made between the mamillary bodies and the infundibular recess.

Open resection has been shown to benefit patients postoperatively by accomplishing removal of most if not all of the tumor.[29, 39] *For patients with benign lesions the surgical resection can prove to be curative. In patients with malignant tumor components there is evidence that surgical debulking may improve the response to postoperative adjuvant therapy.*[98] Gross total tumor resection also provides ample tissue specimen to the neuropathologist for diagnosis. This circumvents the potential problems of sampling error and erroneous diagnosis associated with the small volume of tissue provided by stereotactic biopsy. The bulk of evidence provided by the current literature is derived from retrospective analysis, including cases performed a decade ago. Several advances have been made over the past decade that will likely lower the morbidity and mortality associated with open procedures as well as stereotactic biopsy in future studies.

Tissue diagnosis is a vital part of management in most patients with pineal region tumor. However, nonoperative management of patients with positive tumor markers is a reasonable option for some patients. A markedly elevated level of AFP and β-hCG is pathognomonic for germ cell tumor with malignant components. New strategies currently under study have been aimed at minimizing surgical intervention prior to ascertaining whether a tumor is responsive to radiation and/or chemotherapy. In their 1998 retrospective study, Choi and colleagues described the treatment of 107 patients with primary intracranial germ cell tumor including 60 patients with tumors in the pineal region.[99] Thirty of these patients were managed without surgery on the basis of radiologic findings and tumor markers. Univariant analysis of a response to trial radiation and chemotherapy was shown to correlate with outcome, justifying the administration of trial chemotherapy or radiotherapy without tissue biopsy in this subgroup of patients. These findings match well with a 1997 study by Sawamura and colleagues evaluating the necessity of radical resection in patients with intracranial germino-

mas.[100] Twenty-nine patients treated with irradiation and/or chemotherapy were studied retrospectively, including 10 with solitary pineal region masses. The results showed no significant difference in outcome related to extent of surgical resection, with an overall tumor-free survival rate of 100% with a follow-up of 42 months. This retrospective evidence is compelling in favor of withholding surgical treatment of children with marker-positive germ cell tumors.

SURGICAL MANAGEMENT

Improvements in surgical techniques and neuroanesthesia have significantly lowered the morbidity and mortality associated with pineal region surgery. For those patients for whom primary surgical resection is the best therapeutic and diagnostic option, there are several well-described approaches currently in use.[29] In general, surgical approaches to the pineal region can be divided into supratentorial, infratentorial, and, most recently, a combined supratentorial/infratentorial approach. Supratentorial approaches include the parietal-interhemispheric approach, described by Dandy, and the occipital-transtentorial approach, originally described by Horrax and later modified by Poppen[3, 101, 102] (Fig. 22–10).

The supratentorial approach is best applied to patients with tumors extending supratentorially or laterally into the trigone of the lateral ventricle. The main advantage of the supratentorial approach relates to the wide exposure that can be obtained. The transcallosal interhemispheric approach uses a paramedian trajectory between the falx and the right parietal lobe, with partial resection of the corpus callosum. The occipital-transtentorial approach requires retraction of the occipital lobe and division of the tentorium for adequate exposure. The main disadvantage of supratentorial approaches is the difficulty associated with removing tumor that lies below the convergence of the deep venous system. Complications of the transcallosal interhemi-

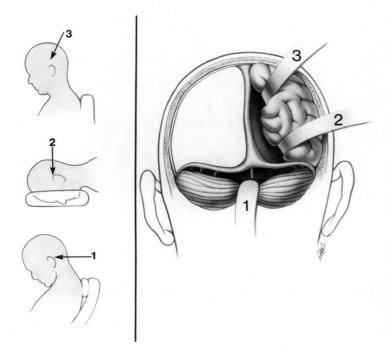

Figure 22–10 Surgical approaches to the pineal region: (1) infratentorial-supracerebellar; (2) occipital-transtentorial; (3) parietal-interhemispheric.

spheric approach may result from excessive retraction of the parietal lobe. The occipital–transtentorial approach can result in visual defects secondary to occipital lobe retraction and associated damage to the calcarine cortex.

The infratentorial approach is a direct midline approach, originally described by Krause and popularized by Stein, that provides an easily recognized orientation for the surgeon.[103–105] A midline trajectory between the tentorium and the cerebellum allows the tumor to be encountered below the deep venous system (Fig. 22–11). When this procedure is performed with the patient in the sitting position, the cerebellum tends to fall away, exposing the pineal region while minimizing pooling of venous blood in the operative field. The main disadvantage associated with this approach is the limited access to tumors that extend above the deep venous complex and anteriorly into the third ventricle. Lateral exposure is also restricted by this approach.

Several different positions have been described for supra- and infratentorial approaches to the pineal region. The sitting-slouch position is generally used for the infratentorial-supracerebellar and transcallosal-interhemispheric approaches. The main complications of this position include subdural and epidural hematoma secondary to ventricular and cortical collapse, pneumocephalus, and air embolus. The three-fourths prone lateral position is used for the occipital-transtentorial approach and avoids many of the complications associated with the sitting-slouch position. A prone position with elevation of the patient's shoulders and the head tilted to the right combines the advantages of the sitting-slouch and three-fourths prone lateral positions. The Concorde position was described by Kobayashi and later modified by Bloomfield and

colleagues for patients with pineal region tumors.[106, 107] The Concorde position is more comfortable for the surgeon and reduces the risk of air embolism, but it can be cumbersome in larger patients. It is often desirable for preadolescent patients.

A combined supra-infratentorial transsinus approach with the patient in a semiprone position has been described for large pineal region tumors.[108, 109] This approach provides wide exposure laterally, superiorly to the posterior third ventricle, and inferiorly to the superior medullary velum. Other advantages include safe visualization of important venous structures and minimal retraction of the cerebellum and occipital lobe. The main disadvantage of this approach is that it entails a very extensive operation, including sacrifice of the nondominant transverse sinus, that may only be suitable for exceptional cases.

The most common complications following pineal region surgery regardless of the approach are extraocular movement dysfunction, ataxia, and altered mental status.[29, 39, 110] Many of these neurologic findings, such as extraocular movement dysfunction and ataxia, are present preoperatively and become transiently worse postoperatively before significantly improving or resolving completely. Some factors that correlate with an increased incidence of surgical complication include prior irradiation, severe preoperative neurologic deficit, malignant tumor pathology, and invasive tumor characteristics. The most devastating complication of pineal region tumor surgery is postoperative hemorrhage into a subtotally resected tumor bed.[110] The hemorrhage may be delayed for several days and is commonly associated with very vascular tumors, such as pineal cell tumors.[29] Venous infarction with or without hemorrhage is another grave complication. Less common postoperative complications include shunt malfunction, hemorrhage

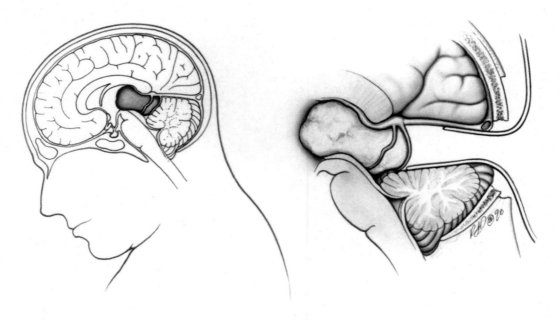

Figure 22–11 The infratentorial-supracerebellar approach exploits the natural corridor between the tentorium and the cerebellum.

during third ventriculostomy following fenestration of the floor of the third ventricle, ventriculostomy closure, and aseptic meningitis. In addition, supratentorial approaches can result in seizures, hemianopsia, or hemiparesis.[29, 102]

BOX 22–10
Potential Surgical Complications

- **Ocular motility dysfunction**
- **Ataxia**
- **Altered mental status**
- **Hemorrhage (subtotal resection)**
- **Venous infarction**
- **Shunt malformation**
- **Aseptic meningitis**
- **Seizure**
- **Hemianopsia**
- **Hemiparesis**

When considering all published series reporting on 20 or more patients in the microsurgical era, pineal region tumor surgery has an overall mortality rate of 0 to 8% and a morbidity rate of 0 to 12%.[29] This is in stark contrast to the mortality rate of 90% reported during the early part of the twentieth century. Long-term outcome after surgical resection depends largely on tumor histology as well as evolving modalities of adjuvant therapy. For patients with malignant tumors, gross total resection in some cases may be associated with a more favorable prognosis. In other patients, such as those with germinoma, initial surgical intervention may become obsolete as preemptive adjuvant therapy becomes more effective.

POSTOPERATIVE STAGING

Once a diagnosis of malignant tumor is made from tissue acquired intraoperatively, the surgeon is obligated to evaluate the patient for spinal metastasis.[110, 111] Prior to widespread use of the MRI, patients were staged postoperatively with CT/myelography. Currently, the most sensitive radiographic modality for screening is a complete spinal MRI with and without gadolinium enhancement.[39] The first MRI scan should be timed at least 2 weeks after surgery, as nonspecific spinal canal enhancement can occur in the early postoperative period.[110] Equivocal findings on the initial postoperative scan warrant a repeat scan within 1 to 2 weeks. Radiographic artifacts secondary to surgery regress, whereas drop metastasis remain stable or increase in size over time (Fig. 22–12). The role for postoperative lumbar puncture and subsequent CSF analysis for cytology is questionable.[112, 113] The presence of abnormal cells postoperatively does not correlate well with spinal metastasis due to spillage during surgery.

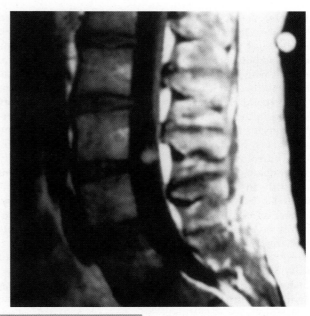

Figure 22–12 Gadolinium-enhanced magnetic resonance image demonstrating drop metastasis in the lumbar region of a 16-year-old boy with a malignant germ cell tumor.

The timing for follow-up cranial MRI varies depending on tumor histology and degree of resection. *To estimate the amount of tumor removed it is advantageous to acquire a postoperative brain magnetic resonance image within 48 hours of surgery.* Postoperative enhancement unrelated to residual tumor may be seen on magnetic resonance procedures done later. The significance of residual tumor depends on tumor histology and the efficacy of available adjuvant therapy. The radioresponsive germinoma is a good example of this phenomenon. Series of patients treated with adjuvant radiation are reported to have a 100% tumor-free survival up to 4 years after diagnosis.[99] This survival rate has been shown to be unrelated to the extent of tumor resection. In contrast, much of the literature evaluating tumor resection and malignant pineal cell tumors and nongerminomatous germ cell tumors suggests that larger resections facilitate adjuvant therapy and long-term survival.[13, 29] Regardless of tumor histology, long-term follow-up is required for all patients with pineal region tumors as recurrences several years after remission are possible.

ADJUVANT THERAPY

Radiation Therapy

Current treatment protocols for children older than 3 years with malignant pineal region tumors include radiotherapy. Early clinical trials with series of patients treated with radiotherapy had significant morbidity.[114, 115] Even low doses of radiation can have significant long-term effects on a child's cognitive development.[116, 117] *Radiation-induced deficits are an important consideration because many children with pineal region tumors enjoy prolonged survival.* Potential complications include hypothalamic and endocrine dysfunction, cerebral necrosis, new-tumor formation, and progression of disease. There have been at least 35 cases of radiation-induced meningioma in children after radiotherapy for pineal region tumors reported in the literature since 1953.[118] Standard radiotherapy protocols for children with malignant pineal cell tumors use 4000 cGy of whole-brain irradiation followed by 1500 cGy to the pineal region.[39, 119, 120] The dose is given in 180-cGy daily fractions. Whole-brain irradiation can cause significant morbidity in prepubescent patients, limiting the recommended initial extended field to between 2500 and 3000 cGy. An additional dose directed at the tumor bed can subsequently be given. Several studies have shown that patients receiving less than 5000 cGy are at risk for recurrence, strongly suggesting that 5000 cGy is the optimal total dose of radiation. For children with malignant germ cell tumors, standard treatment is focal radiotherapy followed by irradiation to the ventricular field.

The application of radiotherapy depends on the histology of the tumor being treated. Germinomas are among the most radiosensitive tumors, with patient response rates and long-term tumor-free survival greater than 90% in most published series. Nongerminomatous malignant germ cell tumors are significantly less responsive to radiation, with a 5-year survival rate between 30 and 40% based on use of this treatment alone.[40, 119] Children with low-grade pineocytomas can be cautiously followed after complete surgical resection without any adjuvant radiation. *There is no clear evidence that radiotherapy benefits patients with low-grade lesions.*[110] The morbid side effects of radiation can be avoided by carefully following these patients with serial MRI to assess tumor recurrence or progression.

The use of prophylactic spinal irradiation is controversial. Early recommendations for postoperative spinal irradiation have been preempted by reports showing the incidence of drop metastasis into the spine to be relatively low.[121, 122] The propensity of a pineal region tumor to metastasize to the spine varies with tumor histology. Estimates of spinal seeding with pineal cell tumors are in the range of 10 to 20%, with significantly higher rates noted for pineoblastoma as compared to pineocytoma.[75] The incidence of spinal metastasis for germinomas has been reported to be as high as 11% and endodermal sinus tumors up to 23%.[123–126] Craniospinal radiotherapy for nongerminomatous germ cell tumors is controversial but routinely used in some countries.[60] As modern improvements in surgical and adjuvant therapy are reflected in present-day long term survival, the rates of spinal metastasis will likely drop significantly, making the need for spinal irradiation obsolete. *Currently, a reasonable approach is to give spinal irradiation only for documented seeding.* For patients with pineoblastomas, some authors suggest the use of preemptive spinal irradiation therapy even if the postoperative surveillance magnetic resonance image is negative.[120]

Chemotherapy

Chemotherapy has evolved as an attractive means to minimize the amount of radiation needed to effectively treat children with pineal region tumors. As with radiotherapy, the response to chemotherapy for patients with pineal region tumors varies according to tumor histology. Germ cell tumors have been historically more sensitive to chemotherapy than pineal cell tumors.

Germinomas and nongerminomatous germ cell tumors have showed response rates ranging from 80% to 100% with platinum-based regimens[40] (Fig. 22–13). Patients with

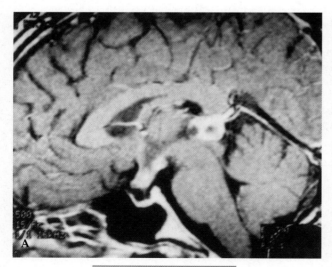 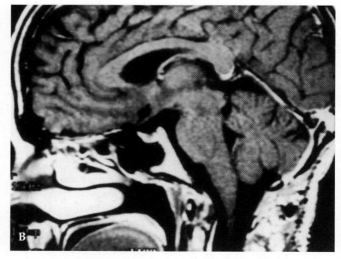

Figure 22–13 Gadolinium-enhanced sagittal magnetic resonance image of a patient with a mixed germ cell tumor before (A) and after (B) treatment with a platinum-based chemotherapy regimen.

extracranial nongerminomatous germ cell tumors respond well to treatment with a wide array of chemotherapeutic agents. Patients with intracranial nongerminomatous germ cell tumors have shown response rates up to 78% with some regimens.[127] The Einhorn regimen, which included cisplastin, vinblastine, and bleomycin, and later substituted etoposide for vinblastine and bleomycin, has been used with some success.[58, 128] Several ongoing studies are attempting to determine the optimal sequence of adjuvant therapy for children with nongerminomatous germ cell tumors.[129] Presently, these children are treated with a course of chemotherapy prior to irradiation.

The dramatic success of radiotherapy in treating children with germinomas has precluded extensive consideration of chemotherapy as a first-line treatment in older children.[99] *Chemotherapy should only be considered a first-line treatment in very young children.* Some authors advocate treating children with chemotherapy prior to irradiation in an effort to reduce radiation exposure and its associated morbidity.[130] Currently, most clinicians advocate that a derivative of Einhorn's regimen be used in patients with recurrent or metastatic germinomas, but not as a first-line treatment. Some clinicians advocate use of chemotherapy as well as radiotherapy after diagnosis of nongerminomatous germ cell tumors.[127] The impetus for adding chemotherapy initially in these patients comes from the 5-year survival rate of 30 to 65% in children with nongerminomatous germ cell tumors treated with radiotherapy alone.[63, 99]

The reported effectiveness of chemotherapeutic regimens for children with pineal cell tumors is limited to anecdotal case reports and reported series involving small numbers of patients.[131] No dominant agent has evolved as the drug of choice, and treatment regimens have included various combinations of vincristine, lomustine, cisplatin, etoposide, cyclophosphamide, actinomycin D, and methotrexate. Recently, high-dose cyclophosphamide has been advocated as a single-agent protocol in the treatment of children with pineoblastomas.[132] In their 1996 study, Ashley and colleagues demonstrated that children treated with high-dose cyclophosphamide had stable or diminishing disease while on protocol. Impaired pulmonary function and thrombocytopenia were notable side effects.

Radiosurgery

Stereotactic radiation or radiosurgery is being increasingly applied to patients with CNS disease.[133–135] Currently, the experience with radiosurgery and pineal region tumor patient is limited. Manera and colleagues have described 11 patients with pineal region tumors treated with stereotactic radiosurgery, all of whom showed a response to treatment without preemptive whole-brain radiation.[136] In the pediatric population, radiosurgery is an attractive potential first-line treatment that merits further investigation. Radiosurgery is currently optimized for targets less than or equal to 3 cm, which would preclude treatment of some patients with larger pineal region tumors. As experience with radiosurgery grows, it might become a useful modality in the treatment of tumor recurrence.

BOX 22–11
Clinical Sequelae of Pineal Region Tumors

- Hydrocephalus
- Parinaud's syndrome (vertical gaze palsy, pupillary paresis)
- Mydriasis
- Convergence spasm
- Pupillary inequality
- Convergence nystagmus
- Ataxia
- Dysmetria
- Diabetes insipidus
- Precocious puberty
- Secondary amenorrhea
- Growth arrest

FOLLOW-UP, PROGNOSIS, AND MANAGEMENT OF RECURRENCES

Lifelong follow-up of children with pineal region tumors is required.[39, 120] These tumors can recur locally or appear distally as late as 5 years after diagnosis. In addition, patients who have received irradiation can present later in life with new tumor formation (i.e., meningioma).[118] MRI scans should be obtained on a periodic basis as determined by tumor histology of original diagnosis, extent of resection, and presence of metastasis at time of diagnosis. Tumor marker studies for patients with germ cell tumors should also be performed on a periodic basis even if markers were normal at diagnosis. The prognosis is dependent on tumor histology and subject to change as more effective adjuvant therapy is developed. In general, patients with intracranial germinomas have an excellent prognosis because of the radiosensitivity of these tumors. *Children with nongerminomatous germ cell tumors have a significantly worse prognosis than children with germinomas, as do children with pineal cell tumors.* There is no conventional approach to managing recurrence. Chemotherapy, radiotherapy, or radiosurgery can be applied if maximal doses have not already been administered. A second surgical procedure is generally reserved for patients with benign lesions who demonstrate recurrence several years later.[39, 137] Recurrent germ cell tumors have been shown to respond to chemotherapy as have some pineal cell tumors, though to a lesser degree.[99] Radiosurgery may be a consideration for all recurrences less than 3 cm in diameter.

SUMMARY

Pineal region tumors represent a rare but challenging problem in pediatric neurosurgery. Therapeutic and diagnostic advances in several disciplines have significantly improved the prognosis of children with these lesions. Current clinical and basic science research will help refine therapies and further augment survival rates while lowering morbidity.

REFERENCES

1. Zulch KJ. Reflections on the surgery of the pineal gland (a glimpse into the past). Gleanings from medical history. *Neurosurg Rev* 1981;4:159–163.
2. Borit A. History of tumors of the pineal region. *Am J Surg Pathol* 1981;5:613–620.
3. Dandy W. Operative experience in cases of pineal tumor. *Arch Surg* 1936;33:19–46.
4. Camins MB, Schlesinger EB. Treatment of tumours of the posterior part of the third ventricle and the pineal region: a long term follow-up. *Acta Neurochir* 1978;40:131–143.
5. Van Wagenen W. A surgical approach for removal of certain pineal tumors: report of a case. *Surg Gynecol Obstet* 1931;53:216.
6. Torkildsen A. Should extirpation be attempted in cases of neoplasms in or near the third ventricle of the brain. Experiences with a palliative method. *J Neurosurg* 1948;5:269.
7. Edwards MS, Hudgins RJ, Wilson CB, et al. Pineal region tumors in children. *J Neurosurg* 1988;68:689–697.
8. Rowland J, Glidewell O, Sibley R, et al. Effects of different forms of central nervous system prophylaxis on neuropsychologic function in childhood leukemia. *J Clin Oncol* 1984;2:1327–1335.
9. Erlich SS, Apuzzo ML. The pineal gland: anatomy, physiology, and clinical significance. *J Neurosurg* 1985;63:321–341.
10. Quest D, Kleriga E. Microsurgical anatomy of the pineal region. *Neurosurgery* 1980;6:385–390.
11. Bruce J, Tamarkin L, Riedel C, et al. Sequential cerebrospinal fluid and plasma sampling in humans: 24-hour melatonin measurements in normal subjects and after peripheral sympathectomy. *J Clin Endocrinol Metab* 1991;72:819–823.
12. Ringertz N, Nordenstam H, Flyger G. Tumors of the pineal region. *J Neuropathol Exp Neurol* 1954;13:540–561.
13. Bruce J, Stein B, Fetell M. Tumors of the pineal region. In: Rowland L, ed. *Merrit's Textbook of Neurology*. Baltimore: Williams & Wilkins; 1995:359–367.
14. Posner M, Horrax G. Eye signs in pineal tumors. *J Neurosurg* 1946;3:15–24.
15. Fetell MR, Stein BM. Neuroendocrine aspects of pineal tumors. *Neurol Clin North Am* 1986;4:877–905.
16. Krabbe K. The pineal gland, especially in relation to the problem on its supposed significance in sexual development. *Endocrinology* 1923;7:379–414.
17. Zondek H, Kaatz A, Unger H. Precocious puberty and choriepithelioma of the pineal gland with report of a case. *J Endocrinol* 1953;10:12–16.
18. Takeuchi J, Handa H, Nagata I. Suprasellar germinoma. *J Neurosurg* 1978;49:41–48.
19. Steinbok P, Dolmen C, Kaan K. Pineocytomas presenting as subarachnoid hemorrhage: report of two cases. *J Neurosurg* 1977;47:776–780.
20. Burres K, Hamilton R. Pineal apoplexy. *Neurosurgery* 1979;4:264–268.
21. Bruce J, Stein B. Supracerebellar approaches in the pineal region. In: Apuzzo M, ed. *Brain Surgery: Complication Avoidance and Management*. New York: Churchill Livingstone; 1993:511–536.
22. Tien RD, Barkovich AJ, Edwards MS. MR imaging of pineal tumors. *Am J Roentgenol* 1990;155:143–151.
23. Smirniotopoulos JG, Rushing EJ, Mena H. Pineal region masses: differential diagnosis. *RadioGraphics* 1992;12:577–596.
24. Zee CS, Segall H, Apuzzo M, et al. MR imaging of pineal region neoplasms. *J Comput Assist Tomogr* 1991;15:56–63.
25. Chang T, Teng MM, Guo WY, Sheng WC. CT of pineal tumors and intracranial germ-cell tumors. *Am J Roentgenol* 1989;153:1269–1274.
26. Bruce JN, Stein BM. Pineal tumors. *Neurosurg Clin North Am* 1990;1:123–138.
27. Muller-Forell W, Schroth G, Egan PJ. MR imaging in tumors of the pineal region. *Neuroradiology* 1988;30:224–231.
28. Zimmerman R. Pineal region masses: radiology. In: Wilkins R, Rengachary S, eds. *Neurosurgery*. Vol. 1. New York: McGraw-Hill; 1985:680–686.
29. Bruce JN, Stein BM. Surgical management of pineal region tumors. *Acta Neurochir* 1995;134:130–135.
30. Sawaya R, Hawley D, Tobler W, et al. Pineal and third ventricle tumors. In: Youmans J, ed. *Neurological Surgery*. Philadelphia: WB Saunders; 1990:3171–3203.
31. Allen JC, Nisselbaum J, Epstein F, Rosen G, Schwartz MK. Alphafetoprotein and human chorionic gonadotropin determination in cerebrospinal fluid: an aid to the diagnosis and management of intracranial germ-cell tumors. *J Neurosurg* 1979;51:368–374.
32. Jooma R, Kendall BE. Diagnosis and management of pineal tumors. *J Neurosurg* 1983;58:654–665.
33. Arita N, Ushio Y, Hayakawa T, et al. Serum levels of alpha-fetoprotein, human chorionic gonadotropin and carcinoembryonic antigen in patients with primary intracranial germ cell tumors. *Oncodev Biol Med* 1980;1:235–240.
34. Yamashita J, Handa H. Diagnosis and treatment of pineal tumours: Kyoto University experience (1941–1984). *Acta Neurochir Suppl* 1988;42:137–141.
35. Allen JC. Controversies in the management of intracranial germ cell tumors. *Neurol Clin* 1991;9:441–452.
36. Shinoda J, Miwa Y, Sakai N, et al. Immunohistochemical study of placental alkaline phosphatase in primary intracranial germ-cell tumors. *J Neurosurg* 1985;63:733–739.
37. Talerman A. Germ cell tumours. *Ann Pathol* 1985;5:145–157.
38. Wilson ER, Takei Y, Bikoff WT, et al. Abdominal metastases of primary intracranial yolk sac tumors through ventriculoperitoneal shunts: report of three cases. *Neurosurgery* 1979;5:356–364.
39. Bruce J. Management of pineal region tumors. *Neurosurg Q* 1993;103–119.
40. Jennings MT, Gelman R, Hochberg F. Intracranial germ-cell tumors: natural history and pathogenesis. *J Neurosurg* 1985;63:155–167.
41. Haase J, Nielsen K. Value of tumor markers in the treatment of endodermal sinus tumors and choriocarcinomas in the pineal region. *Neurosurgery* 1979;5:485–488.
42. Neuwelt EA, Glasberg M, Frenkel E, Clark WK. Malignant pineal region tumors: a clinico-pathological study. *J Neurosurg* 1979;51:597–607.
43. Yoshida J, Sugita K, Kobayashi T, et al. Prognosis of intracranial germ cell tumours: effectiveness of chemotherapy with cisplatin and etoposide (CDDP and VP-16). *Acta Neurochir* 1993;120:111–117.

44. Neuwelt EA, Mickey B, Lewy AJ. The importance of melatonin and tumor markers in pineal tumors. *J Neural Transm Suppl* 1986;21:397–413.

45. Hoffman HJ, Yoshida M, Becker LE, Hendrick EB, Humphreys RP. Experience with pineal region tumours in childhood. *Neurol Res* 1984;6:107–112.

46. Russell DS, Rubinstein LJ. Tumours of specialized tissues of central neuroepithelial origin. In: Russell DS, Rubinstein LJ, eds. *Pathology of Tumours of the Nervous System.* Baltimore: Williams & Wilkins; 1989.

47. Packer RJ, Sutton LN, Rosenstock JG, et al. Pineal region tumors of childhood. *Pediatrics* 1984;74:97–102.

48. Malogolowkin MH, Mahour GH, Krailo M, Ortega JA. Germ cell tumors in infancy and childhood: a 45-year experience. *Pediatr Pathol* 1990;10:231–241.

49. Giovannelli G. Pineal region tumors: endocrinological aspects. *Child's Brain* 1982;9:267–273.

50. Ahmed SR, Shalet SM, Price DA, Pearson D. Human chorionic gonadotrophin secreting pineal germinoma and precocious puberty. *Arch Dis Child* 1983;58:743–745.

51. Scheithauer BW. Neuropathology of pineal region tumors. *Clin Neurosurg* 1985;32:351–383.

52. Shankar SK, Rao TV, Vidyasagar G, Deshpande DH. Yolk sac tumor of the pineal region. *Indian Pediatr* 1981;18:581–584.

53. Bjornsson J, Scheithauer BW, Okazaki H, Leech RW. Intracranial germ cell tumors: pathobiological and immunohistochemical aspects of 70 cases. *J Neuropathol Exp Neurol* 1985;44:32–46.

54. Steno J, Bizik I, Biksadsky P. Pineal region teratomas in children. *Ann N Y Acad Sci* 1997;824:241–244.

55. Matsutani M, Sano K, Takakura K, et al. Primary intracranial germ cell tumors: a clinical analysis of 153 histologically verified cases. *J Neurosurg* 1997;86:446–455.

56. Raaijmakers C, Wilms G, Demaerel P, Baert AL. Pineal teratocarcinoma with drop metastases: MR features. *Neuroradiology* 1992;34:227–229.

57. Russell DS, Rubinstein LJ. Tumours and tumour-like lesions of maldevelopmental origin. In: Russell DS, Rubinstein LJ, eds. *Pathology of Tumours of the Nervous System.* Baltimore: Williams & Wilkins; 1989:664–765.

58. Calaminus G, Bamberg M, Baranzelli MC, et al. Intracranial germ cell tumors: a comprehensive update of the European data. *Neuropediatrics* 1994;25:26–32.

59. Herrmann HD, Westphal M, Winkler K, et al. Treatment of nongerminomatous germ-cell tumors of the pineal region. *Neurosurgery* 1994;34:524–529; discussion 529.

60. Calaminus G, Andreussi L, Garre ML, et al. Secreting germ cell tumors of the central nervous system (CNS). First results of the cooperative German/Italian pilot study (CNS sGCT). *Klin Padiatr* 1997;209:222–227.

61. Salzman KL, Rojiani AM, Buatti J, et al. Primary intracranial germ cell tumors: clinicopathologic review of 32 cases. *Pediatr Pathol Lab Med* 1997;17:713–727.

62. Eberts TJ, Ransburg RC. Primary intracranial endodermal sinus tumor: case report. *J Neurosurg* 1979;50:246–252.

63. Packer RJ, Sutton LN, Rorke LB, et al. Intracranial embryonal cell carcinoma. *Cancer* 1984;54:520–524.

64. Ferraresi S, Angelini L, Solero CL, et al. Endodermal sinus tumor of the pineal region presenting with a radicular pain. *Eur Neurol* 1986;25:458–460.

65. Felix I, Becker LE. Intracranial germ cell tumors in children: an immunohistochemical and electron microscopic study. *Pediatr Neurosurg* 1990;16:156–162.

66. Olsen MM, Raffensperger JG, Gonzalez-Crussi F, et al. Endodermal sinus tumor: a clinical and pathological correlation. *J Pediatr Surg* 1982;17:832–840.

67. Inoue HK, Naganuma H, Ono N. Pathobiology of intracranial germ-cell tumors: immunochemical, immunohistochemical, and electron microscopic investigations. *J Neurooncol* 1987;5:105–115.

68. Fujii T, Itakura T, Hayashi S, et al. Primary pineal choriocarcinoma with hemorrhage monitored by computerized tomography: case report. *J Neurosurg* 1981;55:484–487.

69. Jouvet A, Fevre-Montange M, Besancon R, et al. Structural and ultrastructural characteristics of human pineal gland, and pineal parenchymal tumors. *Acta Neuropathol* 1994;88:334–348.

70. Stefanko SZ, Manschot WA. Pinealoblastoma with retinoblastomatous differentiation. *Brain* 1979;102:221–232.

71. Min KW, Scheithauer BW, Bauserman SC. Pineal parenchymal tumors: an ultrastructural study with prognostic implications. *Ultrastruct Pathol* 1994;18:69–85.

72. Dudgeon J, Lee WR. The trilateral retinoblastoma syndrome. *Trans Ophthalmol Soc U K* 1983;103:523–529.

73. Brownstein S, de Chadarevian JP, Little JM. Trilateral retinoblastoma: report of two cases. *Arch Ophthalmol* 1984;102:257–262.

74. Finelli DA, Shurin SB, Bardenstein DS. Trilateral retinoblastoma: two variations. *Am J Neuroradiol* 1995;16:166–170.

75. Schild SE, Scheithauer BW, Schomberg PJ, et al. Pineal parenchymal tumors: clinical, pathologic, and therapeutic aspects. *Cancer* 1993;72:870–880.

76. Regis J, Bouillot P, Rouby-Volot F, et al. Pineal region tumors and the role of stereotactic biopsy: review of the mortality, morbidity, and diagnostic rates in 370 cases. *Neurosurgery* 1996;39:907–912; discussion 912–914.

77. Fetell MR, Bruce JN, Burke AM, et al. Nonneoplastic pineal cysts. *Neurology* 1991;41:1034–1040.

78. Bodensteiner JB, Schaefer GB, Keller GM, McConnell JR. Incidental pineal cysts in a prospectively ascertained normal cohort. *Clin Pediatr (Phila)* 1996;35:277–279.

79. Di Costanzo A, Tedeschi G, Di Salle F, Golia F, Morrone R, Bonavita V. Pineal cysts: an incidental MRI finding? *J Neurol Neurosurg Psychiatry* 1993;56:207–208.

80. Fain JS, Tomlinson FH, Scheithauer BW, et al. Symptomatic glial cysts of the pineal gland. *J Neurosurg* 1994;80:454–460.

81. Klein P, Rubinstein LJ. Benign symptomatic glial cysts of the pineal gland: a report of seven cases and review of the literature. *J Neurol Neurosurg Psychiatry* 1989;52:991–995.

82. Fleege MA, Miller GM, Fletcher GP, et al. Benign glial cysts of the pineal gland: unusual imaging characteristics with histologic correlation [see comments]. *Am J Neuroradiol* 1994;15:161–166.

83. Goodman R. Magnetic resonance imaging-directed stereotactic endoscopic third ventriculostomy. *Neurosurgery* 1993;32:1043–1047.

84. Wong TT, Lee LS. A method of enlarging the opening of the third ventricular floor for flexible endoscopic third ventriculostomy. *Child's Nerv Syst* 1996;12:396–398.

85. Ellenbogen RG, Moores LE. Endoscopic management of a pineal and suprasellar germinoma with associated hydrocephalus: technical case report. *Minim Invasive Neurosurg* 1997;40:13–15; discussion 16.

86. Devkota J, Brooks BS, el Gammal T. Ventriculoperitoneal shunt metastasis of a pineal germinoma. *Comput Radiol* 1984;8:141–145.

87. Berger M, Baumeister B, Geyer J, et al The risks of metastases from shunting in children with primary central nervous system tumors. *J Neurosurg* 1991;74:872.

88. Cranston PE, Hatten MT, Smith EE. Metastatic pineoblastoma via a ventriculoperitoneal shunt: CT demonstration. *Comput Med Imaging Graph* 1992;16:349–351.

89. Blasco A, Dominguez P, Ballestin C, et al. Peritoneal implantation of pineal germinoma via a ventriculoperitoneal shunt [letter]. *Acta Cytol* 1993;37:637–638.

90. Gururangan S, Heideman RL, Kovnar EH, et al. Peritoneal metastases in two patients with pineoblastoma and ventriculoperitoneal shunts. *Med Pediatr Oncol* 1994;22:417–420.

91. Rickert CH. Abdominal metastases of pediatric brain tumors via ventriculoperitoneal shunts. *Child's Nerv Syst* 1998;14:10–14.

92. Robinson S, Cohen AR. The role of neuroendoscopy in the treatment of pineal region tumors. *Surg Neurol* 1997;48:360–365; discussion 365–367.

93. Ferrer E, Santamarta D, Garcia-Fructuoso G, et al. Neuroendoscopic management of pineal region tumours. *Acta Neurochir* 1997;139:12–20.

94. Colombo F, Benedetti A, Alexandre A. Stereotactic exploration of deep-seated or surgically unamenable intracranial space-occupying lesions. *J Neurosurg Sci* 1980;24:173–177.

95. Broggi G, Franzini A, Migliavacca F, Allegranza A. Stereotactic biopsy of deep brain tumors in infancy and childhood. *Child's Brain* 1983;10:92–98.

96. Dempsey PK, Kondziolka D, Lunsford LD. Stereotactic diagnosis and treatment of pineal region tumours and vascular malformations [see comments]. *Acta Neurochir* 1992;116:14–22.

97. Kreth FW, Schatz CR, Pagenstecher A, et al. Stereotactic management of lesions of the pineal region. *Neurosurgery* 1996;39:280–289; discussion 289–291.

98. Shokry A, Janzer RC, Von Hochstetter AR, et al. Primary intracranial germ-cell tumors: a clinicopathological study of 14 cases. *J Neurosurg* 1985;62:826–830.

99. Choi JU, Kim DS, Chung SS, Kim TS. Treatment of germ cell tumors in the pineal region. *Child's Nerv Syst* 1998;14:41–48.

100. Sawamura Y, de Tribolet N, Ishii N, Abe H. Management of primary intracranial germinomas: diagnostic surgery or radical resection? *J Neurosurg* 1997;87:262–266.

101. Horrax G. Treatment of tumors of the pineal body: experience in a series of twenty-two cases. *Arch Neurol Psychiatry* 1950;64:227–242.

102. Poppen J. The right occipital approach to a pinealoma. *J Neurosurg* 1966;3:1–8.

103. Stein BM. The infratentorial supracerebellar approach to pineal lesions. *J Neurosurg* 1971;35:197–202.

104. Stein BM. Supracerebellar-infratentorial approach to pineal tumors. *Surg Neurol* 1979;11:331–337.

105. Stein BM. Surgical treatment of pineal tumors. *Clin Neurosurg* 1979;26:490–510.

106. Kobayashi S, Sugita K, Tanaka Y, Kyoshima K. Infratentorial approach to the pineal region in the prone position: Concorde position. Technical note. *J Neurosurg* 1983;58:141–143.

107. Bloomfield S, Sonntag V, Spetzler R. Pineal region lesions. *Barrow Neuro Institute Quart* 1985;1:10–23.

108. Sekhar LN, Goel A. Combined supratentorial and infratentorial approach to large pineal-region meningioma. *Surg Neurol* 1992;37:197–201.

109. Ziyal IM, Sekhar LN, Salas E, Olan WJ. Combined supra/infratentorial–transsinus approach to large pineal region tumors. *J Neurosurg* 1998;88:1050–1057.

110. Stein BM, Bruce JN. Surgical management of pineal region tumors (honored guest lecture). *Clin Neurosurg* 1992;39:509–532.

111. Bruce DA, Allen JC. Tumor staging for pineal region tumors of childhood. *Cancer* 1985;56:1792–1794.

112. Waga S, Handa H, Yamashita J. Intracranial germinomas: treatment and results. *Surg Neurol* 1979;11:167–172.

113. Ueki K, Tanaka R. Treatments and prognoses of pineal tumors—experience of 110 cases. *Neurol Med Chir (Tokyo)* 1980;20:1–26.

114. Smith NJ, El-Mahdi AM, Constable WC. Results of irradiation of tumors in the region of the pineal body. *Acta Radiol Ther Phys Biol* 1976;15:17–22.

115. Griffin BR, Griffin TW, Tong DY, et al. Pineal region tumors: results of radiation therapy and indications for elective spinal irradiation. *Int J Radiat Oncol Biol Phys* 1981;7:605–608.

116. Bendersky M, Lewis M, Mandelbaum DE, Stanger C. Serial neuropsychological follow-up of a child following craniospinal irradiation. *Dev Med Child Neurol* 1988;30:816–820.

117. Avizonis VN, Fuller DB, Thomson JW, et al. Late effects following central nervous system radiation in a pediatric population. *Neuropediatrics* 1992;23:228–234.

118. Starshak RJ. Radiation-induced meningioma in children: report of two cases and review of the literature. *Pediatr Radiol* 1996;26:537–541.

119. Fuller BG, Kapp DS, Cox R. Radiation therapy of pineal region tumors: 25 new cases and a review of 208 previously reported cases. *Int J Radiat Oncol Biol Phys* 1994;28:229–245.

120. Kang JK, Jeun SS, Hong YK, et al. Experience with pineal region tumors. *Child's Nerv Syst* 1998;14:63–68.

121. Dattoli MJ, Newall J. Radiation therapy for intracranial germinoma: the case for limited volume treatment. *Int J Radiat Oncol Biol Phys* 1990;19:429–433.

122. Linstadt D, Wara WM, Edwards MS, Hudgins RJ, Sheline GE. Radiotherapy of primary intracranial germinomas: the case against routine craniospinal irradiation. *Int J Radiat Oncol Biol Phys* 1988;15:291–297.

123. Levin CV, Rutherfoord GS. Metastasizing pineal germinoma: a case report and review. *South Afr Med J* 1985;68:36–39.

124. Takakura K. Intracranial germ cell tumors. *Clin Neurosurg* 1985;32:429–444.

125. Ono N, Isobe I, Uki J, et al. Recurrence of primary intracranial germinomas after complete response with

radiotherapy: recurrence patterns and therapy. *Neurosurgery* 1994;35:615–620; discussion 620–621.

126. Wolden SL, Wara WM, Larson DA, et al. Radiation therapy for primary intracranial germ-cell tumors. *Int J Radiat Oncol Biol Phys* 1995;32:943–949.

127. Chang TK, Wong TT, Hwang B. Combination chemotherapy with vinblastine, bleomycin, cisplatin, and etoposide (VBPE) in children with primary intracranial germ cell tumors. *Med Pediatr Oncol* 1995;24:368–372.

128. Einhorn L, Donohue J. Cis-diaminedichloroplatinum, vinblastine, and bleomycin combination therapy in disseminated testicular cancer. *Ann Intern Med* 1977;87:293–298.

129. Robertson PL, DaRosso RC, Allen JC. Improved prognosis of intracranial non-germinoma germ cell tumors with multimodality therapy. *J Neuro-oncol* 1997;32:71–80.

130. Allen JC, DaRosso RC, Donahue B, Nirenberg A. A phase II trial of preirradiation carboplatin in newly diagnosed germinoma of the central nervous system. *Cancer* 1994;74:940–944.

131. Jakacki RI, Zeltzer PM, Boyett JM, et al. Survival and prognostic factors following radiation and/or chemotherapy for primitive neuroectodermal tumors of the pineal region in infants and children: a report of the Children's Cancer Group. *J Clin Oncol* 1995;13:1377–1383.

132. Ashley DM, Longee D, Tien R, et al. Treatment of patients with pineoblastoma with high dose cyclophosphamide. *Med Pediatr Oncol* 1996;26:387–392.

133. Backlund EO. Radiosurgery in intracranial tumors and vascular malformations. *J Neurosurg Sci* 1989;33:91–93.

134. Brada M. Radiosurgery for brain tumours. *Eur J Cancer* 1991;27:1545–1548.

135. Goodman ML. Gamma knife radiosurgery: current status and review. *South Med J* 1990;83:551–554.

136. Manera L, Regis J, Chinot O, et al. Pineal region tumors: the role of stereotactic radiosurgery. *Stereotact Funct Neurosurg* 1996;66:164–173.

137. Stein BM, Fetell MR. Therapeutic modalities for pineal region tumors. *Clin Neurosurg* 1985;32:445–455.

Chapter 23

Phakomatoses

David M. Weitman and Philip H. Cogen

The term *phakoma*, translated from the Greek as "mother spot" or freckle, was first used by Van der Hoeve, a Dutch ophthalmologist, during the 1920s to describe the benign retinal lesions seen in tuberous sclerosis. Subsequently, the term has been expanded to include other lesions of the retina, and those diseases in which retinal hamartomas are commonly seen are now referred to as phakomatoses. This diverse group of syndromes is identified by the presence of both hamartomas and true neoplasms involving all three primary germ layers. All of the phakomatoses associated with intracranial and intraspinal neoplasia demonstrate cutaneous signatures. Neurofibromatosis, the most common phakomatosis, is covered in Chapter 32 of this text. Most of the phakomatoses are hereditable, with a high rate of spontaneous mutation and penetrance (Table 23–1). Tumor suppressor genes appear to play an important role in the onset of tumorigenesis associated with these diseases.

BOX 23–1
The Phakomatoses

- **Tuberous sclerosis (Bourneville's syndrome)**
- **Von Hippel–Lindau disease**
- **Basal cell nevus (Gorlin's syndrome)**
- **Ataxia-telangiectasia (Louis-Bar syndrome)**
- **Neurocutaneous melanosis**

TUBEROUS SCLEROSIS (BOURNEVILLE'S SYNDROME)

Tuberous sclerosis (TS), an autosomal dominant disease, has cutaneous, visceral, ophthalmologic, and neurologic manifestations. Although von Recklinghausen first described the typical complex of symptoms in 1862, the disease bears the name of the French physician who published the first case studies. Bourneville initially used the term "tuberous sclerosis" to describe the firm nodules of the cerebral cortex characteristically associated with the disease. Children with TS may be identified by occurrence of both hamartomas and true neoplasms affecting multiple organs. Neuronal migration anomalies may also contribute to developmental and central nervous system (CNS) impairment.

Although TS is an autosomal dominant disorder, as many as 60% of cases arise via spontaneous mutations. Variable penetrance may be identified even in a single kinship. There have been several reports of clinically and radiographically normal parents with two affected children, suggesting that the gene may be nonpenetrating in some cases.[1,2] The prevalence of TS is difficult to ascertain due to symptom variability, but studies suggest a frequency of 1 in 9400 and a yearly incidence of 0.56 cases per 100,000.[3] Children with few of the clinical stigmata of TS who represent a *forme fruste* of the disease may lead to underreporting of actual prevalence.

The diagnosis of TS was initially based on clinical findings. *The classic triad described by Vogt*[4] *includes adenoma sebaceum, seizures, and mental retardation.* Subsequent studies

---

TABLE 23–1 Genetics of the Phakomatoses Associated with CNS Tumors, Excluding Neurofibromatosis

Disease	Inheritance pattern	Genetic loci		Ref.
Tuberous sclerosis	Autosomal dominant	TSC-1	9q34	19
		TSC-2	16p13.3	40
von Hippel–Lindau disease	Autosomal dominant	VHL	3p25–26	67
Basal cell nevus syndrome	Autosomal dominant	BCNS	9q	76
Ataxia-telangiectasia	Autosomal recessive	ATM	11q23	80

have shown that fewer than one third of patients show these signs as the sole manifestation of their TS. The factors identified by the Diagnostic Criteria Committee of the National Tuberous Sclerosis Association[4] include primary, secondary, and tertiary features of the disease (Table 23–2). Thus, the diagnosis of TS is based on the fulfillment of primary, secondary, and/or tertiary criteria.

Clinical Presentation

Cutaneous Signs

TS is most frequently identified in late childhood because some of the most typical criteria for diagnosis do not develop until then. These factors include facial angiofibromas, ungual fibromas, and renal angiomyolipomas. Earliest disease manifestations, which may be present at birth, include hypomelanocytic macules on the trunk,[5] tufts of white scalp hair,[6] and depigmented areas of the iris,[7] although none of these signs is specific for TS. The forehead plaque, a lesion similar to the raised subepidermal fibrous proliferation called a shagreen patch, may be identified at birth and is more specific for TS; however, it occurs less often than other skin manifestations.[8]

Cardiac Signs

Some children may present initially with symptoms referable to their visceral lesions. *Large intraventricular cardiac rhabdomyomata may present with heart failure*[9] *and smaller lesions may cause arrhythmias.*[10] Two children have been reported with cardiac rhabdomyomata who developed heart block after carbamazepine administration,[11, 12] and two neonates have been described who died during craniotomies for tumor resection from refractory arrhythmias caused by cardiac rhabdomyomas.[13] There is also a case reported of a cerebral embolus with brain infarction secondary to cardiac tumor(s) in a 19-month-old.[14] Cardiac rhabdomyomata identified by fetal ultrasonography may identify TS prenatally.[15]

Renal Signs

Children with TS rarely present with renal symptoms; in a series of 139 patients, 61% were found to have renal angiomyolipomas (49%), cysts (32%), and carcinoma (2.2%).[16] Isolated tumors of the kidney have also been reported as a *forme fruste* of TS.[17] Cysts in the kidney are more prevalent in children and may present with obstructive nephropathy and renal failure.[18]

Neurologic Signs

The myriad of neurologic signs and symptoms in TS include seizures, hemiplegia, and hemianopsia. Up to 80% of children with TS manifest developmental delay. Cognitive delay in children with TS correlates strongly with an early onset of seizures, although the causal relationship between these findings is unclear. Associated abnormalities of behavior include autism, attention deficit–hyperactivity disorder, and learning disabilities.[19] Seizure types seen in children with TS include infantile spasms and/or partial motor or complex partial epilepsy with or without secondary generalization. Infantile spasms are generally associated with a poor prognosis.

TABLE 23–2 Diagnostic Criteria for Tuberous Sclerosis Complex

Primary features
    Facial angiofibromas[a]
    Multiple ungual fibromas[a]
    Cortical tuber (histologic confirmation)
    Subependymal nodule or giant cell astrocytoma (histologic confirmation)
    Multiple calcified subependymal nodules protruding into the ventricle (radiographic evidence)
    Multiple retinal astrocytomas[a]

Secondary features
    Affected first-degree relative
    Cardiac rhabdomyoma (histologic or radiographic confirmation)
    Other retinal hamartoma or achromatic patch[a]
    Cerebral tubers (radiographic confirmation)
    Noncalcified subependymal nodule (radiographic confirmation)
    Shagreen patch[a]
    Forehead plaque[a]
    Pulmonary lymphangiomyomatosis (histologic confirmation)
    Renal angiomyolipoma (radiographic or histologic confirmation)
    Renal cysts (histologic confirmation)

Tertiary features
    Hypomelanotic macules[a]
    "Confetti" skin lesions[a]
    Renal cysts (radiographic confirmation)
    Randomly distributed enamel pits in deciduous and/or permanent teeth
    Hamartomatous rectal polyps (histologic confirmation)
    Bone cysts (radiographic confirmation)
    Pulmonary lymphangiomyomatosis (radiographic confirmation)
    Cerebral white-matter "migration tracts" or heterotopias (radiographic evidence)
    Gingival fibromas[a]
    Hamartoma of other organs (histologic confirmation)
    Infantile spasms

Definite TSC: Either one primary feature, two secondary features, or one secondary plus two tertiary features
Probable TSC: Either one secondary plus one tertiary feature, or three tertiary features
Suspect TSC: Either one secondary feature or two tertiary features

[a] Histologic confirmation is not required if the lesion is clinically obvious.
TSC, tuberous sclerosis complex
Reprinted from Roach ES, Smith M, Huttenlocher P, et al. Diagnostic criteria: tuberous sclerosis complex. *J Child Neurol* 1992;7:223, with permission.

A study of 24 patients with infantile spasms showed that all but one developed chronic epilepsy, and none had normal development.[20] Seizures associated with TS may be medically refractory.[21] Isolated hemiparesis and hemiplegia without mass effect appear infrequently, seen in only 2 of 8 patients in one series[3] and 2 of 10 patients in another.[21] A rare presentation of TS in neonates is the early identification of an intracranial tumor. These infants may be relatively asymptomatic, presenting with megalencephaly, or manifest signs and symptoms of raised intracranial pressure or seizures.[13, 22, 23] The development of acute hydrocephalus and intracranial hypertension from intraventricular lesions is uncommon in older children[24] because tumor growth tends to be slow.

BOX 23–2
Neurologic Presentation

- **Seizures**
- **Hemiplegia**
- **Hemianopsia**
- **Developmental delay**
- **Behavioral abnormalities including autism, attention deficit–hyperactivity disorder**
- **Intracranial tumor**
- **Hydrocephalus**

Ocular Signs

Both microphthalmos and exophthalmos may be seen in children with TS, as may pain from intraocular tumor growth.[25] Retinal tumors rarely affect vision. Retinal phakomas identified fundoscopically have been reported in up to 87% of children with TS.[26] These lesions are characteristically flat pale plaques, but they may also show achromatic areas or astrocytic proliferation ("mulberry astrocytoma").

Diagnosis

The diagnosis of TS has been improved by the use of magnetic resonance imaging (MRI). Prior to the advent of these techniques, skull radiographs were used to identify intracerebral calcifications, and pneumoencephalography or contrast ventriculography revealed subependymal nodules or intraventricular tumors. With current imaging techniques, less than 5% of children with TS will have a normal scan.[27] On computed tomography (CT) (Fig. 23–1), TS typically presents with subependymal nodules that may or may not be calcified, numbering into the twenties. Calcified nodules associated with TS may appear in the first few weeks of life. On nonenhanced CT scans, they appear hyperdense relative to gray matter.[27] They typically do not enhance unless they become subependymal giant cell astrocytomas.[28]

CT Findings

Cortical tubers are often difficult to identify on CT scan. They may be seen as calcifications within an expanded gyrus that does not contrast-enhance. Cortical tubers are usually hypodense in comparison with gray matter.[27] TS lesions seen in the white matter may be calcified and/or hypodense on CT scan (Fig. 23–1). Similar posterior fossa lesions may be seen in approximately 10% of patients, always accompanied by supratentorial findings. Subependymal giant cell astrocytomas are most often hyperdense in comparison with brain on nonenhanced CT scans, and show intense contrast enhancement.[13, 22, 23] These are the lesions most commonly associated with obstructive hydrocephalus. Not infrequently, children with TS show ventriculomegaly without frank obstruction,[29] perhaps the result of impaired absorption due to increased CSF protein or cells.

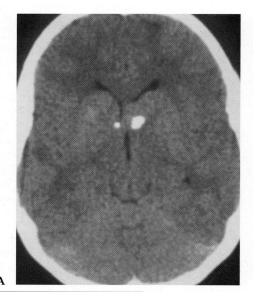
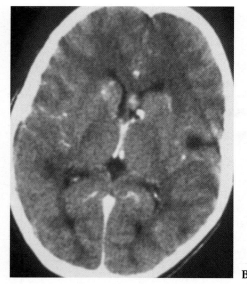

A   B

Figure 23–1 Computed tomography scan without (A) and with (B) the administration of contrast in a 9-year-old girl with tuberous sclerosis. Note the presence of numerous small calcified nodules at both foramen of Monro.

- **Subependymal nodules**
  - **Hypodense**
  - **With or without calcium deposits**
- **Subependymal giant cell astrocytoma**
  - **Enhance**
  - **Hyperdense**
  - **Hydrocephalus**
- **Cortical tubules**
  - **Calcium deposits**
  - **No enhancement**

MRI Findings

The most sensitive radiographic study for the diagnosis of TS is gadolinium-enhanced MRI[30] (Fig. 23–2). Cortical tubers appear as focally expanded gyri, which do not enhance. Frequently, tubers are of high signal intensity on all sequences, although they may appear hypointense compared with gray matter on T1-weighted imaging. Cortical tubers are most common in the frontal lobes, followed by the parietal, occipital, and temporal lobes, and lastly the cerebellum. Subependymal nodules, usually bilateral, are located in the ventricles near the foramina of Monro, measuring 10 to 15 mm in diameter. These non–contrast-enhancing nodules show variable signal intensity on both T1- and T2-weighted sequences. Other white matter lesions in TS are also seen on magnetic resonance images, including bands of abnormal signal intensity radiating from the ventricles to the cortical mantle and/or wedge-shaped lesions with their apex at the ven-

tricle and their base at a cortical tuber. White matter mass lesions appear less often; they are hyperintense on T2-weighted images and hypo- to isointense on T1-weighted images after completion of myelination. A reverse pattern of intensities may be seen in infants owing to immature myelin development.[31] Subependymal giant cell astrocytomas are typically hypointense compared with white matter on T1-weighted images, hyperintense on T2-weighted images, and densely contrast enhancing with gadolinium injection (Fig. 23–2). Signal characterisitics may be changed by intratumoral cyst formation or hemorrhage.[23]

- **Cortical tubers**
  - **Expanded**
  - **No enhancement**
  - **Often high signal**
  - **Frontal > parietal > occipital**
- **Subependymal nodules**
  - **Bilateral**
  - **Intraventricular (near foramen of Monro)**
  - **Variable signal intensity**
- **White matter lesions**
  - **Bands of abnormal signal intensity**
  - **Wedge-shaped lesions**
- **Subependymal giant cell astrocytoma**
  - **Hypointense on T1-weighted images**
  - **Hyperintense on T2-weighted images**
  - **Contrast enhancement**

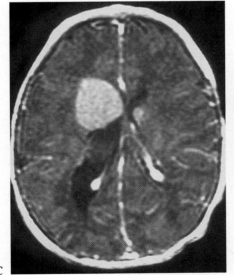 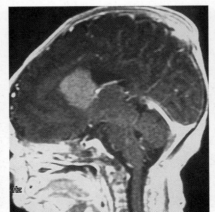 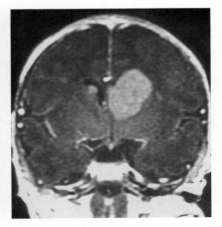

A–C

Figure 23–2   Gadolinium-enhanced T1 images in the axial (A), sagittal (B), and coronal planes of a newborn girl with prenatally diagnosed tuberous sclerosis. The presence of this lesion, a subependymal giant cell astrocytoma, on the fetal ultrasound made the diagnosis.

EEG Findings

Electroencephalographic findings identified in TS may include hyposarrhythmia in children with infantile spasms and/or spike-and-wave patterns as seen in other types of epilepsy. The scalp electroencephalographic and electrocorticographic abnormalities in TS may be more extensive than the radiographic lesions.[21]

Clinical Features

TS, a disorder of cellular migration and differentiation affecting all three germinal layers, is thus identified by the presence of hamartomas in the skin, CNS, and viscera. Although malignancies are rare, an increased incidence of renal cell carcinomas in TS patients has been reported.[32] *The facial angiofibromata (adenoma sebaceum) rarely occur before the age of 3 years, however, they are ultimately present in approximately 50% of patients.* These facial angiofibromata consist of fibrovascular tissue that does not include the sebaceous glands, and they are not adenomata. *The peri-/subungual fibromas are fleshy lesions in the nail beds of the fingers or toes. Present in approximately 15 to 20% of patients, multiple peri-/subungual fibromas are pathognomonic for TS. Shagreen patches, which are raised, irregular lesions of subepidermal fibrous tissue, are most often found on the back or flank in 20 to 35% of adult patients. Earliest cutaneous manifestations of TS are hypopigmented macules of the trunk, identified in 70 to 80% of patients and best seen with a Woods ultraviolet lamp.* The classic "ash leaf" macule is usually found on the trunk, is round or irregularly shape, and is present at times in a confetti pattern. Hypopigmented macular lesions in TS show a normal number of melanocytes, with a decreased amount of melanin in the melanophores.

BOX 23–5
Cutaneous Manifestations

- Facial angiofibroma (30%)
- Subungual fibromas (15 to 30%)
- Shagreen patches (20 to 35%)
- Hypopigmented macules on the trunk (70 to 80%)

Ocular Signs

Retinal hamartomas, common ocular manifestations of TS reported in as many as 87% of patient,[8] consist of a benign astrocytic proliferation. There is a single case report of a histologically confirmed retinal giant cell true astrocytoma.[9] Although solitary retinal hamartomas may be identified either sporadically or in other disorders, multiple retinal hamartomas are pathognomonic for TS. Depigmented regions of the iris, another manifestation of TS, are likely the ocular correlates of hypomelanotic skin macules. TS-associated visceral lesions include cardiac rhabdomyomata, pulmonary lymphangiomyomatosis, renal cysts and angiomyolipomata, hamartomatous rectal polyps, bone cysts, and pitting of the tooth enamel. When identified alone, these abnormalities are not pathognomonic for TS, although some patients with these abnormalities will subsequently develop TS. Multiples of these tumors are also diagnostic of TS. These visceral hamartomas are composed of smooth muscle and mature fat and blood vessels that will enlarge over time and are rarely seen in children. *Renal involvement has been shown in 50 to 80% of patients with TS, and approximately 50% of patients with renal angiomyolipomas will subsequently be diagnosed with TS.[10, 33] The cardiac rhabdomyomata seen in TS generally diminish in size or even disappear with advancing age.[11, 34]* Cardiac rhabdomyomata, the most common tumors of the heart in children, are seen in approximately 50% of children with TS.[35] Fifty to eighty percent of children with cardiac rhabdomyoma will eventually be diagnosed with TS.[10, 36]

Lymphangioleiomyomatosis of the lungs is seen in female patients with TS; the reason for this sexual dimorphism is unknown. Although lesions may be identified as early as age 3 months,[37] they usually present at an older age.

Lymphangioleiomyomatosis consists of proliferation of smooth muscle cells in the lungs and interstitial infiltrates and cystic changes in the air spaces.

Pathologic Features

Grossly, cortical tubers appear as firm, expanded gyri (Fig. 23–3A), and their cut surface shows a homogeneous appearance with loss of the gray/white matter interface.

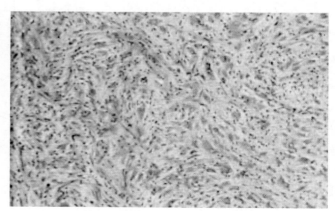

A   B

Figure 23–3 Common pathology in tuberous sclerosis. (A) Cortical tuber. (B) Subependymal giant cell astrocytoma.

Microscopically, tubers also show loss of the normal columnar and lamellated cytoarchitecture. Regions of fibrillary astrocytes alternate with areas of immature neurons, with loss of cellular orientation. Occasionally, giant cells of probable neuronal origin are identified. Subependymal nodules (SENs; Fig. 23–3) frequently calcify and contain primarily glial fibrillary acidic protein (GFAP) staining cells. Large and bizarre-appearing astrocytes may be seen. *The difference between the SEN and the subependymal giant cell astrocytoma (SGCA) is the tendency of the latter to enlarge and to contrast-enhance on both CT and MR images.* The histologic features of these lesions are identical. Six to fifteen percent of patients with TS develop SGCAs.[38, 30] Although a histologically confirmed SGCA has been considered pathognomonic for TS, reports of patients with this tumor who do not manifest any of the other stigmata of the disease[39] suggest a *forme fruste* of TS. SGCAs consist of giant cells, gemistocytic astrocytes, interspersed neurons, and occasional ganglion cells. The cells typically stain positively for GFAP and may contain Rosenthal fibers. These tumors are generally benign, despite their pleomorphic appearance, areas of necrosis, and/or presence of mitoses or endothelial proliferation. Although it has been suggested that SGCAs arise from SENs,[28] it is unclear if postoperative tumor recurrence results from slow regrowth of residual tumor or nascent growth from a SEN. The white matter lesions of TS include focal gray matter heterotopias, hypomyelinated areas, and regions of gliosis, which frequently underlie a cortical abnormality.

BOX 23–6
Pathologic Features

- **Subependymal nodules**
  - **Calcium deposits**
  - **Positive staining for GFAP antibodies**
  - **Large and bizarre astrocytes**
- **Subependymal giant cell astrocytoma**
  - **Giant cells**
  - **Gemistocytic astrocytes**
  - **Interspersed neurons**
  - **Occasional ganglion cells**
- **White matter lesions**
  - **Focal gray matter heterotopias**
  - **Hypomyelination**
  - **Gliosis**

Genetic Localization

There appear to be at least two distinct genetic loci associated with TS. The *TSC-1* gene (tuberous sclerosis complex) has been mapped to chromosome 9q34,[19] whereas *TSC-2* is located at 16p13.3.[40] Genetic linkage studies have shown familial cases to be evenly distributed between the two loci.[41] Although it has been suggested that patients with *TSC-2* mutations show more severe manifestations of the disease,[42] this remains unclear.[43] The 180-kDa product of the *TSC-2* gene, a protein called tuberin, is expressed in many tissue types.[43] Tuberin appears to stimulate the GTPase activity of RAP1A, a RAS-related protein; patients with *TSC-2* mutations may show constitutive activity of the protein.[44] The *TSC-1* gene product has yet to be identified. Both of the TS genes appear to act as tumor suppressors, with inactivation of both copies producing the disease phenotype.[45] Although hamartomas from the same patient may show different gene mutations, they are always in the same TS gene, suggesting that both germline and somatic deletion and/or mutation result in hamartomatous change. It is likely that, in addition to controlling cellular proliferation, both TS genes play a role in cell migration and differentiation.

Treatment

After the diagnosis of TS, it is recommended that children undergo MRI every 1 to 2 years to monitor the progress of hydrocephalus, track previously identified lesions, and detect new structural pathologic processes.[46] While the timing and indications for neurosurgical treatment in TS are variable, surgery is necessary to relieve increased intracranial pressure from tumors. The excision of intracranial neoplasms following a documented growth increase unassociated with significant mass effect or intracranial hypertension may be warranted. Proponents of early surgical intervention have argued that rapid deterioration of patients from obstructive hydrocephalus due to a mass lesion is avoided, and resection more easily achieved, with a smaller bulk.[47] Although prior studies showed a relatively high operative mortality,[48] the institution of newer surgical approaches and techniques and the introduction of the operating microscope have significantly improved the outcome of surgery. Several studies have shown no operative deaths or new neurologic deficits in four patients following resection of SGCAs from the region of the foramen of Monro.[49, 50] Those children whose intracranial tumors are consistent with the diagnosis of TS should undergo a careful examination for other disease stigmata. Children with a high likelihood of TS should also undergo preoperative evaluation to exclude the presence of a cardiac rhabdomyoma.[13]

The two most common approaches to the foramen of Monro are the frontal transcortical approach[51] and the transcallosal approach. Ventricular dilation promotes access to the tumor, and bilateral lesions may be removed through a unilateral craniotomy if there is significant hydrocephalus. Frameless-guided stereotaxy may be an important adjunct to either technique. The transcallosal approach, which avoids a cortical incision and provides direct ventricular access, is preferred by the authors for most tumor resections. Although SGCAs may be highly vascular, complete resection results in hemostasis. Hydrocephalus is frequently encountered in TS with or without obstructing lesions. Ventricular enlargement may result from poor CSF absorption or CSF overproduction. In one series,[29] hydrocephalus in the absence of SGCA was seen in 2 of 18 TS patients, both treated with ventriculoperitoneal shunts. When hydrocephalus is the result of ventricular obstruction by an SGCA, CSF flow is often restored following tumor resection, obviating the need for a permanent shunt. An external ventricular drain may be left following resective surgery prior to the determination of the adequacy of CSF flow. The improvement in operative technique, benign clinical course of these tumors, and unproven efficacy and side effects of ionizing radiation on the developing brain mitigate against the use of therapeutic irradiation.

For children with TS whose seizures are medically refractory and arise from a focal hemispheric lesion, such as a large cortical tuber or dysplasia, surgery may be beneficial. Perot et al.[52] described three patients with a *forme fruste* of TS whose seizures improved following removal of dysplastic cortex. Subsequently, Palmini et al.[53] reviewed the outcome of surgical resection for medically refractory epilepsy associated with cortical migrational lesions: 10 of 26 patients had a *forme fruste* of TS. Of the 8 evaluable patients, however, only 2 had a good or excellent outcome, defined by a major seizure reduction of 90% or greater, and 3 patients showed a less than 50% reduction in frequency. These results are probably due to the observation that the epileptogenic region of the brain defined either by scalp electroencephalography or intraoperative electrocorticography was more extensive than the structural lesions seen on imaging studies. Furthermore, the outcome was better associated with resection of an extensive structural lesion than an epileptogenic area of cortex. *Thus, patients with TS who show extensive brain abnormalities are unsatisfactory candidates for seizure surgery, although a discrete cortical epileptogenic lesion may be amenable to operative management.*

Little has been reported on life expectancy in TS, although the death rate has been shown to be increased for all patients. Of 355 Mayo Clinic patients with TS evaluated by Shepherd et al.,[38] 49 were deceased, 9 of whom expired from unrelated causes. The largest number of TS-related deaths were the result of renal failure (11 patients), followed closely by the complications of SGCAs (10 patients), including 4 who died from treatment. *The most common cause of death in children aged 10 to 19 years was a brain tumor.* Nine of 13 patients with severe mental deficiency died from presumed status epilepticus, ascertained from the death certificate without postmortem examination. Improved diagnostic studies, including prenatal screening, and newer treatment modalities should positively impact the future outcome of TS.

VON HIPPEL–LINDAU DISEASE (VHL)

Von Hippel–Lindau disease (VHL), a rare autosomal dominant genetic disorder with a high degree of penetrance, results in tumors of the CNS and viscera. *Although VHL is included among the phakomatoses because of the ocular and visceral findings, there is no cutaneous signature.* The first two patients were described by von Hippel in 1904, and Lindau was the first to associate retinal tumors with CNS lesions. VHL may be manifest in the kidneys, adrenals, lungs, liver, and pancreas. *The types of lesions associated with VHL include hemangioblastomas, pheochromocytomas (Fig. 23–4), renal and pancreatic cancers and cysts, and epididymal cysts.*

Epidemiologic Factors

The true incidence of the disease has been difficult to estimate because there is clustering of cases within families, and sporadic cases of VHL are rarely diagnosed before the age of 25 years. One study from East Anglia, England, estimates the incidence of VHL to be 1 in 36,000 live births, with a minimum heterozygote prevalence of 1 in 53,000 population,[54] similar to a prevalence of 1 in 39,000 estimated from a series

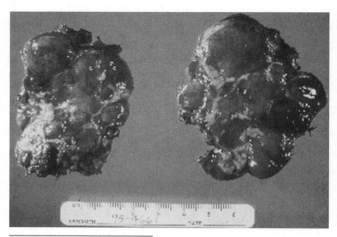

Figure 23–4 Pheochromocytoma is a common peripheral tumor seen in children with von Hippel–Lindau disease.

in Freiberg, Germany.[55] There is no gender difference. Sporadic cases of VHL accounted for approximately 8% of all cases from a large series reported by Maher.[56] CNS hemangioblastomas outside of the retina have been documented in 20 to 75% of patients with VHL,[57] with only a small proportion of these patients presenting before age 20.

Diagnosis

The diagnostic criteria for VHL established by Melmon and Rosen[58] are as follows: presence of two or more hemangioblastomas, one hemangioblastoma with a visceral lesion (pheochromocytoma (Fig. 23–4), pancreatic or renal cyst, or renal cell carcinoma), or one retinal or CNS hemangioblastoma or visceral lesion with a positive family history. Gene penetrance is both tumor type and age-dependent, with virtually complete penetrance by age 60 years.[56] VHL is infrequently diagnosed during childhood and most commonly presents in the third decade of life.

Retinal angioma, the most common initial finding in the disease,[56] may be either symptomatic or identified by fundoscopic examination and/or fluorescein angiography. Persons with retinal angioma typically show loss of vision from hemorrhage, exudates, and retinal detachment. *Hemangioblastoma of the cerebellum is associated with the signs and symptoms of a posterior fossa mass lesion, including headache, vomiting, lethargy, and ataxia. Polycythemia is a common consequence of erythropoietin production by these tumors,[59] and papilledema is often present.[57, 60]* Only 1% of tumors in patients with VHL are located in the supratentorial compartment. *Spinal cord hemangioblastomas account for about 25%[57] of tumors in VHL.* Presenting with neck, chest, or back pain, patients may also show loss of sensation and/or signs of spinal cord compression. Acute decompensation may result from hemorrhage into either cranial or spinal lesions.

Patients with VHL may present primarily with visceral rather than neurologic manifestations: a subgroup of VHL patients have been identified in whom pheochromocytoma is the major feature of the disease, with significant associated hypertension.[61] Pheochromocytoma may be diagnosed by the presence of catecholamine metabolites in the urine and by imaging studies.[62]

Renal cell carcinoma is another systemic manifestation of VHL. To date, the youngest patient with a renal cell carcinoma was a 16-year-old boy, whose asymptomatic tumor was detected with screening ultrasonography.[63]

BOX 23–7
Diagnosis

- ≥2 hemangioblastomas
- 1 hemangioblastoma plus
  - Pheochromocytoma
  - Pancreatic/renal cyst
  - Renal cell carcinoma
- 1 retinal/CNS hemangioblastoma or visceral lesion and a family history of disease

---

Hemangioblastomas typically appear as cystic lesions with a mural nodule on neuroradiologic imaging studies. The nodule is isodense to brain on CT and frequently enhances with contrast administration. On MRI, the cyst has a signal intensity equal to that of CSF, and the mural nodule enhances intensely and homogeneously with contrast administration. There may be flow voids within or close to the mural nodule.

Cerebral angiography, once the diagnostic procedure of choice, is rarely needed for surgical planning, although angiography with embolization may be a useful presurgical adjunct if the nodule is large and extremely vascular. On angiography, the nodule shows a striking blush with delayed contrast washout.

BOX 23–8
Hemangioblastoma
Imaging Findings

- CT
  - Cystic lesion and mural nodule
  - Isodense nodule
  - Contrast enhancement of nodule
- MRI
  - Cyst signal equal to CSF
  - Mural nodule enhances intensely and homogeneously
  - Possible flow voids

Many different imaging techniques are used to diagnose and/or follow the associated visceral lesions of VHL. They include ultrasonography, CT, and MRI, and scanning with meta-iodobenzylguanidine, an isotopic catecholamine analog, may be useful for localizing an extrarenal pheochromocytoma.

Screening guidelines have been developed for patients with multiple lesions and family members of patients with VHL (Table 23–3). The role of further workup of family members of patients who present with only a single lesion associated with disease is unclear.

Experimental studies using polymerase chain reaction (PCR) analysis of DNA markers linked to the VHL gene are being conducted to define whether asymptomatic family members carry germline mutations and are at risk for developing lesions later in life.[64, 65] The results of these studies are also useful for counseling affected individuals on their risk

---

TABLE 23–3 Cambridge Screening Protocol for von Hippel–Lindau Disease in Affected Patients and At-Risk Relatives

Affected patient
1. Annual physical exam and urine testing
2. Annual direct and indirect ophthalmoscopy with fluoroscein angioscopy or angiography
3. MRI (or CT) of brain every 3 years to age 50 and every 5 years thereafter
4. Annual renal ultrasonography, with CT scan every 3 years (more frequently if multiple renal cysts present)
5. Annual 24-hour urine collection for VMA

At-risk relative
1. Annual physical examination and urine testing
2. Annual direct and indirect ophthalmoscopy from age 5. Annual fluorescein angioscopy or angiography from age 10 to age 60
3. MRI (or CT) of brain every 3 years from age 15 to age 40 and then every 5 years until age 60
4. Annual renal ultrasonography, with abdominal CT every 3 years from age 20 to age 65
5. Annual 24-hour urine collection for VMA

VMA, vanillylmandelic acid.

N.B. These guidelines are for asymptomatic individuals; symptomatic patients should be investigated urgently. The frequency of screening may be reduced in relatives in whom DNA linkage studies reduce their risk.

Reprinted from Maher EH, Yates JRW, Harries R, et al. Clinical features and natural history of von Hippel–Lindau disease. *Q J Med* 1990;77:1160, with permission.

of passing the gene to their offspring, for prenatal screening, and for the diagnosis of de novo germ line mutations in patients with solitary lesions.[66]

All of the tumor types associated with VHL can also occur sporadically in patients without the disease. However, the tumors are seen at an earlier age and are frequently multiple and bilateral in VHL. Hemangioblastoma is the primary CNS lesion associated with VHL. Approximately 30 to 40% of patients presenting with hemangioblastoma will be diagnosed with VHL; conversely, approximately 60% of patients with VHL develop hemangioblastoma. Macroscopically, hemangioblastomas appear pink to orange, and are fleshy and very vascular. The exudation of fluid across the fenestrated endothelium of the tumor vessels leads to cyst formation. Microscopically, these tumors are composed of endothelial-lined vascular channels interspersed with lipid-laden ("foamy") stromal cells. Hemangioblastomas may be difficult to distinguish from metastatic renal cell carcinoma, particularly in patients with a primary lesion in the kidney. Immunohistochemistry aids in the identification of the tumor type. Renal cell carcinomas will show positivity with epithelial cell markers that include keratin, epithelial membrane antigen, and Lu-5, which are not expressed in hemangioblastomas. Hemangioblastoma stromal cells will react with antibodies to erythropoietin.[59] The cyst wall of a hemangioblastoma may be mistaken for a benign cerebellar astrocytoma on histologic examination owing to the presence of piloid cells and Rosenthal fibers. Although they may be multifocal at presentation, CNS hemangioblastomas do not metastasize and act as benign tumors.

BOX 23–9
Pathologic Features

- **Endothelial line vascular channels interspersed with lipid-laden stromal cells**
- **May be confused with metastatic renal cell carcinoma**
- **No reaction with keratin, EMA, and Lu-5 markers**

Genetic Features

The molecular genetic data obtained from the study of VHL closely parallel the predictions of Knudsen's tumor suppressor hypothesis. Positional mapping techniques defined the VHL locus at chromosome arm 3p25-26,[67] from which site the associated gene was ultimately cloned. Sporadic cerebellar hemangioblastomas, as well as sporadic renal cell carcinomas and pheochromocytomas, appear to arise from two somatic gene mutations, whereas these same tumors when associated with VHL require only a single somatic mutation as the other mutant gene copy is inherited through the germline. Germline mutations in the VHL gene identified to date include nonsense, missense, microdeletions, and insertions. The type of gene mutation may be associated with the phenotypic severity of the disease.[68, 69] Somatic gene rearrangements tend to be deletions. The product of the VHL gene, identified as a 30-kd protein that binds transcription factors

elongin B and C, has been hypothesized to inhibit cell proliferation by inhibiting transcription elongation.[70] In vitro studies have shown that specific mRNAs for vascular growth factors may be increased in cells lacking normal VHL protein, thus leading to the formation of vascular tumors.[71]

Treatment
Surgery

Complete surgical excison is the treatment of choice for all hemangioblastomas and is generally curative. Small asymptomatic lesions may be followed radiographically, with operative intervention for tumor growth or symptom onset. A gliotic plane surrounding the nodule and the cyst identified at surgery allows resection of the tumor even when located in the brain stem or spinal cord. The cyst wall may be left intact during the initial dissection, aiding in the identification of the resection plane. Partial drainage of the cyst contents allows cerebellar relaxation without anatomical distortion. Intraoperative ultrasonography may be useful if the tumor nodule is deeply situated. As piecemeal resection of the nodule may result in brisk bleeding, dissection around the tumor border with coagulation of feeding vessels is preferable. Complete resection of the nodule is important to prevent both recurrence of the lesion and postoperative hemorrhage from residual neoplastic vessels. Children who present with hydrocephalus due to tumor benefit from perioperative external ventricular drainage, and permanent CSF shunting is rarely required.

Radiation Therapy

Although complete surgical extirpation is curative for hemangioblastoma, multiple small lesions and those located in eloquent areas may not yield to conventional operative intervention without significant morbidity. Thus, alternative therapies have been designed to treat complex or multiple lesions. Conventional fractionated irradiation has been used postoperatively in adults, with disease-free survival data related to total therapeutic dose.[72, 73] Although significant improvement in survival was noted with high-dose focal irradiation (>75 Gy) in one study,[73] VHL patients made up only a small proportion of those treated, and none of them were children. Use of such high doses of conventional fractionated radiation is, in general, contraindicated in children. Stereotactic radiosurgery has also been employed to treat multiple small and/or recurrent cerebellar hemangioblastomas in adult patients with VHL.[74] Control of tumor was achieved in four patients over a 7- to 30-month follow-up period. However, two of these patients required shunts (one cystoperitoneal, one ventriculoperitoneal), and one patient suffered significant radiation necrosis. It is unclear whether this technique will be applicable to the pediatric population.

In 152 patients in whom the natural history of VHL was examined, actuarial survival data revealed a higher mortality at all ages.[56] Mean age at death was 41 years (range 13 to 67 years), with a median survival of 49 years. The most common causes of death were renal cell carcinoma and cerebellar hemangioblastoma. Overall mortality from CNS hemangioblastoma in VHL has also been higher in another series.[57]

However, most of the major sources of morbidity and mortality in VHL are now treatable, and with early diagnosis of patients at greatest risk using molecular genetic screening and close vigilance with imaging studies the outlook of affected patients will improve in the future.

MISCELLANEOUS SYNDROMES

A number of other disorders have also been classified as neurocutaneous. Although they are congenital, these disorders may present later in life. These rare syndromes manifest with cutaneous, visceral, CNS, and ocular anomalies associated with vascular, hamartomatous, and malignant and benign neoplasms of multiple organs.

Basal Cell Nevus Syndrome/Gorlin's Syndrome

Basal cell nevus syndrome (BCNS), or Gorlin's syndrome, is an autosomal dominant disorder with a high spontaneous mutation rate. Approximately 5% of patients will develop *medulloblastoma*, often before the age of 2 years; conversely, 1 to 2% of patients with medulloblastoma will be diagnosed with BCNS.[75] BCNS is most often diagnosed in the second or third decade of life when the cutaneous stigmata of the disease become apparent. The cardinal features of the syndrome are basal and squamous cell carcinomas, craniofacial anomalies including cleft lip and palate, hypertelorism, keratohyaline cysts of the mandible, dystrophic calcification of the falx, frontal bossing, and skeletal anomalies, predominantly scoliosis, bifid ribs, and metacarpal dysplasias. The gene associated with BCNS has been identified on chromosome 9q and behaves as a tumor suppressor.[76] *Cells isolated from BCNS patients show faulty DNA repair when exposed to ionizing radiation.*[77] One patient has been reported with multiple radiation-induced intracranial and extracranial neoplasms following therapeutic irradiation for a medulloblastoma prior to being diagnosed with BCNS.[78] The diagnosis of BCNS may be delayed because the cutaneous manifestations may not be apparent, leading to patients with medulloblastoma who respond to irradiation by developing secondary neoplasms (Fig. 23–5). Molecular genetic diagnostic testing may soon be available to provide information regarding the likelihood of BCNS occurring in a patient with medulloblastoma.

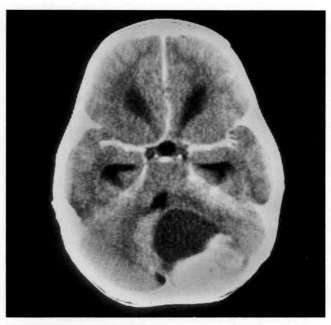

Figure 23–5 Posterior fossa medulloblastoma seen in a 2-year-old boy subsequently identified with basal cell nevus syndrome. The tumor was resected and the child responded to chemotherapy and irradiation witn no recurrence of this lesion. Eleven years later he underwent resection of a second supratentorial lesion that proved to be a meningioma (see Chapter 25).

on chromosome 11q23,[79] which may represent differing forms of the disease. Genetic anomalies in A-T have also been described on chromosome 14.[80] Although the precise biochemical mechanisms have not been fully elucidated, cells from patients with A-T show increased sensitivity to ionizing radiation and are deficient in DNA repair, leading to a high level of chromosome breakage. Truncal ataxia, an early feature of the disease, may be mistaken for cerebral palsy. Oculomotor abnormalities are common and are often the first

---

> ## BOX 23–10
> ### Clinical Features
>
> - **Basal/squamous cell carcinoma**
> - **Craniofacial anomalies**
> - **Skeletal anomalies**

Ataxia-Telangiectasia

Ataxia-telangiectasia (A-T), or Louis-Bar syndrome, is an autosomal recessive disorder characterized by progressive cerebellar degeneration: ocular, conjunctival, and cutaneous capillary telangiectasias (Fig. 23–6); cellular and humoral immune deficiency; and a predisposition to malignancy. Multiple genetic complementation groups have been identified

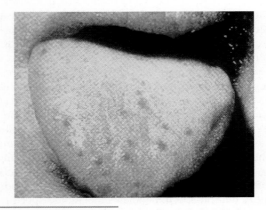

Figure 23–6 Telangiectatic lesions of the tongue in a child with ataxia-telangiectasia.

presenting signs of the disease. Telangiectasias commonly arise in the conjunctiva by age 3 to 5 years and progress in size and number throughout the patient's life. Choreoathetosis and/or dystonia is seen in a large majority of patients, and dystonic posturing combined with atrophy of the intrinsic hand muscles may result in flexion and extension contractures of the fingers.[81, 82] Patients aged 20 to 30 years may also develop spinal muscular atrophy, with loss of deep-tendon reflexes and decreased sensation. Developmental delay and cognitive deficits are not seen in this disease. *Patients with A-T have a tendency to develop cancers, mainly leukemia, although they show an increased incidence of medulloblastoma and glioma.*[83, 84] Owing to the effect of ionizing radiation on A-T cells, reduced craniospinal irradiation has been proposed for patients with medulloblastoma.[85] Magnetic resonance images of patients with A-T show striking atrophy of the cerebellar folia and vermis, associated with an *ex vacuo* increase in the size of the fourth ventricle.[86]

BOX 23–11
Clinical Features

- **Cerebellar degeneration (ataxia)**
- **Ocular/cutaneous capillary telangiectasias**
- **Immune deficiency**
- **Predisposition to malignancy**

Neurocutaneous Melanosis

Neurocutaneous melanosis (NCM) is a rare, sporadic phakomatosis characterized by cutaneous pigmented nevi and leptomeningeal melanocytosis, with or without primary skin or CNS melanomas. Patients with CNS disease frequently present in infancy with hydrocephalus, cranial nerve palsies, seizures, or symptoms of spinal cord compression. Some features of cutaneous nevi have been associated with a higher incidence of CNS involvement; patients exhibiting large lesions (≥ 20 cm) with satellite lesions in a posterior axial location have a higher incidence of CNS melanosis. In contrast, pigmented nevi of the extremities are rarely associated with underlying CNS pathology.[87] Pathologic findings include pigmented melanocytes within the brain, particularly in the deep cerebellar nuclei and brain stem, primary malignant melanoma in the subarachnoid space of the basal cisterns and spinal cord, thickened leptomeninges and posterior fossa cysts, including Dandy-Walker malformation.[88, 89] *Hydrocephalus may be either obstructive or communicating, and is occasionally diagnosed prenatally.* CSF shunting, used for management of hydrocephalus, may result in peritoneal metastasis.[89] MRI is the most sensitive diagnostic modality, and melanin deposits exhibit a characteristic high signal intensity on T1- and T2-weighted images, with diffuse meningeal enhancement following contrast administration. Melanomas also show intense enhancement.[88, 89] Histopathologically, the tumors are composed of sheets of small cells, with larger melanin-producing cells. The cells react with antibodies to vimentin, neuron-specific enolase, melanoma-specific antigen, and S100.[87, 88] Radiotherapy and chemotherapy have not proven useful for patients with disseminated disease, and most children die within a year or two of diagnosis.[90]

BOX 23–12
Clinical Features

- **Cutaneous pigmented nevi**
- **Leptomeningeal melanocytosis**
- **Possible skin/CNS lesions**

SUMMARY

The phakomatoses are genetic syndromes characterized by cutaneous signatures (with the exception of VHL) and CNS manifestations. Their diagnosis depends on clinical and radiologic manifestations typical for the disease and a family history suspicious for the particular entity. Surgical excision of the intracranial tumors associated with these diseases is the treatment of choice in most cases. Their progress is based on treatment outcome and the extent of the disease at presentation.

REFERENCES

1. Flinter FA, Neville BGR. Examining the parents of children with tuberous sclerosis. *Lancet* 1986;2(8516):1167.
2. Connor JM, Stephenson JBP, Hadley MDM. Nonpenetrance in tuberous sclerosis. *Lancet* 1986;2(8518):1275.
3. Wiederholt WC, Gomez MR, Kurland LT. Incidence and prevalence of tuberous sclerosis in Rochester, Minnesota, 1950 through 1982. *Neurology* 1985;35:600–603.
4. Roach ES, Smith M, Huttenlocher P, et al. Diagnostic criteria—tuberous sclerosis. *J Child Neurol* 1992;7:221–224.
5. Jung EG. The cutaneous symptoms of tuberous sclerosis. *J Genet Hum* 1975;23:218–222.
6. McWilliam RC, Stephenson JB. Depigmented hair: the earliest sign of tuberous sclerosis. *Arch Dis Child* 1978;53:961–963.
7. Gutman I, Dunn D, Behrens M, et al. Hypopigmented iris spot: an early sign of tuberous sclerosis. *Ophthalmology* 1982;89:1155–1159.
8. Fryer AE, Osborne JP, Schutt W. Forehead plaque: a presenting skin sign in tuberous sclerosis. *Arch Dis Child* 1987;62:292–293.
9. Geva T, Santini F, Pear W, et al. Cardiac rhabdomyoma: rare cause of fetal death. *Chest* 1991;99:139–142.
10. Webb DW, Thomas RD, Osborne JP. Cardiac rhabdomyomas and their association with tuberous sclerosis. *Arch Dis Child* 1993;68:367–370.
11. Weig SG, Pollack P. Carbamazepine-induced heart block in a child with tuberous sclerosis and cardiac rhabdomyoma: implications for evaluation and follow-up. *Ann Neurol* 1993;34:617–619.
12. Knilans TK. Carbamazepine-induced atrioventricular block in a child with tuberous sclerosis and cardiac rhabdomyoma. *Ann Neurol* 1994;36:804–805.
13. Painter MJ, Pang D, Ahdab-Barmada M, Bergman I. Connatal brain tumors in patients with tuberous sclerosis. *Neurosurgery* 1984;14:570–573.

14. Konkol RJ, Walsh EP, Power T, Bresnan MJ. Cerebral embolism resulting from an intracardiac tumor in tuberous sclerosis. *Pediatr Neurol* 1986;2:108–110.

15. Journel H, Roussey M, Plais MH, et al. Prenatal diagnosis of familial tuberous sclerosis following detection of cardiac rhabdomyoma by ultrasound. *Prenat Diagn* 1986;6:283–289.

16. Cook JA, Oliver K, Mueller RF, Sampson J. A cross-sectional study of renal involvement in tuberous sclerosis. *J Med Genet* 1996;33:480–484.

17. van Baal JG, Fleury P, Brummelkamp WH. Tuberous sclerosis and the relation with renal angiomyolipoma: a genetic study on the clinical aspects. *Clin Genet* 1989;35:167–173.

18. Bernstein J, Robbins TO. Renal involvement in tuberous sclerosis. *Ann NY Acad Sci* 1991;615:36.

19. Haines JL, Short MP. Kwiatkowski DJ, et al. Localization of one gene for tuberous sclerosis within 9q32-9q34, and further evidence for heterogeneity. *Am J Hum Genet* 1991;49:764–772.

20. Riikonen R, Simell O. Tuberous sclerosis and infantile spasms. *Dev Med Child Neurol* 1990;32:203–209.

21. Palmini A, Andermann F, Olivier A, et al. Focal neuronal migration disorders and intractable partial epilepsy: a study of 30 patients. *Ann Neurol* 1991;30:741–749.

22. Hahn JS, Bejar R, Gladson C. Neonatal subependymal giant cell astrocytoma associated with tuberous sclerosis: MRI, CT, and ultrasound correlation. *Neurology* 1991;41:124–128.

23. Oikawa S, Sakamoto K, Kobayashi N. A neonatal huge subependymal giant cell astrocytoma: case report. *Neurosurgery* 1994;35:748–750.

24. Boesel CP, Paulson GW, Kosnik EJ, Earle KM. Brain hamartomas and tumors associated with tuberous sclerosis. *Neurosurgery* 1979;4:410–417.

25. Pascual-Castroviejo I, Patron M, Gutierrez M, et al. Tuberous sclerosis associated with histologically confirmed ocular and cerebral tumors. *Pediatr Neurol* 1995;13:172–174.

26. Kiribuchi K, Uchida Y, Fukuyama Y, et al. High incidence of fundus hamartomas and clinical significance of a fundus score in tuberous sclerosis. *Brain Dev* 1986;8:509.

27. Kingsley DPE, Kendall BE, Fitz CR. Tuberous sclerosis: a clinicoradiological evaluation of 110 cases with particular reference to atypical presentation. *Neuroradiology* 1986;28:38–46.

28. Morimoto K, Mogami H. Sequential CT study of subependymal giant-cell astrocytoma associated with tuberous sclerosis. *J Neurosurg* 1986;65:874–877.

29. Conzen M, Oppel F. Tuberous sclerosis in neurosurgery: an analysis of 18 patients. *Acta Neurochir (Wien)* 1990;106:106–109.

30. Braffman BH, Bilaniuk LT, Naidich TP, et al. MR imaging of tuberous sclerosis: pathogenesis of this phakomatosis, use of gadopentetate dimeglumine, and literature review. *Radiology* 1992;183:227–238.

31. Stricker T, Zuerrer M, Martin E, Boesch C. MRI of two infants with tuberous sclerosis. *Neuroradiology* 1991;33:175–177.

32. Weinblatt ME, Kahn E, Kochen J. Renal cell carcinoma in patients with tuberous sclerosis. *Pediatrics* 1987;80:898–903.

33. Washecka R, Hanna M. Malignant renal tumors in tuberous sclerosis. *Urology* 1991;37:340–343.

34. Nir A, Tajik AJ, Seward JB, et al. Tuberous sclerosis and cardiac rhabdomyoma. *Am J Cardiol* 1995;76:419–421.

35. Smith HC, Watson GH, Palel RG, et al. Cardiac rhabdomyomata in tuberous sclerosis: their course and diagnostic value. *Arch Dis Child* 1989;64:196.

36. Harding CO, Pagon RA. Incidence of tuberous sclerosis in patients with cardiac rhabdomyoma. *Am J Med Genet* 1990;37:443–446.

37. Castro M, Shepherd CW, Gomez MR, et al. Pulmonary tuberous sclerosis. *Chest* 1995;107:189–195.

38. Shepherd CW, Gomez MR, Lie JT, Crowson CS. Causes of death in patients with tuberous sclerosis. *Mayo Clin Proc* 1991;66:792–796.

39. Halmagyi GM, Bignold LP, Alsop JL. Recurrent subependymal giant-cell astrocytoma in the absence of tuberous sclerosis. *J Neurosurg* 1979;50:106–109.

40. European Chromosome 16 Tuberous Sclerosis Consortium: Identification and characterization of the tuberous sclerosis gene on chromosome 16. *Cell* 1993;75:1305–1315.

41. Short MP, Haines JL, Bowe C, et al. Linkage and heterogeneity in tuberous sclerosis: linkage to chromosome 16 and resolution of old problems. *Am J Hum Genet* 1992;51(Suppl):A201.

42. Carbonara C, Longa L, Grosso E, et al. Apparent loss of heterozygosity at TSC-2 over TSC-1 chromosomal region in tuberous sclerosis hamartomas. *Genes Chrom Cancer* 1996;15:18–25.

43. Wilson P, Rameh V, Kristiansen A, et al. Novel mutations detected in the TSC2 gene from both sporadic and familial TSC patients. *Hum Mol Genet* 1996;5:249–256.

44. Wienecke R, Konig A, DeClue JE. Identification of tuberin, the tuberous sclerosis-2 product: tuberin possesses specific RAP1GAP activity. *J Biol Chem* 1995;270:16409–16414.

45. Sepp T, Yates JR, Green AJ. Loss of heterozygosity in tuberous sclerosis hamartomas. *J Med Genet* 1996;33:962–964.

46. Rozkowski M, Drabik K, Barszcz S, Jozwiak S. Surgical treatment of intraventricular tumors associated with tuberous sclerosis. *Child's Nerv Syst* 1995;11:335–339.

47. Waga S, Yamamoto Y, Kojima T. Massive hemorrhage in tumor of tuberous sclerosis. *Surg Neurol* 1977;8:99–101.

48. Holanda FJCS, Holanda GMP. Tuberous sclerosis: neurosurgical indications in intraventricular tumors. *Neurosurg Rev* 1980;3:139–150.

49. Tschuchida T, Kamata K, Kawamata M, et al. Brain tumors in tuberous sclerosis: report of four cases. *Child's Brain* 1981;8:271–283.

50. McLaurin RL, Towbin RB. Tuberous sclerosis: diagnostic and surgical considerations. *Pediatr Neurosci* 1986;12:43–48.

51. Hirsch J-F, Sainte-Rose C. A new surgical approach to subcortical lesions: balloon inflation and cortical gluing. *J Neurosurg* 1991;74:1014–1017.

52. Perot P, Weir B, Rasmussen T. Tuberous sclerosis: surgical therapy for seizures. *Arch Neurol* 1966;15:498–506.

53. Palmini A, Andermann F, Olivier A, et al. Focal neuronal migration disorders and intractable partial epilepsy: results of surgical treatment. *Ann Neurol* 1991;30:750–757.

54. Maher ER, Iselius L, Yates JRW, et al. Von Hippel–Lindau disease: a genetic study. *J Med Genet* 1991;28:443–447.

55. Neumann HPH, Wiestler OD. Clustering of features of von Hippel–Lindau syndrome: evidence for a complex genetic locus. *Lancet* 1991;337:1052–1054.

56. Maher ER, Yates JRW, Harries R, et al. Clinical features and natural history of von Hippel–Lindau disease. *Q J Med* 1990;77:1151–1163.

57. Neumann HPH, Eggert HR, Scheremet R, et al. Central nervous system lesions in von Hippel–Lindau syndrome. *J Neurol Neurosurg Psych* 1992;55:898–901.

58. Melmon KL, Rosen SW. Lindau's disease. *Am J Med* 1964; 36:595–617.

59. Tachibana O, Yamashima T, Yamashita J. Immunohistochemical study of erythropoietin in cerebellar hemangioblastomas associated with secondary polycythemia. *Neurosurgery* 1991;28:24–26.

60. Maher ER, Yates JRW, Ferguson-Smith MA. Statistical analysis of the two stage mutation model in von Hippel–Lindau disease, and in sporadic cerebellar haemangioblastoma and renal cell carcinoma. *J Med Genet* 1990;27: 311–314.

61. Richard S, Biegelman C, Duclos JM, et al. Pheochromocytoma as the first manifestation of von Hippel–Lindau disease. *Surgery* 1994;116:1076–1081.

62. Ein SH, Shandling B, Wesson D, Filler RM. Recurrent pheochromocytomas in children. *J Pediatr Surg* 1990;25: 1063–1065.

63. Keeler LI, Klauber GT. Von Hippel–Lindau disease and renal cell carcinoma in a 16-year-old boy. *J Urol* 1992;147: 1588–1591.

64. Maher ER, Bently E, Payne SJ, et al. Presymptomatic diagnosis of von Hippel–Lindau disease with flanking DNA markers. *J Med Genet* 1992;29:902–905.

65. Crossey PA, Eng C, Ginalska-Malinowska M, et al. Molecular genetic diagnosis of von Hippel–Lindau disease in familial pheochromocytoma. *J Med Genet* 1995;32:885–886.

66. Decker H-JH, Neuhaus C, Jauch A, et al. Detection of a germline mutation and somatic homozygous loss of the von Hippel–Lindau tumor-suppressor gene in a family with a de novo mutation. A combined genetic study, including cytogenetics, PCR/SSCP, FISH, and CGH. *Hum Genet* 1996;97:770–776.

67. Latif F, Tory K, Gnarra J, et al. Identification of the von Hippel–Lindau disease tumor suppressor gene. *Science* 1993;260:1317–1320.

68. Chen F, Kishida T, Yao M, et al. Germline mutations in the von Hippel–Lindau disease tumor suppressor gene: correlations with phenotype. *Hum Mutat* 1995;5:66–75.

69. Zbar B, Kishida T, Chen F, et al. Germline mutations in the von Hippel–Lindau disease (VHL) gene in families from North America, Europe, and Japan. *Hum Genet* 1996; 8:348–357.

70. Duan DR, Pause A, Burgess WH, et al. Inhibition of transcription elongation by the VHL tumor suppressor protein. *Science* 1995;269:1402–1406.

71. Iliopolous O, Levy AP, Jiang C, et al. Negative regulation of hypoxia-inducible genes by the von Hippel–Lindau protein. *Proc Natl Acad Sci USA* 1996;93:10595–10599.

72. Sung DI, Chang CH, Harisiadis L. Cerebellar hemangioblastomas. *Cancer* 1982;49:553–555.

73. Smalley SR, Schomberg PJ, Earle JD, et al. Radiotherapeutic considerations in the treatment of hemangioblastomas of the central nervous system. *Int J Radiat Oncol Biol Phys* 1990;8:1165–1171.

74. Page KA, Wayson K, Steinberg GK, Adler JR Jr. Stereotactic radiosurgical ablation: an alternative treatment for recurrent and multifocal hemangioblastomas. *Surg Neurol* 1993;40:424–428.

75. Evans DGR, Farndon PA, Burnell LD, et al. The incidence of Gorlin syndrome in 173 consecutive cases of medulloblastoma. *Br J Cancer* 1991;64:959–961.

76. Farndon PA, Del Mastro RG, Evans DGR, Kilpatrick MW. Location of the gene for Gorlin syndrome. *Lancet* 1992; 339:581–582.

77. Featherstone T, Taylor AMR, Harnden DG. Studies on the radiosensitivity of cells from patients with basal cell naevus syndrome. *Am J Hum Genet* 1983;35:58–66.

78. O'Malley S, Weitman D, Olding M, Sekhar L. Multiple neoplasms following craniospinal irradiation for medulloblastoma in a patient with nevoid basal cell carcinoma syndrome. *J Neurosurg* 1997;86:286–288.

79. Gatti RA, Berkel I, Boder E, et al. Localization of an ataxia-telangiectasia gene to chromosome 11q22-23. *Nature* 1988;336:577–580.

80. Aurias A, Croquette MF, Nuyts JP, et al. New data on clonal anomalies of chromosome 14 in ataxia telangiectasia: tct(14;14) and inv(14). *Hum Genet* 1986;72: 22–24.

81. Leuzzi V, Elli R, Antonelli A, et al. Neurological and cytogenetic study in early-onset ataxia-telangiectasia patients. *Eur J Pediatr* 1993;152:609–612.

82. Gatti RA, Boder E, Vinters HV, et al. Ataxia telangiectasia: an interdisciplinary approach to pathogenesis. *Medicine* 1991;70:99–117.

83. Miyagi K, Mukawa J, Kinjo N, et al. Astrocytoma linked to familial ataxia-telangiectasia. *Acta Neurochir (Wien)* 1995;135:87–92.

84. Hart RM, Kimler BF, Evans RG, Park CH. Radiotherapeutic management of medulloblastoma in a pediatric patient with ataxia telangiectasia. *Int J Radiat Oncol Biol Phys* 1987;13:1237–1240.

85. Porteous MEM, Burn J, Proctor SJ. Hereditary haemorrhagic telangiectasia: a clinical analysis. *J Med Genet* 1992;29:527–530.

86. Steele JG, Nath PU, Burn J, Porteous ME. An association between migrainous aura and hereditary haemorrhagic telangiectasia. *Headache* 1993;33:145–148.

87. DeDavid M, Orlow SJ, Provost N, et al. Neurocutaneous melanosis: clinical features of large congenital melanocytic nevi in patients with manifest central nervous system melanosis. *J Am Acad Dermatol* 1996;35: 529–538.

88. Poe LB, Roitberg D, Galyon DD. Neurocutaneous melanosis presenting as an intradural mass of the cervical canal: magnetic resonance features and the presence of melanin as a clue to diagnosis: case report. *Neurosurgery* 1994;35:741–743.

89. Craver RD, Golladay SE, Warrier RP, et al. Neurocutaneous melanosis with Dandy–Walker malformation complicated by primary spinal leptomeningeal melanoma. *J Child Neurol* 1996;11:410–414.

90. Byrd SE, Darling CF, Tomita T, et al. MR imaging of symptomatic neurocutaneous melanosis in children. *Pediatr Radiol* 1997;27:39–44.

Chapter 24

Choroid Plexus Tumors

Richard G. Ellenbogen and Daniel J. Donovan

Choroid plexus tumors in children are rare and interesting tumors. They arise from the neuroepithelial lining of the ventricular choroid plexuses.[1, 2] The tumors demonstrate a wide spectrum of histologic and biologic properties, from the well-demarcated benign papilloma to the highly anaplastic, infiltrative carcinoma. The benign subset, choroid plexus papilloma, are resectable and thus potentially curable. The malignant subset, choroid plexus carcinoma, have a prognosis that is poor but slightly less ominous than that normally expected of malignant brain tumors, with reports of selected survivors living more than 5 years.[3–5]

Choroid plexus tumors are uncommon entities, composing 0.4 to 1.0% of all intracranial tumors.[6] Papilloma of the choroid plexus was described in only 0.6% of Cushing's 2023 verified intracranial tumors in 1932 and in only 0.5% of Zulch's review of 6000 intracranial tumors reported in 1956.[7, 8] Among children, however, they are slightly more common, representing 1 to 5% of pediatric brain tumors in various published series and 4 to 12% of brain tumors among patients younger than 1 year.[9–12]

The first description of a primary choroid plexus tumor was in an autopsy specimen of a 3-year-old girl by Guerard in 1833.[13] This case was later cited by Davis and Cushing in 1925.[14] Between 1833 and 1925, publications on neoplasms of the choroid plexus emphasized the rarity of the lesion or its association with hydrocephalus.[14–23] In 1906, Bielschowsky and Unger reported the first surgical resection of a choroid plexus tumor in an adult.[24] However, the patient later died. In 1919, Perthes reported the first long-term survival of an adult with a choroid plexus tumor.[18] With respect to children, in 1930 Van Wagenen[22] reported excision of a tumor from the lateral ventricle of a 3-month-old child, and in 1934 Dandy[25] described the removal of a choroid plexus tumor from a 14-year-old girl. Dandy also pioneered the transcallosal route to the third ventricle and was the first to describe its use for excision of a choroid plexus tumor in 1922. The first successful removal of a third-ventricle papilloma was through a transfrontal approach and was reported by Masson in 1934.[26]

A wide variety of surgical approaches to removal of these surgically formidable neoplasms have been described, and the appropriate choice must be based on the individual characteristics and location of each tumor. Choroid plexus tumor should be included in the differential diagnosis of any intraventricular mass, especially in a young child, and when resectable is often a welcome diagnosis in comparison with others in this location.

CLINICAL FEATURES

Primary choroid plexus neoplasms are found in patients of any age, from birth to the eighth decade of life. More than 70% occur in children, and at least 50% are found in children younger than 2 years.[3, 9, 27–30] Reports of in utero tumors by prenatal ultrasonography seem to indicate a congenital origin for some of these tumors.[31, 32] A preponderance of male patients has been described in several series;[3, 33–37] however, other series show a fairly even distribution between males and females.[6, 38] *There does not seem to be a difference in age at diagnosis, sex, symptoms, or location of tumor in patients with papilloma as opposed to those with carcinoma.*[3]

The patient's initial clinical features can be grouped into four overlapping sets of signs: increased intracranial pressure (ICP), seizures, hemorrhage, and focal neurologic abnormalities. By far, most children are brought to the hospital for an investigation of hydrocephalus or macrocephaly. These patients present with signs of increased ICP, which include tense fontanelle, splayed sutures, vomiting, lethargy, and irritability.[3, 9, 33] The symptoms of choroid plexus tumors are caused predominantly by the hydrocephalus that afflicts approximately 90% of pediatric patients, and the duration of symptoms ranges from several weeks to 6 months. Although most infants present with intracranial hypertension, the presentation in young children may be more nonspecific. Less common but well-documented presentations include head tilt, titubation, weakness, failure to thrive, developmental delay, and "shunt-resistant" hydrocephalus.[39–43] The shunt-resistant hydrocephalus is secondary to a choroid plexus tumor, which can produce many times the normal rate of cerebrospinal fluid (CSF).[44] This overproduction of CSF can be sufficient to cause abdominal ascites if a ventriculoperitoneal shunt is placed prior to surgical removal of the tumor.[43] Even such rare side effects as psychosis and bobble-head doll syndrome have been reported in the literature.[45]

BOX 24–1
General Clinical Features

- **Increased ICP (hydrocephalus)**
  - **Tense fontanelle**
  - **Splayed sutures**
  - **Vomiting**
  - **Lethergy**
  - **Irritability**
- **Seizures**
- **Hemorrhage**
- **Focal neurologic findings**

Children with posterior fossa lesions may exhibit signs of brain stem compression, cranial nerve paresis, and cerebellar dysfunction. The scarcity of tumors in the cerebellopontine angle in children makes it difficult to generalize on their presentation, although hydrocephalus is a prominent finding.[46–48]

BOX 24–2
Clinical Features
of Posterior Fossa Lesions

- **Brain stem compression**
- **Cranial nerve paresis**
- **Cerebellar signs**

Children with third ventricular tumors present with hydrocephalus but may also exhibit endocrine disturbances, precocious puberty, diabetes insipidus, or diencephalic disorders.[23, 49, 50]

BOX 24–3
Clinical Features
of Third-Ventricle Lesions

- **Hydrocephalus**
- **Endocrine disturbances**
  - **Precocious puberty**
  - **Diencephalic syndrome**
  - **Obesity**
  - **Diabetes insipidus**
  - **Failure to thrive**

An interesting feature of choroid plexus tumors is their anatomical distribution. They are most commonly found in the lateral ventricles in children and less commonly in the fourth ventricle, in contrast to adults, in whom the majority of these tumors are found in the fourth ventricle and its lateral recesses.[2, 28, 29, 37, 51–54] No developmental feature adequately explains this unique anatomical distribution. Approximately 75% of tumors in children are found in the lateral ventricles. Most tumors in the lateral ventricle are found in the

atrium/trigone, but they may also be seen in the temporal horn or near the foramen of Monro. Van Wagenen's original report that the majority of lateral ventricular tumors are found in the left ventricle has not been supported by other series, which find a similar number in right and left lateral ventricles.[3, 22] Location in the third ventricle is less common but has been described in both children and adults.[37, 38, 43, 55] Third ventricular choroid plexus neoplasms in pediatric series average approximately 10%[3, 50, 55] and range from 0%[9, 48] to 29%.[33] Primary extraventricular locations are the rarest sites, but tumors have been described in children in the cerebellopontine angle, suprasellar cistern, foramen magnum, and spinal subarachnoid space.[2] Extension of the tumor from one ventricle to another or through a ventricular foramen or into a subarachnoid cistern is occasionally noted.[29, 43] In Rovit's 1970 review of 245 cases of choroid plexus tumor reported in the literature, 9 cases (3.7%) of tumor in multiple locations were discovered, 6 of which were in the lateral ventricle.[56] However, since the advent of advanced imaging techniques, these tumors can be visualized more accurately extending into other CSF spaces and the brain parenchyma. Choroid plexus tumors in children, like other intraventricular tumors in adults, are often quite large by the time of diagnosis; in one series, they averaged 4 cm in diameter at the time of diagnosis.[3]

BOX 24–4
Tumor Location

- **Lateral ventricle**
  - **Atrium/trigone**
  - **Temporal horn**
  - **Foramen of Monro**
- **Fourth ventricle**
- **Third ventricle**
- **Extraventricular**
  - **Cerebellopontine angle**
  - **Foramen magnum**
  - **Spinal subarachnoid space**

Hydrocephalus, which is a cardinal manifestation of choroid plexus neoplasms, can be the result of obstruction of CSF pathways or overproduction of CSF. Overproduction of CSF by these tumors has attracted much interest and been the subject of numerous reports.[20, 29, 44, 57–63] Initially, the resolution of hydrocephalus after complete resection of choroid plexus tumors was the basis for postulating that oversecretion of CSF was responsible for the hydrocephalus.[6] However, an increased rate of CSF production has been unequivocally demonstrated with choroid plexus neoplasms, albeit proven in only a few patients.[28, 44, 60, 62–64] Rekate et al demonstrated that although overproduction of CSF can cause hydrocephalus, a complex combination of CSF overproduction and limited outflow may be the cause in many patients.[65]

Tumor mass, blood products, tumor products, cellular debris, and metastases can mechanically obstruct the normal egress of CSF, thus causing hydrocephalus. Necrosis, tumor hemorrhage, operative hemorrhage, and ependymitis have all been implicated as causes of hydrocephalus in patients with such choroid tumors.[36, 40, 48, 66–69] Elevation of CSF protein is found in the majority of patients, and xanthochromia in the CSF is common; frank hemorrhage is less common.[6] The obstruction of CSF absorptive pathways may also explain why despite a gross total excision of tumor the hydrocephalus may persist. *Approximately one-third to one-half of patients with choroid plexus neoplasms require permanent CSF diversion postoperatively even when the tumor is completely removed.*[3, 33, 48, 67, 68]

Another interesting entity reported is "diffuse villous hypertrophy" of the choroid plexus, a term originally coined by Davis in 1924 to describe a bilateral choroid plexus lesion.[16] As there is little histopathologic difference between papilloma and normal choroid plexus tissue, it is difficult to determine if this entity represents a true neoplasm or simple hypertrophy of the choroid plexuses. Bilateral papilloma is a rare condition, as demonstrated by its absence from series of choroid plexus papilloma.[6, 27, 29, 52–54] The observation that overproduction of CSF can result from villous hypertrophy of the choroid plexus or papilloma has since been reported by several investigators who commented on the difficulty in diagnosis.[16, 28, 40, 63, 64, 70] Placement of a ventriculostomy and measuring CSF formation may help in the documentation of overproduction of CSF. Laurence described six tumors among his own patients but was cautious about their removal.[28] However, several surgeons have shown that resection of these rare bilateral choroid plexus lesions results in resolution of the CSF overproduction and alleviation of the concomitant hydrocephalus.[63, 64, 70]

IMAGING

Plain films may show marked calcification and nonspecific signs of increased pressure, such as splayed sutures.[6, 27, 71] Historically, pneumoencephalography, ventriculography, and angiography were utilized to show these tumors to be intraventricular masses with associated hydrocephalus.[6] Unfortunately, several deaths were associated with the application of pneumoencephalography and ventriculography in the diagnosis of choroid plexus tumors as well.[28, 48] These deaths were probably a result of the large shifts created by placing a brain needle with air or fluid into large ventricles with a large mass.

The introduction of computed tomography (CT) improved the safety and accuracy of diagnosis, and ultimately the outcome, in children harboring these tumors.[29] Both papilloma and carcinoma appear isodense to hyperdense on CT scan, with frequent calcification and usually marked enhancement (Fig. 24–1). Tumors are spherical, multilobular, and sometimes cystic. They may extend to another ventricle or CSF cistern, a finding not entirely specific for choroid plexus tumors (Fig. 24–2).

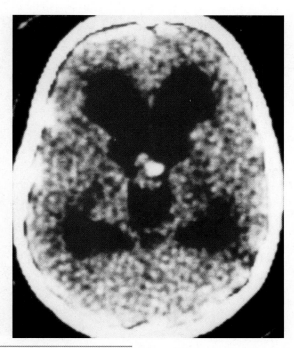

Figure 24–1 CT scan is from a child who presented for an evaluation of macrocephaly. Note the partially calcified choroid plexus papilloma in the third ventricle.

Magnetic resonance imaging (MRI) usually shows a mass that is isointense or slightly hypointense to gray matter on T1-weighted images and hyperintense on T2-weighted images. This tumor is often a lobulated, homogeneous, intraventricular mass on both short TR/TE and long TR/TE sequences.[72] Enhancement with paramagnetic substances, such as gadolinium-DTPA, is markedly bright and usually homogeneous, although various patterns can be seen, including nodular, peripheral, and cyst wall enhancement (Fig. 24–2 and 24–3). A common finding is the presence of serpentine signal voids, indicating that an enlarged blood vessel is supplying the tumor.[73, 74] MRI is the diagnostic imaging study of choice because of its detailed anatomical delineation and triplanar imaging ability. Magnetic resonance angiography may provide additional information regarding the vascular supply of the tumor. The relative ease and availability of magnetic resonance angiography has slowly supplanted the need for transfemoral cerebral angiography in the management of these tumors in children, unless presurgical embolization is required.

BOX 24–5
CT Findings

- Iso- to hyperdense
- Marked enhancement
- Calcification
- Multilobular
- Occasionally cystic

BOX 24–6
MRI Findings

- T1: iso- to hypointense
- T2: hyperintense
- Gadolinium enhancement
- Signal voids indicating enlarged blood vessels

Both papilloma and carcinoma can compress the surrounding brain, although brain invasion is a characteristic of carcinoma.[75]

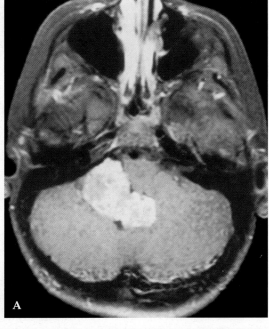

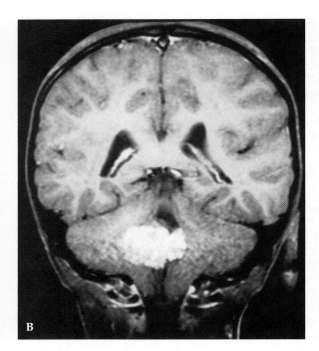

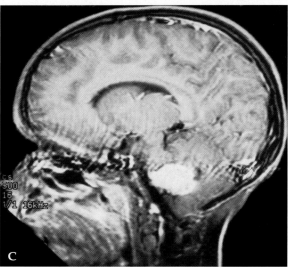

Figure 24–2   MRI T1-weighted axial (A), coronal (B), and sagittal (C) images with gadolinium enhancement in a 7-year-old child with a choroid plexus carcinoma of the fourth ventricle. The tumor demonstrates nodular enhancement as it fills the ventricle and creeps out of the foramen of Luschka.

Some authors have commented on the peritumor vasogenic edema in the surrounding white matter in carcinoma.[73, 75] Carcinoma does have a greater tendency to invade the brain, but it can also be found in an entirely intraventricular location.

The radiologic differential diagnosis of choroid plexus tumors in children includes ependymoma, primitive neuroectodermal tumor, astrocytoma, germinoma, teratoma, meningioma, and metastases to the choroid plexus. Despite the significant difference in histologic appearance, these tumors can appear homogeneous on MRI and quite similar in magnetic resonance appearance to choroid plexus tumors. Other unusual tumorlike masses that can appear similar include inflammatory pseudotumor, choroid plexus cysts, and xanthogranulomas.

BOX 24–7
Radiologic Differential Diagnosis

- **Ependymoma**
- **Primitive neuroectodermal tumor**
- **Astrocytoma**
- **Germinoma**
- **Meningioma**
- **Metastases**
- **Inflammatory pseudotumor**
- **Choroid plexus cysts**
- **Xanthogranuloma**

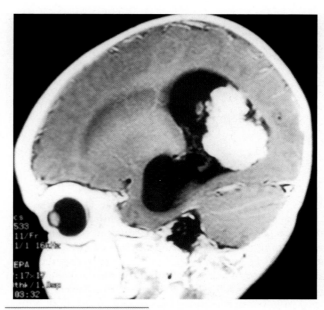

Figure 24–3 Sagittal T1-weighted gadolinium-enhanced image of a choroid plexus papilloma in a 5-month-old shows some of the most common characteristics of these lesions: a bright, homogeneous signal from a large, irregular, cauliflower-shaped mass, located within the atrium of the lateral ventricle, fed by hypertrophied choroidal vessels.

PATHOLOGY AND DIFFERENTIAL DIAGNOSIS

On gross analysis, a choroid plexus papilloma has a cauliflower-like surface and appears as a generally well-circumscribed mass arising from within a ventricle. The papilloma can extend into the brain parenchyma, compressing it along a broad margin. Heavily calcified tumors may be difficult to section without first being decalcified.[2] Microscopically,

choroid plexus tumors typically appear as a single layer of cuboidal epithelial cells surrounding a delicate fibrovascular stalk, arranged in a papillary configuration with fingerlike projections of tissue (Fig. 24–4). A well-formed continuous basement membrane is a prominent feature noted in all cases. Choroid plexus tumors span the histologic spectrum from extremely well-differentiated tumors to anaplastic tumors with minimal epithelial differentiation. Both well-differentiated and poorly differentiated components may be seen in a single tumor.[2] However, the majority of choroid plexus neoplasms lie in the well-differentiated part of the spectrum. It is occasionally difficult to differentiate normal choroid plexus from a papilloma, but the latter contains cells that are more crowded, columnar in shape, pleomorphic, and demonstrating more variation in nuclear size. The nuclear/cytoplasmic ratio is often increased.[2]

Ultrastructural observations include apical microvilli, scattered cilia, and interdigitating lateral cell borders sitting atop a basement membrane seated on a delicate fibrovascular stalk. Stromal calcification or xanthomatous changes may be evident.[2] Atypical microscopic features may be observed in papilloma; these include increased cellularity (two or three cell layers as opposed to one), mitoses, nuclear pleomorphism, and poorly formed papillary structures. These intermediate tumors may possess one or two of these features and are called atypical papilloma, but do not necessarily have a more aggressive natural history and are not classified as carcinoma.[2] However, anaplastic transformation of well-differentiated tumors has been reported to occur over time. Although uncommon, a lesion that is initially well differentiated or atypical can become anaplastic as documented during a subsequent resection.[76,77]

The histologic features of papilloma versus carcinoma have been the subject of both close scrutiny and controversy. The focus in diagnosis often centers on the important question, What characteristics differentiate papilloma from carcinoma? *Review of the literature reveals that from a historical perspective the criteria for differentiation of papilloma from carcinoma has not been uniform.* The definition of choroid plexus carcinoma has varied slightly in several studies based on

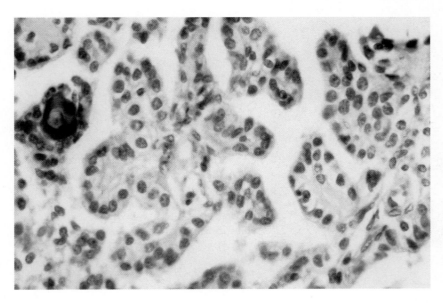

Figure 24–4 Typical papillary appearance of a choroid plexus papilloma that was completely excised from the lateral ventricle of a child. Note the single layer of columnar cells with organized papillary architecture based on a delicate fibrovascular stroma. The cells are more columnar and pleomorphic than normal choroid plexus cells (hematoxylin and eosin; original magnification × 80).

histologic criteria.[3, 11, 36, 78, 79] Dohrmann and Collias,[11] utilizing Russell and Rubinstein's[36] and Lewis's[80] criteria of carcinoma, reviewed 22 cases of primary choroid plexus carcinoma in the literature from 1844 to 1975 and found that only 11 satisfied the criteria of carcinoma. Similarly, Lewis's review of the literature resulted in the dismissal of many other claims of carcinoma.[80]

The consistent histologic features of choroid plexus tumors that unequivocally differentiate carcinoma from papilloma include cellular anaplasia, loss of differentiated papillary choroid architecture, nuclear pleomorphism, mitosis, necrosis, and giant cell formation (Fig. 24–5). At the extreme end of the spectrum are the sheets of anaplastic cells without appreciable papillae. These tumors are very cellular with complex cribriform structures, with a high mitotic index. One issue of contention centers around whether brain invasion either is required or by itself secures the diagnosis of carcinoma. Some authors insist that invasion be demonstrated histologically, whereas others do not.[79] It is noteworthy that not all surgical specimens have brain tissue insinuated within their projections, especially in cases when the surgeon used ultrasonic aspiration or microsurgical suction to remove the specimen at the brain-tumor interface and brain is not included in the surgical specimen. Thus, the absence of fingerlike projections invaginating into the brain parenchyma does not necessarily eliminate the diagnosis of carcinoma. Some tumors may invade the stroma but on careful histopathologic analysis are shown not to have invaded the brain. In addition, some choroid tumors with relatively benign histologic features are invasive, whereas some anaplastic tumors seem to have circumscribed borders.[3, 81] Often, the diagnosis of invasion is inferred by MRI, not by histologic evidence. Thus, although invasion of brain makes the diagnosis of carcinoma highly likely, such diagnosis is not invariably secured unless there are associated malignant cellular features.

BOX 24–8
Pathologic Features of Carcinoma

- **Cellular anaplasia**
- **Loss of differentiated papillary choroid architecture**
- **Nuclear pleomorphism**
- **Mitosis**
- **Necrosis**
- **Giant cell formation**

Some authors maintain that even in choroid plexus papilloma macro- and microscopic implants can be found in the leptomeninges, the subarachnoid space of the spinal cord, and the ventricular system.[82, 83] A rare case of pulmonary metastases from a choroid plexus papilloma was reported in an 11-year-old girl by Vraa-Jensen in 1950. The child developed pulmonary metastasis and lesions in the skull, which demonstrated malignant transformation (carcinoma) at autopsy.[84] Except for this case report, there has not been evidence of clinically symptomatic metastases from papilloma.

The electron microscopic findings are useful for distinguishing choroid plexus carcinoma from ependymoma, which can occasionally share a close histologic appearance. The presence of a basal lamina as seen in choroid plexus tumors often rules out ependymal origin of a tumor.[85]

Some studies have demonstrated the diagnostic utility of immunohistochemical methods. *Immunohistochemical staining of choroid plexus tumors reveals both epithelial and glial characteristics.* Choroid neoplasms are positive for cytokeratin (epithelial), S100 (diffuse staining), and vimentin.[86, 87] Choroid plexus carcinoma retains cytokeratin positivity but decreased S100

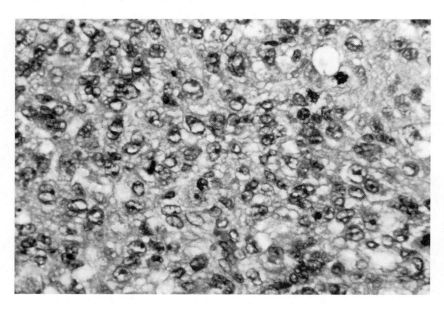

Figure 24–5 Sample taken from a large choroid plexus carcinoma that invaded the wall of the lateral ventricle of a child. Note the loss of differentiated papillary architecture (cf. Fig. 24–4), nuclear pleomorphism with mitoses, and giant cell formation (hematoxylin and eosin; original magnification × 40).

staining.[77] Positivity for carcinoembryonic antigen is more common in carcinoma, whereas S100 positivity is more common in papilloma.[88] Ependymoma is characterized by nonepithelial glial elements as well as epithelial components. Ependymomas lack the prominent basement membrane possessed by choroid plexus tumors and seen on periodic acid–Schiff (PAS) preparations, electron micrographs, or immunohistochemical specimens stained for laminin.[89] Choroid plexus neoplasms are positive for cytokeratin, whereas ependymomas are not; ependymomas are widely glial fibrillary acidic protein (GFAP)–positive, whereas choroid plexus tumors are diffusely but not uniformly GFAP-positive. In an adult with an intraventricular mass, S100 positivity favors a choroid plexus primary tumor versus a metastatic tumor.[2]

BOX 24–9
Immunohistochemical Markers

- **Positive for cytokeratin**
- **Positive for S100**
- **Positive for vimentin**
- **Positive or negative for GFAP**

In an immunohistochemical study of choroid plexus neoplasms, it was noted that a child who survived with a choroid plexus carcinoma had a tumor that stained positive for S100 and negative for epithelial membrane antigen, as often seen in papilloma. This immunohistochemical profile was not present in another child in the series, who died with carcinoma.[90] This outcome and staining profile suggested a biological or genetic variability in carcinoma that may in future help us identify which children are likely to do better than others. *In addition, DNA sequences similar to those found in simian virus 40 (SV40) have been found in choroid plexus tumors.* This provocative finding is supported by the observation that some transgenic mice infected with SV40 have been known to develop choroid plexus neoplasms, which is indicative of the oncogenic properties of polyoma viruses.[91] However, in summary, no clear-cut immunochemical or molecular criteria have emerged with any consistency to separate papilloma from carcinoma or provide for prognostic significance.

PREOPERATIVE PLANNING AND SURGICAL CONSIDERATIONS

Many different surgical approaches have been described to remove choroid plexus tumors specifically and intraventricular tumors in general. The location of these lesions in the ventricle makes passing through neural structures mandatory in all surgical approaches to their extirpation.[92] *The basic principles of tumor removal are an appropriately placed cortical incision, early isolation of the vascular supply (both arterial and venous), mobilization of the tumor, and microdissection and*

resection to reduce blood loss. It is sometimes very difficult to mobilize a choroid plexus neoplasm, especially when it has grown to a large size, as is common in children. Vigorous manipulation of an extremely large tumor in a patient is unwise as the arterial supply may be disrupted prior to its visualization. This is when piecemeal resection is performed. Debulking of the tumor's papillary regions with bipolar electrocautery or ultrasonic suction can make a large tumor more manageable. Once the vascular supply is identified it can be occluded so that the more vascular tumor mass can be excised en bloc or piecemeal.

An appreciation of the relevant anatomy is extremely helpful in surgical approaches to the ventricles. The primary arteries to the choroid plexus are the anterior and posterior choroidal arteries. The arterial supply of these tumors usually arises from hypertrophied branches of these choroidal arteries. The anterior choroidal artery arises from the internal carotid artery, distal to the posterior communicating artery, and courses posteriorly through the choroidal fissure to lie near the posterior choroidal artery. The anterior choroidal artery often supplies tumors in the atrium and temporal horn. Because the choroidal arteries pass through the choroidal fissure, opening of this fissure permits proximal control of the feeding vessels.

The posterior choroidal arteries are grouped into the lateral and medial divisions. The lateral posterior artery arises from the posterior cerebral artery, pierces the ventricle, and traverses the choroidal fissure at the level of the crus of the fornix. This vessel supplies the temporal horn, atrium, and body of the lateral ventricle and tumors contained in those cavities.[92] The medial posterior choroidal artery, which also originates from the posterior cerebral artery, travels through the velum interpositum sending inconstant branches to the lateral ventricles through the choroidal fissure and foramen of Monro. The medial posterior choroidal artery can supply tumors in the third ventricle and the lateral ventricle, as well as the choroid plexus in the roof of the third ventricle. Tumors may be supplied by one enlarged artery or by multiple feeders from the anterior and posterior choroidal arteries simultaneously.[92]

Fourth-ventricle tumors are vascularized by choroidal branches of the posterior inferior cerebellar artery or superior cerebellar arteries.

Venous drainage is often deep, through the subependymal veins, internal cerebral veins, vein of Rosenthal, vein of Galen, quadrigeminal or precentral cerebellar veins. The veins are useful landmarks in directing the surgeon during choroid plexus tumor excision. Many important veins compose the deep lateral and medial groups, but perhaps the best known for surgical and angiographic orientation in tumor removal in the lateral ventricle is the thalamostriate vein.

The appropriate choice of surgical approach is determined by tumor location, vascular supply, and the experience and preference of the surgeon. Extremely large tumors may require a combination of more than one approach so that the cortical excision and retraction is minimal.

The transcortical approaches are powerful ones because they permit access to all five regions of the lateral ventricle through one approach or a combination of approaches. On the other hand, the low risk of neuropsychological sequelae and seizure after a well-performed callosal section makes this route attractive and appropriate for selected patients. Tumors in the frontal horn can become large and cause obstruction of the foramen of Monro, with subsequent ventricular dilatatation. The transcortical middle frontal gyrus approach is an excellent one for tumors in the ipsilateral anterior horn. Tumors that extend interiorly from the lateral ventricle into the third ventricle and require a subchoroidal exposure for removal are better visualized through a transcortical approach than a transcallosal approach. Patients who have small ventricles, tumor in both lateral ventricles, or tumor in the body of the lateral ventricle may often be more easily approached through a transcallosal route.

The superior parietal approach is a natural one for neurosurgeons because it uses a path to the lateral ventricle that is taken when placing a parietal occipital catheter for CSF diversion. It is a reasonable approach for reaching choroid plexus neoplasms in the collateral trigone, posterior part of the body, atrium, and glomus regions of the ventricle. The lateral posterior choroidal artery, which may be obscured by the tumor mass, should be uncovered in the choroidal fissure between the pulvinar and the crus of the fornix and be isolated and secured to devascularize the tumor. This approach is more risky in the dominant than the nondominant hemisphere.

No single middle fossa approach permits early control of both the anterior and the posterior choroidal arteries initially.[93] The middle temporal gyrus approach provides a direct route to the middle fossa choroid plexus neoplasms with minimal morbidity and early control of the anterior choroidal artery feeding vessels. The lateral temporoparietal junction approach is used in rare cases when a large tumor is harbored in the nondominant atrium. With this approach the risk of a field deficit and damage to the angular gyrus is high, but it may be the shortest and most direct route to the tumor below.

Posterior fossa tumors can be removed by a standard posterior fossa craniectomy, retrosigmoid, or extreme lateral approaches. Tumors confined to the fourth ventricle can be reached through a vermal split or cortisectomy through the cerebellar hemisphere. Tumors that exit through the foramen of Luschka or those that creep anterior to the cerebellopontine angle may require a more laterally placed skull base approach.

BOX 24–10
Surgical Approaches

- **Transcortical**
  - **Middle frontal gyrus**
  - **Superior parietal**
  - **Middle temporal gyrus**
- **Transcallosal**
- **Posterior fossa**

PROGNOSIS AND ADJUVANT THERAPY

Prior to 1958, 67 children with choroid plexus neoplasms in all locations were described in the literature. Of these, 24 had been operated on and 13 had survived.[6] In 1979, Fortuna et al reported a 48% surgical mortality in the literature from their review of 25 cases of choroid plexus neoplasms removed from the third ventricle.[94] The intraventricular location, associated hydrocephalus, and an abundant vascular supply are the principal features of all these tumors and are responsible for their associated morbidity and mortality. These lesions present a technical challenge even to the experienced neurosurgeon. *Even in the last three decades, surgical mortality in series has been reported as high as 24%[27,53] and as low as 0%.[48]*

Improved outcomes were achieved by progressive developments in CSF shunting techniques, imaging technology, hemostasis, microsurgical technique, and perioperative care (i.e., the intensive care environment, neuroanesthesia) such that several series report a 100% perioperative survival in patients with papilloma who underwent surgery after 1961.[3,33,48]

The complications of transcortical and transcallosal surgery are specific to the approach, preoperative condition of the patient, location of the tumor, and difficulty encountered in removing the tumor. The risks and potential complications are well described and include hematoma, hemiparesis, seizure disorders, developmental delay, neuropsychological deficits, visual field deficits, and cranial nerve deficits.[38,43]

BOX 24–11
Potential Surgical Complications

- **Hematoma**
- **Hemiparesis**
- **Seizures**
- **Developmental delay**
- **Neuropsychological deficits**
- **Visual field deficits**
- **Cranial nerve deficits**
- **Subdural fluid collections**

All of the series on choroid plexus neoplasms are too small to support general statements concerning neurologic outcome. Histopathologic features do not always correlate with outcome but, not surprisingly, children with papilloma tend to have significantly more favorable outcomes than children with less resectable carcinoma. Eight of 10 infants with choroid plexus papilloma in the third ventricle survived without recurrence after tumor resection in the series reported by Schijman et al in 1990.[43] However, 3 of the 8 survivors had a seizure disorder and mental retardation.[43] Thirteen of 17 of Tomita et al's patients reported in 1988 exhibited normal neurologic and psychomotor development after removal of their choroid plexus papilloma.[33] The majority were younger than 2 years at the time of diagnosis. In a series of 40 patients with choroid plexus neoplasms studied over a 45-year period, only 50% with carcinoma survived, compared with 84% with papilloma. The major morbidity in the survivors was hemiparesis (23%) and seizures (25%). However, 18% of the patients presented with a seizure, thus obscuring the precise incidence of postoperative seizures caused by the surgical intervention. While 23% of patients with papilloma enjoyed an excellent outcome without neurologic deficit, surprisingly, 14% of patients with carcinoma also did.

There is controversy among centers about the prognosis of choroid plexus carcinoma. *There is considerable disagreement on the degree to which surgical excision extends survival in the malignant lesions.* Some groups maintain a pessimistic posture despite survival of patients in their own series, arguing that these tumors possess a uniformly grave outcome.[12, 79] However, the groups who record survivals are no less cautious. In 1982, Carpenter et al reviewed 25 patients in the literature with choroid plexus carcinoma and concluded that only 4 of them enjoyed "relatively good results."[95] The groups with survivors have simply been impressed that aggressive surgical intervention (multiple times if necessary), followed or preceded by adjuvant therapy has yielded a few long-term survivors—an outcome previously considered impossible.[3–5]

The complete removal of a neoplasm of the choroid plexus does not obviate the need for placement of a shunt in all pa-tients.[48, 67, 68] Furthermore, one of the more problematic complications of intraventricular surgery for choroid neoplasms is the development of symptomatic subdural fluid collections, which has been discussed in detail by several authors.[9, 38, 96] While this complication is not merely confined to the removal of choroid plexus tumors, it has been seen with both the transcortical and the transcallosal approach. Jooma and Grant reported two cases of subdural hygromas after transcallosal removal of third ventricular papillomas.[55] In Boyd and Steinbock's surgical series of 11 patients with choroid plexus neoplasm, 2 patients developed postoperative subdural collections requiring a subdural peritoneal shunt after transcortical surgery.[38] The authors argued that this complication may possibly be lessened by making a smaller cortisectomy, filling the ventricles with physiologic saline prior to dural closure, and placing a fine pial suture or tissue glue to close the fistulae.[38]

Extent of surgical resection of choroid plexus tumors remains the single most important determinant of long-term disease-free survival.[3, 5, 30, 37, 97, 98] *Adjuvant therapy may be required for tumors that are incompletely resected, malignant, or have shown neuraxis/leptomeningeal spread.* External-beam irradiation remains a potent form of adjuvant therapy in older children, especially craniospinal irradiation for patients with drop metastases, leptomeningeal spread, and tumors invading the parenchyma.[99] The role of radiation therapy, both conventional and focused-beam, remains undefined in the treatment of this disease. The documented neuropsychological effects of radiation therapy on the developing brain[100] has led to alternative approaches. Patients younger than 3 years have received chemotherapy in lieu of radiation therapy to spare them cognitive dysfunction and short stature associated with radiotherapeutic treatment. Gianella-Borradori et al successfully treated two children with subtotal resected malignant carcinomas with an 8-drugs-in-1-day regimen without radiation therapy. They concluded that chemotherapy may provide long-term survival but that more trials are needed.[101] There are more recent reports of aggressive multimodality therapy that consists of combined pre- or postresection chemotherapy and radiotherapy. This approach is also used during subsequent attempts at radical resection of choroid plexus carcinoma that could not initially be removed. *The conclusion is that pretreatment with chemotherapy shrinks the tumor, resulting in an easier subsequent surgery and a longer disease-free survival period.*[79, 102, 103] A 1995 report from the Pediatric Oncology Group described eight infants with choroid plexus carcinoma who underwent surgery, followed by successful prolonged postoperative chemotherapy and delayed radiation. The conclusion was that this aggressive multimodality approach prolongs survival even in children who underwent subtotal resection of choroid plexus neoplasm. However, the danger of delayed disease recurrence from meningeal carcinomatosis in carcinoma still exists despite this aggressive multimodality therapy.[104]

SUMMARY

Choroid plexus neoplasms are a highly diverse group of tumors. In children, they often reach a large size and are associated with hydrocephalus prior to diagnosis. They are most commonly found in the lateral ventricles. When histologically benign they rarely demonstrate extraneural metastases and are surgically curable.

Regardless of their histologic characteristics, they are challenging lesions from a surgical point of view, possessing an impressive vascular supply often buried deep in the tumor mass. The anatomy of the ventricles and its relationship to the tumor permits a variety of surgical approaches. A combination of approaches or a staged approach is occasionally required to adequately achieve excision of the lesion with minimal morbidity.

The treatment of choroid plexus papilloma has yielded excellent results with exceptionally high survival rates in the microsurgical era. In the majority of cases it is curable by surgical extirpation alone. Rarely does this tumor recur when totally excised. The treatment of postoperative subdural effusions and hydrocephalus is often the most confounding perioperative challenge in the treatment of these lesions. Significant neurologic deficits can and do occur but are probably fewer in the microsurgical era.

The prognosis for prolonged survival after surgical excision of choroid plexus carcinoma was originally thought to be dismal. However, in the last two decades there have been small series and scattered case reports of survival after removal of this malignant form of choroid plexus neoplasm.[3–5] Some groups are encouraged based on an aggressive surgical posture, appropriate adjuvant therapy, and vigilant follow-up. They maintain that there is some hope for survival, albeit limited and guarded. The series of choroid plexus carcinoma are simply too small to yield any conclusive prognostic data on long-term survival. The advances in imaging, microsurgical technique, postoperative care, and adjuvant therapy have been, in part, responsible for a measured improvement over the previously dismal survival statistics. As long as the lesion remains localized and the patient's condition permits, an attempt at an aggressive therapeutic approach is justified.

REFERENCES

1. Rubinstein L. Tumors of the choroid plexus and related structures. In: Firminger HI, ed. *Tumors of the Central Nervous System*. Washington, DC: Armed Forces Institute of Pathology; 1972.
2. Burger PC, Scheithauer BW. Tumors of neuroglia and choroid plexus epithelium. In: Burger PC, Scheithauer BW, eds. *Tumors of the Central Nervous System*. Washington DC: Armed Forces Institute of Pathology; 1994:136–161.
3. Ellenbogen RG, Winston KR, and Kupsky WJ. Tumors of the choroid plexus in children. *Neurosurgery* 1989;25(3):327–335.
4. Lena G, Genitori L, Molina J, et al. Choroid plexus tumors in children: review of 24 cases. *Acta Neurochir* 1990;106:68–72.
5. Packer R, Perilongo G, Johnson D, et al. Choroid plexus carcinoma of childhood. *Cancer* 1992;69:580–585.
6. Matson D. Tumors of the choroid plexus. In: Matson DD, ed. *Neurosurgery of Infancy and Childhood*. Springfield, IL: Charles C Thomas; 1969:581–595.
7. Cushing H. *Intracranial Tumors*. Springfield, IL: Charles C Thomas; 1932.
8. Zulch K. Biologie und Pathologie der Hirngeschwulste. In: Ovecrona H, Tonnis W, eds. *Handbuch der Neurochirurgie*. Berlin: Springer-Verlag; 1956.
9. Matson D, Crofton F. Papilloma of the choroid plexus in childhood. *J Neurosurg* 1960;17:1002–1027.
10. Koos W, Miller M. *Intracranial Tumors of Infants and Children*. St. Louis: Mosby; 1971:239–244.
11. Dohrmann G, Collias J. Choroid plexus carcinoma. *J Neurosurg* 1975;43:225–232.
12. Humphreys R, Nemoto S, Hendrick EB, et al. Childhood choroid plexus tumors. *Conc Pediatr Neurosurg* 1987;7:1–18.
13. Guerard M. Tumeur Fongeuse dans le ventricle droit du cerveau chez une petite fille de trois ans. *Anat Paris* 1832;8:211–214.
14. Davis L, Cushing H. Papillomas of the choroid plexus: a report of six cases. *Arch Neurol Psychiatry* 1925;13:681–710.
15. Boudet G, Clunet J. Contribution a l'etude des tumeurs epitheliales primitives de l'encephale. *Arch Med Exper Anat Pathol* 1910;22:379–411.
16. Davis L. A physiopathological study of the choroid plexus with the report of a case of villous hypertrophy. *Med Res* 1924;44:521–534.
17. Garrod. Papillomatous tumor in the fourth ventricle of the brain. *Lancet* 1873;1:303.
18. Perthes G. Entfernung eines Tumors des Plexus Choriodeus an dem Seitenventrikel des Cerebrums. *Munch Med Wschr* 1919;66:677–678.
19. Rand C, Reeves D. Choroid plexus tumors in infancy and childhood: report of four cases. *Bull Los Angeles Neurol Soc* 1940;5:405–410.
20. Sachs E. Papillomas of the fourth ventricle. *Arch Neurol Psychiatry* 1922;8:379–382.
21. Slaymaker S, Elias F. Papilloma of the choroid plexus with hydrocephalus: report of a case. *Arch Intern Med* 1909;3:289–294.
22. Van Wagenen W. Papillomas of the choroid plexus: report of two cases, one with removal of tumor and one with "seeding" of the tumor in the ventricular system. *Arch Surg (Chicago)* 1930;20:199–231.
23. Turner O, Simon M. Malignant papillomas of the choroid plexus: report of two cases with review of the literature. *Am J Cancer* 1937;30:289–297.
24. Bielschowsky M, Unger E. Kenntnis der primaren Epithelgeschwulste der Adergeflechte des Gehirns. *Arch Klin Chir* 1906;81:61–82.
25. Dandy W. *Benign Encapsulated Tumors of the Lateral Ventricle*. Baltimore: Williams & Wilkins; 1934.
26. Masson C. Complete removal of two tumors of the third ventricle with recovery. *Arch Surg* 1934;28:527–537.
27. Hawkins JCI. Treatment of choroid plexus papillomas in children: a brief analysis of twenty years' experience. *Neurosurgery* 1980;6:380–384.
28. Laurence K. The biology of choroid plexus papilloma and carcinoma of the lateral ventricle. In: Vinken P, Bruyn G, eds. *Tumors of the Brain and Skull*. Part 2, *Handbook of Clinical Neurology*. New York: Elsevier; 1974;555–595.
29. Pascual-Castroviejo I, Villarejo F, Perez-Higueras A, et al. Childhood choroid plexus neoplasms: a study of 14 cases less than 2 years old. *Eur Pediatr* 1983;140:51–56.
30. Johnson DL. Management of choroid plexus tumors in children. *Pediatr Neurosci* 1989;15(4):195–206.
31. Tomita T, Naidich TP. Successful resection of choroid plexus papillomas diagnosed at birth: report of two cases. *Neurosurgery* 1987;20:774–779.
32. Body G, Darnis E, Pourcelot D et al. Choroid plexus tumors: antenatal diagnosis and follow-up. *J Clin Ultrasound* 1990;18:575–578.
33. Tomita T, McLone DG, Flannery AM. Choroid plexus papillomas of neonates, infants and children. *Pediatr Neurosc* 1988;14:23–30.
34. Knierim DS. Choroid plexus tumors in infants. *Pediatr Neurosurg* 1990;16:276–280.
35. Kahn E, Luros J. Hydrocephalus from overproduction of cerebrospinal fluid (and experiences with other papilloma of the choroid plexus). *J Neurosurg* 1952;9:59–67.
36. Russell D, Rubinstein L. *Pathology of Tumors of the Nervous System*. 2nd ed. London: Edward Arnold; 1971.
37. McGirr SJ, Ebersold MJ, Scheithauer BW, et al., Choroid plexus papillomas: long-term follow-up results in a surgically treated series. *J Neurosurg* 1988;69:843–849.
38. Boyd M, Steinbock M. Choroid plexus tumors: problems in diagnosis and management. *H Beyrisyrg* 1987;66:800–805.
39. Shaw J. Papilloma of the choroid plexus. In: Amador L, ed. *Brain Tumors in the Young*. Springfield, IL: Charles C Thomas; 1983;655–670.
40. Ray B, Peck F, Jr. Papilloma of the choroid plexus of the lateral ventricles causing hydrocephalus in an infant. *J Neurosurg* 1956;13:405–410.
41. Abbott K, Rollas Z, Meagher J. Choroid plexus papilloma causing spontaneous subarachnoid hemorrhage. *J Neurosurg* 1957;14:566–570.
42. Ernsting J. Choroid plexus papilloma causing spontaneous subarachnoid hemorrhage. *J Neurol Neurosurg Psychiatr* 1955;18:134–136.

43. Schijman E, Monges J, Raimondi A, et al. Choroid plexus papillomas of the third ventricle in childhood. *Child's Nerv Syst* 1990;6:331–334.

44. Milhorat T, Hammock M, Davis D, et al., Choroid plexus papilloma: proof of cerebrospinal overproduction. *Child's Brain* 1976;2:273–289.

45. Pollack IF, Schor NF, Martinez JA, et al. Bobble-head doll syndrome and drop attacks in a child with a cystic choroid plexus papilloma of the third ventricle. *J Neurosurg* 1995;83:729–732.

46. Hammock M, Milhorat T, Breckbill D. Primary choroid plexus papilloma of the cerebellopontine angle, presenting as brain stem tumor in a child. *Child's Brain* 1976;2: 132–142.

47. Wilkins R, Rutledge B. Papillomas of the choroid plexus. *J Neurosurg* 1961;18:14–18.

48. Raimondi A, Gutierrez F. Diagnosis and surgical treatment of choroid plexus papillomas. *Child's Brain* 1975;1: 81–115.

49. Cassinari V. Tumori della parte anteriore del terzo ventricolo. *Acta Neurochir* 1963;11:236–271.

50. Pecker J, Ferrand B, Javalet A. Tumeurs du troisieme ventricule. *Neurochirurgie* 1966;12:1–136.

51. Aicardi JGJ, Lepintre J, Cherrie JJ, Thieffry S. Les papillomes des plexus choroides chez l'enfant. *Archs Fr Pediatr* 1968;25:673–686.

52. Bohm J, Strange R. Choroid plexus papillomas. *J Neurosurg* 1961;18:493–500.

53. Guidetti B, Spallone A. The surgical treatment of choroid plexus papillomas: the results of 27 years' experience. *Neurosurgery* 1981;6:380–384.

54. Zhang W. Clinical significance of anterior inferior cerebellar artery in angiographic diagnosis of choroid plexus papilloma at the cerebellopontine angle. *Chin Med J (Engl)* 1983;96:275–280.

55. Jooma R, Grant D. Third ventricle choroid plexus papillomas. *Child'sBrain* 1983;10:242–250.

56. Rovit R, Schechter M, Chodroff P. Choroid plexus papillomas—observation on radiologic diagnosis. *Am J Roentgenol* 1970;110:608–617.

57. Fairburn B. Choroid plexus papilloma and its relationship to hydrocephalus. *J Neurosurg* 1958;17:166–171.

58. Johnson R. Clinicopathological aspects of the cerebrospinal fluid circulation. In: Wilstenholme G, O'Conner M, eds. *Ciba Foundation Symposium on Cerebrospinal Fluid Production, Circulation and Absorption.* Boston: Little, Brown and Company; 1957:265–281.

59. Portnoy H, Croissant P. A practical method of measuring hydrodynamics of cerebrospinal fluid. *Surg Neurol* 1976; 5:273–277.

60. Vigouroux A. Ecoulement de liquide cephalorachidien: hydrocephalie papillome des plexus chorides du IV ventricule. *Rev Neurol* 1970;16:281–285.

61. Sahar A, Feinsod M, Beller A. Choroid plexus papilloma: hydrocephalus and cerebrospinal fluid dynamics. *Surg Neurol* 1980;13:476–478.

62. Eisenberg H, McComb G, Lorenzo A. Cerebrospinal fluid overproduction and hydrocephalus associated with choroid plexus papilloma. *J Neurosurg* 1974;40:380–385.

63. Welch K, Strand R, Bresnan M, et al. Congenital hydrocephalus due to villous hypertrophy of the telencephalic

choroid plexuses: case report. *J Neurosurg* 1983;59: 172–175.

64. Gudeman S, Sullivan H, Rosner M, et al. Surgical removal of bilateral papillomas of the choroid plexus of the lateral ventricles with resolution of hydrocephalus. *J Neurosurg* 1979;50:677–681.

65. Rekate HL, Erwood S, Brodkey JA, et al. Etiology of ventriculomegaly in choroid plexus papilloma. *Pediatr Neuroscience,* 1985–86;12:196–201.

66. Husag L, Costabile G, Probst C. Persistent hydrocephalus following removal of choroid plexus papilloma of the lateral ventricle. *Neurochirugia (Stuttgart)* 1984;27:82–85.

67. Jellinger K, Grunert V, Sunder-Plassmann M. Choroid plexus papilloma associated with hydrocephalus in infancy. *Beyrioaeduatrue* 1970;1:344–348.

68. McDonald J. Persistent hydrocephalus following the removal of papillomas of the choroid plexus of the lateral ventricles. *J Neurosurg* 1969;30:736–740.

69. Smith J. Hydrocephalus associated with choroid plexus papillomas. *Neuropathol Exp Neurol* 1933;14:442–449.

70. Hirano H, Hirahara K, Tetsuhiko A, et al. Hydrocephalus due to villous hypertrophy of the choroid plexus in the lateral ventricles. *J Neurosurg* 1994;80:321–323.

71. Crofton F, Matson D. Roentgenologic study of choroid plexus papillomas in children. *Am J Roentgenol Radium Ther Nucl Med* 1950;84:273–311.

72. Vazquez E, Ball WS, Prenger EC, et al. Magnetic resonance imaging of fourth ventricular choroid plexus neoplasms in childhood. *Pediatr Neurosurg* 1991;17:48–52.

73. Coates TL, Hinshaw DB Jr, Peckman N, et al. Pediatric choroid plexus neoplasms: MR, CT, and pathologic correlation. *Radiology* 1989;173:81–88.

74. Schellhas KP, Siebert RC, Heithoff KB, et al. Congenital choroid plexus papilloma of the third ventricle: diagnosis with real-time sonography and MR imaging. *Am J Neuroradiol* 1988;9:797–798.

75. Morrison G, Sobel D, Kelly W, et al. Intraventricular mass lesions. *Radiology* 1984;153:435–442.

76. Gullotta F, de Melo A. Plexus chorioideus: klinishe, lightmikroskopische und elektronenoptische Untersuchungen. *Neurochirurgia (Stuttgart)* 1979;22:1–9.

77. Paulus W, Janisch W. Clincopathologic correlations in epithelial choroid plexus neoplasms: a study of 52 cases. *Acta Neuropathol (Berlin)* 1990;80:635–41.

78. Matsuda M, Uzura S, Nakasu S, et al. Primary carcinoma of the choroid plexus in the lateral ventricle. *Surg Neurol* 1991;36:294–299.

79. St. Clair SK, Humphreys RP, Pillay PK, et al. Current management of choroid plexus carcinoma in children. *Pediatr Neurosurg* 1991;92(17):225–233.

80. Lewis P. Carcinoma of the choroid plexus. *Brain* 1967;90: 177–186.

81. Ausman J, Shrontz C, Chason J, et al. Aggressive choroid plexus papilloma. *Surg Neurol* 1984;22:472–476.

82. Russell D, Rubinstein L. *Pathology of Tumors of the Nervous System.* 2nd ed. Baltimore: Williams & Wilkins; 1963: 141–142.

83. Ringertz N, Reymond A. Ependymomas and choroid plexus papillomas. *J Neuropathol Exp Neurol* 1949;8:355.

84. Vraa-Jensen G. Papilloma of the choroid plexus with pulmonary metastases. *Acta Paychtr (Koln)* 1950;25:299–306.

85. Hirano A. Some contributions of electron microscopy to the diagnosis of brain tumors. *Acta Neuropathol (Berlin)* 1978;43:119–128.

86. Ang L, Taylor A, Bergin D, et al. An immunohistochemical study of papillary tumors of the central nervous system. *Cancer* 1990;65:2712–2719.

87. Cruz-Sanchez F, Rossi M, Hughes J, et al. Choroid plexus papillomas: an immunohistological study of 16 cases. *Histopathology* 1989;15:61–69.

88. Coffin C, Wick M, Braun J, et al. Choroid plexus neoplasms: clinicopathological and immunohistochemical studies. *Am Surg Pathol* 1986;10:394–404.

89. Furness P, Lowe J, Tarrant G. Subepithelial basement deposition and intermediate filament expression in choroid plexus neoplasms and ependymomas. *Histopathology* 1990;16:251–255.

90. Shirakawa N, Kannuki S, Matsumoto K. Clinocopathological study on choroid plexus tumors: immunochemical features and arygyrophilic nucleolar organizer regions values. *Noshuyo Byori* 1994;11(1):99–105.

91. Bergsagel D, Finegold M, Butel J, et al. DNA sequences similar to those of simian virus 40 in ependymomas and choroid plexus tumors of childhood. *N Engl J Med* 1992;326:988–993.

92. Timurkaynak E, Rhoton A, Barry M. Microsurgical anatomy and approaches to the lateral ventricles. *Neurosurgery* 1986;19:685–723.

93. Jun C, Nutic S. Surgical approaches to intraventricular meningiomas of the trigone. *Neurosurgery* 1985;16:416–420.

94. Fortuna A, Celli P, Ferrante L, et al. A review of papillomas of the third ventricle. *J Neurosurg* 1979;23:61–72.

95. Carpenter D, Michelsen W, Hays A. Carcinoma of the choroid plexus. *J Neurosurg* 1982;56:722–777.

96. Shillito J, Matson D. *An Atlas of Pediatric Neurosurgical Operations.* Philadelphia: WB Saunders; 1982.

97. Pierga J, Kalifa C, Terrier-Lacombe MJ, et al. Carcinoma of the choroid plexus: a pediatric experience. *Med Pediatr Oncol,* 1993;21(7):480–487.

98. Sharma R, Rout D, Gupta A, et al. Choroid plexus papillomas. *Br J Neurosurg,* 1994;8(2):169–177.

99. Geerts Y, Gabreels F, Lippens R, et al Choroid plexus carcinoma: a report of two cases and review of the literature. *Neuropediatrics* 1996;27(3):143–148.

100. Duffner P, Cohen M, Thomas P, et al. The long term effects of cranial irradiation in the central nervous system. *Cancer* 1985;56:1841–1847.

101. Gianella-Borradori, Zeltzer PM, Bodey B, et al. Choroid plexus tumors in childhood. *Cancer* 1992;69:809–816.

102. Kumabe T, Tominaga T, Kondo T, et al. Intraoperative radiation therapy and chemotherapy for huge choroid plexus carcinoma in an infant—case report. *Neurol Med-Chir* 1996;36(3):179–184.

103. Araki K, Aori T, Takahashi J. et al. A case report of choroid plexus carcinoma. *No Shinkei Geka-Neurological Surgery* 1997;25(9):853–857.

104. Peschgens T, Stollbrink-Peschgens C, Mertens R, et al. Zur Therapie des Plexus-chorioideus-Karzinomas im Kindesalter: Fallbeispiel und Literaturubersicht. *Klinische Pediatrie* 1995;207(2):52–58.

Chapter 25

Intracranial Meningioma

Leon E. Moores and Philip H. Cogen

The typically benign nature of meningiomas and the importance of surgical resection in their treatment have undoubtedly been responsible for the enthusiasm with which neurosurgeons view these lesions.[1] Since Cushing first described these tumors in 1922 and, together with Eisenhardt, categorized them in 1938, improvements in recurrence-free and overall survival have resulted from advances in imaging and microsurgical technique.[2, 3] In the pediatric population, the longer life expectancy of children demands particular attention to the long-term outcome from therapy. Apart from the male predominance, calvarial deformation, increased incidence of intraventricular location, and tumor growth without dural attachment, pediatric meningiomas differ little from adult meningiomas. Presenting symptoms, tumor histology, and outcome are thus similar in adult and pediatric patients. The current literature suggests that, like adult meningiomas, these tumors in the pediatric age group should be managed with aggressive surgical resection. Radiation therapy should be considered for subtotally resected lesions. Patients should be instructed early on regarding the need for lifetime follow-up imaging.

EPIDEMIOLOGIC FACTORS

Meningiomas are rare in children.[58, 64] A small percentage of all meningiomas are found in patients younger than 21.[52] Several reports since 1980, early on in the magnetic resonance imaging (MRI) era, reviewed a total of 6613 meningiomas in patients of all ages, 1.7% of which were diagnosed in pediatric patients.[4–8] However, the definition of a pediatric patient was inconsistent, as the upper age cutoff varied from 15 to 20 years. Several recent series have revealed that only 2.7% of 3825 aggregate reported childhood brain tumors were meningiomas.[5–11] By comparison, in adults approximately 13 to 20% of intracranial tumors are meningiomas.[12, 13]

The overall annual incidence of pediatric brain tumors in North America has been estimated at 2.5–4/100,000 children.[14] The U.S. Census Bureau data for 1999 estimate that 80 million citizens in the United States are younger than 20 years (www.census.gov). This should translate into approximately 2000 to 3200 newly diagnosed pediatric brain tumors per year. Given a meningioma incidence of 2.7% of pediatric

tumors, 54 to 86 newly diagnosed meningiomas should be identified in children each year.

The association of meningiomas with neurofibromatosis (NF) has been well documented.[4–7, 9, 15, 16] The occurrence of meningiomas in both NF-1 and NF-2 has been described (Fig. 25–1). One series documented 12 patients with meningiomas, reporting that 7 patients had NF-1 and 5 patients had NF-2.[9] In several series, the percentage of patients with meningiomas who also have NF is much higher than the percentage of patients in the general population who have NF. In five aggregate series reviewing 126 pediatric patients with meningiomas, 1 of 4 patients with meningiomas had NF.[4–7] This is significantly higher than the incidence of NF-1 in the general population of 1:2500 or the incidence of NF-2 of 1:40000.

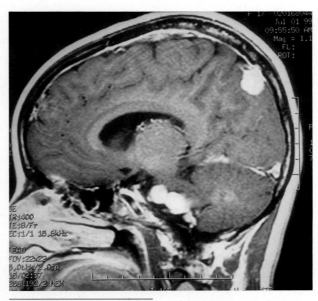

Figure 25–1 A 17-year-old girl with neurofibromatosis type 1 and multiple intracranial meningiomas. One parasagittal meningioma is shown, and a larger parasagittal meningioma was present on the contralateral side. Note the presence of multiple neurofibromas along the cranial nerves anterior to the brain stem.

CLINICAL FEATURES

Data from the computed tomography (CT) and MRI era have shown the peak age for patient presentation is the eighth to ninth decade of life.[17-18] Within the pediatric population, the incidence peaks at age 12 (Table 25–1).

Unlike the male/female ratio of 1:2 in adult meningiomas,[18] there is a distinct male predominance in the pediatric population. Four recent studies clearly document both patient age and sex in detail and allow direct comparison (Table 25–2).[9, 11, 19–21] The resulting male/female ratio is 1.4:1. Although hormonal influences have been postulated as the cause of the male/female ratio in adults, no female predominance after age 12 years was noted in these combined data. However, it is likely that hormonal effects beginning at puberty would not manifest themselves for at least 5 to 10 years.

As with most intracranial mass lesions, the signs and symptoms are dependent on the location of the tumor, the rapidity of growth, and the tendency toward irritation of surrounding tissue. Meningiomas are typically indolent and thus present as slow-growing extra-axial mass lesions with deformity of adjacent neural elements. The average duration of symptoms in several combined reports (43 total patients) was 15 months.[10, 20–22] In ten series reported in the English literature since 1980, 45% (83/184) of children presented with symptoms of increased intracranial pressure, such as headache, nausea, vomiting, and changes in mental status.[4–9, 11, 21, 22] Papilledema may be identified in association with either extraordinarily large masses or secondary hydrocephalus. Motor deficits were seen in 25% (46/184) of these children, cranial nerve palsies in 21% (39/184), and seizures in 20% (38/184). Cranial deformities were reported in 12% (22/184), personality changes in 3% (6/184), and neck pain in 0.5% (1/184) of cases. Table 25–3 compares pediatric and adult series.

The location of pediatric meningiomas differs minimally from that in adults. Several studies have shown an increased frequency of intraventricular (Fig. 25–2) posterior fossa and

TABLE 25–1 Age Data in Pediatric Meningioma Patients

Study	>1 yr	1–5 yr	6–10 yr	11–19 yr	Mean
Erdincler et al.	2	5	4	18	N/A
Baumgartner et al.	0	1	3	8	12
Ferrante et al.	1	1	3	14	12
Davidson et al.	1	1	2	13	12
Kolluri et al.	0	3	5	10	13
Herz et al.	0	1	2	6	N/A
Total	4	12	19	69	12

N/A, not applicable.
References for data included in this table are included within the text.

TABLE 25–2 Age and Sex Data in Pediatric Meningioma Patients

Study	<12 yr old Male	<12 yr old Female	>12 yr old Male	>12 yr old Female
Erdincler et al.	7	3	6	4
Davidson et al.	6	5	12	6
Kolluri et al.	0	3	4	2
Herz et al.	4	4	5	5
Total	17	15	27	17
Ratio	1.1:1		1.6:1	

References for data included in this table are included within the text.

TABLE 25–3 Presentation in Pediatric and Adult Meningiomas (%)[4–8, 11, 18, 22, 23]

Factor	Pediatric population (184 cases)	Adult population (774 cases)
Increase intracranial pressure	45	43
Motor deficit	25	19
Cranial nerve palsy	21	12
Seizures	21	12
Calvarial deformity	12	0

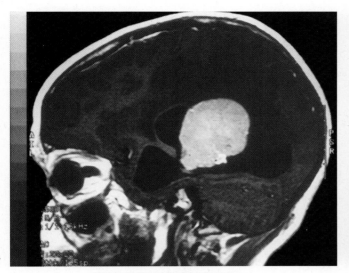
A

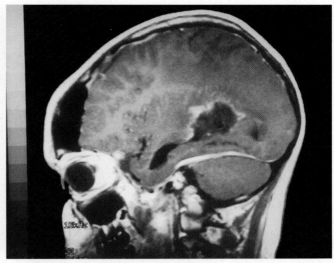
B

Figure 25–2 (A) Pre- and (B) postoperative magnetic resonance image of an 11-year-old boy with a large intraventricular meningioma. Histology was that of typical meningioma.

non-dural-based lesions in children. *In recent reports, intraventricular and non-dural-based meningiomas were more prevalent in children, but the majority of lesions were still located in the supratentorial compartment.*

In the 215 lesions reported since 1980, there were 140 (65%) convexity and supratentorial skull base lesions.[4–11, 20, 21] This is similar to several adult series showing an approximately 75% supratentorial location.[18, 23] Twenty-one (10%) of the pediatric lesions were found in the posterior fossa. This does not differ substantially from reports in which 14% of meningiomas in adults were located in the posterior fossa.[18, 23]

The absence of dural attachment and intraventricular location is more common in children. Twenty-one pediatric lesions (10%) were reported without dural attachment,[4–11, 20, 21] versus no meningiomas without dural attachment in three large adult series reporting on 1431 patients.[18, 23, 24] Intraventricular meningiomas arise from the velum interpositum, choroid plexus, or the floor of the third ventricle. In 215 total pediatric cases, intraventricular lesions accounted for 11% (23 cases). In two adult series, only 2% were intraventricular.[18, 23]

ETIOLOGIC FACTORS

The literature is contradictory concerning trauma as a possible etiologic factor in the formation of meningiomas. A study by Annegers et al. in 1979 found no correlation.[25] In their review of 3587 patients with significant head trauma from 1935 to 1974, they found 2953 survivors without known previous history of a brain tumor. A total of 29,859 person-years of follow-up was recorded. Three meningiomas were found, with 1.85 expected (95% confidence interval 0.3 to 4.7). It is important to consider several factors that may have influenced these results. The inclusion criteria for significant head trauma were loss of consciousness,

perievent amnesia, or skull fracture. These strict inclusion criteria may be responsible for the lower association than that seen in previous studies where patients with meningiomas were asked if they recalled any previous head trauma.[3] In addition, the incidence of meningiomas in the injury group may have been lower due to the relatively short (10-year) average follow-up. When compared to latency data postirradiation, this is a relatively brief period. Finally, the authors made no comment on whether the data were sex-matched. Because men experience more head trauma and women have a higher incidence of meningiomas, the number of meningiomas found in an injury group would be lower (more males) and the expected incidence in a general population would be higher (more females) if the populations were not matched for sex. Barnett et al. reviewed several cases with compelling anatomical and histologic association between known significant head trauma and subsequent meningioma formation, but small numbers rendered the study inconclusive.[26] Schlehofer, et al. reported in 1992 a case control study of 226 intracranial tumors matched with 418 controls without tumors.[27] As part of a detailed survey, patients were asked if they had suffered a head injury that resulted in a physician visit and occurred at least 5 years prior to diagnosis of the tumor. The analysis showed a slightly decreased risk of formation of intracranial tumors in the head trauma cohort. When meningiomas were analyzed separately, the relative risk after head injury was 0.52 (95% confidence interval 0.3 to 1.0).

Radiation to the meninges increases the risk of meningioma formation (Fig. 25–3). Increasing dose or young age at the time of treatment may decrease the latent period for tumor formation.[54, 65] Therapeutic irradiation has been categorized as either low (<10 Gy), moderate (10 to 20 Gy), or high (>20 Gy) dose.[59] The study on meningioma formation after irradiation, which established both a relative risk and a dose response, reviewed 10,834 patients who had undergone low-dose radiation treatment for tinea capitis.[28] These patients were compared to

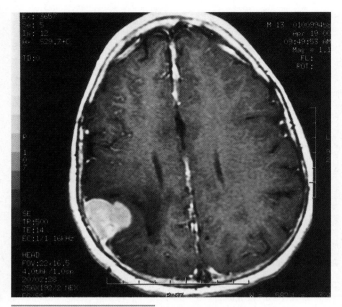

Figure 25–3 13-year-old boy who presented with a right parietal meningioma 11 years after cranial irradiation for a medulloblastoma.

10,834 age and sex-matched controls as well as to 5392 nonirradiated siblings. Low-dose irradiation in this study was associated with a relative risk of meningioma formation of 9.5 (95% confidence interval 3.5 to 25.7%), and this risk increased with dosage from less than 1 Gy to more than 3 Gy. The average time from irradiation to diagnosis of the meningioma was 21 years. Mack and Wilson found in their group of patients receiving high-dose irradiation that the latency to tumor formation was reduced with increased radiation dose and younger age at time of irradiation.[29] Ghim et al. corroborated these findings in 1993 with a review of 15 children aged 2 months to 9 years (mean age 2.5) who had high-dose external-beam irradiation.[30] The mean time to diagnosis of the meningiomas was 13 years (range 5 to 15) and the mean radiation dosage was 41 Gy (range 15 to 80 Gy). Soffer et al. have argued that radiation-induced meningiomas are biologically different from meningiomas in patients who had no previous local irradiation.[31] In comparing 42 radiation-induced meningiomas with 84 meningiomas unassociated with radiation, they noted a statistically significant increase in recurrence rate, number of malignant meningiomas, and number of tumors classified as hypercellular. There was a trend toward increased pleomorphism, mitotic rate, necrosis, and brain invasion in postirradiation tumors, although these data did not reach statistical significance.

Chromosomal abnormalities have also been associated with meningiomas in both adult and pediatric populations.[51] Abnormalities of chromosome 22, from monosomy 22 to 22q− either with or without complex karyotype, have been studied in some detail. Slavc et al. in 1995 studied the chromosomes of three pediatric patients with meningiomas and found two with loss of part of chromosome 22.[16] The single patient without a diagnostic chromosomal abnormality had an anaplastic

meningioma. None of these patients had clinical evidence of NF-2. The investigators reported a 60% sensitivity in the ability to detect chromosomal abnormalities. Cogen et al. noted that the loss of heterozygosity mapped to human meningiomas on chromosome 22 overlapped the NF-2 region but included a distal sequence.[32] Loss of chromosome 22 alleles has been reported in meningioma patients with and without a diagnosis of NF-2.[15] In this work, Biegel et al. found that six of eight pediatric meningioma patients had abnormalities of chromosome 22. The two patients with NF-2 had monosomy of chromosome 22. Certainly the association with chromosome 22 abnormalities that is common to both meningiomas and NF-2 remains of interest and deserves further study. Patients with meningiomas have also been noted to have loss of chromosome 1, 6, 8, 18, or Y, or gain of chromosome 20.[15]

IMAGING

Plain film imaging of meningiomas can show hyperostosis, bone erosion, or calcifications within the tumor. Three reports showed that 60% of plain radiographs performed in 71 pediatric patients with meningiomas had one or more of these findings.[5, 9, 10] However, these abnormalities are quite nonspecific for diagnosis of tumor type.[61]

BOX 25–1 Radiographic Features
• **Hyperostosis**
• **Bone erosion**
• **Calcification**

In many cases CT can be diagnostic of a meningioma. In a mixed adult and pediatric series of 559 CT scans performed at the Mayo Clinic, 94% of meningiomas were correctly diagnosed on preoperative CT scan.[23] The scan typically shows an extra-axial mass that is hyperdense with respect to gray matter. The mass displaces normal neural structures from the dural or ventricular site of origin. There is a characteristic flattening of the sulci and compression of the gyri that are the opposite of the widened gyri of an intrinsic parenchymal mass. In as many as 25% of cases meningiomas have areas of calcification that appear hyperdense on CT scan and may be focal or diffuse. Cystic changes have been reported in pediatric and adult patients; these cysts are hypodense on CT. In 215 patients reported in 10 pediatric series, the incidence of cystic meningiomas was 8%,[4–11, 20, 21] versus adult series with a 3 to 5% incidence of cystic meningiomas.[2, 33] The solid portions of meningiomas typically show strong and homogeneous enhancement. Areas of calcification will not enhance, although the density may rival that of the adjacent enhancing tumor. CT scanning is also exquisitely sensitive in terms of the bony changes that may occur in this disease. Hyperostosis, blistering, scalloping, and thinning of the bone are readily recognizable on high-resolution bone window images.

BOX 25–2
CT Features

- **Hyperdense, extra-axial**
- **25% show calcification**
- **May be cystic**
- **Enhance with contrast**
- **Bone changes**

The angiographic appearance of meningiomas depends on the vascular pattern and on the displacement of adjacent vascular structures. Meningiomas often receive uniform and finely detailed blood supply to their periphery from the adjacent pial vessels. The center of the tumor is supplied by dural branches from the external carotid or the cavernous sinus, with the exception of intraventricular lesions that are supplied by choroidal branches. Vessels fill early in the arterial phase, typically described as a blush and present in 85% of meningiomas. These vessels retain contrast into the venous phase after the adjacent capillaries have washed out their contrast.[18] Currently, CT and MRI have supplanted angiography for diagnosis of meningiomas. The sensitivity of modern MRI is such that both the tumor's relationships to major arteries and the patency and degree of stenosis of those arteries can often be determined. Feeding vessels are typically too small to image with MRI, but the location of the meningioma indicates the origin of the blood supply in the majority of cases. Currently, angiography is most valuable for use as an adjunct to preoperative embolization. In larger tumors or in tumors with a blood supply that cannot be easily accessed early in the case, embolization 24 to 48 hours prior to surgery may result in lower blood loss and better visualization due to decreased bleeding in the operative field. The risks of angiography must be weighed against the benefits in each case, and smaller convexity lesions generally do not warrant angiographic evaluation and preoperative treatment.

BOX 25–3
Angiographic Features

- **External carotid or cavernous sinus feeders**
- **Intraventricular lesions have choroidal feeders**
- **Arterial blush**
- **Late washout**

MRI of meningiomas yields excellent anatomical detail (Figs. 25–1 and 25–2). The extra-axial location of most meningiomas can be confirmed in three planes, allowing much greater certainty that the lesion is actually outside the brain parenchyma. T1-weighted images (T1WI) typically show a lesion isointense to mildly hypointense to adjacent gray matter that compresses the sulci, flattens the gyri, and displaces the brain, brain stem, and/or cranial nerves away from the bone and dura.[53] T2-weighted imaging (T2WI) often demonstrates more of a mixed signal than is apparent on CT or

T1WI. As with CT, tumor enhancement is uniform and striking in its intensity in the absence of cysts and calcium. Unlike CT images, however, calcium is hypointense on MRI and will not visually blend with the contrast-enhanced tumor tissue. One of the most consistent features and one of the often discussed postcontrast findings on MRI is the tapering of enhancement along the periphery of the tumor as the adjacent involved and/or reactive dura is imaged—the "dural tail." Though it is suggestive of meningioma, it is not pathognomonic. Metastatic disease, lymphoproliferative disorders, inflammatory processes, and primary bone lesions, among others, may also demonstrate this finding.

BOX 25–4
MRI Features

- **Three-plane anatomical detail**
- **T1-weighted images: isointense, mildly hypointense**
- **T2-weighted images: mixed signal**
- **Uniformly bad enhancement**
- **Tapers at the periphery**

Nuclear magnetic resonance (NMR) spectroscopy characteristically shows an increased choline peak and decreased N-acetylaspartate (NAA) peak in meningiomas. In a lesion that is difficult to distinguish from astrocytoma, the high NAA and low choline peaks of astrocytomas can help to narrow the differential diagnosis.

BOX 25–5
NMR Spectroscopic Features

- **Increased choline peak**
- **Decreased NAA peak**

HISTOLOGIC FEATURES

Macroscopically, meningiomas are firm, grayish tan to yellow, circumscribed masses with a variable number of lobulations. They typically displace the adjacent neural elements and in doing so preserve an arachnoid plane between the tumor and the normal parenchyma. Malignant meningiomas are an exception, routinely violating the pial barrier and invading the brain tissue.

Many subtypes of meningiomas have been described, and the categorization of patients is documented in many references.[4–11, 20, 21] From a descriptive standpoint, the histologic differentiation is reproducible and often straightforward.[51, 56, 60, 62, 63] However, from a prognostic standpoint, the classifications of meningothelial, fibroblastic, transitional, and psammomatous are less relevant. *For this reason, the World Health Organization*

(WHO) and the Armed Forces Institute of Pathology (AFIP) have classified meningiomas into typical, atypical, and manaplastic/malignant.[34, 35] These categories have prognostic significance. Glaholm et al. reported 5-, 10-, and 15-year actuarial tumor control rates of 84%, 74%, and 68%, respectively, with typical histology; 44%, 13%, and 0% with atypical histology; and 35%, 0%, and 0% with malignant histology[36] (Table 25–4). WHO also stresses that the papillary meningioma is an important prognostic pathologic variant.[35]

Regardless of their clinical implications, the recognition of the various subtypes of *typical meningiomas* is important for diagnosis. In a review of 203 pediatric lesions, 40% (82 tumors) were meningothelial or syncytial.[4–11] This compares with adult literature showing an incidence of 38%.[18] *Meningothelial meningiomas are recognized by indistinct cell borders that produce a sheetlike appearance without recognizable geometrical patterns.* The cells are somewhat monotonous in appearance and have a normal nuclear-to-cytoplasmic ratio.

Thirty-four tumors, or 17% of the pediatric series, were classified as fibroblastic.[4–11] A large adult series found 7% of meningiomas to be fibroblastic.[18] *Fibroblastic meningiomas have elongated cells separated by dense bands of collagen.* The nuclei are hyperchromatic, and psammoma bodies and whorls are uncommonly seen.

The same authors[4–11] reported 33 transitional, or mixed, pediatric lesions (16% of 203 tumors). This is lower than the adult series' percentage of 33%.[18] These tumors are recognized as the classic meningioma. Hemotoxylin and eosin (H&E) stains show whorls, lobules, elongated spindle cells, psammoma bodies, and collagenized blood vessels (Fig. 25–4).

TABLE 25–4 Tumor Control Rate (%)

Tumor type	5-year	10-year	15-year
Typical	84	74	68
Atypical	44	13	0
Anaplastic/malignant	35	0	0

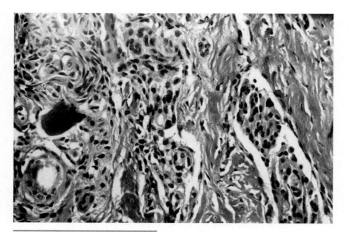

Figure 25–4 H&E-stained section of a typical meningioma. Note the whorling, the elongated spindle cells, a hyalinized vessel, and a psammoma body.

Atypical meningiomas are in the middle of the spectrum of malignant categorization of meningiomas. Their histologic features do not warrant classification as anaplastic, yet they do not appear sufficiently benign to be diagnosed as typical. Twelve pediatric tumors (6%) were found to be atypical based on increased cellularity, a sheetlike growth pattern similar to syncytial meningiomas, a higher nuclear-to-cytoplasmic ratio, prominent nucleoli, and increased mitotic activity.[4–11] A large adult and pediatric series reported that in 319 primary intracranial meningiomas 6% were atypical.[17] Although this series reported all age groups, none of the atypical tumors were present in patients younger than 29 years.

Anaplastic, or malignant, meningiomas can be diagnosed according to gross or histologic criteria. In the reviewed pediatric cases, 2% of meningiomas were anaplastic or malignant.[4–11] Mahmood et al. reported that 1.7% of 319 adult meningiomas were anaplastic or malignant,[17] and 7% of the adults in the series from Manitoba also had tumors of this histology.[18] Gross invasion of brain parenchyma in a histologically benign-appearing lesion would justify a diagnosis of malignancy. In addition, a substantial increase in the mitotic rate, cellular atypia, nuclear/cytoplasmic ratio, or cellularity over that which would be expected for a diagnosis of atypical would increase the grade to anaplastic or malignant. This is the malignant end of the spectrum of histologic diagnosis, and no clear and discrete criteria have been established to differentiate between atypical and anaplastic/malignant lesions.

Papillary meningiomas, characterized by perivascular pseudorosettes separated from the vessels by a fine reticulin border, were found in 2% of pediatric cases (5/203).[4–11] These tumors show uniform nuclei and scattered mitoses in addition to the pseudorosettes. The latest WHO classification of brain tumors stresses the aggressive biological nature of this subtype.[35]

The remainder of the pediatric tumors were sarcomatous (14, or 7%), psammomatous (11, or 5%), angioblastic (7, or 3%), and myxoid (1, or 0.5%).[4–11] In an adult series, the psammomatous type composed 4% and the angioblastic meningiomas 2% of all tumors.[18]

Immunohistochemical stains of meningiomas show positivity for vimentin and epithelial membrane antigen (EMA). Meningiomas are negative for glial fibrillary acidic protein (GFAP) and synaptophysin. Some meningiomas are positive for cytokeratin (CK), S100, and, particularly in secretory meningiomas, carcinoembryonic antigen (CEA).[34]

The electron microscopy of meningothelial and transitional meningiomas is characterized by intercellular junctions, cytoplasmic intermediate filaments, and complex interdigitating processes. Fibrous meningiomas do not demonstrate these intercellular interactions because the cells are separated by collagen.[34, 35]

TREATMENT

As with any disease process, the risk of treatment must be weighed against the natural history of the disease. To a great extent, the location of the meningioma defines both options. A small convexity meningioma may present little risk to the patient, but the risks associated with surgical removal of such a lesion are also minimal. In the case of a pediatric patient who has a long projected life expectancy, the anticipated growth of a meningioma is likely to produce symptoms, and therefore the analysis often falls in favor of removal. Alternatively, a large tumor surrounding the lower cranial nerves in an asymptomatic patient with significant medical comorbidity may warrant observation or stereotactic radiosurgery.

Observation

Although it is not uncommon to observe an indolent asymptomatic meningioma in an older patient who might be expected to expire before the lesion becomes symptomatic, the life expectancy of children precludes this approach in the majority of cases. Observation should be reserved for patients who are asymptomatic or have minimal and nonprogressive symptoms, whose lesion is being followed closely with serial MRI, and who needs to grow to a safer weight for surgery or recover from an acute illness.

Radiation Therapy

Radiation therapy has not superseded surgery as a primary treatment modality for pediatric meningiomas. Several series have demonstrated the efficacy of radiation therapy in meningiomas for stabilization and, in some cases, decreased lesion size.[5, 37–40, 55] However, these series all have limited follow-up, ranging from a median of 22.9 months to 4.9 years. In the setting of a young patient with a life expectancy of 50 to 70 additional years, this interval is significantly less reassuring. However, as an adjuvant treatment radiation therapy has shown promise. Stafford et al., in a retrospective review of 581 adult and pediatric meningioma patients, concluded that radiation therapy should be strongly considered for malignant, papillary, or anaplastic meningiomas regardless of degree of resection and should be used in recurrent tumors either combined with surgery or alone.[23] In subtotally resected benign meningiomas their data was inconclusive, though they noted an increased risk of recurrence in young patients, males, tumors with increased mitotic index (>3), and tumors involving the anterior visual pathway. Goldsmith et al. argued that subtotally resected tumors should be irradiated. In their review of 140 benign tumors with a median follow-up of 40 months, the recurrence-free survival at 5 years was 91%.[41] Radiation therapy should be considered in any patient who is treated with less than a Simpson grade 2 resection[1] or whose tumor has atypical, anaplastic, or malignant histologic characteristics.

Surgery

As discussed above, the majority of pediatric meningiomas are best treated surgically.[50] The long life expectancy of the patient, the relatively short follow-up in published results of radiation treatment, and the potential for surgical cure in many cases mandates surgical intervention in the absence of considerable contraindication. Furthermore, the variability of this tumor in the pediatric population warrants biopsy for histologic confirmation.

Surgery may be enhanced by the use of preoperative embolization. Larger convexity meningiomas, skull base meningiomas, and large intraventricular meningiomas may possess a vigorous blood supply from external or internal carotid sources. The vessels may be located at the depths of the surgical field, creating a situation in which the blood supply is inaccessible surgically until the conclusion of the case. Preoperative embolization can improve visualization during surgery by reducing bleeding and may reduce operative time and intraoperative blood loss. Dexamethasone, oral or intravenous, may be started the evening before surgery and tapered postoperatively as the clinical status permits. Intraoperatively the patient is loaded with anticonvulsants unless therapeutic levels have been established preoperatively. Prophylactic antibiotics are given prior to skin incision and for 24 to 48 hours postoperatively. In the case of larger lesions, or smaller lesions with significant edema, 0.5 to 1 g/kg of mannitol is given at skin incision.

Patient positioning and surgical approaches to each meningioma will vary with the tumor location. Several excellent articles and texts have discussed the skull base techniques for more complex lesions; at least one of these articles was specifically written for pediatric skull base lesions.[42, 43] Small meningiomas can be removed en bloc, circumnavigating the lesion. Careful dissection of the brain–tumor interface, retracting mainly on the tumor, with placement of cottonoid patties around the dissected space often allows preservation of the pial surface and total resection of the extra-axial tumor. When possible, a 1-cm margin of dura that is grossly free of tumor is resected and sent as a separate pathology specimen. Larger tumors, or those with a brain stem or cranial nerve interface, are resected by initial removal of the superficial and accessible capsule. The core of the tumor is then gradually resected from superficial to deep and from the center to the periphery, leaving a "rind" of tumor capsule that is serially dissected from the brain as the thinned capsule becomes more pliable.

Chemotherapy

Currently, chemotherapy has no established role in the management of meningiomas, even in the presence of atypical or malignant histology. Several small series with limited follow-up have been published using antiprogesterone agents, hydroxyurea, or interferon,[44–49] but further work must be done before widespread recommendations for use can be made.

PROGNOSIS

Perioperative morbidity and mortality are comparable in pediatric and adult surgical series. In three studies following 71 patients, 54 (76%) had gross total resections.[6, 7, 9] In seven reports comprising a total of 134 pediatric patients, perioperative mortality was 4% (5 patients). In a series of mainly adults, the total excision rate was 80% and the overall mortality was 1.6%.[23] It is difficult to compare outcome data from recent pediatric series, as resection rates are not always indicated, tumor histology is not always specified, and the incidence of NF is not always correlated with recurrence data. Table 25–5 shows the inclusive dates for case collection, duration of follow-up, histologic data, neurologic outcome, and recurrence data. Hung et al. reported only one recurrence in 10 patients on average 6.1 years follow-up, and this patient was reported to have had a subtotal resection.[10] However, no information about the surveillance methods was given. Baumgartner et al. described six recurrences in their series of

TABLE 25–5 Outcome Data for Pediatric Meningioma Patients

Study (inclusive dates)	Cases	Average follow-up	Malignant histology	Neurologic outcome	Recurrence data
Hung et al. (1980–90)	10	6.1 yr	NR	6 "excellent"	4/10 had STR. 1/10 STR recurred @ 17 mo
Ferrante et al. (not described)	19	7 yr	2 sarcomatous	NR	5/19 MTR 7 yr
Baumgartner et al. (1964–94)	12	5 yr	2 malignant, 2 atypical	NR	6/12 recurred, MTR 3 yr
Erdincler et al. (1968–94)	29	6.5 yr	NR	13 (45%) intact 8 (28%) disability	4/29 recurred, MTR not reported

NR, not reported; STR, subtotally resected.
References for data included in this table are included within the text.

12 patients at a mean time to recurrence of 3 years.[4] All but one recurrence had either less than total resection or atypical/malignant histology. The patient with a total resection of a typical meningioma had a 14-year recurrence-free interval. The high ratio of malignant tumors in this series may reflect referral bias, as the cases were collected at the M.D. Anderson Cancer Center. Erdincler et al. noted only four recurrences in 29 patients with an average 6.5 year follow-up, but the time to recurrence and the histologic characteristics were not described.[9] All of the patients with recurrence had total resection, but no mention of surgical margins was made. Ferrante et al. reported five recurrences in 19 patients with mean time to recurrence of 7 years.[6] Three recurrences were in patients with subtotal resection of typical meningiomas, and two were in patients with gross total resection of sarcomatous meningiomas. These numbers are not dissimilar to those in the adult literature, in which progression-free survival with total resection is 88% and 75% at 5 and 10 years, respectively. In partial removal, the 5- and 10-year progression-free survival rates were, respectively, 61% and 39%.[23] Jääskeläinen et al. showed that the recurrence rate in adults with total resection was 19% at 20 years, but the definition of gross total resection included tumor resection with coagulation of and not resection of involved dura.[24] Direct comparison of adult and pediatric prognosis data is not possible, and more data are needed before definitive treatment algorithms can be developed. However, it is clear that clinical and imaging follow-up should be continued for life. Late recurrences occur in both adult and pediatric meningioma series, and MRI with gadolinium contrast is both minimally invasive and extremely sensitive. Although the imaging interval is subject to debate, we perform follow-up MRI at 3 months, 6 months, and 1 year postoperatively, annually for 3 to 5 years, and then every other year for life. Repeat imaging is done at closer intervals for atypical or malignant meningiomas, and imaging is repeated as needed for any pertinent change in clinical course.

SUMMARY

Pediatric meningiomas mimic adult meningliomas in many ways. When the literature reported after 1980 is analyzed, the presentation, imaging, anatomical location, histologic characteristics, surgical outcome, and prognosis are remarkably similar. In particular, there are no data to support an increased incidence of posterior fossa lesions in children, and the proportion of atypical and malignant histologic characteristics is no different between the two groups. The recurrence rate appears to be similar for both with treatment, though the data are very limited in the pediatric group. *The variance in pediatric patients includes reversal of the male/female ratio, presentation with calvarial deformity, increased frequency of intraventricular location, and development of meningiomas without dural attachment.* Less important clinically, but also noted in published reports, are an increased incidence of fibroblastic histology and a decreased incidence of transitional histology. Aggressive removal of this benign tumor in the pediatric population is warranted because of the long life expectancy of patients and the improved tumor control afforded by complete resection, including dural margins. Owing to the longer life span of children, radiation should be considered as an adjuvant for subtotal resections. Clinical follow-up and repeat imaging at appropriate intervals for the rest of the patient's life are essential. Excellent results are likely if the surgical treatment algorithms employed in adult meningiomas are followed in pediatric patients. Centers that treat significant numbers of these lesions in children should be encouraged to report their approaches to treatment and outcomes in detail to provide a basis for comparison with the limited data currently available.

REFERENCES

1. Simpson D. The recurrence of intracranial meningiomas after surgical treatment. *J Neurol Neurosurg Psychiatry* 1957;20:22–39.
2. Cushing H. The meningiomas (dural endotheliomas): their source, and favoured seats of origin. *Brain* 1922;45:282–316.
3. Cushing H, Eisenhardt L. *Meningiomas: Their Classification, Regional Behavior, Life History, and Surgical End Results.* Baltimore: Charles C Thomas; 1938.

4. Baumgartner JE, Sorenson JM. Meningioma in the pediatric population. *J Neuro-oncol* 1996;29:223–228.
5. Deen HG Jr, Scheithauer BW, Ebersold MJ. Clinical and pathological study of meningiomas of the first two decades of life. *J Neurosurg* 1982;56:317–322.
6. Ferrante L, Acqui M, Artico M, et al. Cerebral meningiomas in children. *Child's Nerv Syst* 1989;5:83–86.
7. Germano IM, Edwards MSB, Davis RL, Schiffer D. Intracranial meningiomas of the first two decades of life. *J Neurosurg* 1994;80:447–453.
8. Sano K, Wakai S, Ochiai C, Takakura K. Characteristics of intracranial meningiomas in childhood. *Child's Brain* 1981;8:98–106.
9. Erdincler P, Lena G, Sarioglu AC, et al. Intracranial meningiomas in children: review of 29 cases. *Surg Neurol* 1998;49:136–141.
10. Hung P, Wang H, Chou M, et al. Intracranial meningiomas in childhood. *Acta Paed Sin* 1994;35:495–501.
11. Kolluri VRS, Reddy DR, Naidu MRC, et al. Meningiomas in childhood. *Child's Nerv Syst* 1987;3:271–273.
12. Longstreth WT, Dennis LK, McGuire VM, et al. Epidemiology of intracranial meningioma. *Cancer* 1993;72:639–648.
13. Pau A, Dorcaratto A, Pisani R. Third ventricular meningiomas of infancy: a case report. *Pathologica* 1996;88:204–206.
14. Miltenburg D, Louw DF, Sutherland GR. Epidemiology of childhood brain tumors. *Can J Neurol Sci* 1996;23:118–122.
15. Biegel JA, Parmiter AH, Sutton LN, et al. Abnormalities of chromosome 22 in pediatric meningiomas. *Genes Chrom Cancer* 1994;9:81–87.
16. Slavc I, et al. Exon scanning for mutations of the NF2 gene in pediatric ependymomas, rhabdoid tumors, and meningiomas. *Int J Cancer* 1995;64:243–247.
17. Mahmood A, Caccamo DV, Tomecek FJ, Malik GM. Atypical and malignant meningiomas: a clinicopathological review. *Neurosurgery* 1993;33:955–963.
18. Rohringer M, Sutherland GR, et al. Incidence and clinicopathological features of meningioma. *J Neurosurg* 1989;71:665–672.
19. Sankila R, Kallio M, Jääskeläinen J, Hakulinen T. Long-term survival of 1986 patients with intracranial meningioma diagnosed from 1953 to 1984 in Finland. *Cancer* 1992;70:1568–1576.
20. Davidson GS, Hope JK. Meningeal tumors of childhood. *Cancer* 1989;63:1205–1210.
21. Herz DA, Shapiro K, Shulman K. Intracranial meningiomas of infancy, childhood and adolescence. *Child's Brain* 1980;7:43–56.
22. Artico M, Ferrante L, Cervoni L, et al. Pediatric cystic meningioma: report of three cases. *Child's Nerv Syst* 1995;11:137–140.
23. Stafford SL, et al. Primarily resected meningiomas: outcome and prognostic factors in 581 Mayo Clinic patients, 1978 through 1988. *Mayo Clin Proc* 1998;73:936–942.
24. Jääskeläinen J. Seemingly complete removal of histologically, benign intracranial meningioma: late recurrence rate and factors predicting recurrence in 657 patients. *Surg Neurol* 1986;26:461–469.
25. Annegers JF, Laws ER, Kurland LT, Grabow JD. Head trauma and subsequent brain tumors. *Neurosurgery* 1979;4:203–206.
26. Barnett GH, Chou SM, Bay JW. Posttraumatic intracranial meningioma: a case report and review of the literature. *Neurosurg* 1986;18:75–78.
27. Schlehofer B, Blettner M, Becker N, et al. Medical risk factors and the development of brain tumors. *Cancer* 1992;69:2541–2547.
28. Ron E, et al. Tumors of the brain and nervous system after radiotherapy in childhood. *N Engl J Med* 1988;319:1033–1039.
29. Mack EE, Wilson CB. Meningiomas induced by high-dose cranial irradiation. *J Neurosurg* 1993;79:28–31.
30. Ghim TT, Seo J, O'Brien M, et al. Childhood intracranial meningiomas after high dose irradiation. *Cancer* 1993;71:4091–4095.
31. Soffer D, Pittaluga S, Feiner M, Beller AJ. Intracranial meningiomas following low-dose irradiation to the head. *J Neurosurg* 1983;59:1048–1053.
32. Cogen PH, Daneshvar L, Bowcock AM, et al. Loss of heterozygosity for chromosome 22 DNA sequences in human meningioma. *Cancer Genet Cytogenet* 1991;53:271–277.
33. Parisi G, Tropea R, Giuffrida S, et al. Cystic meningiomas. *J Neurosurg* 1986;64:35–38.
34. Burger PC, Scheithauer BW. *Atlas of tumor pathology: tumors of the central nervous system*, Washington, DC: Armed Forces Institute of Pathology; 1994:259–286, 442–443.
35. Kleihues P, Burger PC, Scheithauer BW. The new WHO classification of brain tumors. *Brain Pathol* 1993;3:255–268.
36. Glaholm J, Bloom HJG, Crow JH. The role of radiotherapy in the management of intracranial meningiomas: the Royal Marsden Hospital experience with 186 patients. *Int J Radiat Oncol Biol Phys* 1990;18:755–761.
37. Duma CM, Lunsford LD, Kondziolka D, et al. Stereotactic radiosurgery of cavernous sinus meningiomas as an addition or alternative to microsurgery. *Neurosurgery* 1993;32:699–705.
38. Kondziolka D, Flickenger JC, Perez B. Judicious resection and/or radiosurgery for parasagittal meningiomas: outcomes from a multicenter review. *Neurosurg* 1998;43:405–414.
39. Kondziolka D, Levy El, Niranjan A, et al. Long-term outcomes after meningioma radiosurgery: physician and patient perspectives. *J Neurosurg* 1999;91:44–50.
40. Subach BR, Lunsford LD, Kondziolka D, et al. Management of petroclival meningiomas by stereotactic radiosurgery. *Neurosurgery* 1998;42:437–445.
41. Goldsmith BJ, Wara WM, Wilson CB, Larson DA. Postoperative irradiation for subtotally resected meningiomas. *J Neurosurg* 1994;80:195–201.
42. Cogen PH, Donahue DJ. Approaches to the posterior fossa in children. In: Sekhar L, de Oliviera E, eds. *Cranial microsurgery: Approaches and Techniques.* New York: Thieme Medical Publishers; 1998:403–406.
43. Kennedy JD, Haines SJ. Review of skull base surgery approaches: with special reference to pediatric patients. *J Neuro-oncol* 1994;20:291–312.
44. Cassidy LM, et al. Hormonal treatment of bilateral optic nerve meningioma. *Eye* 1997;11:566–568.

45. Coke CC, Corn BW, Werner-Wasik M, et al. Atypical and malignant meningiomas: an outcome report of seventeen cases. *J Neuro-oncol* 1998;39:65–70.

46. Cusimano MD. Hydroxyurea for treatment of meningioma. *J Neurosurg* 1998;88:938–939.

47. Kaba SE, DeMonte F, Bruner JM, et al. The treatment of recurrent unresectable and malignant menigiomas with interferon alpha-2B. *Neurosurgery* 1997;40:271–275.

48. Schrell UM, Rittig MG, Anders M, et al. Hydroxyurea for treatment of unresectable and recurrent meningiomas. II. Decrease in size of meningiomas in patients treated with hydroxyurea. *J Neurosurg* 1997;86:840–844.

49. Sharif S, et al. Non-surgical treatment of meningioma: a case report and review. *Br J Neurosurg* 1998;12:369–372.

50. Altmors N, et al. Intracranial meningiomas: analysis of 344 surgically treated cases. *Neurosurg Rev* 1998;21:106–110.

51. Bhattacharjee MB, Armstrong DD, Vogel H, Cooley LD. Cytogenetic analysis of 120 primary pediatric brain tumors and literature review. *Cancer Genet Cytogenet* 1997;97:39–53.

52. Bowman R, DeLeon G, Radkowski MA, et al. 15-year-old young woman with morning headaches. *Pediatric Neurosurg* 1998;29:46–51.

53. Darling CF, et al. MR of pediatric intracranial meningiomas. *Am J Neuroradiol* 1994;15:435–444.

54. Duffner PK, Krischer JP, Horowicz ME, et al. Second malignancies in young children with primary brain tumors following treatment with prolonged postoperative chemotherapy and delayed irradiation: a pediatric oncology group study. *Ann Neurol* 1998;44:313–316.

55. Hakim H et al. Results of linear accelerator–based radiosurgery for intracranial meningiomas. *Neurosurgery* 1998; 42: 446–454.

56. Katayama Y, Tsubokawa T, Yoshida K. Cystic meningiomas in infancy. *Surg Neurol* 1986;25:43–48.

57. Kobata H, Kondo A, Iwasaki K, et al. Chordoid meningioma in a child. *J Neurosurg* 1998;88:319–323.

58. Molleston MC, Moran CJ, Roth KA, Rich KM. Infantile meningioma. *Pediatr Neurosurg* 1994;21:195–200.

59. Moss SD, Rockswold GL, Chou SN, et al. Radiation-induced meningiomas in pediatric patients. *Neurosurgery* 1988;22: 758–761.

60. Odake G. Cystic meningioma: report of three patients. *Neurosurgery* 1992;30:935–940.

61. Osborne AG. *Diagnostic Neuroradiology.* Baltimore: CV Mosby; 1994:584–603.

62. Pinna G, et al. Cystic meningiomas—an update. *Surg Neurol* 1986;26:441–452.

63. Reddy DR, et al. Cystic meningiomas in children. *Child's Nerv Syst* 1986;2:317–319.

64. Sheikh BY, Siqueira E, Dayel F. Meningioma in children: a report of nine cases and review of the literature. *Surg Neurol* 1996;45:328–335.

65. Waga S, Handa H. Radiation-induced meningioma: with review of the literature. *Surg Neurol* 1997;5:215–219.

Chapter 26

Oligodendroglioma

Robert F. Keating and Lisa Mulligan

EPIDEMIOLOGY

Historically, oligodendrogliomas have been rare tumors in all age groups. First presented by Bailey and Cushing in 1926[1] and later described in greater detail,[2] they remain an enigmatic type of tumor. While accounting for 4 to 7% of all intracranial neoplasms,[3, 4] they represent only 1% of all pediatric brain tumors.[5] When oligodendrogliomas are taken as a group, the pediatric subset accounts for 6 to 12%.[6] The median age of presentation in children is 13.1 years and there is a slight male preponderance.[7] Although the development of an increasingly sophisticated radiologic examination has made it possible to demonstrate the presence of smaller lesions, there is also an improved appreciation of subtle pathologic differences between oligodendrogliomas and dysembryoplastic neuroepithelial tumors (DNETs).

CLINICAL PRESENTATION

Due to their indolent growth characteristics, it is not uncommon for oligodendrogliomas to present with longstanding symptoms. The average length of time to diagnosis is 1.6 years,[4] and the most common presentation is seizures. In one series of 39 pediatric patients with pure oligodendroglioma,[4] 85% of patients presented with seizures; with headaches, evidence of increased intracranial pressure (ICP), precocious puberty, and visual changes presenting in order of decreasing frequency.

BOX 26–1
Presenting Signs/Symptoms

- **Seizure**
- **Headache (increased ICP)**
- **Milestone delay**
- **Precocious puberty**
- **Visual changes**

As would be expected, symptoms depend largely on location of the tumor as well as size. The majority of oligodendrogliomas are supratentorial cortical and subcortical tumors. The most common reported location is frontal, followed by temporal, parietal, hypothalamic, and intraventricular. Not uncommonly, multiple lobes are involved and rarely examples of leptomeningeal spread are observed.[4] Clinically, presentation often varies, depending on the grade of the tumor. *Low-grade indolent tumors more frequently present with seizures, whereas the higher grade lesions manifest increased ICP secondary to their rapid growth.* The experience of Rizk et al[5] with 15 pediatric patients having a pure oligodendroglioma demonstrated that all patients who presented with seizures had benign lesions, whereas seven of eight of children presenting with increased ICP symptoms had anaplastic lesions. They also found that the overall prognosis was strictly related to the histopathology rather than degree of tumor resection.

RADIOGRAPHIC PRESENTATION

Several characteristics are suggestive of the diagnosis of oligodendroglioma but none are pathognomonic. Noncontrast computed tomography (CT) most often manifests tumors as a hypodense area (Fig. 26–1), although these lesions may also

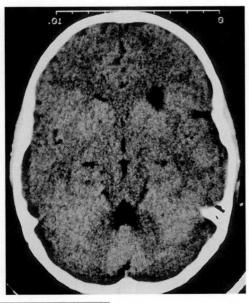

Figure 26–1 CT scan demonstrating a hypodense area at the left caudate nucleus. The patient was a 10-year-old boy who presented with seizures and was later diagnosed with oligodendroglioma.

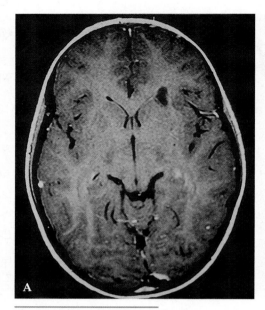
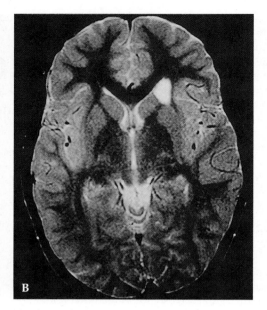

Figure 26–2 (A) T1-weighted magnetic resonance scan of the same patient demonstrating decreased signal in the region of the left caudate. (B) T2-weighted image manifesting an increased signal seen in patients with oligodendrogliomas.

present as hyper- or isodense. Contrast enhancement was seen in 24% of patients in one series,[4] with 40% also demonstrating calcification. In Rizk et al,[5] all four patients with contrast-enhancing lesions had anaplastic tumors. It has also been shown that mixed tumors (oligoastrocytomas) often enhance.

On noncontrast T1-weighted magnetic resonance images (Fig. 26–2A), most tumors present in a hypodense fashion (decreased signal), whereas on T2 studies the signal is increased[8] (Fig. 26–2B). In the series from Tice et al,[4] 80% of their patients had enhancement after gadolinium.

tumors have large numbers of small capillaries running at sharp geometrical angles forming a pattern similar to chickenwire. Nevertheless, although perinuclear halo and chickenwire patterns may be considered classical histologic features, they are unreliable as sole criteria for diagnosis. Fortin et al.[9] comment that nuclear regularity and roundness, as well as an eccentric rim of eosinophilic cytoplasm lacking obvious cell processes, are more constant features. These tumors, like other gliomas, tend to be poorly demarcated and infiltrative. Their uniform cellular density, as well as their nuclear size and calcification, assist in the pathologic characterization. Other sec-

---

BOX 26–2
Radiographic Appearance

- CT
  - More often hypodense
  - Infrequent enhancement
  - Commonly calcify
- MRI
  - Decreased T1 signal
  - Increased T2 signal
  - Frequent gadolinium enhancement

PATHOLOGIC FEATURES

Diagnosis is frequently made by the classic microscopic appearance of "fried-egg" artifact and chickenwire vasculature (Fig. 26–3). Due to a fairly consistent fixation artifact, a perinuclear halo forms yielding a fried-egg pattern. Many of these

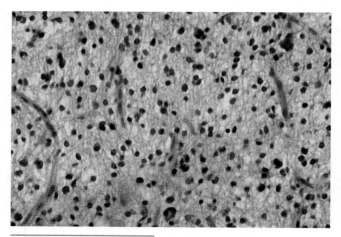

Figure 26–3 Classic microscopic appearance of oligodendroglioma with "fried egg" and "chickenwire" presentation. The fried-egg aspect is secondary to a fixation artifact, whereas the chickenwire expression is due to the presence of many small capillaries running at sharp angles with respect to one another. Neither feature can be considered pathognomonic.

ondary features seen during cortical infiltration, as described by Berger and Scheithauer,[10] are perineural satellitosis, perivascular aggregation, and subpial accumulations.

To date, despite intensive efforts, there are no consistent immunohistochemical markers that selectively stain normal oligodendrocytes. In addition, there are no ultrastructural features that reliably identify these tumors as true oligodendrogliomas. Nevertheless, recent cytogenetic studies have demonstrated occasional *p53* mutations as well as a high incidence of chromosomal loss from 19q and 1p.[11–14] In addition, numerous growth factors have also recently been identified in association with oligodendrogliomas. An overexpression of epidermal growth factor receptor (EGFR) has been reported,[15] although the *EGFR* gene does not appear to be amplified.

GRADING

Oligodendrogliomas, much like their astrocytic counterparts, may present within a spectrum of malignant transformation. Lesions may be low grade or may demonstrate anaplastic or malignant features. In addition, *malignant transformation is not uncommon and often requires long intervals.*[16] Numerous grading systems have been developed. The first grading system to enjoy wide acceptance was devised by Smith et al in 1983[17] and consists of a four-tiered system. Grading levels A through D are based on the presence or absence of five characteristics: *nuclear cytoplasmic ratio, maximal cell density, pleomorphism, endothelial proliferation,* and *necrosis.* The principal shortcoming of the Smith scale is the lack of prognostic difference between groups B and C. The Smith et al data[17] demonstrate a 94-month mean survival for grade A tumors, 51 months for grades B and C, and 17 months for grade D. A more recent grading system by Dumas-Duport et al[18] utilizes only two discriminating features: the presence of contrast enhancement on imaging studies and endothelial hyperplasia. The absence of both features defines a grade A lesion, whereas the presence of either feature denotes a grade B tumor. Outcomes and mean survival were observed for both categories, with a mean survival of 11 years for grade A patients and 3.5 years for grade B. This system was further supported by a 96% interobserver reproducibility.

DIFFERENTIAL DIAGNOSIS

The differential diagnosis for oligodendroglioma includes fibrillary astrocytoma, ganglioglioma and DNETs, as well as nonneoplastic lesions such as infarcts and demyelinating lesions.

BOX 26–3
Differential Diagnosis

- Ganglioglioma
- Fibrillary astrocytoma
- DNET
- Neurocytoma
- Infarct/demyelinating dx

It is not uncommon for oligodendrogliomas to have astrocytic components, and this should not be confused with a fibrillary astrocytoma. Typically, fibrillary astrocytomas have more pleomorphism even at lower grades. Nevertheless, there are some oligodendrogliomas that have significant components of astrocytoma, and it is generally believed that a tumor that is composed of more than 25% of another cell type qualifies as a mixed tumor. Although controversy exists, a number of investigators feel that mixed oligoastrocytomas have a better prognosis than pure astrocytoma.[9, 19]

Recently, the diagnosis of DNET has helped to define the pathology of the oligodendroglioma further and has illuminated some difficulties in previous outcome studies. DNETs are equally rare lesions that present in children, often with epilepsy. Frequently observed in the temporal lobe, they are often in a superficial, cortical location. There are several microscopic similarities, including round and uniform cells with perinuclear clearing, as well as the presence of neuronal elements.[9, 20] Nevertheless, there are structural differences that help in differentiating these tumors. The DNET is a multinodular tumor unlike the oligodendroglioma, which also has neurons within the tumor. However, in contrast to the clustering of cells around a neuron in the satellitosis of an oligodendroglioma, the neurons of a DNET float in a mucoid background. In addition, the DNET often has a distinct basophilic matrix that stains well with Alcian blue.

The difficulty in distinguishing between a DNET and an oligodendroglioma often arises when a small biopsy is sent. This is a particular problem in the setting of a stereotactic biopsy. Often it is imperative to observe the larger architectural patterns to make an accurate differentiation. To date, there is no immunohistochemical stain that conclusively distinguishes between the two tumors.[21] Nevertheless, the distinction between the tumors is important. DNETs are benign tumors without malignant potential that do not require any further adjuvant therapy following complete excision. In general, they have an excellent prognosis. Unfortunately, the accidental inclusion of DNETs in any oligodendroglioma study may skew survival data.

It must be kept in mind that nonneoplastic lesions may also mimic oligodendrogliomas. In areas of infarction as well as demyelination, macrophages laden with lipid-rich material can stain similarly to the fried-egg appearance of an oligodendrocyte. Consequently, it is critical that a careful examination be carried out to reveal the subtle differences in the cell borders.

THERAPEUTIC APPROACHES

Management of oligodendrogliomas involves three modalities: surgery, irradiation, and chemotherapy. The role of surgery is well supported in many studies that have demonstrated that the extent of resection is directly proportional to survival.

Surgery

Surgery is undertaken with two purposes: to yield a diagnosis and to resect as much tumor as possible with minimal morbidity. The best long-term outcomes appear to be associated with the greatest degree of resection. This is particularly so in children, in whom low-grade tumors may behave in a more benign fashion than those in adults. These patients may not require additional therapy. Both Tice et al,[4] who looked specifically at oligodendrogliomas in children, and Pollack et al,[7] who reviewed low-grade hemispheric tumors in children, reported that the extent of surgical excision is a statistically sensitive univariate predictor of outcome. However, both studies point out that the behavior of these tumors in children may differ significantly from that in adults, whereas the percentage of lesions that progress to higher grade tumors is far less in children. In addition, it has been observed that children with subtotal resection still tend to have a good outcome if the lesion is a non-anaplastic oligodendroglioma.

To the contrary, the recent experience of Razack et al[22] did not demonstrate any correlation between extent of resection and survival; however, as expected, it did correlate with histopathology as well as better outcome in the younger patients. Their group of 19 patients followed for an average of 39.7 months manifested a 65% 5-year survival. In an earlier study, Dohrmann et al[23] found no statistical difference between surgical resection and radiation; however, they did not evaluate a correlation with histologic aggressiveness.

Radiation

To date, the optimal use and timing of irradiation in the setting of an oligodendroglioma remains unclear. The data are confusing even among the adult population, although a consensus appears to be emerging condoning the use of postsurgical irradiation for anaplastic stage I lesions and perhaps even for subtotal resection. Nevertheless, the literature on radiation remains clouded. Two studies that were published within a year of each other arrived at opposing conclusions and recommendations. The earlier study, published in 1987 by a group at Duke University,[24] reported results over the years 1940–1983 and involved the treatment of 71 patients with oligodendroglioma. Thirty-seven patients were irradiated following surgery and the remaining 34 were not. The mean survival was 4.5 years for the nontreated group versus 5.2 years for the irradiated patients. However, this was not statistically significant. A comparison of median time to clinical deterioration as well as time to documented recurrence was also not statistically significant. One year later, a different conclusion was reached by a group at the University of California at San Francisco.[25] Their data, taken from the same time period and reviewing the experience of 42 patients, looked not only at irradiation versus nonirradiation but also at the behavior of mixed gliomas following irradiation. A 10-year survival of 56% was demonstrated for irradiated patients, in contrast to 18% for nonradiated patients. Similar results were seen in the mixed-glioma group as well.

A more recent study from Turkey,[26] which reviewed the results of radiotherapy among 77 patients with oligodendrogliomas, suggested that postoperative radiotherapy was necessary to minimize recurrences.

The contradiction in results from these two studies is not unique. There are numerous examples in the literature either supporting or refuting the need for postoperative irradiation. One explanation for this discrepancy is that because the tumor is very rare, it has taken many years to accrue enough clinical data to support a statistically meaningful study.

During that time, standards in care have changed drastically, especially in the fields of radiation therapy, imaging, and surgical therapeutics. A multi-institutional study would help to decrease this variation but would impose additional problems inherent in this type of approach.

In 1997, Allison et al[27] reviewed combined radiation-chemotherapy regimens for the management of both anaplastic and non-anaplastic tumors. Of eight patients who underwent 60-Gy irradiation following surgery without chemotherapy, five remained controlled, whereas three failed and subsequently required salvage therapy. In contrast, patients receiving only 50 Gy or those receiving no radiation required additional therapy. Based on these results, Allison et al[27] thought that many other studies tried to draw conclusions from data on patients who did not receive adequate radiation. That may help to explain the variations in conclusions from some of the previous studies that spanned more than four decades, during which patients received widely divergent doses of radiation.

To complicate matters further, the majority of studies that looked at the benefits of radiation excluded children or had a minimal number of pediatric patients. Furthermore, children are exquisitely sensitive to side effects from radiotherapy. Pollack et al[7] in their analysis of 71 children with low-grade tumors noted that 34% of individuals receiving radiation developed cognitive difficulties, as compared with 8.6% who did not receive radiotherapy. Endocrine function also suffered in 17% of irradiated children, in contrast to 2.9% in the control group. Furthermore, it is commonly believed that these tumors behave differently in the pediatric population and demonstrate a more benign course than that seen in adults. In their series on pediatric and adolescent oligodendrogliomas, Tice et al[4] performed total resection in 20 of 39 patients, subtotal resection in 16 of 39 patients, and partial resection in 3 of 39 patients. In all cases, there was no progression of tumor (mean follow-up of 5.06 years) and none of the patients received postsurgical radiotherapy. The experience of Pollack et al led them to recommend that low-grade tumors with a gross total resection as well as lesions with subtotal resection should be observed initially before the institution of radiation therapy. They acknowledged that there was a greater progression-free interval in children who received radiation but also reported that overall survival was not affected and the only malignant transformations were observed in previously irradiated children. Some groups felt that children with oligodendrogliomas should receive radiation, but even those groups offered more restricted recommendations for children. Allison et al[27] in their review of radiation and oligodendroglioma indicated that radiation therapy should be withheld from children and that chemotherapy should be the only postsurgical adjunct offered until the patient was older. Their series included only three patients younger than 12 years, and they felt that it was important to wait until the children were old enough to receive an adequate dose of 60 Gy, as compared with the 50-Gy dose that had failed consistently.

Chemotherapy

Perhaps the most exciting development in the treatment of oligodendrogliomas was the discovery that anaplastic tumors are often chemosensitive. Since the late 1980s, evidence has been accumulating to support this premise. In 1994, Cairncross and Macdonald[28] implemented a multi-institutional Phase II study to examine the efficacy of PCV (procarbazine, lomustine [CCNU], vincristine) chemotherapy for newly diagnosed as well as recurrent anaplastic oligodendrogliomas. In the study, 24 eligible and 9 ineligible patients were treated. Response was graded as complete when 100% disappearance of tumor had occurred, partial response −1 when more than 90% of the tumor had disappeared, and partial response −2 when 50 to 90% of the tumor had resolved. Cairncross and Macdonald reported that 75% of eligible patients had a response, with 38% demonstrating a complete response, 17% PR-1, and 21% PR-2, whereas 8% of patients progressed through the PCV chemotherapy without showing a response. The remainder of individuals had stable disease. In assessing median time to progression, complete responders had at least 25.2 months with no active disease, whereas the median time was at least 16 months for the PR-1 group and 8 months for the PR-2 group. Patients with progressive disease manifested changes by 1.2 months. However, due to the small numbers in each subgroup, it was not possible to derive any meaningful statistical analysis overall. Nevertheless, it appeared that tumor size correlated with the degree of response, with the best response noted for the smaller lesions. Although these studies were undertaken in an adult population and the efficacy in children is yet to be determined, this may prove to be an effective alternative to radiation, especially in young children.

Cairncross et al[29] have recently demonstrated that there are genetic predictors of chemotherapeutic response as well as survival in patients with anaplastic oligodendroglioma. When analyzing molecular genetic alterations involving chromosomes 1p, 10q, 19q, TP53 (17p), and CDKN2A (9p), it was found that losses involving both chromosomes 1p and 19q were statistically significant in predicting chemosensitivity and longer recurrence-free survival.

In 1996, Kim et al[30] published their results using PCV chemotherapy for mixed oligoastrocytomas with anaplastic features. The overall response rate was 91%, with 10 of 32 patients having a complete response and 19 of 32 demonstrating a partial response. Thus, it would appear that PCV chemotherapy is an effective tool not only for oligodendrogliomas but for mixed tumors as well.

The response of low-grade oligodendrogliomas to PCV chemotherapy was evaluated by Mason et al in 1996.[31] Although the number of patients was small, of the nine patients treated, eight had some response to the chemotherapy, with a mean reduction in tumor size of 51%. Neurologic deficits and seizures were improved in all affected patients. In a larger and more recent Phase II study,[32] the effectiveness of PCV was evaluated in patients with low-grade oliogodendrogliomas as well as recurrent tumors after surgery. Of the 26 patients,[16] (62%) responded to PCV, with 12% manifesting a complete response and 50% demonstrating a partial response. The patients with a complete response harbored pure oligodendrogliomas. The results also suggested that chemotherapy with PCV is effective in the treatment of low-grade oligodendrogliomas and oligoastrocytomas.

In addition to studies of PCV chemotherapy, studies (in vitro) are also being conducted to investigate the potential of tamoxifen in the setting of high- and low-grade pediatric gliomas. Pollack and Kawecki[33] described the effect of tamoxifen on a host of different gliomas, including an oligodendroglioma and a mixed-glioma cell line. A clear dose-dependent inhibition of cell proliferation was seen, and *new clinical trials are planned to examine the effect of tamoxifen on pediatric gliomas.*

SUMMARY

Oligodendrogliomas are rare glial neoplasms that present with numerous treatment challenges in both adult and pediatric populations. The most exciting recent development has been the discovery of the tumor's chemosensitivity, as well as the allelic loss of chromosome arms 1p and 19q as being a possible marker for chemosensitivity and longer survival. Nevertheless, much work is needed to verify the safety and efficacy of these agents in the pediatric population. In addition, whereas the tumor may behave differently in the pediatric patient, the recommendation of when to treat requires additional investigation. Treatment options must also encompass the role of irradiation in view of its delete-rious effects in children. Nevertheless, surgery remains the mainstay of therapy, and each case must be examined individually to determine the appropriate adjuvant therapy for a child with an oligodendroglioma based on the patient's age and on the location and grade of the tumor. New concepts emerging in the literature should help optimize the diagnosis of these lesions and reduce interobserver variability.

REFERENCES

1. Bailey P, Cushing H. A classification of tumors of the glioma group on a histogenetic basis with a correlation study of prognosis. Philadelphia: JB Lippincott; 1926.
2. Bailey P, Bucy PC. Oligodendrogliomas of the brain. *J Pathol Bacteriol* 1929;32:735–751.
3. Nijjar TS, et al. Oligodendroglioma: the Princess Margaret Hospital experience. *Cancer* 1993;71:4002–4006.
4. Tice et al. Pediatric and adolescent oligodendrogliomas. *Am J Neuroradiol* 1993;14:1293–1300.
5. Rizk T et al. Cerebral oligodendrogliomas in children: an analysis of 15 cases. *Child's Nerv Sys* 1996;12:527–529.
6. Peterson K, Cairncross JG, Oligodendrogliomas. *Neurol Clin* 1995;13:861–873.
7. Pollack IF, et al. Low-grade gliomas of the cerebral hemispheres in children: an analysis of 71 cases. *J Neurosurg* 1995;82:536–547.
8. Shimizu KT, et al, Management of oligodendrogliomas. *Radiology* 1993;186:569–572.
9. Fortin et al. Oligodendroglioma: an appraisal of recent data pertaining to diagnosis and treatment. *Neurosurgery* 1999;45(6):1279–1291.
10. Berger PC, Scheithauer BW. *Tumors of the Central Nervous System*. Washington, DC: Armed Forces Institute of Pathology; 1994.
11. Bello MJ, et al. Allelic loss at 1p and 19q frequently occurs in association and may represent early oncogenic events in oligodendroglial tumors. *Int J Cancer* 1995;4:207–210.

12. Kraus JA, et al. Shared allelic losses on chromosomes 1p and 19q suggest a common origin of oligodendroglioma and oligoastrocytoma. *J Neuropathol Exp Neurol* 1995; 54:91–95.

13. Reifenberger J, et al. Molecular genetic analysis of oligodendroglial tumors shows preferential allelic deletions on 19q and 1p. *Am J Pathol* 1994;145:1175–1190.

14. Von Deimling A, et al. Evidence for a tumor suppressor gene on chromosome 19q associated with human astrocytomas, oligodendrogliomas, and mixed gliomas. *Cancer Res* 1992;52:4277–4279.

15. Reifenberger J et al. Epidermal growth factor expression in oligodendroglial tumors. *Am J Pathol* 1996;149:29–35.

16. Saito A, Nakazato Y. Evaluation of malignant features in oliogodendroglial tumors. *Clin Neuropathol* 1999;18(2): 61–73.

17. Smith MT, et al. Grading of oligodendrogliomas. *Cancer* 1983;52:2107–2114.

18. Dumas-Duport C, et al. Oligodendrogliomas. Part II. A new grading system based on morphological and imaging criteria. *J Neuro-oncol* 1997;34:61–78.

19. Shaw EG, et al. Supratentorial gliomas: a comparative study by grade and histological type. *J Neuro-oncol* 1997; 31:273–278.

20. Leung SY, et al. Dysembryoplastic neurepithelial tumor. *Am J Surg Pathol* 1994;18:604–614.

21. Wolf HK, et al. Neuronal antigens in oligodendrogliomas and dysembryoplastic neruoepithelial tumors. *Acta Neuropathol* 1997;94:436–443.

22. Razack N, et al. Pediatric oligodendrogliomas. *Ped Neurosurg* 1998;28(3):121–129.

23. Dohrmann GJ, et al. Oligodendrogliomas in children. *Surg Neurol* 1978;10:21–25.

24. Bullard D, et al. Oligodendrogliomas: an analysis of the value of radiation therapy. *Cancer* 1987;60:2179–2185.

25. Wallner K, et al. Treatment of oligodendrogliomas with and without post-operative irradiation. *J Neurosurg* 1988; 68:684–688.

26. Turgut M, et al. The treatment of cerebral oligodendrogliomas with particular reference to features indicating malignancy: report of seventy-seven cases. *Neurosurg Rev* 1998;21(2-3):138-46

27. Allison RR, et al. Radiation and chemotherapy improve outcome in oligodendroglioma. *Int J Rad Oncol Biolog Phys* 1997;37:399–403.

28. Cairncross JG and Macdonald. Chemotherapy for anaplastic oligodendroglioma. *J Clin Oncol* 1994;12:2013–2021.

29. Cairncross JG, et al. Specific genetic predictors of chemotherapeutic response and survival in patients with anaplastic oligodendrogliomas. *J Natl Cancer Inst* 1998; 90(19):1473–1479.

30. Kim L, et al. Procarbazine, lomustine, and vincristine (PCV) chemotherapy for grade III and grade IV oligoastrocytomas. *J Neurosurg* 1996;85:602–607.

31. Mason WP, et al. Low-grade oligodendroglioma responds to chemotherapy. *Neurology* 1996;46:203–207.

32. Soffietti R, et al. PCV chemotherapy for recurrent oligodendrogliomas and oligoastrocytomas. *Neurosurgery* 1998;43(5):1066–1073.

33. Pollack IF, Kawecki S. The efficacy of tamoxifen as an antiproliferative agent in vitro for benign and malignant glial tumors. *Pediatr Neurosurg* 1995;22:281–288.

Chapter 27

Extraneural Metastasis

David F. Jimenez and Richard Teff

Metastasis of primary central nervous system (CNS) tumors to locations outside the craniospinal axis is uncommon. Although the true incidence in children and adults is not well known, overall rates from 0.4% to 33% are documented in different published series.[1-3] More recent data suggest that higher estimated incidences of 20 to 30% should be expected.

PATHOPHYSIOLOGY

Several theories have been proposed to address why primary CNS tumors rarely metastasize outside of the CNS. The classical theory, introduced by Willis in 1952, postulated four basic premises.[4] The first is that the CNS does not have a lymphatic system and consequently there is no lymphatic pathway between the brain or spinal cord to the surrounding soft tissues or regional lymph nodes, thereby preventing local spread of primary CNS tumors. A second premise is that as rapidly expanding neoplasms compress surrounding tissues, the small venous channels that normally carry hematogenous metastases to distant sites are compressed, subsequently preventing the initiation of systemic metastases from the CNS. Willis's third premise is that patients with malignant brain tumors usually have significantly decreased survival rates. Because patients do not survive longer than a few years following diagnosis, they rarely live long enough to develop visible or symptomatic metastases. Finally, Willis postulated that neural elements do not grow into these tissues outside of the CNS, which could prevent metastases from flourishing in extraneural environments. Willis's original premises and assumptions have been challenged and refuted. The existence of lymphatic drainage of cerebrospinal fluid into the extracranial tissues has been demonstrated.[5] The fact that malignant CNS tumors can invade veins and be recovered from the venous blood of patients during and after surgery has been demonstrated by Morley[6] and Smith.[3] Successful extracranial growth of brain tumor cells has been demonstrated in the tissue model after transplantation of glioma cells into the pleural and peritoneal cavities.[8] Battista et al demonstrated that anaplastic astrocytomas can grow and develop in extraneural sites in humans.[7]

BOX 27–1
Extraneural Metastases

- **Prior surgery**
- **Shunting**
- **Increased long-term survival**

Nevertheless, extraneural metastasis of CNS tumors does occur, and a significant majority of patients who develop metastasis have undergone previous surgery for treatment of the primary tumor. Consequently, surgery has been implicated as a mechanism by which the blood-brain barrier is bypassed by tumor cells.[9] Several theories of how surgery allows for extraneural metastasis have been proposed. The induction of negative atmosphere in the cerebral veins during surgery may possibly develop a suction effect, leading tumor cells to enter the systemic circulation[2] as previously stated, as was demonstrated by Smith et al in 1969.[3] Infiltration by tumor cells into glial scar vessels may also allow systemic dissemination. These vessels have been theorized to be less easily compressible than normal vessels and more patent, allowing easier infiltration by tumor cells.[10] Another possible way for tumor cells to metastasize is by invading the dura's vascular structures at the surgical site.[11, 12] Lastly, disruption of normal anatomical barriers associated with surgery may allow the tumor cells to migrate into the bone and scalp flaps, permitting access to the lymphatic and vascular systemic circulation.[13]

Another important and well-known mechanism for the spread of tumors outside of the CNS is via shunting of cerebrospinal fluid (CSF) to the peritoneum, atrium, or pleural cavity. Wolf in 1954 was the first to propose a causal relationship between extraneural metastasis and CSF shunts.[14] Since then, several authors have reported the association between shunting and extraneural metastasis. Kleinman et al reported on 103 patients with extracranial medulloblastoma metastasis and found that 22% had been shunted.[15] In a series of patients shunted prior to craniotomy for removal of medulloblastomas, the extraneural metastatic incidence was 15%.[16] An autopsy series of patients with ventriculoatrial shunts demonstrated a fourfold increase in extraneural metastasis to the lung.[15] Mechanistically, shunts become open conduits for intracranial neoplasms that have seeded the CSF into the abdominal or pleural cavities or the vascular system via the atrium. Attempts at decreasing the risk of metastasis have been carried out by placing filters in the shunts. However, these filters, increase the rate of shunt obstruction by causing blockage of the shunt by tumor cells. The preoperative shunting of medulloblastomas or ependymomas is not currently recommended.

Another proposed cause of increased reports of extraneural metastasis is the successful treatment of these tumors and the concomitant prolongation of life with aggressive multimodality therapy.[1, 9] Theoretically, the concept of exponential tumor growth suggests that with tumor cells doubling in number, a predictable increase in tumor mass over time can be ascertained.[17]

After 20 doublings, the average cancer cell reaches a volume of 1 mm³. After 30 doublings, it reaches a diameter of 1 cm. The average glioma is diagnosed at 4 doublings and is fatal at 8 doublings. If a CNS tumor metastasizes at surgery, it would take 30 doublings to reach 1 cm³, a size that could be diagnosed. By increasing the patient's longevity with aggressive therapy, the necessary doubling time is achieved for the extraneural metastasis to be detected and diagnosed.

BOX 27–2
Tumors Likely to Metastasize

- **Medulloblastoma**
- **Glioma**
- **Ependymoma**
- **Pineal germinoma**

Aside from postsurgical and shunt-induced metastases, a population still remains with spontaneous extraneural metas-

tases. Several cases of gliomas metastatic to bone marrow and distant lymph nodes prior to any surgery have been reported.[2, 18, 19] In another compelling discussion, the authors question why there is no difference in the sites of metastatic implant in preoperative and postsurgical patients.[2, 18] These rare cases represent spontaneous metastases and warrant further investigation into the mechanisms of primary CNS tumor spread.

INCIDENCE OF EXTRANEURAL METASTASES IN CHILDREN

The reported literature of extraneural metastases is summarized in Table 27–1.[20–35] Hoffman and Duffner reported the known cases prior to 1985.[28] Based on these data, the most common expected lesion is medulloblastoma, followed by astrocytic tumors and ependymoma. As expected, all listed tumors are poorly differentiated and aggressive types. The true incidence of extraneural metastatic medulloblastoma is

TABLE 27–1 Summary of the Literature

Tumor Type	Hoffman	Ono	Shen	Rosemberg	Chamberlain	Lesoin	Cerame	Pang	Couselo
Medulloblastoma	65				7				1
Astrocytoma/GBM	11			1				1	
Meningeal tumor	5		1						
Ependymoma	13								
PNET	2								
Choroid plexus carcinoma	1								
Pinealoblastoma	2					1			
Germinoma	4	1							
Choriocarcinoma	5								
Endodermal sinus tumor	3								
Embryonal carcinoma	1								
Mixed germ cell tumor	1								
Gliosarcoma							1		
Oligodendroglioma									
Total	113	1	1	1	7	1	1	1	1

Tumor type	Tamura	Valladares	Becker	Schnitzler	Sakata	Kanai	Watterson	Grand Total
Medulloblastoma	2			4		1		81
Astrocytoma/GBM								13
Meningeal tumor								6
Ependymoma								13
PNET								2
Choroid plexus carcinoma		1						2
Pinealoblastoma								3
Germinoma								5
Choriocarcinoma								5
Endodermal sinus tumor								3
Embryonal carcinoma								1
Mixed germ cell tumor					1		1	3
Gliosarcoma								1
Oligodendroglioma			1					
Total	2	1	1	4	1	1	1	138

TABLE 27–2   Metastatic Locations of Medulloblastomas

Lymph nodes	Visceral	Osseous	Other
Retroauricular	Peritoneum	Femur	Scalp
Mediastinal	Lung	Ribs	Incisional scar
Abdominal	Pleura	Vertebrae	Buttocks
Cervical	Bowel	Clavicle	Maxilla
Axillary	Liver	Sternum	Bone marrow
Para-aortic	Breast	Mandible	
Inguinal	Retroperitoneum	Tibia	
		Humerus	
		Radius	
		Hip	
		Scapulae	
		Sacrum	
		Pelvis	
		Skull	
		Ulna	

not well known. Different reports estimate ranges from 2 to 20%.[15, 16, 34, 36–38] Although glioblastoma multiforme is the tumor most prone to extraneural metastasis in the adult population,[9] medulloblastoma metastasizes more commonly in children. There is no age-related predilection toward extraneural metastasis of medulloblastoma.[18] In one series, extraneural metastases were seen in patients age 9 months to 43 years.[15] The average age was 13 years.[15] Thirty percent of patients with medulloblastoma and extraneural metastases manifested their metastases by age 3 years.[15] Seventy percent were diagnosed by age 15 years.[15] Males suffer extraneural metastasis of their medulloblastomas twice as commonly as females.[15] This matches the sex-linked incidence of primary medulloblastoma.[39] The most common sites of extraneural metastatic medulloblastoma are bone, bone marrow, and lymph nodes[40] (Table 27–2). In one autopsy series, 82% of metastases were to bone, 65% were to lymph nodes, and 40% were to viscera.[15] Other commonly reported sites include lung, pleura, liver, breast, and peritoneum.[41] Of bony metastases, the most common sites are pelvis, femur, and vertebrae.[15, 42] Other reported bony sites include rib, humerus, tibia, scapula, skull, mandible, clavicle, and sternum.[15]

The astrocytic tumors, glioblastoma multiforme and anaplastic astrocytoma, less commonly produce extraneural metastases in children. One series reports an incidence of 12.5% in the pediatric population.[2] There is no increased incidence based on age or sex.[18] Common sites of extraneural metastasis are lung, lymph nodes, bone, pleura, and liver[2] (Fig. 27–1). In one series involving children and adults, 60% of extraneural metastases were to lungs or pleura (Fig. 27–2), 51% were to lymph nodes, 30% were to bone, and 22% were to liver.[2] Other sites included heart, adrenal gland, kidney, diaphragm, mediastinum (Fig. 27–3), pancreas, thyroid, and peritoneum[2] (Table 27–3). Of lymph node metastases (Fig. 27–4), 62% were to cervical nodes and 32% were to hilar or mediastinal nodes.[2] Of bony metastases 73% were to vertebrae.[2] Roughly parallel to the incidence in the astrocytic tumors, ependymoma accounts for approximately 10% of extraneural metastases in the pedi-

atric population.[28] Incidences match the age and sex predilections of the primary tumor. Common sites of extraneural metastasis include lung, lymph nodes, bone, pleura, and liver.[9] There have been reports of ependymomas mestastazing to the skin (Fig. 27–5). Extraneural medulloblastoma metastases are less common than CNS metastases. Fifty-three percent of all medulloblastomas spread in the CSF pathways.[15] Extraneural metastases may be associated with recurrent primary tumor. An autopsy series found 87% of patients with extraneural medulloblastoma metastases to have recurrent tumor in the posterior fossa.[15] Another series found 6 of 88 patients to have extraneural medulloblastoma metastases an average of 5 months before local recurrence was found.[15] At least one case report discovered an extraneural medulloblastoma metastasis before the primary lesion was diagnosed.[43] Two cases have been reported in which no primary tumor could be found.[15]

Less is known about the remaining tumor types. One series of primary pineal tumors with extraneural metastases reported 93% of these to be germinomas.[44] Patients with primary pineal tumors tended to manifest their extraneural metastases between the ages of 3 and 34 years.[44] In this series, males were seven times more likely than females to suffer extraneural metastases.[44] See Table 27–4 for pineal tumor locations. Meningeal tumors tended to metastasize to lung, pleura, lymph nodes, liver, and bone.[18] Pituitary tumors metastasized to lung, lymph nodes, bone, muscle, and viscera.[44] The remaining tumors with rare extraneural metastases include choroid plexus carcinoma, pinealoblastoma, choriocarcinoma, gliosarcoma, oligodendroglioma, primitive neuroectodermal tumors, and germ cell tumors.[20, 25, 27, 28, 32, 33, 35]

TIME TO RECURRENCE

For all tumor types, the average time between discovery of primary CNS tumors and evidence of extraneural metastasis is 2 years.[17] For medulloblastomas, the range is 3 to 48 (mean 17) months.[25] *Because medulloblastomas more often metastasize*

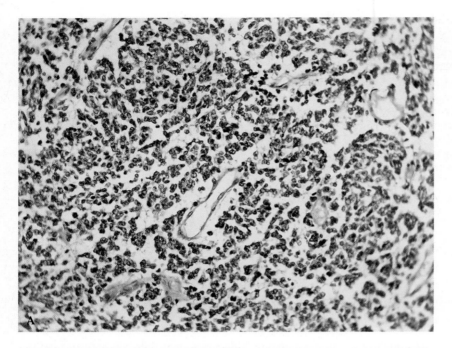

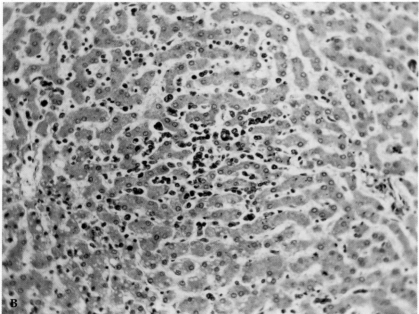

Figure 27–1   (A) Microscopic section of primary medulloblastoma (AFIP Neg 55-20203). (B) Same lesion metastatic to liver (AFIP Neg 55-20204).

through the spinal fluid, CNS metastases are discovered an average of 11 months before the appearance of extraneural metastases.[15]

SURVIVAL

The majority of prognostic data are collected from series involving medulloblastoma patients. Survival in individuals with extraneural medulloblastoma metastases ranges from 2 weeks to 3 years (mean 7 months).[15] Lymph node metas-

tases are a sign of poor prognosis.[15] Individuals with lymphadenopathy due to medulloblastoma metastasis live an average of 4 months.[15] For patients treated with surgery and radiotherapy, the mean survival is 24 months.[45] Additional chemotherapy increases survival time to 38 months.[45]

Survival data of patients with extraneural metastases from tumors other than medulloblastoma are not well documented. One patient with germinoma and extraneural metastases lived 38 months after surgery.[20] Patients with glial extraneural metastases live 1 month to 13 years (mean 18.2

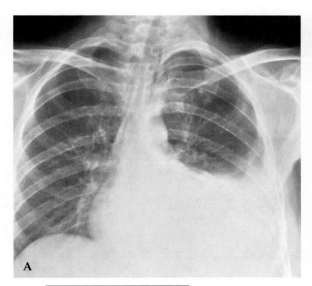
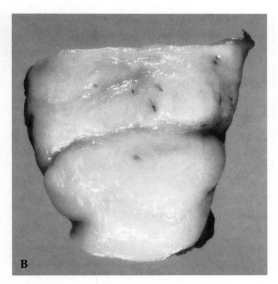

Figure 27–2   Chest radiograph of medulloblastoma metastatic to the chest wall (AFIP Neg 83-568). Gross specimen of medulloblastoma metastatic to the chest wall (AFIP Neg 86-8918).

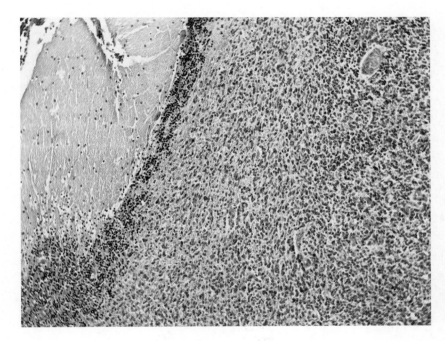

Figure 27–3   Microscopic section demonstrating extraneural medulloblastoma metastasis to the mediastinum.

months).[2] Eighty-three percent of these individuals die within 2 years of metastasis diagnosis.[2] Finally, patients with primary pituitary tumors and extraneural metastases have a life expectancy of only a few months.[44]

DIAGNOSTIC WORKUP

Weiss's criteria are the gold standard to firmly establish the diagnosis of extraneural metastasis. These are based on post-mortem examination and include the following premises.[46]

BOX 27–3
Weiss's Criteria

- **Single histologically characteristic tumor**
- **History consistent with brain tumor**
- **Autopsy to rule out other primary tumor**
- **Identical morphology in primary and metastatic masses**

TABLE 27–3   Metastatic Locations of Astrocytomas and Glioblastomas

Lymph nodes	Visceral	Osseous	Other
Retroauricular	Lung	Ribs	Orbits
Cervical	Liver	Scapula	
Para-aortic	Kidney	Sternum	
Supraclavicular	Heart	Vertebra	
Paratracheal	Adrenal gland	Acetabulum	
Hilar	Pancreas	Arm	
Abdominal	Pericardium		
Mediastinal	Diaphragm		
Peripancreatic	Thyroid		
Intraparotid	Peritoneum		
Bronchial			
Submandibular			

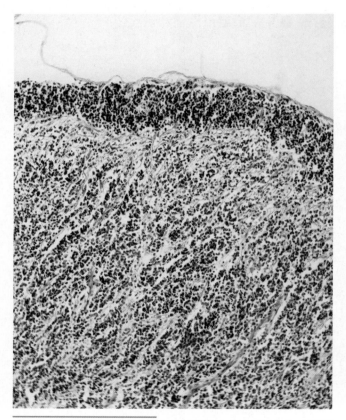

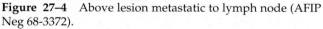

Figure 27–4 Above lesion metastatic to lymph node (AFIP Neg 68-3372).

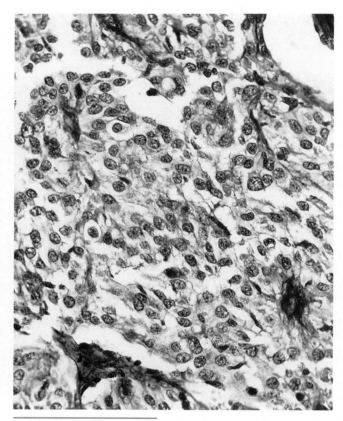

Figure 27–5 Microscopic section of myxopapillary ependymoma metastatic to the skin of the trunk (AFIP Neg 66-5896).

Evaluation of patients with suspected extraneural metastases begins with a high index of suspicion. The single most common complaint seen in these patients is bone pain.[17] As lesions are often found in and near the spinal canal, careful differentiation between bony and radiculopathic pain should be established. Bony pain usually is not exacerbated by Valsalva maneuver and commonly manifests as localized swelling with tenderness to palpation.[47] Patients may also present with weight loss, poor appetite, and malaise. Physical examination may reveal visible or palpable masses, lymphadenopathy, localized swelling, tenderness to palpation, or even pathologic fractures.[15] Patients with liver metastases often have hepatomegaly and right upper quadrant pain. Peritoneal metastases may cause a diffuse, nonspecific, abdominal pain.[17]

TABLE 27–4   Metastatic Locations of Pineal Tumors

Lymph nodes	Viscera	Osseous	Other
Hilar	Lung	Sacrum	Lumbar muscles
Supraclavicular	Liver	Ribs	Cervical muscles
	Kidney	Femur	
	Bladder	Cervical spine	
	Pancreas	Humerus	
	Diaphragm	Scapula	
	Peritoneum	Pelvis	

History and physical examination prompt further studies. Laboratory evaluations should include routine chemistry and hematology panels as well as specialized tests to pursue suspected lesions. Blastic bony metastases often elevate calcium, phosphorus, and acid phosphatase levels.[48] Alkaline phosphatase may be normal, however.[48] Liver metastases usually elevate serum transaminases. Tumor markers such as α-fetoprotein and human chorionic gonadotropin may also be elevated. Bone marrow evaluation may reveal tumor cells or a leukoerythroblastic anemia.[40, 47] One should note, however, that a similar anemia is seen in response to radiation or chemotherapy. Biopsy of palpable lymph nodes is recommended and may be performed open or by fine-needle aspiration.[17]

Finally, radiologic studies can be helpful in characterizing and localizing extraneural metastases. The screening test of choice is a bone scan, which demonstrates osteolytic lesions in 35%, osteoblastic lesions in 60%, and mixed lesions in 5% of patients with bony lesions.[10, 15, 16] Plain roentgenograms demonstrate lytic or blastic lesions,[47] but infiltration of bone marrow may not always result in radiographic abnormalities.[15] Chest X ray is useful in finding lung metastases. Computed tomography is then used to localize lesions for fine-needle aspiration. If needle biopsy is unsuccessful, endoscopic or open biopsy of thoracic or abdominal lesions provides additional tissue for pathologic examination.

TREATMENT

The first treatment of patients at risk for extraneural metastases is prevention and involves a combination of surgery and adjunctive therapies. Because one of the most common avenues of extraneural metastasis is CSF shunts, careful timing of shunting should be considered. Prior to the routine use of computed tomography, patients were routinely shunted to prevent obstructive hydrocephalus secondary to aqueductal effacement. *Recent studies now recommend shunting after gross total resection of the primary tumor unless the patient cannot tolerate waiting.*[49] Patients are observed with serial neurologic examinations and computed tomograms as needed. Several studies have used shunt filters as one method of preventing shunt-related extraneural metastases.[44, 49] These devices have proven to be flawed at best. Failure due to obstruction or unsuccessful filtration of tumor cells often prompts shunt

revisions and may preclude the routine use of these devices. Recent discussions quoting higher incidences of extraneural metastases are evidence that patients are surviving longer and thus may have an increased likelihood of developing metastases.[1, 50, 51] Those who do manifest metastatic disease are treated with chemotherapy and may also receive radiation therapy.

Medulloblastoma metastases are the most common extraneural lesions treated with chemotherapy. Cyclophosphamide and vincristine are the two most commonly employed agents.[25] Together with adriamycin, they have been shown to be most efficacious in treating medulloblastoma metastases.[25] A median time of 17 months to progression of disease (range 4 to 65+ months) has been quoted.[25] Granulocytopenic fever and thrombocytopenia are common side effects of this three-drug combination.[25] Other agents used in treating extraneural medulloblastoma metastases are chloroethylnitrosoureas, methotrexate, procarbazine, platinum compounds, and hexitol epoxides.[25]

The use of chemotherapeutic agents to treat metastases prompts a discussion about whether all patients with aggressive primary tumors should routinely receive chemotherapy and radiation therapy. Chemotherapy destroys proliferating cells and therefore may allow nonproliferating tumor cells to flourish.[17] It also alters one's immune status and may prevent patients from mounting a response to metastatic disease. Similarly, radiation therapy has a known oncogenetic effect and may cause severe neurologic dysfunction in children.[17] Studies have shown drops in IQ, growth retardation, hypopituitarism, sensorineural hearing loss, and neural tissue damage due to radiation necrosis.[49] Despite these drawbacks, patients with both medulloblastomas and germinomas should receive craniospinal radiation (25 to 40 Gy) plus 10 to 15 Gy to the tumor bed after maximum possible surgical resection of the primary tumor. In addition, patients with spinal fluid shunts should be considered for chemotherapy prophylaxis once they reach the age of 3 years.

SUMMARY

The overall incidence of pediatric extraneural metastases is 20 to 30%, and the main mechanisms by which such metastases occur are surgery and shunts. The most common extraneural metastatic primary masses are medulloblastoma, astrocytic tumors, and ependymoma. Of these, medulloblastomas are most commonly metastatic to bone and viscera; astrocytomas and glioblastomas are most commonly metastatic to lymph nodes and viscera; and ependymomas are most commonly metastatic to lymph nodes. In addition, CNS metastases commonly accompany extraneural metastases. The average time to discovery of extraneural metastases is 2 years. The most common presenting complaint is bone pain. The screening test of choice for extraneural metastases is a bone scan, and the treatment of choice is chemotherapy. Most patients with extraneural metastases die within 2 years of discovery.

REFERENCES

1. Duffner PK, Cohen ME. Extraneural metastases in childhood brain tumors. *Ann Neurol* 1981;10:261–265.
2. Pasquier B, Pasquier D, N'Golet A, et al. Extraneural metastases of astrocytomas and glioblastomas: clinicopathological study of two cases and review of literature. *Cancer* 1980;45:112–125.
3. Smith DR, Hardman JM, Earle KM. Metastasizing neuroectodermal tumors of the central nervous system. *J Neurosurg* 1969;31:50–58.
4. Willis RA. *The Spread of Tumors in the Human Body*. 2nd ed. London: Butterworth; 1952:101.
5. McComb JG. Recent research into the nature of cerebrospinal fluid formation and absorption. *J Neurosurg* 1983;59.
6. Morley TP. The recovery of tumor cells from venous blood draining cerebral gliomas: a preliminary report. *Can J Surg* 1959;2:363–365.
7. Battista AF, Bloom W, Loffman H, et al. Autotransplantation of anaplastic astrocytomas into the subcutaneous tissues of mass. *Neurology* 1961;11:977–981.
8. Zimmerman HM. The natural history of intracranial neoplasms with special reference to gliomas. *Am J Surg* 1957;93:913–924.
9. Liwnicz B, Rubenstein L. The pathways of extraneural spread in metastasizing gliomas: a report of three cases and critical review of the literature. *Hum Pathol* 1979;10:453–467.
10. Gyepes MT, D'Angio GJ. Extracranial metastases from central nervous system tumors in children and adolescents. *Radiology* 1966;87:55–63.
11. Drachman DA, Winter TS, Karon M. Medulloblastomas with extracranial metastasis. *Arch Neurol* 1963;9:86–98.
12. Wasser Krug R, Peyser E, Lichtig C. Extracranial bone metastasis from intracranial meningiomas. *Surg Neurol* 1979;12:480–484.
13. Eade OE, Urlich H. Metastasizing gliomas in young subjects. *J Pathol* 1971;103:245–256.
14. Wolf A, Cowen D, Stewart WB. Glioblastoma with extraneural metastasis by way of ventriculopleural anastomosis. *Trans Am Neurol Assoc* 1954;79:140–142.
15. Kleinman GM, Hochberg FH, Richardson EP. Systemic metastases from medulloblastoma: report of two cases and review of the literature. *Cancer* 1981;48:2296–2309.
16. Hoffman HJ, Hendrick EB, Humphreys RP. Metastasis via ventriculoperitoneal shunt in patients with medulloblastoma. *J Neurosurg* 1976;44:562–566.
17. Cohen ME, Duffner PK. Extraneural metastases in childhood brain tumors. In: *Brain Tumors in Children: Principles of Diagnosis and Treatment*. New York: Raven Press; 1984:295–307.
18. Glasauer FE, Yuan RHP. Intracranial tumors with extracranial metastases. *J Neurosurg* 1963;20:474–493.
19. Rubinstein LJ. Development of extracranial metastases from a malignant astrocytoma in the absence of previous craniotomy: case report. *J Neurosurg* 1967;26:542–547.
20. Ono N, Isobe I, Uki J, et al. Recurrence of primary intracranial germinomas after complete response with radiotherapy: recurrence patterns and therapy. *Neurosurgery* 1994;35(4):615–620.
21. Shen WC, Ho YJ, Le SK, Lee KR. [Intracranial germ cell tumors] [Chinese]. *Chinese Med* 1992;49(5):354–364.
22. Kanai H, Nagai H, Mabe H, et al. [A case of extraneural metastasis of medulloblastoma successfully treated with cisplatin and etoposide] [Japanese]. *Jap J Cancer Chemother* 1992;19(4):545–547.
23. Watterson J, Priest JR. Control of extraneural metastasis of a primary intracranial nongerminomatous germ-cell tumor. *J Neurosurg* 1989;71:601–604.
24. Rosemberg S, Lopes MC, Elks L, et al. Extraneural metastasis of brainstem. *Clin Neuropathol* 1988;7(3):131–3.
25. Chamberlain MC, Silver P, Edwards MS, et al. Treatment of extraneural metastatic medulloblastoma with a combination of cyclophosphamide, adriamycin and vincristine. *Neurosurgery* 1988;23(4):476–479.
26. Lesoin F, Cama A, Dhellemmes P, et al. Extraneural metastasis of a pineal tumor. *Eur Neurol* 1987;27(1):55–61.
27. Cerame MA, Guthikonda M, Kohli CM. Extraneural metastases in cliosarcoma: a case report and review of the literature. *Neurosurgery* 1985;17(3):413–418.
28. Hoffman HJ, Duffner PK. Extraneural metastases of central nervous system tumors. *Cancer* 1985;56:1178–1182.
29. Pang D, Ashmead JW. Extraneural metastasis of cerebellar glioblastoma multiforme. *Neurosurgery* 1982;10(2):252–257.
30. Couselo Sanchez JM, Alonso Martin A, Iglesias Diz JL, et al. Extraneural metastasis of medulloblastoma. *Revista Espanola de Oncologia* 1982;29(1):63–68.
31. Tamura M, Kawafuchi J, Ishida Y, et al. [Extraneural metastasis in cerebellar medulloblastomas-report of two cases and review of the literature (author's translation)][Japanese]. *Neuro Medico-Chirurgica* 1980;20(3):257–264.
32. Valladares JB, Perry RH, Kalbag RM. Malignant choroid plexus papilloma with extraneural metastasis. *J Neurosurg* 1980;52(2):251–255.
33. Becker H, Walter GF, Tritthart H, et al. [Extraneural metastasis of an oligodendroglioma in ventriculo-peritoneal shunt]. [German] *Onkologie* 1978;1(5):216–220.
34. Schnitzler ER, Richards MJ, Chun RW. Cerebellar medulloblastoma: an analysis of four cases of extraneural metastasis. *Am J of Dis in Childn* 1978;132(10):1004–1008.
35. Sakata K, Yamada H, Sakai N, et al. Extraneural metastasis of pineal tumor. *Surg Neurol* 1975;3(1):49–54.
36. Das S, Dalby JE. Distant metastases from medulloblastoma. *Acta Radiol Ther* 1977;16:117–123.
37. Patterson E. Distant metastases from medulloblastoma of the cerebellum. *Brain* 1961;84:301–309.

38. Chatty E, Earle K. Medulloblastoma—a report of 201 cases with emphasis on the relationship of histologic variant to survival. *Cancer* 1971;28:977–983.

39. Brutschin P, Culver GJ. Extracranial metastases from medulloblastomas. *Radiology* 1973;107:359–362.

40. Bach M, Simpson WJ, Platts ME. Metastatic cerebellar sarcoma (desmoplastic medulloblastoma) with diffuse osteosclerosis and leukoerythroblastic anemia. *Am J Roentgenol* 1969;103:38–43.

41. Raimondi AJ, Tomita T. Medulloblastoma in childhood. *Acta Neurochir* 1979;50:127–138.

42. Lewis MB, Nunes LB, Powell DE, Shnider BI. Extraaxial spread of medulloblastoma. *Cancer* 1973;31:1287–1297.

43. McComb JG, Davis RL, Isaacs H, Landing BH. Medulloblastoma presenting as neck tumors in two infants. *Ann Neurol* 1980;7:113–117.

44. Galassi E, Tognetti F, Frank F, Gaist G. Extraneural metastases from primary pineal tumors: review of the literature. *Surg Neurol* 1984;21:497–504.

45. Nathanson L, Kovacs SG. Chemotherapeutic response in metastatic medulloblastoma: report of two cases and a review of the literature. *Med Pediatr Oncol* 1978;4:105–110.

46. Weiss L. A metastasizing ependymoma of the cauda equina. *Cancer* 1955;8:161–171.

47. Lassman LP. Diagnosis and management of skeletal metastases from cerebellar medulloblastoma. *Child's Brain* 1976;2:38–45.

48. Ho EP, Lieber A, DeLand FH, Maruyama Y. Generalized osteoblastic bony metastases from medulloblastoma. *Oncology* 1976;33:253–256.

49. Park TS, Hoffman HJ, Hendrick EB, et al. Medulloblastoma: clinical presentation and management. *J Neurosurg* 1983;58:543–552.

50. Alvord EC. Why do gliomas not metastasize? *Arch Neurol* 1976;33:73–75.

51. Hoshino T, Wilson CB. Review of basic concepts of cell kinetics as applied to brain tumors. *J Neurosurg* 1975;42:123–131.

Chapter 28

Infantile Brain Tumors

Concezio Di Rocco, Aldo Iannelli, and Fabio Papacci

Brain tumors occurring in infancy and early childhood are among the most difficult and challenging seen by the neurosurgeon. Traditionally these tumors have been accompanied by great pessimism. In the general opinion, they were associated either with early patient death or, in cases of long-term survival, with greatly impaired psychomotor development. This negative attitude was due to both the difficulties in treating surgically these patients and the limits to providing complete care in patients in whom radiotherapy cannot be applied. The recent development of multidisciplinary clinics and programs where pediatric neurosurgeons, pediatric neurologists, pediatricians, and pediatric oncologists work as a team has reignited interest in this type of pathology. The interest in infantile tumors was further stimulated by the awareness that the prognosis of many neoplasms of infants and toddlers after modern treatment is not necessarily worse and, in some instances, is even better than that of similar tumors occurring in the older pediatric population and in adults.[1-3] Regrettably, in too many countries only a few infants are ever referred to specialized centers. Most continue to be treated in general neurosurgery departments, reflecting the insufficient awareness on the part of medical institutions of the advantages of having these particular patients treated by specialists. Consequently, unjustified pessimism on the outcome, on one side, and dispersion of the experiences, on the other side, combine to make brain neoplasms of infants and toddlers an insufficiently explored field of pediatric neurosurgery.

There are several potential points of interest regarding infantile brain tumors.

1. The information that these tumors may provide with regard to etiology. *Actually, when occurring in utero or soon after birth, these tumors constitute a unique model for human neuro-oncogenesis as exogenous factors may have acted in their development only for the short intrauterine and neonatal periods.*

2. The clinical characteristics, which still need further investigation. Incidence, topographic location, oncotype distribution, clinical presentation, and response to treatment of brain neoplasms in infants and toddlers differ from their counterparts in older pediatric groups.

3. The analysis of the effects generated by the necessity of withholding radiotherapy in this fragile subset of patients

- The possibility of evaluating the results of avoiding, postponing, or decreasing the dosage of radiotherapy

- The reliable appreciation of the specific role of the surgical treatment in controlling the disease in subjects managed with supportive therapy alone after the surgical excision of the tumor

- The design of new, more aggressive or more prolonged regimens of chemotherapy and the evaluation of their application as primary postoperative treatment modalities.

EPIDEMIOLOGY

Prospective epidemiologic studies on brain tumors are not practically feasible in the pediatric population due to the excessive cost and the excessive time that would be required as a result of their low annual incidence (1 to 3 cases per 100,000 births). Consequently, most of the information currently available has been obtained from retrospective studies. These types of studies have the advantage of requiring relatively low efforts and costs, but they also present various kinds of limitations, in particular because most are hospital- rather than population-based. Even when the information is obtained from regional or national cancer registries, the reliability of the statistical evaluation cannot be absolute as it may be exposed to the bias of the long time necessary to collect a sufficient number of cases. During such a period, the inclusive criteria may have changed as a result of the introduction of more refined diagnostic tools. Striking differences exist in already published series depending on the particular method for collecting statistical material utilized by multiple authors in various countries. Furthermore, studies based on autopsy statistics cannot provide absolute data as they are related to the characteristics of the clinical department serviced by a given pathology institute.

In cases of brain tumors of infancy and early childhood, the arbitrary choice of age limits for certain developmental periods in many investigations prevents the reader from obtaining objective figures from the literature. Furthermore, the variable setting of the upper age limits for infantile brain tumor series makes it difficult to compare the different experiences with regard to the incidence as well as the topographic and oncotype distribution of the various nosographic entities in specific patients subgroups.

An additional difficulty is posed by possible racial or/and environmental differences for certain types of tumors in studies performed in different geographic areas (e.g., teratomas in East Asian countries[4, 5] or Mexico,[6] Burkitt's lymphomas in Africa[7]), variable presence of cases due to familial inheritance,[8–12] different histopathologic diagnoses and nosographic classifications (dermoid cysts considered as germ cell tumors, primitive neuroectodermal tumors, or PNETs, as medulloblastomas), and the inclusion or exclusion of certain pathologic entities, such as metastases, angiomas, lipomas, or lymphomas.

General Information

Primary tumors of the central nervous system (CNS) represent nearly 10% of all malignant diseases but compose approximately 20 to 23% of all pediatric neoplasms.[9, 13, 14] More than 90% of them involve the brain, the remainder being confined to the spinal cord.[9, 13]

The incidence of pediatric brain tumors seems to have increased progressively in recent decades, with maximal values in developed countries such as Sweden (32.7 to 34.9 cases per million,[15, 16] Canada, England, New Zealand, and the United States; however, a minor increase seems to characterize series reported in Japan.[13, 17–21] The steady rise in incidence—about a 1% rise per year—appears to be typical for brain tumors, a statistic that differs significantly from other neoplastic diseases, namely, leukemias, Hodgkin's disease, non-Hodgkin's lymphomas, renal tumors, and ocular tumors.[18] Such a finding cannot be explained merely on the grounds of the current improved diagnostic accuracy.

In the early 1990s, the total annual incidence of brain tumors in the United States was estimated to be approximately 22 per million.[22] In the same year, a 20-year survey of patients younger than 20 years undertaken in Europe gave an incidence of 31 per million for males and 26 for females, respectively.[9] In all of the different geographic areas, males outnumber females with a male/female ratio ranging from 1.1 for Europe and the United States to 1.6 for Africa.[16, 18, 22, 23]

Brain Tumors in Early Childhood

Nearly 80% of all childhood brain tumors occur within the first 10 years of life.[24] The risk of brain tumors in children decreases with increasing age.[25] In the study on 3291 children with histologically verified neoplasms of the CNS carried out in 1988 by the Childhood Brain Tumor Consortium, which grouped 10 North American institutions,[26] 7% of all tumors presented during the first 12 months of life. The annual risk in the subsequent years was 7 to 8% until the age of 8 years, after which a decline could be noted.

In our personal series of 558 brain tumors consecutively observed in a period of 15 years (1981–1995), 162 (29%) were treated in children younger than 3 years, which is the age limit for withholding radiotherapy in our institution. Of these patients, 70 (43.2%) subjects were infants younger than 1 year, 43 (26.6%) children in the second year of life, and 49 (30.2%) children in the third year of life, respectively (Fig. 28–1). Males represented 60% of our cases, with a male/female ratio

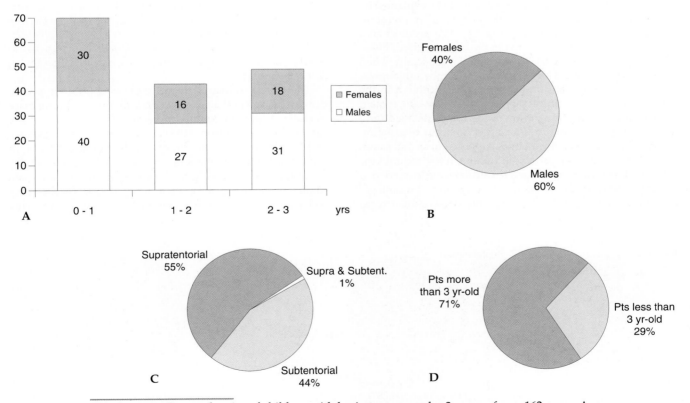

Figure 28–1 Personal series of children with brain tumors under 3 years of age: 162 cases. Age (A), sex (A, B), and topographic (C) distribution. (D) Relative incidence of the group of subjects younger than 3 years and the whole pediatric population with brain tumors (558 cases).

of 1.5 (Fig. 28–1B). This age distribution is different from that of other series dealing with intracranial tumors occurring in early childhood in which the number of cases increases with age[27] and probably reflects the referral pattern of children with brain tumors to a center specialized in pediatric neurosurgical care.

Among infantile brain tumors, those occurring during the first 12 months of life have been the subject of particular interest because of their etiologic implications. In a study performed in East Germany on still-born babies and infants up to 1 year of age, the incidence of brain neoplasms was 1.1 per million births.[28] It has been calculated that brain tumors diagnosed during the first year of life account for about 36 cases per million and their associated mortality for about 0.04 to 0.18% of the deaths recorded in the same period of time.[17, 29, 30] In pediatric neurosurgical series, intracranial tumors in this age group were considered rare before the introduction of the modern diagnostic tools for neuroimaging, with figures indicating values inferior to 3% of the total population of children with intracranial tumors.[31–36] Since the early 1980s, however, a major incidence was reported.[37–40] *Currently, in most pediatric neurosurgical series, brain neoplasms in infants younger than 1 year old correspond to figures around or above 10%,*[26, 41] *with a maximal value of 18% reported by Sakamoto et al.*[39]

In our series, infants aged less than 1 year represented 12.5% of the whole pediatric population under 16 years of age treated in our institution for an intracranial neoplasm (Fig. 28–2).

The age distribution curve of this subgroup of patients indicates two peaks in frequency, with the first corresponding to the first months of life and the second to the end of the first year of life (Fig. 28–3). These peaks could be explained by considering that the diagnosis of an intracranial brain tumor can be obtained during intrauterine life. The presence of a tumor is also frequently detected in the first months of life in cases of particularly marked macrocrania, especially when associated with clinical signs of increased intracranial pressure. On the other hand, mild cranial enlargement in the absence of any other clinical manifestation may long remain underestimated and recognition of the tumor delayed until the end of the first year of life as psychomotor retardation becomes evident when the infant is supposed to sit and stand.

The relative incidence of brain tumors in the second year of life is somewhat more difficult to calculate due to overlap in several series of cases symptomatic in the first 12 months of life and treated surgically later. In some series, similar cases

are regarded as belonging to the first year of life. However, the overall experience seems to indicate that the relative incidence of brain tumors in this specific subset of patients is less than that found in infants up to 1 year of age as the cumulative incidence in the first 2 years of age tends to be a little below or above 16% of all brain tumors occurring in the pediatric population.[1, 21, 42, 43] In our series, however, the incidence of tumors occurring during the second year of life was 7.7% and the cumulative incidence of the first 2 years was 20.2% of the whole population of children with brain tumors (Fig. 28–1).

Congenital Brain Tumors

The proportion of infants with brain tumors appears relatively constant in recent series where the diagnosis of the disease was based on prenatal routine sonographic examinations and postnatal neuroimaging investigations, namely, cerebral ultrasonography, computed tomography (CT), and magnetic resonance imaging (MRI). The phenomenon suggests that preconceptional oncogenic factors do not play a more major role than that in past years.[24]

The prenatal origin of some tumors of infancy is obvious for those that are recognized in utero[41, 44–47] or in the neonatal period.[48–50] However, some authors consider that most brain tumors recognized during the first 24 months of life might have been present at birth,[8, 12, 26] thus extending the definition of congenital tumors beyond the traditionally accepted period of early infancy.[51]

The hypothesis that tumors arise from embryonal cells rather than from a malignant degeneration of already differentiated tissues was propounded in the 1800s. *Congenital brain tumors could provide some evidence for the hypothesis of tumor induction from immature parts of the CNS during intrauterine life because of the limited exposure of the fetus or the newborn to possible oncogenic factors apt to provoke the neoplastic transformation of mature cells.*

There are two main criteria for defining a tumor as congenital: the age of the patient at presentation of clinical manifestations and the histopathologic characteristics of the tumor. The age criterion is the basis of various classifications. In 1951, Arstein and co-workers[31] defined congenital brain tumors as those symptomatic during the first 60 days of life. In 1964, Solitare and Krigman[52] proposed subdividing brain tumors of the first year of life in three groups: (1) definitely congenital tumors, already symptomatic at birth or during

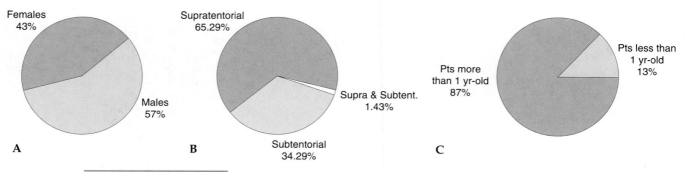

Figure 28–2   Personal series of infants under 1 year of age: 70 cases. Sex (A) and topographic (B) distribution. (C) Relative incidence between infants younger than 1 year and the whole pediatric population with brain tumors (558 cases).

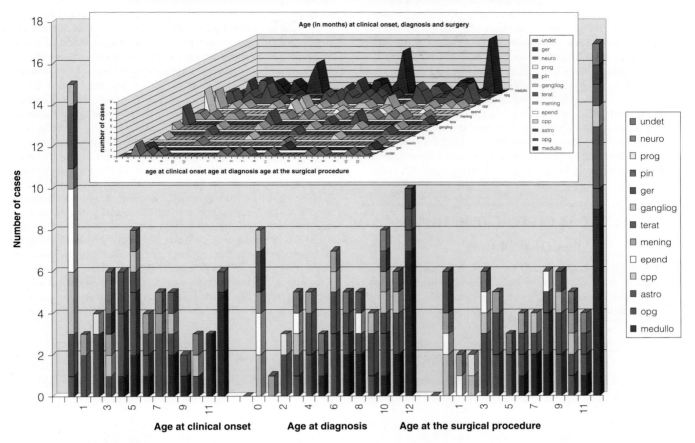

Figure 28–3   Age and oncotype cumulative distribution of 70 infants younger than 1 year with brain tumor at presentation, at diagnosis, and at operation (bottom). The distribution of the singles oncotypes in the same periods is reported in the upper part of the figure.

the first 4 weeks of life; (2) probably congenital tumors, symptomatic during the first year of life; and (3) possibly congenital tumors, symptomatic before but recognized after the end of the first year of life. In the early 1970s, the concept of neonatal tumors was introduced to account for tumors present at birth or recognized during the first 2 weeks of life.[29, 53, 54] In 1986, Ellams and co-workers[55] proposed a three-group classification substantially similar to that of Solitare and Krigman—definitely congenital, probably congenital, and possibly congenital brain tumors—but established age settings for the appearance of the clinical manifestations and recognition of the lesion at 6 weeks from birth, 6 months, and the end of the first year of life, respectively.

The main advantage of classifications based on temporal criteria is that they provide some information concerning the actual clinical incidence of brain tumors in early infancy. Thus, it is possible to calculate that neoplasms developing in utero and detected either at birth or during the first month of life constitute about 0.5 to 1.5% of all childhood brain tumors[30, 43, 56] and 14% of those occurring during the first year of life.[57] They account for 5% of neonatal deaths.[51]

In our series, four tumors—two choroid plexus papillomas, one teratoma, and one ependymoma—were detected in utero and another 11 were detected during the first month of

life. Thus, in our experience, definitely congenital tumors accounted for 21% of the brain tumors occurring in infants younger than 1 year and 2.6% of all brain tumors in the pediatric population.

The different biologic behavior of the various tumors represents the main limit of the temporal classifications of neoplasms as hamartomas, craniopharyngiomas, medulloblastomas, and teratomas: Though originating in fetal life, they may remain asymptomatic in infancy.[30, 39, 58]

For example, teratoma, the most common tumor at birth,[48, 59] represents only 5% of the 886 cases of brain tumors in children younger than 1 year considered in the cooperative study carried out by the Education Committee of the International Society for Pediatric Neurosurgery (ISPN) in 1991.[57] The few cases of teratoma detected in utero were particularly large, sometimes filling the cranial cavity so completely as to make it impossible to establish the exact site of tumor origin.[47] Craniopharyngioma, which accounts for 1.4 to 4% of brain tumors in the general[60, 61] and 10% in the pediatric population,[24] is practically absent in the above-mentioned cooperative study of the ISPN,[57] in spite of its congenital development.[36, 42, 62]

The histogenetic criterion for classifying infantile brain tumors is utilized for tumors such as teratomas, dermoids, epidermoids, chordomas, lipomas, craniopharyngiomas, and colloid cysts, whose origin from abnormally migrated or differentiated cells has been proved. Most of these tumors are characterized by low growth rates, so that their presence in infants may remain undetected for a surprisingly long time. On the other hand, some "embryonal" tumors, namely, retinoblastomas, pinealoblastomas, medulloblastomas, ependymoblastomas, and neuroblastomas,[63-66] which originate from immature cells but with restricted differentiation lines, may present in adulthood.

Cytogenetic classifications explain the relative distribution of central neuroepithelial tumors on the basis of the width of the window of neoplastic vulnerability, identifiable with the number of cells still cycling at the time of an oncogenic insult, which is significantly larger for glial than for neuronal cells.[67]

CLINICAL CHARACTERISTICS

Sex Distribution

The analysis of sex distribution has some relevance to neurooncology because of the obvious sex predilection of certain neoplasms. According to Zülch,[60] there is an overall slight preponderance of males over females among the general population

with brain tumors (53% to 47% in his series, that is, a male-to-female ratio of 11:9). In general terms, the more malignant tumors of neuroepithelial origin have a preponderance in males, whereas the benign tumors of the coverings of the brain occur more frequently in females. Such an association seems to apply also to infants younger than 1 year whose tumors would be characterized by a high incidence of malignant forms and a predilection for males.[8, 27] Actually, the sex distribution is not an absolute feature as it may vary with patient age and tumor location; for example, the male preponderance of craniopharyngiomas reaches a male-to-female ratio of 4:1 in the first two decades versus a ratio of 2:1 in the whole population.

With regards to sex distribution, children do not differ in general from their adult counterparts as the male-to-female ratio in the pediatric population is slightly greater to 1.[16, 18] Higher values for male preponderance are, however, observed for certain tumors, such as medulloblastoma, germinoma, and choroid plexus papilloma[26] (Figs. 28–4 and 28–5).

In the 1991 cooperative study of the ISPN on brain tumors in infants younger than 1 year,[57] males (54.2%) outnumbered females (45.8%), with a ratio of 1.18. Such a ratio, close to 1, is confirmed by the cumulative analysis of various series reported in the literature[27] (Table 28–1). Consequently, series suggesting that brain tumors have a probability of occurring

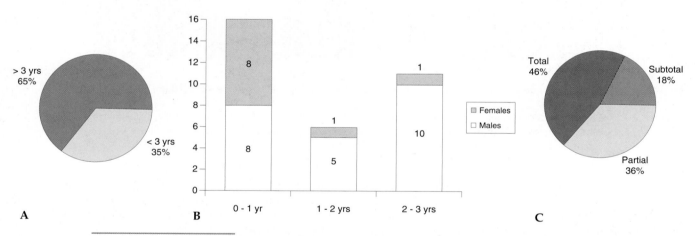

Figure 28–4 Medulloblastomas and primitive neuroectodermal tumors in children under 3 years of age. Relative incidence as referred to the whole pediatric population with this type of tumor (A). Age and sex relative distribution in the first 3 years (B) and the degree of surgical tumor excision (C).

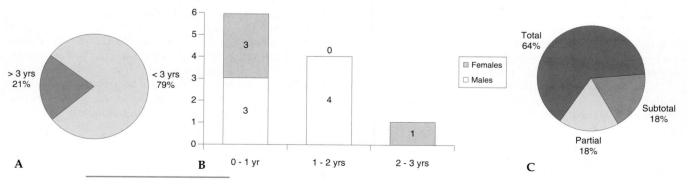

Figure 28–5 Choroid plexus tumors in children younger than 3 years. Relative incidence as referred to the whole pediatric population with this type of tumor (A). Age and sex relative distribution in the first 3 years (B) and the degree of surgical tumor excision (C).

TABLE 28–1 Relative Frequency, Gender Ratio, and Location of the Most Common Pediatric Brain Tumors in the First Year of Life

Country	First author (year)	Cases (no.)	M/F (no.)	S/I (no.)	Astr (no.)	Med (no.)	Epen (no.)	Plex (no.)	PNET (no.)	Tera (no.)
Argentina	Zuccaro[86]	40	0.8 (18/22)	4.0 (32/8)	44.7 (18)	13.2 (5)	5.3 (2)	13.2 (5)	10.5 (4)	2.6 (1)
Austria	Jellinger[73]	56	n.d.	n.d.	21.4 (12)	8.9 (5)	8.9 (5)	3.6 (2)	—	1.8 (1)
Canada	Ventureyra[88]	11	n.d.	4.5 (9/2)	45.5 (5)	—	—	9.1 (1)	9.1 (1)	9.1 (1)
	Asai[89]	41	1.3 (23/18)	2.4 (29/12)	41.5 (17)	2.4 (1)	2.4 (1)	19.5 (8)	12.2 (5)	2.4 (1)
England	Jooma[84]	100	n.d.	1.5 (60/40)	31.0 (31)	20.0 (20)	18.0 (18)	13.0 (13)	3.0 (3)	3.0 (3)
France	Lapras[88]	29	1.6 (18/11)	2.5 (21/8)	24.1 (7)	17.2 (5)	24.1 (7)	3.4 (1)	—	1.3 (?)
	Lellouch[89]	n.d.	1.1 (?)	1.5 (?)	27.0 (?)	14.0 (?)	25.0 (?)	9.0 (?)	9.0 (?)	5.0 (?)
Germany	Ellams[86]	12	0.7 (5/7)	1.0 (6/6)	8.3 (1)	33.3 (4)	—	—	—	—
	Staneczek[94]	130	1.3 (73/57)	n.d.	20.8 (27)	16.2 (21)	16.2 (21)	6.2 (21)	—	6.2 (8)
	Jänish[95]	102	n.d.	n.d.	36.3 (37)	21.6 (22)	11.8 (12)	8.8 (9)	—	5.9 (6)
	Rickert[97]	22	1.0 (11/11)	3.4 (17/5)	13.6 (3)	13.6 (3)	13.6 (3)	—	22.7 (5)	4.5 (1)
Japan	Sato[75]	10	0.4 (3/7)	9.0 (9/1)	30.0 (3)	—	10.0 (1)	10.0 (9)	—	20.0 (2)
	Sakamoto[86]	18	1.0 (9/9)	3.5 (14/4)	22.2 (4)	16.7 (3)	11.1 (2)	5.6 (9)	—	16.7 (3)
	Oi[90]	218	1.0 (109/109)	2.3 (152/66)	24.2 (53)	16.5 (36)	11.3 (25)	12.4 (27)	2.1 (5)	9.3 (20)
Italy	Colangelo[80]	14	1.3 (8/6)	1.8 (9/5)	21.4 (3)	21.4 (3)	21.4 (3)	—	—	7.1 (1)
	Galassi[89]	28	1.8 (18/10)	2.1 (19/9)	33.3 (9)	4.2 (1)	12.5 (3)	20.8 (6)	8.3 (2)	—
	Di Rocco[93]	51	1.2 (28/23)	1.4 (30/21)	36.1 (18)	25.5 (13)	10.6 (5)	8.5 (4)	—	4.3 (2)
Mexico	Rueda-Franco[88]	32	1.0 (16/16)	2.6 (23/9)	25.0 (8)	3.1 (1)	15.6 (5)	3.1 (1)	9.4 (3)	9.4 (3)
	De la Torre[93]	35	1.6 (22/13)	2.3 (24/11)	20.0 (7)	5.7 (2)	17.1 (7)	—	11.4 (4)	20.0 (7)
S. Arabia	Murshid[94]	14	n.d.	1.0 (7/7)	28.6 (4)	35.7 (5)	14.3 (2)	7.1 (1)	14.3 (2)	7.1 (1)
Spain	Gonzalez-Ruiz[89]	29	n.d.	3.1 (22/7)	17.2 (5)	10.3 (3)	6.9 (2)	34.5 (10)	3.4 (1)	6.9 (2)
U.S.A.	Raimondi[83]	39	1.3 (22/17)	1.8 (25/14)	30.8 (12)	23.1 (9)	2.6 (1)	15.4 (6)	2.6 (1)	7.7 (3)
	Tomita[85]	57	n.d.	2.0 (38/19)	29.8 (17)	21.1 (12)	5.3 (3)	17.5 (9)	1.8 (1)	1.8 (1)
	Haddad[91]	22	0.6 (9/13)	2.1 (15/7)	31.8 (7)	—	—	13.6 (3)	27.3 (6)	18.2 (4)
Total		**1110**	**1.1 (392/394)**	**2.1 (561/261)**	**27.7 (308)**	**15.6 (174)**	**11.5 (128)**	**11.6 (129)**	**3.8 (43)**	**6.0 (67)**
ISPN	Oi[90]	307	1.1 (161/146)	2.1 (208/99)	23.3 (72)	17.2 (53)	11.1 (34)	10.7 (33)	4.2 (13)	8.4 (26)
Coop. Study	Di Rocco[91]	886	1.2 (483/403)	2.2 (609/277)	28.6 (253)	11.5 (102)	11.4 (101)	10.6 (94)	6.2 (55)	5.0 (44)
Total		**1193**	**1.1 (644/549)**	**2.1 (817/376)**	**27.2 (325)**	**13.0 (155)**	**11.3 (135)**	**10.6 (127)**	**5.7 (68)**	**5.8 (70)**

Astr, astrocytoma; Med, medulloblastoma; Epen, ependymoma; Plex, plexus tumors; Tera, teratoma; n.d., no data available.

in males twice as great as that in females should be considered as local aberrations.[23, 68–70]

In our series of 70 infants under 1 year of age with brain tumors, boys represented 57% and girls 43% of cases (Fig. 28–2). The slight male preponderance was maintained in subsequent years (Fig. 28–1).

Topographic Distribution

One of the distinguishing features of infantile brain neoplasms in the fetal period and in the first 2 years of life is the prevalence of tumors in the supratentorial compartment. This is in contrast to the predominance of infratentorial tumors in the pediatric population in subsequent ages, starting from the third year of life. The propensity of posterior fossa structures to develop neoplasms after infancy through adolescence has been given various explanations: the persistence at this level of pluripotent cells with DNA that is highly sensitive to environmental insults; the richer vascularization and the slower blood flow of the region, which would permit a higher concentration of a hypothetical blood-borne oncogene factor; or different time spans of certain oncotypes, which would determine the clinical correlation of certain tumors (medulloblastoma, astrocytoma of the cerebellum and brain stem) with certain ages.[73]

The prevalence of the supratentorial location is particularly evident in infants younger than 1 year, in whom supratentorial tumors tend to occur twice as often as infratentorial tumors.[1, 20, 27, 32, 35, 36, 38–40, 42, 71] Only a small percentage of tumors (slightly more than 1%) involve both cranial compartments.[57]

Starting from the second year of life, a progressive reequilibrium between supratentorial and infratentorial tumors can be noted, with a predominance of the infratentorial location characteristic of the older pediatric population (Tables 28–2 and 28–3).[27, 72]

The topographic distribution of our series of 162 cases of brain tumor in children younger than 3 years confirmed this trend, with a predominance of supratentorial (54.8%) over infratentorial (43.9%) tumors and an incidence of 1.3% of tumors developing in both cranial districts (Fig. 28–1). In the first year of life, 65.3% of the tumors were located in the supratentorial and 34.2% in the infratentorial compartment (Fig. 28–2).

A second distinguishing trait of infantile tumors with regard to topographic distribution is their tendency to concentrate along the midline.[74, 75] Indeed, in addition to craniopharyngiomas, pinealomas, and embryonal tumors, which obviously maintain their midline location at any age, infantile neuroectodermal tumors tend to develop near the cerebral ventricles, in contrast to the adult varieties, in relation to the phylogenetically older regions of the CNS. When developing inside neoencephalic structures, such as the cerebral hemispheres, infantile brain tumors are often composed of cell populations of paleoencephalic origin (ependymal tumors, piloid astrocytomas, gangliogliomas, mixed gliomas). The phenomenon may be related to the characteristics of postnatal neurogenesis and gliogenesis; that is, to the cellular proliferation that continues after the fetal period for the first 6 months of postnatal life in some areas of the brain, such as the subependymal layer of the lateral ventricles, the subpial germinal layer,

and the external granular layer of the cerebellum. These structures, which can be distinguished as secondary germinal areas from the primary germinal area of the neuroepithelium, are more exposed to a neoplastic transformation because of their persistent proliferating activity.[73] They correspond topographically to certain tumors of early infancy, namely, medulloblastoma (external granular layer of the cerebellum), PNET (subpial granular layer), and subependymal glioma (subependymal layer).[61, 73, 76]

Midline and paraventricular tumors in our series corresponded to figures of 70% in infants younger than 1 year and 65% in the whole population younger than 3 years.

Oncotype Distribution

The oncotype distribution of infantile brain tumors differs from that of their counterparts in older children, adolescents, and adults. Furthermore, it shows significant variations with age even in the first years of life. Teratoma, which is the most common neoplasm in fetal and connatal series,[30, 59] accounts for one-third to one-half of cases at birth, for 28% in the first 2 months, and for 5% in the first year of life[57] (Figs. 28–3 and 28–6). Similarly, choroid plexus tumors decrease dramatically after the first 2 years of life (Fig. 28–5). On the other hand, neuroepithelial tumors, which prevail in adulthood, become progressively more common, starting from the end of the first year of life to constitute about 89% of the total brain tumors in the pediatric population.

The histologic classification of infantile tumors may present some difficulties because they can exhibit homogeneous patterns of undifferentiated cells (e.g., PNET); relatively homogeneous patterns of immature cells with variable amounts of cells differentiated along neuronal, neuroblastic, ependymal, astrocytic, or oligodendroglial lines (e.g., PNET with clusters of differentiated cells); or patterns of more mature cells, which allows a diagnosis on the basis of the predominant putative cells constituting the bulk of the tumors (e.g., astrocytoma, ependymoma, oligodendroglioma, etc.). Nevertheless, infantile brain tumors may be characterized by the coexistence of various cell populations that justify categorizations such as oligoastrocytoma, astroependymoma, or oligoastroependymoma. In order to interpret such a specific feature it has been propounded that an oncogenic factor could induce the neoplastic transformation of all cell populations of a specific glial line or of their progenitor when acting early, thus giving origin to a mixed glioma, or the transformation of only one glial strain, consequently provoking an isomorphous glioma, when acting late.[77]

There are further histologic and behavioral features that differentiate infantile tumors from the corresponding neoplasms occurring in adults, such as the prevalence of the adamantinomatous variety of craniopharyngiomas or of the sarcomatous form of meningiomas in early childhood[77–79] as well as the prevalence of malignancy in the first year of life (up to 75% of cases) compared to with less than half of these cases in children younger than 2 to 4 years.[8, 27]

In the 1991 cooperative worldwide study of the ISPN involving 886 cases of brain tumor in infants younger than 1 year, the most common oncotypes, in decreasing order of frequency, were astrocytoma (28.6% of the cases), medulloblastoma (11.5 %), ependymoma (11.4%), choroidal plexus

TABLE 28–2 Relative Frequency, Gender Ratio, and Location of the Most Common Pediatric Brain Tumors in the Second Year of Life

Country	First author (year)	Cases	M/F (no.)	S/I (no.)	Astr (no.)	Med (no.)	Epen (no.)	Plex (no.)	PNET (no.)	Tera (no.)
France	Lapras[88]	47	1.0 (23/23)	0.7 (19/28)	17.7 (8)	19.1 (9)	29.8 (14)	2.1 (1)	—	—
	Lellouch[89]	n.d.	1.3 (?)	0.7 (?)	36.0 (?)	14.0 (?)	16.0 (?)	17.0 (?)	3.5 (?)	1.7 (?)
Germany	Rickert[97]	25	1.5 (15/10)	1.1 (13/12)	24.0 (6)	12.0 (3)	24.0 (6)	—	—	—
S. Arabia	Murshid[94]	20	n.d.	1.9 (13/7)	26.3 (5)	10.5 (2)	5.3 (1)	21.1 (4)	—	—
USA	Mapstone[91]	15	n.d.	0.7 (6/9)	40.0 (6)	13.3 (2)	6.7 (1)	6.7 (1)	26.7(4)	—
Total		**107**	**1.2 (38/33)**	**0.93**	**23.6 (25)**	**15.1 (16)**	**20.8 (22)**	**5.7 (6)**	**3.8 (4)**	**0.8 (?)**

Astr, astrocytoma; Med, medulloblastoma; Epen, ependymoma; Plex, plexus tumors; Tera, teratoma; n.d., no data available.

TABLE 28–3 Relative Frequency, Gender Ratio, and Location of the Most Common Pediatric Brain Tumors in the First 2 Years of life

Country	First author (year)	Cases	M/F (no.)	S/I (no.)	Astr (no.)	Med (no.)	Epen (no.)	Plex (no.)	PNET (no.)	Tera (no.)
England	Kumar[90a]	93	n.d.	0.8 (41/52)	20.0 (19)	22.6 (21)	19.4 (18)	6.5 (6)	1.1 (1)	1.1 (1)
France	Fessard[68]	66	n.d.	1.5 (40/26)	31.3 (20)	15.6 (10)	21.9 (14)	9.4 (6)	—	—
	Lapras[88a]	76	1.2 (41/35)	1.1 (40/36)	19.7 (15)	18.4 (14)	27.6 (21)	2.6 (2)	—	1.3 (1)
Germany	Rickert[97]	47	1.2 (26/21)	1.8 (30/17)	19.1 (9)	12.8 (6)	19.1 (9)	—	10.6 (5)	2.1 (1)
Italy	Balestrini[94]	80	1.1 (42/38)	2.0 (53/27)	41.3 (33)	20.6 (16)	14.3 (11)	11.1 (9)	—	1.6 (1)
S. Arabia	Murshid[94]	34	2.4 (24/10)	1.4 (20/14)	27.3 (9)	21.2 (7)	9.1 (3)	15.2 (5)	6.1 (2)	—
Taiwan	Wong[88]	33	n.d.	5.6 (28/5)	32.3 (10)	6.5 (2)	—	19.4 (6)	12.9 (4)	16.1 (5)
USA	Farwell[78a]	54	1.0 (27/27)	0.6 (20/34)	25.9 (14)	29.6 (16)	16.7(9)	5.6 (3)	—	9.3 (5)
	Mapstone[91]	22	1.4 (13/9)	1.0 (11/11)	36.4 (8)	9.1 (2)	4.5 (1)	4.5 (1)	31.8 (7)	4.5 (1)
	Cohen[93]	78	1.5 (47/31)	1.5 (47/31)	38.4 (30)	23.0 (18)	7.7 (6)	10.2 (8)	—	3.8 (3)
	Reed[93]	40	n.d.	0.9 (19/21)	7.5 (3)	27.5 (11)	22.5 (9)	15.0 (6)	5.0 (2)	—
Total		**623**	**1.3 (220/171)**	**1.3 (349/274)**	**27.2 (170)**	**19.7 (123)**	**16.2 (101)**	**8.3 (52)**	**3.8 (21)**	**2.9 (18)**

Astr, astrocytoma; Med, medulloblastoma; Epen, ependymoma; Plex, plexus tumors; Tera, teratoma; n.d., no data available.
[a] First 18 months of life.

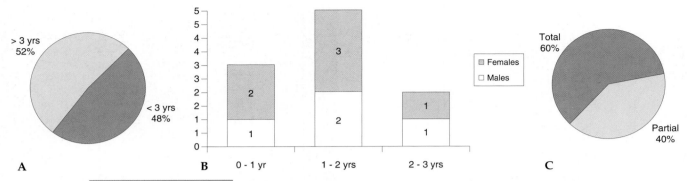

Figure 28–6 Teratomas in children younger than 3 years. Relative incidence as referred to the whole pediatric population with this type of tumor (A). Age and sex relative distribution in the first 3 years (B) and the degree of surgical tumor excision (C).

tumor (11.4%), PNET (6.2%), and teratoma (5%), followed by sarcoma, meningioma, ganglioglioma, neuroblastoma, dermoid, pinealoblastoma, and hamartoma (with an incidence ranging from 1.2% to 0.5%). This distribution has been substantially confirmed by the cumulative analysis of series reported in the literature[27] (Table 28–1).

In the group under 2 years of age, the most obvious changes are the decrease in incidence of choroid plexus tumors (6.6%) and teratomas (2.8%) and the appearance of craniopharyngiomas, which are virtually nonexistent in infants younger than 1 year.[27]

The oncotype distribution of our cases in infancy is reported in Fig. 28–3, together with the relative changes at onset of clinical manifestations, at diagnosis, and at operation. The oncotype and anatomical distributions of brain tumors in our patients younger than 3 years are reported in Table 28–4.

Clinical Presentation

Nonlocalizing signs and symptoms of increased intracranial pressure (macrocrania, full fontanels, split sutures, papilledema), as well as aspecific clinical manifestations such as vomiting, irritability, and behavioral changes, constitute the commonest clinical presentation of infantile brain tumors. Indeed, this kind of clinical picture was observed in more than half of cases at presentation and in more than three-fourths of cases at the time of tumor diagnosis in our population under 3 years of age (Table 28–5).

BOX 28–1
Signs and Symptoms

- **Macrocrania**
- **Full fontanels**
- **Split sutures**
- **Papilledema**
- **Vomiting**
- **Irritability**
- **Behavioral changes**

Rarely, intracranial hypertension rapidly evolves toward a central syndrome composed of agitation, anxiety, torpor, obtundation, and coma in the very young child; more often, it tends to be compensated for by an abnormal increase in head circumference that may progress for a long period of time. Before the introduction of modern diagnostic tools, compensatory macrocrania could be relatively underestimated in the absence of localizing neurologic deficitary signs suggestive of an expanding intracranial lesion. The delay in diagnosis has been shortened, and quite commonly an intracranial brain tumor can be recognized accidentally following neuroimaging studies performed to investigate the nature of aspecific cranial enlargements or unexplained psychomotor retardation. In other cases, the recognition of a brain tumor is the unexpected result of a neuroradiologic examination performed in case of head injury. Rarely, the diagnosis is obtained in utero following a routine ultrasonographic control study during pregnancy.

Seizures are less common in pediatric than in adults patients, probably in relation to the lower incidence of hemispherical lesions in children. However, they represent the second most common revealing clinical manifestation; in our series of patients under age 3, seizures revealed the presence of the tumor in one of seven subjects (Table 28–5)—an incidence similar to that reported for older children.[80]

Failure to thrive, cachexia, or poor feeding are less commonly observed, though these signs usually lead to an early diagnosis because of their known association with hypothalamic tumors.

Visual complaints, on the other hand, are difficult to evaluate in early childhood, when loss of vision can progress quite insidiously and squint may receive scarce attention unless accompanied by head tilt. Visual loss, observed in 3% of our patients at diagnosis, is reported with variable frequency in the literature from values of 4%[75] up to 16 to 19% of cases.[1] Abnormal ocular movements tend to be as common (20%) in patients with supratentorial tumors as in patients with infratentorial tumors.[1] They were noted in 9 of our 70 infants (Figs. 28–7 and 28–8). In infants, nystagmus may be rotatory or may even be substituted by bizarre movements in cases of suprasellar and, less frequently, posterior fossa tumors.

Cranial nerve and pyramidal motor system deficits are considerably less common in infants with brain tumors than

TABLE 28–4 Oncotype and Anatomical Distribution of Brain Tumors in Patients Younger Than 3 Years[a]

Oncotype	Percentage	Site	No. of cases
Glioma	43		
		Parasellar	21
		Brain stem	11
		Frontal	9
		Cerebellar	8
		Temporal	6
		Lateral ventricle	3
		Parietal	3
		Hemispheric	3
		Fourth ventricle	2
		Thalamus	2
		Pineal	1
Medulloblastoma-PNET	35		
		Fourth ventricle	38
		Cerebellar	5
		Frontal	4
		Lateral ventricle	3
		Parietal	1
		Temporal	1
		Pineal	1
Choroid Plexus Tumor	7		
		Lateral ventricle	9
		Third ventricle	2
Teratoma	6		
		Cerebellar	2
		Frontal	2
		Brain stem	1
		Parietal	1
		Temporal	1
		Hemispheric	1
		Lateral ventricle	1
		Pineal	1
Meningioma	3		
		Posterior fossa	2
		Lateral ventricle	1
		Hemispheric	1
Craniopharyngioma	2		
		Parasellar	4
Other	4		
		Orbit	3
		Parasellar	2
		Frontal	2
		Cerebellar	1

[a] Personal series.

SURGICAL TREATMENT

The great majority of infantile brain tumors are amenable to surgical treatment; in other words, it is possible even in newborns, infants, and very young children to reach the main goals of surgery: (1) to establish a tissue diagnosis; (2) to reduce the mass effect exerted by the lesion; (3) to reestablish a possibly impaired cerebrospinal fluid (CSF) circulation, and (4) in some cases to cure the disease. There is an additional objective that is typical of pediatric neurosurgery, that is, to allow patients to reach a normal psychomotor development. Unfortunately, this last goal cannot be obtained in infancy as often as at an older age. A particularly aggressive behavior of a certain infantile brain tumor, an excessive delay in diagnosis resulting in extremely huge neoplasms at

in older children and adults with brain tumors,[57] due to the expansile skull that compensates for an expanding intracranial mass lesion (Table 28–5; Figs. 28–7 and 28–8).

TABLE 28–5   Presenting Clinical Manifestations and Symptomatology at Diagnosis

Sign/Symptom	At Presentation		At diagnosis	
	Cases (no.)	Percentage	Cases (no.)	Percentage
Intracranial hypertension	75	46.3	96	59.3
Seizures	21	13.0	23	14.2
Ataxia	10	6.2	30	18.5
Nystagmus	10	6.2	20	12.3
Cranial nerve deficit	8	4.9	11	6.8
Proptosys	6	3.7	7	4.3
Delayed milestones	5	3.1	18	11.1
Hemiparesys	5	3.1	15	9.3
Torticollis	5	3.1	11	6.8
Subcutaneous mass	3	1.9	3	1.9
Irritability	2	1.2	7	4.3
Lethargy	2	1.2	22	13.6
Ambiopia	2	1.2	5	3.1
No signs	2	1.2	1	0.6
Opistotonus	1	0.6	2	1.2

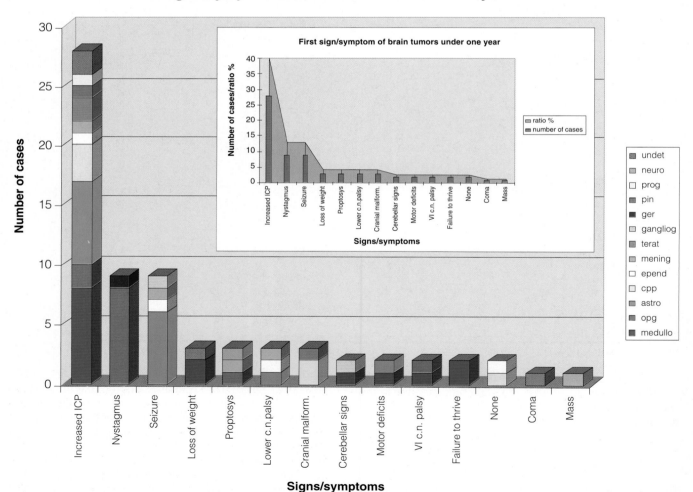

Figure 28–7   Presenting signs and symptoms of brain tumors in infants younger than 1 year. Relative distribution in incidence and correlation with the different oncotypes.

Signs/symptoms of brain tumors in the first year of life at the time of surgery

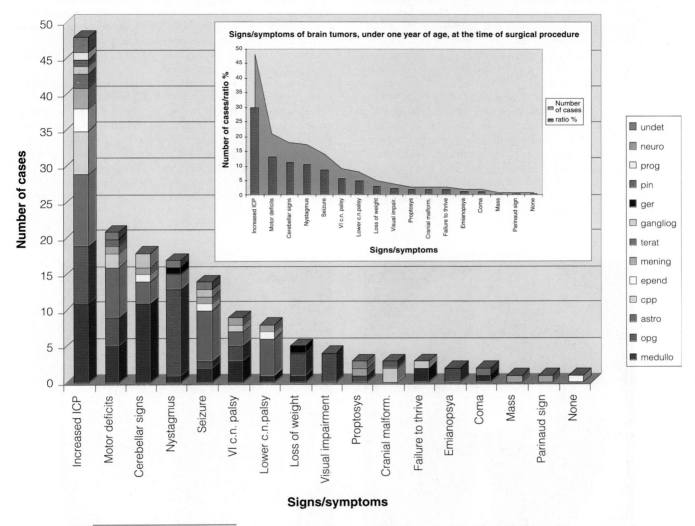

Figure 28–8 Signs and symptoms of brain tumors in infants younger than 1 year at operation. Relative distribution in incidence and correlation with the different oncotypes.

diagnosis, irreversible damage caused by the interference of critically located tumors with the cerebral development, as well as still inadequate therapeutic modalities account for such a limitation.

An experienced surgical and medical team, fully devoted to the care of pediatric patients, is necessary to ensure optimal success, especially when malignancy is present. In fact, though the differences in outcome might be not so obvious for children with benign lesions, there is enough evidence that malignant tumors are significantly better treated in academic specialized centers than in general neurosurgical departments.[81, 82]

The role of the pediatric anesthesiologist is critical for these particularly fragile patients, whose brain is extremely vulnerable to changes in intracranial pressure and cerebral blood flow. Maintenance of body temperature; blood pressure monitoring; frequent controls of electrolytes, hematocrit, and blood gas

levels; careful use of hyperosmolar agents, corticosteroids, and anticonvulsant drugs; and frequent replacement of blood losses are required to minimize cerebral edema and other operative complications.

Preoperative CSF shunting in infants and young children with brain tumors is more often necessary than it is in their adult counterpart. In most pediatric neurosurgical centers, intraoperative external ventriculostomy is utilized to control intracranial pressure during surgery and in the immediate postoperative period; permanent CSF shunting devices are inserted only in those instances in which CSF dynamics are not restored even after tumor removal. More recently, preoperative neuroendoscopic third ventriculostomy has been advocated in cases of posterior fossa tumor and secondary obstructive hydrocephalus for avoiding the implantation of extrathecal CSF shunts and their associated morbidity.

Pre- and postoperative medical control of an excessively elevated intracranial pressure, based on the use of corticosteroids and diuretics, is a mainstay in the management of infantile brain tumors. Similarly, anticonvulsants should be administered in cases of supratentorial tumors in a loading dose during operation and subsequently in a fractioned way for a variable period of time in the postoperative phase to avoid the occurrence of seizures, which in infants may easily result in neurologic deficits. It is worth noting that the risk for seizures in infants and very young children having infratentorial tumors is, in our experience, higher than that recorded in the older pediatric population, though remaining considerably smaller than for the supratentorial location.

Control CT and MRI studies, without and with contrast medium, should be carried out during the first 48 to 72 postoperative hours to evaluate the extent of the surgical excision and eventually differentiate residual tumors from alterations due to hemorrhagic and scarring processes. A second-look operation should be encouraged in all cases in which the immediate postoperative examination reveals the persistence of a residual tumor susceptible to surgical removal. Actually, this second operation does not necessarily carry a major risk and might improve the outcome of subjects in whom radiotherapy cannot be administered.

"Gross" total tumor excision can be carried out in half or more of infantile brain tumors.[41, 57, 83] The best surgical results are obtained in cases of benign tumor (e.g., choroid plexus papilloma or teratoma) (Figs. 28–5 and 28–6) and malignant, though scarcely infiltrating, neoplasm (e.g., medulloblastoma or ependymoma) (Figs. 28–4 and 28–9). On the other hand, infiltrating tumors (e.g., astrocytoma) are not suitable for total resection in a high percentage of cases, unless confined to the cerebellum or to certain areas in the cerebral hemispheres (Figs. 28–10 and 28–11).

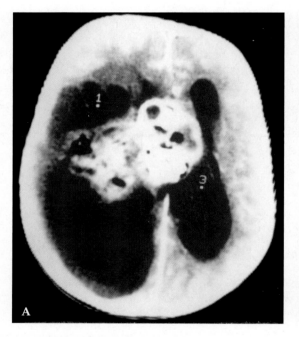

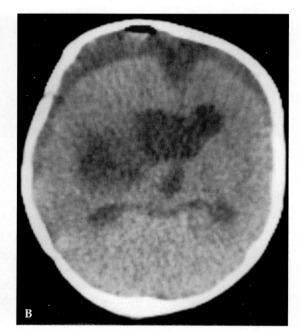

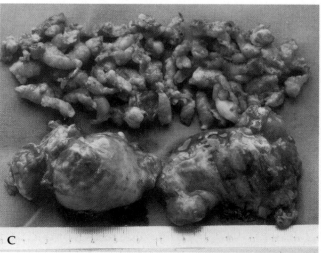

Figure 28–9 Teratoma. Preoperative CT scan examination (A) shows the huge intraventricular mass lesion associated with hydrocephalus. Postoperative CT scan (B) demonstrates the complete surgical excision of the tumor (C) and the volumetric reduction of the ventricular system.

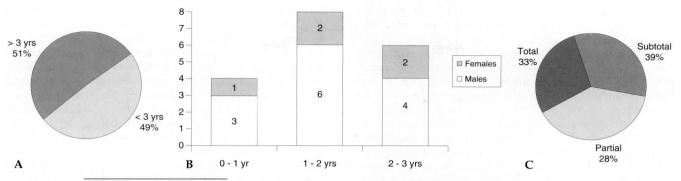

Figure 28–10   Ependymomas in children younger than 3 years. Relative incidence as referred to the whole pediatric population with this type of tumor (A). Age and sex relative distribution in the first 3 years (B) and the degree of surgical tumor excision (C).

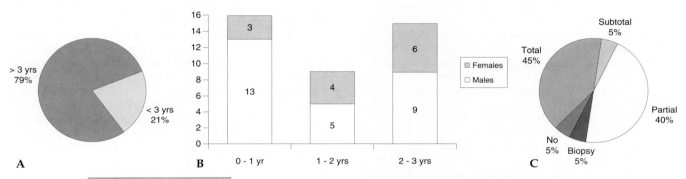

Figure 28–11   Astrocytomas in children younger than 3 years. Relative incidence as referred to the whole pediatric population with this type of tumor (A). Age and sex relative distribution in the first 3 years (B) and the degree of surgical tumor excision (C).

In some malignant, highly vascularized tumors, which may have reached huge dimensions at diagnosis, the surgical resection may be rendered possible or less difficult by the administration of chemotherapy prior to the surgical procedure. Such was, for example, our experience using preoperative chemotherapy with carboplatin alone in some cases of infantile medulloblastoma. The treatment resulted in an obvious tumor regression associated with a decrease in intracranial pressure apparently due to a dual action of the drug: a reduction of the mass effect exerted by the lesion and a dehydration of both the neoplastic tissue and the normal cerebral parenchyma. At the operation, the main induced changes were a higher degree of tumor firmness and its easier anatomical definition from the surrounding nervous structures. The disadvantage for the surgeon in dealing with a firmer tumor (i.e., it became less amenable to suction) was compensated for by the better separation of the pathologic tissue from the intact cerebellar parenchyma, which facilitated tumor radical excision.[84]

OUTCOME

Although still high, the mortality associated with infantile brain tumors has consistently decreased in recent decades from a 17% 1-year survival rate in a series of patients treated between 1958 and 1964[32] to 62 to 80% in some contemporary series.[43, 75, 85]

The neonatal period contributes most to natural and surgical early deaths. Malignant tumors are considered to behave more aggressively in the first 2 years of life, thus raising the question of whether biological aggressiveness of the tumor correlates inversely with host age. It is possible, however, that the generally assumed dismal prognosis of infantile brain tumors depends more on clinical inference generated by the limited experience in treating the very young patient than on an actual higher aggressiveness of the tumor. For example, a major malignancy in the first 2 years of life has been reported for medulloblastoma.[86] Such an oncotype (ependymoma is another) has been said to conform to the Collins rule[87] in the infantile age span; that is, the tumor takes a shorter (or at best equal) time to recur and reach the original size at diagnosis than the period of time required from its development to its recognition (maximum from conception to diagnosis), in spite of any form of therapy. The tendency to infiltrate surrounding nervous structures,[88] the frequent occurrence of metastases,[89, 90] and the common association with severe hydrocephalus were the main features considered to suggest a more aggressive behavior of infantile medulloblastoma and to account for its particularly grim outcome. However, several observations indicate that medulloblastoma may not adhere to the Collins rule even when occurring in infants. Actually, by the late 1970s, the specific aggressiveness of infantile medulloblastoma compared with medulloblastoma found in older age subjects was questioned.[91] More recent reports indicate that the prognosis of totally resected medulloblastoma in infants does not differ from that recorded in older patients; furthermore, long-term survival may be obtained in infants treated with adjuvant chemotherapy alone, without any irradiation treatment or with radiotherapy delayed after the third year of life.[3] There are also authors who postulate that some malignant high-grade gliomas in infants are particularly chemotherapy-sensitive and associated with better outcomes than those of similar tumors occurring in older children and adults.[2]

A further argument against the particular aggressiveness of infantile brain tumors is provided by optic gliomas, a fourth of which occur in the first year of life. In the past, optic gliomas were considered extremely invasive in infants because of the frequent hypothalamic involvement at diagnosis.[38, 92] The large size to which these tumors had grown at the time of clinical recognition induced some authors to consider the possibility of an insufficient immunological response of the very young child.[93] With improvements in diagnostic techniques and neuroimaging surveillance, however, it became obvious that most of the optic pathway tumors could remain indolent for long periods and, in rare cases, regress spontaneously. Optic gliomas appear to carry a better prognosis in younger subjects such that higher cellular loss in infancy that diminishes tumor growth rate in this phase of life

or a minor production of "enhancing antibodies" that protect the tumor has been postulated to explain the phenomenon.[94] In a series of 11 infants with optic pathways glioma treated during the first year of life (Fig. 28–12), we observed spontaneous disappearance of the residual tumor after partial surgical excision in two instances.[95] The surgical mortality in our infantile brain tumor series (36%), though high was significantly lower than that recorded in series prior to the introduction of CTs, which were weighted by long delays in diagnosis.[38]

Analysis of the literature demonstrates unequivocally that the increase in long-term survival of infants with brain tumors corresponds to progress in surgical techniques and adjuvant therapies.[85, 96–98] In the last decade, for example, the operative mortality of brain tumors dropped in the majority of pediatric neurosurgical centers to values of 5 to 15% as compared with surgery-related death rates of 30 to 40% observed as early as 1980.[43, 99–101] In a study review children with brain tumors treated in Britain in the period 1971–1985,[21] the prognosis looked particularly grim. Of the 516 patients considered, 65 (13%) died untreated and an additional 93 (18%) died within a month of surgery, having had no other treatment for their disease. Fewer than half of the children survived more than 1 year. Early deaths occurred significantly more frequently in children younger than 2 years at diagnosis than in those aged 2 to 14 years. Survival rates at 10 years for ependymoma, astrocytoma, and medulloblastoma-PNET ranged around 40%. The contribution of the first 2 years of life to tumoral early mortality was also apparent in a Danish investigation, the results of which were published in 1976,[102] on a population of children aged 0 to 14 years with brain tumors, who survived the surgical treatment for at least a month. The mortality rate was higher in the 0 to 4 years subgroup than in the two additional subgroups 5 to 9 and 10 to 14 years, respectively. However, in this pre-CT series the gap in percentage of survivors of the three age groups at 5 years had become considerably smaller, as deaths had practically reached a plateau (at around 60% of cases) in the 0 to 4 years group. At 10 years, all three age groups showed similar survival rates, which were around 40%.

The favorable effects of modern modalities of treatment, which account for the current higher overall survival rates

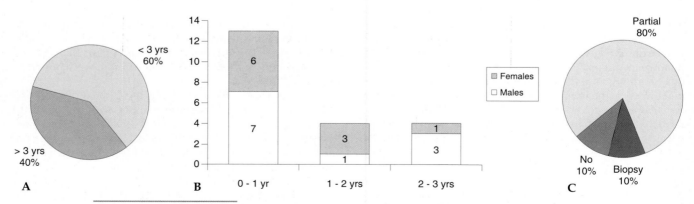

Figure 28–12 Optic-hypothalamic astrocytomas in children younger than 3 years. Relative incidence as referred to the whole pediatric population with this type of tumor (A). Age and sex relative distribution in the first 3 years (B) and the degree of surgical tumor excision (C).

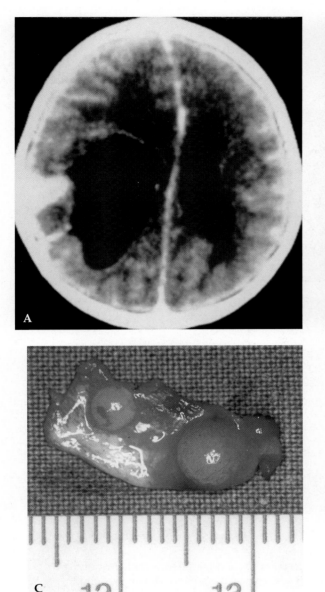

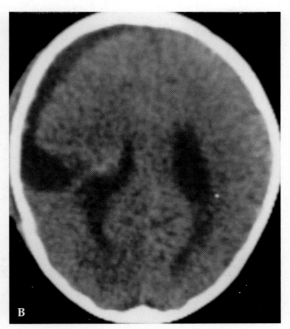

Figure 28–13 Supratentorial ependymoma. Preoperative contrast-enhanced CT scan examination demonstrates the small parietal mass lesion associated with ventricular dilatation (A). In spite of the complete surgical removal, demonstrated by the postoperative CT scan (B), the dismal prognosis of the tumor is heralded by the presence at operation of nodular metastases on the inner face of the dura mater (C).

recorded in the whole pediatric population with brain tumors, as compared with those described in the above mentioned studies, are even more evident when malignant tumors are considered separately. No patient with a highly malignant tumor operated on in the first year of life survived in Lapras's series published in late 1980s.[83] In contrast, long-term survivals were obtained in 8 (42%) of 19 infants with medulloblastoma who were symptomatic in the first year of life and operated on within the first 22 months of life in our institution.[3]

At the end of the 1970s, 25% or fewer 12-month survival rates could be expected in infants younger than 2 years with medulloblastoma; less than one-sixth of the children harboring this kind of neoplasm were alive at 5 years.[103, 104] In the early 1990s, the survival rate at 5 years with the same tumor in the same age group had increased to 36 to 60%.[90, 105]

When series of children with medulloblastoma in the late 1970s and early 1980s were compared with series of pediatric subjects treated in late 1980s at a single institution, it was evident that the worse prognosis for very young children was tenable only for the early series, whereas no statistically significant differences in survival could be observed between younger and older children in the more recent group.[97]

Radical surgical excision of the tumor is the mainstay of treatment for infantile benign tumors as well as for some nondiffuse malignant neoplasms (Fig. 28–13 and 28–14). Up to 75% of infantile benign tumor radical excisions are associated with long-term survival.[1, 41, 43] Neoplasms developing in areas of

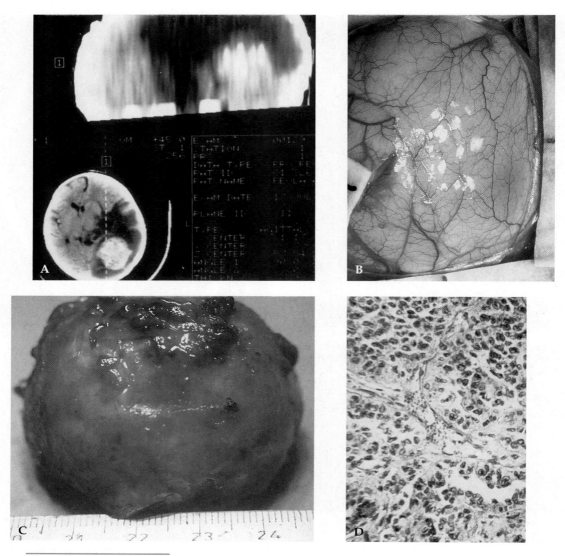

Figure 28–14 Meningioma. Note the intracerebral location (A) and the extreme flattening of the cortical surface. The completely excised tumor and its histological features are shown in C and D, respectively.

the brain that permit their total removal, such as the cerebral hemispheres, the cerebellum, or the orbital segment of the optic nerve, carry the best prognosis. Prognosis is gloomy for midline benign gliomas of the chiasmatic, hypothalamic, and diencephalic regions, which cannot be treated aggressively.[75] Unfortunately, the midline location is particularly common in the pediatric age group (Fig. 28–15).

The high mortality and the difficulties in surgical treatment in the first months of life account for the relatively low survival rates of infants with posterior fossa ependymoma and medulloblastoma. Less than half of patients with these types of tumors are alive at 10 years.[21] However, radical excision can result in a cure even in the case of noninfiltrating malignant tumors, as demonstrated in several series of infantile malignant neoplasms by the presence of long-term survivors who were not given adjuvant therapies.[3, 43] More

frequently, however, long-term survival is obtained by multimodality treatment combining surgery, radiotherapy, and chemotherapy.[1] One characteristic (though rare or even unique) feature of infantile malignant tumors is the possibility of a change in biologic and pathologic pattern toward that of a less aggressive lesion following repeated tumor resections as reported in cases of connatal ependymoma[41] and PNET.[75]

Unfortunately, survival is not the only consideration for children with brain tumors. All of the modalities of treatment traditionally used to achieve long-term survival—surgery, radiotherapy, and chemotherapy—may also damage the developing nervous system substantially. At the present time, a great proportion of survivors remain at risk for late neurologic, intellectual, and endocrinologic sequelae. Some patients may need lifelong assistance, never functioning independently.

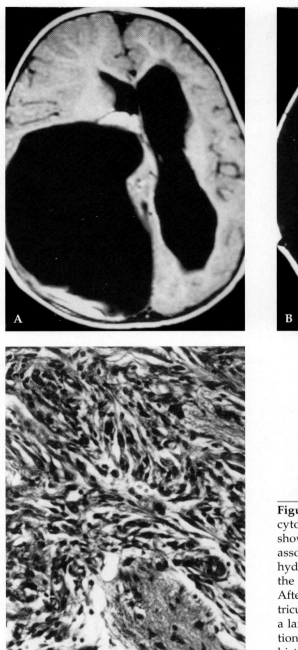

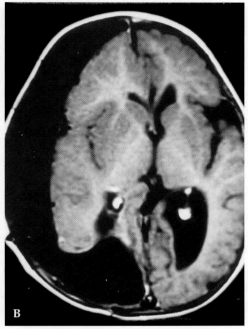

Figure 28–15 Desmoplastic infantile astrocytoma. Preoperative MR examinations (A) shows a solid midline nodular tumoral mass associated with a huge cyst and obstructive hydrocephalus. A further solid component of the tumor is present in the occipital cortex. After the tumor's complete excision, the ventricular anatomy returns to normal easily with a large extra-axial cerebrospinal fluid collection (B). In spite of the apparently aggressive histological pattern (C), this tumor bears an excellent prognosis.

Tumor histology influences outcome in very young children less significantly than in their older counterparts. In fact, even benign lesions in infants may be associated with a dismal prognosis when their precocious occurrence in fetal life and possible associated hydrocephalus may have caused irrepairable injury before the tumor was recognized. Choroid plexus papillomas, for example, are regarded as very benign in nature, and their surgical removal results in a cure in nearly all cases. In infancy, these tumors present usually with associated severe dilatation of the cerebroventricular system, which seems to be well compensated for by the calvarial expansion and functional resilience of the immature nervous system. However, in spite of the complete removal of tumor and early control of secondary hydrocephalus, several of the affected subjects exhibit very poor postoperative psychomotor development.[106] Similarly, teratomas are often accompanied by developmental delay, even in cases of successful surgical excision, because of the interference in brain formation and maturation exerted by the tumor during the intrauterine period.[47]

The effect of surgical maneuvers on late outcome is difficult to evaluate. In several instances the characteristics of the tumor have prevented differentiation of possible damages induced by the operation from those directly attributable to the presence of the tumor, e.g., invasion of midline cerebral structures in cases of benign infiltrating gliomas or, as already mentioned, longstanding compression of periventricular regions in cases of severe associated hydrocephalus.

However, inference from older children seems to indicate that the surgical treatment, unless weighted by complications, has a small role in inducing late sequelae.[107]

The specific role of chemotherapy in determining late neurologic and intellectual deficits is also difficult to assess as this type of treatment has almost always been associated with radiation therapy. Historical experiences with intrathecal chemotherapy (methotrexate) alone and in combination with radiation therapy in children undergoing prophylactic treatment for leukemia seem to support a relatively major role of irradiation because the neurologic deficits resulting from the combination of radiotherapy and chemotherapy do not differ significantly from those induced by radiotherapy alone. There is, however, enough evidence that demonstrates an increased toxicity of the two modalities of treatment when administered in combination. In such an event, some of the late organic lesions, such as mineralizing microangiopathy resulting in dystrophic calcification of cerebral cortex, appear to correlate with the dose of chemotherapy administered, though primarily caused by ionizing radiations.[107]

Radiotherapy in infancy and early childhood undoubtedly exerts detrimental effects on late intellectual performances, the importance of which tends to increase with the duration of follow-up. *Treatment-related neurologic toxicity consists mainly of leukoencephalopathy, cortical atrophy, and microangiopathy.* These anatomopathologic changes are the substratum of clinical manifestations, namely, neurologic and intellectual deficits, growth failure, and various endocrinologic abnormalities.[108–110]

The treatment of infantile brain tumors is a field of constant revision. No single protocol has proven superior for this type of neoplasm; probably radiation therapy is still the most effective treatment. However, the devastating effects of radiation therapy on the immature CNS at the dose required to cure a tumor and the neuropsychological effects of even lower doses administered in combination with chemotherapy justify past and recent attempts by neuro-oncologists to delay, and possibly avoid completely, radiotherapy while utilizing more aggressive and prolonged regimens of postoperative chemotherapy.[111] Preliminary evidence of multi-institutional prospective studies indicates that with this kind of regimen it is possible to prevent disease progression and to delay irradiation for 1 or 2 years in a large proportion of malignant infantile brain tumors.[112] The best results (up to 74 to 90% of the children) have been obtained in cases of localized tumors, such as medulloblastoma. However, encouraging successes have also been recorded in subjects with malignant gliomas and diffuse infiltrating brain stem gliomas. The overall outcome for infants so treated appears to compare favorably with that obtained in older children treated with standard postoperative radiation therapy.[113] Furthermore, the children seem to reach appropriate neurodevelopmental milestones, although this is limited by the still excessively short duration of the follow-up observation.

SUMMARY

Although a cure remains elusive in several cases of infantile brain tumors, survival rates have increased substantially for several types of neoplasms. Progress in diagnosis, better preoperative neuroimaging techniques, more aggressive surgical approaches, intensified regimens of chemotherapy, and radiation withdrawal have radically improved the prognosis of these types of lesions.

Long-term survival now can be achieved in nearly three-fourths of infants and very young children with benign brain tumors. Several of these children can be cured by total excision of the lesion. Unfortunately, the high incidence of benign tumors involving the midline brain structures in this age group prevents the surgeon from carrying out a complete surgical removal in subjects in whom an aggressive treatment would result in unacceptable morbidity. Nevertheless, favorable outcomes can be expected in such patients as many of the tumors may respond to chemotherapy.

Only one-fourth of infantile malignant tumors are associated with long-term survival. Nevertheless, radical excision may still cure some of these tumors, once regarded as untreatable, rarely without any additional therapy but more often with adjuvant postoperative chemotherapy.

Conventional radiotherapy is avoided in infants and very young children. The trend is toward lengthening the time between the surgical operation and the administration of this type of therapy in late childhood. The experience in infants is too limited to support an evaluation of the results of more sophisticated ways of delivering irradiation treatment (radiosurgery, brachytherapy, hyperfractionated radiation) that are widely utilized in older children.

Similar to tumors occurring in older age groups, infantile brain tumors have also benefited from the development of new chemotherapeutic agents and associated treatments, such as autologous bone marrow rescue, hematopoietic growth factors, and interleukins. Intensified chemotherapic regimens have resulted in long-term disease control in infants who did not receive any radiation therapy, apparently without significant secondary neurologic morbidity.

Quality of life remains an important issue in the management of infantile brain tumors. Presently, about one-fourth of survivors enjoy normal life, with few or no neurologic deficits: An additional percentage present a certain degree of neurologic or intellectual impairment. Thirty to forty percent of survivors are severely disabled.

REFERENCES

1. Cohen BH, Packer RJ, Siegel KR, et al. Brain tumors in children under 2 years: treatment, survival and long-term prognosis. *Pediatr Neurosurg* 1993;19:171–179.
2. Duffner PK, Krischer JP, Burger PC, et al. Treatment of infants with malignant gliomas: the Pediatric Oncology Group experience. *J Neuro-oncol* 1996;28:245–256.
3. Di Rocco C, Iannelli A, Papacci F, et al. Prognosis of medulloblastoma in infants. *Child's Nerv Syst* 1997;13: 388–396.

4. Oi S, Matsumoto S, Choi JU, et al. Brain tumors diagnosed in the first year of life in five Far Eastern countries: statistical analysis of 307 cases. *Child's Nerv Syst* 1990;6:79–85.

5. Wong TT, Ho DM, Chi Cs, et al. Brain tumors in the first 2 years of life. *Child's Nerv Syst* 1988;4:184 (abstr).

6. De La Torre-Mandragon L, Ridaura-Sanz C, Reyes-Mujca M, et al. Central nervous system tumors in Mexican children. *Child's Nerv Syst* 1993;9:260–265.

7. Aghadiuno PU, Adeloye A, Olumide AA, et al. Intracranial neoplasms in children in Ibadan, Nigeria. *Child's Nerv Syst* 1985;5:230–233.

8. Kumar R, Tekkok IH, Jones RAC. Intracranial tumours in the first 18 months of life. *Child's Nerv Syst* 1990;6:371–374.

9. Birch JN, Hartley AL, Teare MD, et al. The inter-regional epidemiological study of childhood cancer (IRESCC): case-control study of children with central nervous system tumours. *Br J Neurosurg* 1990;4:17–25.

10. Gold EB, Leviton A, Lopez R, et al. The role of family history in risk of childhood brain tumors. *Cancer* 1994;73:1302–1311.

11. Jones SM, Phillips PC, Molloy PT, et al. Congenital anomalies and genetic disorders in families of children with central nervous system tumours. *J Med Genet* 1995;32:627–632.

12. Farwell JR, Flannery JT. Cancer in relatives of children with central nervous system neoplasms. *N Engl J Med* 1984;311:749–753.

13. Staneczeck W, Janisch W. Epidemiological aspects of primary CNS tumours in childhood and adolescence. *Pathologe* 1994;15:207–215.

14. Bleehen NM. Preface. In: Bleehen NM, ed. *Tumours of the Brain*. Berlin: Springer-Verlag; 1986:V–VI.

15. Ericsson J L-E, Karnstrom L, Mattsson B. Childhood cancer in Sweden 1958–1974. *Acta Pediatr Scand* 1978;67:425–432.

16. Lannering B, Marky I, Nordborg C. Brain tumors in childhood and adolescence in West Sweden 1970–1984: epidemiology and survival. *Cancer* 1990;66:604–609.

17. Preston-Martin S. Epidemiology of primary CNS neoplasms. *Neurol Clin* 1996;14:273–290.

18. Breslow NE, Langholz B. Childhood cancer incidence: geographical and temporal variations. *Int J Cancer* 1983;32:703–716.

19. Desmeules M, Mikkelsen T, Mao Y. Increasing incidence of primary malignant brain tumors: influence of diagnostic methods. *J Natl Cancer Inst* 1992;84:442–445.

20. Mori K, Kurisaka M. Brain tumors in childhood: statistical analysis of cases from the brain tumors registry of Japan. *Child's Nerv Syst* 1986;2:233–237.

21. Stiller CA, Bunch K. Brain and spinal tumours in children under two years: incidence and survival in Britain, 1971–1985. *Br J Cancer* 1992;66(Suppl 18):S50–S53.

22. Bleyer WA. The impact of childhood cancer in the United States and the world. *CA Cancer J Clin* 1990;40:355–367.

23. Izuora GI, Ikerionwu S, Saddegi N, et al. Childhood intracranial neoplasms, Enugu, Nigeria. *West Afr J Med* 1989;8:171–174.

24. Leviton A. Principles of epidemiology. In: Cohen ME, Duffner PK, eds. *Brain Tumors in Children: Principles of Diagnosis and Treatments*. 2nd ed. New York: Raven Press; 1994:27–49.

25. van Hoff J, Schymura MJ, Carnen MG. Trends in the incidence of childhood and adolescents cancer in Connecticut, 1935–1979. *Pediatr Oncol* 1988;16:78–87.

26. The Childhood Brain Tumor Consortium. A study of childhood brain tumors based on surgical biopsies from ten North American institutions: sample description. *J Neuro-oncol* 1988;6:9–23.

27. Rickert Ch, Probst-Cousin S, Gullotta F. Primary intracranial neoplasms of infancy and early childhood. *Child's Nerv Syst* 1997;13:507–513.

28. Jänisch W, Haas JF, Schreiber D, et al. Primary central nervous system tumors in still-born and infants. *J Neuro-oncol* 1984;2:113–116.

29. Jellinger K, Sunder-Palssman H. Connatal intracranial tumors. *Neuropediatrics* 1973;4:46–64.

30. Jänisch W. Brain tumors in infancy. *J Neuropathol Exp Neurol* 1995;Suppl:S55–S65.

31. Arnstein LH, Boldery E, Naffzinger H. A case report and survey of brain tumors during neonatal period. *J Neurosurg* 1951;8:315–319.

32. Fessard C. Cerebral tumors in infancy. *Am J Dis Child* 1968;115:302–308.

33. Keith H, Winchell McK, Kernahan J. Brain tumors in children. *Pediatrics* 1949;3:839–844.

34. Koos WTH, Miller MH. *Intracranial Tumors in Infants and Children*. Stuttgart: Thieme; 1971.

35. Sato O, Tamura A, Sano K. Brain tumors in early infants. *Child's Brain* 1975;1:121–125.

36. Jooma R, Hayward RD, Grant DN. Intracranial neoplasms during the first year of life: analysis of one hundred consecutive cases. *Neurosurgery* 1984;14:31–41.

37. Amacher LA. Intracranial tumefactions in infants. *Conc Pediatr Neurosurg* 1983;4:306–318.

38. Raimondi AJ, Tomita T. Brain tumors during the first year of life. *Child's Brain* 1983;10:193–207.

39. Sakamoto K, Kobayashi N, Ohtsubo H, et al. Intracranial tumors in the first year of life. *Child's Nerv Syst* 1986;2:126–129.

40. Zuccaro G, Taratuto AL, Monges J. Intracranial neoplasms during the first year of life. *Surg Neurol* 1986;26:29–36.

41. Di Rocco C, Iannelli A, Ceddia A. Intracranial tumors in the first year of life: a report on 51 cases. *Acta Neurochirurg* 1993;123:14–24.

42. Tomita T, Mc Lone DG. Brain tumors during the first twenty-four months of life. *Neurosurgery* 1985;17:913–919.

43. Balestrini MR, Micheli R, Giordano L, et al. Brain tumors with symptomatic onset in the first two years of life. *Child's Nerv Syst* 1994;10:104–110.

44. Lipman Sp, Pretorious DH, Ruma CK, et al. Fetal intracranial teratoma: US diagnosis of three cases and a review of the literature. *Radiology* 1985;157:491–494.

45. Alvarez M, Chitkara U, Lynch L, et al. Prenatal diagnosis of fetal brain tumors. *Fet Ther* 1987;2:203–208.

46. Oi S, Tamaki N, Kondo T, et al. Massive congenital intracranial teratoma diagnosed in utero. *Child's Nerv Syst* 1990;6:459–461.

47. Rickert CH, Probst-Cousin S, Louwen F, et al. Congenital immature teratoma of the fetal brain. *Child's Nerv Syst* 1997;13:356–359.

48. Takaku A, Kodama N, Ohara H, et al. Brain tumor in newborn babies. *Child's Brain* 1978;4:365–375.

49. Isaacs H Jr. Perinatal (congenital and neonatal) neoplasms: a report of 110 cases. *Pediatr Pathol* 1985;3:165–216.
50. Oi S, Kokunai T, Matsumoto S. Congenital brain tumors in Japan (ISPN Cooperative Study): specific clinical features in neonates. *Child's Nerv Syst* 1990;6:86–91.
51. Raskind R, Brighel F. Brain tumors in early infancy: probably congenital in origin. *J Pediatr* 1964;65:727–732.
52. Solitare GB, Krigman MR. Congenital intracranial neoplasm. *J Neuropathol Exp Neurol* 1964;23:280–292.
53. Sunder-Plasman M. Supratentorial-Tumoren in ersten Lebenjahr. *Helv Pediatr Acta* 1971;26:449–459.
54. Sunder-Plasman M, Jellinger K. Neuroektodermale Hirngeschwulste in ersten Lebenjahr. *Acta Neurochir* 1971;24:107–120.
55. Ellams ID, Neuhauser G, Agnoli A-L. Congenital intracranial neoplasms. *Child's Nerv Syst* 1986;2:165–168.
56. Jooma R, Kendall BE. Intracranial tumours in the first year of life. *Neuroradiology* 1982;23:267–274.
57. Di Rocco C, Iannelli A, Ceddia A. Intracranial tumors of the first year of life: a cooperative survey of the 1986–1987 Education Committee of the ISPN. *Child's Nerv Syst* 1991;7:150–153.
58. Tabaddor K, Shulman K, Dal Canto MC. Neonatal craniopharyngiomas. *Am J Dis Child* 1974;128:381–383.
59. Wakai S, Arai T, Nagai M. Congenital brain tumors. *Surg Neurol* 1984;21:597–609.
60. Zülch KJ. *Brain Tumors.* Berlin: Springer-Verlag; 1986:102.
61. Rubinstein LJ. *Tumors of the Central Nervous System.* Washington, DC: Armed Forces Institute of Pathology; 1972:292–294.
62. Hurst HW, Mc Ilhenny J, Park TS, et al. Neonatal craniopharyngioma: CT and ultrasonic features. *J Comput Assist Tomogr* 1988;12.858–861.
63. Fujita S. The matrix cell and cytogenesis in developing central nervous system. *J Comp Neurol* 1963;12:37–42.
64. Ehret M, Jacobi G, Hey A. Embryonal brain neoplasms in the neonatal period and early infancy. *Clin Neuropathol* 1987;6:218–223.
65. Hirakawa K, Suzuki K, Ueda S. et al. Fetal origin of the medulloblastoma: evidence from growth analysis of two cases. *Acta Neuropathol (Berlin)* 1986;70:227–234.
66. Taboada D, Fronfe A, Alono A., et al. Congenital medulloblastoma: report of two cases. *Pediatr Radiol* 1980;9:5–10.
68. Jänisch W, Haas JF. Epidemiological investigations in brain tumors in the GDR: possibilities and limits. *Arch Geschwultsforsch* 1984;55:243–247.
69. Colangelo M, Buonaguro A, Ambrosio A. Intracranial tumors in early infancy: under one year of age. *J Neurosurg Sci.* 1980;24:27–32.
70. Galassi E, Godano U, Cavallo M, et al. Intracranial tumors during the 1st year of life. *Child's Nerv Syst* 1989;5:288–298.
71. Ambrosino MM, Hernanz-Schulman M, Genieser NB, et al. Brain tumors in infants less than a year of age. *Pediatr Radiol* 1988;19:6–8.
72. Conti Reed U, Rosenberg S, Dias Gherpelli JL, et al. Brain tumors in the first two years of life: a review of forty cases. *Pediatr Neurosurg* 1993;19:180–185.
73. Giuffre' R. Biological aspects of brain tumors in infancy and childhood. *Child's Nerv Syst* 1989;5:55–59.
74. Koos WT, Pendl G, eds. Lesions of the cerebral midline. *Acta Neurochir* 1985;(Suppl 35).
75. Mapstone TB. Brain Tumors in children less than 24 months old. *Persp Neurol Surg* 1993;4:17–29.
76. Lewis PD. Cell proliferation in the postnatal nervous system and its relationship to the origin of gliomas. *Semin Neurol* 1981;1:181–187.
77. Dickinson JG, Flanigan TP, Kemshead JT et al. Identification of cell surface antigens present exclusively on a subpopulation of astrocytes in human foetal brain cultures. *J Neuroimmunol* 1983;5:111–123.
78. Kahn EA, Gosch HH, Seeger JF, et al. Forty-five years' experience with craniopharyngiomas. *Surg Neurol* 1973;1:5–12.
79. Sano K., Wakai S, Ochiai C, et al. Characteristics of intracranial meningiomas in childhood. *Child's Brain* 1981;8:98–106.
80. Cohen ME, Duffner PK. *Brain Tumors in Children.* 2nd ed. New York: Raven Press; 1994:13–26.
81. Duffner PK, Cohen ME, Flannery JT. Referral patterns of childhood brain tumors in the state of Connecticut. *Cancer* 1982;50:1636–1640.
82. Kramer S, Meadows AT, Pastore G., et al. Influence of place of treatment in diagnosis, treatment, and survival in three pediatric solid tumors. *J Clin Oncol* 1984;2:917–923.
83. Lapras C, Guilburd JN, Guyotat J, et al. Brain tumors in infants: a study of 76 patients operated upon. *Child's Nerv Syst* 1988;4:100–103.
84. Di Rocco C, Iannelli A, La Marca F, et al. Preoperative chemotherapy with carboplatin alone in high risk medulloblastoma. *Child's Nerv Syst* 1995;11:574–578.
85. Brown K, Mapstone TB, Oakes WJ. A modern analysis of intracranial tumors of infancy. *Pediatr Neurosurg* 1997;26:25–32.
86. Choux M., Lena G, eds. *Le medulloblastome.* Neurochirurgie, Suppl 28. Paris: Masson; 1982.
87. Collins VP, Loeffler RK, Tivey H. Observations on growth rates of human tumors. *Am J Roentgenol* 1956;76:988–1000.
88. Allen JC, Epstein F. Medulloblastoma and other primary malignant neuroectodermal tumors of the CNS: the effect of patients' age and extent of disease on prognosis. *J Neurosurg* 1982;57:446–451.
89. Finlay JL, Goins SC. Brain tumors in children: advances in chemotherapy. *Am J Pediatr Hematol Oncol* 1987;9:264–271.
90. Geyer R, Levy M, Berger MS, et al. Infants with medulloblastoma: a single institution review of survival. *Neurosurgery* 1991;29:707–711.
91. Hirsch JF, Renier D, Czernichow P, et al. Medulloblastoma in childhood: survival and functional results. *Acta Neurochir (Wien)* 1979;48:1–15.
92. Kanamory M, Shibuya M, Yoshida J, et al. Long-term follow-up of patients with optic gliomas. *Child's Nerv Syst* 1985;1:272–278.
93. Borit A, Richardson EP. The biological and clinical behaviour of pylocytic astrocytomas of the optic pathways. *Brain* 1982;105:161–187.
94. Alvord EC, Lofton S. Gliomas of the optic nerve or chiasm: outcome by patients' age, tumor site and treatment. *J Neurosurg* 1988;68:85–98.

95. Caldarelli M, Di Rocco C, Papacci F. Gliomi delle vie ottiche ad esordio clinico nel primo anno di vita. *Min Pediatr* 1996;48:535–542.

96. Belza MG, Donaldson SS, Steinberg GK, et al. Medulloblastoma: freedom from relapse longer than 8 years—a therapeutic cure? *J Neurosurg* 1991;75:575–582.

97. Packer RJ, Sutton LN, Goldwein JW, et al. Improved survival with the use of adjuvant chemotherapy in the treatment of medulloblastoma. *J Neurosurg* 1992;74:433–440.

98. Schofield DE, Yunis EJ, Geyer RJ, et al. DNA content and other prognostic features in childhood medulloblastoma. *Cancer* 1992;69:1307–1314.

99. Birch JM, Marsden HB, Morris Jones PM, et al. Significant improvements in survival in children cancer: results of a population based survey spanning thirty years. *Br Med J* 1988;296:1372–1376.

100. Mapstone TB, Warf BC. Intracranial tumors in infants: characteristics, management, and outcome of a contemporary series. *Neurosurgery* 1991;28:343–348.

101. Tomita T. Long-term effects of treatment for childhood brain tumors. *Neurosurg Clin North Am* 1992;3:959–971.

102. Gjerris F. Clinical aspects and long-term prognosis of intracranial tumours in infancy and childhood. *Develop Med Child Neurol* 1976;18:145–159.

103. Farwell JR, Dohrman GJ, Flannery IT. Intracranial neoplasms in infants. *Arch Neurol* 1978;35:533–537.

104. Duffner PK, Cohen ME, Myers MH, et al. Survival in children with brain tumors: SEER program 1973–1980. *Neurology* 1986;36:597–601.

105. Jenkins D, Goddard K, Armstrong D, et al. Posterior fossa medulloblastoma in childhood: treatment, results and proposal for a new staging system. *Int J Radiat Oncol Biol Phys* 1990;19:265–274.

106. Di Rocco C, Iannelli A. Poor outcome of bilateral congenital choroid plexus papillomas and extreme hydrocephalus. *Eur Neurol* 1997;37:33–37.

107. Riva D, Milani N, Pantaleoni C, et al. Combined treatment modality for medulloblastoma in childhood: effects on neuropsychological functioning. *Neuropediatrics* 1991; 22:36–42.

108. Spunberg JJ, Chang CH, Gelman M, et al. Quality of long-term survival following irradiation for intracranial tumors in children under the age of two. *Int J Radiat Oncol Biol Phys* 1981;7:727–736.

109. Shalet SM, Gibson B, Swindell R, et al. Effect of spinal irradiation on growth. *Arch Dis Child* 1987;62:461–464.

110. Suc E, Kalifa C, Brauner R et al. Brain tumors under the age of three: the price of survival, a retrospective study of 20 long-term survivors. *Acta Neurochir (Wien)* 1009;106:93–98.

111. Horowitz ME, Kun LE, Mulhern RK, et al. Feasibility and efficacy of preirradiation chemotherapy for pediatric brain tumors. *Neurosurgery* 1988;22:687–690.

112. Duffner PK, Horowitz ME, Krischer PhD et al. Postoperative chemotherapy and delayed radiation in children less than three years of age with malignant brain tumors. *N Engl J Med* 1993;328:1725–1731.

113. Jeng MJ, Chang TK, Wong TT et al. Preirradiation chemotherapy for very young children with brain tumors. *Child's Nerv Syst* 1993;9:150–153.

Chapter 29

Miscellaneous Brain Tumors

Steven J. Schneider and Salvatore A. Insinga

Tumors of the central nervous system (CNS) are the second most common malignancy in children. The most prevalent types are astrocytoma, medulloblastoma, ependymoma, and craniopharyngioma, which compose at least 90% of all pediatric brain tumors.[1] These have been previously discussed. This chapter will focus on the less common intracranial tumors of childhood. From the authors' own series of over 400 brain tumors in childhood, the following lesions will be discussed in detail: *dysembryoplastic neuroepithelial tumor* (DNT), *pleomorphic xanthoastrocytoma* (PXA), *atypical teratoid/rhaboid tumor* (ATT/rhabdoid), *colloid cyst, neurocytoma,* and *ganglioglioma* (Table 29–1). It is imperative to distinguish these unusual tumors because their prognosis and treatment may differ radically from that of other types of tumors.

DYSEMBRYOPLASTIC NEUROEPITHELIAL TUMOR

Dysembryoplastic neuroepithelial tumor was first described by Daumas-Duport et al in 1988, in a group of young patients with medically refractory epilepsy who were potentially cured by surgical excision. The term *DNT* stressed a possible origin in dysembryogenesis.[2] The World Health Organization (WHO) has classified DNT as a "neuronal and mixed neuronoglial tumor,"[3] but some consider it a malformative or hamartomous lesion.[4–6] DNT remains a relatively rare entity, with approximately 200 reported cases occurring predominantly in the pediatric age group.[7] An incidence of approximately 1% in patients younger than 20 years and 0.25% in patients older than 20 years has been reported, but the true incidence is unknown because many of these lesions were previously erroneously classified.[8] DNT may represent from 5% to 15% of temporal lobe tumors in patients undergoing temporal lobe resections for intractable epilepsy[9, 10] and from 5% to 13% of tumors found in all resections for epilepsy.[6, 10, 11] There appears to be a slight male predominance.[2, 12] DNT in association with neurofibromatosis type 1 (NF-1) has been reported in three cases.[13, 14]

TABLE 29–1 Pathologic Distribution of Pediatric Brain Tumors (Patients <18 years old) in Authors' Series

Tumor	No.
Astrocytoma (grade 1–2)	159
PNET	63
Astrocytoma (grade 3–4)	28
Ependymoma	25
Craniopharyngioma	22
Pineal region tumor	19
Dermoid tumor	16
Brain stem glioma	13
Ganglioglioma	10
Pituitary Adenoma	10
Meningioma	6
Oligodendroglioma	6
Epidermoid tumor	5
Choroid plexus tumor	5
Histocytosis	5
Hemangioblastoma	5
Optic nerve glioma	4
Hypothalamic glioma	4
Pleomorphic xanthoastrocytoma	3
Colloid cyst	3
Teratoma	3
Gliosarcoma	3
Atypical teratoid/rhabdoid tumor	3
Osteogenic sarcoma	3
Dysembryoplastic neuroepithelial tumor	2
Neurocytoma	2
Ectopic germinoma	2
Acoustic neuroma	2
Neuroblastoma	2
Neurofibroma	2
Lymphoma	1
Chondrosarcoma	1
Ependymoblastoma	1
Hemangiopericytoma	1
Total	439

The authors thank the following individuals without whose help and support this chapter would not have been possible: Dr. Peter Farmer, Department of Pathology, North Shore University Hospital; Dr. Elsa Valderama, Department of Pathology, Long Island Jewish Medical Center/Schneider Childrens Hospital; Ms. Sherry Grimm; Ms. Jessica Feijoo; and Dr. Joseph Zito.

Clinical Presentation

Clinically, lesions often present with a longstanding history of a refractory seizure disorder (typically, partial complex) commencing in childhood.[2, 5, 10] The average onset of seizure activity is 9 to 9.5 years (range 1 week to 30 years), and the duration of symptoms can extend over many years (average, 9 years).[2, 12] Rarely do patients present with symptoms of increased intracranial pressure (i.e., headache, nausea, and vomiting). Papilledema, visual field deficit, or prominence of the skull overlying the lesion is only occasionally appreciated, and the neurologic examination and intelligence level are usually normal.[2, 7, 12] Electroencephalography often reveals localized slow activity and may demonstrate interictal spiking. Often seizures are medically intractable and require surgical intervention.[2, 5–7, 10, 12]

Imaging

On neuroimaging, a supratentorial cortical lesion is often seen. The most common location is the temporal lobe in approximately two-thirds of tumors.[9, 11, 15] They may involve other cortical areas, extend subcortically, or involve the caudate nucleus.[7] Infratentorial location, including the cerebellum,[16] and multifocality[17] is rarely reported. On computed tomography (CT), the lesion is sharply demarcated and moderately hypodense, occasionally demonstrating small amounts of calcification or enhancement (Fig. 29–1). It may

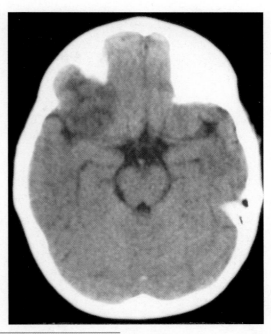

Figure 29–1 CT scan demonstrating a sharply demarcated nonenhancing hypodensity of the inferior frontal lobe in a dysembryoplastic neuroepithelial tumor.

also be markedly hypodense with a more cystic appearance. The overlying calvarium may be remolded due to the longevity of the lesion.[2, 11, 12, 15, 18] Magnetic resonance imaging (MRI) demonstrates low signal intensity on T1-weighted sequences (Fig. 29–2) and increased signal intensity on T2-weighted sequences (Fig. 29–3) with absence of perifocal edema. Proton density–weighted sequences usually reveal

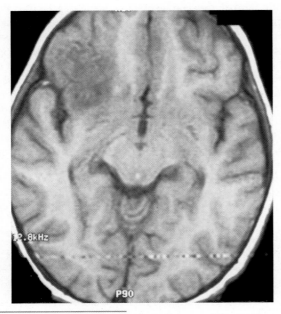

Figure 29–2 Magnetic resonance image of dysembryoplastic neuroepithelial tumor of the inferior frontal lobe with low signal intensity on T1-weighted sequence in a 3-year-old who presented with a seizure disorder. Note the absence of significant mass effect.

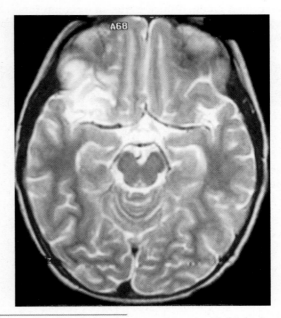

Figure 29–3 Magnetic resonance image with high signal on T2-weighted sequence in dysembryoplastic neuroepithelial tumor with conspicuously absent perifocal edema (see Fig. 29–1).

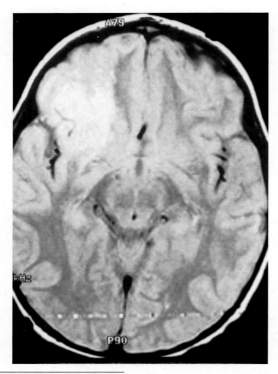

Figure 29–4 Magnetic resonance image utilizing T2-weighted sequence in dysembryoplastic neuroepithelial tumor (see Fig. 29–3), demonstrating a mild hyperintensity on proton density–weighted sequence.

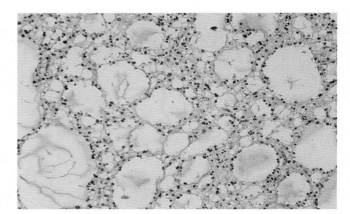

Figure 29–5 Photomicrograph of dysembryoplastic neuroepithelial tumor demonstrating a microcystic component of small blue oligodendroglial-like cells in a myxoid background (H&E × 20).

Pathology

On pathologic examination, DNT classically appears as a multilobular lesion consisting of several elements, including a "specific glioneuronal element," a nodular component, and associated cortical dysplasia. The most consistent finding is the specific glioneuronal element, characterized by small blue oligodendroglial-like cells and neurons in a mucinous background (Fig. 29–5). They tend to align themselves along the neuronal axons, giving the impression that the neurons are floating in the interstitial fluid. The exact nature of the oligodendroglial-like cells remains unclear. The second component is nodules composed of multiple cell types, which include oligodendrocytes, astrocytes, or both. Occasional mitotic figures are seen, as well as some degree of cellular atypia. The third constituent, an associated area of adjacent cortical dysplasia, can also be seen.[2, 14, 21] It has been proposed that these lesions arise from secondary germinal layers, such as the subpial and external granular layers.[2] *It has also been suggested that DNT arises from an associated dysplastic focus and represents an atypical hamartoma due to its location within the white matter, association with cortical dysplasia, cure by surgical excision, and the disorganized neuronal and glial elements that lack significant cellular atypia.*[6] Conversely, the presence of areas of increased cellularity and mitotic figures that express proliferative cell markers supports the view that DNT represents a benign neoplastic process.[6, 12] *Differential diagnoses include oligodendroglioma, mixed oligoastrocytoma, and ganglioglioma, which can be very difficult to discern due to overlapping features.*

an area of variable hyperintensity in relation to the cortex (Fig. 29–4). Gadolinium enhancement is minimal.[2, 11, 12, 15] The presence of a retained thick gyrus–like configuration or a "megagyrus-like" appearance within the lesion expanding the cortex has been described.[9, 19]

BOX 29–2
Imaging Appearance of DNT

- **CT**
  - **Sharp demarcation**
  - **Moderately hypodense**
  - **Hypodense with calcification**
  - **Minimal contrast enhancement**
- **MRI**
  - **T1: low signal intensity**
  - **T2: increased signal intensity**
  - **Proton density: variable hyperintensity**
  - **Negligible gadolinium enhancement**

Serial imaging usually demonstrates a stable lesion. Growth or intratumoral hemorrhage associated with perifocal edema is rare.[11] On iodine I 123 inosine 5′-monophosphate, technetium Tc 99m hexamethyl propyleneamine oxine, and thallium single proton emission computed tomography (SPECT), marked hypoperfusion without uptake is demonstrated.[20]

BOX 29–3
Pathologic Features of DNT

- **Specific glioneuronal element**
  - **Small blue oligodendroglial-like cells**
  - **Neurons in mucinous background**
- **Nodular component: oligodendrocytes, astrocytes, or both**
- **Adjacent cortical dysplasia**

Treatment

The natural history of DNT appears to be that of a stable lesion with little, if any, potential for growth. Malignant transformation has not been reported. Therefore, the main indication for treatment is palliation of symptoms. Surgical excision is often curative and is the treatment of choice for lesions associated with intractable seizures.[2, 6, 7, 10, 12, 18] Gross total resection should be carried out whenever possible, although subtotal resections have also had gratifying results. Asymptomatic lesions in eloquent cortex may be observed. Radiotherapy offers no added benefit and should be avoided.[2, 18] It is imperative that the entity of DNT be recognized so that misdiagnosis and potentially harmful adjunctive radiotherapy and/or chemotherapy can be avoided.

PLEOMORPHIC XANTHOASTROCYTOMA

Pleomorphic xanthoastrocytoma (PXA) is a rare tumor first described in 1979 by Kepes et al in 12 patients who had relatively favorable prognoses despite their having tumors with a pleomorphic and bizarre appearance suggestive of malignancy.[22] These tumors remain rare, with only about 100 cases reported.[23–25] PXA is found primarily in the second and third decades of life.[23] The median age at time of diagnosis is 14 years (range 2 to 62 years), and there is no sexual or racial predominance.[24]

Clinical Presentation

The initial clinical presenting complaint is seizures in up to 80% of patients, and it is the only symptom in 44%. Increased

intracranial pressure and focal neurologic deficits are seen in approximately 20% and 5%, respectively. The median duration of symptoms is 2 years (range 0 to 16 years).[23, 24] An association with NF-1 has also been reported.[26]

PXA is usually a superficial cortical tumor, involving the temporal lobe in 76% of reported cases, but with other cortical, subcortical, and thalamic locations also reported.[23, 27] There are also reports of multicentric, cerebellar, and spinal cord PXA.[28–30] These lesions may contain a solitary cyst (90%), a mural nodule (25%), or appear solid.[24]

> **BOX 29–4**
> **Clinical Characteristics of PXA**
>
> - **Seizures**
> - **Slow growing**
> - **Located in temporal lobe**
> - **Cystic**
> - **Mural nodule**

Imaging

CT usually reveals a very low-density area corresponding to the cystic portion and a less hypodense area corresponding to a mural nodule that enhances intensely.[21, 31] Calcification, significant mass effect, and peritumoral edema are less common.[32] MRI reveals the solid portion as isointense to gray matter on T1-weighted sequences (Fig. 29–6), mildly hyperintense on T2-weighted sequences (Fig. 29–7), and enhancing

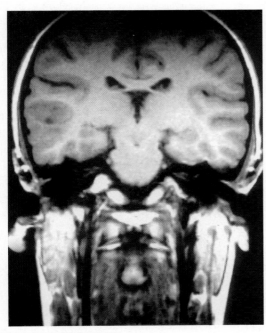

Figure 29–6 Magnetic resonance image demonstrating isointensity in gray matter on T1-weighted sequence in a pleomorphic xanthoastrocytoma of the superficial temporal lobe in a 15-year-old who presented with a seizure disorder.

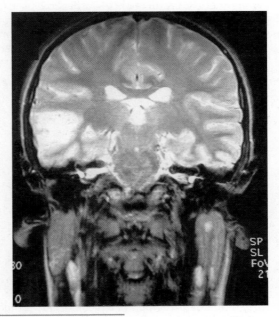

Figure 29–7 Magnetic resonance image utilizing a T2-weighted sequence reveals a mild signal hyperintensity in this pleomorphic xanthoastrocytoma (see Fig. 29–6).

homogeneously post gadolinium.[33] The leptomeninges may be involved, but dural invasion is unusual.[34]

BOX 29-5
Imaging Appearance of PXA

- CT
  - Hypodense
  - Enhancing mural nodule
- MRI
  - T1: isointense solid portion
  - T2: mildly hyperintense
  - Enhances homogeneously with gadolinium

Pathology

Macroscopic examination reveals a tumor containing a mural nodule of yellow or reddish tissue, well circumscribed from the surrounding brain, and encapsulated by a proteinaceous cyst.[21] On histologic examination, PXA demonstrates astrocytic cells with significant cellular atypia, pleomorphism, nuclear hyperchromatism, and bizarre multinucleate giant cell formation. The cells classically are xanthomatous with intracellular lipid but can also be plump eosinophilic granular bodies or elongated in a densely cellular matrix (Fig. 29–8). A reticulin network surrounds individual cells or is aligned along spindle-shaped bundles. Although low mitotic activity can be present, necrosis and endothelial proliferation are rare.[21, 22, 24] Immunohistochemical staining reveals glial fibrillary acidic protein (GFAP) positivity and defines the astrocytic nature of the tumor.[22] Neuronal phenotyping with antibodies, such as synaptophysin, may be positive, as composite forms of PXA-ganglioglioma have been reported.[25, 35, 36] An association of PXA with areas of cortical dysplasia has also been reported, suggesting that it may be linked to other glioneuronal lesions, such as DNT.[37] Anaplastic transformation with areas of necrosis, endothelial proliferation, and high

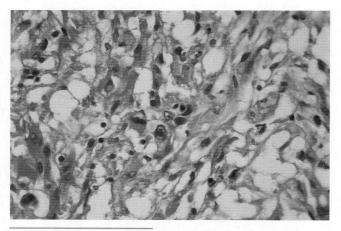

Figure 29–8 Photomicrograph of a pleomorphic xanthoastrocytoma revealing bizarre "lipidized" astrocytes. Note the absence of mitotic figures or necrosis despite the pleomorphic appearance.

mitotic index has been reported.[38] PXA may be mistaken for more aggressive tumors, so it is important that it be recognized and treated appropriately.

BOX 29-6
Pathologic Features of PXA

- Astrocytes
  - Cellular atypia
  - Pleomorphism
  - Nuclear hyperchromatism
  - Bizarre multinucleated giant cells
- Xanthomatous
- Low mitotic activity

Treatment

The natural history of PXA is usually that of a benign, slow-growing tumor, responding well to surgical excision. The treatment of choice is gross total resection, facilitated by its preferred superficial location.[22, 23] Long-term survival of 5, 10 and 15 years in 91%, 82%, and 77% of patients, respectively, with a median survival of 18 years has been reported.[24] This favorable prognosis exists despite the lesion's pleomorphic and bizarre appearance and is not affected by the extent of resection for up to 10 years following resection.[39] Others have suggested that patients with gross total resection appear to fare better than those undergoing partial excision in the absence of necrosis.[24] Anaplastic transformation is associated with a poorer prognosis, and a correlation with increased mitotic activity has been suggested.[39] *In a more recent review, the single most important negative prognostic factor for PXA was the presence of necrosis.* Necrosis was found in 20% of patients initially, or at time of recurrence, and was associated with a median postoperative survival of 1 year. This was not influenced by the degree of resection or radiotherapy.[24] Although radiotherapy has been suggested to reduce the probability of recurrence,[39] whether or not there is a distinct benefit remains controversial.[23, 24, 39] The efficacy of chemotherapy remains unproven. Unfortunately, all data reported have been retrospective due to the rarity of PXA. At present, gross total or subtotal resection of PXA without necrosis on histologic examination can be followed by observation alone. Adjuvant therapy can be considered in the presence of necrosis on histologic examination, recurrence, and/or malignant transformation.

ATYPICAL TERATOID/RHABDOID TUMOR

Malignant rhabdoid tumor (MRT), an uncommon childhood neoplasm, consists of rhabdoid cells typically arising from within the kidney. Its name is derived from its similarity on light microscopy to rhabdomyosarcoma, but it lacks other features of skeletal muscle.[40, 41] It was first described by Beckwith in the kidney in 1978[42] and in the CNS by Briner in 1985.[43] It has subsequently been identified in the CNS as an isolated lesion or associated with a renal tumor.[40, 44–49] Another CNS tumor was described containing rhabdoid cells as part of a mixed population of cells including nests of primitive neuroectodermal tumor–medulloblastoma (PNET-MB) associated with mesenchymal and/or epithelial tissue. Initially, these tumors were considered PNET-MB but did not appear to share the same clinical features. Subsequently, this neoplasm has been called atypical teratoid tumor (ATT) to denote the possibility that the combination of these disparate elements suggests a special type of teratoma. It does not, however, share any of the other typical features of classic teratoma.[50, 51] Whether or not the MRT and ATT represent the same neoplasm is obscure. However, both lesions share several features that have led to their classification together as atypical teratoid/rhabdoid tumor (ATT/rhabdoid). Both contain rhabdoid cells, have a high incidence in infancy, have similar aggressive courses, and abnormalities in chromosome 22 are reported in some cases.[50, 51] The designation of ATT/rhabdoid tumor has been used interchangeably for both tumors and will be used in this chapter.

ATT/rhabdoid tumors of the CNS are rare neoplasms with less than 150 cases reported.[40, 45–53] The exact incidence is unknown, with many occurrences having been previously classified as PNET-MB. The peak incidence is during the first 2 years of life, whereas PNET-MB peaks at age 3 to 5 years.[48, 51] The mean age at diagnosis is 17 to 29 months (range in utero to 14.9 years). There appears to be a slight male predominance (3:2), similar to that in PNET-MB.[50, 51]

BOX 29–7
Clinical Features of MRT

- Rhabdoid cells (kidney)
- Mixed population
- Presentation in infancy
- Aggressive
- Chromosome 22 abnormality
- Located in posterior fossa
- Leptomeningeal spread

Clinical Presentation

The clinical presentation is usually dependent on tumor location at time of diagnosis. Common presenting symptoms in children younger than 3 years include lethargy, vomiting, and/or failure to thrive, with head tilt and cranial nerve palsies, whereas headache and focal neurologic deficits are more prevalent in older children. Tumor location in the posterior fossa and cerebellum are reported in 63 to 69 % of cases, whereas supratentorial, multifocal, and extrame-dullary spinal cord locations have also been cited.[48, 50] It is reported that 70% of children younger than 3 years of age at diagnosis had a posterior fossa tumor, as compared with 33% of older children.[50] Leptomeningeal dissemination, present at diagnosis in 28 to 34% of patients, showed no age correlation.[48, 50]

Imaging

Features on neuroimaging are nonspecific and similar to those found in PNET-MB. The noncontrast CT scan reveals an area of increased density, enhancing inhomogeneously with contrast. Cysts and hemorrhages are common. MRI demonstrates decreased signal intensity on T1-weighted sequence (Fig. 29–9), iso- or decreased intensity on T2-weighted sequence, and isointense relative to gray matter on proton density–weighted relative sequence, typically enhancing with gadolinium.[40, 48, 50–53]

BOX 29–8
Imaging Appearance of MRT

- CT
  - High density
  - Nonuniform enhancement
  - Cysts
  - Hemorrhage
- MRI
  - T1: decreased signal enhancement
  - T2: isodense, with decreased signal enhancement
  - Enhancement with gadolinium

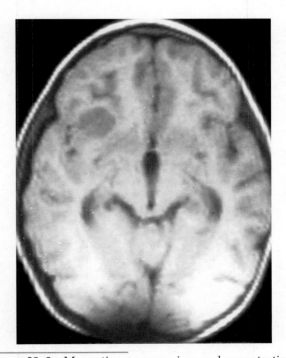

Figure 29–9 Magnetic resonance image demonstrating a decreased signal intensity on T1-weighted sequence in an atypical teratoid/rhabdoid tumor in an 8-year-old who presented with headache. Leptomeningeal dissemination was appreciated during surgical removal and the patient had a coexistent renal tumor that was pathologically consistent with malignant rhabdoid tumor.

Pathology

On macroscopic examination, the tumor is usually described as tan-white and of variable consistency.[46, 48] Histologically, ATT/rhabdoid tumor may appear as a classic MRT, i.e., highly cellular and containing rhabdoid cells that are round to oval epithelioid, with a single, often eccentric nucleus and usually a prominent nucleolus (Fig. 29–10). The cytoplasm is eosinophilic and abundant, with occasional hyaline inclusion bodies. Necrosis and high mitotic activity are common.[41] They may also appear as ATT tumors, possessing rhabdoid cells in combination with nests of PNET-MB. Sometimes mesenchymal and/or epithelial tissue is present.[50, 51] Immunohistochemical stains commonly show a positive reaction for vimentin and epithelial membrane antigen, as well as others including cytokeratin, smooth-muscle actin, and GFAP.[50] Ultrastructural examination demonstrates "whorl-like" cytoplasmic aggregations of filaments probably corresponding to the cytoplasmic inclusions on light microscopy.[45] Cytogenetically, these tumors (both CNS ATT/rhabdoid tumor and peripheral MRT) have shown a propensity toward abnormalities in chromosome 22 and include monosomy, deletions, and reciprocal translocations.[51, 54] The histogenesis of the rhabdoid cell remains unclear and includes the possibility that it may be histiocytic, mesenchymal, neuroectodermal, or meningeal.[55]

BOX 29–9
Pathologic Features of MRT

- **Highly cellular**
- **Rhabdoid cells**
  - **Round or oval**
  - **Eccentric nucleus**
- **Necrosis**
- **High mitotic activity**

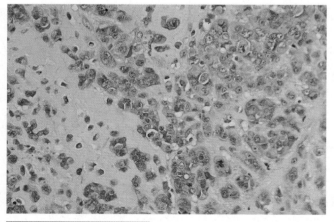

Figure 29–10 Photomicrograph of atypical teratoid/rhabdoid tumor demonstrating prominent rhabdoid cells with vesicular nuclei, prominent nucleoli, and filled with abundant PAS-positive cytoplasm (PAS × 40).

Treatment

The natural history of CNS ATT/rhabdoid tumor is one of local aggressiveness with a propensity for leptomeningeal dissemination. This tumor may be more aggressive and less responsive than PNET-MB.[50, 51] CNS and renal tumors may coexist in a number of cases.[44] Abdominal CT should be carried out in patients with CNS ATT/rhabdoid tumors to determine if a renal tumor is also present.[49] In addition, the entire neuraxis should be examined by MRI for leptomeningeal spread. It is postulated that this enhanced propensity for dissemination may be secondary to increased expression of collagenases by the tumor.[56] Prognosis is poor, with death often occurring within a year despite multimodality therapy, including surgery, irradiation, and chemotherapy.[50, 51] Surgical excision or debulking of these tumors is limited to diagnosis and palliation. Radiotherapy is of limited application due to the young age of these patients. Although tumor growth with large doses of radiation (more than 5000 cGy total) may be partially inhibited,[57] it has not been shown to significantly alter the progression of the disease.[50] Various chemotherapeutic regimes have been utilized but appear to be resistant to any of those offered by the Pediatric Oncology Group.[50] Longer survival has been reported in one small series of patients with CNS ATT/rhabdoid tumors who underwent a rhabdomyosarcoma-directed protocol, but the significance remains obscure.[58]

COLLOID CYST

Colloid cyst is an uncommon lesion located in the anterior third ventricle. In 1858 Wallman reported the first case,[59] and in 1933 Dandy reported the first pediatric case.[60] Although colloid cysts represent 0.5 to 2% of intracranial tumors, occurrence in childhood is rare, with less than 50 cases reported.[59, 60] The mean age at presentation in children is approximately 11 years, with the youngest reported case at 2 months. In contrast, the adult population has a presentation typically between the third and fifth decades of life. Neither group shows a particular sex predominance.[41, 59, 60]

Clinical Presentation

The clinical manifestation of a colloid cyst is secondary to the accompanying hydrocephalus that results from the obstruction of one or both of the foramens of Monro. In childhood, the most common presentation is headache with nausea/vomiting. Other signs of increased intracranial pressure, including papilledema and diplopia, may be present. The onset of symptoms may range from days to months.[59, 60] Sudden death in children associated with acute hydrocephalus has been reported in several cases.[61–64] The adult population appears to manifest similar clinical features but also manifests drop attacks, transient loss of consciousness, and dementia.[65] Both children and adults may present with acute neurologic deterioration. The mortality rate is higher in children than in adults (33% vs. 6–16%).[59]

BOX 29–10
Clinical Features of Colloid Cysts

- **Hydrocephalus common**
- **Sudden death reported**

Spinal Cord Tumors

Section III

Chapter 30

Astrocytoma

Cheryl A. Muszynski, Shlomi Constantini, and Fred J. Epstein

In 1911, Elsberg and Beer reported the first successful removal of an intramedullary spinal cord tumor.[1] Seven years later, Frazier described his technique for removing encapsulated intramedullary neoplasms.[2] However, early attempts at resection of intrinsic intramedullary spinal cord tumors were associated with unacceptably high operative morbidity and mortality. For the next several decades there was little impetus to modify the accepted approach of biopsy, dural decompression, and radiation therapy, even as the latter regimen, used routinely, resulted in a relatively short remission followed by serious disability or death. Although "traditional" views were based on the assumption that extensive removal of tumors from the spinal cord without inflicting neurologic injury was not feasible,[3, 4] in 1954 Greenwood—with the aid of bipolar cautery and loupe magnification—successfully completed resection of intramedullary ependymomas in six patients.[5] During the past 40 years, experience gained by other neurosurgeons worldwide has proved that the majority of intramedullary spinal cord lesions, including astrocytomas, can be radically excised with an acceptable morbidity and mortality, along with a low incidence of recurrence.[6–16]

CLINICAL MANIFESTATIONS

Parents invariably become aware of a problem long before objective signs of neurologic dysfunction surface. *In a significant number of pediatric patients, the onset of symptoms is related to an apparently trivial injury, whereas in others, parents describe exacerbations and remissions.*

Local pain along the spinal axis is the most common early symptom in both children and adults. Other symptoms include motor disturbance, loss of sensation, paresthesias, dysesthesias, and, rarely, sphincter dysfunction. Weakness of the lower extremities is usually first manifested as a subtle alteration of a previously normal gait, which is only obvious to a parent noting a child's tendency to fall more frequently or to walk on the heels or toes. In young children, there is commonly a history of being a "late walker," and in the youngest (under 2 years), there is often a history of motor regression, that is, reverting to crawling rather than walking, or refusing to stand.

BOX 30–1
Clinical Signs and Symptoms

- **Pain**
  - **Local**
  - **Radicular**
- **Motor disturbances**
- **Sensory disturbances (paresthesias)**
- **Gait changes**
- **Spasticity**
- **Reflex changes**
- **Scoliosis**
- **Bowel/bladder difficulty**

Seventy percent of patients experienced severe pain along the spinal axis, which is usually most acute in the bony segments directly over the tumor. *Characteristically, the pain is worse in the recumbent position where venous congestion further distends the dural tube, resulting in typical night pains.* After a nondiagnostic orthopedic evaluation, it is common to discover that adult patients have been chronic users of analgesics, including narcotics.

Radicular pain occurs in about 10% of cases and is usually limited to one or two cervical, thoracic, or lumbar dermatomes (similar to root pain from a variety of disease processes). Paresthesias are occasionally associated with dysesthetic pain, and both symptoms are more common with neoplasms in the cervical than in the thoracic spinal cord.

With both cervical and thoracic tumors, mild spasticity, increased reflexes, extensor plantar signs (with or without clonus), and head tilt with torticollis occur. In the relatively rare group of malignant astrocytomas, symptoms are similar in quality but with a shorter duration and increased intensity.

Mild scoliosis is the most common early sign of an intramedullary thoracic cord astrocytoma. Pain and paraspinal muscle spasm commonly occur prior to objective signs of neurological dysfunction and are assumed to be secondary to the evolving scoliosis. Insidious, progressive motor weakness in the lower extremities was initially manifested by "awkwardness" and only later by frequent falls and an obvious limp. Early sensory abnormalities are uncommon, although dysesthesias and paresthesias are occasionally present.

Sphincter laxity was a very late sign, except for tumors that originate in the conus/cauda equina regions. More rostrally located tumors, even with cystic components extending into the conus, rarely presented with sphincter abnormalities. Unusual and falsely localizing signs and symptoms uncommonly result from subarachnoid hemorrhage,[17, 18] hydrocephalus due to raised cerebrospinal fluid (CSF) pressure,[19] and intramedullary cyst formation.[20]

ETIOLOGY

The cause of glial tumors in general, and of astrocytomas in particular, is unknown. Although chromosomal rearrangements and overexpression of oncogenes have been described in spinal astrocytomas, their significance is still unclear.[21–26]

BIOLOGIC BASIS

For the most part, intramedullary astrocytomas are relatively circumscribed and produce a limited fusiform swelling of the cord. About 40% are cystic. Rostral and caudal cyst walls usually do not harbor neoplastic cells. In asymmetrical and extensive lesions, the cord may be rotated and distorted. In pediatric astrocytomas, the posterior columns may be displaced laterally. Occasionally, adjacent leptomeninges may be infiltrated with tumor tissue.

Microscopically, spinal astrocytomas typically resemble the diffuse fibrillary astrocytoma of the cerebrum but show a considerable disposition to becoming pilocytic.[27] Occasionally, in more benign examples, relatively poor cellularity may raise the differential diagnosis of spinal cord gliosis. Approximately 30% of pediatric,[28] and 25% of adult[10] spinal astrocytomas have anaplastic features.[29]

EPIDEMIOLOGY

Spinal cord tumors are relatively rare neoplasms, accounting for only 4 to 10% of all central nervous system tumors. Earlier series of intraspinal tumors tended to present more extramedullary lesions, whereas modern series—oriented more to surgical "challenges"—emphasize the relative number of intramedullary spinal cord tumors. Therefore, it is difficult to quantify the real incidence of intramedullary versus extramedullary and extradural tumors.[30]

While in adults intramedullary tumors compose only about 20% of all intraspinal neoplasms, at least 35% of the pediatric spinal cord tumors are intramedullary.[27, 31–33] The glioma family accounts for the vast majority of intramedullary spinal cord tumors. Among 436 patients (all ages) with intramedullary spinal cord tumor operated by Dr. Fred Epstein between 1985 and 1999, 49% were in the pediatric age range. Of these 436 patients, 37% presented with ependymomas, 29% with astrocytomas, 14% with gangliogliomas, 7% with mixed gliomas, and 14% with other lesions [e.g., hemangioblastomas, primitive neuroectodermal tumors (PNETs), lipomas, and ganglioneurocytomas]. Whereas astrocytomas and gangliogliomas were especially prevalent in the younger age groups, ependymomas were more frequently observed in the older groups.[34, 35]

BOX 30–2
Authors' Experience with 226 Patients (1985–1999)

- 37% ependymomas
- 29% astrocytoma
- 14% ganglioglioma
- 7% mixed gliomas
- 14% other tumors (hemangioblastoma, PNET, lipoma, etc.)

DIAGNOSTIC EVALUATION

Plain films are relatively insensitive for the evaluation of patients with suspected intradural and especially intramedullary pathology. Even secondary bony changes, such as pedicle erosion or foraminal widening, are better demonstrated with computed tomography.[36] However, plain films are better for the diagnosis of instability and for the quantification of scoliotic and kyphotic deformities (Fig. 30–1).

By providing an excellent image of intramedullary neoplasms, magnetic resonance imaging (MRI) has made most

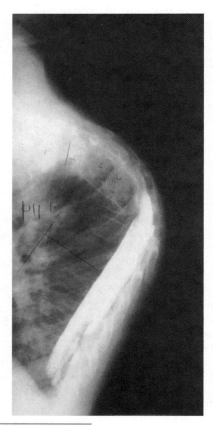

Figure 30–1 Plain radiograph (lateral view) of the thoracic spine demonstrates significant kyphosis.

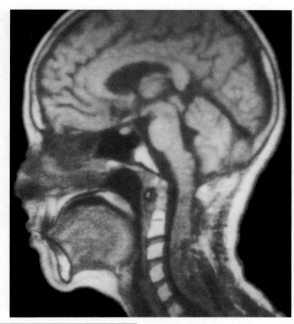

Figure 30–2 Sagittal T1-weighted image demonstrates diffuse widening of the cervical spinal cord. This tumor was resected and histologically proven to be a pilocytic astrocytoma.

invasive neurodiagnostic studies obsolete; additional studies become unnecessary.[37] Exceptions include the necessity to perform myelography in patients either with severe scoliosis, when it may be difficult to obtain the mandatory mid-sagittal images, or with an artificial implant. The T1-weighted images are the most informative (Fig. 30–2), disclosing the presence of rostral and caudal cysts, intramedullary cysts, and the solid component of the tumor. The T2-weighted images provide a "myelographic appearance" to the CSF and cysts. Injection of gadolinium is mandatory for all spinal cord tumors.[38] Gadolinium may enhance the solid component of the tumor and help delineate it from surrounding edema. Unlike ependymomas, which contrast-enhance brightly, astrocytomas give the cord a lumpy appearance, with no or irregular contrast enhancement.

BOX 30–3
MRI Appearance

- T1
  - **Rostral/caudal cysts**
  - **Solid components**
- **T2: cysts/syrinx**
- **Gadolinium enhancement of solid component may be irregular**

MANAGEMENT

Most neoplasms are low grade and surgically curable. Modern neurosurgical aids—the operating microscope, intraoperative ultrasonography,[34, 39] the CO_2 laser,[40] and especially

ultrasonic aspiration[32]—have dramatically improved the outcome, decreasing the operative morbidity associated with spinal astrocytomas.[10]

Spinal cord astrocytomas are relatively firm, occasionally contain microscopic foci of calcium, and only rarely have a cleavage plane to facilitate an "en bloc" resection. In the overwhelming majority of cases, it is necessary to remove the tumor from inside-out until a "glial-tumor interface" is recognized as a change in color and consistency between the tumor and the adjacent normal neural tissues.

In the past, neurosurgeons were limited to traditional suction-cautery techniques for the removal of neoplasms. Although this was often satisfactory for brain tumors, it was extremely hazardous for the spinal cord due to the transmitted heat and movement through the tumor to the adjacent normal cord, which was invariably firmly adherent to it. As a result of these technical limitations, a significant morbidity was associated with intramedullary spinal cord tumor surgery.

The development and application of the Cavitron ultrasonic aspirator (CUSA) system significantly improved the conventional systems and made a major contribution to spinal cord tumor surgery[32] (Fig. 30–3). The ultrasonic aspirator is the ideal instrument to rapidly debulk and remove all but residual fragments of a spinal cord neoplasm.

The neurosurgical laser is equally ideal for removing the residual fragments, as it may be employed with great precision along the length of the glial-tumor interface. Although the laser may be employed in place of the CUSA, it is extremely tedious and time consuming to direct it to a very voluminous intramedullary neoplasm. Furthermore, the resultant laser "char" makes it difficult to recognize the glial-tumor interface, mandating frequent interruptions of the ongoing dissection while the blackened tissues are gently removed with microsuction.

It is desirable to carry out a limited laminectomy over the solid component of the neoplasm but not to unnecessarily extend it over rostrally and/or caudally associated cysts. Transdural ultrasonography is utilized to define the location of the tumor vis-à-vis the area exposed by the laminectomy[39] (Fig. 30–4). With this technique, the spinal

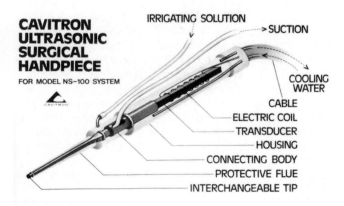

Figure 30–3 The Cavitron ultrasonic surgical aspirator (CUSA), which provides tissue fragmentation within 1 mL of the vibrating tip, suspends the fragmented tissue in the irrigation fluid, and aspirates the emulsion.

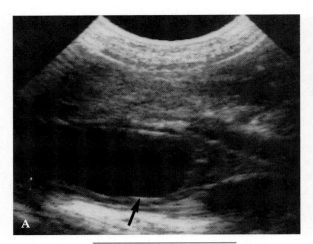 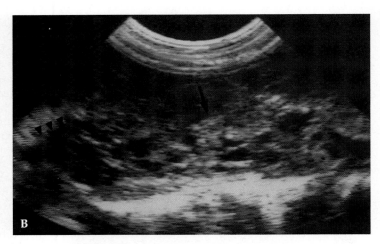

Figure 30–4 (A) Intraoperative transdural ultrasonography (sagittal section) reveals the caudally located cyst (arrow) of an intramedullary astrocytoma. (B) Intraoperative ultrasonography (sagittal section) discloses the solid (arrow) and cystic (arrowheads) components of an intramedullary astrocytoma.

cord is viewed in both sagittal and transverse sections. The rostral and caudal limits of the tumor, as well as the presence or absence of associated cysts, may then be assessed.

For patients not previously operated who need bony openings of more than two segments, we use the Midas-Rex instrument (Midas Rex, Fort Worth, TX) to perform an osteoplastic laminotomy. This allows for subsequent replacement of the lamina, which serves as a nidus for subsequent osteogenesis, posterior fusion, and protection against local trauma in the future.

At this juncture, the dura is opened. In the presence of a rostral and/or caudal cyst, it is not necessary to open the dura widely over the cyst; they are easily drained as the solid component of the neoplasm is excised. *It is vital to emphasize that the expanded spinal cord is commonly rotated and distorted, and it is essential to carefully inspect and identify normal landmarks prior to performing myelotomy.* The latter is best performed under high magnification using sharp dissection.

Following completion of the myelotomy, there is usually 1 to 2 mm of white matter overlying the neoplasm, which is removed using the laser or bipolar cautery with a very fine suction. Next, pial traction sutures are used to facilitate the opening of the myelotomy incision and to improve exposure of the intramedullary tumor. The normal tissue is carefully displaced to the sides using a plated bayonet (Codman and Shurtleff, CD#5256), which is a modified simple bayonet whose tips have been replaced with spherical thin plates.[41] The "plated tips" are placed between the tumor and the adjacent tissues, and the instrument is gently released. The tension is distributed equally over a relatively wide surface area to avoid perforation of tissues.

It must be emphasized that in the presence of an astrocytoma no effort should be exerted to define a plane of cleavage around the tumor. The neoplasms must be removed from the inside to the outside until a glial-tumor interface is recognized by the change in color and consistency of the adjacent tissues. Only very rarely is there a true plane of dissection. Futile efforts to define its presence result in unnecessary retraction and manipulation of functioning neural tissue.

The excision of the solid *noncystic* astrocytoma is initiated in the midportion rather than in the rostral or caudal pole of the neoplasm (Fig. 30–5) because there is no clear rostral or caudal demarcation of the tumor, as occurs when there are rostral or caudal cysts. In addition, the "poles" of the neoplasm are the least voluminous; therefore, removal of this part of the neoplasm may be the most hazardous aspect of the surgery as normal neural tissue may be easily disrupted. The last fragments of the rostral and caudal segments of the tumor are removed by working within the myelotomy and "distracting" the residual neoplasm into the surgical cavity without extending the myelotomy (Fig. 30–6). This is an essential technical point because the tumors characteristically taper, and normal neural tissue is most vulnerable to injury in these areas. It is very helpful to utilize intraoperative ultrasonography to clearly identify the rostral and caudal extent of the tumor and to monitor one's progress during the resection part of the procedure.

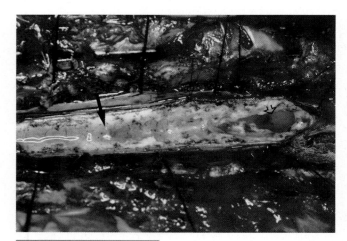

Figure 30–5 Intraoperative appearance of intramedullary astrocytoma with solid noncystic portion of tumor (closed arrow) flanked by caudally located cyst (open arrow).

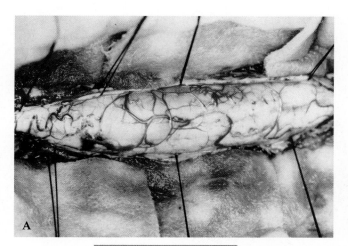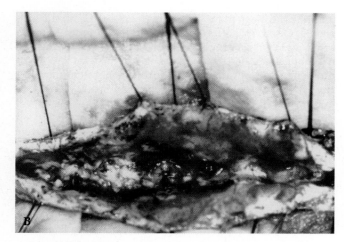

Figure 30–6 (A) Intraoperative photograph of a cervical mixed glioma. Note the expanded cord as well as prominent veins on the surface. (B) Following tumor resection, a large cavity remains, with a thin layer of normal tissue left behind.

INTRAOPERATIVE ELECTROPHYSIOLOGIC MONITORING

During the past decade, intraoperative neurophysiologic monitoring has been infrequently used for spinal cord tumor surgery. However, recently it has become an indispensable adjunct to our surgical practice. This type of monitoring allows one to customize the surgical technique to an individual's baseline electrophysiologic signals. In the past, only sensory evoked potentials (SEPs) were readily available for intraoperative recording. However, advances have now made it possible to monitor motor evoked potentials (MEPs) as well.[42–47] In addition, the electrophysiologic data may be updated every 2 to 3 seconds, providing nearly "real-time" feedback to the surgeon at the time of tumor resection.

To date, Dr. Fred Epstein has used this type of monitoring in more than 300 procedures for intramedullary spinal cord tumor resection. MEPs were elicited with transcortical electrical current stimulation. Spinal epidural MEPs were elicited by giving single square-wave impulses of 500 microseconds duration at intensities of 15 to 160 mA. Epidural recordings were obtained with a dedicated catheter-electrode composed of three platinum-iridium recording cylinders. In the past 2 years, intraoperative limb muscle MEPs were also recorded. Compound muscle action potentials (CMAPs) were obtained from the thenar and anterior tibial muscles bilaterally with stainless-steel electroencephalogram (EEG) needle electrodes inserted in the muscles.

SEPs were recorded after transcutaneous stimulation of the tibial nerves bilaterally with constant current impulses. SEP recordings were obtained in two locations: over the spinal cord rostral to the lesion (spinal epidural SEPs) and over the cerebral cortex (cortical SEPs). In patients with preoperatively impaired proprioception, it was rarely possible to obtain baseline SEPs for monitoring. Typically, SEPs are transiently disrupted when a myelotomy is being done to gain access to the tumor. When SEPs are preserved intraoperatively, joint position sense is preserved postoperatively.

When baseline SEPs were normal but SEPs were lost intraoperatively, a transient loss of joint position sense was observed postoperatively. We have found that spinal epidural SEPs are more reliable predictors of postoperative function than the cortical ones.

Likewise, our recent experience has shown that epidural MEPs are reliable predictors of postoperative neurologic status. More specifically, a less than 50% reduction of intraoperative epidural MEPs portends a transient mono- or paraparesis postoperatively. Amplitude reduction of more than 50% was associated with a more profound postoperative neurologic deficit. In the latter cases, the potential for significant recovery was much less certain. Although the threshold for motor recovery has not yet been scientifically documented, we do not push dissection beyond a 50% decline in the MEPs. If and when such a fall in potentials occurs, we halt dissection and wait for the recovery of potentials.

Muscle MEPs reflect the function of the motor pathways from the subcortical white matter to beyond the neuromuscular junction in each of the patient's extremities. These evoked potentials are particularly useful in the conus medullaris and cauda equina regions, two areas over which the epidural MEPs are nonobtainable. One limitation of muscle MEP monitoring is the inherent sensitivity to the effects of anesthetic agents.[42–47] For this reason, our intramedullary spinal cord tumor patients are anesthetized with a combination of propofol, fentanyl, and nitrous oxide. No muscle relaxants or halogenated agents are used. In general, we have observed that intraoperative muscle MEPs tend to decrease before any changes are noted in epidural MEPs. More specifically, when muscle MEPs are lost without any significant change in epidural D-wave amplitudes, a transient postoperative motor deficit invariably results. Therefore, we now recognize that the loss of muscle MEPs is a warning sign of subsequent change in epidural MEPs.

Routinely, prior to tumor resection, criteria for what constitutes a significant change are set for each patient according to the baseline potentials and the pathology present. In many cases, during dissection of an intramedullary tumor, a minor (i.e., less than 30%) decrement in epidural MEPs occurs. Often, irrigation of the wound with tepid Ringer's solution reverts these signals back to baseline status. This signal change may simply reflect changes in the local ionic environment that occur during tumor resection, rather than disruption of motor pathways (i.e., the "true" loss of signals). In our practice, it is not uncommon to start and stop the dissection many times during the course of tumor resection.

When the laser is employed for more than 20 consecutive seconds, there is often an adverse, probably thermal, effect that is manifested by a decrease in amplitude and increase in latency. When this occurs, the dissection is interrupted and the resection cavity is irrigated with Ringer's solution at a temperature of 30 to 33°C. In most of these cases, electrical activity returns to baseline within 30 to 90 seconds.

Since we have found a consistent correlation between intraoperatively acquired neurophysiologic data and postoperative function, we rely on such monitoring for decision making during intramedullary spinal cord tumor resection.

COMPLICATIONS

Patients with malignant tumors are at a relatively high risk for surgical injury. In fact, patients with severe preoperative disability and extensive noncystic tumors are very likely to deteriorate as a result of surgery. The incidence of significant postoperative motor deficit in an intact patient is below less than 5%. In a patient with a significant preexisting (preoperative) deficit, the morbidity is higher. Therefore, it is essential that patients with known intramedullary spinal cord tumors undergo surgery prior to the evolution of significant neurologic dysfunction.

Impaired position sense, even in the presence of normal motor function, is a serious functional disability that mandates extensive rehabilitative physical therapy. This potential complication is stressed in our preoperative discussion with patients and parents. However, the risk of injury to the posterior columns is significantly smaller when operating on an astrocytoma in a child than it is when operating on one in an adult.

Other postoperative complications include those related to ineffective wound healing and perioperative CSF fistulae. Thus, a specific approach was developed to reduce the morbidity of wound closure following extensive and complicated laminectomy.[48, 49] Special attention is given to the fascia, which is usually the only water-tight layer. Both fascia and muscle are released, first superficially from the subcutaneous tissues and then deeply from the bony elements. If this does not achieve closure without tension, relaxing incisions are performed. The musculofascial layer is closed with "figure of 8" tightly knotted Novafil or Prolene sutures. Any doubt regarding the integrity of the closure may be verified with fluid injection under pressure.

Scoliosis and kyphosis commonly evolve after surgery. In some cases of kyphosis (Fig. 30–7), the deformity is of a sufficient magnitude to cause spinal cord compression and progressive myelopathy.[50] In these patients, recurrent tumor should always be considered before the spinal deformity is identified as being responsible for the neurologic dysfunction. It is imperative that the entity of spinal deformity be appreciated because treatment and prognosis are obviously

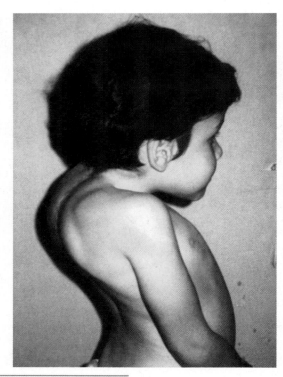

Figure 30–7 Severe kyphosis in a 6-year-old boy who previously underwent a multilevel cervical laminectomy for astrocytoma resection.

very different. Scoliosis usually does not cause spinal cord compression, although it obviously may potentiate a preexisting neurologic disability. It is essential that all children be followed closely by a pediatric orthopedic surgeon experienced in the care of kyphosis and scoliosis. We recommend that the surgical indication for spinal fusion be regarded as more urgent in this group of patients than in those with idiopathic deformities.

BOX 30–4
Complications

- **Motor/sensory deficits**
- **Impaired position sense**
- **Infection**
- **CSF leak**
- **Kyphoscoliosis**

In a recent retrospective study of 45 patients who had undergone surgery for intramedullary spinal cord tumors, we considered the influence of performing an osteoplastic laminotomy (OL) over a simple laminectomy (Lam) for progressive postoperative kyphoscoliosis (PPOKS) in children.[51] In the OL group, the incidence of PPOKS during a mean follow-up period of 3.4 years was 3 in 20. In the Lam group, the incidence was significantly higher at 9 in 25. Because all three patients in the OL group who developed PPOKS also experienced recurrent disease, we concluded that, whenever possible, it is preferable to perform an OL, despite the fact that this technique may not prevent the postoperative evolution of spinal deformity in the presence of recurrent tumor.[52]

ADJUNCTIVE TREATMENT

Although there is no clear evidence that radiation or chemotherapy has a significant impact on the outcome for patients with intramedullary spinal cord tumor, the role of surgery remains uncontested. If a pediatric patient with a low-grade intramedullary spinal cord tumor is treated with radical excision, long-term progression-free survival generally ensues, without the need for adjuvant treatment. Therefore, pediatric intramedullary tumors should be recognized as a "surgical disease," at the time of presentation and again at the time of recurrence. Because low-grade tumors in children possess very little potential to transform into high-grade ones,[53] we do not recommend radiation therapy for the preponderance of patients with residual low-grade intramedullary spinal cord tumors.

For subtotally resected and recurrent high-grade intramedullary spinal cord tumors, postoperative irradiation is advocated. Nonetheless, in children younger than 5 years, radiation should be avoided because of the detrimental effects on the growing central nervous system.[54, 55] Although the spinal cord is 10 to 15% lower than the brain in functional tolerance, susceptibility to the destructive effects of radiation increases with the extent of cord irradiation as well as with the total dose. Therapeutic irradiation in substantial doses over extensive segments of spinal cord may result in myelitis. In addition, irradiation subsequent to spinal surgery predisposes to kyphosis and subluxation. Finally, irradiation may induce the development of a second malignant tumor, with a rate of up to 20% over 30 years of follow-up.[53]

Regarding chemotherapy, present evidence points exclusively to benefits in low-grade gliomas of the brain.[56] Nevertheless, the Children's Cancer Group is evaluating various regimens for intramedullary spinal cord tumors. Ultimately, it is our conviction that this option should be employed only when there is evidence of tumor progression and dissemination, and within the confines of a protocol.

Intramedullary spinal cord glioblastomas invariably progress. The optimal treatment for this entity has yet to be determined.[29] Despite aggressive adjuvant therapy, patients with malignant intramedullary spinal cord tumors have a postoperative median survival of up to 12 months.[29] Most likely, this is the consequence of progressive infiltration of the tumor within the cord and through its pial banks, resulting in paraplegia, quadriplegia, and, eventually, death.

SUMMARY

Though considered inoperable a few decades ago, most intramedullary spinal cord tumors are now surgically curable. Aggressive resection using modern neurosurgical equipment and techniques, including the CUSA system and intraoperative electrophysiologic monitoring, enables the neurosurgeon to successfully excise the majority of these neoplasms. In such cases, patients may have long-term progression-free survival without the need for additional treatment. However, in cases of malignant lesions, the optimal postoperative treatment has not yet been determined.

To ensure likelihood of success, these lesions must be expeditiously diagnosed and treated.

REFERENCES

1. Elsberg CA, Beer E. The operability of intramedullary tumors of the spinal cord: a report of two operations with remarks upon the extrusion of intraspinal tumors. *Am J Med Sci* 1911;142:636–647.
2. Frazier CH. *Surgery of the Spine and Spinal Cord*. New York: D. Appleton & Co; 1918:37.
3. Coxe WS. Tumors of the spinal canal in children. *Am J Surg* 1961;27:62–73.
4. Guidetti B, Mercuri S, Vagnozzi R. Long term results of the surgical treatment of 129 intramedullary spinal gliomas. *J Neurosurg* 1981;54:323–330.
5. Greenwood JJ. Total removal of intramedullary tumors. *J Neurosurg* 1954;11:616–621.
6. Ahyai A, Woerner U, Markakis E. Surgical treatment of intramedullary tumors (spinal cord and medulla oblongata): analysis of 16 cases. *Neurosurg Rev* 1990;13:45–52.
7. Cooper PR. Outcome after operative treatment of intramedullary spinal cord tumors in adults: intermediate and long-term results in 51 patients. *Neurosurgery* 1989;25: 855–859.
8. Cooper PR, Epstein F. Radical resection of intramedullary spinal cord tumors in adults: recent experience in 29 patients. *J Neurosurg* 1985;63:492–499.
9. Epstein F, Epstein N. Surgical treatment of spinal cord astrocytomas of childhood: a series of 19 patients. *J Neurosurg* 1982;685–689.
10. Epstein F, Farmer JP, Freed D. Adult intramedullary astrocytoma of the spinal cord. *J Neurosurg* 1992;77:355–359.
11. Guidetti B. Intramedullary tumours of the spinal cord. *Acta Neurochir* 1967;17:7–23.
12. Guidetti B, Mercuri S, Vagnozzi R. Long term results of the surgical treatment of 129 intramedullary spinal gliomas. *J Neurosurg* 1981;54:323–330.
13. Malis LI. Intramedullary spinal cord tumors. *Clin Neurosurg* 1978;25:512–540.
14. Naidu MR, Dinakar I. Intramedullary mass lesions of the spinal cord. *Clin Neurol Neurosurg* 1989;91:135–138.
15. Rossitch EJ, Zeidman SM, Burger PC, et al. Clinical and pathological analysis of spinal cord astrocytomas in children. *Neurosurgery* 1990;27:193–196.
16. Stein B. Surgery of intramedullary spinal cord tumors. *Clin Neurosurg* 1979;26:529–542.
17. Admiraal P, Hazenberg GJ, Algra PR, et al. Spinal subarachnoid hemorrhage due to a filum terminale ependymoma. *Clin Neurol Neurosurg* 1992;94:69–72.
18. Shen WC, Ho YJ, Lee SK, et al. Ependymoma of the cauda equina presenting with subarachnoid hemorrhage. *Am J Neuroradiol* 1993;14:399–400.
19. Rifkinson-Mann S, Wisoff JH, Epstein F. The association of hydrocephalus with intramedullary spinal cord tumors: a series of 25 patients. *Neurosurgery* 1990;27: 749–754.
20. Tanaka H, Shimizu H, Ishijima B, et al. Myxopapillary ependymoma of the filum terminale with a holocord cyst: a case report [Japanese]. *No Shinkei Geka* 1986;14:997–1003.

21. Barnum SR, Jones JL, Benveniste EN. Interferon-gamma regulation of C3 gene expression in human astroglioma cells. *J Neuroimmunol* 1992;38:275–282.

22. Ransom DT, Ritland SR, Kimmel DW, et al. Cytogenetic and loss of heterozygosity studies in ependymomas, pilocytic astrocytomas, and oligodendrogliomas. *Genes Chrom Cancer* 1992;5:348–356.

23. Tabuchi K, Fukuyama K, Mineta T, et al. Altered structure and expression of the *p53* gene in human neuroepithelial tumors. *Neurol Med Chir (Tokyo)* 1992;32:725–732.

24. Van de Kelft, et al. Loss of constitutional heterozygosity in human astrocytomas. *Acta Neurochir (Wien)* 1992;117:172–177.

25. Von DA, Bender B, Jahnke R, et al. Loci associated with malignant progression in astrocytomas: a candidate on chromosome 19q. *Cancer Res* 1994;54:1397–1401.

26. Wu JK, Chikaraishi DM. Differential expression of ros oncogene in primary human astrocytomas and astrocytoma cell lines. *Cancer Res* 1990;50:3032–3055.

27. Russell DS, Rubinstein LJ. *Pathology of tumours of the nervous system*. Baltimore: Williams & Wilkins; 1989:83.

28. Constantini S, Houten J, Miller D, et al. Intramedullary spinal cord tumors in children under the age of three years. *J Neurosurg* 1996;85:1036–1043.

29. Cohen AR, Wisoff JH, Allen JC, et al. Malignant astrocytomas of the spinal cord. *J Neurosurg* 1989;70:50–74.

30. Raffel C, Edwards MSB. Intraspinal tumors in children. In: Youmans JR, ed. *Neurological Surgery*. Philadelphia: WB Saunders; 1990:3574–3588.

31. Alter M. Statistical aspects of spinal cord tumours. In: Vinken PJ, Bruyn GH, eds. *Handbook of Clinical Neurology*. Vol 19. *Tumors of the Spinal Cord*. Part I. Amsterdam: North-Holland; 1975:1–22.

32. Constantini S, Epstein F. Ultrasonic dissection. In: Wilkins RH, Rengachary SS, eds. *Neurosurgery*. New York: McGraw-Hill, 1995:607–608.

33. Slooff JL, Kernohan JW, MacCarty CS. *Primary Intramedullary Tumors of the Spinal Cord and Filum Terminale*. Philadelphia: WB Saunders, 1964.

34. Constantini S, Epstein F. Spinal ependymoma. In: Gilman S, Goldstein GW, Waxman SG, eds. Neurobase 1994, CD-ROM.

35. Constantini S, Epstein F. Intraspinal tumors in children and infants. In: Youmans JR, Becker DP, Dunsker SB, et al, eds. *Neurological Surgery*. Philadelphia: WB Saunders, 1994.

36. Wang AM, Lin JC, Haykal HA, et al. Ependymoma of filum terminale: metrizamide-enhanced CT evaluation. *Computed Radiol* 1986;10:239–243.

37. Nemoto Y, Inoue Y, Tashiro T, et al. Intramedullary spinal cord tumors: significance of associated hemorrhage at MR imaging. *Radiology* 1992;182:793–796.

38. Shoshan Y, Constantini S, Ashkenazi E, et al. Intramedullary spinal cord renal carcinoma metastasis diagnosed by gadolinium enhanced MRI. *Neuro-orthopedics* 1991;11:117–123.

39. Epstein F, Farmer JP, Schneider SJ. Intraoperative ultrasonography: an important adjunct for intramedullary tumors. *J Neurosurg* 1991;74:729–733.

40. Dam HP, Houidi K, Person H, et al. Contribution of ultrasonic cavitation—CO_2 laser combination in the excision of panmedullary ependymoma [Review] [French]. *Neurochirurgie* 1992;38:376–380.

41. Epstein F, Ozek M. The plated bayonet: a new instrument to facilitate surgery for intra-axial neoplasms of the spinal cord and brain stem. *J Neurosurg* 1993;78:505.

42. Deletis V. Intraoperative monitoring of the functional integrity of the motor pathways. *Adv Neurol* 1994;64:201–214.

43. Loughnan BA, Anderson SK, Hetreed MA, et al. Effects of Halothane on motor evoked potentials recorded in the extradural space. *Br J Anesth* 1989;63:561–564.

44. Deletis V. Intraoperative monitoring of the functional integrity of the motor pathways. In: Devinsky O, Beric A, Dogali M, eds. *Electrical and Magnetic Stimulation of the Brain and Spinal Cord*. New York: Raven Press; 1993:201–214.

45. Lang EW, Chestnut RM, Beutler AS, et al. The utility of motor-evoked potential monitoring during intramedullary surgery. *Anesth Analg* 1996;83:1337–1341.

46. Levy WJ, York DH, McCaffrey M, et al. Motor evoked potentials from transcranial stimulation of the motor cortex in humans. *Neurosurgery* 1984;15:287–302.

47. Zentner J. Noninvasive motor evoked potential monitoring during neurosurgical operations in the spinal cord. *Neurosurgery* 1989;24:709–712.

48. Zide BM. How to reduce the morbidity of wound closure following extensive and complicated laminectomy and tethered cord surgery. *Pediatr Neurosurg* 1992;18:157–166.

49. Zide BM, Wisoff JH, Epstein F. Closure of extensive and complicated laminectomy wounds. *J Neurosurg* 1987;67:59–64.

50. Sim FH, Svien HJ, Bicket WH, et al. Swan neck deformity following extensive laminectomy. *J Bone Joint Surg* 1967;49:564.

51. Costantinini S (personal communication).

52. Leahu D, Abbott R, Wisoff JH, et al. The effect of laminoplasty versus laminectomy in operations for the removal of intramedullary spinal cord tumors. Pediatric Section of the American Association of Neurological Surgeons, 1992.

53. Dirks PB, Jay V, Becker LE, et al. Development of anaplastic changes in low-grade astrocytomas of childhood. *Neurosurgery* 1994;34:68–78.

54. Clayton PE, Shalet SM. The evolution of spinal growth after irradiation. *Clin Oncol* 1991;3:220–222.

55. Duffner PK, Horowitz ME, Krischer JP, et al. Postoperative chemotherapy and delayed radiation in children less than three years of age with malignant brain tumors. *N Engl J Med* 1993;328:1725–1731.

56. Packer RJ, Ater JA, Allen J, et al. Carboplatin and vincristine chemotherapy for children with newly diagnosed progressive low-grade gliomas. *J Neurosurg* 1997;86:747–754.

Chapter 31

Ependymoma

Steven J. Schneider and Alan D. Rosenthal

Ependymoma is a relatively rare neoplasm that accounts for approximately 10% of primary central nervous system (CNS) tumors in children.[1] Although 50% of ependymomas occur in the first two decades of life,[2] it is estimated that in the United States only 100 new cases occur each year in children younger than 15 years.[3] In childhood, 90% of ependymomas are intracranial, whereas 10% are intraspinal. Conversely, in adults, 40% of ependymomas are intracranial and 60% are intraspinal.[4]

These spinal tumors arise from ependymal cells lining the central canal or from cell clusters in the filum terminale. As primary spinal neoplasms, they present either as intramedullary tumors above the conus or as intradural extramedullary tumors of the cauda equina involving the filum terminale, conus medullaris, or both. Rarely are they ectopic in origin, more commonly involving the sacrococcygeal region anterior to the sacrum (presacral) or posterior in the subcutaneous tissues.[5–7] Primary intracranial ependymomas may metastasize distally via the meninges to the spinal axis.[8, 9] Intramedullary and extramedullary tumors represent distinct clinicopathologic entities, and these distinctions are emphasized. The authors have also included their personal experience with the management of seven primary spinal ependymomas between 1987 and 1997.

INCIDENCE

Spinal tumors compose approximately 15% of primary CNS tumors in children, with primary spinal ependymomas representing 10% of those occurring in children 18 years or younger.[10] There is a varied distribution of spinal cord tumors in children, as opposed to adults. In children, approximately 35% are intramedullary, and 30% are intradural and extramedullary.[10–12] In the adult population, approximately 20% are intramedullary, and 60% are intradural and extramedullary.[12, 13] Up to 30% of pediatric intramedullary tumors are ependymomas, whereas in the adult population ependymomas can exceed 50%.[11, 14] In pediatric intramedullary tumors, ependymomas occur two to four times less frequently than astrocytomas. Similarly, intramedullary tumors above the conus in children younger than 10 years have only a 10% incidence of ependymoma versus a 75% incidence of astrocytoma or gangli-

oglioma.[14–16] The highest incidence of intramedullary glioma in childhood is in the 10- to 16-year age group,[14] whereas the highest incidence of astrocytoma and ependymoma is in the 10- to 15-year age group.[17] Primary intradural extramedullary ependymomas, with rare exception, arise from the filum terminale and conus medullaris. Filum terminale ependymomas represent at least 40 to 50% of spinal ependymomas in adults, as opposed to only 8 to 14% in children younger than 16 years.[10, 18, 19] In a review of 26 cases, Gagliardi et al reported a peak incidence for children between 10 and 16 years of age.[20] In adults, the peak incidence remains between the third and fifth decades of life.[13] Spinal ependymomas in children younger than 5 years of age are rare. DiLorenzo et al reported a 75% occurrence rate in children older than 5 years.[10] The literature reports a variable but insignificant sex preference for pediatric intramedullary ependymomas.[10, 14, 17] However, in childhood myxopapillary filum tumors, there is a male-to-female ratio of 1.9:1[20]; the ratio is less pronounced in adult myxopapillary tumors.[13]

In our series conducted between 1987 and 1997, of 7 primary spinal ependymomas occurring in children 18 years or younger similar to other series, 4 were intramedullary and 3 were found in the filum (Table 31–1). There was no sex preference seen in the intramedullary tumors; however, 2 of the 3 filum tumors were found in males. The age distribution correlates with the older peak for ependymoma, as compared with astrocytoma (Fig. 31–1).

TABLE 31–1 Tumor Type

Pathology	Number	Male	Female
Ependymoma	4	2	2
Filum ependymoma	3	2	1
Astrocytoma	16	9	7
Ganglioglioma	2	1	1
Dermoid	1	1	
Lipoma	1		1
Hemangioblastoma	1		1

The authors thank Dr. Joseph A. Epstein and Ms. Sherry Lynn Grimm for their assistance in the editing and preparation of this chapter.

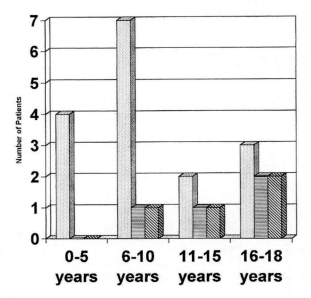

Figure 31–1 Age distribution and tumor type.

LOCATION

Both pediatric intramedullary astrocytomas and ependymomas demonstrate a rostral preference in the spinal axis.[14] Age-related differences remain controversial. In 1982, DiLorenzo et al reported a 31% incidence of cervical cord involvement in children,[10] whereas in 1994 Epstein and Ragheb reported a 46% incidence of cervical cord involvement in childhood, as compared with 28% in adults.[14] In the review by McCormick and Stein, there was a 68% incidence in adults, reflecting the more aggressive surgical approach that has been applied to these lesions.[11] Steinbok et al emphasized that the incidence of cervical cord involvement in children may actually be higher than previously cited for similar reasons.[12] The distribution of intramedullary tumors in our series reflects a 65% cervical cord involvement for ependymomas and astrocytomas (Table 31–2).

Intraspinal ependymomas in childhood are rare and are often grouped with those of adults when reported in the literature. There is a relative paucity of information extracted from case reports and retrospective studies prior to the advent of magnetic resonance imaging (MRI) and advancements in surgical technology. Therefore, the data derived must be interpreted with caution.

TABLE 31–2   Tumor Location

Location	Ependymoma	Astrocytoma
Cervicomedullary	1	5
Cervical	1	3
Cervicothoracic	1	4
Thoracic	1	4
Filum	3	0

TUMOR PATHOLOGY

The histologic classification and grading system for ependymal neoplasms is somewhat controversial; a division prevails between non-anaplastic (benign) and anaplastic malignant lesions.[21] The benign group is composed of two types: classical ependymoma with several variants and myxopapillary ependymoma.[22, 23] Histologically, classical ependymoma is a benign-appearing dense cellular tumor characterized by prominent perivascular pseudorosette formation (Fig. 31–2). True rosette formation is less common. *Infiltration of the surrounding neural tissue does not occur, and a sharp demarcation creates a surgical cleavage plane.* Benign histologic variants most commonly include the cellular, papillary, and clear cell subtypes. Nomenclature varies depending on the classification schema utilized.[22–26] In all age groups, the classical ependymoma and its cellular subtype account for the vast majority of intramedullary tumors above the conus medullaris.[22, 23, 25] These intramedullary tumors rarely, if ever, seed the cerebrospinal pathways or metastasize to other parts of the body. Myxopapillary ependymoma, a unique ependymoma, is usually restricted to the filum terminale.[22, 23, 27] Its rarely reported in the brain or in ectopic locations.[5–7, 28, 29] Although other subtypes of ependymoma may occur in the filum terminale in childhood, immunohistochemical staining has demonstrated that myxopapillary forms account for at least 90% of the pathologic lesions.[27] The same predilection is seen in adults. Myxopapillary ependymoma has become synonymous with filum ependymoma, and the terms are used interchangeably in the literature. It typically possesses a papillary arrangement of columnar cells around a vascularized center of acellular hyalinized connective tissue (Fig. 31–3). There appear to be intracellular and perivascular accumulations of mucin.[22, 23, 27] This imitates the degenerative changes seen in the filum during development.[13] In childhood, these tumors have been reported to metastasize, despite their benign histologic appearance and after gross total resection, whereas in adults this rarely occurs.[20] Metastases outside the CNS are

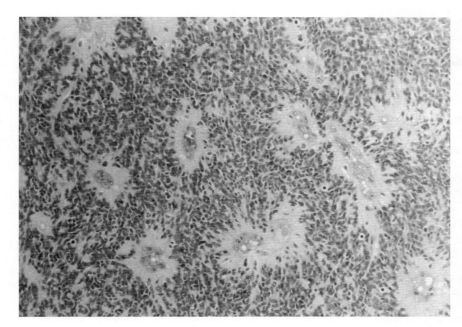

Figure 31–2 Photomicrograph of a classical ependymoma demonstrating pseudorosette formation (33× magnification).

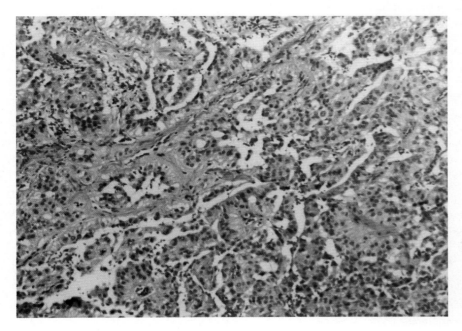

Figure 31–3 Photomicrograph of a myxopapillary ependymoma demonstrating typical papillary arrangement of cells around an acellular hyalinized spinal cord (25× magnification).

extremely rare, but they are more likely to occur in myxopapillary tumors arising ectopically.[20, 27] Anaplastic or malignant ependymoma is rare in the spinal cord.[30, 31] DiMarco et al reported an incidence of approximately 3%.[31] Nuclear pleomorphism, high cell density, necrosis, endothelial proliferation, and increased mitotic figures distinguish this tumor from a benign process.[32] These tumors may recur with an increased incidence and may metastasize within the CNS.[30, 33] Extraneural metastases are extremely rare.[34] Currently, there is significant controversy over the importance of histologic appearance as a prognostic factor. Schiffer et al demonstrated that this correlation for intracranial ependymoma is variable,

but no prognostic factors for spinal ependymoma have been identified.[32] Ross and Rubenstein similarly reported a variable prognosis for malignant ependymoma.[35] In our series, all of the spinal tumors were histologically benign, with four intramedullary tumors being classic ependymomas and three filum tumors being myxopapillary.

Spinal ependymoma may be secondary to a primary intracranial tumor that has metastasized. Approximately 5% of all newly diagnosed intracranial ependymomas will have clinical evidence of spinal metastasis along the cerebrospinal fluid (CSF) pathways.[36, 37] This is more commonly seen in infratentorial high-grade malignant tumors.[21] Surgery plays little, if any, role in their management, and treatment relies heavily on adjunctive radiotherapy and chemotherapy. The prognosis for these children remains poor.

NEUROFIBROMATOSIS

Intramedullary spinal cord ependymoma appears to be associated with neurofibromatosis.[38, 39] Lee et al reported 9 intramedullary tumors, 5 ependymomas and 4 astrocytomas, in patients with neurofibromatosis type 2 (NF-2).[38] *The ependymomas occurred in the patients with NF-2 whereas astrocytomas occurred in association with NF-1.* The gene for NF-2 resides on chromosome 22. The gene product of the NF-2 gene (*merlin* or *schwannomin*) is believed to play a role in the inhibition of cell contact. It is highly homologous to a family of proteins that include moesin, erzin, radixin, and erythrocyte.[40, 41] Some authors postulate that mutations in this gene can cause tumor growth.[39, 40] Research regarding the molecular genetics of ependymoma has revealed deletions or translocation of chromosome 22 in 12 of 30 cases.[4] A familial anaplastic ependymoma has been associated with monosomy 22.[41] More recently, Birch et al demonstrated NF-2 gene transcript mutations occurring in 5 of 7 sporadically occurring spinal ependymomas.[42] There appears to be a relationship between the NF-2 gene and ependymoma, but this has not been clearly defined.

CLINICAL FEATURES

Symptoms

Early diagnosis of spinal ependymoma remains difficult despite the advent of MRI, due in part to the slow growth and evolution of these usually benign tumors. Symptoms may fluctuate relative to peritumoral edema.[16, 18] Occasionally, symptoms are precipitated by mild spinal trauma, further delaying the diagnosis.[18] The mean duration of symptoms for pediatric spinal tumors ranges from 9.2 months to 2 years.[15] Delays in diagnosis for several years are not uncom-

mon. Gagliardi et al reported an average duration of symptoms for childhood myxopapillary ependymomas of 13.3 months.[20] In our series, the mean duration of symptoms for intramedullary ependymoma was 11 months (range 4 to 26 months). The mean duration of symptoms for filum ependymomas was 9 months (range 2 to 19 months). The duration of symptoms may influence outcome,[30] and it is therefore imperative to maintain a high index of suspicion for children with persistent symptomatology. Delayed diagnostic testing is unjustifiable.

The most prevalent symptom found in both intramedullary and filum ependymomas is pain, usually localized to the level of the lesion and less commonly radicular in nature. In our series, pain was a presenting symptom in 6 of 7 (86%) childhood spinal ependymomas (Table 31–3). Epstein and Ragheb reported pain as the presenting symptom in 70% of intramedullary tumors, whereas radicular pain occurred in only 10%.[14] Gagliardi et al reported pain in 80% of pediatric myxopapillary filum ependymomas.[20] Typically, the pain is exacerbated by recumbent positioning and awakens the child at night. Gait disturbance, which is another common symptom, is usually indicative of lower-extremity weakness.[15] It may also be associated with spasticity and/or pain. In our series, gait disturbance was a presenting symptom in 5 of 7 (71%) patients (Table 31–3). DeSousa et al[43] reported gait disturbances in 65% and Lunardi et al[44] in 80% of children with spinal tumors. Other symptoms include weakness, impairment of sensation, torticollis, neck stiffness, scoliosis, and sphincteric disturbance.[12] Bulbar symptoms may be seen with cervicomedullary tumors with significant rostral extension.

Hydrocephalus with increased intracranial pressure may occur in up to 15% of patients with intramedullary tumors. Rifkinson-Mann et al reported on 25 patients with intramedullary spinal cord tumors with hydrocephalus, in which 23 of 25 (92%) were 18 years of age or younger, appearing most commonly with malignant tumors.[45] Only one incident of spinal ependymoma was cited. The mechanism was attributed either to obstruction of CSF pathways by rostral extension of the tumor and cyst or to subarachnoid seeding.[45] Spinal cord tumors rarely present as subarachnoid hemorrhage.[46]

TABLE 31–3 Neurologic Symptoms

Symptom	Intramedullary ependymoma $n = 4$	Intramedullary astrocytoma $n = 16$	Filum ependymoma $n = 3$
Pain	3 (75%)	11 (69%)	3 (100%)
Gait disturbance	3 (75%)	12 (75%)	2 (66%)
Weakness	1 (25%)	4 (25%)	1 (33%)
Sensory loss	1 (25%)	4 (25%)	1 (33%)
Paresthesias	1 (25%)	3 (19%)	0
Torticollis	0	3 (19%)	0
Sphincteric	0	1 (6%)	1 (33%)
Scoliosis	1 (25%)	4 (25%)	0

Signs

Physical examination of a child with a spinal ependymoma usually reveals signs correlating with the level of the tumor. In our series, hyperreflexia and spastic lower-extremity paresis were the most common neurologic signs (Table 31–4).

In the cervical region, neck stiffness, torticollis, and decreased range of motion can be seen secondary to the accompanying pain. Weakness can occur in both the upper and lower extremities. The paresis can reflect upper motor neuron pathology, and atrophy may be associated with spasticity or lower motor involvement. Rostral tumors are associated with weakness late in their course, in contrast to caudal tumors, wherein patients exhibit hand weakness and atrophy early on. Sensory examination consistent with level specificity occurs late in the course.[15, 16] Ependymomas more commonly are associated with a suspended sensory level due to more central locations, in contrast to astrocytomas. Sphincter disturbance is rare and tends to be a late occurrence.[16]

Thoracic tumors commonly present with a neuro-orthopedic deformity, such as scoliosis or kyphosis.[12, 14] Scoliosis with convex to the right is commonly seen with idiopathic cases, whereas that with convex to the left more commonly reflects the presence of a tumor or syrinx.[12] Typically, spastic paraparesis is seen with associated hyperreflexia, increased tone, and positive Babinski responses. Sphincter dysfunction, usually rare and occurring late, is similar to that seen in cervical cord tumors.[16]

Conus and filum tumors may lack objective findings, even late in their course, relative to the ample space in the lumbar thecal sac and the mobile nature of the cauda equina. However, sphincteric dysfunction is more common.[20, 47] A saddle-type sensory loss, decreased sphincter tone, and diminished anal reflexes can be seen. When sphincteric disturbance is part of the initial complaint, it is usually indicative of the presence of a conus lesion.[14]

RADIOLOGY

Plain X Rays

Abnormalities on plain X ray have been noted in up to 63% of ependymomas and 80% of astrocytomas,[12, 48] including scoliosis, canal widening, vertebral body scalloping, and pedicle erosion. Osseous erosion is reported more commonly in ependymomas of the filum and conus, as compared to intramedullary lesions above the conus.[48] However, since the advent of MRI the diagnostic role of X-ray studies has faded. They remain useful for the assessment of spinal alignment and fusion following laminoplasty during the growth of the child.

Computed Tomography/Myelography

Computed tomography (CT) scan following intravenous contrast injection (CT-myelography) may reveal an enhancing solid mass or a blocked spinal canal. However, these imaging modalities have proven ineffective, and thus are rarely utilized for the diagnosis of spinal ependymoma, due in large part to the efficacy of MRI.

TABLE 31–4   Neurologic Signs

Sign	Intramedullary ependymoma $n = 4$	Intramedullary astrocytoma $n = 16$	Filum ependymoma $n = 3$
Hyperreflexia	3 (75%)	14 (88%)	1 (33%)
Spastic paresis, LE	3 (75%)	12 (75%)	1 (33%)
Spastic paresis, UE	1 (25%)	4 (25%)	0
Atrophy (hands)	0	2 (13%)	0
Sensory loss	1 (25%)	4 (25%)	1 (33%)
Decreased sphincter reflexes	0	1 (6%)	1 (33%)
Decreased neck ROM	1 (25%)	4 (25%)	0
Bulbar signs	0	1 (6%)	0

LE, lower extremities; UE, upper extremities; ROM, range of motion.

Magnetic Resonance Imaging

MRI has become the diagnostic procedure of choice for spinal ependymoma, defining the precise location of the tumor and its relationship to the spinal cord and cauda equina. MRI also distinguishes solid from cystic components of the lesion. Localization of the exact levels of the solid portion of the tumor is a considerable aid in preoperative surgical planning.

The MRI appearance of spinal ependymoma is similar in children and adults. In intramedullary tumors, the majority of the T1-weighted images are isointense in comparison with the cord. Occasionally they may be hypointense and rarely may be hyperintense. The cord appears symmetrically expanded over the level of solid tumor.[48, 49] Tumors of the filum and conus are typically hyperintense on T1-weighted images.[49] This has been attributed to the mucinous content of myxopapillary tumors. On the T2-weighted sequences, both tumors usually appear hyperintense, in comparison with the cord. A hypointense rim or cap on T2-weighted images may be seen in 20 to 64% of tumors representing hemosiderin.[49, 50] These appear more frequently in the cervical region and are presumed to result from tumor movement, with a sharp interface creating occult bleeding.[50]

The administration of gadolinium-diethylenetriamine-pentaacetic acid typically reveals a sharply marginated and enhancing centrally located mass[49] (Figs. 31–4 and 31–5).

The enhancement has classically been described as homogeneous, but it can be heterogeneous (Fig. 31–6). Kahan et al reported an incidence of 38% homogeneous, 31% heterogeneous, 19% rim, 6% minimal, and 6% no enhancement.[48]

Cysts can be associated with spinal ependymomas in up to 60% of cases.[48] On MRI they appear hypointense on T1- and hyperintense on T2-weighted images. They may appear intratumoral, rostral/caudal, or as reactive dilatations of the central canal.[48] Lohle et al demonstrated that the fluid in syrinxes associated with spinal cord ependymomas was exudative.[51] Samii and Klekamp reported that the contents of syrinxes associated with intramedullary tumors might be multifactorial, relative to transudate or secretion from the tumor, or due to interference of CSF flow by the tumor creating increased fluid within the cord.[52] The number of segments spanned by a tumor can vary significantly depending on the presence of cysts. Zimmerman and Balaniuk note that ependymomas are usually confined to five segments and that holocord involvement is rare.[53] *Distinguishing intramedullary ependymomas from astrocytomas may be difficult.* However, astrocytomas tend to expand the cord more asymmetrically and are less centrally located than ependymomas. They may not be as sharply marginated as ependymomas[48] and have a greater propensity to involve the holocord.[54] Complete cystic degeneration is more likely to occur in astrocytoma.[55]

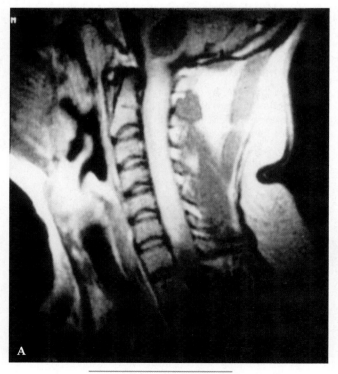
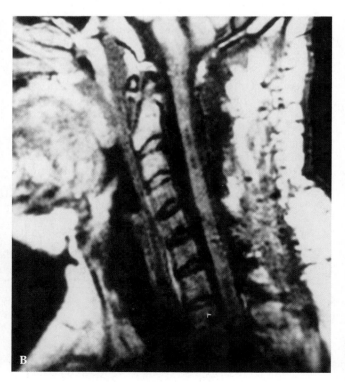

Figure 31–4 (A) Preoperative magnetic resonance image with gadolinium enhancement revealing a sharply marginated ependymoma extending to the upper cervical region with a typical rostral cyst. (B) Postoperative gadolinium-enhanced magnetic resonance image of the same patient revealing gross total resection of tumor.

nosus reflex, providing continuous data during manipulation.[74] This could be particularly useful during tumor removal in the region of the conus. Although the overall benefits are controversial, the authors remain convinced that there have been instances in which neurologic damage has been avoided.

COMPLICATIONS

Neurologic Deterioration

During the immediate postoperative period, most patients demonstrate some degree of neurologic deterioration. This is usually transient and often involves proprioceptive loss that is the result of manipulation of the posterior columns.[11, 17] Initial postoperative neurologic function directly correlates with preoperative function. In a study of 45 patients with intramedullary astrocytomas and ependymomas, who demonstrated moderate neurologic impairment, Innocenzi et al reported an initial postoperative transient worsening in 60% of those with astrocytomas and in 50% of those with ependymomas. The tumor type was also important. At the time of discharge, the proportion of patients whose neurologic status worsened postoperatively was higher in children with astrocytoma than in those with ependymoma, despite similar preoperative functional levels. Long-term follow-up also demonstrated better neurologic condition in patients with ependymomas.[17] Epstein reported an overall 5% incidence of significant motor worsening if spinal cord function was intact preoperatively.[15] *Crisante similarly demonstrated the direct relationship between the preoperative neurologic condition and surgical outcome.*[75] When one includes the adult literature for spinal ependymoma, it becomes evident that patients in good preoperative condition tended to maintain or improve their neurologic status, whereas those in fair condition remained stable and those in poor condition did not improve significantly.[11, 76]

Spinal Deformity

The occurrence of spinal deformities following laminectomy for excision of a spinal tumor is well documented, with kyphotic deformities being most prevalent.[64, 77–79] Such deformities can be new or can be exacerbations of a preoperative condition. Lunardi et al reported new postoperative spinal deformities in 24% of children undergoing laminectomies for intramedullary tumors. In nine patients, preoperative spinal deformities progressed following laminectomy. All patients were treated conservatively with external immobilization for 5 years or until growth was completed. The postoperative incidence of spinal deformities following multilevel laminectomies ranges from 25% to 41%.[44] In younger patients with high-level laminectomies, there is a greater risk even if the facets are left intact.[12, 44] In a series of 45 patients, Epstein compared simple and osteoplastic laminectomies. On review, the incidence of progressive kyphosis was 15% in the osteoplastic group versus 36% in those undergoing simple laminectomies. It is interesting that all of the osteoplastic laminectomized children who had progressive deformity demonstrated recurrent tumor.[15] Some authors[12, 44] have recommended postoperative bracing, but this has no proven benefit.[64] We strongly consider bracing if a significant preoperative deformity exists.

PROGNOSIS AND OUTCOME

The overall 5-year survival for spinal ependymoma is better than that for astrocytomas, ranging from 70% to 100%.[11, 31] Spinal ependymoma has a recurrence rate of 10 to 30%,[27, 30] and the prognosis appears to be dependent on multiple factors.

EXTENT OF RESECTION

Numerous reports have clearly documented the benefits of gross total resection of these tumors.[11, 16, 17, 27, 30, 31, 44, 47, 56–58, 60] Although recurrence may still occur at a rate of up to 10%, the rate following subtotal resection is approximately 20%,[27] with some series reporting a 0 to 5% recurrence rate following gross total resection.[30] The degree of resectability correlates with the clinical appearance of the tumor. Infiltrating and adherent tumors do not lend themselves to gross total resection and hence offer an increased risk for residual or recurrent lesions. This has prompted the current use of radiotherapy to prolong survival of patients with subtotally resected tumors.

CLINICAL HISTORY

Cervoni et al demonstrated that a clinical history of less than 1 year was associated with a recurrence rate of 0%; 12 to 24 months had a risk of recurrence of 22%, increasing to 60% at 60 months.[30] In addition, recurrence of spinal cord tumor correlates with a lower 5-year survival and poorer prognosis, as reported by Cervoni et al.[30] This supports the theory that the demarcation of the tumor is lost over time as it infiltrates the cord,[19] leading to decreased resectability and to a poor neurologic and functional prognosis.

Patients exhibiting a better neurologic condition preoperatively tend to fare better postoperatively.

HISTOLOGY

Some studies have proposed that myxopapillary tumors of childhood have a more aggressive biological process.[20] The review by Cervoni et al, focusing on recurrence, did not bear this out nor did it correlate with age.[30] Whereas anaplastic histology correlates poorly for intracranial ependymomas, this does not appear to be the case for spinal cord ependymomas. Although rare (3%), tumors in this malignant subgroup historically have a more aggressive course,[31, 56] with high recurrence rates despite gross total resection; therefore, radiotherapy is recommended.

LOCATION

The significance of location is controversial insofar as prognosis is concerned. Both Ferrante and Crisante found location in the cervical cord to be a poor prognostic indicator.[75, 80] However, Cervoni et al did not find any correlation with location.[30]

FOLLOW-UP

Patients should be monitored with routine annual postoperative MRI with gadolinium enhancement primarily because of the possibility of delayed recurrence.

SUMMARY

Primary spinal cord ependymomas in childhood are relatively uncommon lesions. They have a long natural history. The tumor is usually benign and sharply demarcated from surrounding neural tissue. Gross total surgical resection is the treatment of choice, and radiotherapy is recommended following subtotal removal, recurrence, or in the presence of malignancy. Prompt diagnosis and surgical intervention is crucial, as it appears that resectability and prognosis decline with delays in treatment.

REFERENCES

1. Dohrman GJ, Farwell JR, Flannery JT. Ependymomas and ependymoblastomas in Children. *J Neurosurg* 1976;5:273–283.
2. Dohrman GJ. Ependymomas. In: Wilkins RH, Rengachary SS, eds. *Neurosurgery*. Vol. 1. New York: McGraw-Hill, 1985:767–771.
3. Chiu JK, Woo SY, Ater J, et al. Intracranial ependymoma in children: analysis of prognostic factors. *J Neuro-oncol* 1992;13:283–290.
4. Hamilton RL, Pollack IF. The molecular biology of ependymoma. *Brain Pathol* 1997;7:807–822.
5. Domingues RC, Mikulis D, Swearingen B, et al. Subcutaneous myxopapillary ependymoma: CT and MR finding (Letter). *Am J Neuroradiol* 1991;12:171–172.
6. Pulitzer DR, Martin PC, Collins PC, et al. Subcutaneous sacrococcygeal ("myxopapillary") ependymal rests. *Am J Clin Pathol* 1988;12:672–677.
7. Helwig EB, Stern JB. Subcutaneous myxopapillary ependymoma: a clinicopathologic study of 32 cases. *Am J Clin Pathol* 1984;81:156–161.
8. Packer RJ, Siegel KR. Leptomeningeal dissemination of primary central nervous system tumors of childhood. *Ann Neurol* 1985;18:217–221.
9. Merchant TE, Haida T, Ming-Hisien W, et al. Anaplastic ependymoma: treatment of pediatric patients with and without craniospinal radiation therapy. *J Neurosurg* 1997;86:943–949.
10. DiLorenzo N, Giuffre R, Fortuna A. Primary spinal neoplasms in childhood: analysis of 1234 published cases (including 56 personal cases) by pathology, sex, age and site: differences from the adult. *Neurochirurgia* 1982;25:153–164.
11. McCormick PC, Stein BM. Intramedullary tumors in adults. *Neurosurg Clin North Am* 1990;1(3):609–630.
12. Steinbok P, Cochrane DD, Poskitt K. Intramedullary spinal cord tumors in children. *Neurosurg Clin North Am* 1992;3(4):931–945.
13. McCormick PC, Post KD, Stein BM. Intradural extramedullary in adults. *Neurosurg Clin North Am* 1990;1(3):591–608.
14. Epstein FJ, Ragheb J. Intramedullary tumors of the spinal cord. In: Cheek WR, ed. *Pediatric Neurosurgery: Surgery of the Developing Nervous System*. 3rd ed. Philadelphia: WB Saunders; 1994:446–457.
15. Constantini S, Epstein FJ. Intraspinal tumors of infants and children. In: Youmans JR, ed. *Neurological Surgery*. 4th ed. Vol. 4. Philadelphia: WB Saunders, 1997:3123–3133.
16. Epstein FJ, Farmer JP. Pediatric spinal cord surgery. *Neurosurg Clin North Am* 1990;1(3):569–590.
17. Innocenzi G, Raco A, Giampaolo C, et al. Intramedullary astrocytomas and ependymoma in the pediatric age group: a retrospective study. *Child's Nerv Syst* 1996; 12:776–780.
18. Arseni C, Horvath L, Iliescu D. Intraspinal tumors in children. *Psych Neuro Neurochir* 1967;70:123–133.
19. Slooff JL, Kernohan JW, MacCarty CS. *Primary Tumors of the Spinal Cord and Filum Terminale*. Philadelphia: WB Saunders; 1964:1–130.
20. Gagliardi FM, Cervoni L, Domenicucci M, et al. Ependymomas of the filum terminale in childhood: report of four cases and review of the literature. *Child's Nerv Syst* 1993;9:3–6.
21. Cobb CS, McDonald JD, Edwards MSB. Ependymomas. In: Youmans JR, ed. *Neurological Surgery*. 4th ed. Vol. 4. Philadelphia: WB Saunders; 1997:2553–2569.
22. Burger PC, Scheithauer BW. Tumors of the central nervous system. *AFIP Atlas of Tumor Pathology*. Third Series. Fascicle 10. Washington, DC: Armed Forces Institute of Pathology; 1994:20–43.
23. Burger PC, Scheithauer BW, Vogel FS. *Surgical Pathology of the Nervous System and Its Coverings*. 3rd ed. New York: Churchill Livingstone; 1991:271–289.
24. Rorke LB, Gilles FH, Davis RL, et al. Revision of the World Health Organization Classification of Brain Tumors for Childhood Brain Tumors. *Cancer* 1985;56: 1869–1886.
25. Russell DS, Rubinstein LJ. Tumours of central neuroepithelial origin. In: Russell DS, Rubinstein LJ, eds. *Pathology of Tumors of the Central Nervous System*. 5th ed. Baltimore: Williams & Wilkins; 1989;192–206.
26. Kleihues P, Burger PC, Scheithauer BW. *Histological Typing of Tumours of the Central Nervous System*. 2nd ed. WHO International Histological Classification of Tumours. New York: Springer-Verlag; 1993:112.
27. Sonneland PR, Scheitauer BW, Onofrio BM. Myxopapillary ependymoma: a clinicopathologic and immunohistochemical study of 77 cases. *Cancer* 1985;56:883–893.
28. Maruyama R, Koga K, Nakahara T, et al. Cerebral myxopapillary ependymoma. *Hum Pathol* 1992;23:960–962.
29. Warbick RE, Raisanen J, Adornato BT, et al. Intracranial myxopapillary ependymoma: case report. *J Neuro-oncol* 1993;15:251–256.
30. Cervoni L, Celli P, Fortuna A, et al. Recurrence of spinal ependymoma (risk factors and long-term survival). *Spine* 1994;19:2838–2841.
31. DiMarco A, Griso C, Pradella F, et al. Postoperative management of primary spinal ependymomas. *Acta Oncologica* 1988;27:371–375.
32. Schiffer D, Chio A, Gordana MT, et al. Histologic prognostic factors in ependymoma. *Child's Nerv Syst* 1991;7:177–182.
33. Fujiyama K, Masao K, Fuji H, et al. Anaplastic ependymoma of the spinal cord in childhood (a case report). *Acta Pathologica Japonica* 1990;40:376–382.
34. Newton JB, Henson J, Walker RW. Extraneural metastasis in ependymoma. *J Neuro-oncol* 1992;14:135–142.
35. Ross GW, Rubenstein LJ. Lack of histopathological correlation of malignant ependymomas with postoperative survival. *J Neurosurg* 1989;70:31–36.
36. Salazar OM, Castro-Vita H, VanHoutte P, et al. Improved survival in cases of intracranial ependymoma after radiation therapy: late report and recommendations. *J Neurosurg* 1983;59:652–659.
37. Salazar OM, Rubin P, Bassano D, et al. Improved survival of patients with intracranial ependymomas by irradiation: dose selection and field extension. *Cancer* 1975; 35:1563–1573.

38. Lee ML, Rezai AR, Freed D, et al. Intramedullary spinal cord tumors in neurofibromatosis. *Neurosurgery* 1996;38:32–37.

39. Rodriguez HA, Berthong M. Multiple primary intracranial tumors in von Recklinghausen's neurofibromatosis. *Arch Neurol* 1966;14:467–475.

40. Troffater JA, MacCollin MM, Rutter JL, et al. A novel moesin-, ezrin-, radixin-like gene is a candidate for neurofibromatosis 2 tumor suppressor. *Cell* 1993;72:791–800.

41. Nijssen PC, Lekanne Deprez RH, Tijssen CC, et al. Familial anaplastic ependymoma: evidence of loss of chromosome 22 in tumor cells. *J Neurol Neurosurg Psychiatry* 1994;57:1245–1248.

42. Birch BD, Johnson JP, Parsa A, et al. Frequent type 2 neurofibromatosis gene transcript mutations in sporadic intramedullary spinal cord ependymomas. *Neurosurgery* 1996;39:135–140.

43. DeSousa AL, Kalsbeck JE, Mealey J, et al. Intraspinal tumors in children: a review of 81 cases. *J Neurosurg* 1979; 51:437–445.

44. Lunardi P, Licastro G, Missori P, et al. Management of intramedullary tumors in children. *Acta Neurochir (Wien)* 1993;120:59–65.

45. Rifkinson-Mann S, Wishoff JH, Epstein FJ. The association of hydrocephalus with intramedullary spinal cord tumors: a series of 25 patients. *Neurosurgery* 1990;27:749–754.

46. Bhandari YS. Subarachnoid hemorrhage due to cervical cord tumor in a child: a case report. *J Neurosurg* 1969;30: 749–751.

47. Schweitzer JS, Batzdorf U. Ependymoma of the cauda equina region: diagnosis, treatment and outcome in 15 patients. *Neurosurgery* 1992;30:202–207.

48. Kahan H, Sklar EM, Post JD, et al. MR characteristics of histopathologic subtypes of spinal ependymoma. *Am J Neuroradiol* 1996;17:143–150.

49. Fine MJ, Kricheff II, Freed D, et al. Spinal cord ependymomas: MR imaging features. *Radiology* 1995;197: 665–658.

50. Nemoto Y, Inoue Y, Tashira T, et al. Intramedullary spinal cord tumors: significance of associated hemorrhage at MR imaging. *Radiology* 1992;182:793–796.

51. Lohle PN, Wurzer HA, Hoogland PH, et al. The pathogenesis of syringomyelia in spinal cord ependymoma. *Clin Neurol Neurosurg* 1994;96:323–326.

52. Samii M, Klekamp J. Surgical results of 100 intramedullary tumors in relation to accompanying syringomyelia. *Neurosurgery* 1994;35:865–873.

53. Zimmerman R, Bilaniuk L. Imaging of tumors of the spinal canal. *Radiol Clin North Am* 1988;26:965–1007.

54. Scotti GM, Scialfa G, Columbo N, et al. Magnetic resonance diagnosis of intramedullary tumors of the spinal cord. *Neuroradiology* 1987;29:130–135.

55. Li MH, Holtas S. MR imaging of spinal intramedullary tumors. *Acta Radiol* 1991;32:505–513.

56. Fischer G, Mansuy L. Total removal of intramedullary ependymomas: follow-up study of 16 cases. *Surg Neurol* 1980;14:243–249.

57. Greenwood J Jr. Surgical removal of intramedullary tumors. *J Neurosurg* 1967;26:276–282.

58. Guidetta B, Mercuri S, Vagnozzi R. Long-term results of the surgical treatment of 129 intramedullary spinal gliomas. *J Neurosurg* 1981;54:323–330.

59. Malis LI. Intramedullary spinal cord tumors. *Clin Neurosurg* 1978;25:512–539.

60. Vijayakumar S, Estes M, Hardy R Jr, et al. Ependymoma of the spinal cord and cauda equina: a review. *Cleve Clin J Med* 1988;55:163–170.

61. Wen BC, Hussey DH, Hitchon PW, et al. The role of radiation therapy in the management of ependymomas of the spinal cord. *Int J Radiat Oncol Biol Phys* 1991;20: 781–786.

62. Whitaker SJ, Bessell EM, Ashley SE, et al. Postoperative radiotherapy in the management of spinal cord ependymoma. *J Neurosurg* 1991;74:720–728.

63. Palmer JJ. Radiation myelopathy. *Brain* 1992;95:1109–1122.

64. Peterson H. Spinal deformity secondary to tumor, irradiation and laminectomy. In: Bradford DS, Hensinger RM, eds. *The Pediatric Spine*. New York: Thieme Medical Publishers; 1985:273–285.

65. Probert JC, Parker BR, Kaplan HS. Growth retardation in children after mega voltage irradiation of the spine. *Cancer* 1973;32:634–639.

66. Rappaport ZH, Loven D, Ben-Aharon U. Radiation-induced cerebellar glioblastoma subsequent to treatment of an astrocytoma of the cervical spinal cord. *Neurosurgery* 1991;29:606–608.

67. Chan HS, Becker LE, Hoffman HJ, et al. Myxopapillary ependymoma of the filum terminale in childhood: report of seven cases and review of the literature. *Neurosurgery* 1984;14:204–210.

68. O'Sullivan C, Jenkin RD, Doherty MA, et al. Spinal cord tumors in children: long-term results of combined surgical and radiation treatment. *J Neurosurg* 1994;81: 507–512.

69. Scott M. Infiltrating ependymoma of the cauda equina: Treatment by conservative surgery plus radiotherapy. *J Neurosurg* 1974;446–448.

70. Nagib MG, O'Fallon MT. Myxopapillary ependymoma of the conus medullaris and filum terminale in the pediatric age group. *Pediatr Neurosurg* 1997;26:2–7.

71. McCormick PC, Stein BM. Comment: Cauda equina ependymoma. *Neurosurgery* 1992;30:207.

72. Epstein FJ, Farmer JP, Schneider SJ. Intraoperative ultrasonography: an important surgical adjunct for intramedullary tumors. *J Neurosurg* 1991;74:729–733.

73. Nagle KJ, Emerson RG, Adams DC, et al. Intraoperative monitoring of evoked potentials: a review of 116 cases. *Neurology* 1996;47:999–1004.

74. Deletis V, Vodusek DB. Intraoperative recording of the bulbocavernosus reflex. *Neurosurgery* 1997;40:88–92.

75. Crisante L, Herrmann HD. Surgical management of intramedullary tumors: functional outcome and sources of morbidity. *Neurosurgery* 1994;35:69–74.

76. Epstein FJ, Farmer JP, Freed DF. Adult intramedullary spinal cord ependymomas: the result of surgery in 38 patients. *J Neurosurg* 1993;79:204–209.

77. Lonstein JE. Post-laminectomy kyphosis. *Clin Orthop* 1977;128:93–100.

78. Winter RB, Hall JE. Kyphosis in childhood and adolescence. *Spine* 1978;3:285–308.

79. Yasuoka S, Peterson HA, MacCarthy CS. Incidence of spinal deformity after multilevel laminectomy in children and adults. *J Neurosurg* 1982;57:441–445.

80. Ferrante L, Mastronardi L, Celli P, et al. Intramedullary spinal cord ependymoma: a study of 45 cases with long term follow-up. *Acta Neurochir (Wien)* 1992;119:74–79.

Chapter 32

Neurofibromatosis

James Tait Goodrich

Neurofibromatosis (NF) is an ancient disease, as evidenced by a recently described votive from the Hellenistic era that represents what has been characterized as neurofibromatosis type 1 (NF-1).[1] In recent times, it has been suggested often but erroneously that Joseph Merrick, Sir Frederick Treves' "elephant man," had neurofibromatosis; it is now thought that the elephant man had the Proteus syndrome[2] (Fig. 32–1).

Few tumors in the pediatric population generate as much emotional turmoil and anguish as NF. It is a common tumor in children, with a high rate of spontaneous mutation. All manifestations of NF occur in cells derived from the neural crest; the NFs are "neural cristopathies." Tumors generated by NF are associated with a notable incidence of brain, spine, and peripheral nerve lesions.[3] Patients tend to have multiple problems that require not only neurosurgical intervention but also medical, ophthalmologic, otolaryngologic, orthopedic, and psychological treatment as well as emotional and social support. At the Montefiore Medical Center/Albert Einstein College of Medicine we have a center that specifically deals with NF. I have been impressed with the range of tumors and clinical manifestations in this disorder. The lack of nonsurgi-cal treatment options is also noteworthy, particularly because it must be admitted that surgery can only be considered palliative. But whereas chemotherapy and radiotherapy have so far proved of minimal efficacy, advances in our understanding of the molecular biological and genetic aspects of the disorder have been among the most exciting in the entire field of tumors in the pediatric age group.

This chapter reviews the clinical characteristics of NF, types of tumors and other disorders seen in patients with NF, and surgical treatment, as well as recent developments in molecular biology.

BACKGROUND

The inheritance pattern in NF is autosomal dominant with a reported 50% spontaneous mutation rate. Although expression of the mutant gene varies widely from individual to individual, its penetrance is complete.[4–6]

NF has been clinically and genetically placed primarily within two categories, although as many as eight have been

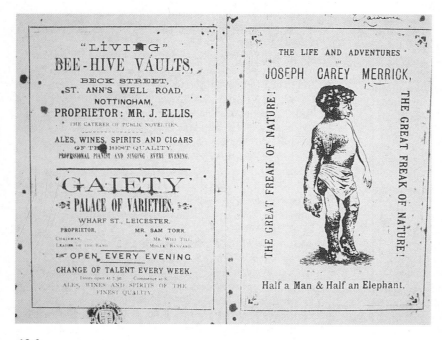

Figure 32–1 A late 19th century advertising broadside presenting Merrick as a freak—"half a man & half an elephant"—hence the term "elephant man."

described.[6-9] In this chapter we use the common designations of neurofibromatosis type 1 (NF-1)—"peripheral," or von Recklinghausen's disease—and neurofibromatosis type 2 (NF-2)—"central," or bilateral acoustic neuroma. Some authors prefer the term "vestibular" to "acoustic," but historical considerations argue the use of "acoustic."[10-12] NF-1 is usually referred to as von Recklinghausen's neurofibromatosis, after Frederick Daniel von Recklinghausen (1833–1910), a professor of pathology at Königsberg who described two patients with NF and introduced the term "neurofibromatosis" in 1882.[13] NF had been described in earlier reports, but it was von Recklinghausen who suggested that its lesions were due to cutaneous fibromas derived from neural tissue. NF-2 is rarely referred to as bilateral acoustic neurofibromatosis; bilateral acoustic schwannomas are the sine qua non for the diagnosis of NF-2.

NEUROFIBROMATOSIS TYPE 1

The incidence of NF-1 ranges from 1 in 3000 to 1 in 4000 individuals.[7-9] Fifty percent of patients diagnosed with NF have no family history of the disorder, confirming that a disturbingly high mutation rate is associated with this tumor.[14] When present, the NF-1 gene has a 100% penetration rate (i.e., at least some clinical manifestations are present). A frustrating aspect for the clinician has been the total unpredictability of gene expression and the eventual severity of the disorder. Within a single family we have seen extraordinary variability in the clinical problems arising in the individual probands.

The diagnostic criteria originally classifed by Riccardi for NF-1 are listed below.[7,8] After much discussion over the years as to what characterizes NF-1, these criteria have recently been accepted as the most predictive.

BOX 32–1
Diagnostic Criteria in NF-1

- **Two or more of the following:**
  - **Five or more café au lait spots (over 5 mm in greatest diameter in prepubertal individuals) or six or more (over 15 mm in greatest diameter in postpubertal individuals).**
  - **Two or more neurofibromas of any type, or one plexiform neurofibroma.**
    - **Freckling in the axillary or inguinal regions, or both.**
    - **Optic glioma.**
    - **Two or more Lisch nodules (see below).**
    - **A distinctive osseous lesion, such as sphenoid dysplasia or thinning of the long bone cortex, with or without pseudoarthrosis.**
    - **A first-degree relative with NF-1 by the above criteria.**

The most characteristic central nervous system (CNS) tumor in NF-1 is the optic and chiasmal glioma. Such a tumor without

other abnormalities can be considered a forme fruste of this disorder;—i.e., it is almost always associated with NF-1. Estimates of the incidence of optic gliomas in patients with NF-1 are in the 15% range,[15,16] though some studies have suggested a greater than 20% incidence.[17,18] These lesions typically present at 5 to 7 years of age with loss of visual acuity, occasionally exophthalmos, and rarely as a diencephalic syndrome with symptoms secondary to increased intracranial pressure (Fig. 32–2).

Optic glioma patients with NF-1 have received considerable attention. Deliganis et al[19] suggested that the occurrence of optic glioma in a child with NF-1 is of prognostic significance. These authors found that the 5- and 10-year survival rates for patients with optic gliomas and NF-1 were 93% and 81%, respectively. In patients with optic gliomas but without NF-1, the 5- and 10-year survival rates were 83% and 76%. However, when evaluated using Kaplan-Meier survival curves, these differences were not significant.

In our experience and that of others,[16] these tumors have variable growth histories, with some showing little or no growth, others remaining quiescent for years, and still others exhibiting rapid growth. An extreme example was a patient whose initial biopsy of an optic glioma disclosed a nonpilocytic low-grade astrocytoma. Fifteen years later, the tumor progressed to glioblastoma multiforme (GBM).[19] Variable courses such as this have led to controversy about treatment.

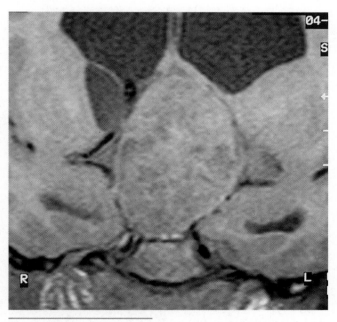

Figure 32–2 Coronal magnetic resonance image of a 14-year-old girl who presented with severe headaches (starting a week prior) vomiting, plus personality changes over the previous 6 months, visual acuity loss over the previous 2 years with loss of color vision in one eye. A magnetic resonance image taken 2 years previously for visual loss was read as normal though a comment was made of possible "increased signal" in one optic nerve. The patient now presents 2 years later with a very large intraventricular tumor arising from the optic chiasm that at surgery proved to be a low-grade juvenile pilocytic astrocytoma.

Pathologically most tumors in NF-1 are pilocytic astrocytomas or low-grade nonpilocytic gliomas; anaplastic astrocytomas and GBM are extremely rare in this group. In addition, these patients have a high survival rate, 75 to 80% after 10 years. The combination of low-grade characteristics and long-term survival makes for an indolent tumor that provides no strong justification for aggressive treatment unless anaplastic changes are present. This has been the view of ophthalmology colleagues for years.

NEUROFIBROMATOSIS TYPE 2

NF-2 is much less common than NF-1, with a reported incidence ranging from 1 in 40,000 to 1 in 100,000 live births, and an autosomal dominant pattern of transmission.[6, 20] The clinical diagnosis is established by the presence of bilateral acoustic schwannomas, seen in 95% of patients (Fig. 32–3). In the absence of these tumors or a family history of them, the diagnosis of NF-2 is difficult. Acoustic tumors present in the younger patient—typically within the second or third decade and usually with a complaint of tinnitus or hearing loss. It is important to differentiate bilateral tumors from the single acoustic schwannoma seen in the older patient, which has no known genetic or inheritance pattern. Exceptions include a patient who presents under the age of 30 years with a unilateral acoustic schwannoma, a child with a recently diagnosed meningioma or schwannoma, and a patient with a unilateral acoustic neuroma with a first-degree relative with NF-2; such persons should be considered highly suspect for NF-2. *In general, NF-2 should be suspected in any pediatric patient who presents with two or more of the following conditions: meningioma, glioma, schwannoma, or juvenile subcapsular lenticular opacity.*[12, 20–23]

A number of other CNS tumors are associated with NF-2, with Schwann cell tumors, meningiomas, and gliomas being the most common. They tend to be multiple and form (with the exception of gliomas) in an en plaque fashion. In one series, meningiomas were reported to be extremely common, found in as many as 50% of patients;[24] this has also been our clinical experience. Due to their clinical indolence, it is sur-

prisingly rare that such tumors require any surgical intervention, the exception being the acoustic neuromas and the spinal cord schwannomas (Fig. 32–4). Ependymoma and astrocytoma are clinically more difficult in that they are most commonly intraspinal, though they also are seen in the brain stem and cerebellum. These lesions have proved much more difficult to treat than the others mentioned, being recalcitrant to chemotherapy and radiotherapy. As discussed above, optic glioma is not seen in NF-2.

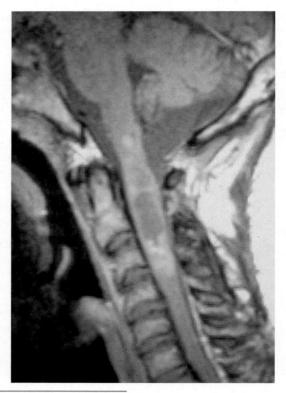

Figure 32–4 A 15-year-old boy who presented with gait difficulty and weakness in the hands. MRI with contrast enhancement revealed this intramedullary tumor that at surgery proved to be a low-grade astrocytoma. Further workup revealed that the patient has NF-2.

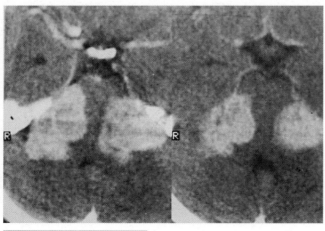

Figure 32–3 A 12-year-old boy who presented initially with only hearing loss on one side. CT (scan) revealed bilateral "kissing" acoustic tumors. Further workup demonstrated that this boy has NF-2.

CLINICAL COURSE AND PROGNOSIS

The clinical course in NF is highly variable. *It has been our impression that the earlier the disease manifests the poorer the prognosis and the more rapid the progression.* Patients who present in the latter teen years or even later have a slower disease progression and hence a better prognosis.

MOLECULAR BIOLOGY

NF has generated much interest on the part of geneticists and molecular biologists. It has been the subject of an early and intensive molecular biologic investigative protocol. In 1939, with great foresight, Worcestor-Drought et al[25] postulated an "evocator" substance in NF; that is, one that brings about the pathologic alterations of NF, including abnormal tissue growth. In fact, more than one evocator has recently been identified.[26, 27] In early work, Riccardi[7] postulated that multiple alleles at a single gene locus or possibly several gene loci account for the closely related but distinct forms of NF. *Contemporary investigations have now mapped the NF-1 locus on chromosome 17 and the NF-2 locus on chromosome 22.*[28–32]

The protein product of the NF-1 gene, neurofibromin, has been characterized.[33, 34] The protein product of the NF-2 gene has also been characterized and is called Merlin.[35] NF-1 and NF-2 are now recognized as belonging to a growing family of tumor suppresser genes. Normal cells contain various genes that suppress neoplastic proliferation. The functional absence of one or more of these genes leads to uncontrolled overproduction of the protein products. Tumor suppresser genes must be deactivated for their growth-suppressing properties to be eliminated. Because these genes appear to operate in a recessive manner, two copies or two mutational events are required in a cell for tumor formation—the so-called two-hit theory.[36] Loss of one copy of the *p53* tumor suppresser gene has been reported in neurogenic sarcomas. This genetic aberration is one of the most common findings in a wide variety of human cancers. Putative tumor suppresser genes have been identified in almost all human cancer cells.[37–53] To date, only a few of the genes involved in aberrations of tumor suppression have been cloned and sequenced.

Neurofibromin, the NF-1 gene product, is a protein with GTPase activity that acts as an inhibitor of the Ras protein.[54–56] Recent work by several groups[57, 58] have shown that the major function of neurofibromin is to down-regulate RasA (p21-Ras) expression and thereby keep cell proliferation in check. One group has also recently identified wild-type RasA proteins in patients with NF-1.[59] It would appear that neurofibromin exerts a key regulatory function on cytoskeletal proteins, limiting cellular proliferation.[54] The recent demonstration of the heterogeneity of gene mutations that can occur within a family prototype is impressive.[60–62] These molecular findings may begin to account for the multiple manifestations of NF observed clinically.[63]

Recent investigations have shown that in at least 60% of NF-2–related tumors (meningioma, sporadic unilateral acoustic neuroma, spinal schwannoma, ependymoma) deletion or rearrangements in chromosome 22 can be detected.[21, 64–67] Definition of the resulting aberrations in cell cycle regulation will eventually lead to better treatment protocols. These gene-linked findings suggest the possibility that preferentially targeting genetically engineered viral vectors at tumor cells may become an effective treatment in the next decade.[68–73]

The recently developed capability for introducing genetic material into mammalian cells by various means has been one of the great technological advances. If one can insert a more "correct" gene, then perhaps the deleterious effects of the NF gene can be reversed. A number of technologies have been used for genome transfer into the nucleus, but the results have been marginally successful. Recently proposed techniques include the "infection" (transfection) of an embryo with a retrovirus encoded with a foreign gene[68, 70, 72] or direct microinjection of genetic material into the nucleus.[69–72] With either technique, success in integrating the transgene into the host genome has been random at best, with a rate of incorporation rarely approaching 20%. Once incorporated, these genes must be induced to express their protein products—a separate and even more difficult problem. Nevertheless, considering the molecular aberrations associated with NF that have been defined to date, this would seem to be an ideal model for a transgenic approach to tumor control.

CLINICAL MANIFESTATIONS

Persons with NF present with a myriad of clinical findings and manifestations (Table 32–1). The clinician will see neoplasms, hyperplasia, and dysplasia. Tissue changes of these types occur in any of the neural and neural supportive structures. Hormones appear to play a strong role in the expression of NF. Puberty and pregnancy are known to aggravate the disorder.[74, 75]

Café au Lait Spots

Café au lait spots are the most common clinical manifestation in NF-1 but are less common in NF-2.[76] A café au lait spot is a small, darkly pigmented lesion that is caused by increased pigmentation in the basal layer of the epidermis. These spots are sometimes present at birth, though not uncommonly they take months to years to appear. They typically increase in number with age and are eventually present in 99% of NF-1 patients. Café au lait spots are also common in unaffected individuals, but the presence of five or more spots is suggestive of NF-1. The presence of five or more spots greater than 5 mm in diameter in a prepubescent patient is considered diagnostic. In the postpubescent patient, the presence of six macules greater than 15 mm is diagnostic. Both the size and the number of café au lait spots tend to increase with hormonal changes, particularly during puberty and pregnancy.

The classic study on café au lait spots is that by Crowe and Schull in 1953.[77] These authors examined 7098 institutionalized patients for spots larger than 1.5 mm. Ten percent of the patients had them, but fewer than 0.2% had three or more. Of the patients within the population, 89.8% of those diagnosed with NF-1 had café-au-lait spots, with 68.3% of this group having six or more. This work led to the Crowe criteria for NF-1; that is, six or more café au lait spots greater than 15 mm in diameter. This was modified in 1966 by Whitehouse[78] to compensate for the pediatric population, in which the spots are clinically manifested later. Whitehouse reviewed 365 children younger than 5 years. NF was diagnosed in children with five or more spots greater than 0.5 cm in diameter.

TABLE 32–1 Clinical Characteristics of NF-1 and NF-2

Characteristic	NF-1	NF-2
Incidence	1 in 3000–4000	1 in 40,000–100,000
Inheritance	Autosomal dominant	Autosomal dominant
Chomosome locus	17q11.2	22q12
Protein	Neurofibromin	Merlin/schwannomin
Protein function	GAP-like function/down-regulates proto-oncogene *RASA*	Links cell membrane to cytoskeleton
Penetrance	100%	95% for VS
Expressivity	Variable	Not variable in VS
Clinical onset	First decade	Second to third decade
Intellectual deficit	> 25%	None
Café au lait	99% by adulthood	Not common
Axillary freckling	Common	Rare
Cutaneous neurofibromas	Frequent	Few
Pachydermatoceles	Uncommon	None
Lisch nodules/iris hamartomas	100% > 20 years of age	None
Buphthalomas	Uncommon	None
Posterior lens opacities	None	> 85%
Skeletal abnormalities (scoliosis, kyphosis, congenital leg bowing, bony erosion, spinal dysraphism)	Not uncommon	Rare
Nervous system tumors		
Acoustic schwannoma	Occasionally	95%
Optic nerve glioma	15%	Very rare
Cerebral glioma	Common	Occasionally
Meningioma	Few	>50%, 30% multiple
Spinal neurofibroma	Common	Absent
Spinal schwannoma	Absent	Common
Plexiform neurofibroma	Common	Uncommon
Other tumors	Not rare	Rare
Herteropia/hemaratoma		
Ependymoma		
Leukemia		
Soft-tissue sarcoma		
Miscellaneous conditions		
Macrocephaly	Common	Rare
Aqueductal stenosis	Not uncommon	None
Endocrine (precocious puberty, diabetes insipidus)	Common	Rare
Developmental delay	Common	Rare
Vascular abnormalities (arterial stenosis, fusiform aneurysms, telangiectasia)	Common	Rare

GAP, guanosine triphosphatase activating protein; VS, vestibular schwannoma.
Table adapted from Dirks PB, Rutka JT. The genetic basis of neurosurgical disorders. In: Youmans J, ed. *Neurological Surgery*. 4th ed. Vol. 4. Philadelphia: WB Saunders; 1996:818.

Axillary and Inguinal Freckling

Though not often present in young children, axillary and inguinal freckling is a hallmark of NF-1, seen in almost all adult patients. Although similar in color to café au lait spots, these freckles are smaller and occur in clusters. They are etiologically distinct from café au lait spots. Freckles virtually never occur in NF-2.

Cutaneous and Subcutaneous Neurofibromas (Fibroma Molluscum)

A diagnostic finding in NF-1 is the presence of two or more cutaneous and subcutaneous neurofibromas arising from distal cutaneous nerve endings. Also referred to as fibroma molluscum, these are soft, rubbery lesions that can either be flush with the skin surface or rise above it. In children they typically are flush with the skin surface when they appear and become pedunculated after puberty.[79] Such fibromas can be highly variable in size, location, and number. Characteristically, these lesions enlarge with age and puberty. During pregnancy they tend to increase in size and number and become intensely pruritic.

Pachydermatoceles

Pachydermatoceles are large folds of excess or loose skin associated with plexiform NF. Some can be quite large and disfiguring, growing in multiple layers (Figs. 32–5 to 32–7).

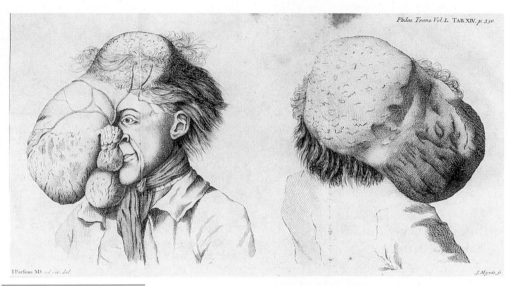

Figure 32–5 An interesting early example of pachydermatocele published in the *Philosophical Transactions of the Royal Society*, Vol. 50 (1777, p. 350).

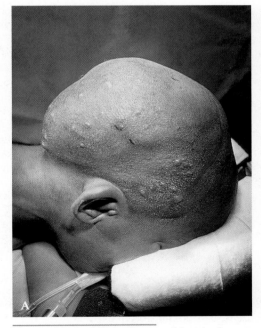
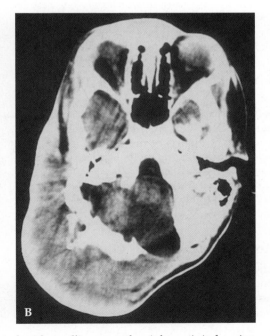

Figure 32–6 **(A)** An 8-year-old girl who presented with swelling over the right occipital region involving the occipital and temporal bone and with infiltration of tumor into the ear. She has since undergone several operations to remove this recurring and disfiguring lesion. In addition, cranioplasties have been done to replace the destroyed skull bone underneath. **(B)** Axial CT of the same patient showing the extent of tumor.

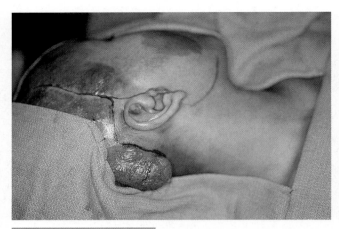

Figure 32–7 Another example of a large disfiguring plexiform neurofibroma of the face and head. A very large café au lait spot can be seen on the right cheek. The neurofibroma essentially encompassed the entire right side of the head, involving the face, ear, and occipital region. A large pedunculated mass can be seen arising from just behind the ear.

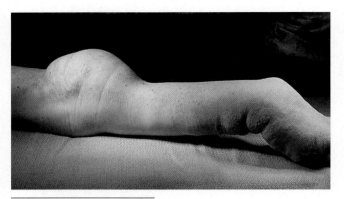

Figure 32–8 A 14-year-old boy with known NF-1 that had been stable. He presented with a rapidly growing (doubled in size in less than 2 months) tumor of the median nerve. At surgery the lesion was removed and revealed sarcomatous changes consistent with malignancy.

Large Peripheral Nerve and Plexus Neurofibromas

Peripheral neurofibromas are commonly found in the larger peripheral nerves (ulnar, radial, and sciatic nerves) and plexus neurofibromas within the larger plexuses (brachical, cervical, and lumbosacral). As opposed to cutaneous neurofibromas, these have a higher potential for undergoing malignant degeneration being reported as 5 to 10%, although this is higher than in our series, in which only one case in 15 years has been recorded (Fig. 32–8).[80–86] In an NF-1 patient with a rapidly expanding peripheral nerve lesion, the diagnosis of malignant degeneration must be ruled out.[87–90]

Lisch Nodules (Ocular Hamartomas)

Lisch nodules are benign lesions that are an important clinical finding in NF-1. These are melanocytic hamartomas that appear as smooth, raised, circumscribed, gelatinous elevations on the surface of the iris of the eye.[91–93] Their color ranges from clear to brown and they are typically bilateral. *In the patient with NF-1 who is older than 20 years, these lesions are universally present; they are rarely present in children younger than 5.*[7] In NF-2 the presence of Lisch nodules has been reported in only one case.[94]

Posterior Capsular Lens Opacities

A characteristic eye lesion seen only in NF-2 is posterior capsular lens opacity, whose distribution typically is bilateral. The prevalence is 85% in patients with NF-2.[95]

Buphthalmos (Ox Eye)

Buphthalmos is a seriously disfiguring disorder that fortunately occurs rarely in NF. Buphthalmos occurs as a result of congenital glaucoma, resulting in a large and deformed globe, optic atrophy, and increased intraocular pressure. It is more common in patients with facial NF and typically is unilateral. It is also associated with François' syndrome (buphthalomas, asymmetrical facial hypertrophy, plexiform neurofibroma of the eyelid).

Skeletal Dysplasia and Other Bone Changes

Orbital osseous dysplasia, a defect in the posterior superior wall of the orbit, typically occurs early in development and may initially be the only clinical manifestation of NF-1. Sphenoid wing dysplasia is reported in 1 to 7% of NF-1 patients.[96–100] Fifty percent of reported cases of orbital osseous dysplasia are in patients with NF-1.[101] Not uncommonly, as a result of a communication of the temporal lobe to the posterior side of the orbit, the sphenoid wing and frontal wing fail to develop completely, causing a pulsatile exophthalmos.[101, 102] Pediatric neurosurgeons may be called on to help correct the bone defect, typically with split-thickness calvarium bone grafts. Interestingly, the first repair of a pulsatile exophtalmos due to orbital osseous dysplasia was reported by Walter Dandy in 1929.[103] This disorder should be recognized early, before long-term injury of the optic nerve or globe has occurred.

Scoliosis and pseudoarthrosis (see below) are additional skeletal findings seen in the older child with NF-1 and should always be kept in mind when following a developing child.[104–106]

Skull Lesions

In neurofibromatosis defects of the calvarium are common. On radiographs round or oval defects (nonsclerotic lucency) are visualized, most frequently over the lambdoid suture.[107] These lesions are seen laterally on the suture, near the squamous suture; a lack of pneumatization can result in the mastoid sinuses.[104] Recently, an ossifying fibroma of the skull in a patient with NF-1 was reported, broadening the range of skull tumors seen in NF-1.[108]

Vascular Abnormalities

Vascular abnormalities are common in NF, often showing up in childhood. Arterial occlusion (often presenting with stroke), telangiectasias, segmental ectasias of large and small vessels, renal artery stenosis (with resultant hypertension), internal carotid artery occlusive disease, and pulmonary arterial stenosis have all been reported.[109–112]

Macrocephaly

Macrocephaly has been reported to be common in NF.[113] Of 34 children with NF-1, 75% were found to have macrocephaly, defined as a head circumference exceeding measurements in the 95th percentile.[113] Similar findings were noted by Holt,[114] who reported that 53 of 69 children with NF-1 had such measurements. The application of magnetic resonance imaging (MRI) techniques has led to the suggestion that macrocephaly is most likely due to increased heterotopias of the brain and abnormal cortical architecture (see below).

Heterotopias/Hamartomas/Unidentified Bright Objects

Interesting magnetic resonance images have been described in NF. UBOs (unidentified bright objects) have been reported with increasing frequency, particularly in T2-weighted studies (in as many as 60 to 70% of NF-1 patients[115–118] (Fig. 32–9). Such UBOs are commonly found in the basal ganglia and brain stem.[119, 120] *They are notable for a lack of mass effect and of surrounding edema and do not enhance in response to gadolinium administration.* Spontaneous regression or disappearance is not uncommon on follow-up studies. Early studies first suggested UBOs to be hamartomas, heterotopias, or dysplastic changes.[119, 120] These conclusions came from an earlier pathologic study by Rosman and Pearce[121] who found "hamartomas" in 10% of brain autopsies. UBOs, rather than being true hamartomas, are now believed to represent sites of vacuolar or spongiotic change.[122]

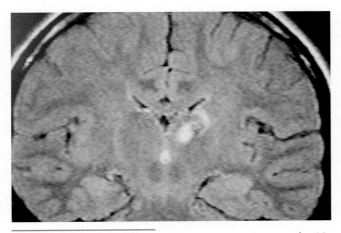

Figure 32–9 Coronal magnetic resonance image of a 10-year-old patient with known NF-1. Bright unidentified objects can be seen here in the basal ganglia. We have followed this patient for 6 years and to date there is no change in size or signal.

Clinical growth histories of UBOs in patients with NF have been poorly documented to date. If anything, magnetic resonance findings may even show radiographic regression. I have followed a number of children with UBOs over the last dozen years without ever detecting a clinically significant radiographic change. It may be that these children do not live long enough for the hamartomas to become clinical problems.

It is of great importance to reach the correct differential diagnosis of brain stem UBOs in NF-1. Such UBOs are frequently confused with low-grade gliomas, which are uncommon in the brain stem. The key feature that distinguishes a glioma or other infiltrative lesion from a UBO is the clinical presence of brain stem dysfunction (e.g., dysarthria, cranial neuropathies, long-tract findings). In NF patients gliomas are more common in the medulla, whereas in non–NF-1 patients they are more common in the pontine region. In patients subjected to biopsy, the common findings have been fibillary or anaplastic astrocytomas.[123] Gliomas in NF-1 patients have a more benign clinical course than those seen in non–NF patients. This was shown in a recent long-term study of 17 NF patients, 14 of whom did not receive adjuvant therapy but were still surviving at the end of 52 months of follow-up.[123]

Other CNS Nonneoplastic Abnormalities Seen in Patients with NF-1

CNS nonneoplastic abnormalities seen in NF-1 patients include gray matter heterotopias, disordered cortical laminations, polymicrogyria, pachygyria, and glial nodules. These pathologic findings all appear to result from errors in neuronal migration and differentiation and their consequences for cortical architecture. It is not surprising that children (and adults) with one or more of these abnormalities have a higher incidence of mild IQ deficits.[124–126] Learning disorders, developmental delay, speech difficulty, and hyperkinetic behavior have all been reported and are common in this group of patients.[79] Fienman and Yakovac[79] found a 24% incidence of developmental delay; Griffith et al[125] reported 16%. Not surprisingly with all these cortical abnormalities, seizures are also more common in the NF-1 population than in the general population.

Non-CNS Tumors Associated with NF-1

Patients with NF-1 have a three to five times greater risk of developing a malignancy than the general population.[3, 82, 89, 127, 128] However, the 30% of NF-1 patients who eventually die of some form of malignancy surpass the general population in this regard by only 5%. The frequency of malignant transformation/degeneration of a neurofibroma is reported as about 5%; rates as high as 29% have been reported in NF-1 patients.[82] It must be remembered that 50% of neurogenic sarcomas are associated with NF-1—hardly an indicator of a good prognosis. It has also been a common observation among clinicians caring for NF-1 patients that, in addition to CNS tumors, they have a higher than expected incidence of non-CNS malignant tumors. A review by Riccardi has borne this out.[129] Associated non-NF tumors reported with a higher than expected incidence include pheochromocytoma, Wilms' tumor, rhabdomyosarcoma, soft-tissue sarcomas, and leukemia. Recent work has shown that children with NF-1 have 200 to 500 times the expected risk of developing a malignant myeloproliferative disease.[130] In children with malignant myeloproliferative disorders (leukemia and related dyscrasias), Side et al[130] found in some NF-1 patients that both alleles in the NF-1 gene are inactivated, suggesting that *NF1* appears to function as a tumor-suppresser gene in immature myeloid cells.

Ganglioneuromas

Ganglioneuromas are rare, slowly growing tumors typically seen in the younger age groups. They occur along the sympathetic nerve chains and most commonly present as posterior mediastinal masses.[124]

Miscellaneous Associated Clinical Disorders

A number of other clinical disorders associated with NF are beyond the scope of this chapter and so are only mentioned in passing. Orthopedic abnormalities are common in patients with NF-1 (and rare in NF-2).[98, 124] They include structural problems, such as congenital bowing or pseudoarthrosis of the tibia or radius (rarer is involvement of the femur and clavicle), focal bone gigantism, fibrocystic lesions, scoliosis, kyphosis (most commonly in the cervical region), short stature, and spinal dysraphism.[20, 104–106] Associated findings include seizures, syringomyelia, and stenosis of the aqueduct.

NEUROSURGICAL MANAGEMENT

Experience with NF-1 and NF-2 over more than 15 years has led me to be extremely conservative in the surgical management of the associated tumors and clinical problems. Early on my policy was to be aggressive in considering virtually any radiographic or clinical evidence of tumor in these children for neurosurgical diagnosis. Cumulative observations indicating that these are typically slowly growing lesions that often achieve impressive size before becoming clinically significant have led me away from early intervention. In addition, these lesions often incorporate functional neurons and nerves, and their removal can lead to an unacceptable proportion of neurologic defects. I have elected to break down the clinical problems seen in NF into several general categories and summarize current neurosurgical management

Acoustic Neuroma

Arising from the vestibular component of the eighth nerve, this tumor is almost always approached by the paramedian suboccipital approach. With the participation of our neurophysiology colleagues, intraoperative monitoring is useful for recording function of both the facial (seventh) and the acoustic (eighth) nerves. Success in preserving facial nerve function has been good, but this has not been the case with the acoustic nerve. The preservation of hearing in non-NF patients with acoustic neuroma is now a common outcome. However, results of this caliber have not been achieved for NF patients with acoustic tumors.[131] The anatomical relationship of the auditory component to the vestibular component

makes it difficult to remove the neuroma without affecting the auditory component. As a result of the high potential for loss of hearing, I now elect to follow patients with known acoustic neuromas with MRI every 6 months until at least a 2-year pattern of growth has been determined. Careful attention is paid during the clinical history to reports of new hearing loss or deterioration of hearing discrimination. *I defer surgery until the patient has presented with any of the following findings: (1) rapid tumor growth, defined as more than 1 cm/year; (2) loss of hearing discrimination in the affected ear; (3) long-tract or brain stem findings thought to be secondary to brain stem compression; (4) presence of hydrocephalus secondary to occlusion of the aqueduct; (5) presence of "kissing" acoustics in which bilateral tumors cause compression of the brain stem.*

Because some children with acoustic neuromas have the potential for spinal cord neurofibromas, the preoperative workup should rule out any significant spinal cord abnormalities. Failure to do so can lead to paralysis from cord compression during operative positioning.

CNS Tumors

Intra-axial lesions of the CNS, particularly those suspected of being UBOs, are followed with serial MRI studies. Gliomas are also followed serially. Often these so-called primary tumors remain quiescent. *If there is a change in the clinical picture or imaging studies that suggests growth, the tumors are resected using intraoperative three-dimensional imaging systems with an attempt at total volumetric radiographic resection.* This attempt can be limited if the tumors occur in eloquent brain areas, such as the motor strip or speech area. Realizing that the life expectancy in patients with progressing gliomas may be short, I emphasize quality-of-life issues, a context in which less is better. The possibility of giving a patient who has a lethal malignant lesion a dense hemiplegia or aphasia has steered me away from aggressive surgical management. When effective molecular therapies surface, more aggressive treatment protocols will become appropriate.

Meningiomas are common in NF-2. Fortunately, they rarely represent a problem to the patient. Experience has shown them to be very slow-growing lesions, requiring surgery in only a handful of cases and then only when the meningioma became large enough (more than 5 cm on average) to cause clinical symptoms. These growths are almost always over the convexity, though occasionally they are found in the cerebellopontine angle and along the spinal column.[132–135] All of these locations are accessible to the surgeon, and the growths are removed in toto, if feasible, with no further treatment advocated.

Optic gliomas/chiasmatic gliomas are common in NF-1 patients.[15, 17, 136–139] They are discussed more appropriately in Chapter 21, but some personal observations may be of interest. I have elected to follow children with these tumors by means of serial imaging studies for the first 2 years post diagnosis; if no growth is seen, then the imaging studies are discontinued. Routine opthalmologic examinations, including visual acuity and visual field tests, are then done on a yearly basis. If any changes are noted in these examinations, then radiologic studies are ordered. As these tumors grow slowly, typically involving the anterior portion of the chiasm and nerve or, occasionally, the posterior chiasm complex, they rarely require surgical intervention.[140] *If the child has lost vision in the eye served by the affected nerve and the tumor has an active growth pattern, then I surgically resect the tumor and nerve. If the tumor is growing rapidly (more than 1 cm/year) and causing compression of surrounding brain structures, then an internal subtotal decompression is done. If the glioma involves the diencephalic structures, then surgery is futile with the exception of a biopsy for diagnosis.* Formerly, radical surgery (gross total resection) of the optic complex was advocated, but factors of high surgical risk, significant loss of visual function, and disturbances of the hypothalamic axis have induced most pediatric neurosurgeons not to apply such aggressive approaches.[140–147] These views were recently reinforced by Sutton's group at the Children's Hospital of Philadelphia[148] when they reviewed the cases of 33 patients treated during a 15-year period. The children each had a globular enhancing mass greater than 2 cm in the hypothalamus/chiasmatic region. These children had either no surgery, conservative surgery (less than 50% biopsy), or a biopsy with adjuvant local radiation therapy, chemotherapy (actinomycin D and vincristine), or both. Tissue diagnosis was pilocystic astrocytoma in every case. At a minimum of 3 years follow-up, 23 of 28 patients were alive, with functional vision in one eye; 12 required no endocrine replacement; and 16 were in regular school environments. Three of 5 patients died from tumor progression, and the other 2 patients died from non–tumor-related events.

Thus, the natural progression of these tumors (typically pilocytic astrocytomas) in the majority of patients is a slow and benign one. The nature of their growth patterns militates against chemotherapy, the exception being those tumors that are showing rapid growth. The risk of malignant degenera-

tion reduces my eagerness to routinely use ionizing radiation as a further adjuvant therapy, the only exception being the child older than 3 years with a rapidly growing lesion.[149–151] Several chemotherapeutic protocols (both Pediatric Oncology Group and Children's Cancer Group) have been suggested, but none has led to improvement in long-term outcome (survival beyond 5 years).[140–143]

Intramedullary tumors of the spine have proved particularly refractory to treatment (Fig. 32–10). With the rare exception of those that present with a tumor nidus and a cystic cavity, which can often be resected safely, most such tumors tend to be diffusely infiltrative and of low-grade character, with no definable margins. Because of their slow growth I have elected to follow this group and have been surprised by their long-term prognosis. Three adults with biopsy-proven intramedullary cervical gliomas have sustained no significant neurologic losses during a more than 5-year follow-up from time of diagnosis. Their MRI findings are much more impressive than their clinical findings. *In the case of intramedullary ependymomas I have opted to remove them when they became clinically significant (i.e., exhibiting tumor progression with loss of function).* Ependymomas are better demarcated and more easily removed without increasing the patient's neurologic deficits than intramedullary cervical gliomas.

Neurofibromas of the Spinal Roots

Any surgeon who has explored the spinal canal of an NF patient has come away impressed by the huge number of lesions present (Fig. 32–11). It is common to find hundreds if not thousands of small fibromas attached to the nerve roots—typically around the dorsal root ganglia and extending along the whole length of the spinal canal. The futility of removing all of them is self-evident; hence the enthusiasm for developing a molecular treatment of this disorder.

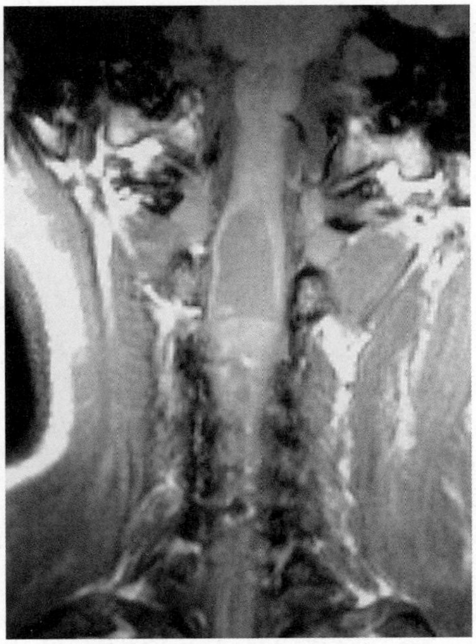

Figure 32–10 Coronal magnetic resonance image of an adolescent boy with an intramedullary tumor that at surgery proved to be a low-grade astrocytoma. The tumor can be seen inferiorly with a large cystic component above.

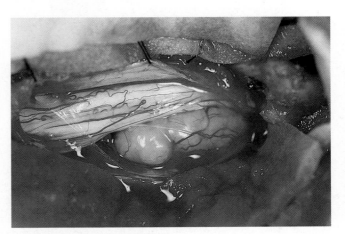

Figure 32–11 An operative view of a 14-year-old girl with known NF-1 who presented with lower-extremity weakness. Workup revealed this large neurofibroma comprising the spinal cord at T8. Visual inspection of the cord revealed multiple small (less than 1–2 mm in diameter) neurofibromas on other roots.

A number of our patients have undergone more than five surgical procedures whose only purpose was to excise spinal cord neurofibromas.

At this point I operate only on "symptomatic" lesions (e.g., those causing severe pain or involving a symptomatic space-occupying lesion). *It is unusual for severe pain alone to constitute an indication for therapy; however, if weakness is progressing or bowel and bladder dysfunction has developed, surgical intervention is indicated.* It can sometimes be extremely difficult to separate the offending neurofibroma from the nerve root without abrogating its neurologic function. Clinically and anatomically the distinct differences between a schwannoma and a neurofibroma are of particular importance to the neurosurgeon. Neurofibromas typically have more fascicles entering and leaving the tumor. When electrophysiologically stimulated, the entering fascicles rarely demonstrate distal motor function (they lack a nerve action potential). The fascicles of schwannomas, on the other hand, run in the capsule surrounding the tumor; intratumoral fascicles are rarer than in neurofibromas. Electrical stimulation of the schwannoma capsule typically shows motor function distally; this technique allows the surgeon to map the tract of the nerve fibers. Any identified functioning fascicle should be spared. Because these lesions are typically attached to the sensory root, loss of sensation is the most common problem.

It has been my impression that conservative therapy preserves neural function and therefore improves quality of life.

Neurofibromas of the Large Plexus and Peripheral Nerves

I have adopted the rationale described for neurofibromas of the spinal roots in the case of large plexus and peripheral nerve lesions (Fig. 32–12). The same anatomical principle applies: such fibromas are intimately associated with the sensory (and sometimes motor) components; they typically arise from a large nerve, and their removal increases the potential for damage to, or loss of, functional nerve tissue—less is more unless function is being lost rapidly[152] (Fig. 32–13). This applies particularly to lesions in the brachial and lumbosacral plexuses. The exception is the rapidly growing neurofibroma. Because of the risk of malignant degeneration and sarcomatous changes, such lesions must be aggressively explored and resected.[153–155] However, for tumors that have demonstated malignant degeneration some have advocated radical forequarter resections with whole-arm (or leg) amputation.[156, 157] However, because there is no evidence that such ultraradical surgery has any significant long-term beneficial effect to the patient, the clinician must factor in surgical morbidity with quality-of-life issues.

Malignant neurofibromas (schwannomas) occur most commonly in NF-1 patients[158, 163] (Fig. 32–14) Between 2% and 5% of patients with NF-1 develop malignant degeneration in their tumors.[80, 129, 158] These malignant tumors can arise either de novo or from an existing neurofibroma. A disturbing number

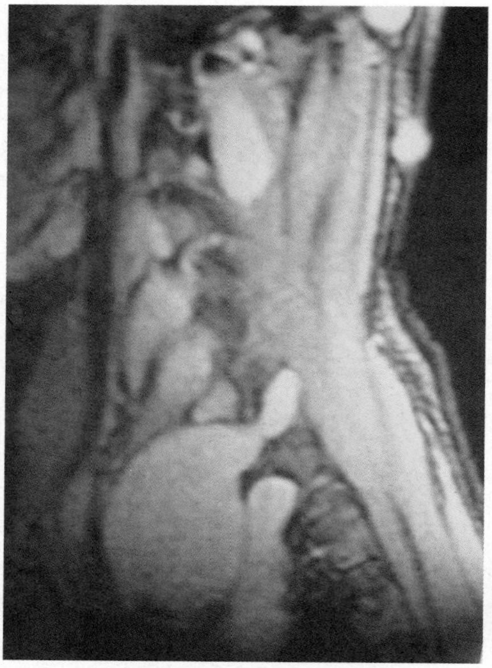

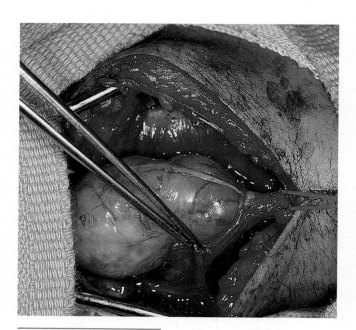

Figure 32–12 Sagittal magnetic resonance image of an 11-year-old boy with known NF-1 who presented with hand weakness. MRI revealed a large, dumbbell-shaped neurofibroma arising from the seventh cervical root, extending into the spinal canal and tracking out along the C7 root into the brachial plexus.

Figure 32–13 Intraoperative view of a dissected ulnar nerve neurofibroma. The "fat" neurofibroma can be seen to the left of the forcep; the forcep is over the exiting distal nerve. The capsule has been opened and is being dissected off. No discrete roots could be located; rather, they blended into the neurofibroma and could not be dissected out. Hence, the entire tumor and nerve had to be resected.

tumors.[87, 164, 165] To date, no efficacious protocols have been developed that have provided any reasonable long-term survivals. Local recurences remain high, and tumor metastases are not uncommon to the lung, liver, bone, and subcutaneous tissues, which further complicates treatment.[163, 166]

Plexiform Neurofibromas

Plexiform neurofibromas involve multiple fascicles. Typically, they are interwoven through the fascicles in long segments of the affected nerve. Consequently, total removal of such lesions is very difficult.[154] Plexiform neurofibromas in the facial region can be seriously disfiguring, particularly those that arise from the facial nerve. Neurosurgeons typically become involved when the growths invade the skull and become intracranial. At Montefiore Medical Center craniofacial surgeons not uncommonly are involved in reconstruction of the soft-tissue losses and of the calvarium. These lesions require the skills of a well-trained craniofacial team (neurosurgeon and plastic, maxillofacial, and otolaryngologic surgeons). Plexiform neurofibromas (particularly those involving the head and neck) can be notoriously vascular, and large blood losses are not uncommon (Fig. 32–15). Because of the involvement of the facial nerve, intraoperative monitoring has proved beneficial in locating the normal branches of the facial nerve. Because it is sometimes impossible to separate normal from abnormal facial nerve branches, the patient should be advised preoperatively of the potential loss of facial nerve function. Plexiform neurofibromas that involve the larger peripheral nerves or plexuses can also be difficult to isolate without significant loss of neural function. Often a partial resection for pain control or removal of mass effect is the treatment of choice, as the option of creating a plegic limb is unacceptable.

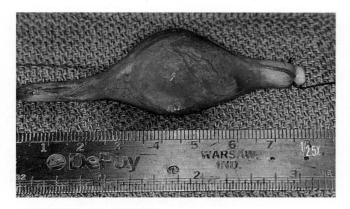

Figure 32–14 A resected neurofibroma lesion from the ulnar nerve of a 15-year-old boy. The lesion was first noted as a painless small nodule 2 years prior to surgery. Over the previous 3 months it underwent rapid growth and at surgery a malignant lesion was found and removed.

of malignancies have occurred in tumors that have been irradiated.[80, 151, 158, 160] Radiation therapy is sometimes advocated as adjunctive therapy after a malignant tumor has been removed, but this is at best a palliative therapy.[161, 162] Malignant degeneration most commonly occurs in older patients, aged 20–50, and therefore is not commonly seen in the pediatric population.[159, 163] Clinically these lesions present as a rapidly growing mass, typically doubling in size within several months. Paresthesias, neurologic deficits, and motor weakness are commonly noted at clinical presentation. Chemotherapy protocols have been tried, typically combinations of doxorubicin, methotrexate, Aleran, and actinomycin D in high-grade

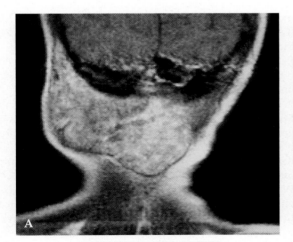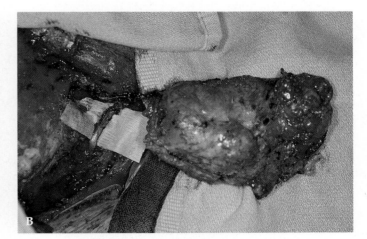

Figure 32–15 **(A)** Coronal magnetic resonance image of the posterior neck region of an 8-year-old boy with known NF-1. A fullness at the base of the neck was noted 2 years previously, and steady but rapid growth occurred over the prior 6 months. At surgery, a large plexiform neurofibroma was found arising from a cervical/occipital nerve root. No malignant changes were found, but the tumor was extremely vascular and tedious to remove. **(B)** Intraoperative view of the same patient with the tumor dissected out. The origin of the nerve that developed this tumor can be seen with a rubber dam placed beneath it.

SUMMARY

The neurofibromatoses are a group of disorders with many manifestations. The high incidence of these lesions makes them a common problem in the practice of the neurosurgeon, neurologist, and oncologist. A better model of neoplasia, with its various mechanisms of dysplasia and neoplasia, does not exist. In addition, patients with NF are likely to have seriously disfiguring abnormalities. No other disorder has repeatedly caused more constant emotional and psychological havoc affecting patient, family, and clinician.

Early recognition in NF is important. Genetic counseling is imperative and may reduce the incidence of the disorder. The use of chemotherapy has been surprisingly unsuccessful. The high risk of malignant sarcomatous degeneration of otherwise benign tumors has reduced enthusiasm for the use of ionizing radiation. No area of tumor research has generated as much excitement as the potential genetic treatment of NF; the search for gene therapy that will enable control of an aberrant or unsuppressed gene appears to be one of the most exciting directions.

REFERENCES

1. Ragga NK, Munier FL. Ancient neurofibromatosis. *Nature* 1994;368:815.
2. Cohen MM Jr. Proteus syndrome: further diagnostic thoughts about the elephant man. *Genetics* 1988;29: 777–782.
3. Cohen BH, Rothner AD. Incidence, types, management of cancer in patients with neurofibromatosis. *Oncology* 1989;3:23–38.
4. Preiser SA, Davenport CB. Multiple neurofibromatosis (von Recklinghausen's disease) and its inheritance: description of a case. *Am J Med Sci* 1918;156:507–540.
5. Barker D, Wright E, Nguyen E, et al. Gene for von Recklinghausen neurofibromatosis is in the pericentric region of the chromosome 17. *Science* 1987;236:1100–1102.
6. Mapstone TB. Neurofibromatosis and central nervous system tumors in childhood. *Neurosurg Clin North Am* 1992;3:771–779.
7. Riccardi VM. Neurofibromatosis: an overview and new directions in clinical investigations. In: Riccardi VM, Mulvihill JJ, eds. *Neurofibromatosis (von Recklinghausen's Disease)*. New York: Raven Press; 1981:1–9.
8. Riccardi VM. *Neurofibromatosis: Phenotype, Natural History and Pathogenesis*. Baltimore: Johns Hopkins University Press; 1992.
9. Mautner V-F, Tatagiba M, Guthoff R, et al. Neurofibromatosis in the pediatric age group. *Neurosurgery* 1993;33: 92–96.
10. Kanter W, Eldridge R, Fabricant R, et al. Central neurofibromatosis with bilateral acoustic neuroma: genetic, clinical and biochemical distinctions from peripheral neurofibromatosis. *Neurology* 1980;30:851–859.
11. Listernick R, Charrow J. Neurofibromatosis type 1 in childhood. *J Pediatr* 1990;116:845–853.
12. Mulvihill JJ, Parry DM, Sherman JL, et al. NIH Conference: Neurofibromatosis-1 (von Recklinghausen disease) and neurofibromatosis-2 (bilateral acoustic neurofibromatosis)—an update. *Ann Intern Med* 1990;133:39–52.
13. Von Recklinghausen F. *Uber die multiplen fibrome der Haut und ihre Beziehung zu den Multiplex Neuromen*. Berlin: A. Hirschwald; 1882.
14. Crowe FW, Schull J, Need JV. *A Clinical Pathological and Genetic Study of Multiple Neurofibromatosis*. Springfield, IL: Charles C Thomas; 1956.
15. Lewis RA, Gerson LP, Axelson KA, et al. Von Recklinghausen neurofibromatosis: incidence of optic gliomata. *Ophthalmology* 1984;91:929–935.
16. Listernick R, Charrow J, Greenwald MJ, Mets M. Natural history of optic pathway tumors in children with neurofibromatosis type 1: a longitudinal study. *J Pediatr* 1994;125:63–66.
17. Lund AM, Skovby F. Optic glioma in children with neurofibromatosis type 1. *Eur J Pediatr* 1991;150:835–838.
18. Menor R, Marti–Bonmati L, Mulas F, et al. Imaging considerations of central nervous system manifestations in pediatric patients with neurofibromatosis type 1. *Pediatr Radiol* 1991;21:389–394.
19. Deliganis AV, Geyer, JR, Berger MS. Prognostic significance of type 1 neurofibromatosis (von Recklinghausen disease) in childhood optic glioma. *Neurosurgery* 1996; 38:1114–1119.
20. Martuzza RL, Eldridge R. Neurofibromatosis 2. *N Engl J Med* 1988;318:684–688.
21. Jacoby LB, Pulaski H, Rouleau GA, et al. Clonal analysis of human meningiomas and schwannomas. *Cancer Res* 1990;50:6783–6786.
22. Flexon PB, Nadol JB, Schuknecht HP, et al. Bilateral acoustic neurofibromatosis (neurofibromatosis 2): a disorder distinct from von Recklinghausen's neurofibromatosis (neurofibromatosis 1). *Ann Otol Rhinol Laryngol* 1991;100:830–834.
23. Thapar K, Fukuyama K, Rutka JT. Neurogenetics and the molecular biology of human brain tumors. In: Laws EL, Kaye A, eds. *Encyclopedia of Human Brain Tumours*. Edinburgh: Churchill Livingstone; 1994.
24. Evans DG, Huson SM, Donnai D, et al. A genetic study of type 2 neurofibromatosis in the United Kingdom. II. Guidelines for genetic counseling. *J Med Genet* 1992;29:847.
25. Worcester–Drought C, Carnegie DW, McMenemey W. Multiple meningeal and perineural tumors with analogous changes in the glia and ependymoma (neurofibroblastomatosis) *Brain* 1939;60:85–117.
26. Krontiris TG, Cooper GM. Transforming activity of human tumor DNAs. *Proc Natl Acad Sci USA* 1981;68:820–823.
27. Westphal M, Herrmann HD. Growth factor biology and oncogene activation in human gliomas and their implications for specific therapeutic concepts. *Neurosurgery* 1989;25:681–684.
28. Cawthon R, Weiss R, Xu G, et al. A major segment of the neurofibromatosis type 1 gene: CDNA sequence, genomic structure and point mutations. *Cell* 1990;62:193–201.
29. Daston M, Scrable H, Nordlund M, et al. The protein product of neurofibromatosis type 1 gene is expressed at highest abundance in neurons, Schwann cells, and oligodendrocytes. *Neuron* 1992;8:415–428.
30. Rouleau GA, Merel P, Lutchman M, et al. Alteration in a new gene enclocding a putative membrane–organizing

protein causes neurofibromatosis type 2. *Nature* 1993; 363:515–521.

31. Rouleau GA, Seizinger BR, Wertelecki W, et al. Flanking markers bracket the neurofibromatosis type 2 (NF2) gene on chromosome 22. *Am J Hum Genet* 1990;46:323–328.

32. Guttman DH, Collins FS. Recent progress toward understanding the molecular biology of von Recklinghausen neurofibromatosis. *Ann Neurol* 1992;31:555.

33. Ballester R, Marchuk D, Bobuski M, et al. The NF–1 locus encodes a protein functionally related to mammalian GAP and yeast IRA proteins. *Cell* 1990;63:851–859.

34. DeClue J, Cohen B, Lowy D. Identification and characterization of the neurofibromatosis type 1 protein product. *Proc Natl Acad Sci USA* 1991;88:9914–9918.

35. Trofatter JA, MacCollin MM, Rutter JL, et al. A novel moesin-, ezrin-, radixin-like gene is a candidate for the neurofibromatosis 2 tumor suppressor. *Cell* 1993;72: 791–800.

36. Knudsen AG. Mutations and cancer: statistical study of retinoblastoma. *Proc Natl Acad Sci USA* 1971:68:820–823.

37. Hollstein M, Sidransky D, Vogelstein B, et al. *p53* mutations in human cancers. *Science* 1991;253:49–53.

38. Levine GA, Momand J, Finlay CA. The *p53* tumor suppressor gene. *Nature* 1991;351:453–456.

39. Menon AG, Anderson KM, Riccardi VM, et al. Chromosome 17p deletions and *p53* gene mutations associated with the formation of malignant neurofibrosarcomas in von Recklinghausen neurofibromatosis. *Proc Natl Acad Sci USA* 1990;87:5435–5439.

40. Nigro JM, Baker SJ, Preisinger AC, et al. Mutations in the *p53* gene occur in diverse tumor types. *Nature* 1989;342: 705–708.

41. Vogelstein B, Kinzler K. *p53* function and dysfunction. *Cell* 1992;70:523–526.

42. Newcomb EW, Lang FF, Koslow M. Molecular biology of brain tumors. In: Tindall GT, Cooper PR, Barrow DL, eds. *The Practice of Neurosurgery*. Baltimore: Williams & Wilkins; 1996:475–493.

43. Pollack IF, Hamilton RL, Finkelstein SD, et al. The relationship between *TP53* mutations and overexpression of *p53* and prognosis in malignant gliomas of childhood. *Cancer Res* 1997;57:304–309.

44. El–Deiry WS, Kern SE, Pietenpol JA, et al. Definition of a consensus binding site for *p53*. *Nature Genet* 1992;1:45.

45. El–Deiry WS, Tokin T, Velculescu VE, et al. WAF 1, a potential mediator of *p53* tumor suppression. *Cell* 1993; 75:817.

46. Dirks PB, Rutka JT. The genetic basis of neurosurgical disorders. In: Youmans JR, ed. *Neurological Surgery*. 4th ed. Vol. 2. Philadelphia: WB Saunders; 1996:811–828.

47. Harris CC, Hollstein M. Clinical implications of the *p53* tumor suppressor gene. *N Engl J Med* 1993;229:1318.

48. Kern SE, Pietenpol JA, Thiagalingam S, et al. Oncogenic forms of *p53* inhibit *p53*–regulated gene expression. *Science* 1992;256:827.

49. Leigus E, Marchuk DA, Collins FS, et al. Somatic deletion of the neurofibromatosis type 1 gene in a neurofibromasarcoma supports the tumour suppressor gene hypothesis. *Nature Genet* 1993;3:122.

50. Malkin D, Jolly KW, Barbier N, et al. Germline mutations of the *p53* tumor suppressor gene in children and young adults with second malignant neoplasms. *N Engl J Med* 1992;326:1309.

51. Seizinger BR. NFI: a prevalent cause of tumorigenesis in human cancers? *Nature Genet* 1993;3:97–99.

52. Skuse G, Kosciolek B, Rowley P. Molecular genetic analysis of tumors in von Recklinghausen neurofibromatosis: loss of heterozygosity for chromosome 17. *Genes Chrom Cancer* 1989;1:36–41.

53. Vogelstein B, Kinzler KW. *p53* function and dysfunction. *Cell* 1992;70:523–526.

54. Guttman DH, Collins FS. The neurofibromatosis type 1 gene and its protein product, neurofibromin. *Neuron* 1993;54:335–343.

55. Xu G, O'Connell P, Viskochil D, et al. The neurofibromatosis type 1 gene encodes a protein related to GAP. *Cell* 1990;62:599–608.

56. Guttman DH, Wood D, Collins FS. Identification of the neurofibromatosis type 1 gene product. *Proc Natl Acad Sci USA* 1991;89:9658–9662.

57. Martin G, Viskochil D, Bollag G, et al. The GAP–related domain of the neurofibromatosis type 1 gene product interacts with ras p21. *Cell* 1990;63:843–849.

58. Basu TN, Gutmann DH, Fletcher JA et al. Aberrant regulation of ras proteins in malignant tumour cells from type 1 neurofibromatosis. *Nature* 1992;356:713–715.

59. DeClue J, Papageorge A, Fletcher J, et al. Abnormal regulation of mammalian p21ras contributes to malignant tumor growth in von Recklinghausen (type 1) neurofibromatosis. *Cell* 1992;69:265–227.

60. Huson SM, Compston DA, Clark P, et al. A genetic study of von Recklinghausen neurofibromatosis in southeast Wales: 1. Prevalence, fitness, mutation rate, and effect of paternal transmission on severity. *J Med Genet* 1989;26:704.

61. Jadayel D, Fain P, Upadhyaya M, et al. Paternal origin of new mutations in von Recklinghausen neurofibromatosis. *Nature* 1990;343:559.

62. Wertelecki W, Rouleau GA, Superneau DW, et al. Neurofibromatosis 2: clinical and DNA linkage studies in a large kindred. *N Engl J Med* 1988;319:278–283.

63. Li Y, Bollag G, Clark R, Stevens I, et al. Somatic mutations in the neurofibromatosis 1 gene in human tumors. *Cell* 1992;69:275–281.

64. Dumanski JP, Rouleau GA, Nordenskjoid M, et al. Molecular genetic analysis of chromosome 22 in 81 cases of meningioma. *Cancer Res* 1990;50:5863–5867.

65. Bianchi AB, Hara T, Ramesh V, et al. Mutations in transcript isoforms of the neurofibromatosis II gene in multiple human tumor types. *Nature Genet* 1994;6:185.

66. Seizinger BR, de la Monte S, Atkins, et al. Molecular genetic approach to human meningiomas: loss of genes on chromosome 22. *Proc Natl Acad Sci USA* 1987;84: 5419–5423.

67. Wolff RK, Frazer KA, Jackler RK, et al. Analysis of chromosome 22 deletions in neurofibromatosis type 2–related tumors. *Am J Hum Genet* 1992;51:478–485.

68. Martuza RL, Malick A, Markert JM, et al. Experimental therapy of human glioma by means of genetically engineered virus mutant. *Science* 1991;252:854–856.

69. Le Gal La Salle G. Berrard JJ, Berrard S, et al. An adenovirus vector gene transfer into neurons and glia in the brain. *Science* 1993;259:988–990.

70. Jaenisch R, Breindle M, Harbers K, et al. Retroviruses and insertional mutagenesis. *Cold Spring Harbor Symp Quant Biol* 1985;50:439–445.

71. Culver KW, Ram Z, Wallbridge S, et al. In vivo gene transfer with retroviral vector–producer cells for treatment of experimental brain tumors. *Science* 1992;256:1550–1552.

72. Gordon JE, Ruddle FH. Gene transfer into mouse embryos: production of transgenic mice by pronuclear injection. *Meth Enzymol* 1983;101:411–433.

73. Hanahan D. Transgenic mice as probes into complex systems. *Science* 1989;246:1265–1275.

74. Lott IT, Richardson EP Jr. Neuropathological findings and the biology of neurofibromatosis. In: Riccardi VM, Mulvihill JJ, eds. *Neurofibromatosis (von Recklinghausen's Disease)*. New York: Raven Press;1981:23–32.

75. Ansari A, Nagamani M. Pregnancy and neurofibromatosis (von Recklinghausen's disease). *Obstet Gynecol* 1976;47: 25S–29S.

76. Mackool BT, Fitzpatrick TP. Diagnosis of neurofibromatosis by cutaneous examination. *Semin Neurol* 1992; 12:358.

77. Crowe FW, Schull WJ. Diagnostic importance of café-au-lait spots in neurofibromatosis. *Arch Intern Med* 1953;91: 758–766.

78. Whitehouse D. Diagnostic value of the café-au-lait spot in children. *Arch Dis Child* 1966;41:316–319.

79. Fienman NL, Yakovac WC. Neurofibromatosis in childhood. *J Pediatr* 1970;76:339–346.

80. Ducatman BS, Scheithauer BW, Piepgras DG, et al. Malignant peripheral nerve sheath tumors: a clinicopathologic study of 120 cases. *Cancer* 1986;57:2006–2021.

81. Guha A, Bilbao J, Kline DG, Hudson AR. Tumors of the peripheral nervous system. In: Youmans JR, ed. *Neurological Surgery*. 4th ed. Vol. 4. Philadelphia: WB Saunders; 1996:3175–3187.

82. Hope DC, Mulvihill JJ. Malignancy in neurofibromatosis. In: Riccardi VM, Mulvihill JJ, eds. *Neurofibromatosis (von Recklinghausen's Disease)*. New York: Raven Press; 1981: 33–56.

83. Hosoi K. Multiple neurofibromatosis (von Recklinghausen's disease) with special reference to malignant transformation. *Arch Surg* 1931;22:258–281.

84. Lefkowitz I, Obringer A, Meadows A. Neurofibromatosis and cancer: incidence and management. In: Rubenstein A, Korf B, eds. *Neurofibromatosis: A Handbook for Patients, Families and Health-Care Professionals*. New York: Thieme-Stratton; 1990:86–92.

85. Rogalski R, Louis D. Neurofibrosarcomas of the upper extremity. *J Hand Surg* 1991;16A:873–876.

86. Sands MJ, McDonough MT, Cohen AM, et al. Fatal malignant degeneration in multiple neurofibromatosis. *JAMA* 1975;233:1381–1382.

87. Sordillo P, Helson L, Hajdu S, et al. Malignant schwannoma—clinical characteristics, survival, and response to therapy. *Cancer* 1981;53:2503–2509.

88. Sorensen SA, Mulvihill JJ, Nielsen A. Long-term follow-up of von Recklinghausen neurofibromatosis: survival and malignant neoplasms. *N Engl J Med* 1986;314: 1010–1015.

89. Storm FK, Eilber FR, Mirra J, et al. Neurofibrosarcoma. *Cancer* 1980;45:126–129.

90. White H. Survival in malignant schwannomas: an 18 year study. *Cancer* 1971;27:720–729.

91. Ragge NK, Falk RE, Cohen WE, Murphree AL. Images of Lisch nodules across the spectrum. *Eye* 1993;7:95–101.

92. Lubs ML, Bauer MA, Formas ME, et al. Lisch nodules in neurofibromatosis 1. *N Engl J Med* 1991;324:1256.

93. Kaiser–Kupfer M. 1. Ophthalmic manifestations. In: Mulvihill JJ, moderator. Neurofibromatosis 1 (von Recklinghausen) and neurofibromatosis 2 (bilateral acoustic neurofibromatosis): an update. *Ann Intern Med* 1990;113:39.

94. Charles SJ, Moore AT, Yates Jr, et al. Lisch nodules in neurofibromatosis type 2. *Arch Ophthalmol* 1989;107:1571.

95. Kaiser-Kufer M, Freidln V, Danles MB, et al. The association of posterior capsular lens opacities with bilateral acoustic neuromas in patients with neurofibromatosis type 2. *Arch Ophthalmol* 1989;107:541–545.

96. Poole MD. Experiences in the surgical treatment of cranio–oribital neurofibromatosis. *Br J Plast Surg* 1989; 42:155–162.

97. White AK, Smith RJ, Bigler CR, et al. Head and neck manifestations of neurofibromatosis. *Laryngoscope* 1986; 96:732–737.

98. Binet EF, Kieffer SA, Martin SH, Peterson HO. Orbital dysplasia in neurofibromatosis. *Radiology* 1969;93:829–933.

99. Harkens K, Dolan KD. Correlative imaging of sphenoid dysplasia accompanying neurofibromatosis. *Ann Otol Rhinol Laryngol* 1990;99:137–141.

100. Macfarlane R, Levin AV, Weksberg R, et al. Absence of the greater sphenoid wing in neurofibromatosis type 1: congenital or acquired: case report. *Neurosurgery* 1995;37: 129–133.

101. LeWald LT. Congenital absence of the superior orbital wall associated with pulsating exophthalmos: report of four cases. *Am J Roentgenol* 1933;30:756–764.

102. Jackson IT, Carbonnel A, Potparic Z, Shaw K. Orbitotemporal neurofibromatosis: classification and treatment. *Plast Reconstr Surg* 1993;92:1–11.

103. Dandy WE. An operative treatment for certain cases of meningocele (or encephaloceles) into the orbit. *Arch Ophthalmol* 1929;2:123–132.

104. Crawford AH Jr, Bagamery N. Osseous manifestations of neurofibromatosis in childhood. *J Pediatr Orthop* 1986;6:72–88.

105. Hunt JC, Pugh DG. Skeletal lesions in neurofibromatosis. *Radiology* 1961;76:1–19.

106. Winter RB, Moe JH, Bradford, DS, et al. Spine deformity in neurofibromatosis. *J Bone Joint Surg* 1979;61:671–694.

107. McNiesch LM. Neurofibromatosis. In: Taveras JM, Ferrucci JT, eds. *Radiology: Diagnosis, Imaging, Intervention*. Vol. 5. Philadelphia: JB Lippincott; 1993:1–10.

108. Ruggier, M, Pavone V, Tiné A, et al. Ossifying fibroma of the skull in a patient with neurofibromatosis type 1. *J Neurosurg* 1996;85:941–944.

109. Halpen M, Currarino G. Vascular lesions causing hypertension in neurofibromatosis. *N Engl J Med* 1965;273: 248–252.

110. Levisohn PM, Mikhael MA, Rothman SM. Cerebrovascular changes in neurofibromatosis. *Devl Med Child Neurol* 1978;20:789–793.

111. Schievink WI, Piepgras DG. Cervical vertebral artery aneurysms and arteriovenous fistulas in neurofibro-

matosis type 1: case reports. *Neurosurgery* 1991;29: 760–765.

112. Schut L, Duhaime AC, Bruce DA, Sutton SN. Von Recklinghausen's Disease. In: Hoffman HJ, Epstein F, eds. *Disorders of the Developing Nervous System: Diagnosis and Treatment.* Boston, Blackwell Scientific; 1986:591–605.

113. Weichert KA, Dine MS, Benton C, Silverman FN. Macrocranium and neurofibromatosis. *Radiology* 1973;107: 163–166.

114. Holt JF. Neurofibromatosis in children. *Am J Roentgenol* 1978;130:615–639.

115. Aoki S, Barkovich AJ, Nishimura K, et al. Neurofibromatosis types 1 and 2: cranial MR findings. *Radiology* 1989;172:525–534.

116. Rubinstein AE, Huang P, Kugler S, et al. Unidentified signals on magnetic resonance imaging in children with neurofibromatosis. *Neurology* 1988;38:282.

117. Shu HH, Mirowitz SA, Wippold FJ. Neurofibromatosis: MR imaging findings involving the head and spine. *Am J Roentgenol* 1993;160:159–164.

118. Di Mario FJ, Ramsby G, Greenstein R, et al. Neurofibromatosis type 1: magnetic resonance imaging findings. *J Child Neurol* 1993;8:32–39.

119. Mirowitz SA, Sartor K, Gado M. High-intensity basal ganglia lesions on T1-weighted MR images in neurofibromatosis. *Am J Roentgenol* 1990;154:369–373.

120. Raffel C, McComb JG, Bodner S, et al. Benign brain stem lesions in pediatric patients with neurofibromatosis: case reports. *Neurosurgery* 1989;25:989.

121. Rosman N, Pearce J. The brain in multiple neurofibromatosis (von Recklinghausen's disease): a suggested neuropathological basis for the associated mental defect. *Brain* 1967;90:829–837.

122. Dipaulo D, Zimmerman RA, Rorke LB, et al. Pathological substrate of high intensity foci in neurofibromatosis type 1. *Radiology* 1995;195:721–724.

123. Molloy PT, Bilaniuk LT, Vaughan SN, et al. Brainstem tumors in patients with neurofibromatosis type 1: a distinct clinical entity. *Neurology* 1995;45:1897–1902.

124. Canale DJ, Bebin J. Von Recklinghausen disease of the nervous system. In: Vinken PJ, Bruyn GW, eds. *Handbook of Clinical Neurology.* Vol 14. *The Phakomatosis.* New York: American Elsevier; 1972:132–162.

125. Griffith BH, McKinney P, Monroe CW, Howell A. Von Recklinghausen's disease in children. *Plast Reconstr Surg* 1972;49:647–665.

126. Ferner RE, Chaudhuri R, Bingham J, Cox T, Hughes RAC. MRI in neurofibromatosis 1. The nature and evolution of increased intensity T2-weighted lesions and their relationship to intellectual impairment. *J Neurol Neurosurg Psychiatry* 1993;56:492–495.

127. National Institutes of Health Consensus Development Conference: conference statement: neurofibromatosis. *Arch Neurol* 1988;45:575–578.

128. Boland R. Neurofibromatosis—the quintessential neurocristopathy: pathogenetic concepts and relationships. In: Riccardi VM, Mulvihill JJ, eds. *Neurofibromatosis (von Recklinghausen's Disease).* New York: Raven Press; 1981: 67–75.

129. Riccardi VM. Von Recklinghausen neurofibromatosis. *N Engl J Med* 1981;305:1617.

130. Side L, Taylor B, Cavouette M, et al. Homozygous inactivation of the *NF1* gene in bone marrow cells from children with neurofibromatosis type 1 and malignant myeloid disorders. *N Engl J Med* 1997; 336:1713–1720.

131. Martuzza RL, Ojemann RG. Bilateral acoustic neuromas: clinical aspects, pathogenesis and treatment. *Neurosurgery* 1982;10:1.

132. Balestri P, Calistri L, Vivarelli R, et al. Central nervous system imaging in reevaluation of patients with neurofibromatosis type 1. *Child's Nerv Syst* 1993;9:448–451.

133. Blatt J, Jaffe R, Detch M, et al. Neurofibromatosis and childhood tumors. *Cancer* 1986;57:1225.

134. Freeman TB, Cahill DW. Management of intradural extramedullary tumors. In: Tindall GT, Cooper PR, Barrow DL, eds. *The Practice of Neurosurgery.* Baltimore: Williams & Wilkins; 1996:1323–1334.

135. Ruttledge MH, Sarrazin J, Rangaratnam S, et al. Evidence for complete inactivation of the NF2 gene in the majority of sporadic meningiomas. *Nature Genet* 1994;6:180.

136. Bataini JP, Delanian S, Ponvert D. Chiasmal gliomas: results of irradiation management in 57 patients and review of literature. *Int J Radiat Oncol Phys* 1991;21: 615–623.

137. Dovalic JJ, Grigsby PW, Shepard MJ, et al. Radiation therapy for gliomas of the optic nerve and chiasm. *J Radiat Oncol Biol Phys* 1990;18:927–932.

138. Hoffman HJ, Humphreys RP, Drake JM, et al. Optic pathway/hypothalamic gliomas: a dilemma in management. *Pediatr Neurosurg* 1993;19:186–195.

139. Jenkin D, Angyalfi S, Becker L, et al. Optic gliomas in children: surveillance, resection, or irradiation? *In J Radiat Oncol Biol Phys* 1993;25:215–225.

140. Packer RJ, Rosenstock JG, Bilaniuk LT, et al. Chiasmatic hypothalamic/thalamic gliomas in childhood: efficacy of treatment in neurofibromatosis. *Ann Neurol* 1984;16:402.

141. Milstein JM, Geyer JR, Berger MS, Bleyer WA. Favourable prognosis for brainstem gliomas in neurofibromatosis. *J Neuro-oncol* 1989;7:367–371.

142. Packer RJ, Nicholson HS, Johnson DL, Vezina LG. Dilemmas in the management of childhood brain tumors: brain-stem gliomas. *Pediatr Neurosurg* 1991;17:37–43.

143. Petronio J, Edwards MSB, Prados M, et al. Management of chiasmal and hypothalamic gliomas of infancy and childhood with chemotherapy. *J Neurosurg* 1991;74: 701–708.

144. Savolardo M, Harwood-Nash DC, Tadmor R, et al. Gliomas of the intracranial anterior optic pathways in children. *Radiology* 1981;138:601–610.

145. Spitzer DE, Goodrich JT. Optic gliomas and neurofibromatosis: neurosurgical management. *Neurofibromatosis* 1988;1:223–232.

146. Wisoff JH, Epstein F. Surgical management of chiasmatic-hypothalamic tumors of childhood. *Conc Pediatr Neurosurg* 1989;9:77–90.

147. Wisoff JH, Abbott R, Epstein F. Surgical management of exophytic chiasmatic–hypothalamic tumors of childhood. *J Neurosurg* 1990;73:661–667.

148. Sutton LN, Molloy PT, Sernyak H, et al. Long–term outcome of hypothalamic/chiasmatic astrocytomas in children treated with conservative surgery. *J Neurosurg* 1995;83:583–589.

149. Kestle JR, Hoffman HJ, Mock AR. Moyamoya phenomenon after radiation for optic glioma. *J Neurosurg* 1993; 79:32.

150. Freeman CR, Krischer JP, Sanford RA, et al. Final results of a study of escalating doses of hyperfractionated radiotherapy in brainsteim tumors in children: a Pediatric Oncology Group study. *Int J Radiat Oncol Biol Phys* 1993; 27:197–206.

151. Newbould M, Wilkinson N, Mene A. Post–radiation malignant peripheral nerve sheath tumors: a report of two cases. *Histopathology* 1990;16:263–265.

152. Seib JP, Schultheiss R. Segmental neurofibromatosis of the sciatic nerve: case report. *Neurosurgery* 1992;31: 1122–1125.

153. Basso–Ricci S. Therapy of malignant schwannomas: usefulness of an integrated radiologic–surgical therapy. *J Neurosurg Sci* 1989;33:253–257.

154. Donner TR, Voorhies RM, Kline DG. Neural sheath tumors of major nerves. *J Neurosurg* 1994;81:362–373.

155. Meis J, Enzinger F, Martz K. et al. Malignant peripheral nerve sheath tumors (malignant schwannomas) in children. *Am J Surg Pathol* 1992;16:694–707.

156. Bolten J, Vauthey J, Farr G, et al. Is limb-sparing surgery applicable to neurogenic sarcomas of the extremities. *Arch Surg* 1989;124:118–121.

157. Healy JH, McCormack RR. Nerve tumors. In: Bogumill CP, Fleegler EJ, eds. *Tumors of the Hand and Upper Limb*. Edinburgh: Churchill Livingstone; 1993:205–223.

158. Ducatman BS, Scheithauer BW. Post-irradiation neurofibrosarcoma. *Cancer* 1983; 51:1028–1033.

159. Enzinger FM, Weiss SW, Benign tumors of peripheral nerves. In: Enzinger FM, Weiss SW, eds. *Soft Tissue Tumors*. 2nd ed. St. Louis: Mosby; 1988:719–780.

160. Foley KM, Woodruff JM, Ellis FT, Posner JB. Radiation induced malignant and atypical peripheral nerve sheath tumors. *Ann Neurol* 1980;7:311–318.

161. Shiu MH, Turnbull AD, Nori D, et al. Control of locally advanced extremity soft tissue sarcomas by function: saving resection and brachytherapy. *Cancer* 1984;47: 1385–1392.

162. Woodruff JM. The pathology and treatment of peripheral nerve tumors and tumor-like conditions. *CA Cancer J Clin* 1993;43:290–308.

163. Enzinger FM, Weiss SW. Malignant tumors of peripheral nerves. In: Enzinger FM, Weiss SW, eds. *Soft Tissue Tumors*. 2nd ed. St. Louis: Mosby; 1988:781–815.

164. Rosenberg AE, Dick HM, Botte MJ. Benign and malignant tumors of peripheral nerve. In: Gelberman RH, ed. *Operative Nerve Repair and Reconstructions*. Philadelphia: JB Lippincott; 1991:1587–1625.

165. Mankin HJ. Principles of soft-tissue tumor managment. In: Gelberman RH, ed. *Operative Nerve Repair and Reconstructions*. Philadelphia: JB Lippincott; 1991:1587–1625.

166. Guccion JG, Enzinger FM. Malignant schwannoma associated with von Recklinghausen's neurofibromatosis. *Virchows Arch* 1979;383:43–57.

Chapter 33

Peripheral Nerve Tumors

Gavin W. Britz, Jang-Chul Lee, Robert Goodkin, and Michel Kliot

Peripheral nerve tumors, which can originate from any of the cellular elements of a peripheral nerve, are rare in the pediatric population.[1–12] Management of these tumors is based on a thorough understanding of the anatomical, pathologic, clinical, radiologic, and biologic nature of these tumors. Recent advances in many fields, including molecular biology, magnetic resonance imaging (MRI), and intraoperative electrophysiology and microsurgery, have led to improvements in the management of this clinical problem.

ANATOMY OF THE PERIPHERAL NERVE

Peripheral nerves connect the central nervous system (CNS) with sensory, motor, and autonomic end organs of the body. Peripheral nerves arise immediately distal to the dural covering of the spinal nerve roots and consist of three basic components: the action potential conducting axons, the insulating ensheathing Schwann cells, and a surrounding extracellular compartment consisting of cells (e.g., fibroblasts, macrophages, endothelial cells, and mast cells) and molecules (e.g., proteins, glycoproteins, and proteoglycans).[13–15]

Nerve fibers are ensheathed by Schwann cells, either individually to form myelinated fibers or as part of a group in unmyelinated fibers (Fig. 33–1). Both myelinated and unmyelinated nerve fibers are then embedded within a connective tissue compartment called the endoneurium. The endoneurium in turn is encircled by a compact layer called the perineurium, composed of concentrically arranged elongated perineural cells that partition nerve fibers into fascicles. These perineural cells are thought to arise from fibroblasts despite their having a pericellular basal lamina, a feature characteristic of Schwann cells but not fibroblasts.[15, 16]

Peripheral nerve fascicles are embedded in a connective tissue layer, the internal epineurium (Fig. 33–1), which in turn is encircled by several layers of concentrically arranged cells that form the external epineurium. The internal and external epineurium contain variable quantities of fat, fibroblasts, macrophages, and blood vessels.

The different cellular and molecular elements of peripheral nerve can also be differentiated by immunocytochemistry.[11] For example, Schwann cells can be visualized using antibodies to S100,[17] Leu-7,[18–20] and the low-affinity receptor to nerve growth factor.[21] Perineural cells can be stained with antibodies to epithelial membrane antigen (EMA).[22]

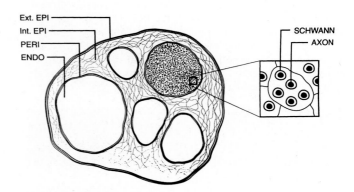

Figure 33–1 Schematic diagram of a cross section of a peripheral nerve. Individual axons are encased by Schwann cells (inset) within the endoneurium (ENDO). The endoneurium is in turn encircled by a connective tissue layer, the perineurium (PERI), composed of perineural cells, which divides the nerve into fascicles. Nerve fascicles are embedded in a layer of connective tissue called the internal epineurium (Int. EPI) which is surrounded by the external epineurium (Ext. EPI). (Reproduced with permission from Grossman RG, Loftus CM, eds. *Principles of Neurosurgery*. 2nd ed. Philadelphia: Lippincott–Raven Publishers.)

We thank Paul Schwartz, Janet Schukar, and Bob Holmberg for their excellent assistance in preparing the figures. We thank Dr. H. R. Winn for his continued generous and enthusiastic support. This work was supported by Training Grant T32NS-07144-15 from the National Institutes of Health, a Royalty Research Fund Grant from the University of Washington, and support from the Seattle Veterans Administration Hospital. MK is the recipient of a Clinician Investigator Development Award from the National Institute of Neurological Disorders and Stroke.

PATHOLOGY

Tumors of the peripheral nerve may originate from any of the intrinsic cellular elements of a peripheral nerve, which include Schwann cells, perineural cells, fibroblasts, endothelial cells, fat cells, and neurons. They may also arise from cell types normally extrinsic to peripheral nerves, such as in the case of metastatic tumors. Pathologic descriptions of the most common types of tumors and nontumor mass lesions involving peripheral nerves are given below.

BENIGN TUMORS ARISING FROM INTRINSIC PERIPHERAL NERVE ELEMENTS

Neurofibromas and Neurofibromatosis Type I

Neurofibromas are the most common type of peripheral nerve tumor, usually occurring sporadically as solitary lesions. In patients with neurofibromatosis type 1 (NF-1), or von Recklinghausen's disease, multiple neurofibromas characterize the disease.[23, 24] The clinical syndrome of NF-1 is characterized by two or more of the following clinical findings[25]: six or more café au lait spots greater than 5 mm in diameter in prepubertal individuals and greater than 15 mm in postpubertal individuals; two or more superficial skin neurofibromas of any type or one plexiform neurofibroma; freckling in the axillary and groin regions; bilateral optic nerve gliomas; two or more Lisch nodules (pigmented hamartomas in the iris of the eye); specific osseous lesions, such as sphenoid wing dysplasia or cortical thinning of a long bone; and a first-degree relative with documented NF-1. These patients may have other clinical features, including macrocephaly, short stature, intellectual handicap, epilepsy, hydrocephalus, and hypertension.[23, 24, 26–28]

BOX 33–1
Clinical Findings of NF-1 (Two or More of the Following)

- Six or more café au lait spots
  - > 5 mm prepubertal
  - > 15 mm postpubertal
- Two or more superficial skin neurofibromas or one plexiform neurofibroma
- Axillary/groin freckling
- Bilateral optic nerve gliomas
- Two or more Lisch nodules
- Osseous lesions
- First-degree relative with documented NF-1

NF-1 is a genetic disease transmitted in an autosomal dominant fashion with almost 100% penetrance. A high spontaneous mutation rate of the NF-1 gene occurs, as half of the patients do not have a positive family history of neurofibromatosis.[29] Genetic studies suggest that the spontaneous mutation involves the paternal gene of the long arm of chromosome 17,[30–38, 131] although phenotypic variation suggests that other genetic loci can modify the expression of the NF-1 gene.[39]

The protein product of the NF-1 gene is called neurofibromin. *Neurofibromin is expressed at high levels in Schwann cells*

and is believed to act as a tumor suppresser gene.[29, 30, 33, 40–43] NF-1 patients start out in life by inheriting one mutant NF-1 allele, and a somatic mutation or "second hit" causes a mutation to the second normal NF-1 allele, leading to the development of these tumors.[45]

Neurofibromin is a member of the Ras–guanosine triphosphatase activating protein (Ras-GAP) family. Ras is an important cytosolic signal transduction proto-oncogene that regulates both cellular proliferation and differentiation.[44, 46–50] In its activated state it is phosphorylated (Ras-GTP), and when it is dephosphorylated it becomes inactive (Ras-GDP). Neurofibromin promotes the inactivation of Ras by converting Ras-GTP to Ras-GDP.[5, 50] *Therefore, a mutation of neurofibromin that impairs its function results in enhanced activation of Ras.*[51, 49] It has been suggested that neurofibromin may modulate two different activities of Ras[36]: first as a negative regulator of the p21Ras-mediated signaling pathway for proliferation[47] and second as a downstream regulator of a p21Ras-mediated signaling pathway for cellular differentiation.[36]

Neurofibromas are often firm and light tan. Since the tumor cells grow between axons and fascicles, neurofibromas often have a fusiform appearance, with single or multiple nerve fascicles entering and exiting the tumor.[52] Tumor cells may also extend through the external epineurium to produce a polypoid lesion. Histologically, their appearance is variable and can consist of assorted cell types, including Schwann cells, fibroblasts, and a cell that has ultrastructural but not immunohistochemical characteristics of the perineural cell and has been referred to as the "neurofibroma cell"[12] (Fig. 33–2). These neurofibroma cells stain with antibodies to the S100 protein[17] and coagulation factor XIIIa,[53] but they do not stain with antibodies to EMA, which normally stain perineural cells.[22] These tumors are usually characterized by spindle-shaped cells surrounded by collagen bundles (Fig. 33–2). Neurofibromas are more likely to undergo malignant transformation than schwannomas and when they do they are characterized by areas of necrosis, cellular pleomorphism, and a high mitotic index.

Schwannomas and Neurofibromatosis Type 2

Schwannomas are tumors that usually occur sporadically, although they may also occur in association with NF-1 and NF-2.[8, 23, 24, 54, 55] Schwannomas usually arise from a single nerve fascicle as solitary tumors. These types of tumor rarely form a "plexiform schwannoma," which occurs when the tumor arises from multiple nerve branches simultaneously.[1] Macroscopically schwannomas are usually globular or multilobulated. They generally arise from peripheral nerves or the parasympathetic nervous system portion of cranial nerves but may rarely occur within the CNS.[10] The cells forming these benign tumors have histologic, ultrastructural, and antigenic characteristics of Schwann cells.[6, 10, 12, 56] These characteristics include broad cytoplasmic processes, a characteristic basal lamina, and immunoreactivity to S100, the low affinity nerve growth factor receptor, and Leu-7 antibodies.[17, 19, 57] The histologic appearance of these tumors is characterized by spindle-shaped cells arranged in a pattern of either densely (Antoni A) or loosely (Antoni B) organized cellular areas (Fig. 33–3). Verocay bodies represent a palisading pattern of densely packed cells within Antoni A areas.

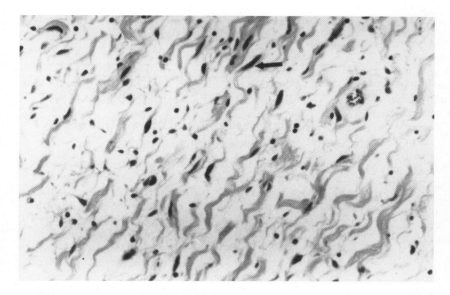

Figure 33–2 Hematoxylin-eosin staining of a neurofibroma demonstrating spindle-shaped cells (black arrow) dispersed in a loose extracellular matrix abundant in mucopolysaccharides. (Reproduced with permission from Grossman RG, Loftus CM, eds. *Principles of Neurosurgery*. 2nd ed. Philadelphia: Lippincott-Raven Publishers.)

NF-2 is a phakomatosis with an autosomal dominant pattern of inheritance with high penetrance.[54] Fifty percent of NF-2 cases represent spontaneous new mutations. The current diagnostic criterion for NF-2[25] consists of the presence of one of the following: (1) bilateral vestibular schwannoma; (2) a first-degree relative with NF-2 and either a unilateral vestibular schwannoma or any schwannoma, neurofibroma, meningioma, glioma, posterior subcapsular lens opacity, or cerebral calcification; (3) two of the following: unilateral vestibular schwannoma, multiple meningiomas, peripheral schwannoma, glioma, neurofibroma, posterior subcapsular lens opacity, or cerebral calcification. The NF-2 gene has been localized to the short arm of chromosome 22.[58–61] The product of the NF-2 gene is the protein Merlin. The function of Merlin is unknown, but it is thought to link the cell membrane to its cytoskeletal components. The inactivation of Merlin results in enhanced cellular growth and proliferation but not malignant transformation.[58]

> ## BOX 33–2
> ## Diagnostic Criterion for NF-2 (One of the Following)
>
> - Bilateral vestibular schwannomas
> - First-degree relative with NF-2 or unilateral vestibular schwannoma
> - First-degree relative with NF-2 any one of the following: schwannoma, neurofibroma, meningioma, glioma, posterior subcapsular lens opacity, or cerebral calcification
> - Two or more of the following: unilateral vestibular schwannoma, multiple meningiomas, peripheral schwannoma, glioma, neurofibroma, posterior subcapsular lens opacity, or cerebral calcification

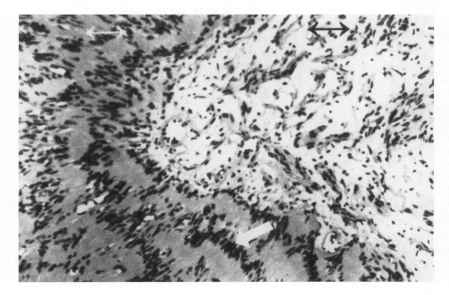

Figure 33–3 Hematoxylin-eosin staining of a schwannoma demonstrating spindle-shaped cells arranged in a characteristic pattern of densely acanged (Antoni A) (left half with white double arrow) or loosely arranged (Antoni B) (right half with black double arrow) cellular areas. The Antoni A areas consist of tightly packed cells in a palisading configuration characterized by the alignment of their nuclei in rows. Verocay bodies are localized areas of densely packed cells within Antoni A areas (large white arrow). (Reproduced with permission from Grossman RG, Loftus CM, eds. *Principles of Neurosurgery*. 2nd ed. Philadelphia: Lippincott-Raven Publishers.)

Perineuromas

Perineuroma is a rare, benign tumor found in adolescents and young adults that usually presents as a mononeuropathy involving an extremity. Perineural cells are found in other peripheral nerve tumors and "localized hypertrophic neuropathy," and therefore controversy exists if a perineuroma represents an abnormal reactive response of the nerve or an actual tumor involving the perineural cells.[62–71] Recent evidence suggests that perineuromas represent, at least in certain clinical cases, a distinct neoplastic entity,[66, 69–72] with the proliferating cells reacting with antibody to EMA but not S100 or Leu-7, suggesting a perineural cell origin.[22, 73] The involved nerve is usually focally or segmentally enlarged, and histologically the perineuroma is characterized by thickening of the perineurium and an "onion bulb" appearance formed from clusters of cells arranged concentrically around axons in a myxoid stroma.

Mucosal Neuroma

Mucosal neuromas are usually found in patients with multiple endocrine neoplasia type 2b. This is a genetic disorder characterized by C-cell hyperplasia and medullary carcinoma of the thyroid, adrenal hyperplasia, pheochromocytoma, and parathyroid hyperplasia.[74–76] It occurs in the lips, tongue, and eyelids and displays clusters of tortuous but separate nerve bundles histologically.[12]

Neurothekeoma

Neurothekeoma is a tumor found in the skin of children and adolescents. The cellular origin of this tumor is unresolved. It has been suggested that it is of peripheral nerve origin,[1] although staining for S100 has been negative.[77] Microscopically, the tumor consists of nests of cells within the dermis that have very prominent cytoplasm, giving them an epithelial appearance.[1]

Granule Cell Tumor

Granule cell tumors present as subcutaneous or submucosal masses in the skin, tongue, and breast.[8, 78] These are benign tumors that rarely demonstrate aggressive behavior and are thought to originate from a normal cellular component of a peripheral nerve. Microscopically, the cells are filled with eosinophilic granules that stain with periodic acid–Schiff, have a basement membrane, and demonstrate variable staining with S100.[78]

Vascular Tumors

Vascular tumors that directly involve peripheral nerves include hemangioblastomas and, less commonly, hemangiopericytomas, hemangiosarcomas, and glomus tumors.[8, 79, 80] Hemangiomas are rare tumors arising from vascular endothelial cells and occur in the younger population.[81–86] Hemangiomas often present with pain and tenderness, as well as sensory-motor neurologic deficits. Histology demonstrates thin-walled vessels filled with erythrocytes.[6, 10]

Neuromuscular Hamartoma

Neuromuscular hamartomas are rare tumors occurring during the first few years of life. These multilobulated masses consist of bundles of disorganized nerve fascicles and muscle fibers. These tumors usually occur in association with peripheral nerves[87, 88] but may be found intracranially.[89]

MALIGNANT TUMORS ARISING FROM INTRINSIC PERIPHERAL NERVE ELEMENTS

Malignant Peripheral Nerve Tumors (Neurogenic Sarcoma)

Malignant neoplasms of peripheral nerves very rarely occur de novo in the first decade, except in patients who have received radiotherapy.[90, 91] In patients with NF-1, transformation of a benign neoplasm, such as a plexiform neurofibroma, may also occur.[92–101] *In such patients, malignant transformation is thought to occur in approximately 4% of cases.*[93, 101] These tumors often affect medium-sized to large nerves, such as those of the brachial and lumbosacral plexus, as well as the sciatic and spinal nerves.[12] The cells of origin of malignant tumors of peripheral nerves are thought to include Schwann cells, fibroblasts, and perineural cells; hence the generic term "neurogenic sarcoma."[102]

On macroscopic inspection, these tumors produce fusiform enlargement of a peripheral nerve with regions of necrosis often found. The microscopic appearance of malignant peripheral nerve tumors is variable, with a herring-bone pattern most commonly encountered.[4] Malignant peripheral nerve tumors may demonstrate metaplastic elements including muscle, bone, cartilage, and epithelial elements.[1, 103] Regardless of the pattern, necrosis, vascular proliferation, and a high mitotic rate are prominent.[6, 10]

TUMORS ARISING FROM EXTRINSIC PERIPHERAL NERVE ELEMENTS

Metastatic and Other Tumors

A variety of tumor types can metastasize to peripheral nerves.[5, 9, 104, 105] Rare tumors that have been found to directly involve peripheral nerves include malignant primitive neuroectodermal tumors (PNETs), thyroid tumors, Ewing's sarcomas, osteochondromas, and bladder tumors.[8, 104, 105]

NONTUMORAL MASSES INVOLVING PERIPHERAL NERVES

Ganglion Cyst

A ganglion cyst appears as a superficial mass that arises from superficial nerves or the synovium of a neighboring joint space.[1, 106] This nonneoplastic cyst is lined by fibrous tissue and filled with a gelatinous matrix. It is believed that repetitive trauma stimulates degenerative or active secretory processes, which give rise to these lesions.[10]

Morton's Neuroma

Morton's neuroma is a reactive process to trauma that occurs typically in the plantar digital nerves between the heads of the third and fourth metatarsal bones.[1, 6, 8] This produces a fusiform enlargement of the entire neurovascular bundle, with atrophy of the nerve and proliferation of the perineurium and epineurium.[6]

DIAGNOSIS

Tumors of the peripheral nervous system are rare and most often found incidentally during the evaluation of a soft-tissue mass. To successfully manage these lesions, the evaluation should include a clinical history and physical examination and a diagnostic workup that encompasses both radiologic and electrodiagnostic studies. Often patients present with pain and/or loss of function in a peripheral nerve distribution. In patients with NF-1, the presence of multiple superficial masses strongly suggests the diagnosis of neurofibromas. An important aspect in the evaluation of any tumor is to assess its malignant potential. In regard to malignant peripheral nerve tumors, this distinction is difficult to make as both the clinical and radiologic features are often indistinguishable from those of benign tumors. The most common presenting complaint is rapid growth of a mass associated with neurologic symptoms, such as pain, paresthesia, numbness, and/or weakness.[7–9, 93, 94]

BOX 33–3
Clinical Presentation

- **Rapid growth of mass**
- **Pain**
- **Paresthesia**
- **Numbness**
- **Weakness**

In addition to assessment of the functional integrity of sensory and motor fibers in peripheral nerves by clinical examination, a variety of electrophysiologic modalities, including electromyography, nerve conduction studies, and studies of somatosensory evoked potential, are available.[8, 9] These are important in that they may reveal subtle peripheral nerve pathology as well as helping to establish baseline function prior to surgical resection.

Imaging studies have become increasingly important in the preoperative evaluation of mass lesions. The advent of computed tomography (CT) and, in particular, magnetic resonance imaging (MRI) has provided information about the local involvement and distant spread of tumors that is critical to the successful management of these clinical problems. Specifically in regard to peripheral nerve mass lesions, MRI with its superior soft tissue imaging characteristics has become particularly important.[107–110] Technical advances have led to the development of *magnetic resonance neurography* (MRN), which generates higher resolution images of nerves, thus permitting the visualization of the normal fascicular structure of nerves and its relationship to both intraneural and extraneural tumors and other types of masses.[111–115] MRN can help the surgeon to preoperatively plan the surgical approach that will allow resection with minimal trauma to

functioning nerve fascicles and thereby maximize the preservation of neurologic function. Another important aspect in obtaining this information is to enable the surgeon to preoperatively estimate the probability of performing a complete surgical resection.

Definitive diagnosis of a malignant peripheral nerve tumor can only be made after surgical biopsy and pathologic examination. The use of imaging studies is less useful in the discrimination of malignant from benign lesions. In malignancy both CT and MRI often demonstrate areas of cavitation and hemorrhage, changes that can also be found in benign tumors such as neurofibromas and schwannomas.[110, 116] The use of gallium 67 citrate scintigraphy may prove useful, as increased uptake has been found preferentially in patients with malignant peripheral nerve tumors.[117] Once a diagnosis of malignancy has been made, chest, abdominal, and pelvic CT scans as well as a bone scan should be obtained for staging. Such information influences treatment decisions and determines the patient's prognosis.

TREATMENT

Benign Peripheral Nerve Tumors and Nontumor Masses

The indication to resect a peripheral nerve tumor depends on the clinical symptoms and findings of the patient, augmented by the electrodiagnostic and/or imaging findings. A mass lesion that is thought to be benign, such as a neurofibroma or ganglion cyst, may be observed clinically, particularly if the patient is asymptomatic. However, when the diagnosis is in question or the patient has severe dysesthesias, progressive loss of sensory or motor function, or rapid enlargement of the tumor, surgical resection is indicated. The goals of the surgical treatment of benign tumors and other mass lesions involving peripheral nerves include establishing a pathologic diagnosis and performing a surgical resection while minimizing the loss of neurologic function.

BOX 33–4
Surgical Indications

- **Questionable diagnosis**
- **Rapid growth**
- **Pain**
- **Neurologic changes**

The tumor should be fully exposed, as should the normal proximal and distal nerve elements when possible. A surgical resection should then be performed using microsurgical technique in combination with intraoperative electrophysiologic stimulation and recording techniques. *The importance of using electrophysiologic monitoring techniques is that these allow the surgeon to differentiate functioning nerve fibers from nonfunctioning tumor, which can be difficult based solely on visual inspection.* These techniques include focal stimulation with recording from muscle, nerve, and spine as well as contralateral scalp in

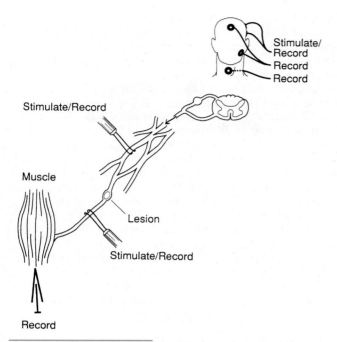

Figure 33–4 Schematic diagram illustrating the various intraoperative electrophysiologic monitoring stimulating and recording techniques available to the surgeon (see text for details). (Reproduced with permission from Kliot M, Slimp J. Techniques and assessment of peripheral nerve function at surgery. In: Loftus C, Traynelis VC, eds. *Intraoperative Monitoring Techniques in Neurosurgery*. New York: McGraw-Hill; 1993:275–285.)

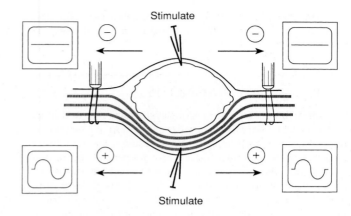

Figure 33–5 Schematic diagram illustrating how focal electrical stimulation of a peripheral nerve containing a mass can help to distinguish functioning nerve fibers (black lines) from nonfunctioning tumor tissue (outlined mass). Focal stimulation of the functioning axons gives rise to an evoked response that propagates away bidirectionally. Focal stimulation of the mass or lesion gives rise to no recordable evoked response. (Reproduced with permission from Kliot M, Slimp J. Techniques and assessment of peripheral nerve function at surgery. In: Loftus C, Traynelis VC, eds. *Intraoperative Monitoring techniques in Neurosurgery*. New York: McGraw-Hill; 1993:275–285.)

the case of SSEP studies[8, 9, 117, 118] (Figs. 33–4 and 33–5). In addition, electromyographic monitoring of injury potentials from muscles can be performed during surgical resection to minimize the risk of a motor deficit.

The tumor may arise from a single nerve fascicle, such as occurs in schwannoma. The remaining fascicles are then often either displaced to one side or uniformly distributed around the tumor. After the imaging studies have been reviewed, the tumor can be approached on the side opposite the fascicles. After the functioning nerve fascicles have been identified with electrophysiologic techniques, the incision can be made in a nonfunctional area oriented within the longitudinal axis of the nerve (Fig. 33–6). Functional nerve fascicles can often then be dissected free and swept circumferentially from the surface of an underlying tumor or other type of mass lesion.[3, 8]

In certain cases, the functional nerve fascicles cannot easily be separated from the tumor, or functioning nerve fibers become incorporated in the superficial capsule of the tumor. In these situations, first internal debulking of the tumor to its capsular margin, often with the use of the cavitron, should be done. The tumor capsule is then mapped using electrophysiologic techniques, distinguishing functional from nonfunctional regions, with the latter undergoing resection (Fig. 33–7). A pathologic diagnosis made intraoperatively by frozen section may also be useful. With the diagnosis of

schwannoma or neurofibroma in a situation where total resection without the risk of inducing a neurologic deficit is not possible, partial resection may be preferable. Growth of these benign tumors can be very slow, and the benefit from obtaining a total resection with neurologic deficit is not warranted. In situations where little or no neurologic function exists in the involved nerve, complete resection followed by nerve grafting may be performed.

Postoperative care should include antibiotics for 24 hours, adequate analgesia, and early mobilization in most cases. Early mobilization promotes gliding of nerve elements and thereby reduces the formation of tethering adhesions. In situations where the resection required anastomoses of nerves with or without nerve grafts, limits on mobilization should be advised to prevent tension on the suture repair site for at least 2 weeks. This should be followed by a gradual and judicious increase in mobilization.

Malignant Peripheral Nerve Tumors

Malignant peripheral nerve tumors are rare and require specialized care that includes complex medical and surgical management.[8, 93, 103, 119, 120] Ideally, the diagnosis would be suspected on clinical evaluation and confirmed by open surgical biopsy. A blind percutaneous needle biopsy is not recommended because damage, with associated functional deficits, may result. A benign pathologic report can be followed by resection using the principles described earlier. If the pathologic diagnosis is indeterminate or demonstrates frank malignancy, simple closure of the wound pending receipt of the definitive pathology report is recommended.

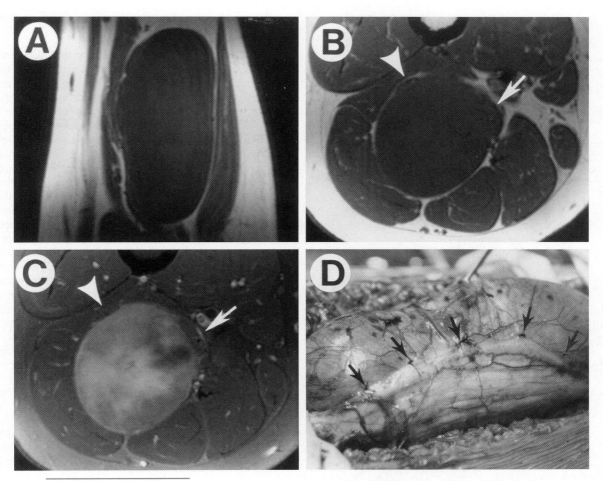

Figure 33–6 MRN images of a 20-year-old woman with neurofibromatosis type 1 and a large right-sided sciatic nerve neurofibroma just above the popliteal fossa. (A) Coronal T1-weighted spin-echo image showing a large oval sciatic nerve neurofibroma displaying low signal. (B) Axial T1-weighted spin-echo image. (C) Axial T1-weighted spin-echo image with gadolinium enhancement showing the fascicular structure of the common peroneal nerve (white arrowhead) and the tibial nerve (white arrow) split apart along the anterior and medial aspect of the tumor, respectively. (D) Intraoperative photograph of the anterolateral aspect of the tumor with proximal to the right and distal to the left. The black arrows overlie the tumor and point to small sutures placed to demarcate the border between tumor and functioning common peroneal nerve fibers (below black sutures). (Reproduced with permission from Kuntz C, Blake L, Britz G, et al. Magnetic resonance neurography of peripheral nerve lesions in the lower extremity. *Neurosurgery* 1996; 39:750–756.)

Management of a biopsy-proven malignant peripheral nerve tumor requires sophisticated surgical planning. This includes staging the disease and obtaining imaging that allows for planning an aggressive surgical resection if possible. An aggressive en bloc surgical resection of the tumor and adjacent soft tissues or limb amputation have been shown to be important in decreasing the local recurrence rate to 10% and in improving the 5-year survival rate to 40 to 50%.[2, 93, 97, 98, 121, 122] This radical resection almost always involves resection of the involved peripheral nerve and repair of the nerve using nerve grafts if a large gap must be bridged.

Adjuvant therapy for malignant peripheral nerve tumors includes both radiotherapy and chemotherapy.[97, 123] Aggressive tumor resection followed by intraoperative and/or postoperative radiation therapy appears to improve patient survival[93, 97, 122, 124] Adjuvant chemotherapy, which has not been proven beneficial, has also been advocated, particularly in cases of disseminated disease,[93, 94, 124] and some results are encouraging.[123, 125] Various other therapeutic protocols have been recommended, including preoperative irradiation and chemotherapy prior to radical surgical resection. Treatment of malignant peripheral nerve tumors remains a challenge as 5-year survival rates are poor, with a median survival of 3 years.[93, 94]

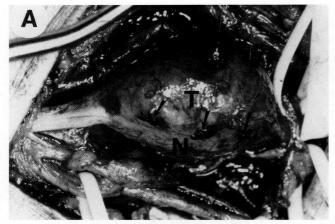
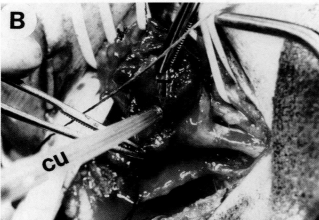
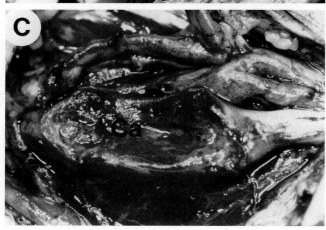

Figure 33–7 Intraoperative photographs demonstrating the surgical removal of an ulnar nerve neurofibroma in the distal forearm. Intraoperative stimulating and recording techniques were utilized to help in delineating the nonfunctional tumor (T) from the functioning ulnar nerve (N). (A) The black arrows point to sutures placed to demarcate the tumor nerve border. (B) Using microsurgical techniques and the cavitron (cu), the nonfunctional tumor is being aspirated away from the parent nerve. (C) Residual tumor cavity (Ca) lined with functioning nerve fibers. (Reproduced with permission from Grossman RG, Loftus CM, eds. *Principles of Neurosurgery.* 2nd ed. Philadelphia: Lippincott-Raven Publishers.)

SUMMARY

Peripheral nerve tumors in the pediatric population are relatively rare, and their management remains a challenge. Although a careful clinical evaluation remains important, scientific advances and technical innovations have greatly enhanced our understanding and management of these tumors. Advancements in electrophysiology have improved both the diagnosis and surgical outcome of these tumors. Improvements in imaging, particularly MRI, have made it possible to preoperatively visualize these lesions in greater detail. It is now possible to preoperatively visualize the relationship of nerve fascicles to nonfunctioning tumor tissue, allowing for better planning of a surgical approach that will minimize the probability of damage to functioning fascicles. Microsurgical techniques have further allowed for safer surgical management of these lesions. Advances in the management of malignant peripheral nerve tumors will likely occur in the area of adjuvant therapy, particularly chemotherapy. Because management of peripheral nerve tumors is complex, it is best carried out in a specialized center with a multidisciplinary approach that includes the skills of radiologists, surgeons, electrophysiologists, oncologists, rehabilitation personnel, neurologists, pathologists, and radiation oncologists.

REFERENCES

1. Burger PC, Scheithauer BW, Vogel FS. Nerve sheath neoplasms. In: *Surgical Pathology of the Nervous System and Its Coverings.* 3rd ed. New York: Churchill Livingstone; 1991:665–730.
2. DasGupta T. Tumors of the peripheral nerves. *Clin Neurosurg* 1978;25:574–590.
3. Donner T, Voorhies R, Kline D. Neural sheath tumors of major nerves. *J Neurosurg* 1994;81:362–373.
4. Enzinger FM, Weiss SW. *Soft Tissue Tumors.* 2nd ed. St. Louis: Mosby; 1988.
5. Guha A, Bilbao J, Kline DG, Hudson AR. Tumors of the peripheral nervous system. In: Youmans JR, ed. *Neurological Surgery.* Philadelphia: WB Saunders; 1996:3175–3187.
6. Harkin JC, Reed RJ. Tumors of the peripheral nervous system. In: *Atlas of Tumor Pathology.* Fascicle 3. Washington, DC: Armed Forces Institute of Pathology; 1969 (reprinted 1982).
7. Kline DG, Donner T, Voorhies RM. Management of tumors of peripheral nerve. In: Tindall G, Cooper P, Barrow D, eds. *The Practice of Neurologic Surgery.* Baltimore: Williams & Wilkins; 1994.
8. Kline DG, Hudson AR. *Operative Results of Major Nerve Injuries, Entrapments and Tumors.* WB Saunders; Philadelphia; 1994.
9. Kline DG, Hudson AR. Surgical management of peripheral nerve tumors. In: Schmidek HH, Sweet WH, eds. *Operative Neurosurgical Techniques.* 3rd ed. Philadelphia: WB Saunders; 1995:2183–2196.
10. Russell DS, Rubinstein LJ. *Pathology of Tumors of the Nervous System.* 5th ed. Baltimore: Williams & Wilkins; 1989.
11. Weiss SW. *Histological Typing of Soft Tissue Tumors.* Berlin: Springer-Verlag; 1994.

12. Woodruff JM. The pathology and treatment of peripheral nerve tumors and tumor-like conditions. *Cancer J Clin* 1993;43:290–308.

13. Lustgarten JH, Avellino AM, Kliot M. Molecular regulation of axonal regeneration in the mammalian nervous system: an overview. In: Hadley MN, ed. *Perspectives in Neurological Surgery*. Vol. 6. Part 2. St Louis: Quality Medical Publishing; 1995:19–43.

14. Mackinnon SE, Dellon AL. *Surgery of the Peripheral Nerve*. New York: Thieme Medical Publisher; 1988:535–549.

15. Thomas PK, Ochoa J, Berthold C-H, et al. Microscopic anatomy of the peripheral nervous system. In: Dyck PJ et al., eds. *Peripheral Neuropathy*. 3rd Philadelphia: WB Saunders; 1993:28–91.

16. Bunge MB, Wood PM, Tynan LB, et al. Perineurium originates from fibroblasts: demonstration in vitro with a retroviral marker. *Science* 1989;243:229–231.

17. Weiss SW, Langloss JM, Enzinger FM. Value of S-100 protein in the diagnosis of soft tissue tumors with particular reference to benign and malignant Schwann cell tumors. *Lab Invest* 1983;40:299–308.

18. McGarry RC, Helfand SL, Quarles RH, Roder JC. Recognition of myelin-associated glycoprotein by the monoclonal antibody HNK-1. *Nature* 1983;306:376–378.

19. Perentes E, Rubinstein LJ. Immunohistochemical recognition of human nerve sheath tumors by anti-Leu-7 (HNK-1) monoclonal antibody. *Acta Neuropathol* 1985;68:319–324.

20. Schuller-Petrovic S, Gebhart W, Lassman H, et al. A shared antigenic determinant between natural killer cells and nervous tissue. *Nature* 1983;306:179–181.

21. Taniuchi M, Clark HB, Schweitzer JB, Johnson EM Jr. Expression of nerve growth factor receptors by Schwann cells of axotomized peripheral nerves: ultrastructural location, suppression by axonal contract, and binding properties. *J Neurosci* 1988;8:664–681.

22. Perentes E, Nakagwa Y, Ross GW, et al. Expression of epithelial membrane antigen in perineural cells and their derivatives: an immunohistochemical study with multiple markers. *Acta Neuropathal* 1987;75:160–165.

23. Riccardi VM. Von Recklinghausen neurofibromatosis. *N En J Med* 1981;305:1617–1627.

24. Riccardi VM. *Neurofibromatosis: Phenotype, Natural History, and Pathogenesis*. 2nd ed. Baltimore: The John Hopkins University Press; 1992.

25. NIH Consensus Development Conference Statement. Neurofibromatosis. *Arch Neurol* 1988;45:575–578.

26. Huson SM. Neurofibromatosis 1: a clinical and genetic overview. In: Huson SM, Hughes, eds. *The Neurofibromatoses*. London: Chapman and Hall; 1988:160–244.

27. Huson SM, Harper PS, Compston DAS. Von Recklinghausen neurofibromatosis: a clinical and population study in south east Wales. *Brain* 1988;111:1355–1381.

28. Senveli E, Altinoers N, Kars Z, et al. Association of von Recklinghausen's neurofibromatosis and aqueduct stenosis. *Neurosurgery* 1989;24:99–101.

29. Von Deimling A, Krone W, Menon AG. Neurofibromatosis type 1: pathology, clinical features and molecular genetics. *Brain Pathol* 1995;5:153–162.

30. Bernards A, Haase VH, Murphy AE, et al. Complete human NF1 cDNA sequence: two alternatively spliced mRNAs and absence of expression in a neuroblastoma line. *DNA Cell Biol* 1992;11:727–734.

31. Cawthon RM, Weiss R, Xu GF, et al. Deletions and a translocation interrupt a cloned gene at the neurofibromatosis type 1 locus. *Cell* 1990;62:187–192.

32. Cawthon RM, Weiss R, Xu GF, et al. A major segment of the neurofibromatosis type 1 gene: CDNA sequence, genomic structure, and point mutations. *Cell* 1990;62:193–201.

33. Gutmann DH, Wood DL, Collins FS. Identification of the neurofibromatosis type 1 gene product. *Proc Natl Acad Sci U S A* 1991;88:9658–9662.

34. Li Y, Bollag, G, Clark R, et al. Somatic mutations in the neurofibromatosis 1 gene in human tumors. *Cell* 1992;69:275–281.

35. Marchuk DA, Saulino AM, Tavakkol R, et al. cDNA cloning of the type 1 neurofibromatosis gene: complete sequence of the NF1 gene product. *Genomics* 1991;11:931–940.

36. Seizinger BR. NF-1: a prevalent cause of tumorigenesis in human cancers. *Nature Genet* 1993;3(2):97–99.

37. Wallace MR, Marchuk DA, Anderson LB, et al. Type 1 neurofibromatosis gene: identification of a large transcript disrupt in three NF-1 patients. *Science* 1990;249:181–249.

38. Jayadel D, Fain P, Upadhyaya M, et al. Paternal origin of new mutations in von Recklinghausen neurofibromatosis. *Nature* 1990;343:558–559.

39. Easton DF, Ponder MA, Huson SM, Ponder BAJ. An analysis of variation in expression of neurofibromatosis type 1: evidence of modifying genes. *Am J Hum Genet* 1993;45:721–728.

40. Gutmann DH, Tennekoon GI, Cole JL, et al. Modulation of the neurofibromatosis type 1 gene product neurofibromin during Schwann cell differentiation. *J Neurosci Res* 1993;36:216–223.

41. Daston MM, Scrable H, Nordlund M, et al. The protein product of the neurofibromatosis type 1 gene is expressed at highest abundance in neurons, Schwann cells, and oligodendrocytes. *Neuron* 1992;8:415–428.

42. DeClue J, Cohen B, Lowy D. Identification and characterization of the neurofibromatosis type 1 protein product. *Proc Natl Acad Sci U S A* 1991;88:9914–9918.

43. Gutmann DH, Collins FS. The neurofibromatosis type 1 gene and its protein product, neurofibromin. *Neuron* 1993;10:335–343.

44. Xu G, O'Connell P, Viskochil D, et al. The neurofibromatosis type 1 gene encodes a protein related to GAP. *Cell* 1990;62:599–608.

45. Skuse G, Kosciolek B, Rowley P. Molecular genetic analysis of tumors in von Recklinghausen neurofibromatosis: loss of heterozygosity for chromosome 17. *Genes Chrom Cancer* 1989;1:36–41.

46. Basu TN, Gutmann DH, Fletcher JA, et al. Aberrant regulation of Ras proteins in malignant tumor cells from type 1 neurofibromatosis patients. *Nature* 1992;356:713–715.

47. Bollag G, McCormick F. Differential regulation of Ras GAP and neurofibromatosis gene product activities. *Nature* 1991;351:576–579.

48. DeClue J, Papageorge A, Fletcher J, et al. Abnormal regulation of mammalian p21ras contributes to malignant

tumor growth in von Recklinghausen (type 1) neurofibromatosis. *Cell* 1992;69:265–273.

49. Guha A, Lau N, Huvar I, et al. Ras-GTP levels are elevated in human NF1 peripheral nerve tumors. *Oncogene* 1996;12:507–513.

50. McCormick F. Ras signaling and NF1. *Curr Opin Genet Dev* 1995;5:51–55.

51. Feldkamp MM, Lau N, Provias JP, et al. Acute presentation of a neurogenic sarcoma in a patient with neurofibromatosis type 1: a pathological and molecular explanation. *J Neurosurg* 1996;84:867–873.

52. Sheela S, Riccardi V, Ratner, N. Angiogenic and invasive properties of neurofibroma Schwann cells. *J Cell Biol* 1990;111:645–653.

53. Gray MH, Smoller BR, Mcnutt NS, Hsu A. Immunohistochemical demonstration of factor XIIIa expression in neurofibromas. *Arch Dermatol* 1990;126:472–476.

54. Evans DGR, Huson SM, Donnai D, et al. A clinical study of type 2 neurofibromatosis. *Q J Med* 1992;304:603–618.

55. Halliday AL, Sobel RS, Martuza RL. Benign spinal nerve tumors: their occurrence sporadically and in neurofibromatosis types 1 and 2. *J Neurosurg* 1991;74:248–253.

56. Kimura H, Fischer W, Schubert D. Structure, expression and function of a schwannoma-derived growth factor. *Nature* 1990;348:257–260.

57. Erlandson RA, Woodruff JM. Peripheral nerve sheath tumors: an electron microscopic study of 43 cases. *Cancer* 1982;49:273–287.

58. Louis DN, Ramesh V, Gusella JF. Neuropathology and molecular genetics of neurofibromatosis 2 and related tumors. *Brain Pathol* 1995;5:163–172.

59. Rouleau GA, Wertelecki W, Haines JL, et al. Alteration in a new gene encoding a putative membrane-organizing protein causes neurofibromatosis type 2. *Nature* 1993;363:515–521.

60. Seizinger BR, Martuza RL, Gusella JF. Loss of genes on chromosome 22 in tumorigenesis of human acoustic neuroma. *Nature* 1986;322:644–647.

61. Trofatter J, MacCollin M, Rutter J, et al. A novel moesin-, ezrin-, radixin-like gene is a candidate for the neurofibromatosis 2 tumor suppressor. *Cell* 1993;72:791–800.

62. Bilbao JM, Khoury NJS, Hudson AR, Briggs SJ. Perineurioma (localized hypertrophic neuropathy). *Arch Pathol Lab Med* 1984;108:557–560.

63. Erlandson R. The enigmatic perineurial cell and its participation in tumors and in tumorlike entities. *Ultrastruct Pathol* 1991;15:335–351.

64. Iyer VG, Garretson HD, Byrd RP, Reiss SJ. Localized hypertrophic mononeuropathy involving the tibial nerve. *Neurosurgery* 1988;23:218–221.

65. Johnson PC, Kline DG. Localized hypertrophic neuropathy: possible focal perineurial barrier defect. *Acta Neuropathol* 1989;77:514–518.

66. Mitsumoto H, Wilbourn AJ, Goren H. Perineurioma as the cause of localized hypertrophic neuropathy. *Muscle Nerve* 1980;3:403–412.

67. Ochoa J, Neary D. Localized hypertrophic neuropathy, intraneural tumor, or chronic nerve entrapment? *Lancet* 1975;1:632–633.

68. Stanton C. Perentes E, Phillips L, Vandenberg SR. The immunohistochemical demonstration of early perineurial

69. Tranmer BI, Bilbao JM, Hudson AR. Perineurioma: a benign peripheral nerve tumor. *Neurosurgery* 1986;19:134–138.

70. Tsang W, Chan J, Chow L, et al. Perineuroma: An uncommon soft tissue neoplasm distinct from localized hypertrophic neuropathy and neurofibroma. *Am J Surg Pathol* 1992;16:756–763.

71. Weidenheim K, Campbell W Jr. Perineural cell tumor. *Virchows Arch A Pathol Anat Histopathol* 1986;408:375–383.

72. Emory TS, Scheithauer BW, Hirose T, et al. Intraneural perineurioma: a clonal neoplasm associated with abnormalities of chromosome 22. *Am J Clin Pathol* 1995;103:696–704.

73. Ariza A, Bilbao JM, Rosai J. Immunohistochemical detection of epithelial membrane antigen in normal cells and perineurioma. *Am J Surg Pathol* 1988;12:678–683.

74. Khairi MRA, Dexter RN, Burzynski, et al. Mucosal neuroma, phaechromocytoma and medullary thyroid carcinoma: MEN type III. *Medicine* 1975;54:89–112.

75. Gorlin RJ, Sedano HO, Vickers RA, Cervenka J. Multiple mucosal neuromas, pheochromocytoma and medullary carcinoma of the thyroid: a syndrome. *Cancer* 1968;54:89–112.

76. Williams ED, Pollack DJ. Multiple mucosal neuromas with endocrine tumors: a syndrome allied to von Recklinghausen's disease. *J Pathol* 1966;91:71–80.

77. Henmi A, Sato H, Wataya T, et al. Neurothekeoma: report of a case with immunohistochemical and ultrastructural studies. *Acta Pathol Jpn* 1986;36:1911–1919.

78. Buley ID, Gatter KC, Kelly PMA, et al. Granule cell tumors revisited: an immunohistological and ultrastructural study. *Histopathology* 1988;12:263–274.

79. Smith K, Mackinnon S, Maccauley R, et al. Glomus tumor originating in the radial nerve: a case report. *J Hand Surg* 1992;17:665–667.

80. Stout AP. Tumors featuring pericytes: glomus tumor and hemangiopericytoma. *Lab Invest* 1956;5:217–223.

81. Bilge T, Kaya A, Atatli M, et al. Hemangioma of the peroneal nerve: case report and review of the literature. *Neurosurgery* 1989;25:649–652.

82. Linde U, Gaap MR. Heamangiom des Nervus Ulnaris. *Hand Chirurgie* 1982;14:20–22.

83. Lusli EJ. Intrinsic hemangiomas of peripheral nerves: report of two cases and review of the literature. *Arch Pathol* 1952;53:266–270.

84. Patel CB, Tsai TM, Kleinert HE. Hemangioma of the median nerve: a report of two cases. *J Hand Surg* (AM) 1986;11A:76–79.

85. Peled I, Iosipovich Z, Rousso M, Wexler MR. Hemangioma of the median nerve. *J Hand Surg* 1980;5A:363–365.

86. Sato S. Ueber das cavernose Angiom des peripherischen Nervensystems. *Arch Klin Chir* 1913;100:553–574.

87. Awasathi D, Kline D, Beckman E. Neuromuscular hamartoma (benign "triton" tumor) of the brachial plexus. *J Neurosurg* 1991;75:795–797.

88. Markel SF, Enzinger FM. Neuromuscular hamartoma—a benign "triton tumor" composed of mature neural and striated muscle elements. *Cancer* 1982;49:140–144.

89. Zwick DL, Livingstone K, Clapp L et al. Intracranial trigeminal nerve rhabdomyoma/choristoma in a child: a case report and discussion of possible histogenesis. *Hum Pathol* 1989;20:390–392.

90. Foley KM, Woodruff JM, Ellis FT, Posner JB. Radiation-induced malignant and atypical peripheral nerve sheath tumors. *Ann Neurol* 1980;7:311–318.

91. Newbould M, Wilkinson N, Mene A. Post-radiation malignant peripheral nerve sheath tumor: a report of two cases. *Histopathology* 1990;16:263–265.

92. Cutler EC, Gross RE. Neurofibroma and neurofibrosarcoma of peripheral nerves, unassociated with von Recklinghausen's disease: a report of 25 cases. *Arch Surg* 1936; 33:733–779.

93. Ducatman B, Scheithauer B, Piepgras D, et al. Malignant peripheral nerve sheath tumors: a clinical pathological study of 120 cases. *Cancer* 1986;57:2006–2021.

94. Hruban R, Shiu M, Senie R, et al. Malignant peripheral nerve sheath tumors of the buttock and lower extremity. *Cancer* 1990;66:1253–1265.

95. Nambison RN, Rao U, Moore R, et al. Malignant soft tissue tumors of nerve sheath origin. *J Surg Oncol* 1984; 25:268–272.

96. Riccardi VM, Powell PP. Neurofibrosarcoma as a complication of von Recklinghausen neurofibromatosis. *Neurofibromatosis* 1989;2:152–165.

97. Sordilla P, Helson L, Hajdu S, et al. Malignant schwannoma: clinical characteristics, survival, and response to therapy. *Cancer* 1981;53:2503–2509.

98. Vieta JO, Pack GT. Malignant neurilemomas in peripheral nerves. *Am J Surg* 1951;82:416–431.

99. Wanebo JE, Malik JM, VandenBerg SR, et al. Malignant peripheral nerve sheath tumors: a clinicopathological study of 28 cases. *Cancer* 1993;71:1247–1253.

100. Wick MR, Swanson PE, Scheithauer BW, Manivel JC. Malignant peripheral nerve sheath tumor: an immunohistochemical study of 62 cases. *Am J Clin Pathol* 1987; 87:425–433.

101. Sorensen S, Mulvhill J, Nielsen A. Longterm followup of von Recklinghausen neurofibromatosis: survival and malignant neoplasms. *N Engl J Med* 1986;314:1010–1015.

102. Hirose T, Samo T, Hizawa K. Heterogeneity of malignant schwannomas. *Ultrastruct Pathol* 1988;12:107–116.

103. Ducatman B, Scheithauer B. Malignant peripheral nerve sheath tumors with divergent differentiation. *Cancer* 1984;54:1049–1057.

104. Brodeur G, Morley J. Biology of tumors of the peripheral nervous system [Review]. *Cancer Metastasis Rev* 1991;10: 321–333.

105. Jaeckle K. Nerve plexus metastasis [Review]. *Neurol Clin* 1991;9:857–866.

106. Tindall SC. Ganglion cysts of peripheral nerves. In: Wilkins R, Rengachary E, eds. *Neurosurgery*. Baltimore: Williams & Wilkins; 1900.

107. Castagno AA, Shuman WP. MR imaging in clinically suspected brachial plexus tumor. *Am J Roentgenol* 1987; 149:1219–1222.

108. Cerfolini E, Landi A, DeSantis G, et al. MR of benign peripheral nerve sheath tumors. *J Comput Assist Tomogr* 1991;15:593–597.

109. Stull M, Moser R. Magnetic resonance appearance of peripheral nerve sheath tumors. *Skel Radiol*. 1991;20: 9–14.

110. Suh J, Abenoza P, Galloway H, et al. Peripheral (extracranial) nerve tumors: correlations of MR imaging and histological findings. *Radiology* 1992;183: 341–346.

111. Britz GW, Dailey AT, West AW, et al. MRI in the evaluation and treatment of peripheral nerve problems. In: Hadley M, ed. *Perspectives in Neurological Surgery*. Vol 6. Part 2. St. Louis: Quality Medical Publishing; 1995: 53–66.

112. Filler AG, Howe FA, Hayes CE, et al. Magnetic resonance neurography. *Lancet* 1993;341:659–661.

113. Filler AG, Kliot M, Hayes CE, et al. The application of magnetic resonance neurography in the evaluation of patients with peripheral nerve pathology. *J Neurosurg* 1996;85:299–309.

114. Howe FA, Filler AG, Bell BA, Griffiths JR. Magnetic resonance neurography. *Magn Res Med* 1992;28:328–338.

115. Kuntz C, Blake L, Britz G, et al. Magnetic resonance neurography of peripheral nerve lesions in the lower extremity. *Neurosurgery* 1996;39:750–756.

116. Levine E, Huntrakoon M, Wetzel L. Malignant-nerve sheath neoplasms in neurofibromatosis: distinctions from benign tumors by using imaging techniques. *Am J Radiol* 1987;149:1059–1064.

117. Kliot M, Slimp J. Techniques and assessment of peripheral nerve function at surgery. In: Loftus C, Traynelis VC, eds. *Intraoperative Monitoring Techniques in Neurosurgery*. New York: McGraw Hill; 1993:275–285.

118. Slimp J, Kliot M. Electrophysiological monitoring: peripheral nerve surgery. In: Andrews RJ, ed. *Intraoperative Neuroprotection*. Baltimore: Williams & Wilkins; 1996:375–392.

119. Bolten J, Vauthey J, Farr G, et al. Is limb-sparing surgery applicable to neurogenic sarcomas of the extremities? *Arch Surg* 1989;124:118–121.

120. Raney B, Schanufer L, Ziegler M, et al. Treatment of children with neurogenic sarcoma: experience at the Children's Hospital of Philadelphia, 1958–1984. *Cancer* 1987; 59:1–5.

121. DasGupta TK, Brasfield RD. Solitary malignant schwannoma. *Ann Surg* 1970;171:419–428.

122. White H. Survival in malignant schwannoma: an 18 year study. *Cancer* 1971;27:720–729.

123. Pinedo HM, Kenis Y. Chemotherapy of advanced soft tissue sarcomas in adults. *Cancer Treat Rev* 1977;4:67–86.

124. Basso-Ricci S. Therapy of malignant schwannomas: usefulness of an integrated radiologic-surgical therapy. *J Neurosurg Sci* 1989;33:253–257.

125. Goldman RI, Jones SE, Heusinkveld RS. Combination chemotherapy of metastatic malignant schwannoma with vincristine, adriamycin, cyclophosphamide, and imidazole carboxamide: a case report. *Cancer* 1977;39: 1955–1958.

Chapter 34

Uncommon Pediatric Spinal Cord Tumors

Caple A. Spence, Russell Buchanan, and Robert Keating

GANGLIOGLIOMA

Incidence

Spinal cord ganglioglioma was first described in 1911 by Pick and Bielschowsky.[1] It is a relatively rare tumor that is seen primarily in adolescents and young adults.[2, 3] Gangliogliomas account for 0.4 to 3.8% of all primary brain tumors,[4-6] and they may account for up to 10% of primary brain tumors in children.[6] In contrast to the incidence of cranial pathology, ganglioglioma affects the spinal cord at a rate of 1.1%.[7] Based on a report from Patel et al,[14] there have been 46 reported cases of spinal cord ganglioglioma.

Epidemiology

Ganglioglioma primarily affects infants or young adults, with the mean age ranging from 8.5 to 31 years.[8-11] Both sexes are almost equally affected.[12, 13] The mean age of patients with spinal cord gangliogliomas is 12 years, whereas the mean age for patients with spinal cord astrocytoma is 4 years.[14]

Pathology

Gangliogliomas are slow-growing, usually benign tumors, corresponding to World Health Organization (WHO) grades I and II.[11, 16, 17] The nomenclature for this tumor has been very confusing. Synonyms have included ganglioglioneuroma, ganglionic neuroma, neuroastrocytoma, neuroganglioma, ganglionic glioma, neuroma gangliocellulare, and neuroglioma.[1, 18, 19] The current classification is based on the relative differentiation of the neuronal components and the presence of glial elements. If the tumor consists solely of large, relatively mature neoplastic neurons or ganglion cells, it is termed gangliocytoma. The additional presence of a neoplastic astrocytic component confers the term "ganglioglioma." The present of additional features, such as a substantial population of small neoplastic mature neurons, bestows the term "ganglioglioneurocytoma."[6]

Gangliogliomas occur anywhere within the central nervous system, with a propensity for the temporal lobe.[20] Locations in decreasing order of incidence are the cerebral hemispheres, the floor of the third ventricle, the brain stem, the cerebellum, and the spinal cord.[3, 21] The most common location in the spinal cord is the cervical region, possibly representing extension from the medulla.[14, 21, 22] Tumors may be located in the cervical, cervicothoracic, thoracic, thoracolumbar, and conus medullaris regions.[23] Spinal gangliogliomas span an average length of eight vertebral body segments, whereas both spinal cord astrocytoma and spinal cord ependymoma span an average length of four vertebral body segments.[14] Despite the focal predilection for the cervical region, spinal gangliogliomas may affect the entire spinal cord in approximately 15% of cases.[14, 17, 24, 25]

> ### BOX 34–1
> ### Locations
>
> - **Hemispheres**
> - **Third ventricular floor**
> - **Brain stem**
> - **Cerebellum**
> - **Spinal cord**

Tumor cysts are seen with a greater frequency in spinal gangliogliomas than in other uncommon spinal cord tumors. Cysts occur in 46% of cases of spinal gangliogliomas as compared with 20% of spinal astrocytomas and 3% of spinal ependymomas.[14]

Microscopically, gangliogliomas are composed of large, mature neurons and neoplastic glial cells (usually astrocytes) (Fig. 34–1). Both cell types show a broad spectrum of histologic features.[3, 6, 8, 26] The neoplastic glial component is composed mainly of glial fibrillary acidic protein (GFAP)–immunopositive fibrillary astrocytes and exhibits various degrees of cellular atypia. Rosenthal fibers as well as eosinophilic granular bodies might be present.[3, 8] The neoplastic neurons are often irregularly oriented, arranged in clusters, and sometimes exhibit anomalous processes, neurofibrillary tangles, myelin sheaths, and synapse formation.[3, 6, 27] Frequently, bi- or multinucleated nerve cells are seen. The neurons are immunopositive for synaptophysin, neurofilament protein, neuron-specific enolase, and chromo-

The authors would like to thank Alann Morrison, M.D., Armed Forces Institute of Pathology for his photographic contributions.

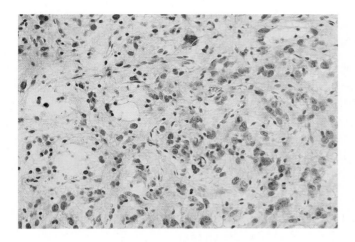

Figure 34–1 This hematoxylin–eosin (H&E) slide of a ganglioglioma contains a mixture of ganglion cells and less differentiated ganglioid elements. The glial component is formed by spindle-shaped cells, which are generally immunoreactive for GFAP.[51] (Courtesy of Alan Morrison, M.D., AFID.)

granin A.[8, 28, 29] Mitoses are usually not seen.[3] Additional histologic changes include a fibrovascular stroma, which is characteristically confined to the neuronal component; small foci of calcification distributed throughout the tumor tissue; and perivascular lymphocytic infiltrates.[3, 6, 8]

BOX 34–2
Pathologic Features

- **Stains positive for GFAP**
- **Cellular atypia**
- **Rosenthal fibers may be present**
- **Clusters of neurons**
- **Neurofibrillary tangles**
- **Binucleated or multinucleated nerve cells**
- **Immunopositive for synaptophysin, NSE, neurofilament protein, chromogranin A, calcium**

The overall potential of spinal ganglionic gangliogliomas for malignant transformation cannot be determined definitively.[17] There have only been a handful of cases described as malignant ganglioglioma.[7, 15, 25, 30, 31] *The significance of anaplastic features in ganglioglioma with respect to their biologic behavior is uncertain, as anaplastic gangliogliomas are not always clinically aggressive.*[2, 7, 15, 16, 32] *To date, no histologic features are known to predict the biologic behavior of ganglio-gliomas.*[2, 7, 15, 16] Tumor grading has not distinguished a prognostically poor group.[2, 12, 15, 29]

Recent work has demonstrated that this tumor has been formerly underdiagnosed, particularly in the spinal cord.[6, 15] One factor leading to this conclusion is the increase in the size of the sample of the biopsy specimens. As surgical techniques and instrumentation have improved, larger biopsy specimens can be safely procured. The increase in sample size decreases inaccuracies in pathologic examination. In addition, immunohistochemical methods have become more reliable and readily available.[6, 28, 33–37] Whereas previous pathologic diagnosis was made solely upon gross examination, light microscopy, and electron micrography, more recent immunohistochemical examination has become routine. This improvement has allowed the disclosure of inconsistencies in a group of tumors that were previously thought of as homogeneous. To make an accurate diagnosis, one must separate ganglioglioma from tumors that have a potential ganglion cell population, large tumor astrocytes, and normal trapped neurons. Immunohistochemical studies aid by staining for glial marker GFAP and for the syntactic vesicle protein synaptophysin. The specificity of the synaptophysin staining pattern has been supported by similar results with antibody staining percent synapsin I.[38] This pattern of immunoreactivity appears to correspond to the ultrastructural observation of axosomatic synapses on the surface of the neoplastic ganglion cells.[39] This pattern does not exist in dysplastic cortex or in hamartomas. No cell has otherwise been demonstrated to be of glial phenotype and show synaptophysin immunoreactivity. *Consequently, synaptophysin staining in this pattern is considered to be specific for gangliogliomas.*

Johannsson et al. attempted to establish a correlation between histologic appearance of ganglioglioma of the spinal cord and clinical course and prognosis.[2] Results indicated a high variability in the histologic appearance of the tumor.[2] They were unable to relate biologic behavior of their cases to any obvious histologic parameters, such as the degree of cell density, cellular pleomorphism, vascular proliferation, necrosis, or hemorrhage.[2] The location of the tumor and its resectability seemed to correlate better with the course of disease.[2] Tumors arising in the midline carry a poor prognosis and result in significant neurologic deficit.[2]

Radiology

Radiographically, gangliogliomas of the spinal cord have no characteristic appearance. Radiographs of the spine may reveal a smooth kyphoscoliosis. On computed tomography (CT) scans, one may appreciate a widened spinal canal. Furthermore, an intramedullary lesion or diffuse enlargement of the spinal cord may be seen.[17, 40] Magnetic resonance imaging (MRI) of the whole spine will also show widening of the spinal cord. T1-weighted magnetic resonance images may show high,[17] low,[41] or irregular signal intensity.[42] The overwhelming majority have mixed signal intensity on T1-weighted images. On T2-weighted images, gangliogliomas present as hyperintense lesions[41–43] (Fig. 34–2). Additionally, T2-weighted images reveal a homogeneous signal in 60% of cases, with the remaining 40% demonstrating a heterogeneous signal. In contrast to T1-weighted images, T2-weighted images did not demonstrate differences in signal characteristics between spinal ganglioglioma, spinal astrocytoma, and spinal ependymoma. Spinal cord

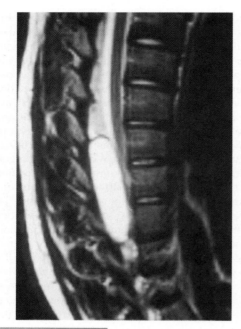

Figure 34–2 Magnetic resonance image from a 10-year-old boy with a 2-month history of vague low back pain as well as lower extremity paresthesias. The tumor has a large extramedullary cystic component with an anterior displacement of the spinal cord. Tumor resection was complete and facilitated by a well-demarcated tissue plane, and was identified as a ganglioglioma by pathologic examination.

ganglioglioma is accompanied by edema very infrequently, in contrast to the other spinal cord tumors. The contrast enhancement, with administration of gadolinium, characteristic of spinal ganglioglioma is primarily patchy in nature as seen in approximately 65% of cases. Approximately 15% of spinal gangliogliomas show no type of contrast enhancement.[42, 43]

BOX 34–3
Radiologic Features

- **T1-weighted images: high, low, irregular signal**
- **T2-weighted images: hyperintense**
- **Infrequent edema**
- **Patchy contrast enhancement (65%)**

Presentation

The presenting symptoms are related to tumor site and include pain, paraparesis, gait disturbances, motor weakness, sensory disturbances, and bowel or bladder dysfunction.[23] The duration of symptoms range from 1 month to 5 years.[23] In contrast to cerebral ganglioglioma, which presents with seizures, the most common presentation of spinal cord ganglioglioma is that of gait disturbance and paraparesis.[2, 3, 20, 21]

Scoliosis and leg length discrepancy are also common findings.[22, 26] The tumor may also be asymptomatic and may be discovered as an incidental finding at autopsy.[2] One review found that up to 77% of patients with spinal cord gangliogliomas present with back pain and appendicular weakness, whereas the remaining had other sensory and motor abnormalities.[15]

BOX 34–4
Clinical Presentation

- **Pain**
- **Weakness**
- **Gait changes**
- **Bowel/bladder changes**
- **Scoliosis**
- **Leg length asymmetry**

Treatment

It has been claimed that the treatment of choice for gangliogliomas, independent of their location, was *total surgical removal* of the lesion. This has been demonstrated to result in good long-term prognosis.[2, 4, 8, 10, 13, 28, 44, 45] Unfortunately, this is not always possible because of the need to preserve functional spinal cord tissue. In gangliogliomas of the spinal cord, the 5-year and 10-year actuarial survival rate after radical resection was reported to be 89% and 83%, respectively.[15]

As these tumors show little propensity for growth, postoperative irradiation should be withheld. When radiation was administered after gross total removal of gangliogliomas, the biologic behavior was no different from that of tumors that were not irradiated.[2, 4, 10, 13, 28, 41] The role for chemotherapy, given adjuvantly after recurrence, for the treatment of gangliogliomas is not clear and cannot be determined definitively.[4, 9, 16, 46, 47] The patient should be followed closely with CT or MRI, and given radiation therapy only when the progression of tumor growth is documented.[2, 4]

Outcome

Long postoperative survival has been documented.[2, 7, 45] The prognosis for ganglion cell tumors is thus generally favorable. On the other hand, tumors that have been diagnosed as gangliogliomas of the spinal cord recurred in roughly 40% of patients after radical resection, whereas those that were called low-grade fibrillary astrocytomas recur in only about 25% of patients. Tumor recurrence has been found to reach 47%.[15] In one large series of 58 patients of gangliogliomas of the cerebral hemispheres, brain stem, and spinal cord, the patients with spinal tumors had a 3.5 higher relative risk of recurrence or death than patients with cerebral tumors.[15] Again, this may be a function of the lack of adequate resection. Furthermore, it is important to point out that many of the series that document outcome were likely following patients who may have had tumors incorrectly diagnosed as ganglioglioma because they were not verified by immunohistochemistry. The reported postoperative results after removal of spinal gangliogliomas range from improvement, to unchanged neurologic status, to severe neurologic deficits.[4, 15, 24, 30, 48–50] The clinical outcome correlated most closely with the patients' preoperative functional status.[15]

Patients who require a second operation have an event-free survival rate following the second operation of almost 70% at 5 years.[15] If recurrence becomes apparent, a second operation should be considered, but radiation therapy may also be an option.

TERATOMA

A teratoma is a true neoplasm composed of all three germ layers, although presence of only two components does not necessarily rule out this diagnosis. The origin of teratoma of the spinal cord is controversial.

Incidence

Recently, approximately 50 cases involving spinal cord teratoma have been reported in the literature.[52–54]

Epidemiology

The number of reported cases is too small for adequate generalizations to be made. However, these tumors seem to affect primarily young adults, males as often as females (Fig. 34–3).

Pathology

Spinal teratomas can be defined as tumors of dysontogenetic origin that are situated in the spinal canal, extradurally or intradurally, and are associated with some sort of spinal malformation. Malformations such as syringomyelia can be seen in the spinal cord, and there may be defects in the development of the neural arches (i.e., spina bifida). Three reported patients had associated congenital anomalies in the spinal axis such as spina bifida and cord dysraphism.[55–57] Most of these lesions have been intradural and extramedullary.[56, 58]

The teratomas found within the spinal canal exist as discrete cystic masses, although they may be attached by a stalk or a tumor nodule. Frequently, an attachment to the spinal cord is not described. The minority of teratomas are intramedullary and in many of the larger tumors the actual site of origin cannot be determined.[59, 60] Teratomas may involve all levels of the cord, but tumors of the lumbar region predominate.[61, 62] Because of the variety of tissue types that have appeared in teratomas, there has been considerable speculation as to their origin. Whether they represent an unsuccessful attempt to form a fetus, either by incorporation of a twin fetus early in development or by growth of the germ cell from the host gonad,[56] the most generally accepted explanation of the origin of teratomas is given by Willis.[63] He states that teratomas arise during early embryonic development from a focus of tissue that escaped the control of inducers, which are believed to be substances that direct and control embryonic growth. Cells can thereby grow freely in a chaotic fashion and yet develop a variety of more or less well-formed tissues. This theory is supported by experimental work and is especially attractive with regard to spinal teratomas because of the complicated process that takes place in the neural tube as it closes.[64] The majority of spinal cord teratomas are mature and therefore benign; however, there has been a report of a case with malignant changes of the adenocarcinomatous type.

Histopathologically (Fig. 34–4) some teratomas are composed of mesodermally derived tissue, whereas others are true teratomas, containing elements of all three germ layers, alien to the structures in which they grow. Spinal cord teratomas are regarded as a tumor rather than a hamartoma due to the presence of tissue components derived from more than one germ cell layer not normal at the site of occurrence. Two types of teratomas exist: mature teratomas, composed of well-differentiated elements, and immature teratomas, which contain elements derived from any or all of the three germ layers.[65] Teratomas may have a cystic component.[65]

Radiology

CT scanning may reveal tumors of different densities within the expanded spinal canal. *This finding, suggestive of heterogeneity of tumor contents, makes it possible to differentiate*

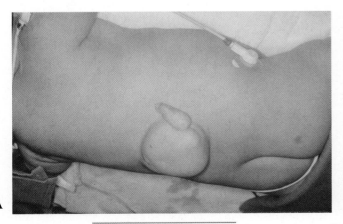
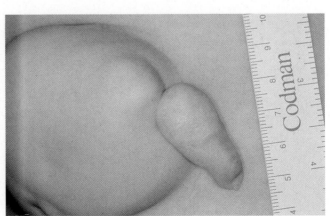

A

B

Figure 34–3 (A) An infant born with a well-formed teratoma over the thoracolumbar region. Note the the appendage (B), which appears to be a digit. (Courtesy of Alan Morrison, M.D., AFIP.)

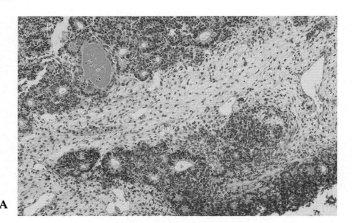

A

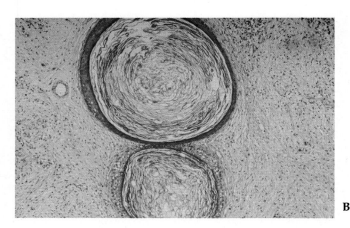

B

Figure 34–4 (A) H&E preparation of an immature teratoma demonstrating undifferentiated mesenchymal tissue as well as elements of the developing nervous system. (B) Cross section of the dermal appendage demonstrating a whorl pattern of fibrous stroma without bone or cartilage. (Courtesy of Alan Morrison, M.D., AFIP.)

teratomas from other types of tumors. MRI is helpful in localizing the lesion in relation to the spinal cord and any possible associated lesions of the spinal cord and column. MRI may also aid in the determination of densities, such as fatty tissue.[54] In addition, cystic components and tethering of the cord may be easily seen.[65]

Presentation

It is not easy to differentiate teratomas from other spinal cord tumors on clinical grounds. Patients may present with back pain, weakness, or gait disturbance.[65–68]

Treatment

Total surgical resection is the treatment of choice (Fig. 34–5). Depending on the extent of disease, this may be difficult without causing damage to surrounding neural tissue. Because of the slow growth of teratomas, partial resection produces long-term improvement in most cases.[66]

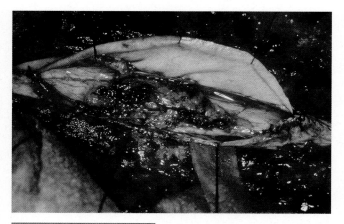

Figure 34–5 Intraoperative photograph of a well-circumscribed teratoma that was totally excised utilizing its defined cleavage plane.

Outcome

The prognosis of spinal cord teratomas is generally favorable. In many reported cases there has been no evidence of recurrence after surgical removal; however, others have reported recurrences.[56, 60–62, 69–72]

HEMANGIOBLASTOMA

Incidence

A spinal cord hemangioblastoma was first reported by Schultze in 1912.[73] The incidence of spinal hemangioblastoma is 1.6 to 2.1% of all spinal cord tumors,[74, 75] 3.3% of intramedullary tumors,[55, 76] 1.7% of extramedullary intradurally tumors, and 3.6% of extradural tumors.[74] Presenting symptoms are seen in 15% of patients before the age of 18 years.[77–79]

Pathology

Von Hippel–Lindau complex is a multicentric disorder of autosomal dominance with incomplete penetrance. Its manifestations have been recognized to include hemangioblastomas of the cerebellum, brain stem, spinal cord, and retina, in addition to renal carcinoma, pheochromocytoma, and cysts of pancreas, kidney, and epididymis.[80, 81] Hemangioblastoma of the spinal cord may be asymptomatic throughout life, and in studies of von Hippel–Lindau disease spinal lesions were found in every patient at autopsy.[82]

There is a strong association between this type of tumor and cyst formation. This is demonstrated in approximately 50 to 70% of patients.[77, 78, 83] Diffuse expansion of the cord is regarded as a characteristic feature[84, 85] and may be secondary to cyst formation or edema/congestion of cord as a result of vascular shunting in hemangioblastoma.[85]

Lesions are singular in 78.7% of cases.[77] The thoracic spinal cord is the most frequently involved (51.2%), with the cervical segments next in frequency (41.2%).[77] Syringomyelia constitutes part of the spinal lesion in 43% of cases, and when only cases of intramedullary spinal hemangioblastoma are considered, the percentage rises to 66.7%.[77] There were no reported cases of syringomyelia arising in a patient whose hemangioblastomas were located exclusively in the extramedullary intradural or extradural space. The majority of spinal hemangioblastomas (60%) are intramedullary and located in the dorsal half of the spinal cord, often near the median septum.[77] Extramedullary intradural hemangioblastomas are often attached to the posterior nerve roots.[77]

Microscopically, the predominant cellular element of hemangioblastoma has characteristics of an endothelial cell. These cells may form masses, chords, and thin-walled blood vessels, only part of which have patent lumens (Fig. 34–6). It is the multiplication of these cells and the vessels to which they give rise that constitutes growth of the tumor. Connective tissue stains may demonstrate an abundant network of reticulin that delineates the outlines of vascular architecture. Between endothelial cells are large numbers of stromal cells containing fat hemosiderin. The cytogenesis of the endothelial and stromal cells of the hemangioblastoma and the origin of associated syringomyelia continue to be debated. There are several opinions regarding the origin of syringomyelia that have been offered. The first hypothesis suggests that the tumor transudes fluid.[86] The second proposes that the tumor cells form plasma in a manner similar to embryonic angioblasts.[87] Finally, it has been suggested that local tissue destruction caused by the tumor gives rise to the cavitation.[88, 89]

Radiology

CT-related artifacts of adjacent osseous structures frequently cause imperfect pictures and may demonstrate opacification of the cyst as well the tumor on immediate or delayed scans.[90, 91] However, MRI has a high specificity, and the enhanced image often demonstrates the cyst clearly. Therefore, in surgical planning, the excellent anatomical demonstration of the lesion by enhanced MRI is essential. Additional information regarding the identification of feeding vessels, particularly the relationship of the tumor to the artery of Adamkiewicz if the lesion lies in the lower thoracic cord, can be critical. At this time, this is possible only by spinal angiogram, which is considered by many to be mandatory.[79]

Presentation

Often the first symptom is back pain; sensory changes are also frequently seen. Radicular pain in addition to sensory loss and posterior column deficits has also been reported. Progressive weakness in the lower extremities results from continued growth and subsequent compression of corticospinal tracts.

Treatment

Lesions should be totally excised. The key to surgical removal, despite the extreme vascularity of the lesion (Fig. 34–7), is the tumor's fiber capsule. If the capsule remains exclusively outside the tumor, total removal is often possible, and complete excision and clinical improvement may be achieved in 72% of patients.[79] Extramedullary and extradural spinal hemangioblastomas are readily removed by surgery. The combination of precise localization of spinal hemangioblastomas by angiography, improved microscopic surgical techniques, and coagulation of pial varicosities with electrocautery will continue to improve the rate of operative success on intramedullary hemangioblastomas.

Radiotherapy is generally thought to be ineffective, though symptomatic improvement has been reported. Of the few patients treated with radiation alone, some experienced some relief of symptoms, whereas others experienced immediate worsening.[92]

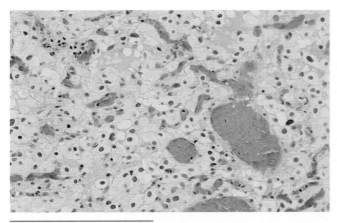

Figure 34–6 H&E slide demonstrating vacuolated, variably lipid-rich stromal cells, which may exhibit nuclear pleomorphism and hyperchromasia but rarely manifest mitoses. Typically, large vessels and cystic spaces are components of the cellular architecture. (Courtesy of Alan Morrison, M.D., AFIP.)

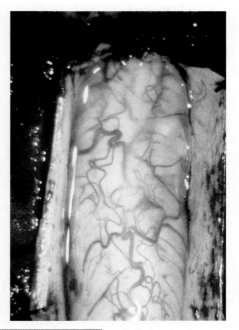

Figure 34–7 Intraoperative photograph demonstrating numerous superficial distended veins as well as enlarged cord secondary to an intramedullary hemangioblastoma.

Outcome

Outcome is often favorable with surgical treatment, and up to 72% of patients experience improvement in their symptoms.[79] Incomplete resection often results in exacerbation of the preoperative symptoms.

OLIGODENDROGLIOMA

Incidence

Primary spinal cord oligodendroglioma is a rare tumor, representing about 2% of all spinal cord tumors and 1.5% of oligodendrogliomas globally.[3, 93] Until Fortuna et al. reviewed the literature, only 38 cases had been reported.[93] The incidence of oligodendroglioma ranges from 0.8 to 4.7% of tumors of the cord and filum,[94–98] and 31.4% of patients affected are under the age of 16.[93]

Pathology

The most common site was the dorsal vertebral region (36.3%),[93] with tumors found in the cervical region (18.2%), lumbar region (18.2%), dorsolumbar region (12.1%), and cervicodorsal region (5.1%). In two cases, both involving patients under 16 years of age, nearly the entire cord was affected.[93]

Microscopically, oligodendroglioma as described in the majority of cases is a soft, gelatinous, infiltrating tumor, white or grayish pink. The classical description of the histologic features of oligodendroglioma was described by Ravens et al. in 1955.[99] The cells are of uniform size and shape, with a clear halo around the nucleus (Fig. 34–8). In addition, there is an absence of glial fibrils in large amounts, as well as a scarcity of coagulation necrosis and a paucity of nuclear abnormalities. Electron micrographs demonstrate that the neoplasm is composed mainly of two types of cellular elements supported by a large homogeneous matrix. A cell of the most abundant type possesses minimal cytoplasm, and the nucleus is frequently irregular and lobulated. Cytoplasmic processes are

short and few, or nonexistent. Identifiable cytoplasm organelles include occasional mitochondria, endoplasmic reticulum rich in ribosomes and prominent Golgi apparatus. The intercellular matrix is a mixture of cell processes and amorphous material, with the latter probably myxoid in nature.[100] Occasionally, a syringomyelic type of cyst may be found.

Radiology

MRI is the procedure of choice in the investigation of this spinal cord tumor. It is imperative for surgical planning. This lesion is hypointense on T1-weighted images and hyperintense on T2-weighted images.

Presentation

Scoliosis, frequently associated with spinal cord tumors,[102] may be the only sign of the tumor and has been seen with whole-cord oligodendroglioma.[101] Clumsiness of gait, paresthesias, and tetraparesis are among the initial symptoms, and impairment of bowel bladder function may follow. The majority of patients complained of pain (69.3%) and muscular disturbance. Fasiculations and contractures were also prominent in 23%.[93] Muscular twitching was reported in 33.3%. Generally, sensory symptoms are uncommon. Under clinical examination most patients were found to have a sensorimotor deficit syndrome, whereas the remaining had motor deficits with no sensory disturbances, decreased reflexes, or nothing at all. Sphincter disturbances were never among the initial symptoms.[93] Six patients had oscillating symptoms with spontaneous remissions involving sensory and motor events.[93]

Treatment

Surgical resection is the only treatment. The natural history of nonmalignant spinal cord gliomas with radiotherapy is one of slow deterioration and eventual death.[103] Some authors

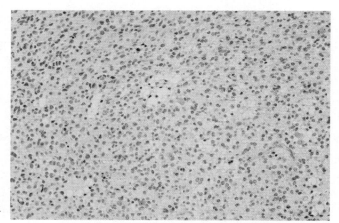
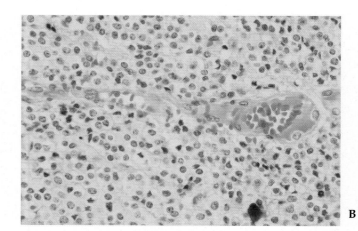

A   B

Figure 34–8   (A) H&E preparation of an oligodendroglioma manifesting the uniformity of nuclear size, delicate nucleoli, as well as (B) surrounding halo artifact from the cytoplasm. Blood vessels are angulated and small in this well-differentiated tumor. (Courtesy of Alan Morrison, M.D., AFIP.)

found that radiotherapy adds to long-term survival in the treatment of spinal cord oligodendrogliomas, though their results were not statistically significant.[93] Radiotherapy following an operation seems to prolong survival. However, the value of whole spine irradiation in the growing child must be based on a weighing of the benefits (or lack of) relative to the risk of spinal cord damage and growth retardation.

Outcome

The outcome of these tumors is directly related to the preoperative neurologic status. Postoperative prognosis in oligodendroglioma cord appears less favorable than that stated for astrocytomas. Indeed, the mean survival of patients following the second operation is lower for oligodendrogliomas at 2.4 years than for astrocytoma (4.6 years).

GERMINOMA

Incidence

Germinoma constitute 0.1% to 3.4% of all intracranial tumors with the highest incidence in Asian patients.[104] Nevertheless, the incidence of spinal cord germinomas is extremely uncommon and predominantly reported in the Japanese literature.[105–108]

Epidemiology

Whereas intra-axial germinomas constitute less than 1% of all germinomas in the United States and Europe, there is a striking incidence of this lesion in Japan. In Japanese patients it accounts for 4 to 19% of all intracranial germinomas. It is not surprising, therefore, that the first primary spinal cord germinoma was recorded in a Japanese patient.[105] Subsequent reports also involved Japanese patients.[106–108] There is no sex predominance for spinal cord germinoma. Furthermore, patients with intramedullary spinal germinoma ranged in age from infant to young adult, and the lesions involved the entire spinal cord, although there was a thoracolumbar predominance.[109]

Pathology

Although the cellular origin of CNS germinoma remains unknown, its most common anatomical locations are the pineal and suprasellar regions. Less common sites include thalamus, basal ganglia, and cerebellar vermis.[104] In the spinal cord, tumors occur most frequently in the lower thoracic region.

CNS germinomas, like their gonadal counterparts, are known to have a propensity to metastasize. This commonly occurs via the CSF through the ventricular system and subarachnoid space. *Therefore, is important to confirm the absence of intracranial germinoma before designating the diagnosis of primary spinal germinoma.* This would include the lack of hypothalamic hypopituitarism or diabetes insipidus in addition to the lack of any radiographic evidence demonstrating intracranial lesions.

Histologically, these tumors present with the two-cell pattern of a germinoma. Multinucleated syncytiotrophoblastic giant cells, which may produce human chorionic gonadotropin, were found in one report.[105] Unlike other germ cell tumors, germinoma cells are negative for α-fetoprotein and for carcinoembryonic antigen. Germ cell tumors arise because of neoplastic changes during embryonic development. Germinomas characteristically infiltrate locally and spread by dissemination through the craniospinal and subarachnoid spaces. Parenchymal metastasis and extradural spread are rare. Grossly, solid tumor tissue can be soft and purplish gray. Microscopically these tumors consist of large polygonal cells surrounded by fibers and connective tissue. Lymphocytic infiltration is most prominent around blood vessels. Cells tend to organize in sheets and lobules and are characterized by large round or oval vesicular nuclei, prominent irregular nucleoli, pale ill-defined cytoplasm, rich stores of glycogen, and coarse or fine granular chromatin.[110–113] Mitotic figures may be present.[110, 114]

Radiology

The MRI findings are variable and include nonenhancing lesions, cystic lesions, and homogeneously enhancing lesions. T1-weighted enhanced images revealed homogeneous tumors of varying iso- or low intensities, depending on the degree of enhancement, that were similar to other intramedullary spinal cord tumors. They may also be associated with syrinx formation.[106]

Presentation

Exclusion of other foci by means of repeated inspection of other spinal cord regions, brain, abdomen, and thorax is mandatory.

Treatment

Because the tumors are radiosensitive, laminectomy and partial decompression with accurate radiation therapy constitute appropriate therapy.[108] It is documented that the total removal of intramedullary tumors has become increasingly more common and that radical or grossly total resections are not affected by higher morbidity than are partial resections. Radiation regimens for germinoma therapy vary. However, prophylactic irradiation of the entire neuraxis is controversial, and some authors[115] have concluded that the risk of spinal metastasis from an intracranial germinoma is too low to warrant routine prophylactic spinal irradiation. Furthermore, the first mode of therapy provided for some patients[115, 116] was local irradiation of cervical cord tumor. However, in these patients, a tumor developed in the spinal cord that was similar to that in the brain.

Only one patient in whom adjuvant chemotherapy was used is reported in the literature; therefore, the use of chemotherapy for intramedullary spinal cord germinomas is still experimental. However, systemic adjuvant chemotherapy may be beneficial for certain intramedullary spinal germinomas that prove refractory to radiotherapy or that recur after radiotherapy.

Outcome

A review of the literature revealed only one patient with the component of syncytiotrophoblastic giant cells who suffered local recurrence following surgical resection.[108] Most patients are free of recurrence during the observation periods.[108]

SUMMARY

Spinal cord tumors in pediatric patients represent a unique and interesting subset of central nervous system pathology. In addition to the more common tumors, ganglioglioma, teratoma, hemangioblastoma, oligodendroglioma, and germinoma should be considered in the differential diagnosis of any pediatric spinal cord lesion. Although discrete distinctions cannot always be made based solely on the demographic or radiologic data, the pathologic examination usually provides the information necessary to classify the tumor and direct further therapy when indicated.

REFERENCES

1. Pick L, Beilschowsky M. Ueber das System der Neurome und Beobachtungen an einem Ganglioneurom des Gehirns. *Z Gesamte Neurol Psychiatry* 1911;6:391–437.
2. Johannsson JH, Rekate HL, Roessmann U. Gangliogliomas: pathological and clinical correlation. *J Neurosurg* 1981;54(1):58–63.
3. Russell D, Rubinstein L. *Pathology of Tumours of the Nervous System*, 5th ed. London: Edward Arnold; 1989.
4. Garrido E, et al. Gangliogliomas in children: a clinicopathological study. *Child's Brain* 1978;4(6):339–346.
5. Zulch K. *Atlas of Gross Neurosurgical Pathology*. New York: Springer-Verlag; 1975:49.
6. Miller DC, Lang FF, Epstein FJ. Central nervous system gangliogliomas. Part 1: Pathology. *J Neurosurg* 1993;79(6):859–866.
7. Kalyan-Raman UP, Olivero WC. Ganglioglioma: a correlative clinicopathological and radiological study of ten surgically treated cases with follow-up. *Neurosurgery* 1987;20(3):428–433.
8. Burger P, Scheithauer B. *Atlas of Tumor Pathology: Tumors of the Central Nervous System*. Series 3, Fascicle 10. Washington, DC: Armed Forces Institute of Pathology; 1994:168.
9. Castillo M, et al. Intracranial ganglioglioma: MR, CT, and clinical findings in 18 patients. *Am J Neuroradiol* 1990;11:109–114.
10. Celli P, et al. Gangliogliomas of the cerebral hemispheres: report of 14 cases with long-term follow-up and review of the literature. *Acta Neurochir* 1993;125(1–4):52–57.
11. Kleihues P, Burger P, Scheithauer B. *Histological Typing of Tumours of the Central Nervous System*, 3rd ed. New York: Springer-Verlag; 1993.
12. Courville C. Ganglioglioma: tumor of the central nervous system: review of the literature and report of two cases. *Arch Neurol Psychiatry* 1930;24:439–491.
13. Demierre B, et al. Intracerebral ganglioglioma. *J Neurosurg* 1986;65(2):177–182.
14. Patel U, et al. MR of spinal cord ganglioglioma [see comments]. *Am J Neuroradiol* 1998;19(5):879–887.
15. Lang FF, et al. Central nervous system gangliogliomas. Part 2: Clinical outcome. *J Neurosurg* 1993;79(6):867–873.
16. Krouwer HG, et al. Gangliogliomas: a clinicopathological study of 25 cases and review of the literature. *J Neurooncol*, 1993;17(2):139–154.
17. Park SH, et al. Spinal cord ganglioglioma in childhood. *Pathol Res Pract* 1993;189(2):189–196.
18. Foerster O, Gagel O. Ein Fall von Gangliocytoma der Oblongata. *Z Gesamte Neurol Psychiatry* 1932;141:797–823.
19. Zhang PJ, Rosenblum MK. Synaptophysin expression in the human spinal cord: diagnostic implications of an immunohistochemical study. *Am J Surg Pathol* 1996;20(3):273–276.
20. Burger P. *Ganglion cell tumor*. Presented at Annual Meeting of the United States and Canadian Academy of Pathology, Boston, Massachusetts, 1990.
21. Wald U, et al. Conus ganglioglioma in a 2 $\frac{1}{2}$-year-old boy: case report. *J Neurosurg* 1985;62(1):142–144.
22. Lichtenstein B, Zeitlin H. Ganglioglioneuroma of the spinal cord associated with pseudosyringomyelia: a histologic study. *Arch Neurol Psychiatry* 1937;37:1356–1370.
23. Hamburger C, Buttner A, Weis S. Ganglioglioma of the spinal cord: report of two rare cases and review of the literature. *Neurosurgery* 1997;41(6):1410–1415; discussion 1415–1416.
24. Albright L, Byrd RP. Ganglioglioma of the entire spinal cord. *Child's Brain* 1980;6(5):274–280.
25. Kitano M, et al. Malignant ganglioglioma of the spinal cord. *Acta Pathol Jpn* 1987;37(6):1009–1018.
26. Ng TH, et al. Ganglioneuroma of the spinal cord. *Surg Neurol* 1991;35(2):147–151.
27. Hori A, Weiss R, Schaake T. Ganglioglioma containing osseous tissue and neurofibrillary tangles. *Arch Pathol Lab Med* 1988;112(6):653–655.
28. Diepholder HM, et al. A clinicopathologic and immunomorphologic study of 13 cases of ganglioglioma. *Cancer* 1991;68(10):2192–2201.
29. Wolf H, et al. Ganglioglioma: a detailed histopathological and immunohistochemical analysis of 61 cases. *Acta Neuropathol* (Berl) 1994;88:166–173.
30. Bevilacqua G, Sarnelli R. Ganglioglioma of the spinal cord: a case with a long survival. *Acta Neuropathol (Berl)* 1979;48(3):239–242.
31. Rodewald L, et al. Central nervous system neoplasm in a young man with Martin-Bell syndrome–fra(X)-XLMR. *Am J Med Genet* 1987;26(1):7–12.
32. Ventureyra E, et al. Temporal lobe gangliogliomas in children. *Child's Nerv Syst* 1986;2(2):63–66.
33. Miller DC, et al. Synaptophysin: a sensitive and specific marker for ganglion cells in central nervous system neoplasms. *Hum Pathol* 1990;21(3):271–276.
34. Isimbaldi G, et al. Ganglioglioma: a clinical and pathological study of 12 cases. *Clin Neuropathol* 1996;15(4):192–199.

35. Jaffey PB, et al. The clinical significance of extracellular matrix in gangliogliomas. *J Neuropathol Exp Neurol* 1996; 55(12):1246–1252.
36. Miller D. The Pathology of gliomas, including tumors of neuronal origin. In: Tindall G, Cooper P, Barrows D, eds. *The Practice of Neurosurgery.* Baltimore: Williams & Wilkins; 1996:601–635.
37. Smith TW, et al. Immunohistochemistry of synapsin I and synaptophysin in human nervous system and neuroendocrine tumors: applications in diagnostic neuro-oncology. *Clin Neuropathol* 1993;12(6):335–342.
38. Hassoun J, et al. Central neurocytoma: an electron-microscopic study of two cases. *Acta Neuropathol* 1982;56(2): 151–156.
39. Rubinstein LJ, Herman MM. A light- and electron-microscopic study of a temporal-lobe ganglioglioma. *J Neurol Sci* 1972;16(1):27–48.
40. Nass R, Whelan MA. Gangliogliomas. *Neuroradiology* 1981;22(2):67–71.
41. Haddad SF, et al. Ganglioglioma: 13 years of experience. *Neurosurgery* 1992;31(2):171–178.
42. Peretti-Viton P, et al. Magnetic resonance imaging in gangliogliomas and gangliocytomas of the nervous system. *J Neuroradiol* 1991;18(2):189–199.
43. Otsubo H, et al. Detection and management of gangliogliomas in children. *Surg Neurol* 1992;38(5):371–378.
44. Hall WA, Yunis EJ, Albright AL. Anaplastic ganglioglioma in an infant: case report and review of the literature. *Neurosurgery* 1986;19(6):1016–1020.
45. Sutton LN, et al. Cerebral gangliogliomas during childhood. *Neurosurgery* 1983;13(2):124–128.
46. Prayson RA, Khajavi K, Comair YG. Cortical architectural abnormalities and MIB1 immunoreactivity in gangliogliomas: a study of 60 patients with intracranial tumors. *J Neuropathol Exp Neurol* 1995;54(4):513–520.
47. Silver JM, et al. Ganglioglioma: a clinical study with long-term follow-up. *Surg Neurol* 1991;35(4):261–266.
48. Bell WO, et al. Leptomeningeal spread of intramedullary spinal cord tumors: report of three cases. *J Neurosurg* 1988;69(2):295–300.
49. Bowles AP Jr, et al. Ganglioglioma, a malignant tumor? Correlation with flow deoxyribonucleic acid cytometric analysis. *Neurosurgery* 1988;23(3):376–381.
50. Kernohan J, Learmonth J, Doyle J. Neuroblastomas and gangliocytomas of the central nervous system. *Brain* 1932; 55:287–310.
51. Berger PaS, BW. *Tumors of the Central Nervous System.* Series 3. *Atlas of Tumor Pathology.* Fascicle 10. Washington, DC: Armed Forces Institute of Pathology; 1994:168.
52. Masten M, Madison W. Teratoma of the spinal cord. *Arch Pathol* (Chicago) 1940;30:755.
53. Hosi K. Intradural teratoid tumours of the spinal cord: report of a case. *Arch Pathol* 1931;10:875–883.
54. al-Sarraj ST, et al. Clinicopathological study of seven cases of spinal cord teratoma: a possible germ cell origin. *Histopathology* 1998;32(1):51–56.
55. Slooff J, Kernohan J, MacCarthy C. *Primary Intra-Medullary Tumors of the Spinal Cord and Filum Terminale.* Philadelphia: WB Saunders; 1946.
56. Ingraham F, Bailey O. Cystic teratomas and teratoid tumors of the central nervous system in infancy and childhood. *J Neurosurg* 1946;3:511–532.
57. VandenBerg S. Neuroenteric cyst or teratomatous cyst (Invited Comment). *J Neurosurg* 1994;8:181.
58. Furtado D, Maeques V. Spinal teratoma. *J Neuropathol Exp Neurol* 1951;10:384–393.
59. Black S, German W. Four congenital tumors found at operation within the vertebral canal: with observations on their incidence. *J Neurosurg* 1950;7:49–61.
60. Lemmen J, Wilson C. Intramedullary malignant teratoma of the spinal cord. *Arch Neurol Psychiatry* 1951;66:61–68.
61. Nicoletti GF, et al. Intramedullary spinal cystic teratoma of the conus medullaris with caudal exophytic development: case report. *Surg Neurol* 1994;41(2):106–111.
62. Rosenbaum TJ, Soule EH, Onofrio BM. Teratomatous cyst of the spinal canal: case report. *J Neurosurg* 1978;49(2): 292–297.
63. Willis R. Teratomas. *Atlas of Tumor Pathology*, Vol. 3. Washington, DC: Armed Forces Institute of Pathology; 1951:3–58.
64. Willis R. *Pathology of Tumors*, 4th ed. New York: Appleton-Century-Crofts; 1967:961.
65. Koen JL, McLendon RE, George TM. Intradural spinal teratoma: evidence for a dysembryogenic origin: report of four cases. *J Neurosurg* 1998;89(5):844–851.
66. Hamabuchi M, Hasegawa R, Murase T. Teratoma of the spinal cord: a case report with CT scans. *J Bone Joint Surg Br* 1989;71(3):390–392.
67. Pickens JM, et al. Teratoma of the spinal cord: report of a case and review of the literature. *Arch Pathol* 1975;99(8):446–448.
68. Garrison JE, Kasdon DL. Intramedullary spinal teratoma: case report and review of the literature. *Neurosurgery* 1980;7(5):509–512.
69. Rhaney K, Barclay G. Enterogenous cyst and cogenital diverticuli of the alimentary canal with abnormalities of the vertebral column and spinal cord. *J Pathol Bacteriol* 1959; 77:457–471.
70. Padovani R, et al. Teratoid cyst of the spinal cord. *Neurosurgery* 1983;13(1):74–77.
71. Bailey O. Intramedullary cystic teratoid tumor of the cervical cord in association with a teratoma of ovary. *Surg Neurol* 1984;267:262–272.
72. Hoefnagel D, Benirschke K, Duarte J. Teratomatous cyst within the vertebral canal observation on the occurrence of sex chromatin. *J Neurol Neurosurg Psychiatry* 1962;25: 159–164.
73. Schultze F. Weitere Beitrage zur Diagnos and operativen Behandlung von Geschwulsten der Ruckenmarkshaute und des Ruckenmarks. *Dtsh. Med. Wochenschr* 1912;36: 1676.
74. Elsberg C. Diagnosis and surgical treatment of tumors of the spinal cord. In: *Proceedings of the Ninth Congress of the International Society of Surgery.* Brussels: Imprimerie Medical et Scientifique; 1932:385–444.
75. Wolf A. Tumors of the spinal cord, nerve roots and membranes. In: Elsberg CA, ed. *Surgical Diseases of the Spinal Cord, Membranes, and Nerve Roots.* New York: Paul B. Hoeber; 1941.
76. Guidetti B. Surgical treatment of vascular tumors and vascular malformations of the spinal cord. *Vasc Surg* 1970;4(3):179–185.
77. Browne TR, Adams RD, Roberson GH. Hemangioblastoma of the spinal cord: review and report of five cases. *Arch Neurol* 1976;33(6):435–441.

78. Yasargil MG, et al. The microsurgical removal of intramedullary spinal hemangioblastomas: report of twelve cases and a review of the literature. *Surg Neurol* 1976;(3):141–148.

79. Murota T, Symon L. Surgical management of hemangioblastoma of the spinal cord: a report of 18 cases. *Neurosurgery* 1989;25(5):699–707; discussion 708.

80. Goodbody RA, Gamlen TR. Cerebellar haemangioblastoma and genitourinary tumours. *J Neurol Neurosurg Psychiatry* 1974;37(5):606–609.

81. Huson SM, et al. Cerebellar haemangioblastoma and von Hippel–Lindau disease. *Brain* 1986;109(6):1297–1310.

82. Michael J, Levin P. Multiple telangiectases of the brain: a discussion of hereditary factors in their development. *Arch Neurol Psychiatry* (Chicago) 1936;36:514–529.

83. Wyburn-Mason R. *The Vascular Abnormalities and Tumors of the Spinal Cord and Its Membranes.* London: Henry-Kimpton; 1943:60–95.

84. Kendall B. Application of angiography to tumours affecting the spinal cord. *Proc R Soc Med* 1970;63(2):185–187.

85. Solomon RA, Stein BM. Unusual spinal cord enlargement related to intramedullary hemangioblastoma. *J Neurosurg* 1988;68(4):550–553.

86. Lindau A. Discussion on vascular tumors of the brain and spinal cord. *Proc R Soc Med* 1931;24:363–370.

87. Stein A, Schilp A, Whitfeld R. The histogenesis of hemangioblastoma of the brain: a review of 21 cases. *J Neurosurg* 1960;17:751–761.

88. Russell D. Capillary haemangioma of spinal cord associated with syringomyelia. *J Pathol* 1932;35:103–112.

89. Davidson C, Brock S, Dyke C. Retinal and central nervous system hemangioblastomatosis with visceral changes (von Hippel–Lindau's disease). *Bull Neurol Inst NY* 1936;5:72–93.

90. Aubin ML, et al. Computed tomography in 75 clinical cases of syringomyelia. *Am J Neuroradiol* 1981;2(3):199–204.

91. Williams AL, et al. Differentiation of intramedullary neoplasms and cysts by MR. *Am J Roentgenol* 1987;149(1):159–164.

92. Kendall B, Russell J. Haemangioblastomas of the spinal cord. *Br J Radiol* 1966;39(467):817–823.

93. Fortuna A, Celli P, Palma L. Oligodendrogliomas of the spinal cord. *Acta Neurochir* 1980;52(3–4):305–329.

94. Chigasaki H, Pennybacker JB. A long follow-up study of 128 cases of intramedullary spinal cord tumours. *Neurol Med Chir* 1968;10:25–66.

95. Kernohan J, Woltman H, Adson A. Intramedullary tumors of the spinal cord: a review of fifty-one cases, with an attempt at histologic classification. *Arch Neurol Psychiatry* 1931;25:679–699.

96. Kernohan J, Woltman H, Adson A. Gliomas arising from the region of the cauda equina: clinical, surgical and histologic considerations. *Arch Neurol Psychiatry* 1933;29:287–305.

97. Norstrom C, Kernohan J, Love J. One hundred primary caudal tumors. *JAMA* 1961;178:1071–1077.

98. Rasmussen T, Kernohan J, Adson A. Pathologic classification with surgical consideration of intraspinal tumors. *Ann Surg* 1940:111.

99. Ravens JR, Adamkiewicz LL, Groff RA. Cytology and cellular pathology of the oligodendrogliomas of the brain. *J Neuropathol Exp Neurol* 1955;14:142–184.

100. Garcia JH, Lemmi H. Ultrastructure of oligodendroglioma of the spinal cord. *Am J Clin Pathol* 1970;54(5):757–765.

101. Arseni C, et al. Spinal dermoid tumours. *Neurochirurgia* (Stuttg) 1977;20(4):108–116.

102. DeSousa AL, et al. Intraspinal tumors in children: a review of 81 cases. *J Neurosurg* 1979;51(4):437–445.

103. Epstein F, Epstein N. Surgical management of holocord intramedullary spinal cord astrocytomas in children. *J Neurosurg* 1981;54(6):829–832.

104. Horowitz MB, Hall WA. Central nervous system germinomas: a review. *Arch Neurol* 1991;48(6):652–657.

105. Hisa S, et al. Intramedullary spinal cord germinoma producing HCG and precocious puberty in a boy. *Cancer* 1985;55(12):2845–2849.

106. Matsuoka S, et al. Intramedullary spinal cord germinoma: case report. *Surg Neurol* 1991;35(2):122–126.

107. Hanafusa K, et al. Intramedullary spinal cord germinoma: case report and review of the literature. *Rofo Fortschr Geb Rontgenstr Neuen Bildgeb Verfahr* 1993;159(2):203–204.

108. Miyauchi, A, et al. Primary intramedullary spinal cord germinoma: case report. *J Neurosurg* 1996;84(6):1060–1061.

109. Itoh Y, et al. Intramedullary spinal cord germinoma: case report and review of the literature. *Neurosurgery* 1996;38(1):187–190; discussion 190–191.

110. Scheithauer BW. Neuropathology of pineal region tumors. *Clin Neurosurg* 1985;32:351–383.

111. Kim K, et al. Pineal germinoma with widespread extracranial metastases. *Diagn Cytopathol* 1985;1(2):118–122.

112. Jennings CD, et al. Suprasellar germ cell tumor with extracranial metastases. *Neurosurgery* 1985;16(1):9–12.

113. Masuzawa T, et al. Germ cell tumors (germinoma and yolk sac tumor) in unusual sites in the brain. *Clin Neuropathol* 1986;5(5):190–202.

114. Jennings MT, Gelman R, Hochberg F. Intracranial germ-cell tumors: natural history and pathogenesis. *J Neurosurg* 1985;63(2):155–167.

115. Shibamoto Y, et al. Treatment results of intracranial germinoma as a function of the irradiated volume. *Int J Radiat Oncol Biol Phys* 1988;15(2):285–290.

116. Nagasawa S, et al. Intracranial and spinal germinomas occurring four years after spinal cord germinoma: case report. *Neurol Med Chir* (Tokyo) 1991;31(11):729–731.

Outcomes and Complications

Section

IV

Chapter 35

Postoperative Considerations

Michael E. Seiff and James Tait Goodrich

Postoperative care begins with emergence from anesthesia. The results of initial neurologic examination obtained after awakening, the first in the succession of frequent neurologic assessments, are compared with those of both the preoperative and subsequent examinations to document steady improvement as the anesthetics are metabolized, or to alert the clinician to an unexpected deficit. Prompt arousal may reduce the apprehension typical of surgeons in the immediate postoperative period. Failure to awaken to satisfaction or demonstration of a focal deficit, such as motor asymmetry or pupillary abnormality, may prompt an imaging study straight from the operating room.

Expectations of timely emergence must be tailored to a number of factors, such as experience of the anesthetist, when the agents were discontinued, or extent of surgery. Tumor size can also influence emergence.[1] Transient neurologic changes known to occur during awakening from anesthesia, such as hyperreflexia, clonus, upgoing plantar responses, and pupillary abnormalities,[2] are seen less often now that the inhalational agents halothane and enflurane have largely been supplanted by isoflurane.

Children and infants are always transported from the operating room with supplemental oxygen, as they are likely at greater risk than adults for postanesthetic desaturation.[3] Once the patient is in the recovery room or pediatric intensive care unit (PICU), standardized neurologic examinations at regular intervals, initially every 15 minutes, remain the most important determinant of the patient's neurologic status. This requires skilled nursing, compulsive documentation, and efficient communication with a team approach of which the physicians, while ultimately responsible, are only a part. Knowledge of the patient's preoperative status is essential for all postoperative caretakers in terms of a detailed history, adequacy of seizure prophylaxis, or existence of a preoperative deficit. Likewise, intraoperative data, such as fluid balance and estimated blood loss, whether brain retraction may increase the risk of brain edema, or if problematic hemostasis may herald a potential bleeding problem, are also key. Thus, all important preoperative and intraoperative information should be documented by the surgeons and disseminated to all physicians and nurses who will have a role in the postoperative care of the child.

In general, the complication rate is lower after surgery for brain tumors than following less elective (i.e., trauma) intracranial procedures. Perioperative morbidity and mortality continue to be a necessary evil with intracranial surgery. A recent review found a postoperative complication in 10% of pediatric and adult patients undergoing a craniotomy for a supratentorial tumor.[4] However, decades of advances continue to improve outcome in this population. As a result of refinements in surgical technique, Cushing in 1932 reported a decrease in mortality from 30.9 to 11.6% in a career-long retrospective of 2000 cases of intracranial tumor.[5] The mortality rate of brain tumor surgery was further reduced by the advent of perioperative steroid use, dropping to less than 3% by the 1960s,[6] and a recent review of nearly 1800 craniotomies for supratentorial tumor resections found a perioperative mortality rate of 2.1%.[4] Clearly, then, the great majority of children who undergo brain tumor surgery should have as their main nemesis the natural history of the disease (and the rigors of adjuvant therapy, if indicated) rather than negative sequelae of the operation itself. Surgery, in a word, should be the least of their problems.

Therefore, the goals in postoperative management (Table 35–1) are recognition of potential systemic, metabolic, or neurologic complications; prevention or minimization of the sequelae of these complications by intervention as necessary; and maintenance or restoration of homeostasis until the patient is stable enough to convalesce in a less vigilant setting. As all complications are considered potentially life threatening if unrecognized or untreated, meticulous attention to detail must be the rule in treatment of the postoperative patient.

BOX 35–1
Goals of Postoperative Management

- **Recognize potential complications: systemic, metabolic, neurologic**
- **Prevent or minimize secondary injury resulting from complications; intervene as necessary**
- **Maintain or restore homeostasis**
- **Follow patient; give meticulous care**

TABLE 35–1   Minimum Postoperative Neurologic Evaluation

Younger child	Older child

Observation
   Level of alertness
   Eye opening
   Facial and limb movement
   Extraocular muscle function
   Respiratory pattern
   Vocal output
Fontanelle palpation (soft, flat, full, bulging, tense)
Elicited responses
   Brain stem reflexes
      Pupillary response to light
      Corneal reflex
      Gag reflex
   Motor response to stimulation
   Vocal response to stimulation
	Observation
	   Level of alertness
	   Eye opening
	   Motor function
	      Spontaneous
	      Purposeful
	Verbal output
	Orientation
	Follow commands
	   Midline
	   Lateralizing
	   3-step midline crossing
	Elicited responses (unconscious)
	   Brain stem reflexes
	      Pupillary response to light
	      Corneal reflex
	      Gag reflex
	      Oculovestibular reflex
	   Motor
	      Response to noxious stimuli
	   Reflexes
	      Extremity tone
	      Deep tendon reflex
	      Plantar reflex (Babinski)

NEUROLOGIC ASSESSMENT

As stated, repeated neurologic evaluation is the first line of defense in early detection of potential problems (Table 35–1). These are performed every 15 min for the first hour on arrival to the recovery room or PICU, and regular hourly assessment is the typical routine once the patient has been stabilized. Although age-related variations exist, the basic approach of clinical observation and response to stimulation (noxious, auditory, visual) remains the mainstay of the neurologic evaluation. Regardless of age, the level of alertness, brain stem reflexes, and motor function can be evaluated in all age groups.

Neurologic Examination
The Younger Patient

There are several modified versions of the Glasgow Coma Scale for application to infants and children (Tables 35–2 to 35–5).[7–11] There is no consensus opinion recommending one system over another, and the pediatric scales are likely subject to more intraobserver variability than the adult scale. The neonate and infant can be observed for spontaneous facial

TABLE 35–2   Glasgow Coma Scale

Category	Response	Score
Eye opening	Spontaneously	4
	To voice	3
	To pain	2
	None	1
Verbal	Oriented speech	5
	Confused speech	4
	Inappropriate speech	3
	Incomprehensible sounds	2
	None	1
Motor	Follows commands	6
	Localizes pain	5
	Withdraws to pain	4
	Abnormal flexion	3
	Abnormal extension	2
	None	1

Range of scores is from 3 to 15.

Modified from Teasdale G, Jennett B. Assessment and prognosis of coma after head injury. *Acta Neurochirurgica* 1976;34:45–55. Reproduced with permission of Springer-Verlag, New York.

TABLE 35–3   Modified Coma Scale for Infants

Category	Response	Score
Eye opening	Spontaneously	4
	To voice	3
	To pain	2
	None	1
Verbal	Coos, babbles	5
	Irritable cries	4
	Cries to pain	3
	Moans to pain	2
	None	1
Motor	Normal spontaneous movements	6
	Withdraws to touch	5
	Withdraws to pain	4
	Abnormal flexion	3
	Abnormal extension	2
	None	1

Range of scores is from 3 to 15.
From James HE, Trauner DA. The Glasgow coma scale. In: James HE, Anas NG, Perkin RM, eds. *Brain Insults in Infants and Children.* Orlando: Grune & Stratton; 1985:179–182. Reproduced with permission of WB Saunders Company, Philadelphia.)

TABLE 35–5   Neonatal Arousal Scale

Best response to bell	
Facial and extremity movements	5
Grimaces/blinks	4
Increase in RR/HR	4
Seizures/extensor posturing	2
No response	1
Best response to light	
Blink and facial/extremity movements	4
Blink	3
Seizures/extensor posturing	2
No response	1
Best motor response	
Spontaneous	
Periods of activity alternating with sleep	6
Occasional spontaneous movements	5
Sternal rub	
Extremity movements	4
Grimace/facial movements	3
Seizures/extensor posturing	2
No response	1

Range of score is from 3 to 15.
RR, respiratory rate; HR, heart rate.
From Duncan CD, Ment LR, Smith B, et al. A scale for the assessment of neonatal neurologic status. *Child's Brain* 1981;8:299–306. Reproduced with permission of S. Karger AG, Basel.

TABLE 35–4   Children's Coma Score

Category	Response	Score
Ocular	Pursuit	4
	Reactive pupils and intact EOM	3
	Fixed pupils or impaired EOM	2
	Fixed pupils and paralyzed EOM	1
Verbal	Cries	3
	Spontaneous respirations	2
	Apneic	1
Motor	Flexes and extends	4
	Withdraws from painful stimuli	3
	Hypertonic	2
	Flaccid	1

Range of scores is from 3 to 11.
From Raimondi AJ, Hirschauer J. Head injury in the infant and toddler. Coma scoring and outcome scale. *Child's Brain* 1984;11:12–35. Reproduced with permission of S. Karger AG, Basel.

and limb movements, eye opening and extraocular muscle function, respiratory pattern, and vocal output. With respect to motor function, the detection of asymmetry is the most important abnormal finding, alerting the clinician to a possible hemiparesis.[12] Responses can be elicited with tactile or noxious stimuli, and the character of cry can also be assessed. Pupillary response and other brain stem reflexes can be tested. The ability to palpate an open fontanel cannot be overemphasized as a means of directly and rapidly providing a gross clinical assessment of intracranial pressure (ICP), with descriptions such as "flat," "soft," "full," "bulging," or "tense" often utilized. Table 35–6 lists a number of findings that may be considered abnormal in older children and adults but normal in patients younger than 2 years.

The Older Patient

The neurologic assessment of older children and adolescents follows that used with adults. Typically, the level of alertness is assessed first, concurrent with notation of the presence or absence of spontaneous or purposeful movements. If not spontaneously open, the ability of the patient to open his or her eyes to vocal or noxious stimuli is observed. Orientation and verbal responses are then gauged. The ability to follow commands can be graded, with a midline command (i.e., tongue protrusion) considered simpler or more primitive than a lateralizing command (i.e., the showing of two fingers). Having the patient touch the opposite ear with a specified finger, such as the thumb, is useful as a more complex three-step midline-crossing command. If the patient is not conscious, testing of the brain stem reflexes, including pupillary response, corneal and gag reflexes, is mandatory. Likewise the motor response to noxious stimuli and assessment of long-tract signs, including tone and deep tendon and plantar

TABLE 35–6   Neurologic Findings in Patients Younger than 2 Years

Normal	Abnormal
Asymmetrical blink	Handedness <18 months
Indistinct or slightly elevated disk margins	Motor asymmetry
Disconjugate gaze	Unilateral fisting
Irregular tongue movements	Hypertonia
Plantar reflexes (up to 1 year)	Flaccidity
Absent or brisk deep tendon reflexes	Anisocoria
Clonus	Failure to attend to auditory or visual stimuli
Brisk pupillary response	
Flexor dominance	

Data from Venes JL, Linder SL, Eiterman RD. Neurological examination of infants and children. In: Youmans JR, ed. *Neurological Surgery*. 3rd ed. Philadelphia: WB Saunders: 37–43; and Andrews BT, Hammer GB. The neurological examination and neurological monitoring in pediatric intensive care. In: Andrews BT, Hammer GB, eds. *Pediatric Neurosurgical Intensive Care*. American Association of Neurological Surgeons; 1997:1–11.

reflexes, is basic to the evaluation of an unconscious patient. The Glasgow Coma Scale Table (Table 35–2) can be useful under these conditions. Though initially validated as a prognosticator for head-injured patients,[7, 8] the scale has found widespread utility in the evaluation of neurologically compromised patients regardless of etiology.

Often the postoperative neurologic examination is tailored to the surgery performed. The examiner may pay closer attention to tests for ataxia or dysarthria in patients who have undergone posterior fossa surgery. The visual fields may warrant closer inspection after cases of suprasellar or hypothalamic tumor surgery, whereas after supratentorial tumor resection the examiner may focus more on tests for motor function. In all cases, it is the early detection of neurologic deterioration through regular examination that offers the patient the best chance of optimizing outcome.

Vital Signs

In the postoperative patient, vital signs should be considered an essential component of the complete neurologic evaluation rather than a separate set of parameters to follow. These include body temperature, heart rate and rhythm via surface electrocardiography, respiratory rate and pattern, and arterial blood pressure (see Boxes 35–2 through 35–5). Pulse oximetry is always followed as well. Knowledge of the age-related and diurnal variations of the normal range for heart rate, respiratory rate, and blood pressure is a prerequisite.

Temperature

Younger patients can experience wide fluctuations in core temperature; esophageal or rectal probes are commonly used. Both elevated and depressed temperatures can influence the level of consciousness and the neurologic exam, and patients with compromised cerebral function are likely more sensitive to these changes.[13] The definition of hypothermia varies from source to source, ranging from below 32.2°C[14] to 35°C[15] to any temperature significantly below 37°C.[16] It may occur following general anesthesia, especially after prolonged surgery, and is seen commonly, with untoward effects resulting if not addressed. Prolongation of emergence secondary to hypothermia can delay the subsequent detection of a deficit; shivering and rewarming can increase oxygen consumption and potentially exacerbate an hypoxemia; and the pressure of air trapped intracranially can increase as the air warms.[17] Arrhythmias, dehydration, and lactic acidosis can also result if hypothermia goes untreated.[18] Hypothermia can also be seen with posterior hypothalamic dysfunction following resection of tumors near this region, such as glioma or craniopharyngioma,[14, 17, 19] or as a syndrome associated with agenesis of the corpus callosum (Shapiro's syndrome).[20] Therapy generally consists of use of heat lamps, blankets, humidified oxygen, and, if necessary, warmed intravenous fluids. *Hypothermia is one of the major causes of postoperative morbidity in infants and neonates and as such is aggressively treated as outlined.*

Postoperative fevers are relatively common. Fever can negatively influence the neurologic status of the patient, even leading to coma if greater than 42°C;[21] hence, a search for a treatable source is always initiated. If fever occurs early in the course in an older patient, it is commonly attributed to atelectasis secondary to general anesthesia. However, there is little experimental support for a causal relationship.[22] A recent survey of nosocomial infection in the PICU found bloodstream, pulmonary, urinary tract, and surgical sites to be the predominant sources.[23] Meningitis is always a concern in the postoperative patient for whom another source cannot be found, and the workup may eventually lead to a lumbar puncture for cerebrospinal fluid (CSF) evaluation. Drug-induced fever by phenytoin is a well-known phenomenon,[14, 24] usually diagnosed by exclusion, as is tumor fever.[22] Fevers secondary to anterior hypothalamic dysfunction (neurogenic or central) are usually high, approaching 40°C.[14] The postictal state is also commonly associated with elevated temperature. Every attempt should be made to aggressively lower the temperature below 38.5°C[18] with cooling blankets or more aggressive measures if antipyretics and source-specific treatment plans are not effective. This is necessary because *fever is known to increase CO_2 concentration and cerebral blood flow (CBF), which can exacerbate increased ICP.*[25, 26]

reversible and titrated to effect to minimize dosing. Physiologic disturbances that may manifest as restlessness or agitation, such as hypoxia or increased ICP, are first ruled out prior to initiation of a regimen to avoid masking of signs and symptoms.[105]

Differentiation of pain, anxiety, or agitation may dictate choice of drug. *Benzodiazepines*, for example, provide anxiolysis and amnesia but not analgesia.[105] Diazepam and midazolam are shorter acting than lorezepam due to differences in lipid solubility. Intermittent or continuous therapy are both utili zed as clinically warranted. Flumazenil is a new benzodiazepine antagonist that can reverse the effects of oversedation.[106] In general, benzodiazepines have limited effect on systemic vascular tone, but hypotension can occur due to inhibition of endogenous catecholamines.[105]

Morphine, the most commonly used opioid for sedation, is primarily an analgesic. Concerns over respiratory depression influence decisions regarding dosage. It is easily reversible with the antagonist naloxone. There is no convincing data to support the suggestion that sedating doses of opioids can increase the risk of seizures in patients.[105]

Propofol is structurally distinct from the above sedative classes and behaves most like a short-acting barbiturate. It provides no analgesia but produces sedative-hypnotic effects in a rapid, dose-dependent manner with equally rapid elimination kinetics. Thus, it allows for uncompromised neurologic assessment within 10 to 15 minutes of cessation of infusion, even after prolonged maintenance of therapy.[107, 108] Propofol can cause respiratory depression as well as affect systemic vascular tone, resulting in significant hypotension, especially after the initial bolus.[105] However, its quick onset, titratable sedating effects, and rapid elimination profile make it an ideal drug for the neurosurgical patient.

In patients requiring paralysis, the non-depolarizing muscle relaxants have no intrinsic effect on CBF, $CMRO_2$, or ICP.[73] *Vecuronium* is the agent most commonly used. It has no cardiovascular effects,[109] as opposed to pancuronium, which may cause hypertension and tachycardia due to vagolytic effects, or atracurium, which may induce histamine-mediated hypotension and increase CBF.[27] The depolarizing agent succinylcholine may cause bradycardia or tachycardia, hyperkalemia, or trigger malignant hyperthermia in susceptible patients.[27] As paralysis dissipates rapidly, usually within 5 to 7 minutes, the use of succinylcholine should be reserved only when brief and transient blockade is required.

CSF Drainage

As stated previously, rapid reduction in ICP can occur as CSF is drained from a patient with increased ICP. Drainage is most effective with hydrocephalus, but usually improves high ICP secondary to edema as well. The slope of the pressure-volume curve is steeper in children than in adults; therefore, the response can be pronounced, with drainage of just a few milliliters substantially lowering the pressure.

Typically, the system is left opened to drainage if the patient has hydrocephalus, with a set point (the positive pressure above which CSF will drain) of 5 or 10 cm H_2O depending on the age of the patient. The volume of CSF drained, the clinical status, the set point, and the size of the ventricles on imaging are all considered while caring for the patient through what is hopefully a transient requirement for an external CSF shunt.[110] With prolonged drainage of CSF it is necessary to replace the lost volume with equal amounts of normal saline to maintain a positive fluid balance and normovolemia in young patients.

When the cause of high ICP is edema, the system is usually continuously transduced and opened for drainage as necessary when ICP exceeds a treatment threshold. Typically a few milliliters drain over a minute or two, the ICP is lowered, and the fluid column is redirected from the drainage bag to the transducer with a flip of the stopcock. Although fiberoptic systems exist which allow simultaneous measurement and drainage, most systems in common use allow one or the other, and clinically there are reasons why intermittent drainage may be preferable. Leaving the system open to drainage increases the risk for obstruction, whether due to coaptation of the ventricle against the catheter tip or occlusion of the catheter lumen by necrotic debris or blood.[110] Also, the ICP measured in an open system will be equal to the set point, possibly leading to falsely low readings or missing significant ICP spikes.[98, 110]

Mannitol and Diuretic Therapy

There is little evidence to support the traditional contention that mannitol lowers ICP by producing an osmotic gradient between the brain and blood that promotes brain dehydration. Some studies have found no significant reduction in normal or edematous brain water content after mannitol administration.[111, 112] Another study was able to show marked brain water losses with urea, an osmotic agent used before mannitol was popularized, but was unable to correlate ICP changes.[113, 114] Others have been able to correlate ICP reduction and brain water effects,[115] but only after increasing mannitol to very high levels from the lower, clinically relevant doses that previously failed to show such an effect.[116] In short, studies attempting to show such a relationship, whether with mannitol or with other agents, are conflicting or have significant discrepancies, suggesting that mechanisms other than brain dehydration may be responsible for mannitol's action on ICP.

An intravenous bolus of mannitol acts as a plasma volume expander; the osmotic load induces a fluid shift from the extravascular to the intravascular compartment. Water is preferentially drawn from the systemic circulation as compared with the brain, with the rate or hydraulic conductivity being several orders of magnitude greater in muscle or intestinal capillaries than brain capillary endothelium.[114, 117, 118] This influx can have several key effects. First, volume expansion increases blood pressure and CPP. This may lead to vasoconstriction as proposed by the vasoconstriction cascade, lowering CBV and ICP.[32, 35, 119] Second, the hemodilution decreases the viscosity of blood,[120] which improves blood flow. In a mechanism similar to autoregulation, vasoconstriction may then occur in order to maintain the same CBF, again leading to a reduction of CBV and ICP.[28, 35, 114, 118] Third, mannitol leads to a deformation of red blood cells—they shrink.[120] This improves oxygen delivery, which likewise may encourage vasoconstriction.[119, 121]

Hence, current theories of mannitol (Table 35–8) and its ability to lower ICP focus on three possible mechanisms: volume

TABLE 35–8 Mannitol Use

> *Mechanisms*
>   Volume expansion improves blood pressure
>   Hemodilution decreases blood viscosity
>   RBC deformation improves O_2 delivery
>   Allows vasoconstriction, reducing CBV and ICP
>   Cerebral dehydration controversial
> *Indications*[a]
>   ICP monitored: high ICP
>   ICP unmonitored: transtentorial herniation or
>   neurologic deterioration
> *Implementation*
>   Initial 1 g/kg bolus over 10–15 min (avoid very rapid
>   infusions)
>   Subsequent dosing 0.25–0.5 g/kg boluses
>   Titrate frequency to duration of effect (frequent serum
>   osmolality determinations)
>   Smaller more frequent dosing preferred over larger
>   less frequent dosing
> *Complications*
>   Closely follow renal status for nephrotoxicity
>   Cumulative dose-dependent risk
>   Maintain serum osmolality <310–320
>   Avoid hypotension and hypovolemia
>   Strict fluid balance monitoring
>   Foley catheter
>   Replace urinary losses

[a] Assumes head position, sedation/paralysis, temperature, and volume status are optimized.
RBC, red blood cell count; CBV, cerebral blood volume; ICP, intracranial pressure.

expansion improving blood pressure, hemodilution decreasing blood viscosity, and red blood cell deformation improving oxygen delivery. Hemodynamic and rheologic interactions may then allow the same CBF and oxygen delivery to be maintained by smaller vessels, allowing vasoconstriction, reducing CBV, and lowering ICP.[28, 35, 114, 119]

The indications for mannitol in the postoperative setting include (1) a patient with a functioning ICP monitor who is otherwise optimized with respect to head position, sedation, volume status, and temperature, with a progressive or pathologic increase in ICP, or (2) a patient without an ICP monitor, systemically optimized as stated, who shows signs of transtentorial herniation or progressive neurologic deterioration, with results of imaging and placement of an ICP monitor pending. The recommended dose varies between 0.25 and 1 g/kg, given as an intravenous bolus over 10 to 15 minutes. Rapid infusions of 5 minutes or less have been reported to cause paradoxical increases in ICP.[119, 122] Frequency is titrated to duration of effect, typically 90 minutes to 6 hours or more,[92] rather than scheduling every 4 or 6 hours. Smaller, more frequent dosing has been advocated over larger, less frequent regimens to minimize side effects; single-dose therapy may be effective.[98, 123] Typically, the initial dose is closer to the 1 g/kg level, and subsequent doses, if required, are smaller, in the 0.25 to 0.5 g/kg range, though this may vary from center to center.

Avoidance of adverse affects of therapy requires vigilant monitoring of various physiologic and metabolic parameters. Renal failure from acute tubular necrosis is known to occur with high serum osmolalities, generally after days of prolonged administration in a cumulative dose-dependent manner.[124] The risk is increased if other nephrotoxic drugs are being used simultaneously.[92] Frequent serum osmolality determinations to keep the level below 310 mOsm[32, 98] or 320 mOsm[92] reduce this risk. Mannitol can accumulate in brain tissue after multiple-dose therapy in a time-dependent manner, extravasating through damaged blood-brain barriers and exacerbating edema.[112] The most serious complication of therapy is hypotension secondary to hypovolemia. Hypotension can compromise CPP, leading to vasodilatation, increased CBV, and increased ICP.[35, 119] Hypovolemia may increase viscosity, which may also lead to vasodilatation.[114] Fluid and electrolyte status is closely followed in all patients receiving mannitol therapy; a bladder catheter is essential, and central venous pressure monitoring may be helpful.[32] It is recommended that urinary losses be replaced to maintain euvolemia.[32, 35, 92, 119]

Nonosmotic diuretics have been given in conjunction with mannitol therapy. The loop diuretic furosemide is thought to have synergistic effects in combination with mannitol,[125, 126] yet the enhanced diuresis can impair the ability to maintain euvolemia and exacerbate electrolyte disturbances.[28, 73]

Hyperventilation

Shortly after the first study correlating hyperventilation and ICP reduction in 1959,[127] physicians automatically administered hypocarbic therapy for the treatment of intracranial hypertension. The lower $PaCO_2$ leads to an alkalosis in the perivascular brain extracellular space that mediates a rapid cerebral arteriolar and pial vasoconstriction.[41, 128] This decreases CBV, which lowers ICP. The response is immediate, peaks at approximately 30 minutes, and can effect an initial reduction in ICP of 25 to 30% or more.[59, 129] Effectiveness is short-lived, however, likely due to buffering activity in the extracellular space.[41] The vasculature soon equilibrates to the hypocarbia, returning to baseline diameter within 20 hours in laboratory animals[41] and restoring CBF to 90% of baseline by 4 hours in healthy adult volunteers.[129]

The benefits of prolonged hyperventilation have therefore been called into question. Indeed, it can lead to potentially harmful situations by several mechanisms. As mentioned earlier, when normocapnea is eventually restored, the vessels, having accommodated to the hypocarbia, can vasodilate in response to the higher $PaCO_2$, leading to potentially dangerous elevations in CBV and ICP.[34, 41, 129] This same accommodation can also limit the effectiveness of additional or more aggressive hyperventilation should further decreases in $PaCO_2$ be desired. High tidal volumes and respiratory rates can decrease preload and cardiac filling pressures in ventilated patients, causing a reduction in blood pressure and compromising CPP.[35, 59] In some cases, ICP has been noted to paradoxically increase with hyperventilation, due to transmission of high pulmonary pressures, exacerbation of ischemia, or unknown mechanisms.[59, 130] *Most importantly, overly aggressive hyperventilation and excessive vasoconstriction can cause or exacerbate ischemia, shown in a number of trials with head-injured adults and children.*[131–134] The diffuse swelling and cerebral hyperemia that may exist as a unique feature in children after head injury is often cited as justification for hyperventilation in that setting,[135, 136] yet this rationale should not be applied to postoperative children in whom the development of high ICP is nontraumatic.

Therefore, as no benefit to prolonged hyperventilation has ever been demonstrated, and out of concern about ischemia, routine use of hyperventilation (Table 35–9) has been curtailed in recent years. However, most authorities agree that there is short-term utility when increased ICP requires acute intervention.[35] This may be especially true in the postoperative setting, as opposed to after head injury where CBF is known to significantly decrease in the immediate postinjury phase.[92, 137] Likewise, mechanical trauma has also been shown to increase the vulnerability of the brain to ischemia.[138, 139] Therefore, when hyperventilation is used to reduce an acute rise in ICP, the risk for causing or exacerbating ischemia in the postoperative setting may be less than that after head injury, where CBF is already compromised and the brain may be more susceptible to ischemic injury. However, this should not obviate concerns for provoking ischemia in the postoperative setting.

The indications for hyperventilation in the postoperative setting therefore include (1) a patient with a functioning ICP monitor who is otherwise optimized with respect to head position, sedation, volume status, and temperature, with a pathologic increase in ICP refractory to mannitol and, if applicable, ventricular CSF drainage; or (2) a patient without an ICP monitor, systemically optimized as stated, who shows signs of transtentorial herniation or progressive neurologic deterioration, results of imaging and placement of an ICP monitor pending. This is a general guideline; the point at which hypocarbic

TABLE 35–9 Hyperventilation Use

Mechanisms
  Low PaCO$_2$ mediates cerebral vasoconstriction
  Reduces CBV and ICP
  Immediate effect, 30-min peak
  Short-lived effect, vasculature equilibrates to low PaCO$_2$
Indications[a]
  ICP monitored: high ICP refractory to mannitol/CSF drainage
  ICP unmonitored: transtentorial herniation or neurologic deterioration
Implementation
  PaCO$_2$ 30–35 mm Hg initially
  Jugular venous saturation monitor for lower PaCO$_2$
  Optimize hematocrit and FIO$_2$
Complications (avoid prolonged hyperventilation)
  Ischemic injury
  Rebound vasodilatation
  Hypotension from decreased preload
  Paradoxical increase in ICP
  Ineffectiveness of additional hypocarbia against subsequent rise in ICP

[a]Assumes head position, sedation/paralysis, temperature, and volume status are optimized.
PaCO$_2$, partial pressure of carbon dioxide, arterial; CBV, cerebral blood volume; ICP, intracranial pressure; CSF, cerebrospinal fluid; FIO$_2$, fraction of inspired oxygen.

therapy is initiated will vary. Combination therapy is common. After manifesting an acute rise in ICP a patient may receive a mannitol bolus and hyperventilation simultaneously while en route to the CT scanner. The cause of the problem as revealed by imaging may then dictate more directed therapy, as in placement of a ventriculostomy for acute hydrocephalus. Hyperventilation would then be discontinued. Prophylactic hyperventilation in patients at risk for neurologic decline in the absence of increased ICP is not recommended.

The recommended target for PaCO$_2$ with hyperventilation is 30 to 35 mm Hg initially. These levels are thought to carry minimal risk for ischemia, are usually effective in lowering ICP, and decrease the risks associated with mechanical ventilation.[32, 35, 98] If more aggressive treatment to lower PaCO$_2$ levels is warranted, it is usually recommended that the degree of hyperventilation be titrated with technical adjuncts, such as jugular bulb venous saturation measurements.[32, 74, 98] With aggressive hyperventilation it has also been recommended that oxygen delivery to the brain be maximized by raising the hematocrit with transfusion as necessary, and increasing the inspired oxygen concentration (FiO$_2$).[73, 140] The temptation to manually and aggressively hyperventilate a patient to rapidly reduce acutely raised ICP ("bag the patient down") should be resisted, as hypotension and ischemia can both ensue.

Barbiturate Therapy

High-dose barbiturate therapy has been used to lower ICP in patients refractory to all other measures. It is very effective, but it does not appear to affect outcome. Due to serious risks and side effects, a lack of efficacy in two randomized trials for head-injured patients,[141, 142] and questionable efficacy in a third,[143] it should truly be considered a last resort. It would be unusual to have to initiate barbiturate therapy in a patient after brain tumor surgery; most cases are posttraumatic.

Sodium pentobarbital (Table 35–10) is the agent used for inducing barbiturate coma. Its effectiveness in lowering ICP is based on its ability to lower the brain's metabolic requirements—it suppresses brain metabolism. A lower CBF will be required to meet the lower metabolic demands, allowing for a decrease in CBV, thereby reducing ICP. High-dose therapy can cause significant cardiovascular depression, especially in inadequately hydrated patients. Prior to initiation of therapy patients are well hydrated, but they still may require inotropic agents and/or vasopressors for hemodynamic instability.[32] A pulmonary artery catheter is usually placed. Immunosuppression leads to increased risk for pneumonia and sepsis; patients are appropriately monitored.[98]

Typically a loading dose of 10 mg/kg is infused over 30 minutes, followed by three additional hourly doses of 5 mg/kg, and a maintenance of 1 mg/kg per hour.[143] Because there is poor correlation between serum level, therapeutic benefit, and complications,[92] dose is titrated to electroencephalographic burst suppression rather than serum level. Patients are usually withdrawn from therapy after 48 hours of ICP control. Often the ICP will rise back up as therapy is withdrawn—a poor sign.

The indication for barbiturate coma in the postoperative setting is a salvageable patient, as judged by overall radiologic, neurologic, and clinical status, with a functioning ICP monitor who is otherwise optimized with respect to head position, sedation, paralysis, volume status, and temperature,

TABLE 35–10 Sodium Pentobarbital Use

Mechanism
  Brain metabolic requirements suppressed
  Lowers CBF, decreases CBV, lowers ICP
Indications[a]
  ICP monitored: high ICP refractory to mannitol, CSF
  drainage, and hyperventilation; salvageable patient
  ICP unmonitored: not indicated
Implementation
  Hydrate patient, pulmonary artery catheter placed
  10 mg/kg load over 30 min, 5 mg/kg doses q 1 × 3,
  1 mg/kg/h maintenance
  Titrate dose to EEG burst suppression
  Withdraw therapy after 48 h
Complications
  Cardiovascular depression
    Hemodynamic instability
  Immunosuppression
    Sepsis
    Pneumonia

[a] Assumes head position, sedation/paralysis, temperature, and volume status are optimized.
CBF, cerebral blood flow; CBV, cerebral blood volume; ICP, intracranial pressure; CSF, cerebrospinal fluid; EEG, electroencephalogram.

with sustained pathologic elevations of ICP refractory to mannitol, ventricular CSF drainage, and hypocarbic therapy, preferably titrated to jugular bulb venous saturation. In the absence of signs of herniation, if the CPP were successfully maintained above 50 mm Hg for a child or 70 mm Hg for an adolescent, despite elevated ICP, we would likely not institute a barbiturate coma unless the patient was undergoing progressive neurologic deterioration.

OTHER COMPLICATIONS

Seizures

At our institution, all children undergoing resection of supratentorial brain tumors receive perioperative seizure prophylaxis. Seizures rarely occur following posterior fossa surgery, possibly due to intraoperative manipulation of supratentorial structures.[144] The incidence of seizures in the immediate postoperative period ranges from 4% to 19%,[144] not stratified for after tumor surgery. Adverse effects on the brain include neuronal injury and increased ICP secondary to increased CBF.[144] This may theoretically increase the risk for hemorrhage. Causes include inadequate prophylaxis, with an 83% incidence in one review;[145] metabolic disturbances, including electrolytes (particularly low sodium), hypoglycemia, and hypoxia; and structural abnormalities, such as hemorrhage, edema, and pneumocephalus.[98] Therefore, an emergency CT scan is indicated in all children who seize postoperatively.

Phenytoin is usually used in patients older than 5 years. The loading dose is usually given preoperatively. Oral admin-

istration is preferred, allowing for slower absorption and fewer side effects, but intravenous dosing is often necessary. This should be limited to 50 mg/min due to risks for cardiac arrhythmias and hypotension.[98] Levels should be obtained immediately after surgery and supplemented as needed. Electrolytes are followed at least daily as well, as perturbations can cause seizures. Younger children often receive phenobarbitol because of fewer side effects as compared with phenytoin. Dose-related adverse effects of phenytoin include drowsiness, nystagmus, ataxia, slurred speech, visual changes, nausea, vomiting, choriothetosis, and megaloblastic anemia.[24] Idiosyncratic or hypersensitivity reactions to phenytoin are also known, the most common being skin rash.[98] Other reactions include fever, lymphadenopathy, eosinophilia, and, in severe cases, hepatitis or desquamation syndromes,[24] such as Stevens-Johnson syndrome. The development of a reaction warrants discontinuation and switching to another anticonvulsant agent. Second agents may be added if monotherapy is unsuccessful in controlling seizures. Therapy is generally continued for 3 months in our institution, or up to 12 months if postoperative seizures have occurred. However, there is considerable geographic variability in seizure prophylaxis. In some European centers, patients receive only 5 days of prophylaxis postoperatively or none at all.

**BOX 35–12
Postoperative Seizures**

- Supratentorial tumor surgery prophylaxis
- Seizures increase CBF, ICP, risk for hemorrhage; damage neurons
- Inadequate levels and metabolic disturbances predispose
- Phenytoin if older than 5 years
- Phenobarbitol if younger than 5 years
- Oral administration preferred
- Levels obtained immediately postoperatively
- Electrolytes followed daily

Hydrocephalus

CSF is produced in the ventricular system. It flows into the posterior fossa and circulates to the subarachnoid spaces of either the spinal canal or the cerebral convexities, where it is absorbed into the systemic venous circulation via the arachnoid granulations. Three types of hydrocephalus can occur following resection of a brain tumor. *Communicating hydrocephalus implies continuity between the ventricular and subarachnoid spaces, usually due to impaired absorption at the level of the arachnoid granulations. Noncommunicating or obstructive hydrocephalus implies a block to ventricular outflow, as in the case of hemorrhage or edema compressing the sylvian aqueduct between the third and fourth ventricles. These terms derive from the ability of a dye (such as indigo carmine) placed in the ventricular*

Infants and Children. Orlando: Grune & Stratton; 1985: 179–182.

10. Raimondi AJ, Hirschauer J. Head injury in the infant and toddler: coma scoring and outcome scale. *Child's Brain* 1984;11:12–35.

11. Duncan CD, Ment LR, Smith B, et al. A scale for the assessment of neonatal neurologic status. *Child's Brain* 1981;8:299–306.

12. Venes JL, Linder SL, Elterman RD. Neurological examination of infants and children. In: Youmans JR, ed. *Neurological Surgery.* 3rd ed. Philadelphia: WB Saunders; 1990: 37–43.

13. Waas TC, Lanier ML, Hofer RE, et al. Temperature changes of ≥1°C alter functional neurologic outcome and histopathology in a canine model of complete cerebral ischemia. *Anesthesiology* 1995;83:325–335.

14. Andrews BT, Hammer GB. The neurological examination and neurological monitoring in pediatric intensive care. In: Andrews BT, Hammer GB, eds. *Pediatric Neurosurgical Intensive Care.* American Association of Neurological Surgeons; 1997:1–11.

15. Petersdorf RG. Hypothermia and hyperthermia. In: Wilson JD, Braunwald E, et al, eds. *Harrison's Principles of Internal Medicine.* 12th ed. New York: McGraw-Hill; 1991:2198.

16. *Stedman's Medical Dictionary.* 24th ed. Baltimore: Williams & Wilkins; 1982.

17. Roselund RC. Postanesthetic care of the neurosurgical patient. *Anesthesiol Clin North Am* 1987;5(3):639–651.

18. Obana WG, Andrews BT. The neurologic examination and neurologic monitoring in the intensive care unit. In: Andrews BT, ed. *Neurosurgical Intensive Care.* New York: McGraw-Hill; 1993:31–42.

19. Brazis PW, Masdeu JC, Biller J. The localization of lesions of the hypothalamus and pituitary gland. In: *Localization in Clinical Neurology.* 2nd ed. Boston: Little, Brown and Company; 1990:306.

20. Noel P, Hubert JP, Ectors M, et al. Agenesis of the corpus callosum associated with relapsing hypothermia: a clinicopathological report. *Brain* 1973;96:359.

21. Plum F, Posner JB. *The Diagnosis of Stupor and Coma.* 3rd ed. Philadelphia: FA Davis Company; 1982:32–39.

22. Marino PL. *The ICU Book.* Philadelphia: Lea & Febiger; 1991.

23. Jarvis WR, Shay DK. Infections associated with hospitalization. In: Long SS, Pickering LK, Prober CG, eds. *Pediatric Infectious Diseases.* New York: Churchill Livingstone; 1997:656–684.

24. Powers NG, Carson SH. Idiosyncratic reactions to phenytoin. *Clin Pediatr* 1985;26(3):120–124.

25. Meyer JS, Handa J. Cerebral blood flow and metabolism during experimental hyperthermia (fever). *Minnesota Med* 1967;50:37–44.

26. Busija DW, Leffler CW, Pourcyrous M. Hyperthermia increases cerebral metabolic rate and blood flow in neonatal pigs. *Am J Physiol* 1988;255:H343–H346.

27. Hammer G, Lindsay JN. The neurosurgical pediatric patient. In: Andrews BT, ed. *Neurosurgical Intensive Care.* New York: McGraw-Hill; 1993:391–413.

28. Shalmon E, Caron MJ, Becker DP. Intracranial pressure: pathology and pathophysiology. In: Tindall GT, Cooper PR, Barrow DL, eds. *The Practice of Neurosurgery.* Baltimore: Williams & Wilkins; 1996:45–70.

29. Cushing H. Concerning a definite regulatory mechanism of the vaso-motor centre which controls blood pressure during cerebral compression. *Johns Hopkins Hosp Bull* 1901;12:290–292.

30. Cushing H. Some experimental and clinical observations concerning states of increased intracranial pressure. *Am J Med Sci* 1902;124:375–400.

31. Hoff JT, Reis DJ. Localization of regions mediating the Cushing response in CNS of cat. *Arch Neurol* 1970;23: 228–240.

32. Luerssen TG, Wolfa CE. Pathophysiology and management of increased intracranial pressure in children. In: Andrews BT, Hammer GB, eds. *Pediatric Neurosurgical Intensive Care.* American Association of Neurological Surgeons; 1997:37–57.

33. Marsh ML, Shapiro HM, Smith RW, et al. Changes in neurologic status and intracranial pressure associated with sodium nitroprusside administration. *Anesthesiology* 1979;51:336–338.

34. Harris ME, Barrow DL. Neuroendocrine physiology and management. In: Andrews BT, ed. *Neurosurgical Intensive Care.* New York: McGraw-Hill; 1993:179–199.

35. Rosner RJ. Pathophysiology and management of increased intracranial pressure. In: Andrews BT, ed. *Neurosurgical Intensive Care.* New York: McGraw-Hill; 1993: 57–112.

36. Duus P. *Topical Diagnosis in Neurology.* 2nd revised edition. New York: Thieme Medical; 1989:130–159.

37. Carpenter MB. *Core Text of Neuroanatomy.* 4th ed. Baltimore: William & Wilkins; 1991:141, 213.

38. Phillipson EA. Disorders of hyperventilation. In: Wilson JD, Braunwald E, et al, eds. *Harrison's Principles of Internal Medicine.* 12th ed. New York: McGraw-Hill; 1991:1116–1121.

39. Brazis PW, Masdeu JC, Biller J. The localization of lesions causing coma. In: *Localization in Clinical Neurology.* 2nd ed. Boston: Little, Brown and Company; 1990:461–463.

40. Plum F. Mechanisms of "central" hyperventilation. *Ann Neurol* 1982;11:636–637.

41. Muizelaar JP, van de Poel HG, Li ZC, et al. Pial arteriolar vessel diameter and CO_2 reactivity during prolonged hyperventilation in the rabbit. *J Neurosurg* 1988;69:923–927.

42. Kennedy SK. Airway management and respiratory support. In: Ropper AH, ed. *Neurological and Neurosurgical Intensive Care.* 3rd ed. New York: Raven Press; 1993:69–95.

43. Gallagher TJ. Pulmonary care and complications. In: Youmans JR, ed. *Neurological Surgery.* 3rd ed. Philadelphia: WB Saunders; 1990:765–789.

44. Monro A. *Observations on the Structure and Function of the Nervous System.* Creech and Johnson, 1783.

45. Kellie G. An account of the appearances observed in the dissection of two of three individuals presumed to have perished in the storm of the 3rd, and whose bodies were discovered in the vicinity of Leith on the morning of the 4th November 1821, with some reflections on the pathology of the brain. *Trans Med Chir Sci Edinb.* 1824;1:84–169.

46. Ryder HW, Espey FF, Kimball FD, et al. The mechanism of the change in cerebrospinal fluid pressure following an induced change in the volume of the fluid space. *J Lab Clin Med* 1953;41:428–435.

47. Shapiro K, Morris WJ, Teo C. Intracranial hypertension: mechanisms and management. In: Cheek WR, ed. *Pedi-*

atric Neurosurgery. 3rd ed. Philadelphia: WB Saunders; 1994:307–319.

48. Ingvar DH, Lassen NA. Regulation of cerebral blood flow. In: Himwich HE, ed. *Brain Metabolism and Cerebral Disorders*. New York: Spectrum Publications; 1976:181–206.

49. Strong A, Pollay M. Cerebral blood flow. In: Tindall GT, Cooper PR, Barrow DL, eds. *The Practice of Neurosurgery*. Baltimore: Williams & Wilkins; 1996:13–22.

50. Lindsay KW, Bone I, Collander R. *Neurology and Neurosurgery Illustrated*. 2nd ed. Edinburgh: Churchill Livingstone; 1991:75.

51. Bilsky M, Posner JB. Intensive and postoperative care of intracranial tumors. In: Ropper AH, ed. *Neurological and Neurosurgical Intensive Care*. 3rd ed. New York: Raven Press; 1993:309–329.

52. Lundberg N. Continuous recording and control of ventricular fluid pressure in neurosurgical practice. *Acta Psychiatr Neurol Scand* 1960;36(Suppl 149):1–193.

53. Fisher CM. Brain herniation: a revision of classical concepts. *Can J Neurol Sci* 1995;22:83–91.

54. Rosner MJ, Becker DP. Origin and evolution of plateau waves. experimental observations and a theoretical model. *J Neurosurg* 1984;60:312–324.

55. Kishore PRS, Lipper MH, Becker DP, et al. Significance of CT in head injury: correlation with intracranial pressure. *Am J Roentgenol* 1981;137:829–833.

56. Teasdale E, Cardoso E, Galbraith S, et al. CT scan in severe diffuse head injury: physiological and clinical correlations. *J Neurol Neurosurg Psychiatry* 1984;47:600–603.

57. Eisenberg HM, Gary HE, Aldrich EF, et al. Initial CT findings in 753 patients with severe closed head injury: a report from the NIH Traumatic Coma Data Bank. *J Neurosurg* 1990;73:688–698.

58. Tasker RC, Matthew DJ, Kendall B. Computed tomography in the assessment of raised intracranial pressure in non-traumatic coma. *Neuropediatrics* 1990;21:91–94.

59. Ropper AH. Treatment of intracranial hypertension. In: Ropper AH, ed. *Neurological and Neurosurgical Intensive Care*. 3rd ed. New York: Raven Press; 1993:29–52.

60. Salmon JH, Hajjar W, Bada HS. The fontogram: a noninvasive intracranial pressure monitor. *Pediatrics* 1977;60(5)721–725.

61. Pareicz E. Introduction. *Monogr Paediatr* 1982;15:1–7.

62. Vidyasagar D, Raju TNK. A simple noninvasive technique of measuring intracranial pressure in the newborn. *Pediatrics* 1977;59:957–961.

63. Welch K. The intracranial pressure in infants. *J Neurosurg* 1980;52:693–699.

64. Menke JA, Miles R, McIlhany M, et al. The fontanelle tonometer: a noninvasive method for measurement of intracranial pressure. *J Pediatr* 1982;100:960–963.

65. Raju TNK, Doshi UV, Vidyasagar D. Cerebral perfusion pressure studies in healthy preterm and term newborn infants. *J Pediatr* 1982;100(1):139–142.

66. Hill A. Intracranial pressure measurements in the newborn. *Clin Perinatol* 1985;12:161–178.

67. Rochefort MJ, Rolfe P, Wilkinson AR. New fontanometer for continuous estimation of intracranial pressure in the newborn. *Arch Dis Child* 1987;62:152–155.

68. Wayenberg JL, Raftopoulos C, Vermeylen D, et al. Noninvasive measurement of intracranial pressure in the newborn and the infant: the Rotterdam teletransducer. *Arch Dis Child* 1993;69:493–497.

69. Kaiser AM, Whitelaw AGL. Normal cerebrospinal fluid pressure in the newborn. *Neuropediatrics* 1986;17:100–102.

70. Mehta A, Wright BM, Shore C. Clinical fontanometry in the newborn. *Lancet* 1988:1(8588):754–756.

71. Horbar JD, Yeager S, Philip AGS, et al. Effect of application force on noninvasive and direct measurements of intracranial pressure. *Pediatrics* 1980;65:455–461.

72. Minns RA. Intracranial pressure monitoring. *Arch Dis Child* 1984;59:486–488.

73. Avellino AM, Berger MS. Intensive care management of children with brain tumors. In: Andrews BT, Hammer GB, eds. *Pediatric Neurosurgical Intensive Care*. American Association of Neurological Surgeons; 1997:235–257.

74. Duhaime AC, O'Rourke M. Intensive care management of children with head injuries. In: Andrews BT, Hammer GB, eds. *Pediatric Neurosurgical Intensive Care*. American Association of Neurological Surgeons; 1997:125–138.

75. Colditz PB, Williams GL, Berry AB, et al: Fontanelle pressure and cerebral perfusion pressure: continuous measurement in neonates. *Crit Care Med* 1988. 16(9)876–879.

76. Yordy M, Hanigan WC. Cerebral perfusion pressure in the high-risk premature infant. *Pediatr Neurosci* 1985–86; 12:226–231.

77. Goitein KJ, Fainmesser P, Sohmer H. Cerebral perfusion pressure and auditory brain-stem responses in childhood CNS diseases. *Am J Dis Child* 1983;137:777–781.

78. Sarnaik AP, Preston G, Lieh-Lai M, et al. Intracranial pressure and cerebral perfusion pressure in near-drowning. *Crit Care Med* 1985;13(4)224–227.

79. Hume A, Cooper R. The effects of head position and jugular vein compression (JVC) on intracranial pressure (ICP): a clinical study. In: Becks JWF, Bosch DA, Brock M, eds. *Intracranial Pressure*. Vol. 3. Berlin: Springer-Verlag; 1976: 259–263.

80. Shapiro HM. Intracranial hypertension: therapeutic and anesthetic considerations. *Anesthesiology* 1975;43:445–471.

81. Lipe HP, Mitchell PH. Positioning the patient with intracranial hypertension: how turning and head rotation affect the internal jugular vein. *Heart Lung* 1980;9:1031–1037.

82. Durward QJ, Amacher AL, Del Maestro FR. Cerebral and cardiovascular responses to changes in head elevation in patients with intracranial hypertension. *J Neurosurg* 1983; 59:938–944.

83. Davenport A, Will EJ, Davison AM. Effect of posture on intracranial pressure and cerebral perfusion pressure in patients with fulminant hepatic and renal failure after acetominophen self-poisoning. *Crit Care Med* 1990;18: 286–289.

84. Rosner MJ, Coley IB. Cerebral perfusion pressure, intracranial pressure, and head elevation. *J Neurosurg* 1986;65:636–641.

85. Rosner MJ, Daughton S. Cerebral perfusion management in head injury. *J Trauma* 1990;30:933–941.

86. Feldman Z, Kanter MJ, Robertson CS, et al. Effect of head elevation on intracranial pressure, cerebral perfusion pressure, and cerebral blood flow in head-injured patients. *J Neurosurg* 1992;76:207–211.

87. Rosner MJ, Rosner SD, Johnson AH. Cerebral perfusion pressure: management protocol and clinical results. *J Neurosurg* 1995;83:949–962.

88. Ropper AH, O'Rourke D, Kennedy SK. Head position, intracranial pressure, and compliance. *Neurology* 1982;32:1288–1291.

89. Emery JR, Peabody JL. Head position affects intracranial pressure in newborn infants. *J Pediatr* 1983;103:950–953.

90. French LA, Galicich JH. The use of steroid for control of cerebral edema. *Clin Neurosurg* 1964;10:212–223.

91. Renaudin J, Fewer D, Wilson CB, et al. Dose dependency of decadron in patients with partially excised brain tumors. *J Neurosurg* 1973; 39:302–305.

92. Bullock R, Chestnut RM, Clifton G, et al. Recommendations for intracranial pressure monitoring technology. In: *Guidelines for the Management of Severe Head Injury*. Brain Trauma Foundation, 1995.

93. Pappius HM, McCann WP. Effects of steroids on cerebral edema in cats. *Arch Neurol* 1969;20:207–216.

94. Weiss MH, Nulsen FE. The effect of glucocorticoids on CSF flow in dogs. *J Neurosurg* 1970;32:452–458.

95. Maxwell RE, Long DM, French LA. The effects of glucosteroids on experimental cold-induced brain edema: gross morphological alterations and vascular permeability changes. *J Neurosurg* 1971;34:477–487.

96. Yamada K, Ushio Y, Hayakawa T, et al. Effects of methylprednisolone on peritumoral brain edema. *J Neurosurg* 1983;59:612–619.

97. Morita M, Andrews BT, Gutin PH. The intensive care management of patients with brain tumors. In: Andrews BT, ed. *Neurosurgical Intensive Care*. New York: McGraw-Hill; 1993:375–389.

98. Kelly DF. Neurosurgical postoperative care. *Neurosurg Clin North Am* 1994;(5)4:789–810.

99. Brunton LL. Agents for control of gastric acidity and treatment of peptic ulcers. In: Gilman AG, Rall TW, Nies A, et al, eds. *Goodman and Gilman's The Pharmaceutical Basis of Therapeutics*. 8th ed. New York: Pergamon Press; 1990:901.

100. American Medical Association Department of Drugs, Division of Drugs and Technology. Agents used in disorders of the upper gastrointestinal tract. In: Lampe KF, McVeigh S, Rodgers BJ, eds. *Drug Evaluations*. 6th ed. Chicago: American Medical Association; 1986:944.

101. Shapiro WR, Heisiger EM, Cooney GA, et al. Temporal effects of dexamethasone on blood-to-brain and blood-to-tumor transport of 14C-alpha-aminoiso-butyric acid in rat C6 glioma. *J Neuro-oncol* 1990;8:197–204.

102. Mellergard P. Changes in human intracerebral temperature in response to different methods of brain cooling. *Neurosurgery* 1992;31:671–677.

103. Shenkin HA, Bezier HS, Bouzarth WF. Restricted fluid intake: rational management in the neurosurgical patient. *J Neurosurg* 1976;45:432–436.

104. Robertson CS, Goodman JC, Narayan RK, et al. The effect of glucose administration on carbohydrate metabolism after head injury. *J Neurosurg* 1991;74:43–50.

105. Mirski MA, Muffelman B, Ulatowski JA. Sedation for the critically ill neurologic patient. *Crit Care Med* 1995;23(12):2038–2053.

106. Bodenham A. reversal of prolonged sedation using flumazenil in critically ill patients. *Anaesthesia* 1989;44:603–605.

107. Harris CE, Grounds RM, Murray AM, et al. Propofol for long-term sedation in the intensive care unit. *Anaesthesia* 1990;45:366–372.

108. Farling PA, Johnston JR, Coppel DL. Propofol sedation for sedation of patients with head injuries in intensive care. *Anaesthesia* 1989;44:222–226.

109. Miller RD. Skeletal muscle relaxants. In: Katzung BG, ed. *Basic and Clinical Pharmacology*, 4th ed. Norwalk, CT: Appleton and Lange; 1989:323–330.

110. Rosner MJ. Techniques for intracranial pressure monitoring. In: Tindall GT, Cooper PR, Barrow DL, eds. *The Practice of Neurosurgery*. Baltimore: Williams & Wilkins; 1996:95–119.

111. Takagi H, Saitoh T, Kitihara T, et al. The mechanism of ICP reducing effect of mannitol. In: Ishii S, Nagai H, Brock M, eds. *Intracranial Pressure*. Vol. 5. New York: Springer-Verlag; 1983:729–733.

112. Kaufmann AM, Cardoso ER. Aggravation of vasogenic cerebral edema by multiple-dose mannitol. *J Neurosurg* 1992;77:584–589.

113. Reed DJ, Woodbury DM. Effect of hypertonic urea on cerebrospinal fluid pressure and brain volume. *J Physiol (Lond)* 1962;164:252–264.

114. Muizelaar JP, Wei EP, Kontos HA, et al. Mannitol causes compensatory cerebral vasoconstriction and vasodilation in response to blood viscosity changes. *J Neurosurg* 1983:59:822–828.

115. Albright AL, Latchaw RE, Robinson AG. Intracranial and systemic effects of osmotic and oncotic therapy in experimental cerebral edema. *J Neurosurg* 1984;60:481–489.

116. Albright AL, Phillips JW. Oncotic therapy of experimental cerebral oedema. *Acta Neurochir (Wien)* 1982;60:257–264.

117. Renkin EM. Multiple pathways of capillary permeability. *Circ Res* 1977;41(6):735–743.

118. Fenstermacher JD. Volume regulation of the central nervous system. In: Staub ND, Taylor EA, eds. *Edema*. New York: Raven Press; 1984:383–404.

119. Rosner MJ, Coley I. Cerebral perfusion pressure: a hemodynamic mechanism of mannitol and the postmannitol hemogram. *Neurosurgery* 1987;21(2):147–156.

120. Burke AM, Quest DO, Chien S, et al. The effects of mannitol on blood viscosity. *J Neurosurg* 1981;55:550–553.

121. Jones MD Jr, Traystman RJ, Simmons MA, et al. Effects of changes in arterial O_2 content on cerebral blood flow in the lamb. *Am J Physiol* 1981;240:H209–H215.

122. Ravussin P, Archer DP, Tyler JL, et al. Effects of rapid mannitol infusion on cerebral blood volumes: a positron emission tomographic study in dogs and man. *J Neurosurg* 1986;64:104–113.

123. Marshall LF, Smith RW, Rauscher LA. Mannitol dose requirements in brain-injured patients. *J Neurosurg* 1978;48:169–172.

124. Dorman HR, Sondheimer JH, Cadnapaphornchai P. Mannitol-induced acute renal failure. *Medicine* 1990;69:153–159.

125. Cottrell JE, Robustelli A, Post K, et al. Furosemide- and mannitol-induced changes in intracranial pressure and serum osmolality and electrolytes. *Anesthesiology* 1977;47:28–30.

126. Roberts PA, Pollay M, Engles C, et al. Effect on intracranial pressure of furosemide combined with varying

doses and administration rates of mannitol. *J Neurosurg* 1987;66:440–446.

127. Lundberg N, Kjallquist A, Bien C. Reduction of increased intracranial pressure by hyperventilation. *Acta Psychiatr Neurol Scand* 1959;34(Suppl 139):4–64.

128. Kontos HA, Raper AJ, Patterson JL. Analysis of vasoactivity of local pH, PCO_2 and bicarbonate on pial vessels. *Stroke* 1977;8:358–360.

129. Raichle ME, Posner JB, Plum F. Cerebral blood flow during and after hyperventilation. *Arch Neurol* 1970;23:394–404.

130. Crockard HA, Coppel DL, Morrow WF. Evaluation of hyperventilation in treatment of head injuries. *Br Med J* 1973;4:634–640.

131. Muizelaar JP, Marmarou A, Ward JD. Adverse effects of prolonged hyperventilation in patients with severe head injury: a randomized clinical trial. *J Neurosurg* 1991;75:731–739.

132. Obrist WD, Langfitt TW, Jaggi JL, et al. Cerebral blood flow and metabolism in comatose patients with acute head injury: relationship to intracranial hypertension. *J Neurosurg* 1984;61:241–253.

133. Muizelaar JP, Marmarou A, DeSalles AAF, et al. Cerebral blood flow and metabolism in severely head-injured children. Part 1. Relationship with GCS score, outcome, ICP, and PVI. *J Neurosurg* 1989;71:63–71.

134. Skippen P, Seear M, Poskitt K, et al. Effect of hyperventilation on regional cerebral blood flow in head-injured children. *Crit Care Med* 1997;25(8):1402–1409.

135. Bruce DA, Raphaely RC, Goldberg AI, et al. Pathophysiology, treatment, and outcome following severe head injury in children. *Child's Brain* 1979;5:174–191.

136. Chestnut RM. Hyperventilation in traumatic brain injury: friend or foe? *Crit Care Med* 1997;25(8)1275–1278.

137. Bouma GJ, Muizelaar JP, Stringer WA, et al. Ultra-early evaluation of regional cerebral blood flow in severely head-injured patients using xenon-enhanced computerized tomography. *J Neurosurg* 1992;77:360–368.

138. Jenkins LW, Lyeth BG, Lewelt W, et al. Combined pre-trauma scopolamine and phencyclidine attenuate post-traumatic increased sensitivity to delayed secondary ischemia. *J Neurotrauma* 1988;5:275–287.

139. Jenkins LW, Moszynski K, Lyeth BG, et al. Increased vulnerability of the mildly traumatized rat brain to cerebral ischemia. the use of controlled secondary ischemia as a research tool to identify common or different mechanisms contributing to mechanical and ischemic brain injury. *Brain Res* 1989;477:211–224.

140. Matta BF, Lam AM, Mayberg TS. The influence of arterial oxygenation on cerebral venous oxygen saturation during hyperventilation. *Can J Anaesth* 1994;41(11):1041–1046.

141. Schwartz M, Tator C, Towed D, et al. The University of Toronto head injury treatment study: a prospective randomized comparison of pentobarbitol and mannitol. *Can J Neurol Sci* 1984;11:434–440.

142. Ward JD, Becker DP, Miller JD, et al. Failure of prophylactic barbiturate coma in the treatment of severe head injury. *J Neurosurg* 1985;62:383–388.

143. Eisenberg HM, Frankowski RF, Contant CF, et al. High-dose barbiturate control of elevated intracranial pressure in patients with severe head injury. *J Neurosurg* 1988;69:15–23.

144. Krauss WE, Post KD. General complications in neurologic surgery. In: Post KD, Friedman ED, McCormick P, eds. *Postoperative Complications in Intracranial Neurosurgery*. New York: Thieme Medical; 1993:2–26.

145. Kvam DA, Loftus CM, Copeland B, et al. Seizures during the immediate postoperative period. *Neurosurgery* 1983;12:14–17.

146. Schmid UD, Seiler RW. Management of obstructive hydrocephalus secondary to posterior fossa tumors by steroids and subcutaneous ventricular catheter reservoir. *J Neurosurg* 1986;65:649–653.

147. Rekate H. Treatment of hydrocephalus. In: Cheek WR, ed. *Pediatric Neurosurgery*. 3rd ed. Philadelphia: WB Saunders; 1994:202–220.

148. Raimondi AJ, Tomita T. Hydrocephalus and infratentorial tumors: incidence, clinical picture, and treatment. *J Neurosurg* 1981;55:174–182.

149. Albright AL, Wisoff JH, Zeltzer PM, et al. Current neurosurgical treatment of medulloblastomas in children: a report from the Children's Cancer Study Group. *Pediatr Neurosci* 1989;15:276–282.

150. Dias MS, Albright AL. Management of hydrocephalus complicating childhood posterior fossa tumors. *Pediatr Neurosci* 1989;15:283–290.

151. Papo I, Caruselli G, Luongo A. External ventricular drainage in the management of posterior fossa tumors in children and adolescents. *Neurosurgery* 1982;10:13–15.

152. Rappaport ZH, Shalit MN. Perioperative external ventricular drainage in obstructive hydrocephalus secondary to infratentorial tumours. *Acta Neurochir (Wien)* 1989;96:118–121.

153. Lee M, Wisoff JH, Abbot R, et al. Management of hydrocephalus in children with medulloblastoma: prognostic factors for shunting. *Pediatr Neurosurg* 1994;20:240–247.

154. Cochrane DD, Gustavsson B, Poskitt KP, et al. The surgical and natural aggressive resection for posterior fossa tumors in childhood. *Pediatr Neurosurg* 1994;20:19–29.

155. Partington MD, Tadanori T. Choroid plexus papilloma of the fourth ventricle. In: Cohen AR, ed. *Surgical Disorders of the Fourth Ventricle*. Cambridge: Blackwell Scientific; 1996:235–244.

156. Singh-Naz N, Sprague BM, Patel KM, et al. Risk factors for nosocomial infection in critically ill children: a prospective cohort study. *Crit Care Med* 1996;24:875–878.

157. Jarvis WR. Epidemiology of nosocomial infections in pediatric patients. *Pediatr Infect Dis J* 1987;6:344–351.

158. Blomstedt GC. Craniotomy infections. *Neurosurg Clin North Am* 1992;3(2):375–385.

159. Dickinson LD, Hoff JT. Infectious disease in neurosurgical intensive care. In: Andrews BT, ed. *Neurosurgical Intensive Care*. New York: McGraw-Hill; 1993:201–226.

160. Blomstedt GC. Infections in neurosurgery. a retrospective study of 1143 patients and 1517 operations. *Acta Neurochir* 1985;78:81–90.

161. Buckwold FJ, Hand R, Hansebout RR. Hospital-acquired bacterial meningitis in neurosurgical patients. *J Neurosurg* 1977;46:494–500.

162. Steinberg JP, Farley MM. Bacterial meningitis. In: Tindall GT, Cooper PR, Barrow DL, eds. *The Practice of Neurosurgery*. Baltimore: Williams & Wilkins; 1996:3335–3369.

163. Ross D, Rosegay H, Pons V. Differentiation of aseptic and bacterial meningitis in postoperative neurosurgical patients. *J Neurosurg* 1988;69:669–674.

164. Carmel PW, Fraser RAR, Stein BM. Aseptic meningitis following posterior fossa surgery in children. *J Neurosurg* 1974;41:44–48.

165. O'Brien MS, Krisht Ali. Cerebellar astrocytomas. In: Cheek WR, ed. *Pediatric Neurosurgery*. 3rd ed. Philadelphia: WB Saunders; 1994:356–361

166. Allen MB, Jr., Johnston KW. Preoperative evaluation. complications, their prevention and treatment. In: Youmans JR, ed. *Neurological Surgery*. 3rd ed. Philadelphia: WB Saunders; 1990:833–900.

167. Berger MS, Geyer JR. Ependymomas of the fourth ventricle. In: Cohen AR, ed. *Surgical Disorders of the Fourth Ventricle*. Cambridge: Blackwell Scientific; 1996:209–211.

168. Mollman HD, Haines SJ. Risk factors for postoperative neurosurgical infections. *J Neurosurg* 1086;64:902–906.

169. Spetzler RF, Zabramski JM. Cerebrospinal fluid fistulae: their management and repair. In: Youmans JR, ed. *Neurological Surgery*. 3rd ed. Philadelphia: WB Saunders; 1990:2269–2289.

170. Sen CN, Sekhar LN. Complications of cranial base surgery. In: Post KD, Friedman ED, McCormick P, eds. *Postoperative Complications in Intracranial Neurosurgery*. New York: Thieme Medical; 1993:111–131.

171. Markham TJ. The clinical features of pneumocephalus based on a survey of 284 cases with report of 11 additional cases. *Acta Neurochir* 1967;15:1–78.

172. Gower DJ, Pollay M. Adverse postoperative events. In: Tindall GT, Cooper PR, Barrow DL, eds. *The Practice of Neurosurgery*. Baltimore: Williams & Wilkins; 1996:1691–1698.

173. Greenberg MS. *Handbook of Neurosurgery*. 3rd ed. Lakeland FL: Greenberg Graphics; 1994:534–535.

174. Blevins LS, Wand GS. Diabetes insipidus. *Crit Care Med* 1992;20:69–79.

175. Sotos JF, Bello F. Diabetes insipidus. In: Bardin CW, ed. *Current Therapy in Endocrinology and Metabolism*. 4th ed. Philadelphia: B. C. Decker; 1991:1–8.

176. Reeves WB, Bichet DG, Andreoli TE. The posterior pituitary and water metabolism. In: Wilson JD, Foster DW, Kronenberg HM, et al, eds. *Williams Textbook of Endocrinology*. 9th ed. Philadelphia: WB Saunders; 1998:341–387.

177. Richardson DW, Robinson AG. Desmopressin. *Ann Intern Med* 1985;103:228–239.

178. Robertson GL, Harris A. Clinical use of vasopressin analogues. *Hosp Pract* 1989;24(10):114–139 passim.

179. Kappy MS, Sonderer E. Sublingual administration of desmopressin. Effectiveness in an infant with holoprosencephaly and central diabetes insipidus. *Am J Dis Child* 1987;141:84–85.

180. Williams TDM, Dunger DB, Lewis RJ, et al. Antidiuretic effect and pharmacokinetics of oral 1-desamino-8-D-arginine vasopressin. 1. Studies in adults and children. *J Clin Endocrinol Metab* 1986;63:129–132.

181. Fjellestad-Paulsen A, Laborde K, Kindermans C, et al. Water-balance during long-term follow-up of oral dDAVP treatment in diabetes insipidus. *Acta Paediatr* 1993;82:752–757.

182. Crutchfield JS, Sawaya R, Meyers CA, et al. Postoperative mutism in neurosurgery: report of two cases. *J Neurosurg* 1994;81:115–121.

183. Rekate HL, Grubb RL, Aram DM, et al. Muteness of cerebellar origin. *Arch Neurol* 1985;42:697–698.

184. Ferrante L, Mastronardi L, Acqui M, et al. Mutism after posterior fossa surgery in children: report of three cases. *J Neurosurg* 1990;72:959–963.

185. Dietze DD, Parker JP. Cerebellar mutism after posterior fossa surgery. *Pediatr Neurosurg* 1990–91;16:25–31.

186. Herb E, Thyen U. Mutism after cerebellar medulloblastoma surgery. *Neuropediatrics* 1992;23:144–146.

187. Asamoto M, Ito H, Suzuki N, et al. Transient mutism after posterior fossa surgery. *Child's Nerv Syst* 1994;10:275–278.

188. Aguiar PH, Plese JPP, Ciquini O, et al. Transient mutism following a posterior fossa approach to cerebellar tumors in children: a critical review of the literature. *Child's Nerv Syst* 1995;11:306–310.

189. Koh S, Turkel SB, Baram TZ. Cerebellar mutism in children: report of six cases and potential mechanisms. *Pediatr Neurol* 1997;16:218–219.

190. Liu GT, Phillips PC, Molloy PT, et al. Visual impairment associated with mutism after posterior fossa surgery in children. *Neurosurgery* 1998;42(2):253–257.

191. Gaskill SJ, Marlin AE. Transient eye closure after posterior fossa tumor surgery in children. *Pediatr Neurosurg* 1991–92;17:196–198.

192. Wisoff J, Epstein F. Pseudobulbar palsy after posterior fossa operation in children. *Neurosurgery* 1984;15:707–709.

193. Constantini S, Epstein F. Complications of fourth ventricular surgery. In: Cohen AR, ed. *Surgical Disorders of the Fourth Ventricle*. Cambridge: Blackwell Scientific; 1996:412–423.

194. Sutton LN, Phillips PC, Molloy PT. Surgical management of medulloblastoma. *J Neuro-oncol* 1996;29:9–21.

Chapter 36

Rehabilitation

Subhadra L. Nori and David Magill

Childhood malignancy accounts for approximately 1% of all cancers diagnosed in the United States each year. Approximately 7000 new cases of cancer in children younger than 15 years occur annually. Cancer is the second most common cause of death, exceeded only by injury. A dramatic decrease in cancer deaths has occurred as a result of the benefits of surgery, chemotherapy, and radiation therapy.[1]

It is estimated that 45,000 long-term survivors exist today; one in 1000 young adults is a cancer survivor.[2, 4] Central nervous system (CNS) cancer is the second most common cancer in children, seen mostly in 5- to 10-year-olds. Embryonal tumors and heritable tumors are more common. Because childhood tumors are not as amenable to screening as tumors in adults, and their incidence is low, a high index of suspicion should be exercised.[1]

Most childhood survivors will have deficits that require rehabilitation. Such deficits may be the result of cancer or its treatment.[5, 6] Physicians who are cognizant of these needs and deficits will be able to provide a better service to these patients by referring them to rehabilitation therapy.

Rehabilitation is defined as adaptation of the patient to the disabilities, in terms of emotional and functional changes, that result from the effects of the disease and/or its treatment.[3]

TYPES OF CANCER REHABILITATION

The general goal for cancer patients is to potentiate independent mobility and autonomy in activities of daily living. Assessment of individuals, or their disease and treatment will determine preventive, restorative, supportive, and palliative goals.[1]

1. *Preventive rehabilitation:* Achievement of maximal function in patients with a good prognosis for cure or remission (e.g., respiratory therapy preoperatively and crutch walking instruction to an amputee).
2. *Supportive rehabilitation:* When no residual major disability is expected. Supportive rehabilitation can be offered to offset a steady decline in function [e.g., provision of activities of daily living (ADL) devices, adaptive self-care equipment, range-of-motion (ROM) exercises, etc.].
3. *Palliative rehabilitation:* To maintain comfort and function during terminal stages of the disease.[7] Periodic assessment of patient's progress and response should be made. Appropriate goals should be selected at different stages of

the disease.[8] Especially with pediatric patients, family, parents, and close friends must be included in the instruction and treatment. Only by gaining the confidence of the patient, especially the young, can therapy be successful.

EFFECTS OF CANCER ON FUNCTION

General Immobility

Cancer in itself causes weakness, pain, and lethargy, thereby making the patient prone to bed rest. The functional recovery is affected by metabolic and physiologic changes associated with bed rest.[9] Bone loss leads to hypercalcemia.[10] Muscle atrophy follows rapidly after bed rest, leading to an inability to walk. Changes in muscle physiology and fiber type have been documented.[11, 12] Pressure ulcers follow as a result of depletion of soft tissue. Bed rest alone depletes the patient's strength by 3% per day. Total immobilization causes a 7% loss of strength per day in immobilized parts. Contractures may soon follow. Other medical complications, such as deep venous thrombosis and pulmonary embolus, are common.[13] Another important impairment is pressure palsy. Peroneal mononeuropathy and ulnar mononeuropathy are commonly seen in cachectic patients on prolonged bed rest.

Joint Contractures

A majority of patients with cancer suffer from pain. To avoid the pain these patients tend to position their joints in a fixed way, which leads to formation of joint contractures. Collagen fibers, ligaments, and tendons undergo a shortening contracture. Heel cords, hips, knees, elbows, and shoulders are the most common areas affected. Therapeutic exercises and joint ROM exercises should be prescribed for these patients. Other modalities, soch as heat and cold, may be used to release these contractures. Motor point blocks with phenol have been helpful in some chronically contracted patients. Splinting of the upper extremity by an occupational therapist will help maintain a hand or foot in its anatomical position. Other orthotic devices are also in use.

Bleeding Problems

Thrombocytopenia can be a side effect of both chemotherapy and radiotherapy. A platelet count below 10,000 mm^3 is hazardous because of potential intra-articular bleed below this level.[14, 15] Exercises should be performed only under careful vigilance in patients with thrombocytopenia. Some centers do not allow any activity for platelet counts below 10,000.[16]

SPECIFIC DEFICITS IN CHILDREN WITH CNS TUMORS

Many problems stemming from cancer or its treatment can be seen in children suffering from brain and spinal cord tumors. Treatment-related complications can arise from surgery, irradiation, or chemotherapy.

Effects of the Tumor

The motor and sensory deficits at the time of presentation depend on the location of the tumor.

Cerebellar Astrocytomas

Up to 95% of children first present with ataxia, described as clumsiness in an older child and unsteady gait in a younger one. Dysmetria is present in a majority, causing deficits with feeding, dressing, or other activities of daily living (ADLs) and may interfere with fine motor coordination.

Nystagmus is usually of the lateral gaze type to the side of the lesion.[17] Cranial neuropathy (most commonly of the sixth nerve) causes diplopia, which in turn causes problems with depth perception and image formation, thus indirectly affecting the gait. Seventh-nerve lesion is seen in 6%,[18] causing dysphagia. Medulloblastomas classically present in the region of the fourth ventricle, vermis, or cerebellar hemisphere. Children with medulloblastoma typically present with the midline syndrome of headache, lethargy, and vomiting. Later on, symptoms of truncal ataxia, nystagmus, and sixth-nerve paralysis due to hydrocephalus develop.[18–21]

Spinal Cord Tumors

Intradural extramedullary tumors, such as epidermoid and dermoid tumors if present in the lumbar area, can cause lower back pain or sciatic pain with radiation of symptoms and pain to the lower extremities. Motor sensory and sphincter changes occur later. Lesions involving the higher spinal segments present with hypertonia, hyperreflexia, and motor sensory and sphincter changes. Gait deficits, such as spastic gait, can be seen in intramedullary tumors.

Cerebral Lesions

Tumors can be supratentorial. For example, primitive neuroectodermal tumors (PNETs) account for 30 to 55% of pediatric brain tumors.[22] Approximately one-third of these involve the cerebral hemispheres.[19] Approximately 20% of supratentorial tumors are malignant neoplasms, such as anaplastic gliomas and glioblastomas, predominantly seen in the first 2 years of life. In addition to headache and vomiting, these children present with intermittent visual disturbances and blindness. Focal signs depend on the location of the tumor. If the motor cortex or basal ganglia is involved, monoparesis or hemiparesis is seen. Subtle changes, such as sensory loss, altered personality and deteriorating school performance, and seizures are also common.[19, 22]

Brain Stem Tumors

Brain stem tumors may cause visual depth perceptual deficits, dysphagia, and mono- or hemiparesis and dysarthria due to multiple cranial nerve involvement of nerves V, VI, VII, IX, and X. Due to associated vomiting and poor weight gain, as well as apathy, debility, disuse atrophy, and other negative effects of immobility ensue, thus forming a vicious circle.

Cognitive Deficits

Supratentorial brain tumors cause three times more cognitive deficits than infratentorial tumors. Mental retardation has been known to occur in survivors of brain tumors. Johnson and McCabe et al,[23] studied 32 patients with medulloblastoma of whom 13 underwent detailed neuropsychological and neurologic evaluations. The investigators concluded that intelligence quotient (IQ) was less than 90 for all patients tested, and patients diagnosed before age 3 years had lower IQ scores than those diagnosed later. Shunting seemed to have a beneficial influence on mean IQ and achievement in math, spelling, and reading.

SEQUELAE OF TREATMENT
Sequelae of Radiation Therapy

Surgical resection is a mainstay for most brain tumors. Radiation therapy often follows in the treatment of primative neuroectodermal tumors (PNETs) of the cerebellum (medulloblastomas), high-grade astrocytomas, ependymomas, and brain stem gliomas.[24] The dose of radiation ranged from 2520 to 4500 cGy. Radiation therapy has been implicated as a cause of long-term neuropsychological and neuroendocrinologic deficits. Cranial irradiation at doses of 1800 to 2400 cGy has been used for the treatment, though the precise risk of irradiation is unknown because of multifactorial occurrence.[25–27] Diffuse white matter abnormalities are found in 80% of these children.[28]

In 1985, Copeland[29] reviewed 74 long-term survivors of brain tumor who were disease-free for more than 5 years. The study found that patients who received cranial irradiation had significantly lower IQ scores than those who did not. Associated with this was a decrease in visual, motor, and fine motor skills, spatial memory, and arithmetic skills. Nonlanguage skills were also affected.

A study by Ellenberg et al[30] in 73 children with brain tumors showed that irradiation of the whole brain was associated with cognitive decline, particularly in children younger than 7 years.

In a study of children younger than 3 years, Mulhern et al[31] concluded that irradiation is not the sole cause of decline in cognitive functioning, but rather that the problem is secondary to the tumor itself and the particular combination of therapies implemented. In this study, chemotherapy was given several months prior to radiation therapy. The majority of patients had declining cognitive function at the beginning of chemotherapy. After radiation therapy, none had improvement in their adaptive status. None of these children were found to function at the normal range.

Myelopathy

A transient myelopathy is known to occur in patients receiving radiotherapy to the spinal cord, typically developing after a latent period of 1 to 30 months with a peak at 4 to 6 months after radiation therapy. These symptoms subside quickly over the next 2 to 9 months.[32] Typically, the patient complains of an electric shock–like feeling radiating from the cervical spine to the extremities. These paresthesias are symmetrical (Lhermitte's sign) and are caused by tension on demyelinated and hypersensitive fibers of the spinal cord.[32]

Delayed radiation myelopathy is a permanent and irreversible condition that is reported in 1 to 12% of patients. The onset is between 9 and 18 months after completion of treatment. The dose and schedule of radiotherapy seems not to have any bearing on this condition.[33] With higher doses the latent period can be shortened in children.[34] Signs and symptoms may be acute or insidious, and may include paresthesias in the lower extremities, sphincter dysfunction, partial Brown-Séquard syndrome, paraplegia and quadriplegia.[35] The posterior columns and superficial lateral tracts are involved. Vascular changes, including arteriolar necrosis and vascular occlusion, occur. A partial Brown-Séquard type of syndrome has also been reported.[32]

Pain is usually central and occurs in the midback region. Motor weakness as well as bowel and bladder involvement can be also seen. Severe injury to the anterior horn cells and plexus can cause lower motor neuron signs and dysfunction.

Endocrine Deficiencies

Endocrine deficiencies occur after radiation therapy for tumors of the CNS, including the hypothalamic-pituitary axis. Growth hormone disorders are common if the ventromedial nucleus of the hypothalamus, the site of growth hormone–releasing factor, is included in the treatment port. Following radiation treatment of posterior fossa neoplasm, panhypopituitarism is also seen.[36] Thirteen to forty percent of children with brain tumor suffer from short stature (height less than the third percentile for age and sex).[37, 38]

Hypothyroidism occurs less often than growth hormone deficiency and may be primary, secondary, or tertiary. Thyroid function testing every 6 months is recommended for the first 3 years in children receiving cranial radiation therapy.[37]

Radiation may cause spinal injury if administered during periods of rapid growth or during puberty; spinal deformities may be severe.[39] Vertebral body deformities, kyphosis, and scoliosis are seen.

Sequelae Related to Chemotherapy

A variety of different drugs and drug combinations have bean shown to be effective in the treatment of brain tumors. Active drugs include vincristine, cisplatin, cyclophosphamide, and methotrexate. Methotrexate may cause significant leukoencephalopathy, especially when used after radiation therapy. Chemotherapy-induced neuropathies are generally distal and symmetrical. Autonomic neuropathies are caused by vincristine and cisplatin[40, 41] and may be severe enough to mimic spinal cord involvement.[42] Cytarabine (Ara-C) is also known to cause brachial plexopathy.[43]

Because of distal axonal degeneration, vincristine neuropathy tends to be prolonged.[44] Sensory complaints of paresthesias, numbness, neuropathic pain, and foot drop have been associated with vincristine toxicity. Peripheral neuropathies and plexopathies are also a result of vincristine or cisplatin toxicity.[44, 45] Encephalopathies, cerebellar syndromes, myopathies, and strokelike syndromes may also occur after the administration of various chemotherapeutic drugs.[46]

Post-Surgical Sequelae

Irritability, confusion, lethargy, and sometimes seizures are known to occur in the immediate postoperative phase. *Postoperative neurologic morbidity may be correlated with the segment of spinal cord that is involved with the neoplasm.* Dissection within the cervical spinal cord may be associated with significant morbidity. Anterior-born cell dysfunction evidenced by atrophy of the muscle groups of upper extremity is not uncommon.

Tumors that are located in the lower spinal segments from T9 to T12 have the greatest incidence of postoperative neurologic morbidity. This is due to compression of gray matter. If the tumor extends into conus medullas, significant postoperative sphincteric dysfunction follows. In children who have undergone extensive laminectomy, postoperative muscle retraction, paraspinal muscle denervation, and spinal deformities may develop.

SPECIFIC REHABILITATION ISSUES OF CHILDREN WITH BRAIN TUMORS

Physiatric evaluation of a child with brain tumors can be a lengthy and time-consuming process. The child may be irritable and uncooperative. Personality changes and headache are common in persons with brain tumors. The evaluation should include parents and siblings; friends and school teachers may be included if necessary.

Frontal Lobe Tumors

Patients with tumor in the frontal lobes may present with personality changes as well as mild slowing of fine motor coordination of the contralateral hand. Drawing a person, writing one's name, buttoning and unbuttoning one's shirt, and similar activities of daily living may be used to uncover and assess fine motor deficits. Primitive grasp and sucking reflexes may even be seen in this syndrome. Dysphagia to liquids can be assessed during drinking of water. Left frontal lobe tumors can also cause nonfluent dysphasia and apraxia of lip, tongue, or hand movements.

Temporal Lobe

Impairment in recent memory, homonymous quadrant anopsia, perceptuals, problem, and spatial disorientation can be seen. Fluid Wernicke-type aphasia is commonly seen when the dominant temporal lobe is involved.

Parietal Lobe

Sensory and perceptual functions are affected to a greater extent than motor functions. Hemianesthesia and hemisensory abnormalities occur with deep-seated tumors. Agnosia and apraxia for dressing is also common.

Brain Stem

Multiple cranial nerve abnormalities associated with ataxia and hemiparesis is the presentation picture.

Spinal Cord Tumor

As discussed in previous paragraphs, signs and symptoms depend on the location of the tumor.

REHABILITATION INTERVENTIONS
Hemiparesis-Hemiplegia

Activities that enhance or maintain the musculoskeletal status of the affected side, including passive ROM, positive and sensory education, should be implemented by the therapist.

Facilitation techniques are used to promote motor recovery. Inhibition techniques discourage abnormal posturing and other unwanted reflex patterns commonly seen in upper motor neuron deficits. Ambulation training can be achieved by the use of pediatric walkers, crutches, canes, and wheelchairs.

Cognitive-Perceptual Interventions

Remediation is provided, via handling that incorporates stimulation of the cortical tracts, involving the use of different tasks to improve visual perception.

Early programmed activities designed to minimize inactivity and disuse, and to maintain proprioceptive and sensory stimuli, should be started.

Adaptive Equipment

The therapist should teach adaptive techniques and prescribe adaptive devices to support patient function. *These adaptive aids include dressers, reachers, dressing aids, and bathroom equipment.* Positioning of upper extremities by means of slings, splints, and orthotic devices is important because these aids prevent contractures. Upper-extremity orthotics may aid in substituting for lost function.

Therapeutic Exercises

These patients have increased metabolic demands and impaired protein-sparing mechanism. Inactivity and the effect of chemotherapy and other treatment modalities further decreases lean body mass and muscle endurance. Therefore, any method that spares protein breakdown and enhances incorporation of protein into lean muscle is beneficial.[47]

Butterfield[48] found that 40 to 50% of submaximal exercise maintains nitrogen equilibrium. *High-intensity endurance programs with high VO_2 max increase protein needs and therefore are unsuitable for cancer patients.*[49]

Carefully selected aerobic, ROM, stretching, isokinetic, isometric, and isotonic exercises can be used in patients with cancer. These exercises are generally safe. Some guidelines for precautions are given in Table 36–1.

Spinal Cord Impairment

Spinal cord damage due to tumor or effect of treatment may result in paraplegia, quadriplegia, or weakness of the involved spinal segments. The therapist should teach assisted mobility to these patients. Use of the wheelchair, manual or

TABLE 36–1 Exercise Guidelines and Precautions for Cancer Patients *(continues on next page)*

Medical problems	Laboratory values	Recommendations
Thrombocytopenia Normal values Platelets 150,000–450,000/mL	30,000–50,000/mL	Active exercise/ROM Light weights (1–2 lb) (no heavy resistance/isokinetics) Ambulation Self-care activity
	20,000–30,000/mL	Gentle exercise (passive or active) Ambulation and self-care with assistance as needed for endurance/balance safety
	Less than 20,000/mL	Minimal or cautious exercise/activity Essential ADLs only
Anemia Normal values: (6m–6y) Hematocrit 37–47% Hemoglobin 12–16 g/dL	Hematocrit < 25% Hemoglobin < 8 g/dL Hematocrit 25–35% Hemoglobin 8–10 g/dL Hematocrit > 35% Hemoglobin > 10 g/dL	Light ROM exercise, isometrics Avoid aerobic or progressive programs Essential ADLs: assistance as needed for safety Light aerobics, light weights (1-2 lb) Ambulation and self-care as tolerated Resistive exercise, ambulation, self-care as tolerated

TABLE 36–1 Exercise Guidelines and Precautions for Cancer Patients (continued)

Medical problems	Laboratory values	Recommendations
Bony Metastasis		
Plain X-ray findings	> 50% cortex involved	No exercises
High risk indicated by following:	25–50% cortex involved	Touch down: not weight bearing, use crutches, walker
Cortical lesions > 2.5–3 cm		Active ROM exercise (no twisting)
> 50% cortical involvement		No stretching
Painful lesions, unresponsive to radiation	0–25% cortex involved	Partial weight bearing
		Light aerobic exercise
		Avoid lifting/straining activity
		Full weight bearing
Pulmonary Dysfunction		
Pulmonary function tests	< 50% of predicted FEV_1 or diffusion capacity	No aerobic exercise
Chest radiograph	50–75% of predicted FEV_1 or diffusion capacity	Light aerobic exercise
	75% + of predicted FEV_1 or diffusion capacity	Most programs fine
	Large plural effusions or pericardial effusions or multiple metastases to lungs	ROM
		Few submaximal isometrics
		Consult cardiologist and oncologist
Cardiac Dysfunction		
Ejection fraction	Low	Low aerobics
Electrocardiogram	Recent premature ventricular contractions	No aerobics
	Fast atrial arrhythmia	Consult cardiologist
	Ventricular arrhythmia	
	Ischemic pattern	
Electrolyte Abnormalities		
Na^+ (133–148 mEq/L)	< 130	No exercise
K^+ (3–6 mEq/L)	< 3.0 (hypokalemic) requires treatment	No exercise
Ca^{2+} (8.8–10.4 mg/100mL?)	> 6.0 (hyperkalemia)[a] requires treatment	
Endocrine Dysfunction		
Diabetes on insulin	Monitor carefully as exercise may potentiate response to insulin	

[a] Often associated with arrhythmias and muscle weakness.

ROM, range of motion; ADL, activities of daily living; FEV_1, forced expiratory volume in 1 second.

Adapted with permission from Gerber LH. Rehabilitation of cancer patient. In: DeVita, Hellman, Rosenberg, eds. *Cancer: Principles and Practice of Oncology.* 5th ed. Philadelphia: Lippincott-Raven Publishers; 1997: table 56-15.

motorized, may be required. Pediatric wheelchairs are available in different sizes and types, and made of durable metal to sustain wear-and-tear. These chairs are light-weight, allowing transportation, and are "growable" to accommodate the growth of a child. They are also available in different colors to suit the likes of a child (Fig. 36–1).

Pediatric walkers are also available in colors and are available in light weight with or without gliding devices to allow a debilitated child to walk with a broad base of support. Adding weights to these walkers aids in the ambulation of a child with ataxia by providing a fixed point of stability and proprioceptive feedback. The degree of functional impair-

ment usually corresponds to the level of spinal segment involvement, as is shown in (Table 36–2).

A patient with C5 quadriplegia will be able to bring food to mouth but needs assist for most ADLs. A patient with C8T1 quadriplegia will have intact hand function. For safe ambulation the hip and knee extension strength should be at least 3/5. Extensive bracing crossing the knee should be avoided in the cancer patient, because the brace consumes a great deal of energy for ambulation, which will be taxing to the already debilitated child with cancer. Ankle-foot orthosis made of light-weight polypropylene or laminated plastic can be used in children with lower extremity weakness.

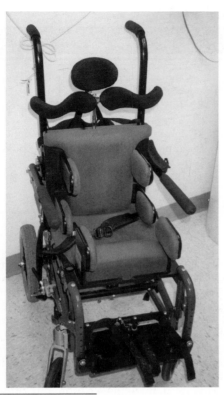

Figure 36–1 Pediatric custom-made light-weight wheel-chair components include lateral support for the spine, head support, leg rests, and reclinable back.

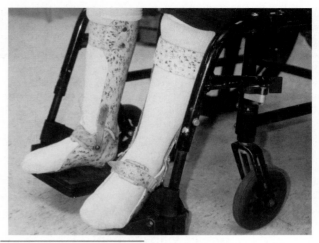

Figure 36–2 Custom-made ankle-foot orthosis provides support to the ankle-joint ligaments and prevents subluxation of bones. Positions anatomically. Provides dorsiflexion assist.

These braces limit plantar flexion and thereby cause an extension moment at the knee to aid in progression of the leg (Fig. 36–2).

Upper Extremity Orthotics and Splints

A detailed discussion of the orthotic devices that are available will not be presented here. Interested readers may obtain information on this subject from textbooks of orthotics (e.g., the chapter by Michael A. Alexander, Maureen R. Nelson, and Anjali Shah in *Pediatric Rehabilitation* 2nd ed).

BOX 36–1
Goals for Orthotics

- **Aid or substitute weak muscles.**
- **Stabilization of the joints (e.g., AFOS).**
- **Prevention of contractures (e.g., A Frame).**
- **Relief of weight bearing from metastatic bone lesions.**
- **Functional training pre- and post-operative.**
- **Positioning of proximal part of limb to gain control over the distal limb to aid in function.**

Bladder Management

Spinal cord damage results in either upper motor neuron bladder or lower motor neuron bladder, depending on the level of involvement. In a flaccid or lower motor neuron bladder, the goal should be to keep the bladder as empty as possible to avoid infection caused by retention of urine or even

TABLE 36–2   Spinal Cord Levels: Functional Relationships

Level of involvement	Intact key muscle	Function
C4	Neck muscles	Unassisted breathing
C5	Biceps	Able to bring hand to mouth
C6	Wrist extensors	Light grasp through tenodesis effect
C7	Elbow extensors	Lift self weight
		Shift during transfers
C8T1	Hand intrinsics	Hand function
Lower thoracic	Hip-knee extensors	Ambulation possible with long leg braces
Lower lumbar	Ankle dorsiflexion	Ambulation with ankle-foot orthosis

hydronephrosis and pyelonephrosis. As early as possible the child and the mother and/or father should be taught to do intermittent catheterization as frequently as every 3 to 4 hours. A child can be taught to self-catheterize by age 10. At this age other methods, such as manipulation, can also be taught.

Outlet obstruction can be managed by an α-adrenergic blocking agent, such as phenoxybenzamine. A parasympathomimetic agent may be of use in flaccid bladder. A patient with both flaccid bladder and outlet obstruction may need both medications. Consultation with a urologist may be necessary in a patient who requires urodynamic evaluation. If all else fails, a suprapubic cystostomy or intraurethral resection or external sphincterotomy may become necessary. By keeping the urine pH acidic, stone promotion and infection can be avoided.

Bowel Management

Bowel management can be instituted by the use of laxatives, stool softeners, and bulking agents. A selected time either in the morning or the evening, after food intake, takes advantage of the gastrocolic reflex and establishes a bowel regimen.

Spasticity

Spasticity is a disabling component of many nervous system diseases of children, including cerebral palsy, traumatic encephalopathy with spinal cord involvement,[50] congenital abnormalities, and degenerative disorders of the CNS. Spasticity is defined as a velocity-dependent increase in resistance to passive stretch seen in concert with the other components of the upper motor neuron syndrome.[51–53]

Spasticity has been of interest for more than 100 years. Because it can cause disabling impairments in function, patients experience muscle tone abnormalities coupled with shortening contractures of the joints. This may lead to progressive joint subluxation and dislocations. Whether or not spasticity needs to be treated depends on its effect on functional impairment. In many cases, although clinically present, spasticity may contribute very little to the disability, and elimination of spasticity may provide no functional advantage to the patient.

Evaluation of spasticity may be performed using the Ashworth Scale (Table 36–3) or the Assistance Scale (Table 36–4).[54]

TABLE 36–3   Ashworth Scale

Grade	
Grade 1	No increased tone.
Grade 2	Slightly increased tone, manifested by a catch and release or minimal resistance when the affected part is moved in flexion or extension.
Grade 3	Marked increase in tone through most of range of motion, but affected parts are easily moved.
Grade 4	Considerable increase in tone; passive movement is difficult.
Grade 5	Affected parts rigid in flexion and extension.

TABLE 36–4   Assistance Scale

Grade	
Grade 5	Maintains independently without assistance.
Grade 4	Maintains with unilateral upper extremity support or requires intermittent contact by therapist for balance only.
Grade 3	Maintains with bilateral upper extremity support or requires constant contact by therapist for balance only.
Grade 2	Full external support of one person.
Grade 1	Cannot be placed.

The WEEFIM (wee little kids functional independence measure) Functional Index measures specific childhood performance of selected ADLs, whereas the Tufts Assessment of Motor Performance (TAMP) assesses motor performance.[55]

Treatment: A wide variety of options are available for the treatment of spasticity; physical therapy, occupational therapy, assistive devices, and orthopedic and neurosurgical procedures all aid in the reduction of spasticity (Fig. 36–3).

Drug therapy using baclofen orally and even intrathecally via an infusion pump is now a common clinical practice. Baclofen inhibits both monosynaptic and polysynaptic reflexes at the spinal level, and decreases excitatory neurotransmitter release from primary afferent terminals.[56] Other medications, such as diazepam and danthrolene sodium, may also be beneficial.

Surgical procedures, such as selective dorsal rhizotomy, may offer permanent alleviation of spasticity.[57]

Metastatic Brain Tumors

Of children with malignant solid tumors, 6 to 12% develop brain metastasis. The tumors that metastasize frequently are

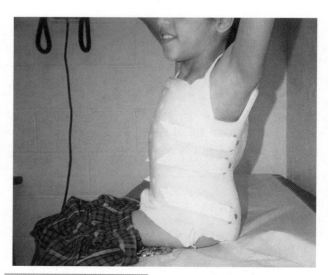

Figure 36–3 Thoracic lumbosacral orthosis. Custom-made plastic body jacket provides external support and aids in healing by preventing forward flexion and rotation.

nephroblastoma (Wilms') and osteogenic and embryonal rhabdomyosarcoma.[58, 59] Onset of symptoms in children is more abrupt than that in adults; 20% present with catastrophic symptoms related to intracerebral hemorrhage. The rehabilitative interventional approach is the same as that for primary tumors.

SUMMARY

It is of prime importance to consider the effects of tumors and residual secondary deficits caused by various treatment modalities on the child suffering from CNS malignancy. An assessment of these disabilities requires knowledge and awareness so that adjustment for motor, cognitive, and other disabilities can be made. A well-planned treatment program must be based on the guidelines outlined in this chapter.

Childhood CNS tumors are not a single disorder but a confluence of factors. Children suffer not only from the effect of the tumor but also from the effects of its management. Because of their youth children do not have a good insight or understanding of the disease or its ramifications. Rehabilitation professionals should be sensitive to this fact and incorporate the parents in the treatment plan. The therapists should be creative and devise techniques that attract the young individual and make the process more enjoyable. Exercise sessions should be tailored to each patient because the metabolic demands and nutritional needs are variable. Any equipment ordered should be carefully tailored to the patient keeping social demands in mind. The equipment should be assessed for malfunction periodically.

Rehabilitation of a child requires a team approach, as with any patient undergoing rehabilitation. Younger children are more susceptible to radiation toxicity and experience more cognitive deficits than adults. Therefore, occupational therapy assistance should be sought for these children for cognitive remediation. Chemotherapy can potentially cause peripheral neuropathies, resulting in such impairments as foot drop and wrist drop. Timely identification and orthotic management will ensure optimal functional results.

As cancer is diagnosed at earlier stages and more survivors are seen today than ever before, rehabilitation intervention may improve the functional outcome of children with CNS tumors.

REFERENCES

1. Ryan BR. Principles of pediatric oncology. In: Lewis MM, ed. *Musculoskeletal Oncology: A Multidisciplinary Approach.* Philadelphia: WB Saunders; 1992:73–86.
2. Herold AH, Roetzheim HG. Cancer survivors. *Prim Care* 1992;4:779–791.
3. Dietz JH. Rehabilitation of cancer patient. *Med Clin North Am* 1969;53:607–624.
4. Peckham CV. Learning disabilities in long term survivors of childhood cancer: concern for parents and teachers. *Int Disabil Stud* 1991;141–145.
5. O'Connor L, Smith-Blesch K. Life cycles issues affecting cancer rehabilitation. *Semin Oncol Nurs* 1992;8:174–185.
6. Ganz PA. Current issues in cancer rehabilitation. *Cancer* 1990;65:742–751.
7. Hinterbuchner C. Rehabilitation of the disability cancer. *N Y State J Med* 1978;78:1066–1069.
8. Ragnarsson KT. Principles of cancer rehabilitation medicine. In: Holland JF, ed. *Cancer Medicine.* Philadelphia: Lea & Febiger; 1993:1054.
9. Wilmore DW. Catabolic illness: strategies for enhancing recovery. *N Engl J Med* 1991;325(10):695.
10. Vico L, Chappard D, Alexandre C, et al. Effects of a 120 day period of bed-rest on bone mass and bone cell activities in man: attempts at countermeasure. *Bone Mineral* 1987;2:383.
11. Booth FW. Physiologic and biochemical effects of immobilization on muscle. *Clin Orthop Rel Res* 1987;219:15.
12. Haggmark T, Eriksson E, Jansson E. Muscle fiber type changes in human skeletal muscle after injuries and immobilization. *Orthopedics* 1986;9(2):181.
13. Mohr DN, Ryu JH, Litin SC, III ECR. Recent advances in the management of venous thromboembolism. *Mayo Clin Proc* 1988;63:281.
14. Andrykowsky MA, Henslee PJ, Farrall MG. Physical and psychosocial functioning of adult survivors of allogenic bone marrow transplantation. *Bone Marrow Transpl* 1989; 4:75–81.
15. Jones AL, Miller JL. Bone marrow morbidity of chemotherapy. In: Plowman PN, McElwain TJ, Meadows AT, et al, eds. *Complications of Cancer Management.* Oxford: Butterworth-Heinemann; 1991:371.
16. O'Brian M, Krrisht A. Cerebellar astrocytomas. In: Cheek W, Marlin A, eds. *Pediatric Neurosurgery.* 3rd ed. Philadelphia: WB Saunders Company; 1994:356–361.
17. Davis CH, Joglekar VM. Cerebellar astrocytomas in children and young adults. *J Neurol Neurosurg Psychiatry* 1981;44:820.
18. Mason DD. Gliomas of the cerebral hemispheres. In: Matson DD, Ingraham FD, eds. *Neurosurgery of Infancy and Childhood.* 2nd ed. Springfield, IL: Charles C Thomas; 1969:480–522.
19. Hoffman HJ. Supratentorial brain tumors in children. In: Youman JR, ed. *Neurological Surgery.* Philadelphia: WB Saunders; 1982.
20. Jooma R, Hayward RD, Grant DN. Intracranial neoplasms during the first year of life: analysis of one hundred consecutive cases. *Neurosurgery* 1984;14:31.
21. Dohrman GJ, Farwell JR, Flannery JT. Astrocytomas in childhood: a population based study. *Surg Neurol* 1985; 23:64.
22. Warnick RE, Edwards MSB: Pediatric brain tumors. *Cur Probl Pediatr* 1991;21:129.
23. Johnson DL, McCabe M, Nicholson S, Joseph A, et al. Quality of long term survival in young children with medulloblastoma. *J Neurosurg* 1994;80:1004–1010.
24. Kadota RP, Allen JB, Hartman GA, et al. Brain tumors in children. *J Pediatr* 1989;114:511–551.
25. Mulhern RK, Crisco, JJ, Kun LE. Neuropsychological sequelae of childhood brain tumors: a review. *J Clin Child Psychol* 1983;12:66.
26. Kun LE, Mulhern RK, Crisco JJ. Quality of life in children treated for brain tumors. *J Neurosurg* 1983;58:1.
27. Silverman CL, Palkes H, Talent B, et al. Late effects of radiotherapy on patients with medulloblastoma. *Cancer* 1984;54:825.

28. Spunberg JJ, Chang CH, Goldman M, et al. Quality of long-term survival following irradiation for intracranial tumors in children under the age of two. *Int J Radiat Oncol Biol Phys* 1981;7:727.

29. Copeland DR, Fletcher JM, Pfefferbaum-Levin B, et al. Neuropsychological sequelae of childhood cancer and long term survivors. *Pediatrics* 1985;75:745–753.

30. Ellenberg L, McComb JG, Siegel SE, et al. Factors affecting intellectual outcome in pediatric brain tumor patients. *Neurosurgery* 1987;21:638–644.

31. Mulhern RK, Horowitz ME, Kovnar EH, et al. Neurodevelopmental status of infants and young children treated for brain tumors with pre-irradiation chemotherapy. *J Clin Oncol* 1989;7:1660–1666.

32. Leibel SA, Guten PH, Davis RL. Tolerance of the brain and spinal cord. In: Guten PH, ed. *Radiation Injury to the Nervous System*. New York: Raven Press; 1991:239–256.

33. Albers JW. Adverse effects of antineoplastic therapy on the peripheral nervous system. *J Am Assoc Electromyogr Electrodiag* 1985;C:37–47.

34. Schultheiss TE, El-Mahdi AM. Statistical analysis of two hundred radiation myelopathy cases. *Proc 7th Int Cong Radiat Res* 1983;D:3–41.

35. Garden FH. Radiation injury to the spinal cord and peripheral nerves. In: *Physical Med and Rehab State of the Art Reviews*. Vol 8. No. 2. Philadelphia: Hanley and Belfus; June 1994.

36. Duffner PK, Cohen ME, Voorhess ML, et al. Long-term effects of cranial irradiation on endocrine function in children with brain tumors. *Cancer* 1985;56:2189.

37. Li FP, Winston KR, Gimbere K. Follow-up of children with brain tumors. *Cancer* 1984;54:135.

38. Shalet SM. Growth and hormonal status of children treated for brain tumors. *Child's Brain* 1982;9:284.

39. Byrd R. Late effects of treatment of cancer in children. *Pediatr Clin North Am* 1985;32:835–851.

40. Wheeler JS Jr, Siroky MB, Bell R, et al. Vincristine-induced bladder neuropathy. *J Urol* 1982;130(2):342.

41. Rosenfeld CS, Broden LE. Cisplatin-induced autonomic neuropathy. *Cancer Treat Rep* 1984;68(4):659.

42. Raphaelson MI, Steven JC, Newman RP. Vincristine neuropathy with bowel and bladder atony, mimicking spinal cord compression. (Letter) *Cancer Treat Rep* 1983;67(6):604.

43. Scherokman B, Filing-Katz MR, Tell D. Brachial plexus neuropathy following high-dose cytarabine in acute monoblastic leukemia. *Cancer Treat Rep* 1985;69(9):1005.

44. Ryan JR, Emami A. Vincristine neurotoxicity with residual equinocavus deformity in children with acute leukemia. *Cancer* 1983;51(3):423.

45. Salner AL, Botnick LE, Herzog AG, et al. Reversible brachial plexopathy following radiation therapy for breast-cancer. *Cancer Treat Rep* 1981;65(9–10):797.

46. Forman A. Peripheral neuropathy in cancer patients: clinical types, etiology, and presentation. *Oncology* 1990;4:85–89.

47. Gollick PD. Metabolism of substrates: energy substrates metabolism during exercise as well as modified training. *Fed Proc* 1985;44:353–357.

48. Butterfield GE, Galloway DH. Physical activity improves protein utilization in young men. *Br J Nutr* 1984;51:171–187.

49. Lemon PWR, Dolly DG, Yaraseske KE. Effect of intensity on protein utilization during prolonged exercise (abstract). *Med Sci Sports Exerc* 1984;16:157.

50. Barolat G. Surgical management of spasticity and spasms in spinal cord injury: an overview. *J Am Paraplegia Soc* 1988;ll(1):9.

51. Young RR. The physiology of spasticity and its response to therapy. *Ann NY Acad Sci* 1988;531:146.

52. Katz RT. Management of spasticity. *Am J Phys Med Rehabil* 1988;67(3):108.

53. Delwaide PJ. Spasticity: from pathophysiology to therapy. *Acta Neuro Chir (Wien)* 1987;39 Suppl 31.

54. Ashworth B. Preliminary trial of carisoprodol in multiple sclerosis. *Practitioner* 1964;192:540.

55. Haley SM, Ludlow LH. Applicability of the hierarchical scales of the Tufts assessment of motor performance for school aged children and adults with disabilities. *Phys Ther* 1992;72(3):191.

56. Latash ML, Penn RD, Corcos DM, et al. Short-term effects of intrathecal baclofen in spasticity. *Exp Neurol* 1989;103(2):165.

57. Peacock WJ, Stahdt LA. Selective posterior dorsal rhizotomy: evolution of theory and practice. *Pediatr Neurosurg* 1991/92;17:128.

58. Vannucci RC, Baten M. Cerebral metastatic disease in childhood. *Neurology* 1974;24:981.

59. Grams F, Walker RW, Allen JC. Brain metastasis in children. *J Pediatr* 1983;103:558.

60. Alexander MA, Nelson R, Shah A. Orthotics: adaptive seating and assistive devices. In: *Pediatric Rehabilitation*. 2nd ed. Molnar G, ed. Baltimore: Williams & Wilkins; 1992.

Chapter 37

Cooperative Group Trials

Roger J. Packer, Richard Sposto, Henry Friedman, and Giorgio Perilongo

The management of primary central nervous system (CNS) tumors in children has become increasingly complex. There is general acceptance that optimum treatment, especially for children with malignant tumors, is multidisciplinary and that the long-term outcome for children with aggressive tumors is improved by treatment at a tertiary referral (usually "academic") center.[1, 2] As therapies evolve, the use of multiple modalities of therapy for an individual patient has become commonplace. In addition, as survival rates rise, the need for evaluation of the quality of life of survivors and the longterm effects of treatment increase. As newer forms of treatment are purported to improve survival and quality of life, it is necessary to determine rigorously if such treatments are more efficacious and/or cause fewer sequelae than conventional treatments. This type of evaluation often requires that more patients be followed than can be accomplished at one institution or, for that matter, at multiple institutions working in concert. This has led to larger national or international studies that evaluate patients in a standardized fashion.

Since the 1960s, there have been multi-institutional groups within North America and Europe evaluating children with cancer.[1, 2] Initially these groups focused on leukemia and other lymphoreticular malignancies. Soon after, when the benefits of such group studies became evident, other pediatric tumors were evaluated. Trials for children with brain tumors have been coordinated by these cooperative groups since the mid- to late 1970s, although the involvement of such cooperative groups in pediatric brain tumor studies lagged behind activities for other pediatric cancers. The reasons for the relative delay of multi-institutional study groups being involved in childhood brain tumor studies are manifold. They include (1) the standard practice, until recently, of considering treatment of brain tumors to be the domain of the neurosurgeon or, less commonly, another lone caretaker (? neurologist); (2) the neolistic mind set of many who care for children with brain tumors, often derived from their experience of caring for adults with brain tumors, that therapy other than surgery is usually futile and only adds to the discomfort of the patient; (3) the lack of expertise within the cooperative group of physicians knowledgeable in the nuances of primary CNS tumors and the CNS in general; and (4) the reluctance of oncologists and other cancer specialists to focus on brain tumors because of their relative rarity, as regards individual tumor types, and the lack of effective treatments.

> ## BOX 37-1
> ## Weaknesses of Cooperative Groups
>
> - **Not initially designed as "brain tumor" groups**
> - **Variability in expertise of institutions**
> - **Loss of individual institution control**
> - **Need for central review**
> - **Design of studies to (? lowest) common denominator of institutions**
> - **Slower incorporation of new techniques not widely available**
> - **Somewhat cumbersome (? delay) in study initiation**
> - **Somewhat less interest in less common brain tumor**

Recently, many of these obstacles have been overcome, as the multidisciplinary needs of the patients and encouraging survival rates in some subsets of patients have led to the wider willingness of referral to academic cancer centers. The cooperative groups have greatly expanded their expertise in pediatric brain tumors and have actively recruited neurosurgeons, neurologists, and other neuroscientists to join the group and participate in the creation of treatment protocols.

> ## BOX 37-2
> ## Strengths of Cooperative Groups
>
> - **Multi-institutional**
> - **Multidisciplinary**
> - **Larger numbers (can do Phase III studies)**
> - **Statistical office (funded)**
> - **Data monitoring in place**
> - **Ability to do central reviews**
> - **Rapid incorporation of advances in oncology**
> - **Orderly review of studies**
> - **Increased interest in brain tumors**

The potential power of such groups is highlighted by the patterns of referral of children with cancer. Although cancers in patients older than 21 years greatly outnumber those occurring in pediatric patients, nearly 20% of all patients entered on cooperative treatment trials in the United States are of the pediatric age.[1, 2] In 1996, pediatric accruals on National Cancer Institute–sponsored trials composed 18.6% of all patient studies, whereas pediatric cancers represented less than 2% of all cancers. Nearly 95% of children with cancer are referred to an academic cancer center participating in one of the two major cooperative groups in the United States. It is estimated that more than 80% of patients seen at an institution that is affiliated with one of the cooperative groups will be eligible for entry in an appropriate study. Over the past decade, there has been an exponential rise in the number of patients with brain tumors entered in cooperative group studies. These studies, which initially focused on the more common childhood brain tumors, such as medulloblastoma, have increasingly encompassed "rarer" forms of brain tumor. Initially, there was a reluctance on the part of the cooperative groups to evaluate patients with benign tumors, such as low-grade gliomas; but more recently, these studies have been developed and, to a degree, successfully completed. Probably even more importantly, it has been accepted that a major reason for the lack of progress in the management of childhood brain tumors is the lack of understanding of the basic neurobiologic underpinnings of these tumors. Given the histologic heterogeneity of childhood brain tumors, individual institutions are hard pressed to gather a significant number of specimens, from well-characterized and homogeneously treated patients, on which to perform biologic studies. Centralized reference or resource laboratories have been developed by the cooperative groups to promote and facilitate neurobiologic studies of childhood tumors.

More important than the other concerns are the potential benefits to individual patients of entry in cooperative-group protocols. Studies in children with leukemia, lymphoma, Wilms' tumor, rhabdomyosarcoma, and medulloblastoma have shown stepwise increases in survival result from well-formed, sequential studies.[1, 2] Children with such tumors have a significant survival advantage when treated at with well-defined protocols tertiary care centers, compared with pediatric patients not enrolled on protocols and not treated at pediatric cancer centers.[1, 2] These results do not detract from important information to be gained from single institutional or smaller multi-institutional studies. Smaller studies are an important avenue for new approaches to be tested, and, because of complexity and availability of resources and new technologies, some treatment approaches can only be performed by a group of dedicated investigators and are probably not suitable, especially in initial testing, for cooperative group trials. Also, cooperative group studies by design are often compromised studies, and if treatments are performed in a groupwide basis, there may be the tendency to make the study less "cutting edge" or complex so as to allow more uniform group participation. An alternative view of the need to make studies performable by the majority of investigators is that this creates studies that are potentially beneficial to more patients than are smaller, new technology–based approaches.

A major focus of group studies is the development of treatments that can be compared with standard treatments and proven, in a statistical fashion, to be superior or inferior. In a sense, this limits the type of studies that can be undertaken in that extremely rare tumors, of which sufficient numbers probably cannot be accrued to result in statistical differences in overall survival, are better not evaluated by groups. However, even with rarer tumors, there is increased pressure by investigators to attempt multi-institutional studies because this may be the only means of accruing enough patients to address management issues.

A major asset of cooperative group studies, as financial resources for academic studies shrink in the United States and probably around the world, is the ability of the groups to provide data management and statistical support to address important management issues in pediatric brain tumors.

GROUPS AND GROUP STRUCTURE

In North America, two major pediatric cancer cooperative groups, the Pediatric Oncology Group (POG) and the Children's Cancer Group (CCG), evaluate up to 95% of patients younger than 15 years with cancer.[1, 2] Both are federally funded (National Cancer Institute; NCI) cancer groups dedicated to the control and treatment of childhood and adolescent tumors. Both groups design, conduct, and evaluate clinical and laboratory studies and are increasingly involved in the treatment of children with brain tumors (Table 37–1).

The Society of Pediatric Oncology (SIOP), initially primarily composed of European cancer centers is an international organization that acts as a professional society for individuals involved in the management of childhood cancer. Although created as a professional society, SIOP has been involved for many years in the development of studies for children with brain tumors. SIOP helps organize multi-institutional and multi-national trials, depending primarily on the cancer groups already in place in different countries. The bulk of the funding for these studies comes from the individual cancer groups rather than from a centrally funded organization, in contrast to CCG or POG. Many of the cooperative groups in Europe are well organized and have an excellent track record in the management of pediatric cancer.

Other cooperative groups have been formed and have organized trials for children with cancer outside of North America and Europe. Study groups in Japan and in multiple countries in South America have developed important clinical trials. However, by and large these study groups are younger and tend to have fewer resources than CCG, POG, or SIOP.

Children's Cancer Group

CCG is an international research organization, primarily funded by the National Cancer Institute, that was founded in 1955.[1] Known as the Children's Cancer Study Group between 1965 and 1990, CCG consists of academic cancer centers throughout the United States and Canada. More recently, there have been affiliated members added to the group from regions including South America (Brazil) and Australia. CCG members include more than 2500 pediatric cancer specialists located in 36 full-member institutions, 80 affiliated members, and 43 corresponding members (in 23 countries). Its primary statistical and operations office is located in the Los Angeles area, with a group chair's office in Houston, Texas.

TABLE 37–1 Cooperative Groups for Childhood Brain Tumors

Name	Origin	Geographic issues	Headquarters
Children's Cancer Group (CCG)	Founded 1955	United States; Canada; international affiliates	Statistical office: Los Angeles, CA Chairman's office: Houston, TX
Pediatric Oncology Group (POG)	Independent 1981; was division of Southwest Oncology Group (SWOG)	United States; Canada	Statistical office: Gainesville, FL Operations office: Chicago, IL
Children's Oncology Group (COG)	Founded 2000	United States; Canada	To be determined
International Society of Pediatric Oncology (SIOP)	Founded as a professional society	Worldwide; member cooperative groups such as United Kingdom, Italian, German, and French pediatric cancer groups	No statistical office President's office moves with president
Pediatric Brain Tumor Consortium (PBTC)	Founded 1999	Nine institutions in the United States	Statistical office: Memphis, TN

Since 1982, the CCG has had a formal brain tumor strategy group whose primary responsibility is to help guide studies that improve the rates of survival and the quality of life of children with primary CNS tumors. Up to then, the CCG has focused on clinical trials for children with the more common forms of brain tumor. The Brain Tumor Strategy Group of CCG is a multidisciplinary group, comprising neurosurgeons, neurologists, oncologists, radiation oncologists, neuroradiologists, neuropathologists, psychologists, and statisticians. Studies that are approved for development by the Strategy Group are then formally developed by specific study groups and approved by all participating institutions and the NCI Institute review board before initiation. A recent addition to the brain tumor efforts of the CCG has been the development of the Brain Tumor Resource Laboratory. This, at present, is a three-pronged laboratory effort with research and resource laboratories in Philadelphia, Seattle, and Pittsburgh performing basic neurobiologic expefiments and preparing tissue for molecular biologic studies.

The Brain Tumor Strategy Group of CCG works closely with various discipline committees within CCG, such as the Neurosurgery Discipline Committee, the Epidemiology Committee, and the Tumor Imaging Committee, to develop studies. These studies are prioritized within the CCG, with the highest priority given to Phase III randomized studies, which usually have the highest potential to advance brain tumor therapy significantly.

Pediatric Oncology Group

POG, like CCG, is a multi-institutional group with centers in both America and Canada. POG is somewhat younger than CCG, submitting its first grant request for approval in 1981. It began as a part of the Southwest Cancer Chemotherapy Study Group and later the pediatric division of the Southwest Oncology Group. Later, other institutions joined the Southwest Oncology Group division to form POG in 1980. Its initial operations office was in St. Louis, Missouri, with the statistical office in Gainesville, Florida. As of 1993, the operations office moved to Chicago, Illinois.

POG is similar in size to CCG. It has a Brain Tumor Committee that serves a purpose similar to that of the CCG Brain Tumor Strategy Group. The committee is also multidisciplinary and is aided by the Neuroscience Committee, which is composed predominantly of neuroscientists, including neurosurgeons, neurologists, neuropathologists, and neuroradiologists. The overall directions of POG are similar to those of CCG. POG has a brain tumor tissue bank at St. Jude Research Hospital. Many of its clinical trials have derived from the basic pediatric brain tumor research studies performed at Duke University.

Intergroup (CCG and POG) Activities

During the past decade, there has been increased effort to combine the clinical activities of POG and CCG. This has led to the development of intergroup studies, jointly developed by the cooperative groups and handled by the representative statistical offices in an alternating fashion. This has allowed studies to be completed that could not have been done otherwise due to the small numbers of patients available for entry from the individual groups.

Children's Oncology Group (COG)

In the late 1990s, the Children's Cancer Group and Pediatric Oncology Group agreed to merge into one pediatric cancer cooperative group, the Children's Oncology Group. It is expected that by the early 2000s the two groups will be fully merged, with one operations office and statistical center. As regards activities relating to brain tumors, as of 1999 the two cooperative groups have had fully integrated sessions with a Brain Tumor Core Committee, comprised of members from the Children's Cancer Group and from the Pediatric Oncology Group.

International Society of Pediatric Oncology

As stated previously, SIOP is both a professional society and a cooperative group that attempts to coordinate multi-institutional and, by design, multinational studies. Because of this overall design, the coordination of the studies performed by groups under the SIOP umbrella is more flexible because national cooperative groups can choose to participate in studies as they wish. This is primarily due to the lack of centralized funding and the need for countries to be essentially self-supporting in the performance of these studies. Most countries in Europe have well-organized cancer study groups that may or may not participate in SIOP studies and perform brain tumor investigations. Cooperative groups that have been especially prominent in the performance of clinical trials for children with brain tumors in collaboration with SIOP include the United Kingdom Children's Cancer Study Group (UKCCSG), the French Pediatric Oncology Group, and the German Pediatric Oncology Group. The German Pediatric Oncology Group was formerly a West German organization but has evolved into a study group accruing patients from Germany (including former East Germany) and Austria. The involvement of Italian groups within the SIOP has been somewhat more fragmented, as regional geographic study groups are more prominent in Italy.

The exact mechanism of study development for SIOP varies depending on the type of tumor being studied and the interests of individual investigators. SIOP has a subcommittee whose primary responsibility is the development of clinical trials for children with CNS cancer. Researchers from each of the individual study groups involved in the development of the national studies bring new ideas and approaches to the meeting; then a decision is made as to who will participate and who will lead the clinical research effort. SIOP does not have a central resource laboratory accruing specimens from studies, nor does it have a statistical office to coordinate all studies.

Pediatric Brain Tumor Clinical Trials Consortium (PBTC)

In a reply to a request for application by the National Cancer Institute in the United States, the Pediatric Brain Tumor Trials Consortium was formed in 1998. The objectives of this consortium are to tie well-established pediatric brain tumor centers in the United States into a formal cooperative group and to have such centers perform innovative, often technologically demanding, clinical trials for children with brain tumors. In theory, such trials are too complex to be expeditiously conducted through the large number of institutions that are members of COG. The PBTC has been formed to supplement the efforts of the Children's Oncology Group by developing and completing Phase I and, possibly, Phase II clinical trials for children with brain tumors, which can then be incorporated into the Children's Oncology Group efforts for nationwide Phase II or Phase III participation. The initial programs chosen for inclusion in the PBTC include:

Children's National Medical Center, Washington, DC
Children's Hospital of Philadelphia, Philadelphia, PA
Dana Farber Cancer Institute/Children's Hospital/

Massachusetts General Hospital, Boston, MA
Children's Hospital of Pittsburgh, Pittsburgh, PA,
Duke University, Durham, NC
St. Jude Children's Research Hospital, Memphis, TN
Children's Hospital of Texas, Houston, TX
Children's Hospital and Research Medical Center, and
Seattle, WA
University of California at San Francisco, San Francisco, CA

The initial studies undertaken by the PBTC include the evaluation of new means of drug delivery; the development of a pilot protocol utilizing intrathecal therapy for children less than three years of age with malignant central nervous system tumors; studies evaluating antiangiogenesis agents; and studies evaluating new biologic therapies, including oral farnyseal transferase inhibitors. A major component of this group will be to incorporate innovative neuroradiographic means and detailed pharmacokinetic studies into treatment protocols. Biologic studies will also be included in treatment protocols, whenever possible.

CLINICAL TRIAL STRUCTURE

Study Types

Clinical trials, which are the major effort of the groups and are designed to identify more beneficial treatments, are typically classified as Phase I, Phase II, or Phase III. Each has a different primary objective. Cooperative groups often also design and conduct nontherapeutic studies addressing other objectives, such as biologic research and epidemiology. Phase I and II trials are used to screen new treatments for toxicity and feasibility (Phase I) and effectiveness (Phase II) before they are studied in larger Phase III trials. In practice, the classification of trials as Phase I, II, or III is not as straightforward. A trial can address Phase I and Phase II or Phase II and Phase III objectives simultaneously. Nevertheless it is beneficial to understand the difference between Phase I, II, and III trials in the usual sense (Table 37–2).

Phase I Studies

Phase I trials are used to evaluate toxicity and feasibility of new treatments or treatment components in a small number of relapsed or refractory patients.[3] Often these studies employ a statistical rule to determine a maximum tolerated dose (MTD). *An important part of the design of these trials is the definition of dose-limiting toxicity (DLT).* These can be one toxicity or a constellation of toxicities whose occurrence in a large proportion of patients would make the treatment unacceptable. In a standard design, several increasing dose levels are used, and patients are recruited in cohorts of three starting with the lowest dose level. Patient entry is suspended until the toxicity evaluation of all patients in the cohort is complete. If 0/3 DLTs occur, three patients are recruited at the next highest level; if 1/3 occur, three more are recruited to the current level; and if 2/3 or more occur, the dose level is rejected as too toxic. Six patients must be treated at the final dose level, and a level is acceptable only if no more than 1/6 DLTs have occurred. *The MTD is defined as the highest dose level with no more than 1/6 DLTs.*

TABLE 37–2   Cancer Clinical Study Types

Type	Aim	Means
Phase I	Evaluate toxicity and feasibility; define dose-limiting toxicity	Dose escalation study; Rule of 3 (small number of patients needed)
Phase II	Estimate effectiveness of treatment	Studies per disease type; minimum of 10—maximum 20–30 per arm (moderate number of patients)
Phase III	Compare two or more treatments	Ideally randomized with control group; at times, historical or concurrent nonrandomized control (large number, prospectively determined)

Although this is a reasonable rule in the first investigation of a treatment, only a small number of patients are involved, and hence the true toxicity of the selected MTD is variable. For example, with six dose levels with true DLT rates of 2%, 5%, 10%, 20%, 30%, and 40%, respectively, dose level 4 is the most likely to be selected, with a DLT rate of 20%. It is almost as likely that level 3 or level 5 would also be selected, with DLT rates of 10% and 30% respectively, and it is possible (7% chance) that level 6 will be selected, with a 40% DLT rate. Although the standard Phase I design provides a crude screen for treatments that are excessively toxic, continued monitoring of toxicities in subsequent studies is essential.

Phase II Studies

The objective of Phase II trials is to estimate effectiveness of new treatments as reflected in acutely measurable disease outcomes, such as tumor response rate. As in Phase I trials, usually small numbers of relapsed or refractory patients are used; however, Phase II trials also may be performed in newly diagnosed patients. In a modified Chang design currently used in some CCG studies, 10 patients initially are recruited.[4] If 0/10 responses are observed, the treatment is considered ineffective, and if 6/10 are observed, the treatment is considered effective enough for further study. If 1/10 to 5/10 responses are observed, 10 more patients are recruited. At least 4/20 responses are required for the treatment to be accepted for further study. With this rule, ineffective treatments will be rejected, and moderately effective treatments (response rate 20 to 30%) accepted, with high probability. As for Phase I trials, the results for a single Phase II trial can are variable. A treatment giving 8/20 responses will have an estimated response rate of 40% ± 11%, or a 95% confidence interval of roughly 18 to 61%. Hence, the data suggest only that the treatment is not totally ineffective; they do not give a precise idea of the true efficacy as measured by response rate or guarantee a high response rate.

For the Phase II design described above, treatments with a low target response level (20 to 30%) in selected groups of patients with resistant disease are potentially valuable additions to the modern, multiagent, multimodality approach to newly diagnosed patients. On the other hand, a treatment with response rates of 20 to 30% in previously untreated tumors would not be expected to effect a large improvement in outcome in diseases that have been shown to respond to

other therapies. Thus, it is important to consider the context in which a particular statistical rule is being applied. The exception would be for disease in which no treatment has yet proved effective.

Phase III Studies

Phase III trials compare two or more treatments in sufficient numbers of patients to estimate with precision the differences in treatment effectiveness.[5] In this discussion, Phase III trials include historical controlled trials, concurrent nonrandomized controlled trials, and concurrent randomized controlled trials, although typically only the last type is considered to be a true Phase III trial.

Historical controlled trials use as a control group a cohort of patients treated at a previous time, comparing them with a cohort of patients given a new treatment. In these trials, it is prudent to assume that there are inequalities in the two patient cohorts in important prognostic factors, resulting in bias in the comparison. One tries to control for this by a posteriori adjustment during statistical analysis, but it may be impossible to adjust adequately for these imbalances. Because the old and new cohorts were treated at different times, there can be unquantified differences between the care received, the histologic or stage definition of disease, ind the quality of the data that make unbiased comparison between treatments impossible. The case of medulloblastoma in CCG is a good example. If one were to mount an historically controlled trial in high-risk (metastatic or more than 1.5 cm^3 residual disease) medulloblastoma, two possible cohorts of patients could be identified: Study CCG-942, performed in the late 1970s and early 1980s, and Study CCG-921, performed in the late 1980s to early 1990's.[6,7] Both studies provide data about two important prognostic factors—degree of dissemination (M stage) and extent of tumor resection—that can be used to define the control group. In fact, the meaning of these data has changed with time. During CCG-942, computed tomography (CT) was not universally available, so that staging was based primarily on surgical impression, cerebrospinal fluid (CSF) analysis, and myelography. Because this trial was open to all medulloblastoma patients, CSF cytology and myelography were not strict eligibility criteria and hence were not performed in a proportion of patients classified as M0 on data flowsheets. During CCG-921, CT scan was available but magnetic resonance imaging (MRI) was not universally available. Today minimally acceptable staging for these patients would require brain and spine MRI and lumbar CSF analysis. Furthermore, given the dramatic improvements in neurosurgery and imaging since the late 1970s, it is clear that patients with "total resection" in 1978 must include those who today would be considered incompletely resected, and that patients with "incomplete resection" today may have on average smaller residual tumor volume than similarly classified patients in 1978. There usually is no way to correct for these real biases in analysis because the qualitative differences in staging and treatment were never captured as part of the original study data. For these reasons, conclusions drawn from historically controlled treatment comparisons may not be convincing unless the observed differences in efficacy are far larger than could be attributed to bias.

The second type of Phase III trial is a concurrent nonrandomized controlled trial. Here the treatment is selected by both patient and physician. Although the time biases discussed above are not an issue, there will still be unquantified differences between the treatment groups. Information of wich only the treating physician is aware, such as poor performance status or degrees of disease spread not reflected in the collected data, will affect outcome and may also influence the choice of treatment. Because these differences are unknown to the study investigators and therefore not available at the time of analysis, concurrent controlled nonrandomized studies share with historically controlled trials many problems of interpretability.

The last type of Phase III trial, the concurrent randomized controlled trial, has become an accepted standard for comparing treatments because the problems noted above in connection with historical or nonrandomized uncontrolled trials are largely avoided. Treatments are randomly assigned to patients who are willing and able to accept either experimental or control treatments. It is presumed at the start of a randomized trial that there is no convincing scientific evidence that one treatment is superior to the other. Such information will accumulate during the trial, and thus *all randomized clinical trials should be designed with interim analysis rules to stop the trial when convincing evidence of a difference between treatments exists or, for that matter, when convincing evidence of no difference exists.*[8] Because of the random assignment, treatment groups will most likely be comparable with respect to unquantified prognostic factors. The randomization does not guarantee comparability, but the chance of important differences between groups is known and is expressed as the p value in the reports of these comparisons. For example, when a difference in outcome between groups is reported with $p < 0.05$, this means that if in fact the two treatments are equally effective, it is unlikely (less than 5% chance) that the difference would have been observed. $p < 0.05$ is no guarantee that the observed difference is due to the treatment and not due to chance. However, if one uses this criterion to judge evidence in all trials, only 5% of trials involving equally effective treatments will show erroneously significant results.

It is important in Phase III trials also to consider the sample size of the trial. Large trials are necessary, if they can be performed in a reasonable time, because they ensure that if there is a difference in treatment effectiveness, the trial will likely provide evidence of it at the level of $p < 0.05$. Small trials are unconvincing when they yield negative results because moderate but important improvements in treatment effectiveness are not likely to be significant.

Statistical Implications

As the above discussion implies, the generally accepted minimum evidentiary criterion for judging treatment differences is $p < 0.05$ in randomized Phase III trials that have 80% power against small, clinically meaningful differences. Treatments that show benefit by this criterion are usually adopted. There are circumstances, however, when this stringent evidentiary requirement may be counterproductive. If the disease is by nature rare, such as in many pediatric cancers, then even a trial recruiting all incident cases in the United States for 10 to 15 years may not achieve 80% power against a moderate improvement in effectiveness. In cases like this there is the real concern that conducting a large and therefore very long trial would result in answers that will be irrelevant when they are obtained, or that the opportunity to study other promising therapies will have been missed, or that the trial simply will fail to reach its accrual goal as participating investigators lose interest. In these circumstances it is justifiable, provided certain conditions are met, to relax these typically stringent evidentiaiy requirements, to perform somewhat smaller trials, and to require less compelling evidence than $p < 0.05$ before adopting a new treatment.[5, 9] Hence, one may decide to adopt a treatment that appears better in a smaller trial even though $p = 0.20$, or possibly larger, and this in the long term may result in larger gains in treatment efficacy after a series of trials. It is important to understand that this does not mean that small trials are justified when large trials can be done through collaboration, but only that when large trials truly cannot be performed in a reasonable time, performing smaller trials with less stringent evidentiary requirements is a reasonable strategy to adopt.

Finally, it is sometimes argued that it is unethical to randomize patients to current treatment when there is a strong belief that a new treatment must be an improvement or, in any case, could not be worse. This is a valid argument when current treatment outcome is poor and when previous treatments have not resulted in clear improvement (e.g., childhood brain stem tumors).[10] It is almost never valid when there has been past success in treatment and further improvements are sought. One must honestly ask whether there is clear and convincing evidence that the new treatment cannot be worse. One must also ask whether it is ethical to expose patients to an unknown experimental treatment in a nonrandomized trial when, because of inherent biases, it is unlikely that a clear picture of the true benefit of the treatment will emerge.

TREATMENT DIRECTIONS OF THE COOPERATIVE GROUPS (SEE TABLE 37–3)

Medulloblastomas and Other Primitive Neuroectodermal Tumors

Studies performed in the mid- to late 1970s by the CCG and SIOP for children with medulloblastomas were the foundation for treatment trials carried out over the ensuing two decades. Two randomized trials were performed concurrently by the CCG and SIOP documenting the importance of

TABLE 37–3   Major Directions of Cancer Groups

Tumor	CCG	POG	SIOP
Medulloblastoma (poor risk)	Complete pre-RT chemo trials (Phase II); pursue concurrent chemo and RT; post-RT high-dose chemo with PSCR (Phase I/II)	Pre-RT chemo (Phase II)	Evaluate pre-RT chemo (Phase II)
Medulloblastoma (average risk)	Prospective randomized Phase III of 2400 cGy CSRT plus one of two chemo arms; intergroup; evaluation of reduction in radiation therapy local volume of craniospinal dose	As CCG, intergroup	Prospective randomized Phase III pre-RT chemo vs. immediate RT
High-grade glioma	Complete pre-RT chemo (Phase II); Radiosensitizers (Phase I/II); Evaluate efficacy of post RT high-dose chemo with PSCR vs. standard chemo (Phase III); Phase III randomized evaluation of efficacy of temozolomide and thalidomide	Pre-RT chemo (Phase II); dose escalation RT (Phase I/II); Phase III, as CCG	Pre-RT thiotepa (Phase II)
Brain stem glioma	Concurrent RT plus radiosensitizers (Phase I/II)	Pre-RT chemo (Phase II)	Per national study groups
Ependymoma	Pre-RT chemo in partially resected (Phase II); Natural history in totally resected; utility of second-look surgery	As CCG, for second-look surgery	Per national study groups
Low-grade glioma	Two different chemos in children younger than 10 y (Phase III); ? In older children	Evaluate cyclophospha-mide prior to other chemo (Phase II) in children younger than 10 y; ? in older children	Evaluate carboplatin and vincristine in young children (Phase II); observation arm for totally resected patients; ? in older children
Malignant tumors in infants	Dose intensification of chemo with PSCR (Phase I/II); ? role of RT (local)	Randomized (Phase III) of two chemo regimens; ? role of RT (local)	Intensive pre-RT chemo (Phase II); ? role of RT
Germ cell	Under discussion	Under discussion	Feasibility study

RT, radiation therapy; CCG, Children's Cancer Group; POG, Pediatric Oncology Group; SIOP, International Society Pediatric Oncology.

prognostic factors for children with posterior fossa primitive neuroectodermal tumors (medulloblastomas) and led to the general separation of patients with such tumors into two risk groups: (1) average-risk patients, who had medulloblastomas that were localized and were extensively resected at the time of diagnosis; and (2) poor-risk patients, who harbored medulloblastomas that had disseminated throughout the leptomeninges at diagnosis or were amenable only to subtotal resection. Subsequent studies have not dramatically clarified these risk groups.[6, 11] *Extent of dissemination remains the single most predictive factor of outcome, whereas other factors,* *such as brain stem involvement and extent of resection, have been shown to be of less predictive importance when the degree of dissemination is taken into account.* The first generation of CCG and SIOP studies also demonstrated for the first time that chemotherapy had a role in the management of medulloblastoma; as in patients with poor-risk disease, the addition of lomustine (CCNU) and vincristine chemotherapy (with or without prednisone) resulted in improved 5-year, disease-free survival. However, for patients with average-risk disease, the addition of chemotherapy did not clearly improve outcome.

Based on these findings, studies performed by the major cooperative groups focused on the intensification of chemotherapy for children with poor-risk disease, whereas, due to concerns over treatment-related sequelae, the major cooperative groups mounted studies that reduced the amount of craniospinal irradiation in patients with nondisseminated disease at the time of diagnosis.

For patients with poor-risk disease, the CCG completed a study in the late 1980s and early 1990s that randomized patients between treatment with craniospinal radiation therapy and either adjuvant CCNU and vincristine chemotherapy during and after radiotherapy, or adjuvant treatment with pre- and postirradiation 8-drugs-in-1-day therapy. This study once again demonstrated the utility of separation of patients into risk categories based on the extent of dissemination at the time of diagnosis and found that for the patients with localized disease the extent of tumor resection was an independent predictive parameter of outcome.[7] Nonposterior fossa primitive neuroectodermal tumors were found to have a poorer prognosis than posterior fossa tumors. However, the use of preirradiation and postirradiation 8-in-1 chemotherapy resulted in poorer overall disease control than treatment with CCNU and vincristine during and after irradiation. A SIOP study performed during the same time period that compared outcome in patients receiving both preirradiation and postirradiation chemotherapy or those receiving postirradiation chemotherapy could not demonstrate a difference in survival for patients who received preirradiation chemotherapy.[12] Although these results are somewhat disappointing, questions were raised concerning the choice of preirradiation chemotherapy, as the drug regimens utilized by both CCG and SIOP were of relatively low intensity, in comparison with other potential drug therapies. POG has attempted to address the issue of whether preirradiation chemotherapy improved the clinical course for children with high-risk medulloblastoma by mounting a study comparing patients treated with preirradiation chemotherapy utilizing cisplatin and etoposide (VP-16) followed by radiation therapy and chemotherapy with patients treated similarly except for the deletion of preirradiation chemotherapy. This study, performed in the early 1990s, was closed for study accrual in March 1996, and information concerning efficacy of treatment is still being analyzed.

More recently, CCG took a somewhat more aggressive approach by piloting the use of high-dose chemotherapy prior to hyperfractionated craniospinal and local radiation therapy for children with poor-risk medulloblastoma.[13] In this study, a four-drug combination of cyclophosphamide, vincristine, VP-16, and cisplatin was alternated with carboplatin and VP-16 for five cycles prior to the initiation of radiotherapy. This study also was closed and is being analyzed. Preliminary results suggest that there may be difficulties with this approach, as nearly 40% of patients had to begin radiation therapy earlier than planned due to excessive toxicity or treatment failure.

Studies in Europe, performed primarily by the German Pediatric Oncology Group, have also attempted to determine the efficacy of more aggressive preirradiation chemotherapy by comparing treatment of children with high-risk medulloblastoma and non–posterior fossa primitive neuroectodermal tumors with either (1) craniospinal irradiation plus CCNU, vincristine, and cisplatinum chemotherapy during

vincristine administration and after irradiation; or (2) intensive preirradiation chemotherapy utilizing ifosfamide, VP-16, methotrexate, cisplatin, and cytosine arabinoside, followed by craniospital radiotherapy. This study has been closed and results are being analyzed.

Future directions for children with high-risk medulloblastoma and non–posterior fossa primitive neuroectodermal tumors are partially dependent on the final analysis of the studies performed to date. The usefulness of preirradiation chemotherapy approaches is still open to debate, and such treatment cannot be recommended until one of the completed studies shows an overall benefit in survival, with tolerable toxicity. In the interim, CCG is exploring two alternative means to improve survival for children with high-risk disease. The first is the use of potentially more effective chemotherapy (carboplatin) concomitantly with radiation therapy, with the added goal of evaluating carboplatin as a radiosensitizer. The second is the utilization of high-dose chemotherapy, with peripheral stem cell rescue, following radiation therapy.

As regards the treatment of children with nondisseminated medulloblastoma, studies performed by the cooperative groups have not demonstrated unequivocally that chemotherapy improves survival. CCG and POG collaborated on a study of children with nondisseminated disease that compared outcome in those treated with conventional doses of craniospinal radiation (3600 cGy) with outcome in those receiving reduced-dose craniospinal radiation (2400 cGy).[14] In this randomized trial, chemotherapy was not given. *The study was closed prior to the expected closure date, as interim analysis disclosed a poorer disease-free survival rate and a higher rate of isolated neuraxis relapses in patients who had received a reduced dose of craniospinal radiation.* Unfortunately, the number of patients entered in this study was somewhat lower than trial design, and follow-up at 5 to 6 years has shown a questionable difference in overall survival between the two treatment arms at the $p = 0.058$ level.

A cooperative group study performed by SIOP utilizing four arms, including two receiving preirradiation chemotherapy, did not demonstrate a difference in overall survival between those patients receiving reduced doses compared with conventional doses of craniospinal radiation.[15] In this trial, the only arm that performed poorly was the study group receiving chemotherapy followed by reduced-dose craniospinal radiotherapy. It was believed that this arm fared less well because of the use of an ineffective preirradiation chemotherapy regimen. In an attempt to address the question of whether the use of preirradiation chemotherapy resulted in poorer overall survival, the UKCCSG, on behalf of SIOP, coordinated a multicenter trial for patients with nonmetastatic medulloblastoma that randomized patients either to immediate craniospinal radiotherapy (3600 cGy) or to chemotherapy with vincristine, carboplatin, and cyclophosphamide for 70 days before commencing radiotherapy at day 100.[16] Although this is a randomized trial, patients who were treated as per one of the two protocol arms, but not randomized, were followed. The study is still accruing patients and as of August 1997, 208 patients had been treated but only 144 randomized. There was no apparent difference between the two therapies at a median follow-up of 17 months.

While these studies have been analyzed, a pilot study was completed by the CCG utilizing 2400 cGy of craniospinal irradiation, a standard local dose of posterior fossal irradiation (5580 cGy), and adjuvant CCNU, vincristine, and cisplatin chemotherapy during and after radiotherapy.[17] At 3 years, the progression-free survival in 68 children between the ages of 3 and 10 treated with this approach was approximately 80%.

In the mid-1990s, an attempt was made by CCG and POG to mount a trial comparing full-dose craniospinal radiotherapy (3600 cGy) to reduced-dose craniospinal radiotherapy (2400 cGy), plus CCNU, vincristine, and cisplatin chemotherapy for children with nondisseminated posterior fossa primitive neuroectodermal tumors. This study was closed after 18 months due to poor accrual rates. A variety of factors were responsible for the poor accrual rates, including the reluctance of some physicians to enter patients in a trial not utilizing chemotherapy; concern about the use of full-dose radiotherapy in young children; and the lack of data to support the benefits and safety of reducing radiotherapy in children older than 10 years at diagnosis. In 1996, a new study was begun by CCG and POG that essentially accepted 2400 cGy as the standard craniospinal dose for children with nondisseminated medulloblastoma. This study is utilizing 2400 cGy of craniospinal irradiation, 5580 cGy of local radiation therapy, and one of two chemotherapeutic arms (CCNU, vincristine, and cisplatin, or CCNU, vincristine, and cyclophosphamide) in an attempt to determine which chemotherapeutic approach utilized during (vincristine) and after radiotherapy results in a better overall rate of survival and less toxicity. This trial was also designed to determine the long-term sequelae of such an approach on a variety of parameters, including neuropsychological function and endocrinologic status.

The randomized, prospective study is targeted for completion by the end of 2000 or early 2001. Discussions are underway concerning the next approach for children with nondisseminated medulloblastomas, while the data on the 2400 cGy of craniospinal irradiation therapy plus one of two chemotherapy arms are being analyzed. An approach under serious consideration is a Phase III randomized evaluation of the safety and efficacy of reducing the volume of radiation delivered to the posterior fossa. An alternative approach is to attempt to reduce the dose of craniospinal radiation.

An important aspect of this intergroup study is the focused biologic investigation. It is clear that current means of stratification of patients with medulloblastoma are suboptimal, as some patients with average-risk disease will develop early treatment failure, often with associated leptomeningeal disease spread. The neurobiologic factors underlying these differences are poorly understood, thus highlighting the need for biologic studies in a large number of patients.

High-Grade Gliomas

The role of cooperative groups in the management of high-grade gliomas has been less prominent than that for medulloblastomas. Given the smaller relative numbers of patients available for study and the poorer overall survival in studies that have been completed, randomized Phase III studies have been difficult to mount. In the mid- to late 1970s, CCG completed a study in a relatively small number of patients that suggested that the addition of CCNU and vincristine

chemotherapy to standard radiotherapy, as compared with treatment with standard radiotherapy alone, improved the overall rate of survival for children with glioblastoma multiforme.[18] This study has been criticized because of its relatively low accrual rate, the inclusion of "aggressive" low-grade glioma patients on protocol, the changes in neuropathologic classification of these tumors, and the seemingly high overall survival rate (approximately 40% at 5 years) for patients with glioblastoma multiforme. *A recent reassessment of these data, including neuropathologic re-review, still substantiates that the addition of CCNU and vincristine chemotherapy, albeit in a very small group of patients with glioblastoma multiforme, results in a better overall survival rate than treatment with radiation therapy alone.* In a subsequent study, the CCG compared preirradiation and postirradiation 8-in-1 chemotherapy with treatment with radiation therapy plus CCNU and vincristine chemotherapy for children with anaplastic glioma and glioblastoma multiforme.[19] In this study, there was no survival advantage for the more aggressive pre- and postirradiation chemotherapy approach. This study demonstrated that extent of resection is an important predictor of outcome, as patients with totally resected tumors fared better than those with subtotally resected lesions.

Because of the limited proven treatment alternatives for patients with malignant gliomas, CCG, POG, and SIOP have decided not to exclusively pursue randomized Phase III studies at this time. A phase III randomized trial is being planned to evaluate the efficacy of temozolomide and thalidomide in children with newly diagnosed high-grade gliomas. The groups are also performing pilot protocols in attempts to define more effective means of treatment. CCG has recently completed a study evaluating couplets of high-dose chemotherapeutic agents prior to irradiation in an attempt to identify more effective agents that later can be incorporated into Phase III trials. The UKCCSG, on behalf of SIOP, is performing a study evaluating 7-day thiotepa administration prior to irradiation. POG is also performing preirradiation chemotherapy studies. At the same time, the POG is evaluating the efficacy of dose escalation of hyperfractionated irradiation therapy for children with supratentorial malignant gliomas. The CCG, after its current preirradiation studies have been completed, will pursue a somewhat different direction; it is planning to use agents, including chemotherapeutic agents, concurrently with radiotherapy in an effort both to increase the efficacy of radiation therapy and to take advantage of the antineoplastic properties of the agents chosen. Presently, a trial utilizing topotecan during radiotherapy is being finalized.

Recent studies have suggested that high-dose chemotherapy, especially with a thiotepa-based regimen, has some efficacy in children with recurrent high-grade gliomas. In one study, performed partially in collaboration with CCG by Finlay and co-workers, 28% of patients with recurrent high-grade gliomas were long-term survivors after treatment with a thiotepa-based myeloablative chemotherapy protocol and autologous bone marrow rescue.[20] This type of approach, utilized prior to radiotherapy, was attempted on a group basis by the CCG but was closed due to unacceptable toxicity after the first 10 patients were treated. The CCG plans to mount a study evaluating the efficacy of high-dose chemotherapy, as consolidation therapy, for children with malignant gliomas. In this study, all patients who are treated with radiation or with radiation and chemotherapy either prior to or during irradiation will be randomized to treatment with either standard CCNU and vincristine chemotherapy or high-dose chemotherapy utilizing a thiotepa-based regimen and peripheral stem cell rescue. In only this way can the true utility of high-dose chemotherapy be determined for children with malignant glioma.

Similarly to the approaches taken for children with medulloblastoma, specimens from patients entered on both POG and CCG studies are being sent to centralized resource laboratories for extensive neurobiologic study.

Brain Stem Gliomas

The treatment of patients with brain stem gliomas has been extremely frustrating, as there is little evidence that any treatment other than conventional radiotherapy is even of transient benefit. Both CCG and POG studied the possible efficacy of hyperfractionated radiation therapy. Dose escalation studies, with doses as high as 7800 cGy, did not demonstrate improved efficacy as compared with historical series of patients treated with standard radiation alone.[21–23] The addition of β-interferon to radiotherapy also did not improve outcome in newly diagnosed patients.[24] A POG study, comparing outcome in children treated with either conventional or hyperfractionated radiation therapy and cisplatin chemotherapy as a radiosensitizer, has been completed for children with brain stem gliomas in an attempt to determine once and for all whether hyperfractionated radiation therapy is of benefit.

Future approaches to management of this disease are problematic. POG is planning to evaluate a series of drugs given prior to irradiation in order to identify better agents for use in patients with newly diagnosed disease. CCG completed a study evaluating couplets of high-dose chemotherapy agents given prior to radiotherapy that did not demonstrate a significant objective response rate. For this reason, before attempting to mount a large randomized trial, CCG will pursue a series of pilot studies evaluating the toxicity and potential efficacy of chemotherapeutic agents and other agents administered during radiation therapy to serve as radiosensitizers and independent antineoplastic agents. Because the use of high-dose chemotherapy at the time of disease relapse or prior to radiation therapy, with or without peripheral stem rescue or autologous bone marrow rescue, has not shown any clear-cut efficacy, CCG will not pursue this approach in children with newly diagnosed brain stem glioma.

Ependymomas

Management of ependymomas also remains problematic. *Single-institution trials have demonstrated that patients with totally resected ependymomas have a better prognosis than those with partially resected disease.* In the one cooperative group trial performed by the CCG, the addition of CCNU and vincristine chemotherapy during and following radiation therapy was not more effective than radiation therapy alone for patients with ependymomas.[25] Single-institution trials have demonstrated that local radiotherapy seems to be as effective as craniospinal plus local radiotherapy in patients with ependymomas.

Based on these results, Phase III trials have been difficult to mount for children with ependymomas. The POG performed a study of surgery and radiation therapy between 1985 and 1990, indicating the benefit of complete resection and demonstrating a low rate of neuraxis dissemination following limited volume irradiation in posteror fossa ependymomas. A second study, conducted between 1991 and 1994, evaluated hyperfractionated irradiation for posterior fossa ependymomas. Preliminary analysis shows no apparent increase in tumor control with high-dose hyperfractionated irradiation; a low but significant proportion of patients had neuraxis dissemination at initial failure. This study is still under analysis. POG is presently pursuing a study in which all patients with totally resected ependymomas, are being registered and observed after treatment with local radiation therapy. Patients with partially resected tumors are treated with two cycles of preirradiation chemotherapy followed by a standard dose (5580 cGy) of localized radiation to the tumor site and more chemotherapy. For those patients with initially partially resected tumors, a second attempt at total tumor resection is an integral part of the protocol, as after the first two cycles of chemotherapies all patients are to be re-evaluated for the possibility of surgical re-resection.

Malignant Tumors in Infants

Over the past decade, all cooperative groups have agreed that alternative treatment approaches are needed for infants with malignant tumors. These tumors are rare and standard treatment, especially with craniospinal irradiation, results in unacceptable long-term sequelae as a result of the proclivity of such tumors to disseminate in the nervous system. Based on the innovative ground-breaking studies of van Eyes and co-workers at MD Anderson, which demonstrated long-term survival after MOPP (meclorethamine, vincristine, procarbazine, and prednisone) chemotherapy in nearly half of a small group of children with medulloblastoma, studies have been performed by all of the major cooperative groups to evaluate the efficacy of chemotherapy for children, younger than 3 years, with malignant tumors.[26]

POG performed studies in the late 1980s utilizing the four-drug regimen of cisplatin, CCNU, vincristine, and VP-16.[27] These studies demonstrated that a subgroup of children could be treated with chemotherapy alone for 2 years or until age 3. In this study, all patients went on to receive radiation at the completion of chemotherapy or at age 3, so that the long-term benefits of chemotherapy as a sole treatment approach could not be evaluated. A somewhat different approach, utilizing the 8-in-1-day regimen, was used by CCG in that after chemotherapy patients with no evidence of residual disease were not given chemotherapy.[28] The 8-in-1-day therapy approach may have resulted in a slightly lower overall short-term disease control rate than the POG four-drug regimen, but direct comparison is difficult.

Presently, CCG, POG, and different study groups within SIOP are involved in protocols utilizing intensified preradiation chemotherapy, with or without radiation therapy, for children with malignant glioma. CCG has recently completed a randomized Phase II study comparing an intensified cyclophosphamide, VP-16, cisplatin, and vincristine approach to an ifosfamide, carboplatinum, VP-16, and vincristine drug regimen. A study just begun by CCG is utilizing an even more intensified treatment approach, incorporating thiotepa and peripheral stem cell rescue, for children younger than 3 years with malignant tumor. In both of these studies, patients who had a complete response to chemotherapy or maintained no evidence of residual disease after surgery received maintenance chemotherapy, but not radiotherapy, after chemotherapy. POG attempted to intensify their four-drug regimen by the use of a brief window of thiotepa prior to the four-drug regimen. This study was halted due to an excessive rate of disease progression prior to beginning the four-drug regimen. POG is presently involved in a randomized trial comparing their initial drug regimen to a similar regimen with intensified cyclophosphamide. In this newer study, patients without residual disease at the end of chemotherapy will not go on to receive radiation. The SIOP groups have investigated a variety of different chemotherapeutic agents for infants with malignant tumor. The UKCCSG is presently coordinating a study utilizing vincristine, carboplatin, methotrexate, cyclophosphamide, and cisplatin for children younger than 3 years with malignant brain tumor. To date, 99 patients have been entered in this study and the study remains open. However, the study was recently closed for children with primitive neuroectodermal tumors.[16] Of the 36 children with primitive neuroectodermal tumors (including medulloblastoma) entered in the study, 31 had metastatic disease at the time of diagnosis, and all progressed during treatment.

The largest European experience has been that of the German Pediatric Brain Tumor Study Group, which has used a combination of cyclophosphamide, vincristine, intravenous methotrexate, intraventricular methotrexate, carboplatin, and VP-16. Preliminary results with this regimen have been encouraging, as the majority of patients remained free of progressive disease after treatment with chemotherapy alone (irradiation is not a standard part of this treatment). However, those patients with leptomeningeal disease at the time of diagnosis had a much poorer overall rate of disease control.

A major issue for all of the cooperative groups, given that chemotherapy seems to benefit only a subgroup of patients with malignant tumors, is how to further improve survival. Recent studies have suggested that for patients with localized disease, focal radiation therapy may result in improved disease control. All groups are looking into the possibility of reintroducing focal radiation therapy in patients with localized disease at the time of diagnosis. It is becoming increasingly recognized that malignant infant tumors are even more histologically and biologically heterogeneous than once believed. There are some tumors, such as atypical teratoid tumors, that carry a horrendous prognosis independent of the type of treatment given. New neurobiologic insights are desperately needed for infants with malignant brain tumors, and both CCG and POG studies have incorporated intensive neurobiologic components into their management protocols.

Low-Grade Gliomas

The development of treatment guidelines for patients with low-grade gliomas has been extremely frustrating. More than any other pediatric brain tumor, these tumors have been historically primarily treated by neurosurgeons, who then decide whether patients are candidates, after surgery, for irradiation, another form of treatment, or observation. Although, in toto, low-grade gliomas are the most common form of childhood brain tumor, they can arise in many different areas within the nervous system, and optimal treatment requires individualization for tumor location, histology, degree of resection, and the age of the patient. Until recently, other than handling registration of patients for demographic reasons, the large cooperative groups had not been involved in the development of protocols for patients with low-grade gliomas.

In the mid-1980s, POG and CCG performed an intergroup study attempting to determine the efficacy of radiotherapy in children with partially resected low-grade gliomas. In this protocol, all patients with totally resected tumors were to be entered in the study and followed. Those patients with partially resected tumors were to be randomized to either immediate treatment with local radiation therapy or observation. After 2 years, the randomized portion of the study was closed due to poor patient accrual. Despite very little information confirming the efficacy or lack of efficacy of radiotherapy, biases were so strong that patients could not be entered in the randomized trial. The natural history arm of the study accrued patients extremely well, and over a 5-year period of accrual more than 700 patients were entered in the study. This information is being analyzed.

Over the past two decades, there has been increased interest in the possible use of chemotherapy for children with low-grade tumors, especially deep infiltrative tumors in very young children.[29] *Single-institution investigations and multi-institutional trials have demonstrated that drugs or drug combinations, such as actinomycin D and vincristine, carboplatin alone, carboplatin and vincristine, and a five-drug nitrosourea-based regimen, controlled progressive disease for some patients with low-grade gliomas.* The largest multi-institutional trial to date, performed by Packer and co-workers, reported an objective tumor shrinkage rate of approximately 60% in 78 children with low-grade tumors and a 3-year, progression-free survival rate of nearly 70%.[30] Based on such information, the cooperative groups are now attempting to study the efficacy of chemotherapy for young children with low-grade glioma. CCG is involved in a study randomizing all children younger than 10 years with progressive, newly diagnosed, low-grade glioma (who have not received previous radiation therapy) to treatment with either a carboplatin and vincristine drug regimen or the five-drug University of California–San Francisco drug regimen, which includes CCNU, vincristine, procarbazine, DBD, and 6-thioguinine. The POG group has added two cycles of high-dose cyclophosphamide, prior to carboplatin and vincristine, in an attempt to determine the response rate of low-grade gliomas to high-dose cyclophosphamide and to determine whether addition of this drug improves long-term disease control. However, the study utilizing high-dose cyclophosphamide was halted because of an excessive rate of disease progression after treatment with two doses of the high-dose cyclophosphamide. The Pediatric Oncology Group has recently joined the Children's Cancer Group in the randomized study.

Study groups throughout Europe are also beginning to investigate the role of chemotherapy in low-grade glioma. At this point, there is no uniform consensus within these study groups over which study to pursue, but a partial group study is under way that is observing patients after total resection and treating those with progressive disease with carboplatin and vincristine. This is being studied by the Italian, German, and United Kingdom strategy groups.

Germ Cell Tumors

Germinomas and other nongerminomatous germ cell tumors of the CNS are a heterogeneous group of tumors that have been evaluated primarily by single-institution and small multi-institutional studies. Due to results of these studies suggesting that intracranial germ cell tumors are responsive to chemotherapy, but possibly slightly less so than non-CNS histologically identical tumors, and the relative rarity of such lesions, it has become evident that large studies are required to determine the role of chemotherapy for germinomas or other nongerminomatous tumors. The majority of trials on germ cell tumors have been published by single institutions in Japan and Japanese cooperative groups. Recently, a multi-institutional international study was organized in an effort to avoid irradiation in germinomas and nongerminomatous germ cell tumors by the use of high-dose combination chemotherapy.[31] This study was only partially successful and this strategy is being reassessed. POG has opened a protocol attempting to determine the feasibility of carrying out a groupwide germinoma trial and to determine the response of germinomas and mixed germ cell tumors to preirradiation chemotherapy utilizing cisplatin and VP-16 in alternation with cylophosphamide and vincristine. This study is also attempting to evaluate the pattern of failure after chemotherapy and radiation therapy. SIOP is planning a study that will treat all secreting intracranial germ cell tumors with pre-irradiation cisplatin, VP-16, and ifosfamide followed by local-field (5400 cGy) radiotherapy for children with nondisseminated disease.

Given the small numbers of patients available for study and the histologic heterogeneity of germ cell tumors, evaluation of these types of studies is expected to be extremely difficult.

Recurrent Disease

CCG and the POG have been actively evaluating a variety of approaches for children with recurrent primary CNS tumors. Both groups are evaluating the potential efficacy of high-dose chemotherapy at time of recurrence, supplemented with either autologous bone marrow rescue or peripheral stem cell rescue, in children with malignant tumors. The groups have taken the lead in evaluating a variety of new agents, in a Phase II setting, for patients with recurrent disease. Drugs such as ifosfamide alone, ifosfamide with VP-16 and vincristine, carboplatin, taxol, fazarabine, topotecan, and temozolomide have either been studied by the cooperative groups or will soon be studied.

In patients with recurrent disease, the efforts of the cooperative groups have been greatly aided by single-institution and small multi-institutional trials. An NCI working group has been actively involved in the evaluation of innovative agents for patients with recurrent disease. If preliminary results suggest efficacy, larger Phase II trials are pursued either in concert with one of both cooperative groups or in

NCI-centered, smaller, multi-institutional groups. Multi-institutional trials, often with drug company support, have been mounted for children with recurrent disease using immunologic agents, new chemotherapeutic agents, new anti–growth factor agents, and gene therapy. The cooperative groups are increasingly working with the pharmaceutical and research companies exploring new biologic approaches for children with recurrent tumors.

SUMMARY

As can be concluded from the above review, the cooperative groups, such as CCG, POG and SIOP, have played an important role in the evaluation of new treatments for children with brain tumors. The groups are extremely effective in determining the efficacy of a particular approach in a Phase III setting. Recently, they have become more involved in primary CNS tumors other than medulloblastoma, brain stem glioma, or high-grade glioma. The fact that the cooperative groups have an extremely important role does not supersede the need for single-institution or smaller multi-institutional studies to gather pilot data for testing in larger group settings. The PBTC may be an important mechanism for expeditiously obtaining pilot information on new means of treatment for childhood brain tumors. In addition, the cooperative groups have recently agreed on the need of resource laboratories dealing with childhood brain tumors to investigate the neurobiologic underpinnings of childhood brain tumors and facilitate translational research for these tumors.

REFERENCES

1. Bleyer WA. The US pediatric cancer clinical trials programmes: international implications and the way forward. *Eur J Cancer* 1997;33:1439–1447.
2. Murphy SB. The national impact of clinical cooperative group trials for pediatric cancer. *Med Pediatr Oncol* 1995;24:279–280.
3. Korn EL, Midthune D, Chen TT, et al. A comparison of two phase I trial designs. *Stat Med* 1994;13:1799–1806.
4. Chang MN, Therneau TM, Wieand HS, Cha SS. Designs for group sequential phase II clinical trials. *Biometrics* 1987;43:865–874.
5. Simon R. Size of phase III cancer clinical trials. *Cancer Treat Rep* 1985;69(10):1087–1093.
6. Evans AE, Jenkin RDT, Sposto R, et al. The treatment of medulloblastoma: results of a prospective randomized trial of radiation therapy with and without CCNU, vincristine, and prednisone. *J Neurosurg* 1990;72(4):572–582.
7. Zeltzer P, Boyett J, Finlay JL, et al. Tumor staging at diagnosis and therapy type for primitive neuroectodermal tumors (PNET) determine survival: report from Children's Cancer Study CCG-921. In SIOP XXVII. 1995.
8. Pocock SJ. Interim analyses for randomized clinical trials: the group sequential approach. *Biometrics* 1982;38(1):153–162.

9. Sposto R and Stram DO. A strategic view of randomized trial design in low-incidence cancer. *Stat Med* 1999 (in review).

10. Packer RJ, Boyett JM, Zimmerman RA, et al. Outcome of children with brain stem gliomas after treatment with 7800 cGy of hyperfractionated radiotherapy: a Children's Cancer Group Phase I/II trial. *Cancer* 1994;74(6):1827–1834.

11. Tait DM, Thorton-Jones H, Bloom HJG, et al. Adjuvant chemotherapy for medulloblastoma: the first multicenter control trial of the International Society of Pediatric Oncology (SIOP I). *Eur J Cancer* 1990;26:464–469.

12. Bailey CC, Gnekow A, Welleck S, et al. Prospective randomized trial of chemotherapy given before radiotherapy in childhood medulloblastoma. International Society of Pediatric Oncology (SIOP) and the (German) Society of Pediatric Oncology (GPO): SIOP II. *Med Pediatr Oncol* 1995;25:166–178.

13. Packer RJ, Allen JC, Geyer F, et al. Childhood primitive neuroectodermal tumors/medulloblastoma: treatment directions of the Children's Cancer Group. *Ann Neurol* 1997;42:536.

14. Deutsch M, Thomas PRM, Krischer J, et al. Results of a prospective randomized trial comparing standard dose neuraxis irradiation (3,600 cGy/20) with reduced neuraxis irradiation (2,340 cGy/13) in patients with low-stage medulloblastoma: a combined Children's Cancer Group–Pediatric Oncology Group study. *Pediatr Neurosurg* 1996; 24:167–177.

15. Bailey CC, Gnekow A, Wellek S, et al. Prospective randomised trial of chemotherapy given before radiotherapy in childhood medulloblastoma. International Society of Paediatric Oncology (SIOP) and the (German) Society of Paediatric Oncology (GPO): SIOP II. *Med Pediatr Oncol* 1995;25:166–178.

16. Bailey CC, Imeson J, Robinson K, et al. Randomized clinical trial of pre-radiotherapy chemotherapy vs. radiotherapy alone for medulloblastoma (PNET III). *J Neuro-oncol* 1997;35:554.

17. Packer RJ, Goldwein JW, Boyett J, el al. Early results of reduced-dose radiotherapy plus chemotherapy for children with non-disseminated medulloblastoma (MB): a Children's Cancer Group study. *Ann Neurol* 1995;38:518.

18. Sposto R, Ertel IM, Jenkin RDT, et al. The effectiveness of chemotherapy for treatment of high-grade astrocytoma in children: results of a randomized trial. *J Neuro-oncol* 1989;7:165–177.

19. Finlay J, Boyett J, Yates A, et al. Randomized phase III trial in childhood high-grade astrocytoma comparing vincristine, lomustine and prednisone with eight-drug-in-1 day regimen. *J Clin Oncol* 1995;13:112–123.

20. Finlay JL, Goldman S, Wong MC, et al. Pilot study of high-dose thiotepa and etoposide with autologous bone marrow rescue in children and young adults with recurrent CNS tumors. *J Clin Oncol* 1996;14:2495–2503.

21. Freeman CR, Krischner JP, Sanford A, et al. Final results of a study of escalating doses of hyperfractionated radiotherapy in brain stem tumors in children: a Pediatric Oncology Group study. *Rad Oncol Biol Phys* 1993; 27:197–206.

22. Packer RJ, Boyett JM, Zimmerman RA, et al. Hyperfractionated radiation therapy (72 Gy) for children with brain stem gliomas: a Children's Cancer Group Phase I/II trial. *Cancer* 1993;72(4):1414–1421.

23. Packer RJ, Boyett JM, Zimmerman et al. Brain stem gliomas of childhood: outcome after treatment with 7800 cGy of hyperfractionated radiotherapy: a Children's Cancer Group Phase I/II trial. *Cancer* 1994;74: 1827–1834.

24. Packer RJ, Prados M, Phillips P, et al: Treatment of children with newly diagnosed brain stem gliomas with intravenous recombinant-interferon and hyperfractionated radiation therapy: a Children's Cancer Group Phase I/II study. *Cancer* 1996;77(10):2150–2156.

25. Lefkowitz I, Evans A, Sposto R, et al. Adjuvant chemotherapy of childhood posterior fossa (PF) ependymoma: craniospinal radiation with or without CCNU, vincristine (VCR) and prednisone (P). *Proc Am Soc Clin Oncol* 1989; 8:87.

26. Van Eys J, Cangir A, Coody D, Smith B. MOPP regimen as primary chemotherapy for brain tumors in infants. *J Neuro-oncol* 1985;3:237.

27. Duffner PK, Horowitz M, Krischer J, et al. Postoperative chemotherapy and delayed radiotherapy in children less than 3 years of age with malignant brain tumors. *N Engl J Med* 1993;328:1725–1731.

28. Geyer JR, Zeltzer PM, Boyett JM, et al. Survival of infants with primitive neuroectodermal tumors or malignant ependymomas of the CNS treated with eight drugs in 1 day: a report from the Children's Cancer Group. *J Clin Oncol* 1994;12:1607–1615.

29. Packer RJ, Lange B, Ater J, et al. Carboplatin and vincristine for recurrent and newly diagnosed low-grade gliomas of childhood *J Clin Oncol* 1993;11:850–856.

30. Packer RJ, Ater J, Allen J, et al. Carboplatin and vincristine chemotherapy for children with newly diagnosed progressive low-grade gliomas. *J Neurosurg* 1997;86:747–754.

31. Balmaceda C, Heller G, Rosenblum M, et al. Chemotherapy without irradiation—a novel approach for newly-diagnosed CNS germ cell tumors: results of an international cooperative trial. *J Clin Oncol* 1996;14:2908–2915.

Chapter 38

Chemosensitivity Testing

Paul L. Kornblith and Dennis R. Burholt

Primary CNS tumors have posed a formidable therapeutic challenge that has yet to be fully overcome. Advances in surgical techniques, radiotherapy, and chemotherapy have made significant improvements possible. Most often, effective therapy involves a combined-modality approach.[1-3] In the multimodality treatment approach, the choice of chemotherapeutic agents is based on clinical trials. Even following this extensive experience, the success rate for chemotherapeutic agent–based protocols often is low.[4-6] In vitro–based chemosensitivity protocols have been developed with the rationale of planning treatment management on an individual patient basis. For the patient with a malignant tumor, knowing the cellular basis of treatment response can be an important factor influencing the choice of therapy. The refinement of chemotherapy for human brain tumors will provide momentum for the adopting of individualized chemotherapy testing to identify those agents most likely to produce a clinical response. The use of individualized chemosensitivity testing will also identify those patients who will not respond to chemotherapy and spare them the systemic toxicity of agents to which their tumors will most probably be resistant.

Brain tumors are the leading form of cancer in children, affecting 33 children per million per year.[7] Modern surgical techniques, pediatric intensive care techniques, and radiation therapy have substantially increased survival in children with brain tumors.[8-10] As new chemotherapeutic agents are identified that are effective against brain tumors and new methods of drug delivery become available to overcome the problem of the blood-brain barrier, the therapeutic choices for brain tumor patients will increase. A more directed approach for selecting among chemotherapeutic agents shown to be effective in at least a percentage of the brain tumor population may be afforded by the use of in vitro chemosensitivity testing.

In this chapter, we briefly examine the role of chemo-therapy in the management of pediatric brain tumors, review the use of chemosensitivity testing for the direction of treatment for brain tumor patients, describe a tissue culture–based chemosensitivity assay for the assessment of tumor cell response, and give examples of the use of the tissue culture–based assay in pediatric brain tumor specimens.

USE OF CHEMOTHERAPY FOR PEDIATRIC BRAIN TUMORS

The number and types of chemotherapeutic agents administered in the treatment of primary CNS tumors has increased substantially in recent years (e.g., refs. 11, 12). In addition to the traditional treatment modalities for brain tumors, a number of innovative therapeutic approaches are now becoming available. These include adoptive immunotherapy, antisense oligonucleotide therapy, gene insertion, and use of differentiating agents. The selection of chemotherapeutic drugs for the treatment of primary brain tumors is largely based on the agent's capacity to cross the blood-brain barrier. To date, this approach in adults has not yielded significant survival prolongation following surgery for high-grade astrocytomas and has not added substantially to radiation therapy in this patient population. However, these agents appear to hold promise in the treatment of pediatric brain tumors. In addition, the identification of new agents and those used for other histologic tumor types, as well as improved methods of drug delivery, have increased the success rate of chemotherapy in the pediatric brain tumor population.

BOX 38–1
New Therapies

- **Immunotherapy**
- **Antisense oligonucleotides**
- **Gene therapy**
- **Differentiating agents**

Until recently, surgery and radiation therapy were the major treatment modalities for childhood brain tumors. However, the use of radiation therapy for childhood brain tumor control has often been associated with untoward sequelae.[13] Radiation-induced neurologic toxicity in the developing child has led to a number of protocols in which adjuvant postsurgical chemotherapy is administered prior to radiation therapy.[14-19] In these protocols, irradiation is often delayed in

The laboratory work presented in this chapter was performed at Precision Therapeutics, Inc., Pittsburgh, PA. No patient identifiers are presented with the data.

the infant population for up to 2 years following surgery and chemotherapy. The potential benefits of delayed irradiation for infants include reduction of late effects, particularly cognitive- and endocrine-related toxicity.

The number of agents being used for the treatment of childhood brain tumors has been expanding continuously (for a review, see 18). Currently, a number of agents other than those historically used for treatment of CNS malignancies [such as carmustine (BCNU), lomustine (CCNU), procarbazine, and vincristine] are in clinical trials. These include cyclophosphamide,[20–22] carboplatin,[23, 24] topotecan,[25, 26] thiotepa,[21] and methotrexate.[24] These agents are often administered in high doses with stem cell support[20–22] or with osmotic disruption of the blood-brain barrier.[24, 27]

CHEMOSENSITIVITY TESTING FOR BRAIN TUMORS

All chemosensitivity assays have four distinct phases.[28, 29] (1) The initial stage is the acquisition and preparation of the tissue. This involves the preparation of the tissue by either mechanical separation or enzymatic digestion of cells. The cells from the tumor specimen are then placed into tissue culture. (2) The next phase of the assay is exposure of the tumor cells to chemotherapeutic agents. The length of drug exposure for a variety of types of chemosensitivity assays varies from acute (1 to 2 hours), to intermediate (4 to 24 hours), to long term (2 to 4 days). The relationship between drug levels attained in vivo following standard clinical doses of an agent and those administered in vitro must be considered. In vitro drug concentration ranges need to be established that bracket the levels reasonably expected to be reached clinically, with a sufficient margin to take into account the individual variations in drug levels that occur within the patient population. (3) The third phase of a chemosensitivity assay is the posttreatment incubation period. This period must be sufficiently long for optimal damage expression to take place. However, if this period is too long a dilution of the measured end point may occur. (4) The final aspect of a chemosensitivity assay is the measurement of end point. A considerable number of end points have been used for the determination of in vitro chemosensitivity of tumor cells; however, the main criterion for an optimal end point is that it accurately measure the number of cells killed by the administered agent.

BOX 38–2
Phases of Chemosensitivity Assays

- **Acquisition and preparation of tissue**
- **Exposure of tumor cells to chemotherapeutic agents**
- **Posttreatment incubation period**
- **Measurement at end point**

The initial attempts at determining in vitro chemosensitivity for brain tumor specimens used a visual assessment of morphologic damage.[30, 31] Although interpretations of these results were somewhat subjective, a wide range of in vitro responses were observed for drugs with a variety of modes of action. This early observation is a recurring theme for a variety of methodologies used to evaluate the in vitro chemosensitivity of cells from brain tumor specimens. Although the data often reflect the overall patient population response to a given agent, the strength of the assay results from the ability to obtain a differential response on an individual patient basis. Other methodologies that has been applied to the analysis of in vitro chemosensitivity include the clonogenic assay,[32] tritiated thymidine incorporation following supraphysiologic drug doses,[33] short-term tritiated thymidine incorporation,[34] the fluorescent cytoprint assay,[35] the adenosine triphosphate luminescence assay,[36] MTT (tetrazolium) assay,[37] radioactive protein precursor incorporation,[38] three-dimensional microorgan culture system,[39] and sister chromatid exchange.[40] Tissue culture–based assays have also been used to evaluate other therapeutic modalities, such as radiotherapy and high-dose tamoxifen therapy.[41]

In a large retrospective study of in vitro chemosensitivity of malignant glioma specimens, Thomas et al[38] examined the response of patients receiving CCNU, procarbazine, and vincristine following whole-head irradiation. The cells from the tumor specimens did not respond uniformly to the application of the chemotherapeutic agents in tissue culture. It was possible to divide the patients into two groups: those who responded to CCNU and procarbazine in vitro and those who did not. The relapse-free interval for those patients with positive cellular responses was significantly longer than the relapse-free interval of those patients whose cells did not respond in culture. As a result of a previous study,[37] Tonn et al[42] used the MTT assay to design a prospective correlative trial comparing cellular response to either BCNU or nimustine (ACNU) with the clinical response to these agents. The results demonstrated a predictive value of in vitro chemosensitivity testing for gliomas. A number of studies have addressed the issue of phenotypic and genotypic heterogeneity within individual glioma specimens.[43, 44] Cellular response to BCNU has been shown to be influenced by DNA content and chromosome number.

TISSUE CULTURE–BASED MICROCYTOTOXICITY ASSAY

The established role of tissue culture studies for the analysis of the biologic behavior of brain tumors has been clearly defined.[45] As a result of a series of tissue culture–based studies, Kornblith et al established a microcytotoxicity assay to detect a humoral immune response in astrocytoma patients.[46] This assay was later used to examine the effect of chemotherapeutic agents on cultured primary glioma cells[47, 48] and to investigate morphologic changes produced by chemotherapeutic agents in vitro.[49, 50] The microcytotoxicity assay was utilized to determine therapeutic predictive relevance for glioma patients.[51] Tumor size increased following treatment in all of the patients who did not respond to BCNU in the tissue culture–based assay; two-thirds of the patients who responded to BCNU in tissue culture had a significant clinical response.

For in vitro chemosensitivity testing, a tumor specimen is transported to the laboratory in a bottle of medium under sterile conditions. The tumor chunk is then minced into small explant segments and transferred to a tissue culture flask. The outgrowth of cells from the explant segment into a monolayer culture is monitored. When a sufficient cell number is present in the growth flasks, cells are trypinized and plated in the wells of a 60-well microtiter plate. Following a 24-hour period to allow for cell adherence and the initiation of cell proliferation, the cells in the microtiter plates are given an acute exposure to chemotherapeutic agents (1 hour for the nitrosoureas and 2 hours for all other agents). For each drug tested, a complete dose-response curve is generated with six drug concentrations per agent. Following drug exposure, the cells are allowed to incubate for another 72 hours. The cells in the microtiter wells are then fixed and stained with Giemsa. The number of cells per well is then determined through the use of an operator-controlled, computer-assisted imaging system. Each microtiter plate contains cells exposed to each of six drug doses as well as untreated control wells. The data are expressed as the cytotoxic index (CI). The higher the CI the greater the cell kill produced by a given agent.

IN VITRO CHEMOSENSITIVITY OF PEDIATRIC BRAIN TUMORS

We have applied the microtiter-based tissue culture chemosensitivity assay to a number of childhood brain tumor primary cell cultures. These data illustrate the differential in vitro response to chemotherapeutic agents observed among pediatric brain tumor specimens. Each of the figures provides a complete dose-response curve for each of the agents tested. (Fig. 38–1) illustrates the results from a pilocytic astrocytoma from a 7-year-old child. As would be expected from historical data, the tumor cells were unresponsive to chemotherapy, with only a slight effect produced by the nitrosoureas in the high-dose region. (Fig. 38–2) presents data from another pilocytic astrocytoma that exhibited a moderate in vitro response to the majority of agents tested. The results from a childhood glioblastoma multiforme are presented in (Fig. 38–3). Unlike the majority of high-grade astrocytomas in adults, the cells from this tumor specimen were very responsive to chemotherapy. Results from another low-grade astrocytoma responsive to in vitro chemotherapy are presented in (Fig. 38–4). (Figs. 38–5 and 38–6) present results obtained from an ependymoma and a medulloblastoma specimen, respectively.

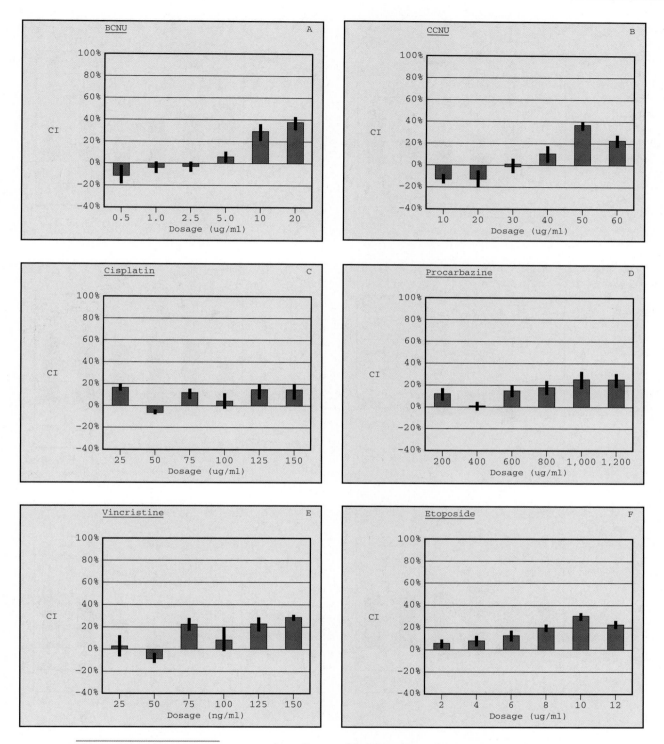

Figure 38–1   Dose-response curves for a 7-year-old child who underwent multimodality therapy for pilocytic astrocytoma. (A) BCNU; (B) CCNU; (C) cisplatin; (D) procarbazine; (E) vincristine; (F) etoposide.

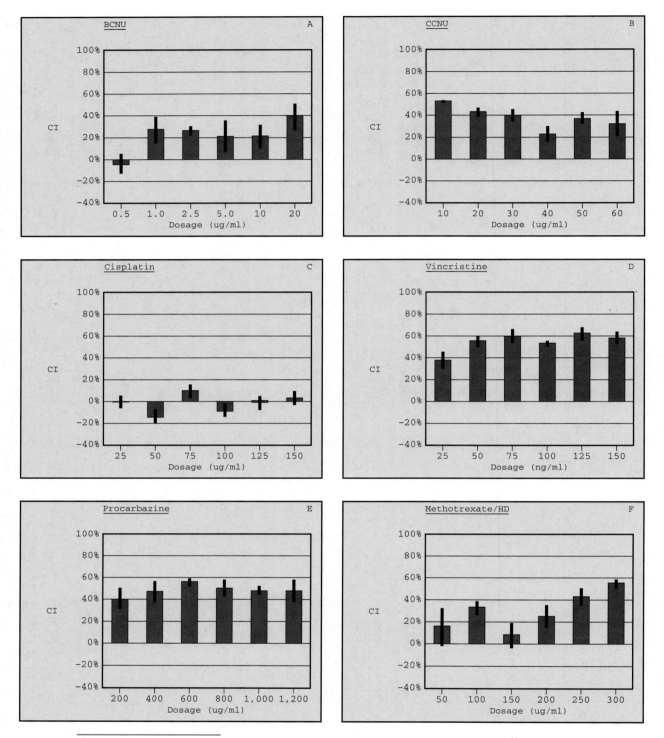

Figure 38–2 Dose-response curves for another child who underwent multimodality therapy for pilocytic astrocytoma. (A) BCNU; (B) CCNU; (C) cisplatin; (D) vincristine; (E) procarbazine; (F) methotrexate/HD.

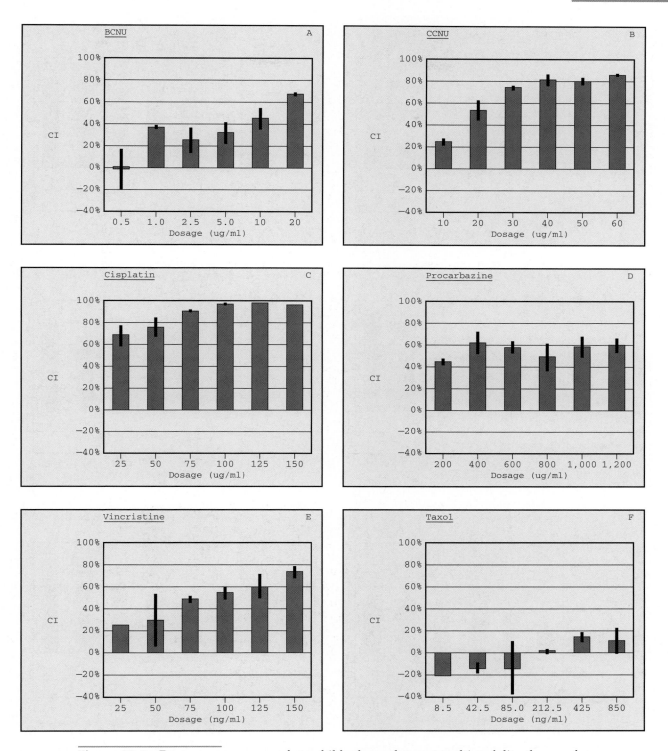

Figure 38–3   Dose-response curves for a child who underwent multimodality therapy for glioblastoma multiforme. (A) BCNU; (B) CCNU; (C) cisplatin; (D) procarbazine; (E) vincristine; (F) taxol.

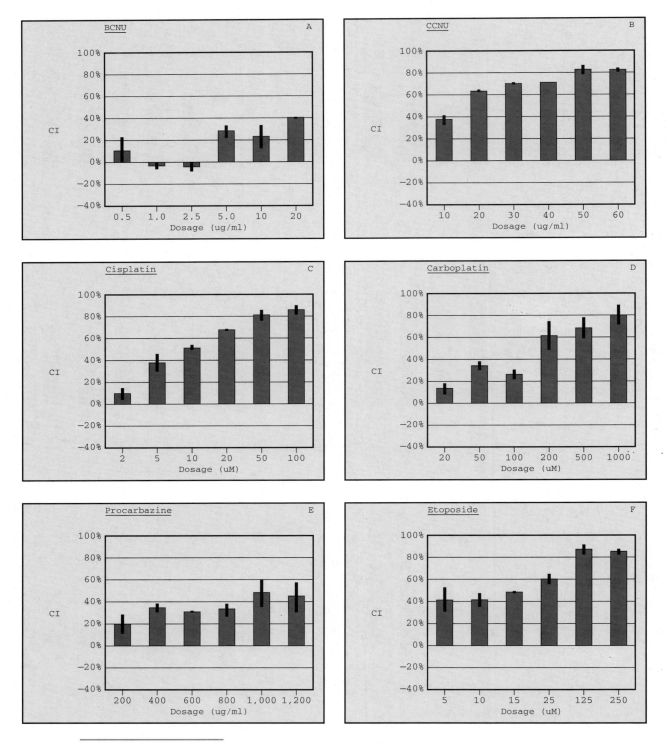

Figure 38–4 Dose-response curves for a child who underwent multimodality therapy for low-grade astrocytoma. (A) BCNU; (B) CCNU; (C) cisplatin; (D) carboplatin; (E) procarbazine; (F) etoposide.

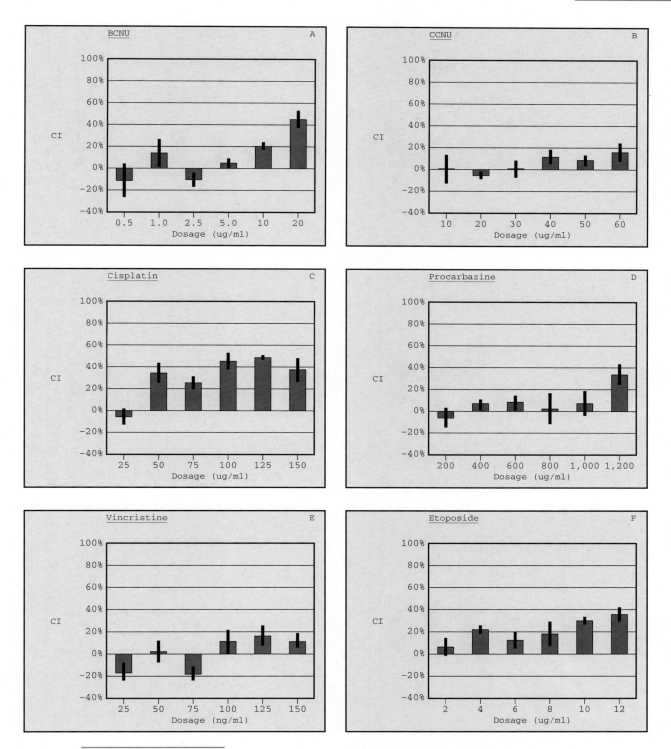

Figure 38–5   Dose-response curves for a child who underwent multimodality therapy for ependymoma. (A) BCNU; (B) CCNU; (C) cisplatin; (D) procarbazine; (E) vincristine; (F) etoposide.

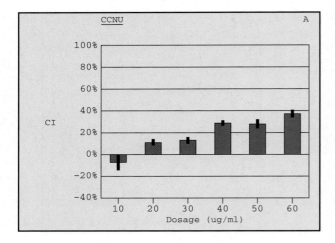

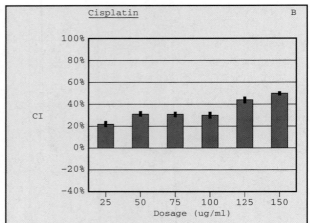

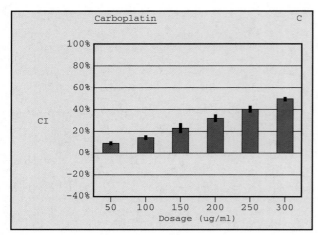

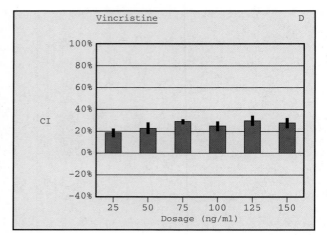

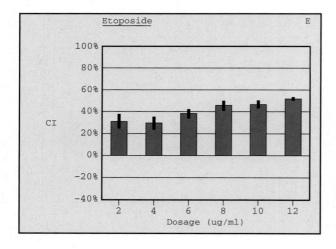

Figure 38–6   Dose-response curves for a child who underwent multimodality therapy for medulloblastoma. (A) CCNU; (B) cisplatin; (C) carboplatin; (D) vincristine; (E) etoposide.

SUMMARY

The data presented here illustrate the use of a tissue culture–based microcytotoxicity assay producing quantitative data that may aid the treatment of the child with brain cancer. Furthermore, the continued growth of these samples into established cell lines might provide valuable material for the screening of new therapeutic agents.

REFERENCES

1. Kornblith PK, Welch WC, Bradley MK. The future of therapy for glioblastoma. *Surg Neurol* 1993;39:538–543.
2. Berger MS: The impact of technical adjuncts in the surgical management of cerebral hemispheric low-grade gliomas of childhood. *J Neuro-oncol* 1996;28:129–155.
3. Garvey M, Packer RJ. An integrated approach to the treatment of chiasmatic-hypothalamic gliomas. *J Neuro-oncol* 1996;28:167–183.
4. Kornblith PL, Welch WC. Principles and application of chemotherapy in brain tumors. In: Vecht Ch J, ed. *Handbook of Clinical Neurology*. Vol. 23(67): *Neuro-Oncology*, Part I. Amsterdam: Elsevier; 1997:277–290.
5. Lyden DC, Mason WP, Finlay JL. The expanding role of chemotherapy for pediatric supratentorial malignant gliomas. *J Neuro-oncol* 1996;28:185–191.
6. Brown K, Mapstone TB, Oakes WJ. A modern analysis of intracranial tumors of infancy. *Pediatr Neurosurg* 1997;26(1):25–32.
7. Tomita T. Neurosurgical perspectives in pediatric neurooncology. *Child's Nerv Syst* 1998;14:94–96.
8. Wisoff JH, Boyett JM, Berger MS, et al. Current neurosurgical management and the impact of the extent of resection in the treatment of malignant gliomas of childhood: a report of the Children's Cancer Group Trial No. CCG-945. *J Neurosurg* 1998;89:52–59.
9. Kalapurakal JA, Thomas, PRM: pediatric radiotherapy: an overview. *Radiol Clin North Am* 1997;35(6):1265–1287.
10. Alekhteyar KM, Glatstein E. Radiotherapy management of brain tumors. In: Kornblith PL, Walker MD, eds. *Advances in Neuro-Oncology*. Vol. 2. Armonk, NY: Futura Publishing Company; 1997:307–329.
11. Kornblith PL, Walker M. Chemotherapy for malignant gliomas. *J Neurosurg* 1988;68:1–17. [published erratum appears in *J Neurosurg* 1988;69(4):645.]
12. Nicholas MK, Prados MD. Chemotherapy of brain tumors. In: Kornblith PL, Walker MD, eds. *Advances in Neuro-oncology*. Vol. 2. Armonk, NY: Futura Publishing Company; 1997:331–362.
13. Tarbell NJ, Loeffler JS. Recent trends in the radiotherapy of pediatric gliomas. *J Neuro-oncol* 1996;28:233–244.
14. Packer RJ, Sutton, LN, Bilaniuk LT, et al. Treatment of chiasmatic/hypothalamic gliomas of childhood with chemotherapy: an update. *Ann Neurol* 1988;23:79–85.
15. Allen JC, Walker R, Rosen G. Preradiation high-dose intravenous methotrexate with leucovorin rescue for untreated primary childhood brain tumors. *J Clin Oncol* 1988;6:649–653.
16. Duffner PK, Horowitz ME, Krischer JP, et al. Postoperative chemotherapy and delayed radiation in children less than three years of age with malignant brain tumors. *N Engl J Med* 1993;328:1725–1731.
17. Vats TS. Adjuvant chemotherapy of pediatric brain tumors. *Ann N Y Acad Sci* 1997;824:156–166.
18. Siffert J, Allen JC. Chemotherapy and pediatric brain tumors. In Kornblith PL, Walker MD, eds. *Advances in Neuro-Oncology*. Vol. 2. Armonk, NY: Futura Publishing Company; 1997:363–412.
19. Prados MD, Russo C. Chemotherapy of brain tumors. *Semin Surg Oncol* 1998;14:88–95.
20. Abrahamsen TG, Lange BJ, Packer RJ, et al. A phase I and II trial of dose-intensified cyclophosphamide and GM-CSF in pediatric malignant brain tumors. *J Pediatr Hematol Oncol* 1995;17(2):134–139.
21. Jakacki RI, Jamison C, Heifetz SA, et al. Feasibililty of sequential high-dose chemotherapy and peripheral blood stem cell support for pediatric central nervous system malignancies. *Med Pediatr Oncol* 1997;29:553–559.
22. Yule SM, Foreman NK, Mitchell C, et al. High-dose cyclophosphamide for poor-prognosis and recurrent pediatric brain tumors: a dose-escalation study. *J Clin Oncol* 1997 Oct; 15(10):3258–3265.
23. Walter AW, Gajjar A, Ochs JS, et al. Carboplatin and etoposide with hyperfractionated radiotherapy in children with newly diagnosed diffuse pontine gliomas: a phase I/II study. *Med Pediatr Oncol* 1998;30(1):28–33.
24. Dahlborg SA, Petrillo A, Crossen JR, et al. The potential for complete and durable response in nonglial primary brain tumors in children and young adults with enhanced chemotherapy delivery. *Cancer J Sci Am* 1998;4(2):110–124.
25. Blaney SM, Phillips PC, Packer RJ, et al. Phase II evaluation of topotecan for pediatric central nervous system tumors. *Cancer* 1996;78(3):527–531.
26. Tubergen DG, Stewart CF, Pratt CB, et al. Phase I trial and pharmacokinetic (PK) and pharmacodynamics (PD) study of topotecan using a five-day course in children with refractory solid tumors: a pediatric oncology group study. *J Pediatr Hematol Oncol* 1996;18(4):352–361.
27. Ruffer JE, Glatstein E. The blood-brain barrier disruption controversy: does it hold water? *Cancer J Sci Am* 1998;4:84–85.
28. Darling JL, Lewandowicz GM, Thomas DGT. Chemosensitivity testing human malignant brain tumors. In: Kornblith PL, Walker MD, eds. *Advances in Neuro-oncology*. Vol. 2. Armonk, NY: Futura Publishing Company; 1997:413–434.
29. Kimmel DW, Shapiro JR, Shapiro WR. In vitro drug sensitivity testing in human gliomas. *J Neurosurg* 1987;66:161–171.
30. Wilson CB, Barker M. Sensitivity of cell cultures of neural tumors to vinblastine sulfate (NSC-49842). *Cancer Chemother Rep* 1965;44:9–13.
31. Wilson CB, Barker M. Relative cytotoxicity of mithramycin and vinblastine sulfate in cell cultures of human neural tumors. *J Natl Cancer Inst* 1967;38:459–463.
32. Von Hoff DD. He's not going to talk about in vitro predictive assays again, is he? *J Natl Cancer Inst* 1990;82: 96–101.
33. Kern DH, Weisenthal LM. Highly specific prediction of antineoplastic drug resistance with an in vitro assay using suprapharmacologic drug exposures. *J Natl Cancer Inst* 1990;82:582–588.

34. Hayward, IP, Hurst T, Parsons PG, et al. Combination chemotherapy tested in a short-term thymidine incorporation assay in primary cultures of ovarian adenocarcinomas. *Int J Cell Cloning* 1992;10:182–189.

35. Leone LA, Meitner PA, Myers TJ, et al. Predictive value of the fluorescent cytoprint assay (FCA): a retrospective correlation study of in vitro chemosensitivity and individual responses to chemotherapy. *Cancer Invest* 1991; 9(5):491–503.

36. Andreotti PE, Cree IA, Kurbacher CM, et al. Chemosensitivity testing of human tumors using a microplate adenosine triphosphate luminescence assay: clinical correlation for cisplatin resistance of ovarian carcinoma. *Cancer Res* 1995;55:5276–5282.

37. Nikkhah G, Tonn JC, Hoffmann O, et al. The MTT assay for chemosensitivity testing of human tumors of the central nervous system. Part II: Evaluation of patient- and drug-specific variables. *J Neuro-oncol* 1992;13:13–24.

38. Thomas DGT, Darling JL, Paul EA, et al. Assay of anti-cancer drugs in tissue culture: relationship of relapse free interval (RFI) and in vitro chemosensitivity in patients with malignant cerebral glioma. *Br J Cancer* 1985;51:525–532.

39. Jung HW, Berens ME, Krouwer HG, et al. A three-dimensional micro-organ culture system optimized for in vitro growth of human malignant brain tumors. *Neurosurgery* 1991;29:390–398.

40. Deen DF, Kendall LE, Marton LJ, et al. Prediction of human tumor cell chemosensitivity using the sister chromatid exchange assay. *Cancer Res* 1986;46:1599–1602.

41. Zhang W, Hinton DR, Surnock AA, et al. Malignant glioma sensitivity to radiotherapy, high-dose tamoxifen, and hypericin: corroborating clinical response in vitro: case report. *Neurosurgery* 1996;38(3):587–590.

42. Tonn JC, Schachenmayr W, Kraemer HP. In vitro chemosensitivity test of malignant gliomas: clinical relevance of test results independent of adjuvant chemotherapy. *Anticancer Res* 1994;14(3B):1371–1375.

43. Kobayashi S, Hoshino T, Dougherty DV, et al. Variable response to 1,3-bis(2-chloroethyl)-1-nitrosourea of human glioma cells sorted according to DNA content. *J Neuro-oncol* 1984;2(1):5–11.

44. Shapiro JR, Pu PY, Mohamed AN, et al. Chromosome number and carmustine sensitivity in human gliomas. *Cancer* 1993;71(12):4007–4021.

45. Kornblith PL. Role of tissue culture in prediction of malignancy. *Clin Neurosurg* 1978;25:346–376.

46. Kornblith PL, Pollock LA, Coakham HB, et al. Cytotoxic antibody responses in astrocytoma patients: an improved allogeneic assay. *J Neurosurg* 1979;51:47–52.

47. Kornblith PL, Rosa L, Bona JD, et al. Response variability of human brain tumors to AZQ in tissue culture. *J Neuro-oncol* 1986;4:49–54.

48. Kornblith PL, Szypko PE: Variations in response of human brain tumors to BCNU in vitro. *J Neurosurg* 1978; 48:580–586.

49. Smith BH, Vaughan M, Greenwood MA, et al. Membrane and cytoplasmic changes in 1,3-bis(2-chloroethyl)-1-nitrosourea (BCNU)–sensitive and resistant human malignant glioma-derived cell lines. *J Neuro-oncol* 1983;1: 237–248.

50. Oberc-Greenwood MA, Smith BH, Cooke C, et al. Selective cytoplasmic and membrane changes induced by cisplatinum. *J Neuro-oncol* 1990;9:191–199.

51. Kornblith PL, Smith BH, Leonard LA. Response of cultured human brain tumors to nitrosoureas: correlation with clinical data. *Cancer* 1981;47(2):255–265.

Chapter 39

Late Effects of Therapy in Long-Term Survivors

H. Stacy Nicholson and Robert Butler

Improvements in survival rates for children and adolescents with central nervous system (CNS) tumors have lagged behind those for most other major pediatric malignancies. However, due to improvements in therapy over the past two decades, most children and adolescents with CNS tumors will be long-term survivors.[1] In particular, children now diagnosed with medulloblastoma or low-grade astrocytoma are most likely to survive long term. Therefore, concerns about late complications of therapy are increasingly important to survivors and their families. In addition to the late consequences of radiation therapy and chemotherapy, which may affect all survivors of childhood cancer, the singular susceptibility of the brain and spinal cord to injury causes several late consequences that are unique to long-term survivors of CNS tumors.

Late complications can be caused by the tumor itself, radiation therapy, chemotherapy, or the psychological trauma of dealing with a malignancy. The late effects in survivors of CNS tumors are diverse and include medical, psychological, and psychosocial problems. Some of these can be life threatening. In fact, long-term survivors of CNS tumors are more likely to die than are other cancer survivors, even when the problem of late relapses is not considered.[2,3] Thus, long-term medical surveillance of these survivors is critically important so that late effects of therapy may be detected while still possibly amenable to intervention.

MEDICAL LATE COMPLICATIONS

Late Mortality

Although 5-year disease-free survival is the measure most often used in clinical trials as a surrogate for cure, it may not correlate with a normal life expectancy. In a large cohort study of adult survivors of childhood cancer,[2] survivors of CNS tumors were much more likely to die during their twenties and thirties than were survivors of all other childhood and adolescent cancers, except for those with Hodgkin's disease. In fact, during their thirties, survivors had a 9.2-fold [95% confidence interval (CI) 3.2 to 26.2] excess risk of death from causes other than the primary cancer. Of the 23 deaths in CNS tumor survivors not due to a relapse or persistence of the primary cancer, the most common causes of death were trauma (4), pneumonia (4), other respiratory diseases (4), cerebrovascular disease (3),

and aspiration of emesis (2). Survivors in this study had been treated between 1945 and 1974; thus, as treatment has changed in the past two decades, fatal late complications may differ for patients who are being treated currently.

BOX 39–1
Causes of Death Other Than Primary Tumor

- **Trauma**
- **Pneumonia**
- **Other respiratory disease**
- **Cerebrovascular disease**
- **Aspiration**

SECOND MALIGNANCIES

Perhaps the late complication of therapy feared most by any cancer survivor is the development of a subsequent cancer. Because of the relatively recent improvements in survival for children with malignant brain tumors, little is known about the actual risk of secondary cancers following brain tumors. However, as more children with brain tumors survive, secondary cancers have become an increasingly common problem.[4] In long-term survivors of CNS tumors, the most common secondary malignancy is another type of brain tumor, usually due to radiation therapy. Radiation therapy is particularly associated with the induction of high-grade astrocytomas, gliomas, and meningiomas. In addition, as pediatric oncologists have increasingly used alkylating agents, platinators, and epipodophyllotoxins (such as etoposide) as chemotherapy for children with brain tumors, there is now also a risk of secondary leukemia in long-term survivors. The most common types of chemotherapy-induced leukemia are myelogenous leukemias (AML). Currently, most reports of secondary malignancies in CNS tumor survivors are case reports; however, as earlier clinical trials mature, secondary cancers are beginning to appear as a late complication.[5]

BOX 39–2
Secondary Malignancies

- Radiation-induced
  - High-grade astrocytoma
  - Glioma
  - Meningioma
- Leukemia

BOX 39–3
Genetic Syndromes Associated with Pediatric CNS Tumors

- Gorlin's
  - Medulloblastoma
  - Basal cell carcinoma
- Turcot's
  - Brain tumor
  - Multiple colonic polyps

Estimates of the risk of a subsequent cancer after CNS tumors are best based on epidemiologic studies. In a population-based study of 1262 histologically confirmed cases of medulloblastoma in the United States and Sweden,[4] 20 secondary malignancies occurred. This corresponded to a 5.4-fold excess of secondary neoplasms (95% CI: 3.3 to 8.4) relative to the number expected based on population data. The median latency between the medulloblastoma and the secondary malignancy was 73 months (range 8 months to 36 years). Types of cancer that occurred in excess of the expected rates (based on population data) included cancers of the salivary glands, cervix uteri, CNS, thyroid gland, and acute lymphoblastic leukemia (ALL). Forty-six percent of secondary malignancies that occurred in patients with adequate treatment data occurred in or near the radiation field. The risk may increase with time as survivor cohorts age. Some case reports have noted latency periods of more than 6 decades for radiation-induced CNS tumors.[6] Future epidemiologic studies in ultralong-term survivors will be critically important to further define the lifetime risk of secondary malignancies.

Also, as clinical trials mature, long-term follow-up beyond the usual 5-year disease-free survival will be important because severe late effects, such as secondary cancers, may impact future treatment decisions. In a study that showed an excellent treatment outcome for 63 children with medulloblastoma treated with lomustine (CCNU), cisplatin, and vincristine as well as craniospinal radiotherapy, three patients developed secondary malignancies (two CNS tumors and one AML).[5] Further follow-up of this and other clinical trials will be critically important in establishing the secondary-cancer risk for specific treatments.

The risk of a secondary malignancy may also be due to factors other than the anticancer therapy,[7, 8] such as an underlying genetic predisposition to malignancy. For such patients, the risk of a secondary cancer will likely be greater than for other children with the same primary cancer. Although most children with brain tumors do not have a known genetic predisposition to cancer, there are known examples of genetic syndromes associated with pediatric brain tumors.[8, 9] These include Gorlin's syndrome, in which children tend to be diagnosed with medulloblastoma at a particularly young age. These children are particularly susceptible to basal cell carcinomas in the radiation fields. Turcot's syndrome includes brain tumors and multiple colonic polyps.[9] A family history can be particularly helpful in ascertaining which patients are at increased risk of secondary malignancies. The family history should be updated at each annual follow-up visit for long-term survivors because relevant new information for the survivor's secondary cancer risk may only become apparent with the passage of time.

Cardiac Complications

The most common late cardiac complications in survivors of childhood cancer are attributable to anthracycline-induced cardiomyopathy.[10] As anthracyclines do not readily cross the blood-brain barrier, these agents are not used to treat children with brain tumors. Therefore, children who have survived brain tumors are not generally at risk for anthracycline cardiotoxicity. *However, other chemotherapeutic agents, such as cyclophosphamide, have also been associated with cardiac dysfunction.* Radiation is also known to damage the heart and lead to premature atherosclerosis. This is particularly true for long-term survivors of Hodgkin's disease treated with high doses of radiation.[11] Children with brain tumors who received spinal irradiation have had some cardiac abnormalities documented, presumably due to the exit beam. In one study that included 26 patients who had received spinal radiotherapy, cardiac evaluations included electrocardiography, 24-hour ambulatory electrocardiography, echocardiography, and exercise testing. Of the 16 patients who were exercise-tested, 75% achieved a maximal cardiac index below the fifth percentile. In addition, 31% had pathologic Q waves, and there was an excess of elevated posterior wall stress.[12] *Although the long-term significance of these findings is not yet known, this study points out that cardiac function must be followed in survivors who received spinal radiotherapy.* Furthermore, precise risk estimates of clinically significant cardiac problems in CNS tumor survivors are not currently available; thus, the long-term cardiac health of CNS tumor survivors requires further study.

Pulmonary Complications

Few data exist regarding late pulmonary complications in long-term survivors of pediatric CNS tumors. *However, many patients, including those with astrocytoma and medulloblastoma, are exposed to the nitrosoureas, which are known to be associated with pulmonary fibrosis.* The risk apparently does not decline with time, and fatal pulmonary fibrosis has been described as long as 17 years after exposure.[13] In addition to the nitrosoureas, other chemotherapeutic agents are known to have pulmonary fibrosis as a potential complication, including cyclophosphamide. The risk from agents other than the nitrosoureas in not likely to be high.

There also appears to be a risk of pulmonary fibrosis associated with spinal radiotherapy. In a study of 28 survivors of childhood brain tumors, half had significant pulmonary fibrosis. Although the numbers were small, only 1 of 7 patients (14%) who received CCNU without spinal radiotherapy, compared with 13 of 21 of those (62%) who received spinal radiotherapy (with or without CCNU), developed pulmonary fibrosis.[14] This included 4 of 8 who did not receive CCNU. In this study, pulmonary fibrosis was associated with a history of spinal irradiation and not with CCNU exposure. Thus, survivors who received spinal radiotherapy for their CNS tumor have a risk of late pulmonary complications. However, similar to the cardiac late effects, more precise estimates of risk are needed, and further follow-up will be required to ascertain how many survivors develop clinically significant pulmonary complications.

Endocrine Disorders

The most commonly affected organ system in long-term survivors of childhood brain tumors is the endocrine system.[15-18] The cause of endocrine problems can be the tumor itself, surgery, or radiotherapy. Tumors of the pituitary or hypothalamic region often present with pituitary dysfunction. Furthermore, the surgical treatment of tumors in this region also posess a risk of pituitary damage. Either the tumor itself or surgery may result in panhypopituitarism. However, by far the most common cause of late endocrinologic sequelae is radiotherapy.[18] Focal radiotherapy that includes the pituitary gland, whole-brain radiotherapy, and/or craniospinal radiotherapy all involve the pituitary and carry a risk of hormonal deficiencies. The deficiencies, which are dose-dependent, most commonly include growth hormone deficiency. In addition, low-dose cranial irradiation (18 Gy) may be associated with the premature onset of puberty, and higher doses of irradiation (more than 40 Gy) may lead to deficiencies of gonadotropins and thyroid hormone–releasing hormone, as well as hyperprolactinemia.[16] Furthermore, the risk of developing hormonal complications of irradiation does not decrease with time. Thus, careful follow-up of growth, pubertal development, and thyroid function is critical because hormonal deficiencies are universally treatable.

BOX 39–4
Hormonal Disorders

- **Growth disorder**
- **Premature puberty**
- **Thyroid function disorder**
- **Gonadotropin deficiency**
- **Hyperprolactinemia**
- **Panhypopituitarism**

In addition, thyroid function should be followed for life, with thyroid function studies performed in all children who received irradiation to the thyroid gland, regardless of whether or not the brain was irradiated, and regardless of the radiotherapy dose to the pituitary gland.[18] As with other hormonal deficiencies, the risk of hypothyroidism does not appear to decrease over time.[19] In addition, radiation therapy may be associated with both benign and malignant thyroid nodules. Thus, as part of the annual checkup, these patients should have careful thyroid palpation.

Hormones that are found to be deficient can be treated with replacement therapy.[15-20] In fact, children with growth hormone deficiency due to radiation therapy respond to replacement therapy as well as children with idiopathic growth hormone deficiency.[20] Consultation with an endocrinologist is important if endocrine deficits are known or suspected. Although there has been some controversy about the use of growth hormone in children with brain tumors,[21] there are no precise estimates of the risk of relapse, if any, posed by its use. Epidemiologic studies will be required to establish risk, if any, and to reassure patients, their families, and their physicians when there is no risk associated with the use of growth hormone.

Hearing Disorders

Depending on the location of the primary tumor, both hearing and sight can be affected. *In addition, chemotherapy with cisplatin can also cause sensorineural hearing loss.*[22] The hearing loss associated with cisplatin is irreversible and is likely to be exacerbated by radiation therapy that includes the ear. Virtually all children receiving cisplatin will have some loss of hearing. However, severe cisplatin ototoxicity in the speech frequencies can be largely prevented with careful monitoring of hearing throughout therapy. Most chemotherapy clinical trials that include cisplatin contain specific guidelines for decreasing or deleting the cisplatin dose based on ototoxicity.

As part of routine follow-up, all children who received cisplatin should have their hearing tested because hearing loss can occur as a late complication even when hearing was previously documented to be sufficient and because many survivors can benefit from amplification. Also, as hearing impairment may affect school performance, the results of the hearing evaluation should be shared with the neuropsychologist so that educational recommendations can include information about hearing.

Renal Complications

Some chemotherapeutic agents used in the treatment of CNS tumors are nephrotoxic, such as cisplatin and ifosfamide.[23] Cisplatin can both decrease the glomerular filtration rate and cause electrolyte abnormalities. Also, wasting of magnesium and potassium are common in children who receive cisplatin. Although most patients will have resolution of these electrolyte abnormalities, some may require long-term supplementation. Similarly, patients who receive ifosfamide may develop renal Fanconi's syndrome, including renal tubular acidosis, phosphaturia, and glucosuria. The initial development of electrolyte abnormalities long after chemotherapy has ended is not expected, and whether the glomerular filtration rate decreases with time is not yet known.

Gastrointestinal and Hepatic Complications

There is generally little risk of late gastrointestinal sequelae in long-term survivors of brain tumors. As noted above, rarely patients may have their brain tumor as the initial manifestation of Turcot's syndrome;[9] therefore, any patient with obstructive symptoms or bloody stool should be considered to be at risk for colonic polyps. As with other cancer survivors who received blood products, there is a small risk of blood-borne infections, including hepatitis. Patients transfused prior to 1992, when routine screening for hepatitis C was implemented, should be screened for hepatitis C.[24]

Neurologic Complications

Children with brain tumors have tumors and therapy that both directly affect the brain, and neurologic sequelae are common. These include seizures, paralysis, radiation necrosis, and migraine-like symptoms.[25, 26] Some of the neurologic complications may be severe and life threatening.[2, 3]

BOX 39–5
Neurologic Sequelae

- **Seizures**
- **Weakness**
- **Radiation necrosis**
- **Migraine**
- **Vascular changes**
  - **Stroke**
  - **Moyamoya syndrome**

Although the tumor and surgery can also cause neurologic damage, most late neurologic complications can be traced to radiation therapy.[27] Whether injuries result from direct radiation damage to neurons and/or glial cells, or to the vasculature, or to a combination of both is not well understood. Radiation necrosis can be a particular problem for the survivor of CNS tumors, requiring steroids or surgery.[25] These lesions often mimic a tumor, and whether a new mass in the radiation bed represents recurrent tumor versus radiation necrosis can often be difficult to ascertain by computed tomography or magnetic resonance imaging. This complication usually occurs between 9 months and 2 years after radiation, and symptoms vary, depending on the location in the brain. Radiation necrosis can cause headache, behavioral changes, seizures, lethargy, hemiparesis, ataxia, and/or increased intracranial pressure.

In addition, vascular changes may occur following radiation and in the most severe cases may cause a stroke.[28] Moyamoya syndrome, in which the small blood vessels have the abnormal appearance of a "puff of smoke," can also occur in this setting.

BOX 39–6
Radiation Necrosis

- **Appears between 9 months and 5 years after radiation**
- **Variable symptoms**
  - **Headache**
  - **Behavioral changes**
  - **Seizures**
  - **Lethargy**
  - **Weakness**
  - **Ataxia**
  - **Increased intracranial pressure**

NEUROPSYCHOLOGICAL AND PSYCHOSOCIAL SEQUELAE

Of all childhood cancers, brain tumors have been associated with the most significant neurocognitive and psychological sequelae. Because of increases in the survival of patients with these tumors, the effects of this disease and its treatment on the patient's functional status have become important issues in pediatric oncology. Quality-of-life–related long-term effects of childhood brain tumors fall into two primary areas: neuropsychological and psychological/social.

Neuropsychological Effects

Brain tumors alter neuropsychological functioning by two processes. The tumor itself can damage CNS tissue by infiltration and pressure. Secondarily, treatments, including resection, irradiation, and chemotherapy, can have an adverse effect on neurologic functions. These include neuropsychological effects that refer to the end product of CNS activity: thought and behavior.

There have been recent advances in our knowledge on the neuropsychological effects of childhood brain tumors and their treatment. Supratentorial tumors are generally associated with the greatest degree of dysfunction, including deficits in intellectual functioning and new learning,[29] as well as executive functions.[30] Executive functions refer to higher cortical processes, such as planning and the inhibition of response. These negative effects can be reasonably independent of treatment and may be partly due to associated pressure changes from hydrocephalus. Infratentorial tumors are also accompanied by neuropsychological deficits that can be relatively mild in nature if CNS irradiation is avoided,[31] but nevertheless present in many children.[32] Finally, diencephalic region brain tumors have been reported to also spare many neuropsychological functions; however, the encoding of new memory engrams can be disrupted in these patients.[29]

Of all treatments used to combat childhood brain cancer, cranial irradiation therapy (CRT) has been associated with the greatest neuropsychological impairment. Whole-brain CRT often results in attentional disturbances, reductions in information processing efficacy, nondominant hemisphere dysfunction, and nonverbal learning disabilities in many children.[33–35] Chemotherapy, on the other hand, appears to be reasonably well tolerated by many children, and the incidence of cognitive impairment secondary to these treatments may be much less than that with CRT.[36] However, recent data from breast cancer survivors suggest that chemotherapy may not spare neuropsychological functioning entirely.[37]

BOX 39–7
Potential Long-Term Effects of Whole-Brain Irradiation

- **Attentional disturbances**
- **Reduced information processing**
- **Nondominant hemisphere dysfunction**
- **Nonverbal learning disabilities**

In addition to the above factors, it has been noted that brain tumors in younger children typically result in greater neuropsychological impairment and that rapidly growing brain tumors are more disruptive to cognition.[38] Although further research is needed on the variables that impact neurocognitive functioning in childhood brain tumors, the above summary has made it apparent that much has already been learned. There is a rapidly growing need for effective methods of cognitive rehabilitation for children who have suffered neuropsychological impairment from a brain tumor and/or its treatment. Recently, preliminary results from a therapeutic program designed to improve neurocognitive functioning in this population have been published.[39] This is an exciting new development that may have a significant positive impact on the quality of life that these children can and should enjoy.

Psychological/Social Effects

In comparison with the neurocognitive effects of childhood brain tumors, relatively little is known about the psychological and social correlates of these diseases. Most studies on the psychosocial impact of childhood cancer have grouped brain tumor patients with all other childhood cancers. Initially, it was reported that pediatric oncology survivors were characterized by high levels of psychological distress and maladjustment.[40] However, more recent studies have concluded that a childhood cancer experience does not necessarily result in significant psychopathology.[41, 42] On the other hand, less severe adjustment problems, such as anxiety reactions and deficits in social competence, have been documented in this population. Treatments commonly used for brain tumors, CRT in particular, have been implicated as possibly precipitating events.[33, 43] Interestingly, though it appears likely that neuropsychological deficits secondary to CNS cancer and their treatment may mediate many psychosocial problems, the severity of these deficits is not necessarily correlated with the extent of the child's psychological reaction.[29]

While significant psychopathology is now generally not thought to be a common correlate of CNS brain tumors, the disease can clearly have a negative impact on quality of life.[44] Neuropsychological deficits secondary to these tumors introduce roadblocks and obstacles into the survivor's life that can become more pronounced and apparent as the child enters adulthood. In addition to problems associated with the aforementioned cognitive disabilities, childhood CNS tumor survivors are at increased risk for unemployment, health problems, and being prohibited from driving.[3] Thus, there appears to be evidence that independence is compromised as a result of surviving a childhood brain tumor. As with cognitive remediation effects, psychological therapies designed to treat these adjustment disorders, socialization problems, and dependency issues are needed so that survivors of childhood brain tumors can enjoy optimal life benefits.

SUMMARY

As therapy for children and adolescents with CNS tumors improves, more patients will become long-term survivors. Therefore, pediatric oncologists, neurosurgeons, endocrinologists, psychologists, and primary care providers need to be familiar with the late sequelae of brain tumors and the anti-cancer therapies used to treat them. These include both medical and psychological late complications, some of which can be life threatening. *Thus, CNS tumor survivors must be followed closely for life.* In addition to routine physical and neurologic examinations, a careful family histories, with emphasis on malignancies, and screening for endocrine dysfunction must be done. Furthermore, careful neuropsychological testing, educational interventions, and counseling regarding vocational rehabilitation and job placement will likely improve the quality of life for survivors of childhood and adolescent CNS tumors.

REFERENCES

1. Pollack I. Brain tumors in children. *N Engl J Med* 1994;332:1238–1239.
2. Nicholson HS, Fears TR, Byrne J. Death during adulthood in survivors of childhood and adolescent cancer. *Cancer* 1994;73:3094–3102.
3. Mostow EN, Byrne J, Connelly RR, Mulvihill JJ. Quality of life in long-term survivors of CNS tumors of childhood and adolescence. *J Clin Oncol* 1991;9:592–599.
4. Goldstein AM, Yuen J, Tucker MA. Second cancers after medulloblastoma: population-based results from the United States and Sweden. *Cancer Causes Control* 1997;8:865–871.
5. Packer RJ, Sutton LN, Elterman R, et al. Outcome for children with medulloblastoma treated with radiation and cisplatin, CCNU and vincristine chemotherapy. *J Neurosurg* 1994;81:690–698.
6. Kleinschmidt-DeMasters BK, Lillehei KO. Radiation-induced meningioma with a 63-year latency period. Case report. *J Neurosurg* 1995;82:487–488.
7. Robison LL. Survivors of childhood cancer and risk of a second tumor. *J Natl Cancer Inst* 1993;85:1102–1103.
8. Goldstein AM, Pastakia B, DiGiovanna JJ, et al. Clinical findings in two African-American families with the nevoid basal cell carcinoma syndrome (NBCC). *Am J Med Genet* 1994;50:272–281.
9. Hamilton SR, Liu B, Parsons RE, et al. The molecular basis of Turcot's syndrome. *N Engl J Med* 1995;332:839–847.
10. Lipshultz SE, Colan SD, Gelber RD, et al. Late cardiac effects of doxorubicin therapy for acute lymphoblastic leukemia in childhood. *N Engl J Med* 1991;324:808–815.
11. Donaldson SS, Kaplan HS. Complications of treatment of Hodgkin's disease in children. *Cancer Treat Rep* 1982;66:977–989.
12. Jakacki RI, Goldwein JW, Larsen ROL, et al. Cardiac dysfunction following spinal irradiation during childhood. *J Clin Oncol* 1993;11:1033–1038.
13. O'Driscoll BR, Hasleton PS, Taylor PM, et al. Active lung fibrosis up to 17 years after chemotherapy with carmustine (BCNU) in childhood. *N Engl J Med* 1990;323:378–382.
14. Jakacki RI, Schramm CM, Donahue BR, et al. Restrictive lung disease following treatment for malignant brain tumors: a potential late effect of craniospinal irradiation. *J Clin Oncol* 1995;13:1478–1485.
15. Sklar CA. Growth and neuroendocrine dysfunction following therapy for childhood cancer. *Pediatr Clin North Am* 1997;44:489–503.

16. Overfield SE, Soranno D, Nirenberg et al. Age at onset of puberty following high-dose central nervous system radiation therapy. *Arch Pediatr Adol Med* 1996;150:589–592.

17. Sklar CA. Growth following therapy for childhood cancer. *Cancer Invest* 1995;13:511–516.

18. Sklar CA, Constine LS. Chronic neuroendocrinological sequelae of radiation therapy. *Int J Radiat Oncol Biol Phys* 1995;31:1113–1121.

19. Hancock LS Cox RS, McDougall IR. Thyroid diseases after treatment of Hodgkin's disease. *N Engl J Med* 1991;325:599–606.

20. Vassilopoulou-Sellin, Klein MJ, Moore BD III, et al. Efficacy of growth hormone replacement therapy in children with organic growth hormone deficiency after cranial irradiation. *Hormone Res* 1995;43:188–193.

21. Hindmarsh P, Brook CG. Growth hormone and recurrence of tumour. *Br Med J* 1992;305:254.

22. Skinner R, Pearson AD, Amineddine HA, et al. Ototoxicity of cisplatinum in children and adolescents. *Br J Cancer* 1990;61:927–931.

23. Daugaard G, Abildgaard. Renal morbidity of chemotherapy. In Plowman PN, McElwain T, Meadows A, eds. *Complications of Cancer Management*. Oxford: Butterworth–Heinemann; 1991:213–231.

24. Luban NL. An update on transfusion-transmitted viruses. *Curr Opin Pediatr* 1998;10:53–59.

25. Martins AN, Johnston JS, Henry JM, et al. Delayed radionecrosis of the brain. *J Neurosurg* 1977;47:336–345.

26. Shuper A, Packer RJ, Vezina LG, et al. "Complicated migraine-like" episodes in children following cranial irradiation and chemotherapy. *Neurology* 1995;45:1837–1840.

27. Kramer S, Lee KF. Complicatioins of radiation therapy: the central nervous system. *Semin Roentgenol* 1974;9:75–83.

28. Reinhold HS, Calvo W, Hopewell JW, et al. Development of blood vessel-related radiation damage in the fimbria of the central nervous system. *Int J Radiat Oncol Biol Phys* 1990;18:37–42.

29. Butler R, Jones G, Finlay J. The differential neuropsychological effects of infratentorial, supratentorial and diencephalic childhood brain tumors. *J Int Neuropsychol Soc* 1998;2:69.

30. Brookshire B, Copeland DR, Moore B, Ater J. Pretreatment neuropsychological status and associated factors in children with primary brain tumors. *Neurosurgery* 1990; 27:8870–8891.

31. Packer RJ, Sposto R, Atkins TE, et al. Quality of life in children with primitive neuroectodermal tumors (medulloblastoma) of the posterior fossa. *Pediatr Neurosci* 1987; 13:169–175.

32. LeBaron S, Zeltzer PM, Zeltzer LK, et al. Assessment of quality of survival in children with medulloblastoma and cerebellar astrocytoma. *Cancer* 1998;62:1215–1222.

33. Butler RW, Hill JM, Steinherz, PG, et al. Neuropsychologic effects of cranial irradiation, intrathecal methotrexate, and systemic metehotrexate in childhood cancer. *J Clin Oncol* 1994;12:2621–2629.

34. Packer RJ, Sutton LN, Atkins TE, et al. A prospective study of cognitive function in children receiving whole-brain radiotherapy and chemotherapy: 2-year results. *J Neurosurg* 1989;70:707–713.

35. Radcliffe J, Packer RJ, Atkins TE, et al. Three and four-year cognitive outcome in children with noncortical brain tumors treated with whole-brain radiotherapy. *Ann Neurol* 1992;32:551–554.

36. Copeland DR, Moore BD III, Francis DJ, et al. Neuropsychologic effects of chemotherapy on children with cancer: a longitudinal study. *J Clin Oncol* 1996;14:2826–2835.

37. Van Dam FS, Schagen SB, Muller MJ, et al. Impairment of cognitive function in women receiving adjuvant treatment for high-risk breast cancer: high-dose versus standard-dose chemotherapy. *J Natl Cancer Inst* 1998;90: 210–218.

38. Ris, MD, Noll RB. Long-term neurobehavioral outcome in pediatric brain-tumor patients: review and methodological critique. *J Clin Exp Neuropsychol* 1994;16:21–42.

39. Butler RW. Attentional processes and their remediation in childhood cancer. *Med Pediatr Oncol* 1998;(suppl 1):75–78.

40. Koocher GP, O'Malley JE. *The Damocles Syndrome: Psychosocial Consequences of Surviving Childhood Cancer*. New York: McGraw-Hill; 1981.

41. Teta MJ, DelPo MC, Kasl SV, et al. Psychosocial consequences of childhood and adolescent cancer survival. *J Chron Dis* 1986;39:751–759.

42. Butler RW, Rizzi LP, Bandilla EB. The effects of childhood cancer and its treatment on two objective measures of psychological functioning. *Childrens Health Care* 1999;28:311–327.

43. Mulhern, RK, Wasserman AL, Friedman AG, Fairclough D. Social competence and behavioral adjustment of children who are long-term survivors of cancer. *Pediatrics* 1989;83:18–25.

44. Johnson DL, McCabe MA, Nicholson HS, et al. Quality of long-term survival in young children with medulloblastoma. *J Neurosurg* 1994;80:1004–1010.

Chapter 40

Ethical Issues in Pediatric Neuro-oncology

Ann-Marie Yost

In no field of medicine are the issues surrounding decision making so emotionally charged as those in pediatric oncology. Traditional ethical concepts—beneficence, nonmaleficence, autonomy, and justice—are modified when applied to pediatric patients. As children have no legal or moral autonomy, concepts such as incompetence,[1] substituted judgment,[1] proximate personhood,[2] and mature minors[1] have evolved to create a concept of autonomy for children. The definition of beneficence has focused on preservation of life, often without consideration of quality of life. A child has not had the life experience necessary to inform decisions about treatment, resuscitation, or cessation of therapy. When decisions about treatment, or the withdrawal of treatment, must be made for children, who should make them? The parents, the medical team, or the courts?

This is a difficult question that has not been fully resolved. Different answers may be given when the issues are viewed from a legal versus a moral or a religious perspective.

Ethics is not a philosophical system that exists in isolation from the rest of human experience. Religious, ethnic, and other sociological factors will influence the physician's and family's decisions. If racial, religious, or other factors are perceived by the family as impediments to shared decision making, the ensuing lack of trust may make even the smallest decisions impossible. Educational barriers may prevent families from fully understanding the information they need to make informed decisions for their child.

This chapter explores the principles of ethical decision making. It examines the roles of members of the health care team and hospital ethics committee (HEC). Case studies are used to illustrate the complexities involved in the making of treatment decisions for children with brain tumors.

Setting goals and establishing communication are key components of this chapter. The multidisciplinary approach to pediatric brain tumors can contribute to the development of conflict if the focus remains on individual team members' areas of concern rather than on the total picture. Conflicts of opinion should be addressed within the team so that the team speaks with one voice to the family. Parents may "double-check" questions, hoping to eventually get a more palatable answer.

Lastly, before beginning the discussion of individual ethical precepts, it is worth emphasizing that it is the physician's responsibility to act ethically, despite any obstacles. In no other career is an individual invested with so much authority over the lives of others. The choice of words in an explanation can often determine the parents' choice. It is morally impera-tive that physicians ensure that decisions stem from the patient's or parents' beliefs and desires, even if these are in conflict with the physician's own.[3-5]

BENEFICENCE

Beneficence is defined as acting in a way that benefits the patient. An adult patient is free to decide what he or she feels will be of benefit. However, in pediatrics, the decision is often made by a third person. In 1979, *Parham v JR* elucidated the right of parents to make medical decisions for minors "absent abuse or neglect." The court attempted to guide parents by creating the "best interests" standard for medical decision making.[1] This is the legal equivalent of beneficence and is at best a vague guide. Subsequent court decisions have added that "medically indicated" and "life-saving" therapies must be provided for children, even in the absence of parental consent.[1]

A type of cost/benefit analysis is often applied to determine beneficence in medical decision making. Is the therapy in question more likely to produce good outcome than to cause negative side effects? Although this would seem easy enough to decide, there is an element of uncertainty in medicine that precludes definitive prognosis. As the degree of uncertainty increases, so does the complexity of the calculation. Is a 60% chance of surviving 5 years with a 90% chance of significant cognitive deficits more beneficent than a therapy offering a 40% chance for 5-year survival with a 40% chance of cognitive deficit? What if the therapy is experimental and no clear-cut analysis can be performed?[6]

The permutations are myriad. The ultimate decisions will depend on the goal set. Is the parents' goal to preserve life? What weight do they place on quality of life? What resources do they have to care for a significantly impaired child? All of these factors may bear on what the parents decide would be in the best interests of the child. The above-mentioned court decisions show a societal bias toward the preservation of life as the standard of best interest for the pediatric patient. A calculation of potential years of life lost is the usual rationale for this approach, but once again, this concept does not encompass quality of life.

There is little discussion in the literature of a quality-of-life standard for best interest.[7] How should the health care provider react if faced with parents who feel that a 60% chance of keeping their child alive didn't balance the risk of serious cognitive, emotional, and behavioral impairment inherent in the therapy? How should the health care provider deal with parents who believe that living with an IQ below 80 is not in keeping with their definition of "best interests" for their child and therefore are refusing therapy? What about the parents of a child who is failing therapy who wish to continue the therapy while hoping for a miracle?

The possible clashes of opinion are easy to see. The medical profession's bias toward preservation of life is underscored by a recent survey in which 25% of doctors and medical students polled stated that withdrawing medical intervention is "murder."[8] It is not difficult to see how personal feelings and belief systems influence the way decisions are made.

Communication in the context of beneficence would involve a frank explanation of what is known about the risks and benefits of therapy for the specific tumor as well as what is known about prognosis. Then the parents must decide on their goal and begin to consider the limits of what they will do to achieve it. Communication must be ongoing and requires constant input and reevaluation from the medical team. The parents' attention should be brought to focus on long-term goals early on, even while they are being helped to cope with the day-to-day trauma of surviving their child's illness.

NONMALEFICENCE

Premum non nocere—"First do no harm." This concept is intimately bound to beneficence. *When ambiguity of prognosis makes it difficult to determine "best interests," then nonmaleficence dictates that the health care team minimize the negative impact of therapy.* This may involve physicians refusing to participate in treatment whose risks outweigh its benefits.[9] Nonmaleficence may also justify treatment that conveys no benefit (other than a psychological one for the family), if the therapy will not harm the child. Counseling and support for the parents is often necessary, especially when decisions involving the use of experimental therapy may have to be made. This counseling may end in discussions of futility. Nonmaleficence, by definition, contains some assessment of quality of life in the sense that its application may determine that prolonging life constitutes doing harm to the child.

Goals and communication here often involve the later stages of the decision making process. Nonmaleficence should be integral to discussions about cardiopulmonary resuscitation and ventilation. A recent essay on the subject of ethics proposed that if family members were informed of the poor outcome of in-hospital resuscitation they would refuse it, especially when their family member is terminally ill.[10]

AUTONOMY

Autonomy is the ethical principle that defines an individual's right to govern his or her own existence. Legal support for the moral concept of autonomy in medical decision making began in 1905. When the Illinois Supreme Court in *Pratt v Davis* ruled that physicians cannot violate the "bodily integrity" of a patient without permission.[4] In 1914, the U.S. Supreme Court defined procedures performed without consent as assault.[4] The subsequent *Salgo v Leland Stanford Jr. University Board of Trustees* decision made information the basis for adequate consent.[4] Therefore, informed consent is the legal standard used to enforce a patient's right to autonomy or self-determination in medical decision making.

Children are a special case in the consideration of autonomy. In both ethical and legal terms, children are recognized to have inadequate experience on which to base decisions regarding their own care. A short anecdote illustrates this point. A 6-year-old boy, when informed that the source of his headaches was a brain tumor, drew a third-person representative named Mr. Angry during play therapy. Mr. Angry let everyone know that the headaches weren't severe enough to need surgery and that they should all just go home. The exception to pediatric incompetence is the "mature minor" (a child over the age of 12 who has rights to decision making that vary from state to state).[1]

The parents' right to make decisions for minors was established in 1925 by *Pierce v Society of Sisters*. The court ruled that parents had "the liberty ... to direct the upbringing and education of children under their control."[1] The previously mentioned *Parham v JR* included medical decision making in parents' rights with the requirement of the best-interests standard.[1]

Society accepts that parents are the best decision makers for their children. The courts' requirement for "indicated" and "life-saving" therapies was a result of challenges to parental authority in cases involving Jehovah's Witnesses and Christian Scientists.[11, 12] In 1925, the U.S. Supreme Court stated that parents were not allowed to "make martyrs of their children."[1] However, the law still tends to favor the rights of parents and the autonomy of mature minors in all but the most egregious cases.[11, 12] Subsequently, physicians have worked to develop new techniques to avoid blood transfusions in Jehovah's Witnesses. The objections of Christian Scientists to medical therapy have been harder to overcome,[12] and it is a testament to society's commitment to autonomy that children can still die because of their parents' religious beliefs.

Informed consent is a legal standard. Ethically speaking, informed consent should be considered a process. This starts with discussion of prognosis, possible therapy, and risks and benefits at the time of diagnosis and workup, and should continue until discontinuation of follow-up or death. Informed consent involves giving parents the information they need to reach decisions. It should not center on an individual therapy or surgery in isolation from the ongoing treatment plan but rather as an integral part of the medical team's efforts to achieve the goals it has set in cooperation with the parents.[4]

Communication in this section must also extend to the child. Consideration must be given to chronological and emotional age, intelligence, education, and coping skills when deciding how to inform the child. Discussion of options prior to informing the child should take place out of earshot because children often understand more than they let on.

A patient of any age suffers from feelings of loss of control. This can be mitigated in older children by including them in discussions and soliciting their thoughts and feelings. Younger children benefit greatly from the use of play therapy. Dolls can be incorporated in the explanation of procedures, and play allows children to vent their anxieties in a safe setting.

JUSTICE

Distributive justice applies the principles of utilitarianism to moral decision making. In medical decision making, distributive justice is often used strictly in an economic sense. It is offered as philosophical justification for cost cutting, rationing, and allocation of scarce resources.

Despite the focus in health care systems on universal coverage and cost cutting, Americans have typically wanted to have their cake and eat it too. The rationing concept applied to experimental therapies and to more established treatments, such as organ transplantation, has yet to be fully applied to the fields of neurosurgery and oncology. Warner and Luce emphasized that a review of the literature shows very little written about CBA or CEA in cancer therapy.[13] They concluded that "the social and political response to cancer seems to preclude consideration of alternatives to [poorly effective] therapies."[13] So the needs of the many lie secondary to the needs of the few if the few are stricken with cancer.

It is erroneous to limit the idea of distributive justice simply to economics. The weight that Americans have given to autonomy has been responsible for relative injustices in several areas,[8] not only in terms of access to health care for some but also in terms of deprivation of attention, affection, and resources for other family and community members of brain tumor patients.

Communication here must address the effect of a patient's treatment course on the family as a whole. Is the prognosis of the disease or expected outcome of the therapy good enough to justify the economic, physical, and emotional toll on the other members of the family unit? Once again, if our goal is preservation of life, then the answer will be yes with greater frequency than if a quality-of-life standard is applied.

To show once again that there are at least two sides to every issue, distributive justice can be used to argue against experimental therapy because of the large outlay of resources (time, money, medicines, emotion). It can also be used to argue for it if the gain in knowledge may potentially benefit many people down the line.

FUTILITY

The concept of futility is relatively new in the field of ethics. It arises from a growing feeling that preservation of life is not always the most appropriate goal. *Futile therapy is defined as treatment that has no chance of benefiting the patient and is, in fact, prolonging an inadequate existence.*

Recognizing futility is a difficult task for both the health care team and the parents. The emotional commitment to the child's therapy and outcome can lead all involved to continue trying, even to a point of greatly diminished returns.

It remains to be seen whether medical futility will become an established end point of treatment protocols.[14, 15] Once again, the potential differences of opinion are staggering.

Ideally, an acknowledgment of futility would be made jointly by the parents and the medical team. The medical team would inform the parents that the child is failing to respond to any of the treatments used and would not benefit medically from additional therapy. The parents would incorporate this information into the ongoing process of goal setting and recognize that the standards of beneficence, nonmaleficence, and justice are no longer being satisfied. The focus would then center on providing the child with a comforting environment in which to die as painlessly as possible.

THE HEALTH CARE TEAM AND THE HEC

Participation of the entire health care team is crucial to the process of ascertaining the parents' goals, expectations, and religious and ethical beliefs. In the early stages of the workup, parents often feel overwhelmed by shock and an overabundance of information. They may feel more comfortable sharing their feelings or revealing concerns to members of the health care team other than the primary surgeon. *Multidisciplinary round or direct communication among team members will ensure that every team member is formulating recommendations based on the same information.*

The special services of chaplains may greatly aid in parent education and goal setting when the parents' religious beliefs have a major impact on decision making. Chaplains offer emotional support of a different type than others on the health care team. They can also discuss differing interpretations of scripture when parents' interpretations either favor futile therapy or reject necessary therapy.[16, 17]

The early involvement of rehabilitation services where appropriate can help orient the parents to the long-term nature of recovery as well as reinforce a goal-directed process.

There is not room within the scope of this chapter to fully address the role of the HEC. It is usually composed of members from all facets of the health care team as well as ethicists and, sometimes, lawyers. Ideally, it would seldom be recruited to influence the decision making process. However, when conflict arises in decision making, the HEC can apply the principles of ethics to help clarify issues.[18]

APPLICATIONS

Application of ethical principles to real-life scenarios relies on communication. This consists of an ongoing open exchange of information between the health care providers and the family. Discussions should be goal-oriented and reflective of the beliefs of the parents. The health care team can best act ethically by helping the parents to become rational decision makers.

This should begin with a discussion of the parents' understanding and expectations based on the diagnosis and prognosis during the initial workup. Advances in some areas of pediatric oncology may artificially elevate parental expectations. Economic competition among hospitals has encouraged this trend. A recent *HEC Forum* report revealed that a significant percentage of literature mailed on request from U.S. children's hospitals used the word "miracle" to describe the available medical care.[19] Early identification of goals can help the health care team steer the family away from unrealistic expectations while determining how the parents' belief systems will influence future decisions.

Discussion of goals and end points will also help the physician to identify his or her feelings about the parents' decisions and how this will influence wording in future discussions. Think again about the previous example: how should a health care provider deal with a family who wants to limit therapy based on an expectation of a poor quality of life when the team's goal was preservation of life, or vice versa? What about a family that places a child's life at risk by refusing recommended and effective therapy? Part of an ethical physician's responsibility is to accept different goals when they are rational, consistent, and do not violate ethical premises, even when such goals are in conflict with the physician's own.

CASE STUDIES

Ethical principles can be best understood through their application to real clinical situations. The following case studies are based on actual clinical material. What should the health care team do in each case? How would the decision be supported or not supported by an analysis based on beneficence, nonmaleficence, autonomy, and justice?

Case One

JY, an 11-year-old boy with one sibling and a very supportive family, presents to the emergency room following two craniotomies for a surgically incurable brain tumor that is poorly responsive to adjuvant therapy. He has headache, worsening hemiparesis, and decreased level of consciousness. Hematocrit reveals massive regrowth of the residual tumor. The parents are opposed to ICU admission because of its negative psychological impact. JY is admitted to the general neurosurgical unit. His improvement after mannitol and increased steroid administration is clearly only palliative. However, surgery will not be curative, and it is unclear how much longer he will survive with this aggressive tumor, even if another surgery is performed. The resection would likely return him in the short term to his current level of functioning, which has constituted an adequate quality of life for him and his parents. The health care team supports the parents whatever their decision.

Prior to his illness, one of JY's greatest joys was playing football. The quarterback of his favorite team has agreed to meet JY during a game to be played 6 weeks hence. The parents are aware that there are no further protocols in which to enroll their son, but they would like to see him achieve this dream.

How does the parents' wish fit in with our ethical schema? The parents have a clear goal that is probably achievable. The risk of negative side effects from the surgery (infection, worsened neurologic deficit, death) is small compared with the benefits of an improved level of consciousness and a possible improvement in motor function and psychological well-being. The pain would be both minimal and familiar to the boy from his previous surgeries. So the cost/benefit analysis of beneficence/nonmaleficence weighs to the side of giving the child this opportunity. Because the parents appear to be realistic and acting in the interests of the child, no challenge to their autonomy is appropriate at this time. However, distributive justice may not be well served because resources are being expended on a therapy that will not alter the ultimate outcome and parental time, money, energy, and affection are being diverted from the patient's sibling.

It would be equally justifiable for the parents to refuse the surgery. The rapid regrowth of the tumor and its poor response to therapy virtually guarantees that this is a limited reprieve at best. The decision would be nonmaleficent as it would avoid prolongation of suffering, and beneficence would be satisfied by a relatively painless death. This could also be interpreted as serving the child's best interests because, as a result of his hemiparesis, he is unable to participate in activities that bring him joy and he will avoid the side effects of the massive steroid doses that would be required. Distributive justice would be served by using the saved resources for a child with potential for a better outcome and the family could begin the process of getting on with their lives without the emotional and economic strain of caring for a dying child.

The decision was made to operate on the patient. What else should be done at this time? Prior to discharge, an outpatient management plan consistent with the stated goal should be arranged. This should focus on the location and type of palliative care, including inpatient versus outpatient hospice and do-not-resuscitate (DNR) status as an outpatient.

Case Two

AZ is an 8-year-old child of Jehovah's Witnesses. He has a rare, surgically incurable tumor that has been previously operated on and is poorly responsive to adjuvant therapy. His parents are requesting a radical cranial procedure to debulk the tumor, with the ultimate goal of prolonging the boy's life. They will not consent to the transfusion of blood products despite their knowing that this will limit the extent of the surgery. The child is given a preoperative course of erythropoietin.

Surgery is attempted but must be aborted due to blood loss. Postoperative complications result in the necessity of a blood transfusion to save the boy's life. The mother, faced with the threat of imminent death, consents to the transfusion. Neither her husband nor any church member is present at the time. The child survives.

What should have been said to the family preoperatively? The application of any of the principles of ethics to this case would yield the same conclusion: no surgery. The surgery carries significant risk of pain and neurologic deficit without any hope of cure. The child was asymptomatic, so that no improvement in his quality of life could be offered. The parents' request for a futile therapy while placing serious limitations on the physician's options is not rational or in the best interests of the child. Justice is not served because little or no benefit is gained despite the expenditure of economic and emotional resources that would be better utilitized in a child with a hope of benefit.

Postoperatively, the emotional and psychological consequences of the mother's violation of religious precepts are not inconsiderable. Their philosophical basis for future decision making is called into question because a blood transfusion was allowed in extremis yet refused when needed for a therapy that might have prolonged life (the parents' goal).

What else could be done? The provision of a risky therapy with no clear benefit to the patient violates all of the doctrines of ethics. However, this should not lead to abandonment of the patient. A thorough exploration of other options in consultation with an oncologist should take place. It is possible that therapies with less risk of negative side effects might be available and could possibly be justified in a risk/benefit analysis. Because no surgical procedure would cure the child, there is no benefit to challenging the parents' autonomy, and it is doubtful that the courts would agree to do so.

Whether or not viable options present themselves, counseling should be initiated early. There should be a discussion about decisions at the end of life. Counseling may also be needed to help the parents cope with any after-effects of the mother's violation of the family's religious precepts.

Case Three

SB is a 5-year-old girl with a rapidly recurrent medulloblastoma status post several previous resections. Several weeks after a gross total resection and course of chemotherapy, she presents again with a massive recurrence with hydrocephalus and obtundation. Her parents, in consultation with the neurosurgeon, decide that further surgery would be of no benefit and the child is admitted to the ICU and made a DNR.

The parents' decision not to submit SB to further surgery is consistent with their goal of maintaining an acceptable quality of life and satisfies the ethical precepts.

What else could be done? Given the decision to allow SB to die, the remaining ethical issue is how she will die. It is questionable that the child's best interests are served by dying in the ICU. If the decision not to resuscitate is made, then there are no interventions requiring ICU care. If the child had been intubated by the emergency medical services system, then stable ventilator care in a non-ICU setting or extubation with cessation of therapy can be offered as options.

The resources being used—nurses, equipment, social worker, chaplain, money—would be better allocated to a critically ill child who is not terminal. In addition, the presence of a dying child and her grieving family takes an emotional toll on the medical staff as well as on other patients and their families.

Support of this child and her family could be well served with better distributive justice if SB were allowed to die in a private room or a hospice unit, if available. The best death for this child would likely be in a hospice setting, preferably at home. Arrangements for this, with support and recognition of the difficulty of this option for the family, could have been planned at the time the child's symptoms began to recur.

SUMMARY

It is important to recognize the forces at play in medical decision making for the pediatric patient. The goal of serving the child's best interests must be maintained while the needs of the family as a whole are addressed. Communication between the family and the health care team is the primary means of educating the family so that they can make informed and ethical decisions.

REFERENCES

1. Cooper R, Koch KA. Neonatal and pediatric critical care ethical decision making. *Crit Care Clin (Med Ethics)* 1996;12(1):149–164.
2. Walters JW. Proximate personhood as a standard for making difficult treatment decisions: imperiled newborns as a case study. *Bioethics* 1992;6(1):12–22.
3. Crausman RS, Armstrong JD. Ethically based medical decision making in the intensive care unit residency teaching strategies. *Crit Care Clin (Med Ethics)* 1996;12(1):71–83.
4. Smith DH. Ethics in the doctor–patient relationship. *Crit Care Clin (Med Ethics)* 1996;12(1):179–198.
5. Lowe F. Ethics in neurosurgery. *Acta Neurochir* 1992;116:187–189.
6. The Presidential Commission recommends respecting the parents in experimental therapy if there is no harm to the child. See ref. 1.
7. Silverman WA. Medical decisions: an appeal for reasonableness. *Pediatrics* 1996;98(6):1182–1184.
8. Koch KA. The language of death: euthanatos et mors the science of uncertainty. *Crit Care Clin (Med Ethics)* 1996;12(1):1–14.
9. Yeoh C, et al. Unproven treatment in childhood oncology: how far should paediatricians co-operate? *J Med Ethics* 1994;20(2):75–76 and commentary on 77–79.
10. Hook CC, Koch KA. Ethics of resuscitation. *Crit Care Clin (Med Ethics)* 1996;12(1):135–148.
11. Catlin A. The dilemma of Jehovah's Witness children who need blood to survive. *HEC Forum* 1996;8(4):195–207.
12. May L. Challenging medical authority: the refusal of treatment by Christian Scientists, 15–21.
13. Warner KE, Luce BR. Cost-Benefit and Cost-Effectiveness Analysis in Health Care. Ann Arbor, MI: Health Administration Press; 1982.
14. Youngner SJ. Medical futility. *Crit Care Clin (Med Ethics)* 1996;12(1):165–178.
15. Tomlinson T, Czlonka D. Futility and hospital policy. *Hastings Center Rep* 1995;25(3):28–35.
16. Connors RB, Smith ML. Religious insistence on medical treatment: Christian theology and re-imagination. *Hastings Center Rep* 1996;26(4):23–30.
17. Wagner JT, Higdon TL. Spiritual issues and bioethics in the intensive care unit: the role of the chaplain. *Crit Care Clin (Med Ethics)* 1996;12(1):15–28.
18. Kelly D, Hoyt JW. Ethics Consultation. *Crit Care Clin (Med Ethics)* 1996;12(1):49–70.
19. Manning S, Schneiderman LJ. Miracle or limits: what message from the marketplace? *HEC Forum* 1996;8(2):103–108.

Page numbers followed by "f" indicate figures.
Page numbers followed by "t" indicate tables.